Equine Laminitis

Equine Laminitis

Editor

James K. Belknap

Professor of Equine Surgery
Department of Veterinary Clinical Sciences
College of Veterinary Medicine
The Ohio State University
Columbus, OH

Associate Editor

Raymond Geor

Professor
Pro Vice-Chancellor College of Sciences
College of Sciences
Massey University
Palmerstone North
New Zealand

WILEY Blackwell

Editorial offices: 1606 Golden Aspen Drive, Suites 103 and 104, Ames, Iowa 50010, USA
The Atrium, Southern Gate, Chichester, West Sussex, PO19 8SQ, UK
9600 Garsington Road, Oxford, OX4 2DQ, UK

For details of our global editorial offices, for customer services and for information about how to apply for permission to reuse the copyright material in this book please see our website at www.wiley.com/wiley-blackwell.

Library of Congress Cataloging-in-Publication Data applied for.

9781119944713 (hardback)

A catalogue record for this book is available from the British Library.

Wiley also publishes its books in a variety of electronic formats. Some content that appears in print may not be available in electronic books.

Cover image: mfto/Gettyimages

Set in 9.5/12pt MinionPro by Aptara Inc., New Delhi, India

1 2017

Contents

Part 4: Diagnostic Evaluation of Equine Laminitis

Part 5: Medical Treatment of the Laminitic Patient

Part 6: Treatment of Laminitis: Digital Support and Stabilization of the Distal Phalanx

Part 7: Treatment of the Laminitis Case

Part 8: Management of Chronic Laminitis

Part 9: Prevention of Laminitis

Contributors

Dominique Alfandari
University of Massachusetts
Department of Veterinary and Animal Sciences
Amherst
MA 01003
USA

Simon R. Bailey
Associate Professor and Reader
Faculty of Veterinary and Agricultural Sciences
University of Melbourne
Victoria
Australia

Gary M. Baxter
Associate Dean for Clinical Services, Director
Veterinary Teaching Hospital
University of Georgia
Athens
GA
USA

James K. Belknap
Professor of Equine Surgery
Department of Veterinary Clinical Sciences
College of Veterinary Medicine
The Ohio State University
Columbus
OH
USA

Samuel J. Black
University of Massachusetts
Department of Veterinary and Animal Sciences
Amherst
MA 01003
USA

Raul J. Bras
Rood and Riddle Equine Hospital
Podiatry Department
Lexington
KY
USA

Teresa A. Burns
Clinical Assistant Professor
Equine Internal Medicine
Department of Veterinary Clinical Sciences
College of Veterinary Medicine
The Ohio State University
Columbus
OH
USA

Hans Castelijns
Equine Podiatry Consultant
Cortona
Tuscany
Italy

Helen Davies
Associate Professor in Veterinary Anatomy
Faculty of Veterinary and Agricultural Sciences
The University of Melbourne
Victoria
Australia

Thomas J. Divers
Cornell University
College of Veterinary Medicine
Ithaca
NY
USA

Bernd Driessen
Professor of Anesthesiology
Section of Anesthesia
Department of Clinical Studies-New Bolton Center
School of Veterinary Medicine
University of Pennsylvania
Kennett Square, Pennsylvania
USA

Andy E. Durham
The Liphook Equine Hospital
Forest Mere
Liphook
Hampshire
UK

Susan C. Eades
Department of Veterinary Clinical Sciences
School of Veterinary Medicine
Louisiana State University
Baton Rouge
LA
USA

Randy B. Eggleston
Clinical Professor of Large Animal Surgery
Department of Large Animal Medicine
College of Veterinary Medicine University of Georgia
Athens
GA
USA

Rafael R. Faleiros
Escola de Veterinária
Universidade Federal de Minas Gerais
Belo Horizonte
Brazil

Andrea E. Floyd
Serenity Equine Hospital
AuroraSeren Equine
Evington
VA
USA

Pat Harris
Equine Studies Group
WALTHAM Centre for Pet Nutrition
Waltham-on-the-Wolds
Leicestershire
UK

Susan J. Holcombe
Professor
Department of Large Animal Clinical Sciences
College of Veterinary Medicine
Michigan State University
East Lansing
MI
USA

Robert J. Hunt
Hagyard Equine Medical Institute
Lexington
KY
USA

Samuel D. A. Hurcombe
Cornell Ruffian Equine Specialists
College of Veterinary Medicine
Cornell University
Elmont
NY
USA

Philip J. Johnson
College of Veterinary Medicine
University of Missouri
Columbia
MO
USA

Britta Leise
Assistant Professor, Equine Surgery
Veterinary Clinical Sciences
Louisiana State University
Baton Rouge
LA
USA

John Loftus
Cornell University College of Veterinary Medicine
Ithaca
NY 14853
USA

Richard A. Mansmann
Equine Podiatry and Rehabilitation Practice
Chapel Hill
NC
USA

Harry J. Markwell
Goulburn Valley Equine Hospital
Congupna
Victoria
Australia

Dianne McFarlane
Professor, Department of Physiological Sciences
Center for Veterinary Health Sciences
Oklahoma State University
Stillwater, OK USA

Catherine McGowan
Professor of Equine Internal Medicine
Institute of Ageing and Chronic Disease
Faculty of Health and Life Sciences
University of Liverpool
Leahurst CH64 7TE
UK

Gabriel J. Milinovich
School of Medicine
The University of Queensland
St Lucia
Queensland 4072
Australia

Stephen E. O'Grady
Virginia Therapeutic Farriery
In Assoc. with: Palm Beach Equine Clinic
Keswick
VA
USA

Andrew H. Parks
Professor Large Animal Surgery
Department of Large Animal Medicine
College of Veterinary Medicine
University of Georgia
Athens
GA
USA

Janet Patterson-Kane
Senior Pathologist
Flagship Biosciences Inc.
Westminster, CO 80021
USA

A.H. Parks
Professor of Large Animal Surgery
Department of Large Animal Medicine
College of Veterinary Medicine
University of Georgia
Athens
GA
USA

Erica Pawlak
University of Massachusetts
Department of Veterinary and Animal Sciences
Amherst
MA 01003
USA

John F. Peroni
Associate Professor Large Animal Surgery
Department of Large Animal Medicine
College of Veterinary Medicine
University of Georgia
Athens
GA
USA

Christopher C. Pollitt
Emeritus Professor of Equine Medicine
Australian Equine Laminitis Research Unit
School of Veterinary Science
The University of Queensland
Gatton Campus
Queensland 4343
Australia

Jeff Ridley
Farrier, AFA, CJF, TE
Leighton
IA
USA

Amy Rucker
Midwest Equine
Columbia
MO
USA

Harold C. Schott, II
Professor
Department of Large Animal Clinical Sciences
College of Veterinary Medicine
Michigan State University
East Lansing
MI
USA

Debra Taylor
Associate Professor
Department of Clinical Sciences
College of Veterinary Medicine
Auburn University
AL
USA

Ramiro E. Toribio
Professor of Equine Medicine
Department of Veterinary Clinical Sciences
College of Veterinary Medicine
The Ohio State University
Columbus
OH
USA

Andrew van Eps
Associate Professor of Equine Medicine
Australian Equine Laminitis Research Unit
School of Veterinary Science
The University of Queensland
Gatton Campus
Queensland 4343 Australia

Richard Wayne Waguespack
Southeastern Veterinary Surgery Center
Columbus
GA
USA

Donald M. Walsh
Founder, Animal Health Foundation
Director of Clinical Research, Homestead Veterinary Hospital
Villa Ridge
MO
USA

Le Wang
National Institute of Arthritis and Musculoskeletal and Skin Diseases (NIAMS)
National Institutes of Health (NIH)
Bethesda
MD 20892
USA

Laura Zarucco
Dipartimento di Scienze Veterinarie
Scuola di Agraria e Medicina Veterinaria
Università degli Studi di Torino
Grugliasco
Italy

Fengqiu Zhang
University of Massachusetts
Department of Veterinary and Animal Sciences
Amherst
MA 01003
USA

Foreword

I was once asked to introduce Professor James Belknap and present to him an award at a prestigious International Equine Conference on Laminitis. The award was for scientific excellence in the field of laminitis research, and the venue was a noisy gala dinner in West Palm Beach, USA. I thought it best not to elaborate too grandly about his already numerous and excellent contributions to the science of laminitis, so without much preamble I happily presented the award with acclamation from the audience. That was over 10 years ago and could have been the culmination of his career if he had slipped into university administrative roles as so many top academics do. However, fortunately for us, his hunger to decipher laminitis prevailed and his scientific production continued setting him apart from his peers and placing him at the forefront of the laminitis scientific community. He is the pre-eminent thinker and instigator of cutting-edge laminitis research, so it is entirely appropriate that he contributes to and edits this important first in the laminitis literature. Jim has the historical background and vision to choose the appropriate authors and rigorously oversee their contributions to deliver an historic, first of its kind publication; a multiauthor text with the scope to deliver new information on nearly every aspect of Equine Laminitis. This ranges from the latest molecular perturbations at the cellular level, state-of-the-art radiography, to the effectiveness of various clinical shoeing techniques applied to horse's feet.

I try to keep abreast of the laminitis literature and didn't expect to learn much by reading the chapters of this book, but I was agreeably shocked to discover how little I knew and much that was new and interesting. It was like meeting old friends and colleagues and talking 'laminitis.' In a book of this sort, the rigours of peer review are relaxed a little and the authors are able to not only present the expert details of their specialization, but to speculate and 'think outside the box.' Thus, we learn of visions for future research, why certain procedures failed or succeeded, and exciting – yet to be published – data.

Reading this book will bring you up to date with the latest information on the horse's foot and its major affliction, laminitis. It will help you better understand the disease and thus formulate effective preventive and treatment strategies. It will even help you deliver improved lecture and workshop material. I was recently lecturing internationally and, stuck with the habit of updating my lecture material at the last minute and with early access to the chapters of the book, I was able to quickly add new, pertinent material (referenced of course) to my PowerPoints. Thus, the text is a timely and essential 'must-have' addition to the bookshelf or computer/tablet of all who work with and are fascinated by the horse's foot.

Although long overdue, a book such as this, written after we have struggled with laminitis into the modern era of molecular biology and veterinary diagnostics, can at last capture important progress that has arisen from peer-reviewed, validated basic and clinical research (all of which is presented by the chief investigators and their teams in the chapters that follow). An example is the recognition that three different categories of laminitis exist: *sepsis-related*; *endocrinopathic*; and *supporting limb laminitis*. Knowing that treatment should be anti-inflammatory, insulin-reducing or circulation-promoting, respectively, has translated into more effective clinical management. Another realization is that, regardless of the laminitis category, the essential clinical problem is displacement of the distal phalanx and its wide-ranging anatomical consequences. Chapters devoted to digital radiographic imaging that can be enhanced with contrast media show how to assess the new laminitis case, monitor the effects of therapeutic farriery on the position of the distal phalanx, and follow the progression of laminitis into its chronic phase. It was refreshing to read that nonsteroidal anti-inflammatory drugs (NSAIDs), while having many useful properties for laminitis therapy, likely have little or no efficacy in directly preventing the condition (Dr J Divers, Medical treatment of the laminitic patient – anti-inflammatory therapy; see Chapter 31). Dr Divers' personal insight that prognosis after sepsis-related laminitis can be correlated to the positive or negative analgesic response to initial phenylbutazone dosing is noteworthy, therapeutic prognostication.

Many teachers of laminitis and certain textbooks still hold with some form of blood supply problem being central to the pathophysiology of all types of laminitis. This long-held tenet has endured long after publication of evidence to the contrary, and I anticipate this textbook will accelerate revision towards more evidence-based pathogenesis. Indeed, Professor Belknap in his introduction to this book states "*Lamellar ischemia, originally thought to be the driving force behind all types of laminitis, only appears to play a primary role in supporting limb laminitis.*" Perhaps the documented presence of vasoconstrictive agents that has been the focus of extensive laminitis research plays only a contributing, synergistic role, in combination with the overwhelming inflammatory mechanisms as suggested by Dr Simon Bailey in his chapter, 'Vasoactive drug therapies for laminitis – pharmacological and clinical aspects.' Recent research indicates that drugs used to promote digital vasodilation for decades, including acepromazine (likely the second most commonly used drug in laminitis therapy after phenylbutazone) are ineffective, and that lamellar blood flow is probably more responsive to dynamic loading/unloading of the foot than to any pharmacological intervention.

A novel focus of the book are chapters devoted to a single cell; the lamellar basal epithelial cell (LBEC), the building block of hoof lamellae. Ultimately, layers of LBECs are responsible for the suspension of the distal phalanx by the hoof wall, and these chapters suggest that dysregulation of the LBEC and its intimate attachments to its neighbors and to the lamellar dermis via its basement membrane is at the heart of the laminitis lesion. It is now clear that the LBEC is not just a casualty of the events occurring within the lamellae, but is likely to be an active participant in the events leading to its structural failure (Dr Leise's chapter 'Inflammation'). In other words, any current hierarchical description of laminitis should start with the LBEC and progress to failure of the suspensory apparatus of the distal phalanx. This concept makes the term laminitis redundant, since the only category of laminitis with a proven inflammatory basis is the sepsis-related form. For clarity, laminitis descriptors should be enrolled to ensure meaning (e.g., clinical laminitis, hyperinsulinemic laminitis, histopathologic laminitis, etc.).

Balance is essential in a book such as this, and it is important that readers should be presented with views counter to those generally accepted. This applies particularly to the question of raising the heels of horses with chronic laminitis. This common practice, deemed beneficial to reduce the pull of the deep flexor tendon, is challenged in the chapter 'Digital Biomechanics Relevant to Laminitis' by Professors Merritt and Davies. By increasing the angle of the hoof, more shear loading may be applied to the lamellar junction and despite the force of the deep digital flexor tendon being reduced, this may be more likely to cause tearing of the lamellar junction and promote its failure. Thus, the mechanical benefits of raising or lowering the heels are currently in dispute, and the reader will benefit from reading the complete chapter and that of Dr A. Parks 'Anatomy and Function.' Likewise, deep flexor tenotomy surgical technique is put into perspective as a salvage procedure, rather than a treatment, and an option only likely to increase the comfort of the animal for a variable amount of time, and rarely to allow the animal to return to a low level of athletic activity (Dr W. Waguespack, 'Deep Digital Flexor Tenotomy'). On the other hand. other well-respected authors in this text promote both heel elevation and deep flexor tenotomy. giving the reader the opportunity to question these techniques and formulate therapeutic options for their own laminitis patients based on reasonable hypotheses.

Finally, as the editor points out in his introduction, a thorough understanding of the different parameters of the diseases leading to lamellar injury and the biomechanics of the foot are required to successfully treat the wide variety of clinical scenarios grouped under laminitis. This text will serve Dr Belknap's vision and amply promote an understanding of laminitis and enable clinicians (veterinarians, farriers, and trimmers) to work together with new information at their disposal to approach each individual laminitis case.

At the American Association of Equine Practitioners Annual Convention (New Orleans) in 2003, I concluded my 'Laminitis – In-Depth' presentation by stating: "*The biological basis of laminitis has become molecular and the discipline of molecular biology has laminitis in its cross-hairs. These are exciting times to be involved in equine research – we now have tools our forefathers would not have thought possible. A coherent body of knowledge will soon emerge that will demystify laminitis.*" Professor Belknap has taken up the molecular biology toolset, and a true understanding of laminitis is indeed emerging from the mist. To achieve this, he created multicenter, international research teams (including Australia), and the outcomes of his work – and that of his collaborators – are presented within the pages of this book.

Ten years ago at the International Equine Conference on Laminitis, at West Palm Beach, I awarded Professor Belknap the award for scientific excellence in the field of laminitis research. I'm certainly glad I did because, as this text proves, there is no doubt that James Belknap has gone on to become the preeminent laminitis researcher of our time. We are fortunate indeed that he has dedicated time and effort away from his research to put together an encyclopedia of laminitis information to benefit us all in our efforts to comfort horses and ponies with the bane of laminitis.

Christopher C. Pollitt
Brisbane, Australia
Author of *The Illustrated Horse's Foot – a Comprehensive Guide*, 2016, Elsevier, MO.
ISBN: 9780702046551.

Abbreviations

α-MSH	alpha-melanocyte-stimulating hormone
β-MSH	β-melanocyte-stimulating hormone
β-END	β-endorphin
γ-MSH	γ-melanocyte-stimulating hormone
11β-HSD	11β-hydroxysteroid dehydrogenase
2-ITT	two-step insulin tolerance test
5-HT	5-hydroxytryptamine
AA	arachidonic acid
ACTH	adrenocorticotrophic hormone
ADAMTS4	a disintegrin and metalloprotease with thrombospondin motifs 4
ADP	adenosine 5′-diphosphate
AGE	advanced glycation end-product
AIRg	acute insulin response to glucose
AJ	adherens junction
AMP	adenosine monophosphate
AMPK	adenosine monophosphate-activated protein kinase
APC	adenomatous polyposis coli
APTT	activated partial thromboplastin time
ATF3	activating transcription factor-3
ATP	adenosine 5′-triphosphate
AUC	area under the curve
AVA	arteriovenous anastomosis
BCS	body condition score
BEC	basal epithelial cell
BM	basement membrane
BMZ	basement membrane zone
BWHE	black walnut heartwood extract
cAMP	cyclic adenosine monophosphate
CD	cluster differentiation
CGITT	combined glucose-insulin tolerance test
cGMP	cyclic guanosine monophosphate
CGRP	calcitonin gene-related peptide
CHO	carbohydrate overload
CIVD	cold-induced vasodilation
CK1α	casein kinase 1α
CLIP	corticotropin-like intermediate lobe peptide
CLP	cecal ligation and puncture
CNS	central nervous system
CNS	cresty-neck score chapter 23
COP	center of pressure
COPr	colloid osmotic pressure
COR	center of rotation
COX-2	cyclooxygenase-2
CP	calprotectin
CP	coronary plexus
CPNB	continuous peripheral nerve blockade
CRI	constant rate infusion
CV	circumflex vessel
DAMP	damage-associated molecular pattern
DDF	deep digital flexor
DDFT	deep digital flexor tendon
DGGE	denaturing gradient gel electrophoresis
DI	disposition index
DIC	disseminated intravascular coagulation
DIP	distal interphalangeal
DIPJ	distal interphalangeal joint
DKK	Dickkopf
DM	diabetes mellitus
DM	dry matter
DMSO	dimethyl sulfoxide
DoP	degree of polymerization
DP	distal phalanx
DRG	dorsal root ganglia
DST	dexamethasone suppression test
DTO	di-tri-octahedral
DTP	developmental time point
ECF	extracellular fluid
ECGF	endothelial cell growth factor
ECM	extracellular matrix
EGF	epidermal growth factor
EHC	euglycemic–hyperinsulinemic clamp
EHSS	equine hindgut streptococcal species
EMS	equine metabolic syndrome
EMSAL	equine metabolic syndrome-associated laminitis
EMT	epithelial to mesenchymal transition
eNOS	endothelial nitric oxide synthase
ESC	ethanol-soluble carbohydrate
ET-1	endothelin-1
EVA	ethyl vinyl acetate
FEA	finite element analysis

FFA	free fatty acid
FISH	fluorescence *in-situ* hybridization
FSIGTT	frequently-sampled intravenous glucose tolerance test
GABA	γ-aminobutyric acid
GH	growth hormone
GIP	glucose-dependent insulinotropic polypeptide
GLP-1	glucagon-like peptide 1
GLUT-4	glucose transporter 4
GP	glycoprotein
GRF	ground reaction force
GSHPx	glutathione peroxidase
GSK3β	glycogen synthase kinase 3β
H&E	hematoxylin and eosin
HCt	hematocrit
HD	hemidesmosome
HDL	high-density lipoprotein
HIF-1α	hypoxia-inducible-factor 1α
HLI	hoof–lamellar interface
HMS	human metabolic syndrome
HMW	high-molecular-weight
HOMA-IR	homeostatic model assessment of insulin resistance
HPAA	hypothalamic–pituitary–adrenal axis
HSD	3-beta-hydroxysteroid dehydrogenase
HSS	hypertonic saline solution
HWST	hoof wall surface temperature
ICAM-1	intercellular adhesion molecule-1
ID	insulin dysregulation
IF	intermediate filament
IFN	interferon
IGF-1	insulin-like growth factor-1
IGF-1R	IGF-1 receptor
IHC	immunohistochemistry
IL	interleukin
IM	intramuscular
iNOS	inducible nitric oxide synthase
IRc	insulin receptor
IR	insulin resistance
IRS	insulin receptor substrate
IRT	insulin response test
ITT	insulin tolerance test
IV	intravenous
IVGTT	intravenous glucose tolerance test
KA	keratinized axis
LBEC	lamellar basal epithelial cell
LCJ	lamellar–circumflex junction
LDH	lactate dehydrogenase
LM	light microscopy
LMW	low-molecular-weight
LMWH	low-molecular-weight heparin
Ln 332	laminin-332
LPS	lipopolysaccharide
LRP	lipoprotein receptor-related protein
LTF	laminitis trigger factor
MAA	macroaggregated albumin
MAPK	mitogen-activated protein kinase
MCG	membrane-coating granule
MCM	membrane-coating material
MCP-1	monocyte chemoattractant protein 1
MDA	malondialdehyde
MIRG	modified insulin-to-glucose ratio
MMP	matrix metalloproteinase
MODS	multiple organ dysfunction syndrome
MPO	myeloperoxidase
MRI	magnetic resonance imaging
MT	membrane-type
NADH	reduced nicotinamide adenine dinucleotide
NF-κB	nuclear factor kappa-B
NIR	near-infrared
NMDA	*N*-methyl-D-aspartate
NO	nitric oxide
NOS	nitric oxide synthase
NPY	neuropeptide Y
NSAID	nonsteroidal anti-inflammatory drug
NSC	nonstructural carbohydrate (WSC + starch)
OCT	optimal cutting temperature
OF	oligofructose
OGTT	oral glucose tolerance test
OIH	opioid-induced hyperalgesia
OST	oral sugar test
PAA	penta acetic acid
PAI	plasminogen activator inhibitor
PAL	pasture-associated laminitis
PAMP	pathogen-associated molecular pattern
PAR	protease-activated receptor
PAS	periodic acid–Schiff
PBC	parabasal epithelial cell
PCR	polymerase chain reaction
PCV	packed cell volume
PDGF	platelet-derived growth factor
PDK1	phosphoinositide-dependent kinase-1
PEL	primary epidermal lamella/lamellae
PGK1	phosphoglycerate kinase 1
PHF	Potomac Horse Fever
PI	pars intermedia
PI3K	phosphatidylinositol 3-kinase
PIP	proximal interphalangeal
PIP2	phosphatidylinositol 4,5-bisphosphate
PMAT	plasma membrane monoamine transporter
PMB	polymixin B
PMN	polymorphonucleocyte
PO	per os (oral)

POA	post oligofructose administration
POMC	proopiomelanocortin
PP1	protein phosphatase 1
PPAR-α	peroxisome proliferator-activated receptor-α
PPID	pituitary pars intermedia dysfunction
PRR	pattern recognition receptor
PSH	plasma thiol
PT	prothrombin time
PU:PD	polyuria/polydipsia
PV	pars ventralis
QUICKI	quantitative insulin sensitivity check index
RBC	red blood cell
RISQI	reciprocal of the square root of insulin
RNS	reactive nitrogen species
ROS	reactive oxygen species
RPS6	ribosomal protein S6
RT-qPCR or qRT-PCR	real-time quantitative PCR
RTX	resiniferatoxin
SAA	serum amyloid A
SADP	suspensory apparatus of the distal phalanx
SC	subcutaneous
SDFT	superficial digital flexor tendon
SDL	secondary dermal lamella/lamellae
SDS–PAGE	sodium dodecylsulfate–polyacrylamide gel electrophoresis
SEL	secondary epidermal lamella/lamellae
Sg	glucose effectiveness
SGLT-1	sodium glucose transporter-1
SI	insulin sensitivity index
siRNA	small interfering RNA
SIRS	systemic inflammatory response syndrome
SIS	skin immune system
SLL	supporting limb laminitis
SLRP	small leucine-rich proteoglycan
SLVB	sublamellar vascular bed
SOD	superoxide dismutase
SP	Substance P
SRL	sepsis-related laminitis
STAT	signal transducing activators of transcription factors
T3	triiodothyroidine
T4	thyroxine
TA	terminal arch
TAT	thrombin–antithrombin
TB	tuberculosis
TCF	T-cell factor
TEM	transmission electron microscopy
TGFβ	transforming growth factor-β
TIMP	tissue inhibitor of metalloproteinases
TLR	toll-like receptor
TNFα	tumor necrosis factor alpha
TP	total protein
t-PA	tissue-type plasminogen activator
TRH	thyrotropin-releasing hormone
TRPV-1	transient receptor potential cation channel, subfamily V, member 1
TUNEL	terminal deoxynucleotidyl transferase dUTP nick end labeling
TxA_2	thromboxane A_2
TZD	Thiazolidinedione
UFH	unfractionated heparin
VEGF	vascular endothelial growth factor
VLDL	very low-density lipoprotein
vWF	von Willebrand factor
WBC	white blood cell
WSC	water-soluble carbohydrate

PART 1

Overview: From Basic Research to Caring for the Laminitis Patient

Equine Laminitis, First Edition. Edited by James K. Belknap and Raymond Geor.

CHAPTER 1

Historical Perspective on Equine Laminitis

Donald M. Walsh and Teresa A. Burns

Historical records reveal considerable well-documented evidence of Equine Laminitis as mankind has used horses throughout history. An excellent review of the entire history of laminitis was published by Wagner and Heymering in 1999 [1], and it is the purpose of this discussion to examine the history of Equine Laminitis as seen in the veterinary medical literature from 1800 to the present day.

Mention of laminitis associated with pasture exposure is conspicuously absent from the veterinary literature before approximately 1940. Absent also is reference to any particular breed predisposition to laminitis, or of obesity leading to the disease. Hormone-related endocrinopathic laminitis, the most common form of the disease today, is a relatively recently described veterinary diagnosis [2] and follows closely the first description of human metabolic syndrome in 1988 [3]. In industrialized countries during the 1900s, large numbers of horses were in daily use, and observations regarding the perceived primary causes of laminitis and response to treatments are recorded in detail [4]. In 1906, an observation was recorded that "…laminitis has been described as occurring when the animal is at grass, and when all causes – at any rate, active ones – have appeared to be absent." H. Caulton Reeks was a Fellow of the Royal College of Veterinary Surgeons and, quoting a case history attributed to W. Stanley Carless (*Veterinary Journal*, vol. **ix**, p. 176) in his classic 1906 "Diseases of the Horse's Foot" [5], he describes an obese mare developing severe laminitis on pasture:

"On July 3 an interesting case of laminitis came under my notice. The subject was a mare, eight years old, which had been running on the common here for some months, and was taken up on the night of July 2 by a boy, who did not observe anything amiss with her. The following morning, on the owner going to the stable, he found the animal in great pain, and at once sent for me. I discovered her to be suffering from laminitis, and saw her again in the evening, when she was much worse. The attack proved to be a most severe one. The owner informed me that she had not been allowed any corn for two months, and that she had no distance to travel on the road from the common. Though on such a poor pasture, the mare was very fat she had never been unwell before this attack. This is the first case I have seen of laminitis occurring when the animal was on grass."

This may be the first recorded reference to pasture-associated laminitis (and laminitis associated with obesity). Relatively rare 110 years ago, this classic association between clinical laminitis and horses and ponies grazing pasture was not generally made until recently. Many causes are listed pre-1940, but not pasture.

By 1800, the terms 'founder' and 'laminitis' were both used in the literature. While the exact mechanism(s) resulting in laminitis were not understood, the conditions associated with it were well documented [6]. One of the primary causes listed was excessive concussion to the feet of exhausted horses. What seemed perplexing was that an animal doing the same work and receiving the same care and feed as other horses could develop the disease while others did not. It was thought by some authors that an unknown 'excitatory factor' must have affected the animal's physiology, such as a core temperature change brought on by drinking cold water while very hot, or a cold draft that cooled a hot, standing horse too quickly [7].

The earliest reports of adverse effects from a particular feed are attributed to the Hittites in 1350 BC, where feeding barley was observed to result in 'foot problems' [8]. It was later established that feeding excessive barley, wheat, or corn could cause laminitis. Early authors also recognized that fever from infections could bring on the disease, and that laminitis was seen often seen after a horse had a severe illness resulting in diarrhea or pneumonia. This was commonly referred to as 'metastatic laminitis.' The use of cathartic medication was also reported to result in laminitis, as well as retained placental membranes in mares [9]. Additionally, it was well known that a horse with a severe injury to a limb could develop laminitis in the foot of the opposite limb if a sling was not used for support of the animal during recovery [4].

In 1915, the population of horses, ponies and mules in the United States peaked at 26.5 million [10]. This equated to one equid for every three people in the nation. With the advent of mechanized farming and the introduction of the automobile, the horse rapidly became functionally redundant. No longer needed for their role in war and as a 'beast of burden' in agriculture, the horse population declined dramatically and breeds of working horses virtually disappeared.

Equine Laminitis, First Edition. Edited by James K. Belknap and Raymond Geor.

Following World War II, horses became 'leisure animals,' relegated principally to sport and recreational purposes. In the *USDA Yearbook of Agriculture* (1942), mention is made of laminitis being caused by over-feeding, chiefly on grains but also green plants or any palatable feed consumed to excess [11]. A lifestyle lacking routine strenuous exercise along with ready access to abundant feed was imposed on a population of horses and ponies genetically predisposed to be 'easy keepers,' ones that required less food than others to maintain and exceed their optimum weight. No longer 'working horses,' these animals were now susceptible to a new form of laminitis linked to obesity and insulin resistance [12].

Equine Laminitis Treatments from the 1800s to the Present Day

Treatments for laminitis described throughout the nineteenth century cited bleeding via jugular, toe, or coronary band phlebotomy in volumes of up to 6–8 quarts (ca. 7–9 liters) as absolutely essential [13]. Some practitioners monitored the digital pulse in the foot and bled the animal until the pulse was no longer palpable over the palmar digital artery. It was believed that if bleeding was performed sooner rather than later, less damage would occur within the foot. Even after 1900, when the practice of bleeding was for the most part abandoned by veterinarians, some still insisted it was indicated for acute laminitis [14]. The stated purpose was to lower blood pressure in the extremity, which then reduced the pressure inside the hoof capsule.

Other early practices to treat acute laminitis were to dose orally with diuretics such as potassium nitrate in the water three times a day [15]. Saltpeter was also used as a diuretic aimed at lowering blood pressure. Removing all cereal grain from the diet and feeding only forage was a recommended treatment [16]. If the case involved over-consumption of grain, a cathartic such as tartar emetic was given or a bran mash fed to evacuate the bowel. Caution was recommended, however, as excessive use of cathartics was suggested to actually *cause* laminitis in horses [4].

Treatment of the feet during a bout of laminitis usually included the removal of shoes when possible. Most early authors advocated using cold water on the feet [11]. It was suggested that this could be accomplished by standing the horse in a tub with ice, if available. Some described using warm water for 20 minutes, then switching to cold. Early in the twentieth century, the US Calvary used ice if available up to the knees and hocks [16]. When the affected horse was not standing in cold water, it was encouraged to lie down by providing it with a well-bedded stall. Bran or linseed oil poultices and ointments such as arnica were applied to the feet to soften them and reduce inflammation [4, 14].

Pain control was of great interest to early health providers working with laminitic horses. Many authors stated that the pain of laminitis was greatly relieved by the horse lying down [15]. To help control pain, Dadd recommended using hops or poppy heads (opium) [17]. Youatt recommended using digitalis as a sedative and nitre (potassium nitrite) to cool the feet in acute laminitis [13]. The 1918 *U.S. Manual for Stable Sergeants* recommends administering an oral tincture of *Cannabis indica* for the control of excessive pain. Interestingly, it was also the drug of choice for the control of colic pain in cavalry horses [16].

Exercise was then, as it is today, a controversial issue. By the early 1900s exercise was encouraged after recovery had started and the horse was willing to move on its own. It was then recommended that the exercise be gradually increased until soundness returned [4, 16].

From 1800 to 1920, the main cause of laminitis cited in the literature was that due to excessive concussion to the feet. Horses worked long hours pounding their feet on very hard surfaces, unlike our sport horses today, which perform on very controlled surfaces to protect their limbs. It is interesting to note that horsemen believed it to be important to condition horses' feet before working them intensely to prevent this form of the disease. They knew that exercise made the foot stronger and the lamellae less likely to be injured by concussive impact. Perhaps coincidentally, the only reference to obesity found in this 1800–1920 literature was advice to "…not work a plethoric horse hard before the feet are in condition" [18]. Plethoric means 'large or excessive,' so this statement is assumed to refer to a horse that was heavy and out of condition and therefore without feet in good condition for work [4]. Authors also cautioned against over-working a green horse until its feet were conditioned to hard work. This concept that exercise strengthens the foot seems to have been lost on many horsemen today, who often allow animals to largely stand idle in stalls. From 1920–1940, little new information about laminitis is found in the literature. The sections on acute laminitis and its treatment in the *USDA Diseases of the Horse* are virtually identical in the 1911, 1928, and 1942 editions.

Changes in Pasture from 1920 to the Present Day

The first reference to pasture as a suspected cause of laminitis was published in the *Yearbook of Agriculture 1942*. In fact, pasture was cited in that reference as the most frequent cause of the disease: "Overeating and consumption of green plants…is the most common cause…" [11]. This seems to signal the start of an era in which the most common form of laminitis is what we now call the 'pasture-associated laminitis' form of endocrinopathic laminitis.

The factors that increased either the incidence and/or the reporting of cases of pasture-associated laminitis after 1942 are unclear, but the following factors may have played a role. Widespread pasture improvement in the United States through advances in agronomy practices may have increased exposure of horses to pastures that were primarily meant to provide forage for production animals (especially cattle). These pastures frequently contain cultivars of grass species that have been selected for higher levels of nonstructural carbohydrates than native grasses. Elevation in the nonstructural carbohydrate content of these grasses is observed primarily in the spring and the fall seasons, which is the same pattern of seasonality that is noted in pasture-associated laminitis in horses and ponies.

Another major change that occurred was to the horse itself. No longer a work animal, horses began to lead a more sedentary lifestyle. The greatly reduced workload, along with an increase in caloric intake from abundant rich grass, may have contributed to the burgeoning rate of equine obesity. Overweight horses are prone to develop insulin resistance and laminitis when grazing spring and fall grasses. Thus, horses may have been put at risk for laminitis from eating heavily improved grass by way of a newly described pathway referred to as endocrinopathic laminitis. This form of the disease is associated with elevated blood insulin levels; laminitis can occur repeatedly, eventually crippling the horse [19]. By the 1960s, the literature commonly lists grass as a cause of laminitis [20]. It is interesting to note that feral horses living on unimproved pastureland in the west seem to be spared this form of laminitis (D. Hyde, personal communication to D. Walsh).

It appears that this form of laminitis could be a man-made problem, one which science should be able to correct using responsible agricultural husbandry practices. Research to understand the pathophysiology of equine metabolic syndrome (EMS) and pituitary pars intermedia dysfunction (PPID) – both disorders that result in endocrinopathic laminitis – is ongoing and described in detail in the following chapters.

Modern Advances in Equine Laminitis Research: Development of Experimental Models

Equine Laminitis has been described since antiquity as an often fatal and therapeutically intractable disease of the equine foot [21, 22]. For several hundred years, information about Equine Laminitis has been gleaned from the observation and treatment of naturally occurring cases (as described above); advances in knowledge of the disease via this mechanism were painstakingly slow and yielded little conclusive information about how laminitis developed or how the condition could be effectively treated.

It was not until the development of several experimental models of laminitis over the past 40 years that major insights have been gained into the pathophysiology of the condition [23–26]. Reliable, consistent induction of laminitis in a controlled fashion has allowed modern researchers not only to investigate the mechanisms and pathways by which laminitis develops but also to evaluate the efficacy of various treatment modalities that have been suggested to be effective for the condition. In fact, one model in particular – the alimentary carbohydrate overload model (discussed further below [23]) – has been instrumental in this regard, as this model has been used to document the efficacy of one of the only consistently effective strategies for the treatment and prevention of sepsis-related laminitis, distal limb cryotherapy [27–29].

With the development of experimental laminitis models and the observation of pathophysiological differences between them, laminitis is now understood to be a heterogeneous condition, with structural failure of the digital lamellae as a 'final common pathway' that can result from diverse inciting etiologies. When comparing the current literature on experimental sepsis-related laminitis and that induced by hyperinsulinemia (as described elsewhere in this text), it appears that these two manifestations of laminitis are quite different. Future studies using these established models of disease are anticipated to exploit these differences to develop novel therapies for the two – now separate – diseases.

Models of Sepsis-Related Laminitis

Laminitis is most classically associated with sepsis and endotoxemia in adult horses, often observed as a complication of diseases such as gastrointestinal strangulation, colitis, pleuropneumonia, and septic metritis [30]. In 1975, Garner and colleagues published a protocol for the reliable experimental induction of laminitis with enteral starch overload [23], and, with this paper, modern laminitis research began to accelerate. This model involves a single-bolus intragastric administration of a mixture of 85% cornstarch and 15% wood flour (17.6 g kg^{-1} body weight); treated horses were observed to become laminitic (Obel grade 3) within 32–48 h, as well as febrile and endotoxemic. Approximately 20–30% of horses dosed according to this model would fail to develop laminitis, which over time became to be seen as a major limitation of the model [31]. That said, an entirely new line of inquiry was opened when some investigators became interested in looking at these 'non-responders' to identify factors that conferred protection [32]. A more consistent and possibly clinically relevant model of alimentary carbohydrate overload has been developed recently [26], involving the administration of a single intragastric dose of 10 g kg^{-1} body weight of oligofructose. Using this model, laminitis can be consistently induced in dosed horses, mitigating the question of how to best deal with non-responding horses. Both models appear to induce disease which closely approximates the sepsis-related laminitis observed clinically in adult horses. Therefore, using these models, several research groups have investigated the roles of inflammation, the digital vasculature, metabolic pathways, and weight bearing on the pathophysiology of sepsis-associated laminitis. Krueger and colleagues [33] noted that acute enteral carbohydrate overload was associated with severe typhlitis/typhlocolitis and mucosal disruption, potentially leading to exposure of the systemic circulation of the affected horse to luminal contents that might predispose to laminitis. Additional studies later documented significant alterations in cecal and colonic microflora and pH associated with this model – changes which were suggested to increase the transmural absorption of several postulated laminitis 'trigger factors,' including bacterial endotoxin and vasoactive amines [31, 34–39]. Later attempts were made at modifying the oligofructose model in an attempt to replicate a suspected 'two-hit' model of end-organ damage in sepsis (in which an initial sublethal 'priming' insult, such as hemorrhage or infection, alters immune responsiveness and is followed quickly by a second – often lethal – insult that induces inappropriate inflammatory responsiveness and organ dysfunction). These modifications did not enhance the severity of disease in experimental horses [40], and the original grain starch and oligofructose models remain the best experimental models of clinical sepsis-associated laminitis that are available to investigators today.

Black Walnut Extract Model

Historical and modern anecdotal observations of laminitis developing in horses bedded on wood shavings containing black walnut tree heartwood (*Juglans nigra*) led to the development of another experimental model of sepsis-associated laminitis [24]. Indeed, concerns about the inconsistency of the enteral carbohydrate overload models, along with the severe pain and systemic illness that they induced, led many investigators to pursue studies involving the black walnut heartwood extract (BWHE) model from 1990–2010. In this model, an extract made from soaking approximately 1 kg of black walnut heartwood overnight in 5 liters of deionized water is filtered and administered via a nasogastric tube to the horse. This model is considered to more closely approximate a single intravenous bolus of endotoxin [41], as horses can be observed to become febrile and leukopenic within 4 h of dosing, and mildly laminitic (Obel grade 1) within 12 h; if no additional doses of BWHE are administered, horses typically recover fully without sustaining significant structural damage to their feet. Critics of this model rightly state that laminitis induced by BWHE does not accurately mimic naturally occurring sepsis-associated disease for this reason. However, this model has contributed greatly to the current understanding of the early pathophysiological events occurring in sepsis-associated laminitis, including the documentation of lamellar inflammation [42–48].

Models of Endocrinopathic Laminitis

Laminitis occurring secondary to EMS/insulin resistance (IR), PPID, or exogenous corticosteroid administration has collectively been referred to as *endocrinopathic laminitis* in horses and ponies. This category of laminitis, which is the most common form afflicting equids currently, has been long assumed to share pathophysiologic characteristics with other forms of laminitis (notably, sepsis-associated disease). However, with the recent discovery that iatrogenic hyperinsulinemia for a period of days can precipitate laminitis [25], studies of this form of laminitis have suggested that it may differ from other forms of the disease. The hyperinsulinemic–euglycemic clamp technique used by Asplin and colleagues has been used as an experimental model of equine metabolic syndrome–associated laminitis (EMSAL) [25, 49, 50]; however, consistent models of laminitis associated with PPID or exogenous corticosteroid administration remain to be described (attempts to experimentally induce laminitis in normal horses with exogenous steroid administration have been unsuccessful). Knowledge of whether these forms of endocrinopathic laminitis are pathophysiologically similar will depend on the development of consistent, repeatable models of the respective diseases, as has been done for sepsis-related laminitis.

Supporting Limb Laminitis

Laminitis is known to be a significant complication of prolonged unilateral weight-bearing in adult horses, and the few publications that exist in the scientific literature regarding supporting limb laminitis are epidemiologic or descriptive in nature [51–53]; however, very little information is currently available regarding the underlying pathophysiologic mechanisms that lead to this condition. Current attempts to develop a consistent experimental model of the disease will hopefully close this knowledge gap, as this is a problem currently receiving attention from the laminitis research community.

Pathophysiology Elucidated Through Study of Experimental Models: Shifting Hypotheses

Equine Laminitis – be it associated with sepsis, endocrine disease, or unilateral lameness – is unlikely to be caused by a single, linear exposure or molecular event. Rather, the pathogenesis of laminitis is likely to be complex, and moreover, it is likely to vary among the clinical circumstances in which the disease is most frequently encountered. The investigation of several hypothetical mechanisms thought to be involved in the development of laminitis over the past 40 years has resulted in shifting attitudes regarding their relative importance; current research strategies favor an integration of many of these mechanisms.

One of the first mechanisms to receive vigorous research attention was that of altered vasomotor tone and resultant ischemia. During the 1970s, Garner and colleagues evaluated the role of hypertension in Equine Laminitis [54]; this same group was also one of the first to describe the angiographic appearance of the laminitic equine foot [55]. Hood *et al.* [22] likened Equine Laminitis to Raynaud's phenomenon (a recurrent ischemic condition of the human digit); later investigations have evaluated the role of thrombosis [56, 57], the role of the veins/venules in lamellar vascular dysfunction [58–62], and the role of insulin [63, 64] on vascular dysfunction and lamellar ischemia in the setting of laminitis. Current investigations of vascular pathophysiology are moving away from simple lamellar ischemia and substrate deprivation toward endothelial dysfunction (as might be associated with insulin resistance).

During the 1990s, the results of several investigations into the role of altered lamellar enzymatic activity were published, and this led to intense interest in the potential therapeutic utility of this mechanism. Pollitt and colleagues, through their studies with gelatin zymography, suggested that the activation of several matrix metalloproteinases (most notably MMP-2 and MMP-9) might result in the degradation of lamellar extracellular matrix components and the attachment of the lamellar basal epithelial cell to its basement membrane, thereby contributing to the structural changes within the hoof capsule that commonly occur in laminitis [65–67]. Later studies by Black and colleagues emphasized the role of other lamellar proteases [68–72]; the majority of work has applied to sepsis-related laminitis, and the role of MMP activation in endocrinopathic laminitis appears insignificant [73]. Additionally, while MMP activation in laminitis has been documented, the cause(s) of this activation remain elusive. As these enzymes can be inhibited pharmacologically in many cases, this mechanistic category remains an attractive therapeutic target for laminitic equids; additional information regarding target and timing, however, is required before widely recommending their use.

During the early to mid-2000s, lamellar inflammation in sepsis-associated laminitis was described comprehensively for the first time by Belknap and colleagues [45, 74]. Several studies were subsequently reported describing the presence of infiltrative leukocytes and elevated concentrations of several pro-inflammatory cytokines and chemokines in the digital lamellae of horses subjected to both BWE and carbohydrate-overload models of laminitis [42–44, 47, 75–77]; these changes were also shown to affect the fore and hind feet of experimental animals [32]. In spite of strong experimental evidence for lamellar inflammation in sepsis-related laminitis, systemic anti-inflammatory therapy has been somewhat disappointing in its attenuation of inflammation associated with laminitis [78]. The only therapy found to effectively block lamellar inflammatory signaling is cryotherapy, with little apparent effect of nonsteroidal anti-inflammatory drugs (NSAIDs) at this point in time [79].

Most recently, investigations of metabolic changes in the digital lamellae, particularly related to glucose and insulin dysregulation, have attracted intense attention. Insulin resistance has been identified as a risk factor for Equine Laminitis, and effects on lamellar metabolism were thought to be involved. Early work focused on the effects of substrate (especially glucose) deprivation, which was shown to encourage the detachment of lamellar basal epithelial cells (LBECs) from their basement membrane *in vitro* [65]; subsequent studies performed by this same group and others showed that glucose uptake by the digital lamellae was insulin-independent, suggesting that glucose deprivation was not a primary mechanism involved in EMSAL [80, 81]. The effects of systemic metabolic dysfunction on both vascular supply to the digit and the LBECs themselves is a primary focus of laminitis research currently, and will likely remain so in the near future, as EMSAL is the most common form of the disease observed clinically.

The advent of the molecular era has resulted in a rapid expansion of knowledge of the pathophysiology of laminitis. Most research groups acknowledge that laminitis likely represents a heterogeneous group of disease states (or a common end result of such states), and there is unlikely to be a singular inciting cause or pathophysiologic mechanism. Rather, the disease is complex and multifactorial, a fact which has been established over the past 40 years of modern laminitis research. The laminitis research community is well-positioned to make rapid advances in knowledge of this disease; the equine genome is published and available, as are rapid molecular screening techniques (such as transcriptome and kinome analyses). Finally, cohesion and cooperation between laminitis research laboratories internationally, including the formation of a laminitis tissue bank [82] and the wide sharing of tissues from animals subjected to experimental models, has advanced – and will continue to advance – the knowledge of this disease and the ability to treat affected animals in the future.

Equine Laminitis Farriery from 1800 to the Present Day

The literature of the 1800s and early 1900s offers very little description of special shoeing techniques for either acute or chronic stages of Equine Laminitis. A common treatment at the sudden onset of the disease advocated removing the shoes if possible, bandaging the feet, and applying cold water to the bandages. The cold was meant to reduce inflammation, and it was also thought that water would soften the horn of the hoof in order to allow the foot to expand (reducing pressure within the hoof capsule).

During recovery from acute (and flares of chronic) laminitis, when the affected horse started to move again, the farrier would attempt to provide support to the foot with a bar shoe, with the bar applied at the heel [5]. The horse with chronic laminitis presented a 'pumiced foot' (a dropped sole and dished anterior hoof wall). Horses with the chronic form, which could be the result of incomplete recovery from the initial attack or from gradual insults to the foot over time, were shod with a thicker bar shoe for support. Acute and chronic cases were also shod in wide-web shoes, with the area over the sole beveled to reduce pressure on the dropped sole. The frustration in trying to help animals with chronic laminitis (similar to today's frustration with shoeing the laminitic horse) can be appreciated by the following description:

"All that can be done in the way of palliation is by shoeing. Nothing must press on the projecting and pumiced part. If the projection be not great, a thick bar shoe is the best thing that can be applied, but should the sole have much descended, a shoe with a wide web,

beveled off so as not to press on the part, may be used. These means of relief, however, are only temporary, the disease will proceed; and, at no great distance of time, the horse will be useless." [6]

By the early 1900s it was recommended that, by 10 days to three weeks after the onset of laminitis, the hoof wall at the toe should be shortened, the sole trimmed if necessary, flat shoes rolled at the toe placed on the feet, and the animal allowed to exercise for a short time daily [5]. Authors recognized that the foot grew rapidly and required trimming and the shoes be reset every three weeks. "The wall at the toe should be short, but excessive thinning of the sole should be avoided" [83]. It seemed to be generally understood that the success of the treatment and recovery was directly related to how much damage had occurred during the acute phase of laminitis.

Modern podiatric treatment of laminitic horses remains in many ways very similar to that described over the past two hundred years. Many of the principles described over 100 years ago are still used today (i.e. heel elevation and increasing ease of breakover), but the mechanics of how these goals are accomplished have evolved over time, with many prefabricated shoeing systems available commercially for use by farriers and equine veterinarians who treat these patients. Popular devices include the NANRIC Ultimate cuff, the Equine Digital Support System/Four-Point Rail Shoe, and the Steward Clog, the use of all of which has anecdotally increased in recent years. However, clinical trial data describing the relative efficacy of these devices is virtually absent currently and sorely needed in order to guide the effective treatment of laminitic horses.

Regarding medical treatment and farriery, both early and modern-day horsemen recognize that preventing laminitis from occurring is far better than attempting to treat the disease once it occurs. The end results of laminitis are too often still ruinous to the horse, a situation that will hopefully be improved in the future through both basic research and well-controlled clinical trials.

Acknowledgments

The authors gratefully acknowledge the skilled assistance of Mr C. Trenton Boyd, BS, MA, AHIP, FMLA, Distinguished Librarian and Curator of the Medical and Veterinary Historical Collections, University of Missouri, Columbia MO, in the research and preparation of this chapter.

References

1. Wagner, I.P. and Heymering, H. (1999) Historical perspectives on laminitis. *Vet. Clin. North Am. Equine Practice*, **15** (2), 295–309.
2. Johnson, P.J. (2002) The equine metabolic syndrome: peripheral Cushing's syndrome. *Vet. Clin. North Am. Equine Practice*, **18** (2), 271–793.
3. Reaven, G.M. (1988) Role of insulin resistance in human disease. *Diabetes*, **37** (12), 1595–1607.
4. Holcombe, A. (1911) Laminitis or Founder, in *Diseases of Horses*. United States Department of Agriculture, pp. 414–430.
5. Reeks, H.C. (1906) Inflammatory affectations of keratogenous apparatus. A. Acute laminitis, in *Diseases of the Horselaminiti* Alex Eger, Chicago, pp. 256–.03.
6. Miles, W.J. (1860) The Feet. *Modern Practical Farrier*. pp. 342–344.
7. Stewart, R. (1867) Acute Founder or Laminitis. *The American Farmer's Horse Book*. pp. 113–117.
8. Rooney, J.R. and Robertson, J.L. (1996) *Equine Pathology*. Iowa State University Press, Ames IA, pp. 188.
9. Reynolds, M.H. (1929) Laminitis (Founder). *Veterinary Studies for Agriculture Students*. pp. 224–226.
10. Kilby, E.R. (2007) The demographics of the US equine population, in *The State of the Animals 2007*. (eds D.J. Salem and A.N. Rowan), Humane Society Press, Washington, DC, pp. 175–205.
11. Mott, L.O., Shahan, M.S., Glintner, L.T., and Frank, A.H. (1942) Founder (Laminitis). *Keeping Livestock Healthy: Yearbook of Agriculture*. United States Department of Agriculture, pp. 455–456.
12. Coffman, J.R. and Colles, C.M. (1983) Insulin tolerance in laminitic ponies. *Can. J. Comp. Med.*, **47** (3), 347–351.
13. Youatt, W. (1856) Inflammation of the Foot or Acute Founder. *On Structures and Diseases of the Horse*. pp. 302–305.
14. Dadd, G.H. (1910) Laminitis (Fever in the Feet or Feet Founder). *American Reformed Horsebook*. pp. 350–351.
15. Youatt, W. (1870) *Youatt's History, Treatment and Diseases of the Horse*, pp. 291.
16. Anonymous (1917) Acute Laminitis (Founder). *The Manual for Stable Sergeants*. United States War Department, pp. 150.
17. Dadd, G.H. (1865) Acute Inflammation of the Feet (Laminitis). *Modern Horse Doctor*. pp. 352–354.
18. Bailliere, Tindall, and Cox (1885) *Veterinary Journal and Annals of Comparative Pathology*, Vol. 20, pp. 422.
19. Walsh, D.M., McGowan, C.M., McGowan, T., *et al.* (2009) Correlation of plasma insulin concentration with laminitis score in a field study of equine Cushing's disease and equine metabolic syndrome. *J. Equine Vet. Sci.*, **29**, 87–94.
20. Miller, R. (1967) How to Prevent Founder. *Health Problems of the Horse: Western Horseman Book*. pp. 14.
21. Smithcors, J. (1957) *Evolution of the Veterinary Art*. Veterinary Medicine Publishing Co, Kansas City, pp. 57–162.
22. Hood, D.M., Amoss, M.S. and Grosenbaugh, D.A. (1990) Equine laminitis: a potential model of Raynaud's phenomenon. *Angiology*, **41** (4), 270–277.
23. Garner, H.E., Coffman, J.R., Hahn, A.W., Hutcheson, D.P., and Tumbleson, M.E. (1975) Equine laminitis of alimentary origin: an experimental model. *Am. J. Vet. Res.*, **36** (4 Pt.1), 441–444.
24. Galey, F.D., Whiteley, H.E., Goetz, T.E., Kuenstler, A.R., Davis, C.A., and Beasley, V.R. (1991) Black walnut (*Juglans nigra*) toxicosis: a model for equine laminitis. *J. Comp. Pathol.*, **104** (3), 313–326.
25. Asplin, K.E., Sillence, M.N., Pollitt, C.C., and McGowan, C.M. (2007) Induction of laminitis by prolonged hyperinsulinaemia in clinically normal ponies. *Vet. J. (London 1997)*, **174** (3), 530–535.
26. Van Eps, A.W. and Pollitt, C.C. (2006) Equine laminitis induced with oligofructose. *Equine Vet. J.*, **38** (3), 203–208.
27. Van Eps, A.W., Pollitt, C.C., Underwood, C., Medina-Torres, C.E., Goodwin, W.A., and Belknap, J.K. (2013) Continuous digital hypothermia initiated after the onset of lameness prevents lamellar failure in the oligofructose laminitis model. *Equine Vet. J.*, **46** (5), 625–630.

28. Van Eps, A.W., Leise, B.S., Watts, M., Pollitt, C.C., and Belknap, J.K. (2012) Digital hypothermia inhibits early lamellar inflammatory signalling in the oligofructose laminitis model. *Equine Vet. J.*, **44** (2), 230–237.
29. Van Eps, A.W. and Pollitt, C.C. (2009) Equine laminitis model: cryotherapy reduces the severity of lesions evaluated seven days after induction with oligofructose. *Equine Vet. J.*, **41** (8), 741–746.
30. Belknap, J.K., Moore, J.N., and Crouser, E.C. (2009) Sepsis – From human organ failure to lamellar failure. *Vet. Immunol. Immunopathol.*, **129** (3-4), 155–157.
31. Sprouse, R.F., Garner, H.E., and Green, E.M. (1987) Plasma endotoxin levels in horses subjected to carbohydrate-induced laminitis. *Equine Vet. J.*, **19** (1), 25–28.
32. Leise, B.S., Faleiros, R.R., Watts, M., Johnson, P.J., Black, S.J., and Belknap, J.K. (2011) Hindlimb lamellar inflammatory response is similar to that present in forelimbs after carbohydrate overload in horses. *Equine Vet. J.*, **44** (6), 633.
33. Krueger, A.S., Kinden, D.A., Garner, H.E., and Sprouse, R.F. (1986) Ultrastructural study of the equine cecum during onset of laminitis. *Am. J. Vet. Res.*, **47** (8), 1804–1812.
34. Garner, H.E., Moore, J.N., Johnson, J.H., Clark, L., Amend, J.F., Tritschler, L.G., Coffmann, J.R., Sprouse, R.F., Hutcheson, D.P., and Salem, C.A. (1978) Changes in the caecal flora associated with the onset of laminitis. *Equine Vet. J.*, **10** (4), 249–252.
35. Moore, J.N., Garner, H.E., Berg, J.N., and Sprouse, R.F. (1979) Intracecal endotoxin and lactate during the onset of equine laminitis: a preliminary report. *Am. J. Vet. Res.*, **40** (5), 722–723.
36. Milinovich, G.J., Klieve, A.V., Pollitt, C.C., and Trott, D.J. (2010) Microbial events in the hindgut during carbohydrate-induced equine laminitis. *Vet. Clin. North Am. Equine Practice*, **26** (1), 79–94.
37. Bailey, S.R., Adair, H.S., Reinemeyer, C.R., Morgan, S.J., Brooks, A.C., Longhofer, S.L., and Elliott, J. (2009) Plasma concentrations of endotoxin and platelet activation in the developmental stage of oligofructose-induced laminitis. *Vet. Immunol. Immunopathol.*, **129** (3-4), 167–173.
38. Bailey, S.R., Cunningham, F.M., and Elliott, J. (2000) Endotoxin and dietary amines may increase plasma 5-hydroxytryptamine in the horse. *Equine Vet. J.*, **32** (6), 497–504.
39. Elliott, J. and Bailey, S.R. (2006) Gastrointestinal derived factors are potential triggers for the development of acute equine laminitis. *J. Nutrition*, **136** (7 Suppl.), 2103S–2107S.
40. Tadros, E.M., Frank, N., Newkirk, K.M., Donnell, R.L., and Horohov, D.W. (2012) Effects of a 'two-hit' model of organ damage on the systemic inflammatory response and development of laminitis in horses. *Vet. Immunol. Immunopathol.*, **150** (1-2), 90–100.
41. Belknap, J.K. (2010) Black walnut extract: an inflammatory model. *Vet. Clin. North Am. Equine Practice*, **26** (1), 95–101.
42. Blikslager, A.T., Yin, C., Cochran, A.M., Wooten, J.G., Pettigrew, A., and Belknap, J.K. (2006) Cyclooxygenase expression in the early stages of equine laminitis: a cytologic study. *J. Vet. Intern. Med./Am. Coll. Vet. Intern. Med.*, **20** (5), 1191–1196.
43. Loftus, J.P., Black, S.J., Pettigrew, A., Abrahamsen, E.J., and Belknap, J.K. (2007) Early lamellar events involving endothelial activation in horses with black walnut-induced laminitis. *Am. J. Vet. Res.*, **68** (11), 1205–1211.
44. Waguespack, R.W., Cochran, A., and Belknap, J.K. (2004) Expression of the cyclooxygenase isoforms in the prodromal stage of black walnut-induced laminitis in horses. *Am. J. Vet. Res.*, **65** (12), 1724–1729.
45. Waguespack, R.W., Kemppainen, R.J., Cochran, A., Lin, H.C., and Belknap, J.K. (2004) Increased expression of MAIL, a cytokine-associated nuclear protein, in the prodromal stage of black walnut-induced laminitis. *Equine Vet. J.*, **36** (3), 285–291.
46. Stewart, A.J., Pettigrew, A., Cochran, A.M., and Belknap, J.K. (2009) Indices of inflammation in the lung and liver in the early stages of the black walnut extract model of equine laminitis. *Vet. Immunol. Immunopathol.*, **129** (3-4), 254–260.
47. Belknap, J.K., Giguere, S., Pettigrew, A., Cochran, A.M., Van Eps, A.W., and Pollitt, C.C. (2007) Lamellar pro-inflammatory cytokine expression patterns in laminitis at the developmental stage and at the onset of lameness: innate vs. adaptive immune response. *Equine Vet. J.*, **39** (1), 42–47.
48. Black, S.J., Lunn, D.P., Yin, C., Hwang, M., Lenz, S.D., and Belknap, J.K. (2006) Leukocyte emigration in the early stages of laminitis. *Vet. Immunol. Immunopathol.*, **109** (1-2), 161–166.
49. De Laat, M.A., Kyaw-Tanner, M.T., Nourian, A.R., McGowan, C.M., Sillence, M.N., and Pollitt, C.C. (2011) The developmental and acute phases of insulin-induced laminitis involve minimal metalloproteinase activity. *Vet. Immunol. Immunopathol.*, **140**, 275–781.
50. De Laat, M.A., McGowan, C.M., Sillence, M.N., and Pollitt, C.C. (2010) Equine laminitis: induced by 48 h hyperinsulinaemia in Standardbred horses. *Equine Vet. J.*, **42** (2), 129–135.
51. Baxter, G.M. and Morrison, S. (2008) Complications of unilateral weight bearing. *Vet. Clin. North Am. Equine Practice*, **24** (3), 621–342, ix.
52. Virgin, J.E., Goodrich, L.R., Baxter, G.M. and Rao, S. (2011) Incidence of support limb laminitis in horses treated with half limb, full limb or transfixation pin casts: a retrospective study of 113 horses (2000–2009). *Equine Vet. J. Suppl.*, **40**, 7–11.
53. Bowman, K.F., Leitch, M., Nunamaker, D.M., Fackelman, G.E., Tate, L.P., Jr, Park, M.I., Boles, C.L., and Raker, C.W. (1984) Complications during treatment of traumatic disruption of the suspensory apparatus in Thoroughbred horses. *J. Am. Vet. Med. Assoc.*, **184** (6), 706–715.
54. Garner, H.E., Hahn, A.W., Salem, C., Coffman, J.R., Hutcheson, D.P., and Johnson, J.H. (1977) Cardiac output, left ventricular ejection rate, plasma volume, and heart rate changes in equine laminitis-hypertension. *Am. J. Vet. Res.*, **38** (6), 725–729.
55. Ackerman, N., Garner, H.E., Coffman, J.R., and Clement, J.W. (1975) Angiographic appearance of the normal equine foot and alterations in chronic laminitis. *J. Am. Vet. Med. Assoc.*, **166** (1), 58–62.
56. Weiss, D.J., Trent, A.M., and Johnston, G. (1995) Prothrombotic events in the prodromal stages of acute laminitis in horses. *Am. J. Vet. Res.*, **56** (8), 986–991.
57. Weiss, D.J., Geor, R.J., Johnston, G., and Trent, A.M. (1994) Microvascular thrombosis associated with onset of acute laminitis in ponies. *Am. J. Vet. Res.*, **55** (5), 606–612.
58. Robertson, T.P., Bailey, S.R., and Peroni, J.F. (2009) Equine laminitis: a journey to the dark side of venous. *Vet. Immunol. Immunopathol.*, **129** (3-4), 164–166.
59. Robertson, T.P., Moore, J.N., Noschka, E., Lewis, T.H., Lewis, S.J., and Peroni, J.F. (2007) Evaluation of activation of protein kinase C during agonist-induced constriction of veins isolated from the lamellar dermis of horses. *Am. J. Vet. Res.*, **68** (6), 664–669.
60. Noschka, E., Moore, J.N., Peroni, J.F., Lewis, T.H., Lewis, S.J., and Robertson, T.P. (2010) Evaluation of the possible role of

prostaglandin F(2 alpha) in laminitis induced in horses by nasogastric administration of black walnut heartwood extract. *Am. J. Vet. Res.*, **71** (2), 186–193.
61. Peroni, J.F., Moore, J.N., Noschka, E., Grafton, M.E., Aceves-Avila, M., Lewis, S.J., and Robertson, T.P. (2006) Predisposition for venoconstriction in the equine lamellar dermis: implications in equine laminitis. *J. Appl. Physiol. (Bethesda)*, **100** (3), 759–763.
62. Noschka, E., Moore, J.N., Peroni, J.F., Lewis, S.J., Morrow, J.D., and Robertson, T.P. (2009) Thromboxane and isoprostanes as inflammatory and vasoactive mediators in black walnut heartwood extract induced equine laminitis. *Vet. Immunol. Immunopathol.*, **129** (3-4), 200–210.
63. Venugopal, C.S., Eades, S., Holmes, E.P., and Beadle, R.E. (2011) Insulin resistance in equine digital vessel rings: an in vitro model to study vascular dysfunction in equine laminitis. *Equine Vet. J.*, **43** (6), 744–749.
64. Eades, S.C., Stokes, A.M., Johnson, P.J., Leblanc, C.J., Ganjam, V.K., Buff, P.R., and Moore, R.M. (2007) Serial alterations in digital hemodynamics and endothelin-1 immunoreactivity, platelet-neutrophil aggregation, and concentrations of nitric oxide, insulin, and glucose in blood obtained from horses following carbohydrate overload. *Am. J. Vet. Res.*, **68** (1), 87–94.
65. French, K.R. and Pollitt, C.C. (2004) Equine laminitis: cleavage of laminin 5 associated with basement membrane dysadhesion. *Equine Vet. J.*, **36** (3), 242–247.
66. French, K.R. and Pollitt, C.C. (2004) Equine laminitis: glucose deprivation and MMP activation induce dermo-epidermal separation in vitro. *Equine Vet. J.*, **36** (3), 261–266.
67. Kyaw-Tanner, M.T., Wattle, O., Van Eps, A.W., and Pollitt, C.C. (2008) Equine laminitis: membrane type matrix metalloproteinase-1 (MMP-14) is involved in acute phase onset. *Equine Vet. J.*, **40** (5), 482–487.
68. Black, S.J. (2009) Extracellular matrix, leukocyte migration and laminitis. *Vet. Immunol. Immunopathol.*, **129** (3-4), 161–163.
69. Coyne, M.J., Cousin, H., Loftus, J.P., Johnson, P.J., Belknap, J.K., Gradil, C.M., Black, S.J., and Alfandari, D. (2009) Cloning and expression of ADAM-related metalloproteases in equine laminitis. *Vet. Immunol. Immunopathol.*, **129** (3-4), 231–241.
70. Black, S.J. (2009) Cartilage and lamina vs. the rest: diversity of equine extracellular matrix components. Proceedings of the 5th International Equine Conference on Laminitis and Diseases of the Foot, West Palm Beach, FL.
71. Loftus, J.P., Johnson, P.J., Belknap, J.K., Pettigrew, A., and Black, S.J. (2009) Leukocyte-derived and endogenous matrix metalloproteinases in the lamellae of horses with naturally acquired and experimentally induced laminitis. *Vet. Immunol. Immunopathol.*, **129** (3-4), 221–230.
72. Loftus, J.P., Belknap, J.K., and Black, S.J. (2006) Matrix metalloproteinase-9 in laminae of black walnut extract treated horses correlates with neutrophil abundance. *Vet. Immunol. Immunopathol.*, **113** (3-4), 267–276.
73. De Laat, M.A., Van Eps, A.W., McGowan, C.M., Sillence, M.N., and Pollitt, C.C. (2011) Equine laminitis: comparative histopathology 48 hours after experimental induction with insulin or alimentary oligofructose in Standardbred horses. *J. Comp. Pathol.*, **145** (4), 399bred.
74. Fontaine, G.L., Belknap, J.K., Allen, D., Moore, J.N., and Kroll, D.L. (2001) Expression of interleukin-1beta in the digital laminae of horses in the prodromal stage of experimentally induced laminitis. *Am. J. Vet. Res.*, **62** (5), 714–720.
75. Faleiros, R.R., Nuovo, G.J., and Belknap, J.K. (2009) Calprotectin in myeloid and epithelial cells of laminae from horses with black walnut extract-induced laminitis. *J. Vet. Intern. Med./Am. Coll. Vet. Intern. Med.*, **23** (1), 174–181.
76. Faleiros, R.R., Leise, B.S., Watts, M., Johnson, P.J., Black, S.J., and Belknap, J.K. (2011) Lamellar chemokine mRNA concentrations in horses with carbohydrate overload-induced laminitis. *Vet. Immunol. Immunopathol.*, **144** (1-2), 45–51.
77. Leise, B.S., Faleiros, R.R., Watts, M., Johnson, P.J., Black, S.J., and Belknap, J.K. (2011) Lamellar inflammatory gene expression in the carbohydrate overload model of equine laminitis. *Equine Vet. J.*, **43** (1), 54–61.
78. Williams, J.M., Lin, Y.J., Loftus, J.P., Faleiros, R.R., Peroni, J.F., Hubbell, J.A., Ravis, W.R., and Belknap, J.K. (2010) Effect of intravenous lidocaine administration on lamellar inflammation in the black walnut extract model of laminitis. *Equine Vet. J.*, **42** (3), 261–269.
79. Paes Leme, F.O., Bonna, F.A.B., De Marval, C.A., Xabier, S.H.L.N., Santos, R.L., Faleiros, R.R., and Alves, G.E.S. (2010) Histopatologia das lâminas do casco de equinos com laminite aguda induzida e tratados com ketoprofeno, fenilbutazona e flunixin meglumine [Histopathology of the digital laminae from horses with acute induced laminitis treated with ketoprophen, phenylbutazone, and flunixin meglumin]. *Arq. Bras. Med. Vet. Zootec.*, **62** (2), 241–250.
80. Asplin, K.E., Curlewis, J.D., McGowan, C.M., Pollitt, C.C., and Sillence, M.N. (2011) Glucose transport in the equine hoof. *Equine Vet. J.*, **43** (2), 196–201.
81. Burns, T.A., Watts, M.R., Weber, P.S., McCutcheon, L.J., Geor, R.J., and Belknap, J.K. (2013) Distribution of insulin receptor and insulin-like growth factor-1 receptor in the digital laminae of mixed-breed ponies: An immunohistochemical study. *Equine Vet. J.*, **45** (3), 326stoch
82. Kane, E. (2009) Advancing laminitis research – a collaborative effort. *DVM360 Magazine,* (May 1). http://veterinarynews.dvm360.com/advancing-laminitis-research-collaborative-effort.
83. Craig, R.A. (1915) Diseases of the Foot, in *Common Diseases of Farm Animals*. Lippincott's Farm Manual, pp. 170–173.

CHAPTER 2
Laminitis: An Overview

James K. Belknap

Few diseases bring more of an emotional response from owners, trainers, veterinarians, and farriers than Equine Laminitis due to the devastating nature of the disease, exemplified by the excruciating pain suffered by many of the afflicted animals. In spite of intensive therapy, the loss of an athletic career or the life of the animal occurs all too-frequently. In the professional world of veterinary medicine and farriery, few topics can stir up a more boisterous argument than the discussion of which treatments are the most effective for laminitis. As in most diseases fraught with controversy in either equine or human medicine (e.g., human sepsis, cancer), the conflict is often a result of the grave nature of the disease combined with the frustration of health professionals confronted with inadequate knowledge regarding the pathogenesis – and therefore the effective treatment – of the disease. Similar to human medicine, veterinary research workers have been able to take advantage of the many rapid advancements in biomedical research during the past two decades to greatly broaden the current understanding of the pathophysiologic mechanisms in laminitis that take place systemically and locally in the lamellar tissue. This progress has not only allowed us to delineate the disease into three general categories – endocrinopathic, sepsis-related, and supporting limb laminitis – but has also begun to greatly change the available treatments of the different types of the disease. When looking back at the literature over the past two decades, many of the earlier advances in scientific investigation moved the field forward by refuting the efficacy of the medical therapies regarded as standards of treatment for the disease. More recently, however, it has become possible to apply new knowledge of pathophysiologic mechanisms and advanced research tools to establish new therapeutic targets and to rapidly assess novel therapies. Although the present understanding of Equine Laminitis is still evolving, the reader will be able to employ the information in this book to develop a current evidence-based knowledge of the disease and therapies.

Advances in imaging technology have greatly enhanced both the clinical and investigative side of laminitis. The ease of use and high resolution of digital radiography markedly enhances our ability to initially assess the laminitis case, to immediately assess the effects of therapeutic farriery on distal phalanx positioning, and to follow the progression of disease in laminitis cases. As discussed in the following text, the results of recent studies using the high-resolution images of digital radiography now allow us to use objective measurements to diagnose and closely monitor the laminitis case. Whilst magnetic resonance imaging (MRI) has been of more value for research than for clinical management at this point in time, it is becoming a valuable tool for clinical management in complex laminitis cases. In addition to advances in imaging, advances in biochemistry have translated into a more effective clinical management of the systemic components of laminitis cases, especially in endocrinopathic laminitis where rapidly improved testing and more accurate interpretation of the test results are available for the management of insulin dysregulation and pituitary dysfunction. This has been a major asset to the clinical management of these types of patients.

The biomechanical component of the disease remains a challenge, however, and has not benefitted as much from recent technological advances. The lamellae, as part of the hoof capsule, are truly a specialized integumentary structure with many similarities on a cellular level to the skin. The hoof evolved as a vital structural component of the musculoskeletal system, with the lamellar attachments suspending the distal phalanx (and therefore supporting the weight of the horse) within the hoof capsule. The end result is that the biomechanics of the foot is as important a factor in the pathogenesis and treatment of laminitis as is the establishment of pharmaceutical targets (discussed above). The structural integrity of the digital lamellae appears to depend on both the maintenance of the cell shape of all lamellar epithelial cells and the maintenance of adhesion of the innermost layer of epithelial cells, the lamellar basal epithelial cell (LBEC) layer, to the underlying dermis. Although the forces sustained by the lamellar epithelium are phenomenally greater than those sustained by any other epithelial cell in the body (including the skin), the lamellar epithelium appears to have only similar mechanisms to the skin epithelium (a similar cytoskeleton and the same protein adhesion complexes to adhere the basal layer to the underlying dermis) to counteract these forces. As described in the following chapters, lamellar failure appears to be a mixture

Equine Laminitis, First Edition. Edited by James K. Belknap and Raymond Geor.

of stretching of the lamellar epithelium which is likely due to the dysregulation of epithelial cytoskeletal dynamics, and dysadhesion from the underlying dermis, which likely occurs through the dysregulation of cell adhesion complexes. Once lamellar failure occurs, these same distractive forces will result in the displacement of the distal phalanx. The unique and critical role of the lamellar epithelium in providing structural stability to an anatomical structure exposed to immense physical forces is most likely the reason that multiple systemic diseases which may have mild to no signs in other organs of the body result in structural breakdown of lamellar integrity and thus are lumped under the term *laminitis*. In order to successfully treat the disorders that cause lamellar failure, we therefore not only need to define and treat the systemic and cellular events leading to dysregulation of the lamellar cells, but also – and just as importantly – we need to mitigate the distracting forces leading to lamellar stretching and separation. To further our ability to successfully treat this disease, we are reliant on ongoing studies in physiology and cellular biology, as well as in equine digital biomechanics and the ability of therapeutic shoeing to address biomechanical concerns. Due to the complex nature of the structure of the equine foot, we still have limited scientific data to accurately define the biomechanical forces at play in both the normal and laminitic equine digit. Without scientific methodology to define these forces, we are also still unable to precisely establish the efficacy of different farriery and shoeing techniques to support and address the biomechanical aspect of the disease. Thus, we still rely on anecdotal reports and the combined veterinary and farrier clinical experience in the management of laminitic feet. Advances have been made primarily due to the ingenuity of farriers; however, due to an inability to objectively test different types of shoeing, a great deal of controversy persists in the care of the foot as part of management of the laminitis case. In this book, we present the current understanding of biomechanical principles taking place in the equine digit, and have attempted to provide a general overview of the current options for foot management for the different types of displacement. In the management of laminitis cases, vigilance is required not only in attempting to avoid complications, but also being able to rapidly diagnose and treat complications when they occur. Therefore, we have dedicated chapters to patient and environmental management for the avoidance of complications, and diagnostic and therapeutic techniques for the management of complications when they occur.

Finally, we need to acknowledge the pioneering efforts of many individuals, and the support of many institutions that have allowed advances in our understanding and treatment of the disease. Although the chapters related to the pathophysiology are written primarily by research workers who have conducted much of the cutting edge research over the past decade to expand our knowledge of the disease, we need to recognize many of the investigators of the past 30–50 years, many of whom had an impact on training current research teams in the field; these experts include Harold Garner (University of Missouri), Jim Moore (University of Georgia), and Chris Pollitt (University of Queensland). We must also give credit to the funding agencies around the world who have provided millions of dollars for laminitis research during the past few decades; these include (but are certainly not limited to) the Grayson Jockey Club Research Foundation, Animal Health Trust, Morris Animal Foundation, U.S. Department of Agriculture, and the Rural Industries Research and Development Corporation (Australia) and Mars Equine (UK/Australia). The Dorothy Havemeyer Research Foundation and American Association of Equine Practitioners must also be mentioned for funding international workshops on laminitis research, bringing together investigators from around the world to not only share data but also to chart the course of future research. On the hoof care side, credit must also be given to individuals such as Robert Eustace, Ric Redden, Burney Chapman, Gene Ovnicek, and Mike Steward, all of whom have played important roles in promoting innovative changes to our treatment of this devastating disease.

CHAPTER 3

Anatomy and Function of the Equine Digit

A.H. Parks

Introduction

The object of therapeutic hoof care for horses with laminitis is to stabilize as best as possible the distal phalanx (DP) within the hoof capsule by minimizing the forces that place excessive tension on the lamellae. To best understand the distribution of forces within the foot, and how they change with movement, it is important to understand the anatomic relationship between the structures of the foot, kinetic events that occur between the ground and the hoof, and the moments that occur about the distal interphalangeal joint. The distal limb contains all the main elements of the musculoskeletal system except muscles, and is covered by highly specialized integument. As such, it is a mechanical system for conveying forces to support weight and provide locomotion. At the core of this system are the bones, joints, and ligaments of the foot.

Anatomy

For this discussion, we are going to use terminology relating to the front feet (i.e., palmar). The foot contains a portion of the middle phalanx, the DP, and the navicular bone. The DP has three surfaces – the articular surface, solear surface, and parietal surface (Fig. 3.1). The junction of the parietal and solear surfaces forms the solear margin; the junction of the articular and parietal surface at the dorsal aspect of the foot forms the proximal or coronary border, part of which forms the extensor process, and the third border is formed on the palmar aspect of the bone by the junction of the solear and articular surfaces. The three surfaces converge at their medial and lateral palmar extremities to form the palmar processes of the distal phalanx. The parietal surface has a roughened texture with multiple perforations; the roughened surface is adapted for soft tissue attachments (primarily the sublamellar dermis) and the perforations permit passage of blood vessels into the adjacent soft tissues (sublamellar and lamellar dermis) of the hoof wall. The solear surface can be divided into two functional surfaces: (i) the larger planum cutaneum, which corresponds to the solear surface of the hoof (this surface does not have perforations and is smooth except where it forms the palmar processes); and (ii) the flexor surface (facies flexoria) (Fig. 3.1), which is a smaller area adjacent to the articular surface on which the deep digital flexor tendon and the distal sesamoidean ligament insert. The articular surface is divided into two functional areas also for two separate articulations – a large one (facies articularis) that articulates with the middle phalanx, and a much smaller one (facies articularis sesamoidea) located in the palmar central aspect that articulates with the navicular bone. The larger facies articularis is divided into two shallow cavities, divided by a low ridge, that articulate with the condyles of the distal middle phalanx.

Attached to the dorsal border of the palmar processes of the distal phalanx are the paired, approximately rhomboid-shaped ungual cartilages (commonly termed 'collateral cartilages'; Fig. 3.2). Approximately 50% of each cartilage extends palmar to the DP. Additionally, approximately 30–50% of the cartilages extend proximal to the coronary band. Each cartilage is thicker distally than proximally, and the medial surface incorporates numerous channels through which veins of a vascular plexus run [1]. The thicker distal portion of the cartilages projects axially so that it is positioned immediately proximal to the bars of the solear surface of the hoof capsule in healthy horses. Additionally, fibrocartilage from the distal axial border of the cartilage blends with the digital cushion. The exact function of these cartilages is unknown, but they are believed to be important in both the normal expansion of the foot that occurs with ambulation and the related function of providing a mechanism for the distal limb to absorb the shock of impact (functioning in conjunction with the venous plexus within the ungual cartilages).

The navicular bone is spindle-shaped, with two surfaces and two borders. The dorsally located articular surface, covered with hyaline cartilage, is further divided into a main surface that articulates with the palmar aspect of the distal articular surface of the middle phalanx and a much smaller articular surface that articulates with a corresponding surface on the DP. The flexor surface on the palmar aspect of the bone, covered with fibrocartilage, facilitates passage of the deep digital flexor tendon. The proximal border is rough and approximately straight. The distal border is also roughened and perforated by several synovial invaginations.

Equine Laminitis, First Edition. Edited by James K. Belknap and Raymond Geor.

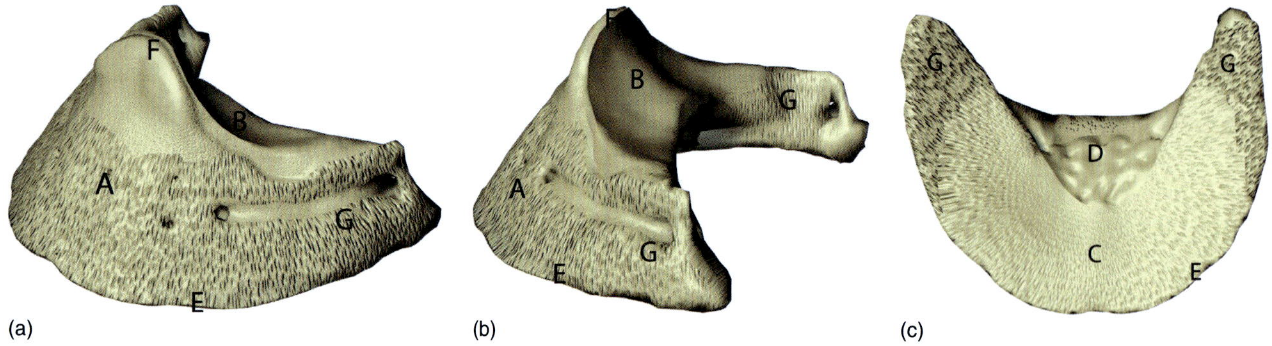

Figure 3.1 (a–c) The distal phalanx. Parietal surface (A), articular surface (B), and the solear surface subdivided into the planum cutaneum (C) and the flexor surface (D); solear margin (E), proximal border and extensor process (F); palmar process (G). Image reproduced with permission from The Glass Horse: Elements of the Distal Limb; courtesy of ScienceIn3D.com.

The distal interphalangeal joint is formed by three separate articulations: one between the middle phalanx and the DP; another between the middle phalanx and the navicular bone; and the third between the DP and the navicular bone. Functionally, the DP and the navicular bone move in tandem so that together they function as a singular articular surface that rotates about the distal articular surface of the middle phalanx. The structure of the articular surfaces are such that the joint is a ginglymus joint (i.e., the primary direction of movement permitted is flexion and extension). However, the saggital ridge on the articular surface of the DP is low and broad, as is the opposing intercondylar groove of the distal middle phalanx, so that the joint permits a modest amount of rotation and a lesser amount of movement in the frontal plane (mostly lateral to medial movement with a minor component of rotation) termed collateromotion (Fig. 3.3).

The ligaments of the distal limb maintain the position of the bones and ungual cartilage in the appropriate relationship to each other, and restrict the range of motion of the bones in relation to each other. The two most important groups of ligaments in the distal limb are the collateral ligaments of the distal interphalangeal joint (Fig. 3.4), which hold the middle and distal phalanx in opposition to each other) and the suspensory ligaments of the navicular bone which, in conjunction with the distal sesamoidean impar ligament, maintain the position of the navicular bone adjacent to the palmar aspect of the middle and distal phalanges). In addition to the ligaments supporting the distal interphalangeal joints, there are a series of ligaments that attach the ungual cartilages to the adjacent structures, including the adjacent bones.

Flexion and extension of the distal interphalangeal joint occurs both actively and passively. Active flexion follows contraction of the deep digital flexor muscle, which increases the tension in the deep digital flexor tendon (Fig. 3.5). The digital portion of the deep digital flexor tendon passes down the palmar aspect of the pastern around the flexor surface of the navicular bone to insert on the flexor surface of the distal phalanx. Active extension/dorsiflexion of the distal interphalangeal joint follows contraction of the common digital extensor muscles mediated via the common digital extensor tendon (Fig. 3.5) through its insertion on the extensor process of the distal phalanx (Fig. 3.1). Passive flexion of the distal interphalangeal joint and dorsiflexion of the metacarpophalangeal joint occur in the course of load-bearing at rest and during the first half of the stride.

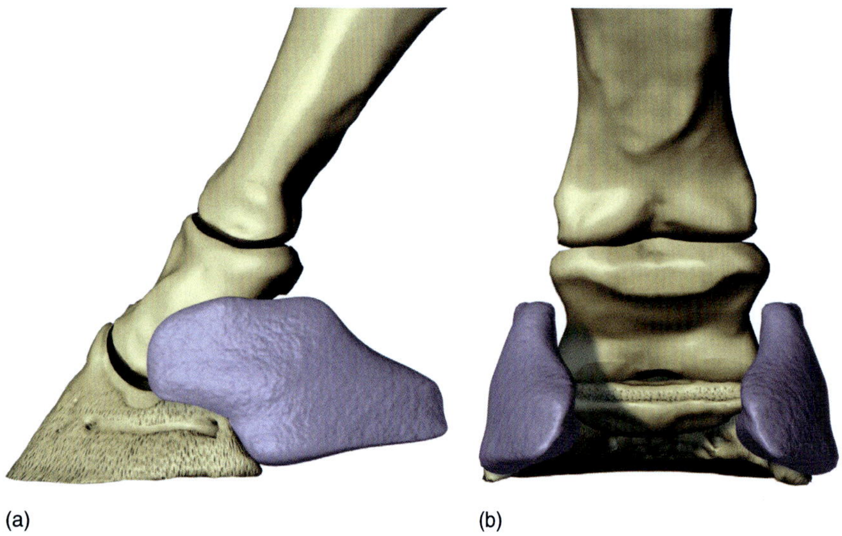

Figure 3.2 (a,b) Ungual cartilages. Images reproduced with permission from The Glass Horse: Elements of the Distal Limb; courtesy of ScienceIn3D.com.

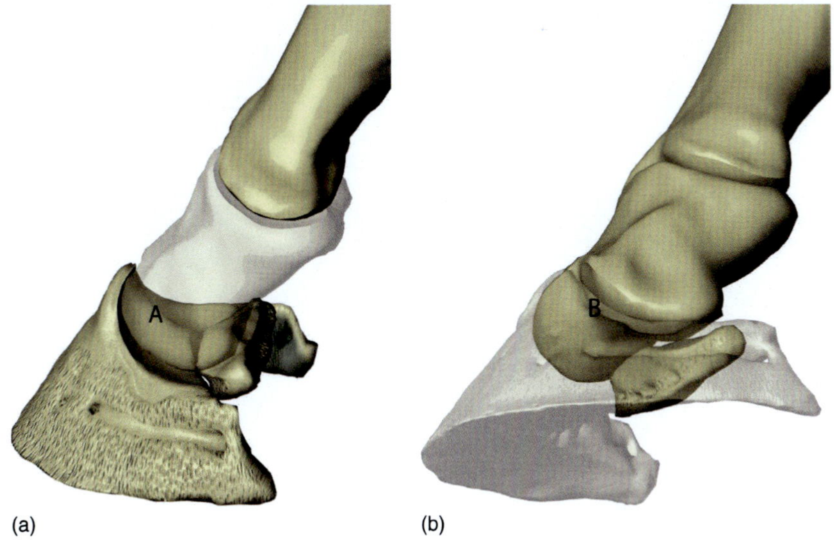

Figure 3.3 (a,b) Distal interphalangeal joint. Low saggital ridge on articular surface of the distal phalanx (A), which articulates with a correspondingly shallow groove (B) situated between the condyles of the distal middle phalanx. Image reproduced with permission from The Glass Horse: Elements of the Distal Limb; courtesy of ScienceIn3D.com.

The vascular supply to the foot (Fig. 3.6) is through the paired palmar digital vessels (arteries and veins). From each of the palmar digital arteries, branches extend to the dorsal and palmar surfaces of each of the phalanges and anastomose with their opposite number. Additionally, there are paired coronary arteries that extend dorsally deep to the coronary band to anastomose with each other. On the palmar surface of the distal digit, there are paired branches of the palmar digital artery that extend distally to the heel bulbs and digital cushion. The paired palmar digital arteries terminate in the terminal arch within the substance of the distal phalanx. From this terminal arch, numerous vessels perforate the parietal surface of the distal phalanx to supply the overlying nonkeratinized soft tissues within the hoof capsule (primarily the lamellar epithelial cells and the lamellar and sublamellar dermis (also termed 'deep dermis' in recent publications). Overall, the blood supply to the foot can be divided into three main zones; the proximal dorsal, distal dorsal, and palmar zones [2]. The blood supply for the proximal dorsal zone is largely derived from the coronary artery and the dorsal artery of the second phalanx, and supplies the soft tissues of the coronary band and those on the proximal parietal surface of the distal phalanx (lamellar and sublamellar dermis). The blood supply to the distal dorsal zone is supplied primarily from the vessels that originate from the terminal arch and perforate the distal phalanx, and also from the dorsal arteries of the distal phalanx which runs through the parietal grooves on the abaxial aspect of the palmar processes; this zone supplies the distal lamellae and the dorsal/abaxial portion of the sole. The proximodorsal and distodorsal blood supplies anastomose within the sublamellar dermis of the wall. Lastly, the third (palmar) blood supply zone is derived from branches of the palmar digital arteries to the heel bulbs, frog, and palmaroaxial aspect of the sole; there are no anastomoses between the dorsal and palmar arterial blood supplies to the sole.

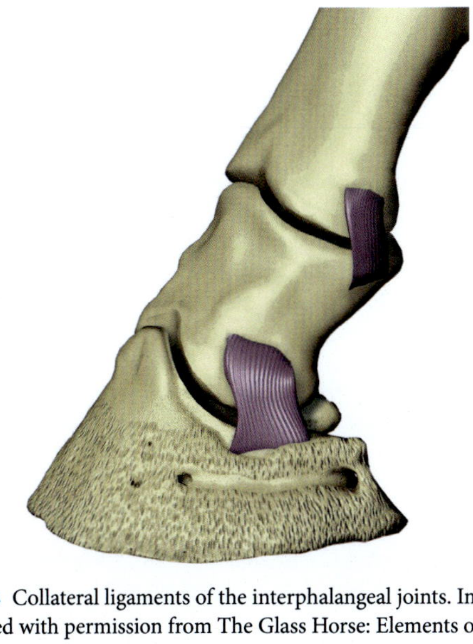

Figure 3.4 Collateral ligaments of the interphalangeal joints. Image reproduced with permission from The Glass Horse: Elements of the Distal Limb; courtesy of ScienceIn3D.com.

The venous return from the digit largely parallels the arterial supply. However, there are significant differences within the foot, which are related to the presence of venous plexuses in the dermis of the coronary band, wall, sole, and frog. Additionally, there are numerous venovenous anastomoses within the axial substance of the ungual cartilages [1]. The majority of veins in the foot do not have valves, but there are valves at the level of the palmar digital vessels.

The classical anatomical study indicates that the palmar digital nerves innervate the majority of the foot, but that the dorsal branch of the palmar nerve innervates the dermis of the dorsal coronary band (Fig. 3.7) [3]. This same study indicates that there is overlap in the innervation of the collateral (abaxial) coronary dermis and of the parietal (lamellar) collateral and heel dermis. A recent physiologic study [4] that examined the response to noxious stimuli at several discreet locations along the coronary band, dorsal lamellae, and sole are largely consistent with the

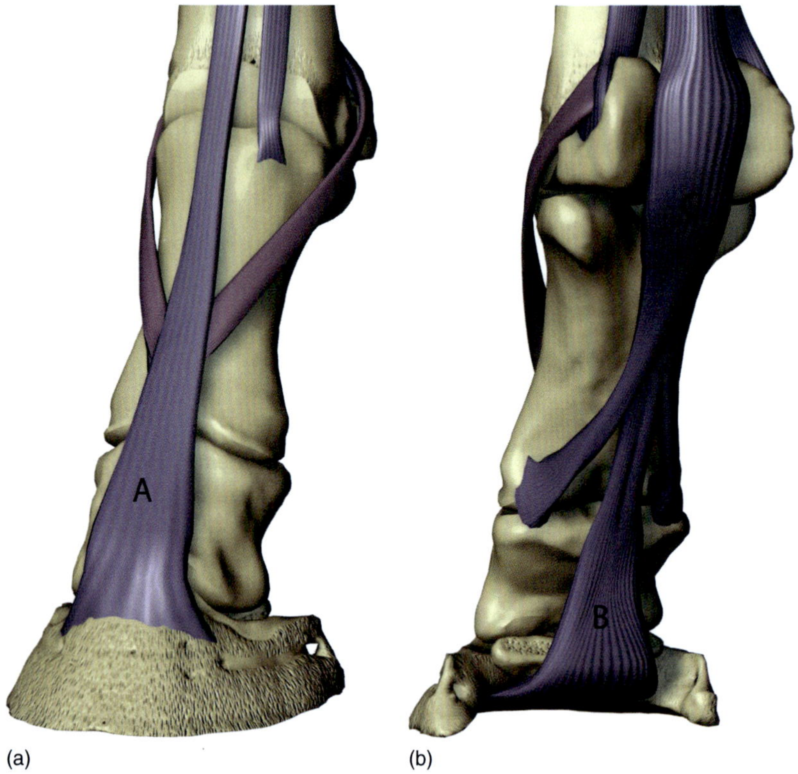

Figure 3.5 (a,b) Tendons. Common digital extensor tendon (A), deep digital flexor tendon (B), and superficial flexor tendon (C). Image reproduced with permission from The Glass Horse: Elements of the Distal Limb; courtesy of ScienceIn3D.com.

prior anatomic study. The physiologic study confirms that the solear dermis and dorsal lamellae are innervated by the palmar digital nerves [4], and that the dorsal coronary band is innervated by the dorsal branch of the palmar nerve. Slight differences between the studies exist regarding the abaxial coronary band; the anatomic study indicating that there was innervation overlap between the two nerves whereas the physiologic study indicates that they are innervated by the dorsal branch. The physiologic study did not address the innervation of the collateral (abaxial) and heel lamellar dermis, which the anatomic study

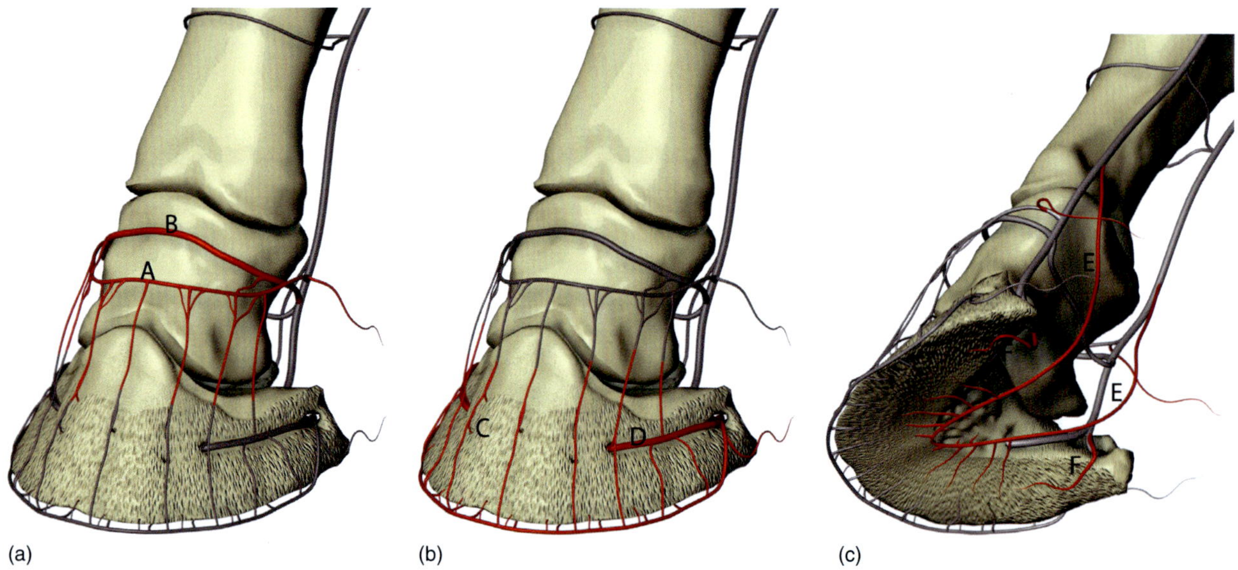

Figure 3.6 (a–c) Arterial supply to the foot. Proximodorsal blood supply from coronary artery (A) and dorsal artery of the middle phalanx (B); dorsodistal blood supply from the vessels originating from terminal arch (C) and the dorsal artery of the distal phalanx (D); palmar blood supply from the branch to the heels (E) and from the palmar artery of the distal phalanx (F). Image reproduced with permission from The Glass Horse: Elements of the Distal Limb; courtesy of ScienceIn3D.com.

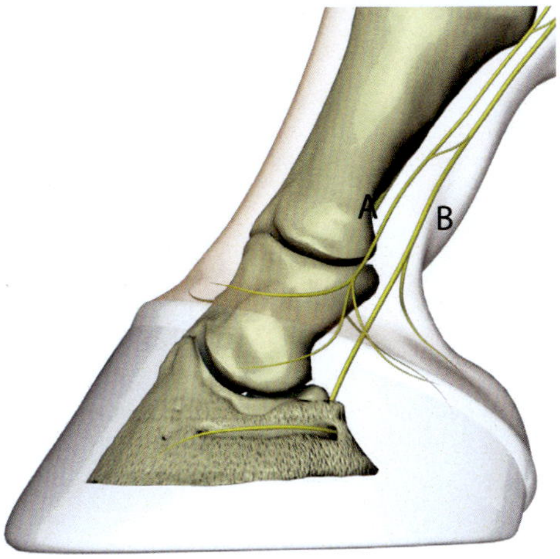

Figure 3.7 Nerves of the foot. Dorsal branch of the palmar nerve (A) and palmar digital nerve (B). Image reproduced with permission from The Glass Horse: Elements of the Distal Limb; courtesy of ScienceIn3D.com.

suggests are areas of overlap in innervation. Also, the point at which the innervation of the coronary band changes from the dorsal branch to the palmar digital nerve is undetermined.

The hoof is the integument of the horse's foot (Figs 3.8 and 3.9). As part of the integument, it is composed of three layers – the epidermis, dermis (or corium), and hypodermis (or subcutaneous tissue). As elsewhere in the integument, the epidermis is further divided into layers. In the hoof, these layers are the stratum basale, stratum spinosum, and stratum corneum; however, the stratum basale (commonly termed the lamellar basal epithelial cell layer in the parietal integument) and stratum spinosum (cellular constituents commonly termed parabasal cells) are frequently collectively referred to as the stratum germinativum. Although the stratum germinativum is usually described as the layer in which the cells divide and develop into mature keratinocytes, there is an extremely low replication rate in the majority of the lamellar tissue. The stratum corneum of the integument of the foot forms the hoof capsule.

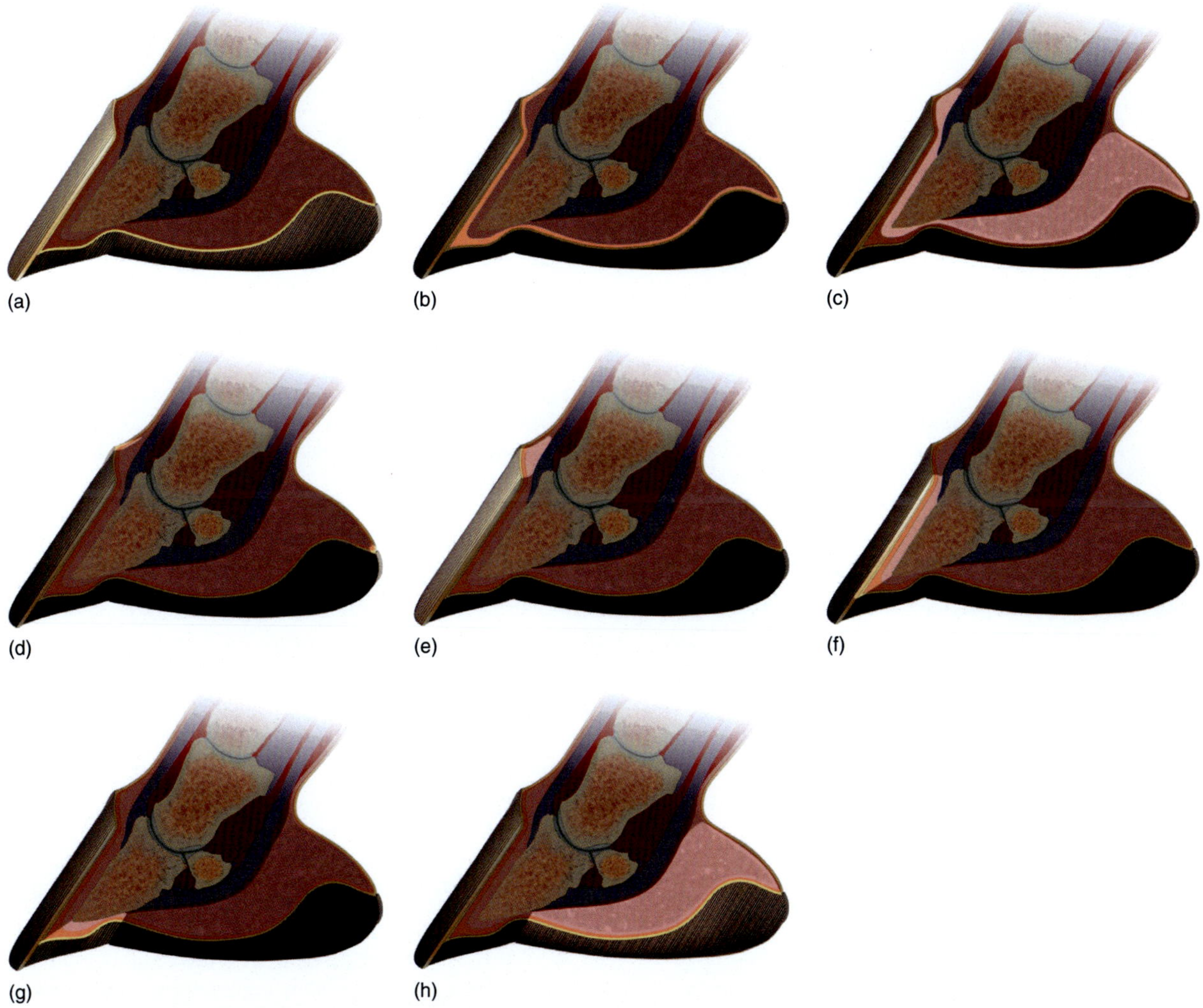

Figure 3.8 (a–h) Integument of the foot by layer: epidermis (A), dermis (B), and subcutaneous tissue (C). Integument of the foot by region: limbic integument (D), coronary integument (E), parietal integument (F), solear integument (G), cuneate and bulbar integument (H). Image reproduced with permission from The Glass Horse: Elements of the Distal Limb; courtesy of ScienceIn3D.com.

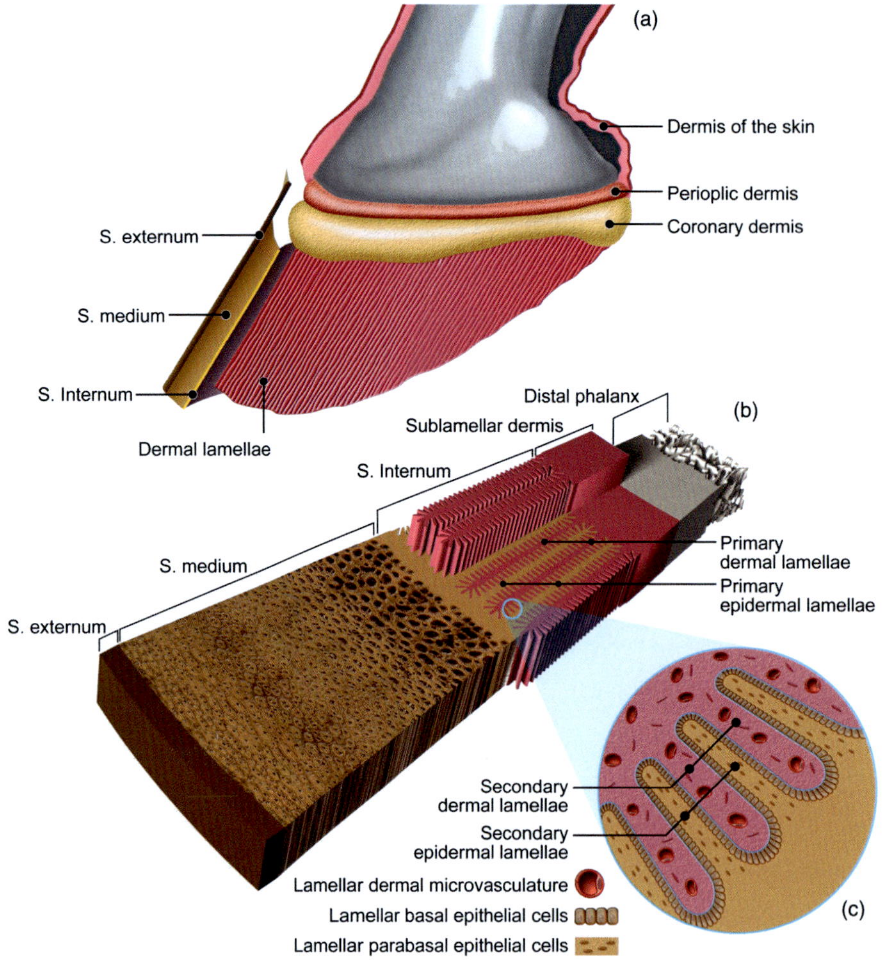

Figure 3.9 Schematic diagram of the anatomic relationship between the hoof capsule, the digital lamellae, and the distal phalanx. The parietal integument responsible for suspension of the distal phalanx within the hoof wall. Note the primary dermal lamellae (A) which interdigitate with the epidermal lamellae of the stratum internum (B), there being approximately 550–600 of each. Note also, on a 'slice' of the digit in a frontal plane (B and C), the increased surface area of the interface between the dermal and epidermal lamellae due to interdigitation of the secondary epidermal and dermal lamellae. Suspension of the distal phalanx within the hoof wall is dependent on the attachment of the lamellar basal epithelial cells (C) to the underlying basement membrane continuous with the lamellar dermis. Illustration courtesy of Tim Vojt, The Ohio State University; The Ohio State University.

As well as being composed of layers, the integument of the foot is divided into several regions or zones that reflect the structure of the integument; limbic (perioplic); coronary; parietal (lamellar); solear; cuneate (related to the frog); and toric (bulbar) integument. The limbic and coronary integuments are adjacent and similarly structured to some degree, and may therefore be considered together. Similarly, the cuneate and toric integument are continuous with each other without a well-defined demarcation between them and thus can be also considered together.

The subcutaneous tissue of the hoof attaches the overlying dermis and epidermis to the underlying distal phalanx and ungual cartilages. The subcutaneous tissue is further specialized deep to the frog to form the digital cushion and at the coronary band where it forms the coronary cushion. There is minimal subcutaneous tissue on the parietal aspect of the distal phalanx. The dermis is the highly vascularized and innervated layer between the subcutaneous tissue and epidermis. Its superficial surface is covered in papillae in the limbic, coronary, solear, and cuneate/bulbar integument, and is folded into lamellae in the parietal integument. The lamellae of the parietal integument (Fig. 3.9) are divided into primary lamellae of which there are approximately 550–600 (Fig. 3.9a) and secondary lamellae, which are foldings of the surface of the primary lamellae (approximately 150–200 secondary lamellae for each primary lamella) [5]. The secondary epidermal lamellae interdigitate with the secondary dermal lamellae (Fig. 3.9b,c); this arrangement of the parietal dermis greatly increases the surface area of the dermal–epidermal interface. The attachment of these interdigitating epidermal and dermal lamellae at this interface is primarily dependent on the attachment of the basal epithelial cell layer (Fig. 3.9c) to the underlying basement membrane continuous with the lamellar dermis. The suspension of the distal phalanx (and therefore the entire appendicular skeleton and weight of the horse) by the hoof wall is dependent on this

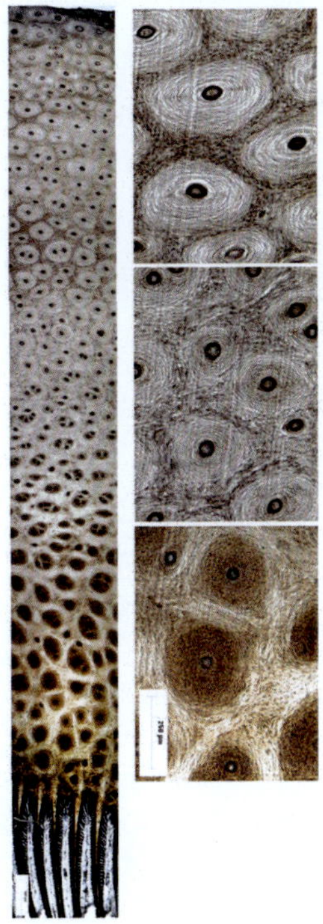

Figure 3.10 Shape, size, density, and structure of horn tubules changes with location in the hoof wall from the stratum internum to the stratum externum. This corresponds to changes in physical properties of the wall, though the exact function of the horn tubules still has to be determined. (Stratum tectorium is synonymous with stratum externum, as used in the chapter text). Illustration courtesy of Dr Chris Pollitt, University of Queensland.

attachment; displacement of the distal phalanx in laminitis occurs due to a failure of this attachment and/or failure of the structural integrity of the lamellar epithelial cells.

The epidermis overlying the coronary and limbic integument forms the horn tubules and intertubular horn (Fig. 3.10); more specifically, the epidermal cells that line the surface of the papillae divide and differentiate into the keratinocytes to form the tubules, while those epidermal cells in the intervening spaces form the intertubular horn. Similarly, the parietal epidermis follows the contours of the parietal dermis forming interdigitating primary and secondary epidermal lamellae. The primary epidermal lamellae contain keratinized cells, but the secondary epidermal lamellae do not.

The hoof capsule, defined as the keratinized integument of the foot, is divided into topographical regions: the coronary band; the wall; the sole; the frog; and the heel bulbs. The keratinized tissues of the frog, sole, and heel bulbs directly reflect the immediately underlying germinal epithelium. Thus, the youngest cells/tissue is directly superficial to the cells from which they were derived. In contrast, the hoof wall is a composite of three layers derived from three different types of epithelium (see Figs 3.8–3.10). The outer layer (stratum externum) is a very thin layer derived from the limbic germinal epidermis, while the middle layer (stratum medium) is derived from the coronary germinal epidermis. Therefore, the most recently formed stratum medium and stratum externum form the proximal wall and the oldest, the most distal wall. The inner layer (stratum internum) is derived from the parietal germinal epidermis (i.e., the lamellar epidermis). The pattern of growth of the hoof wall is very different that of other integumentary tissues of the foot and the skin, in that the outer two layers (stratum externum and medium) of the hoof wall grow in a proximal to distal direction from the coronary band and appear to 'slide' over the underlying layers. Whether this occurs between the stratum medium and the stratum internum, or between the keratinized epithelium of the primary epidermal lamellae and the underlying unkeratinized epithelium, is unknown. This is in sharp contrast to the other integumentary tissues in which the keratinized outer layers are produced by the cells in the statum germinativum immediately beneath the outer layers; that is, the cells move from deeper to more superficial layers.

Function

As part of the integument, the hoof serves several of the functions of healthy skin – that is, it protects the underlying tissues from pathogens, contains sensory organs, and limits the movement of water in either direction. For the most part' the hoof does not contain glands, the exception being the frog, which contains merocrine glands. Its protective function is clearly more important than elsewhere on the body because it is in constant contact with the ground – an environment that frequently contains sharp and/or hard objects. In addition, it has a unique structural function, which is critical in weight-bearing and locomotion (the biomechanics of the foot are discussed in more detail in Chapter 5). Furthermore, the highly specialized nature of the different regions of the integument are important not just in the way that it grows, but also in the way that it heals following injury.

The relationship between the structure of the hoof wall at both the microscopic and molecular level and mechanical properties is a fascinating example of design meeting function in nature. Submicroscopically, the stratum medium of the hoof wall resembles a fiber-reinforced composite [6]; that is, the wall is composed of tubules derived from the germinal epithelium overlying the coronary papillae, which are parallel to the direction of hoof wall growth and in between is the intertubular horn. The horn tubules vary in size, shape, and helical alignment of the cells from the inner to the outer surface of the wall (Fig. 3.10) [7]. The keratin fibrils of the intertubular horn are aligned almost perpendicular to the horn tubules for most of the thickness of the wall [6]. This structural arrangement of the tubules and the fibrils of the intertubular horn of the wall means that the wall behaves almost in an isotropic manner through most of the thickness of the stratum medium, even though the tubules are only oriented in the direction of growth (though it is weakest in the plane parallel to the intertubular horn keratin fibrils) [6]. In the most outer layer of the wall, the intertubular keratin fibrils are much more closely aligned with the horn tubules, while, near the junction of the stratum medium and the stratum internum, there appears to be little to no orderly alignment of the intertubular horn fibrils [7].

When strains are applied to pieces of hoof, the stiffness increases with increased strain rates, which is characteristic of viscoelastic materials [8]. When deliberate cracks made in the hoof wall are forced to propagate, the hoof uniformly fractures between fibrils of the intertubular horn, going across the horn tubules and not between them. This indicates that it is the direction of the intertubular horn keratin fibrils that is the greatest determinant of the response to stress within the wall. The orientation of these intertubular keratin fibrils forces fissures in the hoof wall to become redirected to the outer surface away from sensitive tissues. Those fissures that do propagate to the inner wall reach the zone of intertubular keratin fibrils that are not as orderly aligned. This zone offers minimal resistance to crack propagation and may act as a final mechanism to redirect cracks away from the underlying sensitive tissues [6, 7].

In addition to changes in structure, the mechanical properties of the hoof wall vary with hydration, and the hoof is most fracture-resistant at approximately 75% hydration, which is the level found in the naturally occurring hoof wall [9]. Such is this fracture resistance, that the hoof requires more energy to fracture than bone [7]. Furthermore, across the thickness of the hoof wall is a moisture gradient, with the least hydrated on the outermost layer and the most hydrated in the innermost layer [9]. Correspondingly, the outer layer is stiffest and the inner layer most flexible [7]. This gradual reduction in the stiffness of the wall towards the inside optimizes the transfer of force from the wall to the distal phalanx, while minimizing the likelihood of high shear stresses in any given layer.

The hoof wall is subject to deformation under load. Deformation is, at least in part, the result of the viscoelastic properties of the hoof wall. Viscoelastic materials such as the hoof behave differently depending on the rate of application of force. When deformed abruptly by a rapidly applied force, the hoof behaves elastically, but, when it is subject to a prolonged force, the affected portion of the hoof capsule flows in relation to the adjacent wall – that is, it moves proximally. If the force is removed, the wall has a tendency to return to its original shape. The extent to which an abnormally shaped foot returns to normal is also subject to the state/health of the underlying structures that support the wall. This appears to be subject to limitations, because following prolonged excessive load, longer-lasting (plastic) deformation of the hoof wall occurs.

Load also influences hoof growth. The hoof grows continuously so that, in a healthy state, wear is balanced by new growth. This applies to both the sole and the wall. As previously discussed, the bulk of the substance of the wall (the stratum medium) is formed from the germinal layer of the coronary integument, which glides over the surface of the parietal epithelium as it migrates distally. The basal layer of the parietal epithelium appears to proliferate only minimally. The sole grows distally from the immediately underlying germinal epithelium; the sole and the distal wall are mechanically united at the white line. Although details of the regulation of hoof growth are unknown, various general factors are thought to influence it, including ambient temperature, nutrition, and genetics. The regulation of growth of one part of the hoof in relation to another is also undetermined, though clinical evidence suggests that growth of both wall and sole is in some manner inversely related to the load exerted on them. That is, if one side of the hoof is under reduced load it will grow faster, while a side that is subject to an increased load will grow slower; the evidence to the clinician is visible in the spacing of growth rings. The role of static loading and the different parts of the load cycle during locomotion (e.g., at rest, mid-stride, breakover) are unknown. Furthermore, localized inflammation also appears to selectively cause an increase in local hoof wall growth compared to uninflamed areas.

The structure of the hoof also plays a marked role in damping the vibrations associated with impact. The very shape of the hoof capsule suggests that it is designed so that the wall at the heel and quarters can move in both an abaxial and axial direction because the continuity of the wall is interrupted by the frog; this would suggest that the frog acts, at least in part, as an expansion joint. The principal structures that are thought to play a role in damping vibrations are the hoof capsule, the subcapsular components of the integument, the ungual cartilages, and the frog and digital cushion. It is known that the majority of these impact vibrations are dampened before they reach the osseous skeleton. As discussed above, the viscoelastic composition of the capsule, and movement within the lamellar and sublamellar integument, is likely to be important. Additionally, the deep digital flexor tendon is likely to play a role in supporting the palmar DP and modifying impact vibrations through it's attachment to the flexor surface of the DP. Supporting the palmar aspect of the distal phalanx is likely to play a role. The arrangement of the veins and venules in the body of the ungual cartilage have been proposed to dampen forces exerted on the foot by a hydraulic mechanism, in conjunction with movement of the ungula cartilages and the elastic nature of the digital cushion. It is postulated that blood is forced into numerous veins and venules during impact, providing resistance to blood flow so as to reduce the transmission of high-impact vibrations. Later in the stride, the negative pressure within the digital cushion and adjacent tissues causes the vessels to fill in preparation for the next impact [1].

Foot wounds may be either partial thickness or full thickness. As such, they heal much like their counterparts elsewhere on the horse's body. In partial thickness defects of the hoof wall, the surface defect heals rapidly by epithelialization, without fibroplasia (see Chapter 4 for more detail on wound healing of the hoof wall) [10]. In response to full thickness wounds, the hoof wall exhibits the same phases of wound healing as the integument of the body, except for a lack of retraction of wound margins at the time of injury or during the repair phase because of the rigid nature of the wound margins. The principal differences between the healing of integumental wounds of the hoof wall versus the skin occurs because the different types of integument and their arrangement can affect the functional outcome, particularly with regard to structure. The simplest foot wound involves a single type of integument – for example, a wound that only involves the sole. In this example, the bed of the wound granulates from the margins and underlying subcutaneous tissue/bone surface, and epithelializes from the margins of the wound; the migrating cells of the advancing layer are all derived from the solear epithelium. Once the epithelial cells that have been migrating from the periphery over the granulation tissue cease to migrate, they proliferate and mature into keratinocytes. As the outer cells cornify and the layer of cornified keratinocytes thickens, the full thickness of the defect and normal function of the sole is restored. Grossly, there is no evidence that the wound had occurred, though undoubtedly, there would be some deeper scarring visible histologically.

However, many foot wounds span the boundaries of two or more types of integument. Although they heal by the same processes as more simple wounds, there are at least two consequences that do not affect simpler wounds. The type of horn that forms at the surface of the wound is dependent on the source of the epithelium that covers the defect; therefore, the appearance and structure of the new integument may not resemble the original, either cosmetically or functionally. For example, if a wound involving the coronary band is covered by cells derived from the adjacent parietal/lamellar epithelium, the new horn that grows from that location with not be structurally the same as the adjacent normal wall, but will be somewhat weaker. Any wound that involves the full thickness of the hoof wall without involving either the sole or the coronary band has created a defect in all three strata of the wall and the deeper layers of the parietal (lamellar) integument. As the germinal epithelium surrounding the defect is all derived from the parietal integument, it will completely cover the defect after it has granulated. However, the parietal epithelium will only generate a new thin stratum internum, which serves the normal functions of the skin, but will not replace the structural capacity of the missing wall. The defect in the stratum medium and externum will only be replaced as a new wall grows from the coronary and limbic integument. Therefore, the wall will neither appear nor function normally until this new wall has reached the ground surface of the foot and completely replaced the defect. The veterinarian relies on this type of healing if any type of hoof wall resection is performed on a laminitis case (see Chapter 44 for further discussion of hoof wall resection).

Although the hoof capsule evolved into an impressive, multifaceted tissue capable of withstanding insults ranging from constant impact as the animal travels to the functional healing of superficial wounds to the capsule, the hoof capsule does not appear as well suited to 'bounce back' from the sequelae of loss of lamellar integrity, as occurs in laminitis. One reason for this may be an overall lack of evolutionary pressure as domestication of the horse has likely led to many of the causes of laminitis. As will be addressed elsewhere in this book, one of the largest challenges to the veterinarian and farrier is to attempt to return the anatomic derangements (e.g., displacement of the distal phalanx) and abnormal forces sustained by germinal tissues in the coronary band and sole in order to obtain a hoof capsule with the qualities described above.

References

1. Bowker, R.M., Van Wulfen, K.K., Springer, S.E., *et al.* (1998) Functional anatomy of the cartilage of the distal phalanx and digital cushion in the equine foot and a hemodynamic flow hypothesis of energy dissipation. *Am. J. Vet. Res.*, **59**, 961–968.
2. Goetz, T.E. (1987) Anatomic, hoof, and shoeing considerations for the treatment of laminitis in horses. *J. Am. Vet. Med. Assoc.*, **190**, 1323–1332.
3. Sack, W.O. (1975) Nerve distribution in the metacarpus and front digit of the horse. *J. Am. Vet. Med. Assoc.*, **167**, 298–305.
4. Paz, C.F.R., Magalhaes, J.F., Mendes, H.M.F., Rocha Junior, Sds, Belknap, J.K., Alves, G.E.S., and Faleiros, R.R. (2016) Mechanical nociceptive thresholds of dorsal laminae in horses after local anaesthesia of the palmar digital nerves or dorsal branches of the digital nerve. *Vet. J.*, **214**, 102–108.
5. Pollitt, C.C. (204) Anatomy and physiology of the inner hoof wall. *Clin. Tech. Equine Practice*, **3**, 3–21.
6. Bertram, J.E. and Gosline, J.M. (1986) Fracture toughness design in horse hoof keratin. *J. Exp. Biol.*, **125**, 29–47.
7. Kasapi, M.A. and Gosline, J.M. (1997) Design complexity and fracture control in the equine hoof wall. *J. Exp. Biol.*, **200**, 1639–1659.
8. Kasapi, M.A. and Gosline, J.M. (1996) Strain-rate-dependent mechanical properties of the equine hoof wall. *J. Exp. Biol.*, **199**, 1133–1146.
9. Bertram, J.E. and Gosline, J.M. (1987) Functional design of horse hoof keratin: the modulation of mechanical properties through hydration effects. *J. Exp. Biol.*, **130**, 121–136.
10. Pollitt, C.C. and Daradka, M. (2004) Hoof wall wound repair. *Equine Vet. J.*, **36**, 210–215.

CHAPTER 4

Lamellar Function at the Cellular Level

Christopher C. Pollitt

Cellular Events Important in the Normal Function of the Equine Digit

A basal epithelial cell (BEC) situated in any location other than equine hoof lamellae can essentially be taken for granted. Skin and hair BECs reliably divide in a lifelong, orderly fashion so as to replace the squamous layer of the skin and generate hair respectively, generally without incident. In contrast, the lamellar BECs (LBECs) have been tasked by evolution to participate in a unique suspensory function that is critical to the core survivability of the horse. Disruption of the suspensory attachments that the LBECs make with their immediate extracellular matrix (ECM), and failure of the proteins that link the cytoskeleton to its neighbors, can cause downstream consequences that lead to the condition known as laminitis that cripples horses. The current understanding of laminitis pinpoints the status of the innocuous-looking LBECs as the critical factor in determining whether or not the distal phalanx will descend into the hoof capsule and present the clinical signs of laminitis. In other words, the hallmark pathology of laminitis is a compromise of the suspensory apparatus of the distal phalanx (SADP), and can range in severity from mild to catastrophic.

Amongst mammals, the equine hoof is the most complex and specialized integumentary structure [1]. The distal rim of the hoof wall is the load-bearing border and, based on clear anatomic differences, the hoof wall can be divided into three sections: the *stratum externum* (periople); the *stratum medium* (the tubular bulk of the hoof wall); and the *stratum internum* (the primary and secondary epidermal lamellae). The term *stratum lamellatum* is sometimes used interchangeably with *stratum internum*, but used correctly 'lamellatum' refers to both dermal and epidermal lamellae [2]. An alternate nomenclature notates the hoof wall according to the tissues from which it has proliferated. Thus, coronary horn (the stratum medium) derives from the coronary segment, periople from the perioplic segment, terminal horn (the white line) from the terminal papillae, and the epidermal lamellae from the wall segment [3].

The epidermal and dermal lamellae are integral components of the SADP. The latter is a hierarchical continuum of different tissues and molecules suspending the distal phalanx (DP) by attaching it to the expanded inner surface of the hoof capsule [4–7]. The SADP origin is a dense, reticular network of stout collagen bundles (*stratum reticulare*) that is firmly embedded in the parietal cortex of the DP. The bundles cross the sublamellar dermis at angles aligned with strain, and ultimately insert as fine collagenous filaments into the lamellar basement membrane (BM) (see Fig. 4.1). Projecting from the inner hoof wall and bars are proximodistally oriented leaflets (epidermal lamellae) that interface with complementary dermal lamellae. The (mean ± SEM) number of macroscopically visible epidermal lamellae (primary epidermal lamellae; PELs) in the front feet of 20 Standardbred horses was 561.82 ± 7.02 [8]. The surface area of the lamellar layer is vastly expanded by subdivisions of the PELs into microscopically visible secondary components or secondary epidermal lamellae (SELs see Fig. 4.1). The mean number of SELs of five Standardbred horses assessed at ten dorsal lamellar levels was 134.43 ± 6.21, emanating from each PEL. Fewer SELs are present on each PEL at the heels and bars – 94.70 ± 3.95 and 82.33 ± 4.10, respectively [8]. The perimeter of a typical SEL in the dorsal mid-wall region is approximately 50,111.46 μm (50.0 mm), a considerable increase over the total PEL length of 3622 ± 103 μm (3.6 mm) [9]. Based on several approximations, the surface area of the lamellae of the inner hoof wall of Standardbred horses is 0.82 m^2 [8].

Between the epidermal lamellae are the complementary dermal lamellar components; the primary dermal lamellae (PDLs) and secondary dermal lamellae (SDLs). Within every PDL are bundles of collagenous fibers which subdivide and branch (arborize) into smaller and smaller elements. Fine, collagenous branches from the PDL enter SDLs, and penetrate to the furthest extremities of the SDL, integrating with the reticular layer on the dermal aspect of the LBEC BM to form, collectively, an infinitely large matrix attachment from the distal phalanx to the LBEC. Functioning in concert with other components of the ECM, this collagenous network spanning from the distal phalanx to the LBEC BM provides the physical structure allowing for suspension of the distal phalanx by the inner hoof capsule. SELs characterize the hoof lamellae of the Equidae, and their absence

Equine Laminitis, First Edition. Edited by James K. Belknap and Raymond Geor.

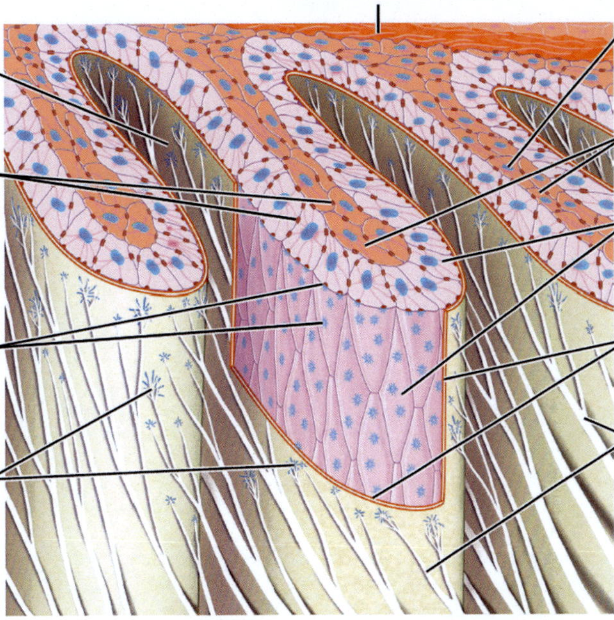

Figure 4.1 Diagram of secondary epidermal lamellae and the suspensory apparatus of the distal phalanx (SADP). The collagen filaments of the SADP insert on the lamellar basement membrane at hemidesmosome attachment sites. Note the oblique angle of the SADP collagen bundles as they insert on the basement membrane-covered surface of the secondary epidermal lamellae. The lamellar basal epithelial cells (LBECs) are fusiform, and the long axes of the LEBCs are aligned proximodistally, similar to the load-bearing collagen bundles of the SADP. Desmosomes link adjoining LEBCs to each other and to the more keratinized parabasal cells forming the central backbone of the SEL. Reproduced with permission from Ref. [53]; © 2015, Elsevier Health Sciences.

in cloven-hooved ungulates such as cattle and sheep suggests a unique, functional adaptation to the equine soliped existence.

The BECs form a layer (*stratum basale*) covering the epidermal lamellae, as well as all other internal surfaces of the hoof capsule. However, LBECs appear to be specialized for maintaining attachment to the distal phalanx; they differ from BECs elsewhere in the foot, which proliferate to form the tubular horn of the hoof wall, the periople, the white line, the sole and the frog. BEC proliferation (cell division to create new cells) is constant in the latter epithelial structures of the foot but, except for the most proximal and distal regions, is almost nonexistent in the majority of the epidermal lamellae. Despite being labeled the *stratum germinativum* in some texts [10], most LBECs reserve their proliferative potential to repair injury (e.g., when the hoof wall is avulsed [11], in the presence of foreign bodies [12], and following laminitis [13,14]. Many LBECs are reportedly stem cells [13], staining positive for the transcription factor P63 (which is essential for the maintenance and proliferative potential of epidermal stem cell populations) [15]. The greatest frequency of lamellar p63-positive BECs was detected in the proximal regions of the hoof, where the rate of cell proliferation is highest (see below).

The presence of stem cells among the LBEC population explains the extraordinary lamellar response after the entire hoof wall is avulsed or surgically stripped (resected). Remarkably, physically stripping away the hoof wall takes with it the epidermal lamellae, but does not remove the lamellar BM. The majority of the lamellar BM survives intact on the surface of the dermal lamellae, and becomes a template over which rapidly proliferating and migrating LBECs reconstruct functional lamellae, with near-normal anatomy, within four days of wall stripping [11]. Thus, lamellar wounding triggers LBEC proliferation amongst the otherwise nonproliferative LBEC population. The activation of proliferation among the normally quiescent LBEC, in response to wounding, may reside with the P63-positive stem cells apparently maintained for just such a purpose [13].

Certainly, the term *stratum germinativum* correctly describes a key activity of all nonlamellar BECs of the hoof. Production of the tubular horn of the periople, hoof wall and bars, white line (terminal horn), sole and frog is constant throughout the life of the horse. In the adult horse, mitosis (in the form of mitotic figures) is observed frequently in sections of tubular horn tissues prepared for light microscopy (LM). Mitosis occurs equally frequently in lamellar sections, but only in a short proximal zone on the inner shoulders of the coronary groove (Fig. 4.2). In the proliferative proximal zone, PELs are generated and subsequently cornify [16] to form the keratinized backbone of each of the approximately 560 primary lamellae. Just as in the coronary tubular horn, the daughters of proliferating LBECs migrate away from the BM and progressively differentiate into corneocytes. They lose their nuclei, condense their intermediate filament cytoskeleton into crosslinked keratin macrofilaments, form a highly crosslinked, insoluble proteinaceous

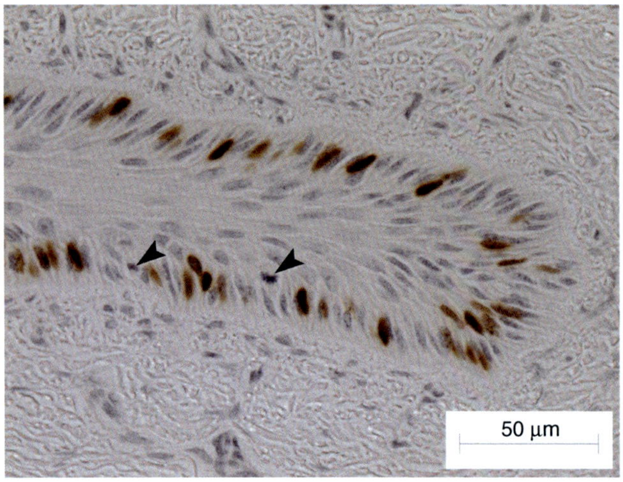

Figure 4.2 Photomicrograph of transverse section a proximal epidermal lamella from a horse euthanized 60 min after the start of an intravenous infusion of bromodeoxyuridine (BRdU), a thymidine analogue that is incorporated into cells undergoing DNA replication. In this proximal lamella, no secondary epidermal lamellae have yet formed, and many of the basal cells show dark brown positive BRdU immunostaining and some mitotic figures (arrowheads), both consistent with intense proliferation. Reproduced with permission from Ref. [16]; © Wiley.

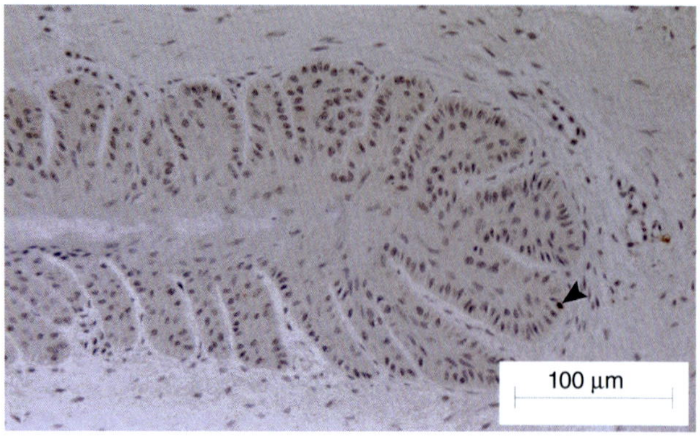

Figure 4.3 Photomicrograph of a transverse section of a lamella distal from the proximal proliferative zone from a horse euthanized 60 min after the start of an intravenous BRdU infusion. Only a single lamellar basal cell (arrowhead), in a secondary epidermal lamella shows black brown positive BRdU immunostaining consistent with proliferation. Reproduced with permission from Ref. [16]; © Wiley.

envelope, creating in each PEL a keratinized axis (KA). The lamellar KA is continuous with the keratinized intertubular horn of the hoof wall, and can be considered an axial extension of it. Lamellar KAs 'grow' down at approximately the same rate as the stratum medium, and with it form an anatomic and functional unit ameliorating the tensile and compression forces between bone and hoof that are encountered during weight-bearing and locomotion [17]. In the proximal lamellar proliferative zone, LBEC proliferation is coordinated to produce invaginations and folds in the LBEC layer that enlarge and become SELs.

Distal to the proximal proliferative zone, proliferation is profoundly diminished and the remaining distal lamellae (Fig. 4.3) retain their morphology, virtually unchanged until, close to the solear surface, a resurgence of LBEC mitosis transforms them into white-line tubular and intertubular horn (terminal horn). This new horn integrates with the KA carried down attached to the continuously downward-migrating intertubular coronary horn. Thus, two separate age classes of epidermis are conjoined; the KA (presumably as old as the 8- to 10-month-old stratum medium at this location) and the newly created, nonpigmented terminal horn. The white line tubular horn merges with the tubular horn of the sole. This describes the situation in the adult foot, and presumably the blueprint of hoof anatomy is laid down in the embryo and added to by incremental growth until maturity.

The hoof SEL consists of basal epidermal (*stratum basale*) and suprabasal (*stratum spinosum*) cell layers that abut the fully keratinized axis or *stratum corneum* of the primary epidermal lamellae. Absent are the *stratum granulosum* and *stratum lucidum,* both of which are present in the skin [1] and in the periople [18].

At least two unresolved questions pertain to lamellar biology.

1. Are the LBECs permanent and immobile residents on the lamellar BM? This is an important question because the KA of the PEL *does* migrate distally along with the contiguous 'downward-growing' *stratum medium.* If it moves distally, and the BECs do not, then considerable remodeling and rearrangement of the parabasal cells, situated between the BEC layer and the KA, must occur. The SEL parabasal cells (PBCs) are nucleated and firmly attached to their neighbors by desmosomes, forming a spiny cell layer or *stratum spinosum.* Precisely where detachment and reattachment (or perhaps sliding) amongst these cell types occurs is speculative.
2. Are the LBECs, between the short, proximal lamellar proliferative zone and the distal, terminal white line horn, proliferating and contributing to the downward journey of the lamellar KA? Lamellae between the known proliferative zones have a very low rate of lamellar mitosis (Fig. 4.3), as confirmed by three different immunohistochemistry (IHC) methods [13,16,19]. The low rate of proliferation seems to preclude a flow of new cells sufficient to drive the lamellar KA downwards.

The fully keratinized axis provides a relatively rigid structural backbone to each lamella. The cells of the KA have no nuclei, their cytoplasm is mainly condensed keratin [18], and their cell membranes are cemented together by the extrusion into the intercellular space of previously manufactured membrane-coating granules (MCGs). Thus, the cells are cemented together with carbohydrate-rich, membrane-coating material (MCM) [20]. This process is initiated and likely completed in the lamellar proximal proliferative zone, when the keratinocytes forming the KA are still metabolically active but are programmed to subsequently 'die' during the cornification process. The dimensions of KAs remain essentially unchanged during their proximodistal journey through the white line to their ultimate destination, the bearing border of the hoof [9]. Stages of progressive keratinization were not observed in cells adjacent to the KA in one study [21], but were observed in another, later study [22]. Without significant LBEC mitosis, the KA seems to be fixed in size as it descends proximodistally. Being fully keratinized and anchored to the hoof wall, the *stratum medium* protects the KA during laminitis pathogenesis [9].

The end-to-end connections between the cells of the KA have been studied using periodic acid–Schiff (PAS)-stained longitudinal sections of lamellae. There are more interdigitations on the end-to-end connection than on the less-burdened cell flanks [20]. The zones of interdigitation contain more carbohydrate-rich MCM and react strongly with the PAS stain. No desmosomes are present amongst cells in the KA, but perhaps these are displaced by the intercellular influx of MCM [20]. Nevertheless, no matter how rigid and cemented together the KA cells are, they have to interact with the parabasal cells of their SEL neighbors and allow differential movement of one against the other. Perhaps the interdigitated boundary between the hardened cornified KA cells and the adjacent, desmosome-rich SEL parabasal cells resembles a morticed joint, and MCM is sufficiently slippery to facilitate a slide-contact mechanism [22]. The low rate of distal LBEC mitosis reported [16, 19, 22] may incrementally add some cells to the KA.

A thin, unbroken, proteinaceous sheet of extracellular BM partitions the dermis from the epidermis, and lines the entire inner hoof wall, sole, and frog. All dermal papillae of the periople, coronary groove, white line, sole and frog, as well as the dermal lamellae of the inner hoof wall and bars, have a BM lining.

The LBECs are in intimate contact with this underlying BM, the various roles of which include providing barrier and structural functions to the LBECs, as well as being involved in the regulation of cell activities such as attachment, growth, migration, differentiation, and signaling [23]. The major components of the BM are collagen type IV, laminin, nidogen/entactin, and perlecan. The latter are glycoproteins and give the BM its strong PAS staining propensity (Fig. 4.4). Collagen type IV is the major form of collagen in the BM, where it forms a highly covalently crosslinked network.

LBEC Attachment

The LBEC is attached to its epidermal cell neighbors and to its underlying BM by different protein complexes (cell junctions). There are three important cell junctions in the context of laminitis, namely desmosomes, adherens junctions, and hemidesmosomes (HDs) (Figs 4.5–4.7). All epidermal cell junctions consist of three elements. The first element is one or more transmembrane proteins. Desmosomes and adherens junctions bridge the membranes of two cells using a cadherin-based transmembrane protein, while HDs, located on the basal surface (adjacent to the lamellar dermis) of the LBECs, have several transmembrane

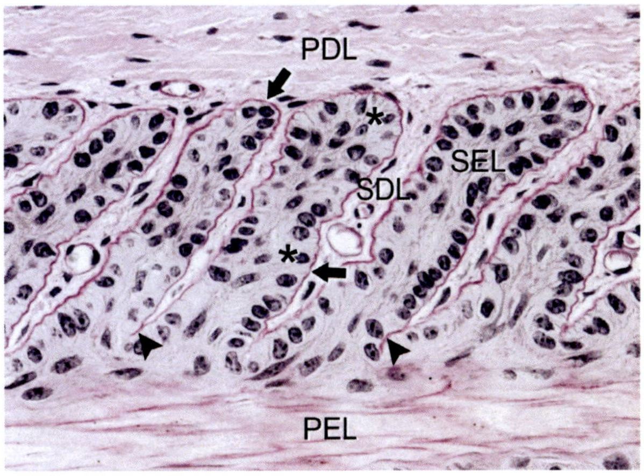

Figure 4.4 Transverse section photomicrograph of periodic acid–Schiff (PAS)-stained normal hoof secondary dermal (SDL) and epidermal lamellae (SEL). The basement membrane (arrowed) of each SEL shows as a dark magenta line closely adhered to the SEL basal cells. Between the bases of each SEL the BM penetrates deeply (arrowheads) and is close to the anuclear, keratinized axis of the primary epidermal lamella (PEL). The SEL tips are rounded and club-shaped. The basal cell nuclei are oval in shape (asterisks) and positioned away from the BM at the apex of each cell. The long axis of each basal cell nucleus is at right-angles to the long axis of the SEL. The SDL are packed with filamentous connective tissue right to their tips, between the SEL bases.

proteins that attach to the BM via an anchoring filament, laminin-332 (Ln 332), anchoring the LBEC plasma membrane, via the HD, to the BM. The second element is the cytosolic 'cytolinker protein' that links the transmembrane proteins to the third component, the cytoskeleton. The cytolinker protein for desmosomes is desmoplakin, for adherens junctions it is β-catenin, and for HDs it is plectin.

The Cytoskeleton

The LBEC cytoskeleton is a meshwork of filaments that criss-crosses the cell in all directions, cradling the nucleus and attaching to the cell plasma membrane by the three types of cell junction mentioned above. It bestows not only mechanical stability to each cell but, by being interconnected to all other LBECs and the surrounding lamellar dermis, stability also to the entire epidermal lamellar system. The main filaments composing the LBEC cytoskeleton are keratin intermediate filaments (IFs) (85%) and actin microfilaments (11%) [24]. The keratin IF network connects not only to HDs at the cell base (adjacent to the BM) but also to the nuclear envelope of the LBEC nucleus. Plectin, which is well-known as the cytolinker protein of the HD, also binds to an outer nuclear envelope protein (nesprin-3), enabling the attachment of IFs to the nucleus [25]. Thus, IFs stabilize the nucleus within the cell cytoplasm by anchoring the nucleus to the basal plasma membrane, via HDs, and to the remaining plasma membrane via desmosomes. Together, the keratin and actin cytoskeleton of the basal and parabasal epidermal cells (epidermal cells between the LBEC layer and the KA of the

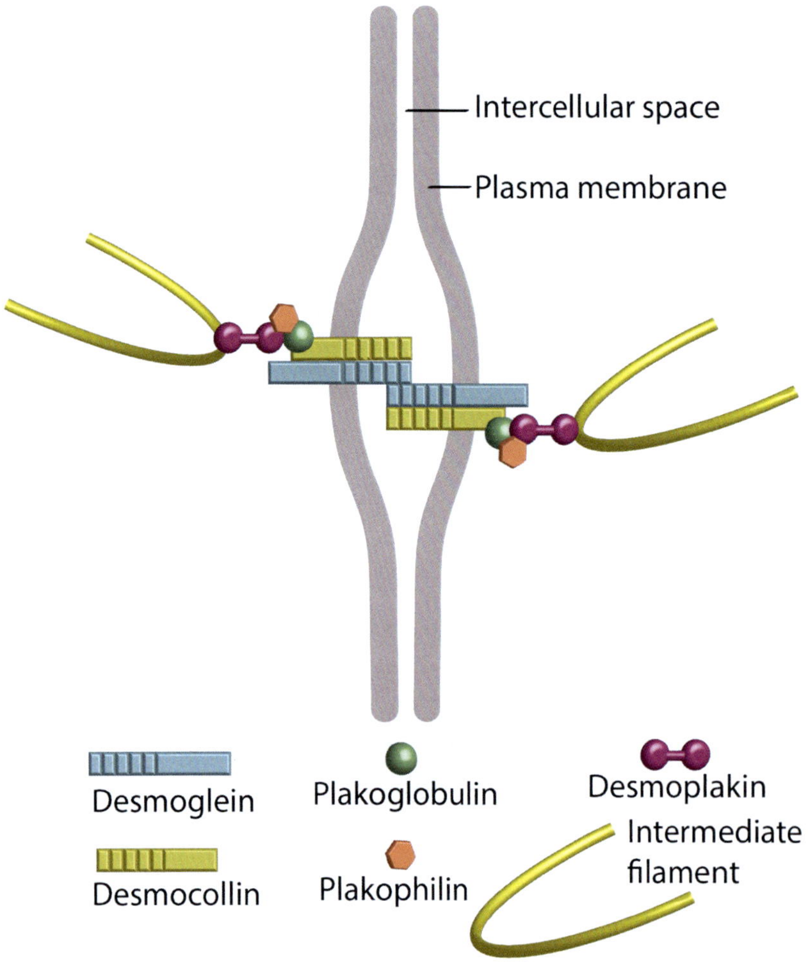

Figure 4.5 Desmosome molecular blueprint. The major desmosomal proteins from three families are superimposed on a schematic desmosome bridging adjacent LBEC plasma membranes. Transmembrane desmosomal cadherins (desmogleins and desmocollin bind the armadillo family protein plakoglobulin, which in turn anchors the plakin family members desmoplakin and plakophilin. Desmoplakin links the keratin intermediate filament cytoskeleton to the desmosome.

primary epidermal lamella) of the SEL and their junctional complexes form a conjoined, functional unit within the SADP.

Keratin Intermediate Filaments, Desmosomes, and Hemidesmosomes

The LBEC nucleus is suspended within the cell cytoplasm by a filamentous scaffold of keratin IFs [26]. This dense, pan-cytoplasmic network anchors the nucleus to two types of cell junction embedded in the LBEC plasma membrane. Desmosomes link adjacent LBECs and parabasal cells to each other (Fig. 4.8), while HDs link the basal LBECs to their underlying BM (Fig. 4.9). Intermediate filaments interact with the actin cytoskeleton to establish a stable cytoskeletal network throughout the cell and tissue. The structure and stability of the whole cytoskeletal network is regulated by signaling proteins (e.g., kinases, phosphatases and heat-shock proteins) belonging to diverse signaling cascades that affect cytoskeleton turnover [26]. Thus, the cytoskeleton should be viewed as not only a static structural entity, maintaining cell architecture, but also as a dynamic entity that can be built or broken down to enable diverse cellular processes such as adhesion or cell migration. The cytoskeleton is also a key regulator of cellular and molecular signaling, modulating cellular pathways by controlling the activity and/or subcellular localization of signaling proteins and their targets. There is a functionally important interaction between the cytoskeleton and the translational machinery; polysomes and ribosomes are physically linked to the cytoskeleton and cytoskeletal perturbations adversely affect protein synthesis [26].

The LBEC keratin IF network is chemically very stable, consisting of long, unbranched filaments approximately 10 nm in diameter [27]. In LBECs, the IFs are normally organized into conspicuous bundles called *tonofilaments* (Fig. 4.10). A unique feature of keratins is the pairing of one type I keratin with one type II keratin, such that the resultant heterodimers and tetramers form the basic building units of the keratin filaments. In LBECs, bundled filaments of tonofilaments are built up from keratinocyte-type keratins such as K5/K14, and with even more pronounced bundling of K1/K10 in the suprabasal epithelial cells. When hoof lamellae are immunostained with K14 antibodies only basal cells stain positive, thus differentiating basal from adjacent parabasal cells (Fig. 4.11). The pattern of K14 staining shows the entire cell cytoplasm to be occupied by keratin IFs; from the basal plasma membrane with its constituent HDs to

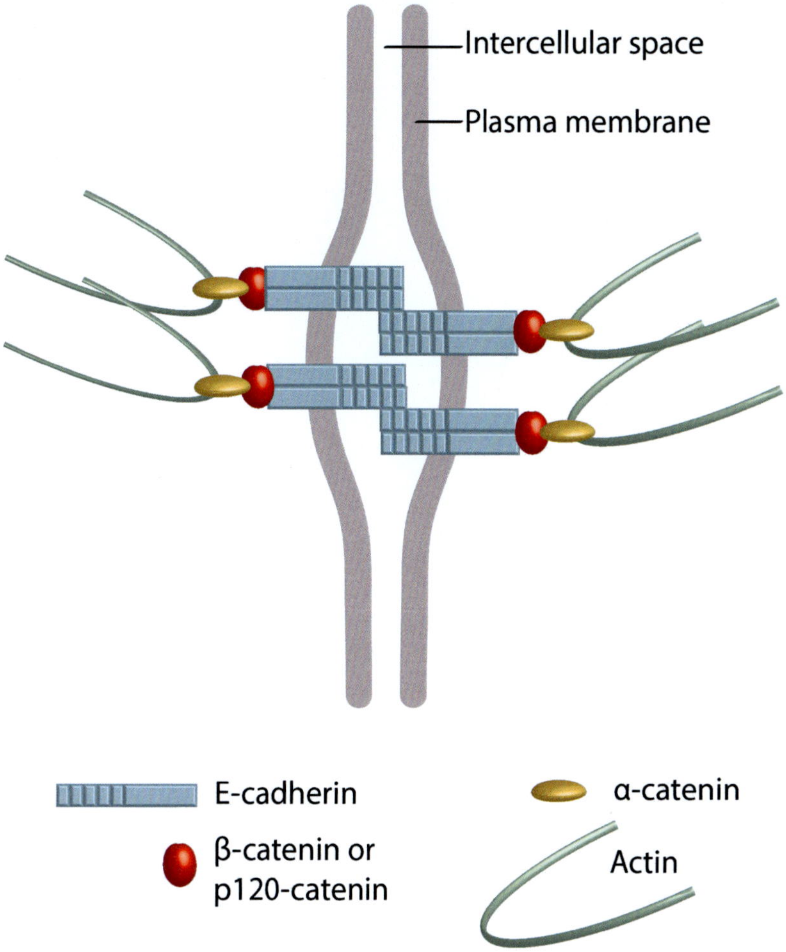

Figure 4.6 Adherens junction (AJ) molecular blueprint. The major proteins from three families are superimposed on a schematic adherens junction bridging adjacent LBEC plasma membranes. In the intercellular space between adjoining cell membranes a pair of E-cadherin molecules bind homotypically with an opposite pair from the adjoining cell. The cytoplasmic tail of E-cadherin links to β-catenin which in turn binds to α-catenin bringing cytoskeletal actin to the cytoplasmic plaque.

the lateral walls and apex where the IFs are attached to desmosomes bridging adjacent cells. The IF cytoskeleton also attaches to the nuclear envelope to create a stable nuclear cage; a dense meshwork of crosslinked filaments surrounds the nucleus and suspends it to all points within the cell [28].

The IF cytoskeleton, with the multitude of attachment plaques which anchor it, is vitally important to the mechanical integrity of the LBEC. The SEL dimensions stay within tight limits because the LBECs are fixed in shape by their cytoskeleton, and are attached to each other and to the underlying BM. The dysregulation of cytoskeleton physiology has significant downstream consequences and is likely to be critically involved in laminitis cellular pathology.

Keratinocytes with 'knocked out' (a specific gene made inoperative in the cells in experimental research) keratin gene clusters, and therefore totally lacking keratin IFs are about 40% 'softer,' more easily deformable, and about 40% less viscous than normal keratinocytes [29]. Neither actin nor microtubule protein levels, nor corresponding cytoskeletal structures, are affected. Interestingly, the cytoskeleton network is fully restored if the *K14* gene is re-expressed in the keratinocytes; normal cellular rigidity, viscosity, and elastic properties are regained showing the vital significance of an intact IF cytoskeleton to cell mechanical integrity [29]. Without keratin filaments, keratinocytes are biomechanically deficient with compromised Young's moduli, and are unable to resist stretching. The implication for laminitis is that a wholesale breakdown and/or release of IFs from their intracellular attachments may similarly reduce LBEC elasticity, making them soft and deformable where once they were resistant. In more simplistic terms, disruption of the IFs of the LBEC cytoskeleton in laminitis likely converts the LBEC 'brick' into an easily deformable 'marshmallow.'

Desmosomes and Keratin IFs

Desmosomes are more than physical bridges between cells; they also interact with signaling cascades to: (i) activate or suppress pathways important to establishing cell polarity; (ii) regulate cell shape and motility; and (iii) influence cell proliferation and differentiation. Interference with these functions results in defective cell differentiation and altered polarity [30]. The major desmosome building blocks are members of three gene families, namely cadherins, armadillo proteins, and plakins (Fig. 4.5).

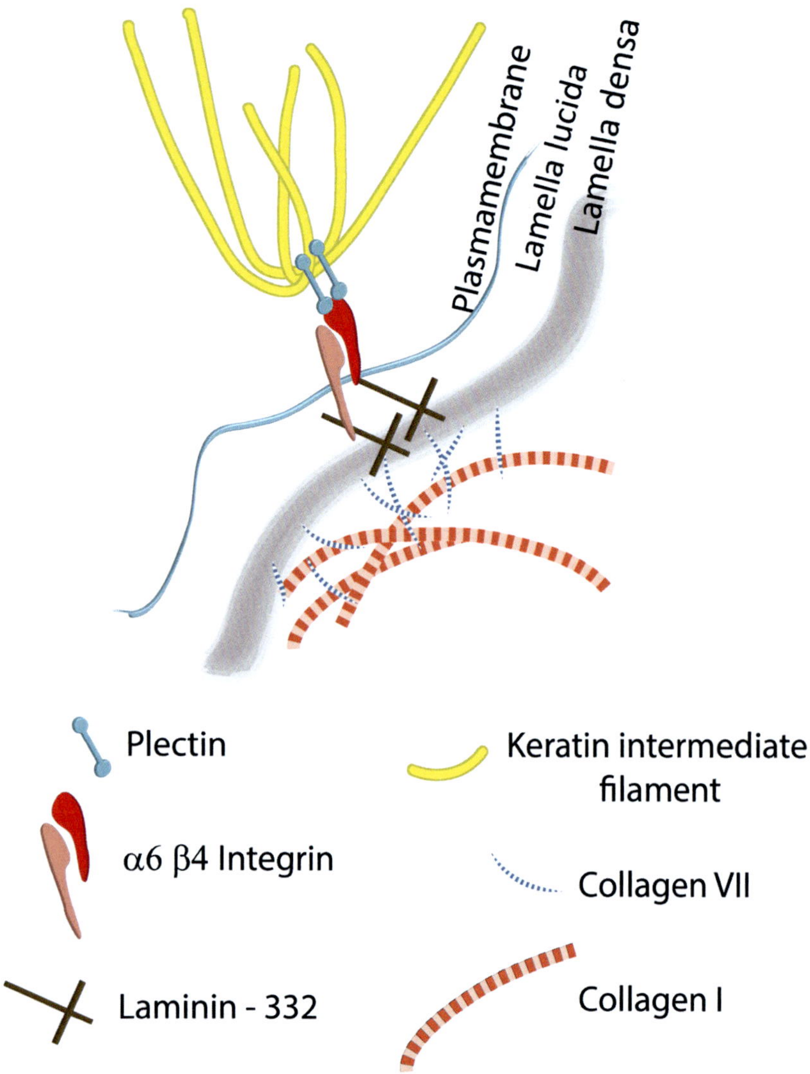

Figure 4.7 LBEC hemidesmosome molecular blueprint of normal lamellar basement membrane (BM) zone. Keratin intermediate filaments link to plectin in the HD intracytoplasmic dense plaque. Plectin is linked to integrin $\alpha_6\beta_4$ which in turn links to the cross-shaped Laminin-332 molecule which, as the anchoring filament, spans the lamella lucida of the BM and embeds in the lamella densa. Also embedded in the lamella densa, but on its dermal side, are loops of banded collagen VII that, as anchoring fibrils, intertwine securely with banded collagen I of the extracellular matrix of the lamellar dermis.

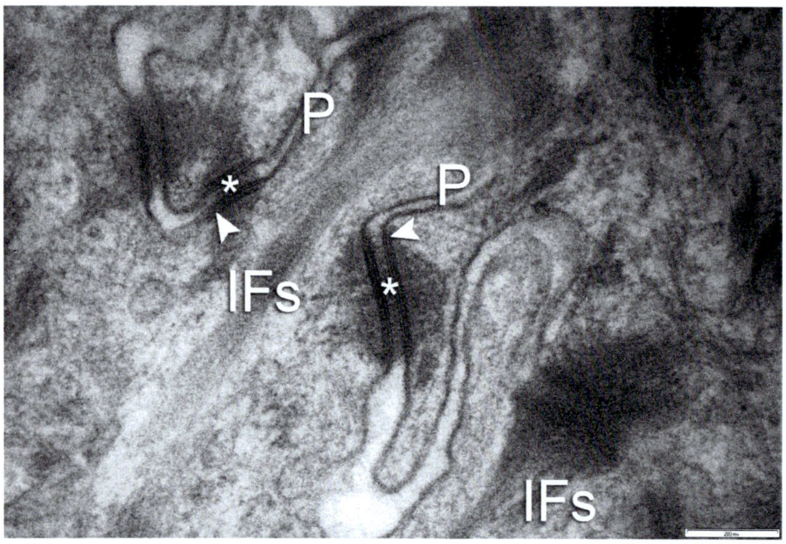

Figure 4.8 Transmission electron micrograph (TEM) of lamellar tissue showing desmosomes bridging the plasma membranes (P) of adjacent LBECs. Intermediate filaments (IFs) merge and anchor to the electron-dense cytoplasmic plaques (arrowheads) of each desmosome. Transmembrane proteins called cadherins (asterisks) bridge the intercellular space between cell plasma membranes creating a tough, biological 'spot-weld.'

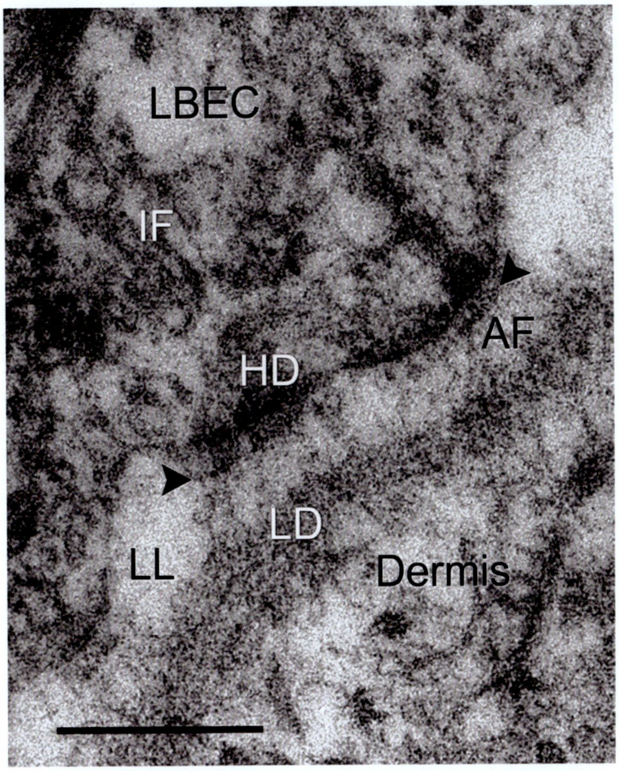

Figure 4.9 Transmission electron micrograph of lamellar tissue showing hemidesmosomes (HD) at the lamellar basal epithelial cell (LBEC) dermoepidermal junction. The electron-dense lamella densa (LD), a meshed sheet of collagen IV, is the major structural component of the basement membrane. Between the LBEC plasma membrane and the LD is the lamella lucida (LL), a clear zone spanned by anchoring filaments (AF). Each HD is constructed of several electron-dense proteins that form the intracytoplasmic dense plaque. The intermediate filament (IF) cytoskeleton attaches via plectin to the intracytoplasmic dense plaque of all hemidesmosomes. The sub-basal dense plate (arrowheads) consists of $\alpha_6\beta_4$ integrins that link to the AFs that are anchored in the LD. Each filament consists of a single glycoprotein molecule called laminin-332 that is unique to hemidesmosomes. Scale bar = 10 nm.

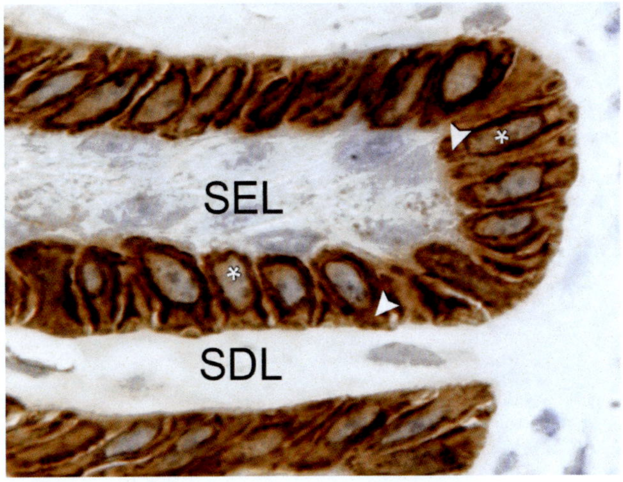

Figure 4.11 Cytokeratin 14 (K14) immunostaining of normal LBECs in transverse section. The dark positive K14 immunostaining (arrowheads) is exclusive to LBECs – adjacent SEL parabasal cells contain a different cytokeratin and thus are K14-negative. The intermediate filament (IF) cytoskeleton spans both poles of each cell suspending the oval-shaped nucleus (asterisks) at the apical pole (the pole furthest from the basement membrane) of the basal cell. The IF cytoskeleton is tethered to the basal plasmalemma by hemidesmosomes and to the apical and lateral plasmalemma by desmosomes. Scale bar = 50 μm.

The transmembrane, extracellular proteins of desmosomes – the cadherins (desmogleins and desmocollins) – mediate cell–cell adhesion and serve as a scaffold for assembly of the desmosomal plaque through their cytoplasmic domains. They form an electron-dense line (Fig. 4.8) where they overlap in the intercellular space [31]. The intracytoplasmic tails of cadherin proteins associate with armadillo family members, plakoglobin and plakophilin, which in turn associate with desmoplakin, the desmosome cytolinker protein. The C terminus of desmoplakin

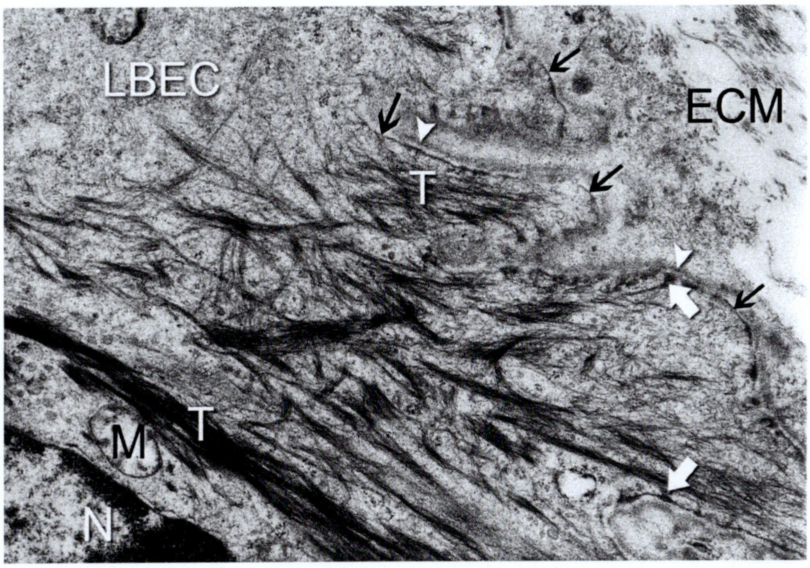

Figure 4.10 Transmission electron micrograph of a lamellar basal epithelial cell (LBEC) showing the keratin intermediate filament cytoskeleton. Intermediate filaments are bundled into dark-staining tonofilaments (T) that crosslink to form a dense, pan-cytoplasmic network. Tonofilaments merge and anchor to hemidesmosomes (white arrows) in the basal plasma membrane (black arrows) that are bridged to the adjacent lamella densa (white arrowheads) of the basement membrane and hence to the dermal extracellular matrix (ECM). M, mitochondria.

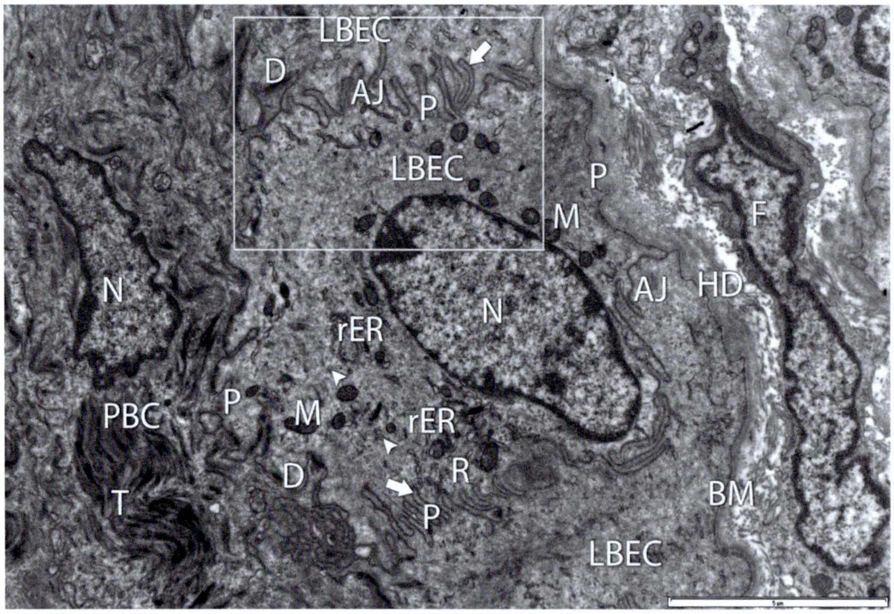

Figure 4.12 Transmission electron micrograph of immersion-fixed normal lamellar basal epithelial cells (LBECs). The nucleated parabasal cell (PBC) on the left is packed with wavy, dark-staining, keratin tonofilaments (T) and is attached to adjacent LBECs by numerous electron-dense desmosomes (D). The lamellar basement membrane (BM) demarcates the lamellar dermoepidermal junction and numerous hemidesmosomes (HD) attach the LBEC plasma membrane (P) to the BM. The plasma membranes between adjacent LBECs is remarkably plicated, forming multiple interdigitations (arrows) between cells. The plasma membranes are tightly apposed, moderately electron-dense and surrounded by fine filamentous material, presumably F-actin. The plicated membranes appear to be a zone of near-continuous adherens junctions, part of the actin-rich zona adherens that encircles the basilateral and apical walls of each cell. The area within the inset is described in more detail below. N, nucleus; M, mitochondria; AJ, adherens junction; R, ribosome (arrowheads); rER, rough endoplasmic reticulum; F, fibroblast.

links with the keratin IFs of the cytoskeleton to create the tensile strength essential for tissue keratinocyte integrity [30].

Adherens Junctions and Actin

Located at cell–cell borders, adherens junctions (AJs) are mildly electron-dense transmembrane structures associated with the actin cytoskeleton, and function as a principal mediator of cell- cell adhesion. Their disassembly correlates with a loss of cell–cell contact and an acquisition of migratory potential [32]. They perform multiple functions, including the initiation and stabilization of cell–cell adhesion, regulation of the actin cytoskeleton, intracellular signaling, and transcriptional regulation [33]. Transmission electron microscopy (TEM) studies have shown AJs to consist of opposing, mildly electron-dense plaques where LBECs contact one another (Figs. 4.12 and 4.13).

Actin filaments are the main cytoskeletal components of the AJ intracellular plaque, while the intercellular space is filled with cadherins (E-cadherin in LBECs), molecular 'spokes' that connect the opposing cell membranes (see Fig. 4.6). The cadherins of AJs were the first to be described and are the 'classic' cadherins. Desmosomal cadherins are the closest to the classic cadherins, and desmosomes, in fact, are similar in appearance to AJs, though not identical [34]. Multiple AJs form the *zonula*

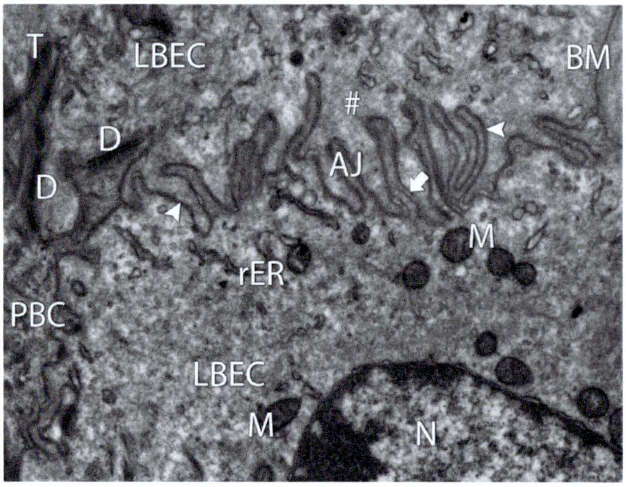

Figure 4.13 Transmission electron micrograph of immersion-fixed control tissue showing the plicated boundary between two adjacent lamellar basal epithelial cells (LBECs). Most of the adjacent plasma membranes are close together and mildly electron-dense (arrowheads) resembling classic adherens junctions (AJs). Other, less frequent, zones are more widely separated (arrowed). Fine actin-like filaments (#) enshroud the plicated plasma membrane zone. Classic desmosomes (D) with tonofilaments (T) join the LBECs to a parabasal cell (PBC). In the cytoplasm, adjacent to the plicated zone, rough endoplasmic reticulum (rER) is relatively abundant. N, nucleus; M, mitochondria; BM, basement membrane.

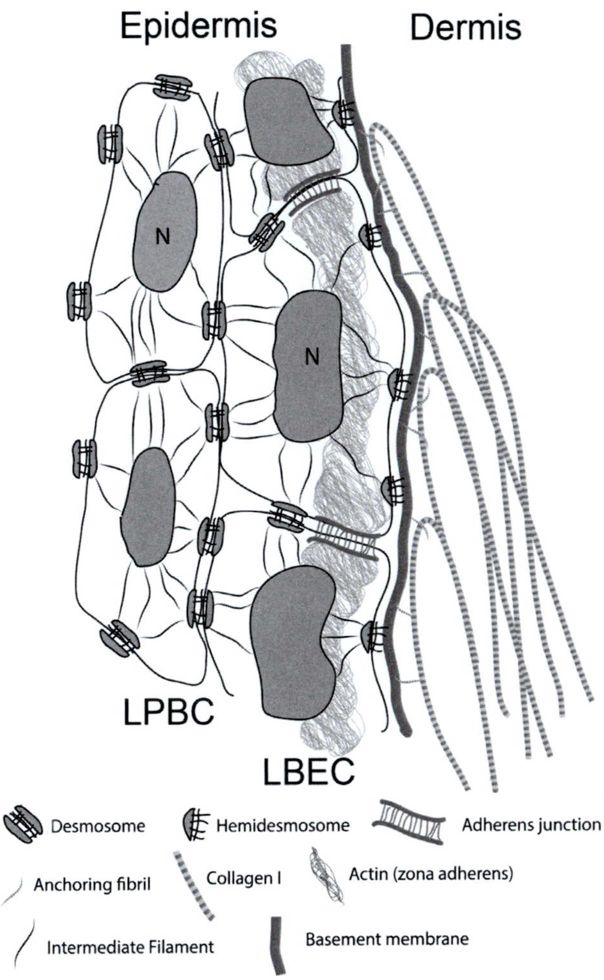

Figure 4.14 Schematic diagram of the cytoskeleton and major cell junctions of lamellar epidermal cells. Hemidesmosomes attach lamellar basal epithelial cells (LBECs) to the basement membrane via anchoring filaments. Desmosomes and adherens junctions connect adjacent cells via transmembrane cadherins. Keratin intermediate filaments span the cytoplasm linking the nucleus to hemidesmosomes and desmosomes. Actin links to adherens junctions via β-catenin and forms the zona adherens, a broad belt of interconnected, contractile actin filaments that encircles the lateral walls of each LBEC. On the dermal side of the basement membrane bundles of collagen I connect to the basement membrane via hook-like anchoring fibrils (collagen VII). LPBC, lamellar parabasal cell; N, nucleus.

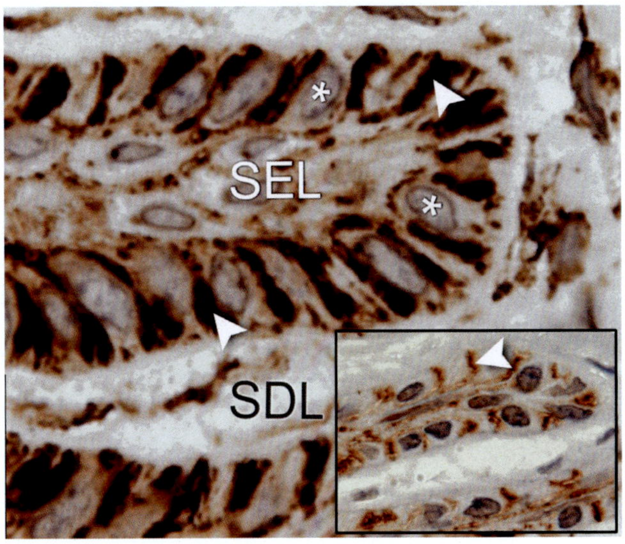

Figure 4.15 Actin and β-catenin immunostaining of normal LBECs in transverse section. In the main picture the dark brown immunostaining (arrowheads) shows actin localized to adherens junctions in the lateral and apical borders of LBECs. It is conspicuously absent at the basal LBEC border, which lacks adherens junctions. The cell boundaries of adjacent SEL parabasal cells are lightly stained, suggesting the presence of adherens junctions. The actin cytoskeleton network occupies the periphery of the LBEC cytoplasm and, unlike the keratin IF cytoskeleton, does not connect to the nucleus (asterisks). β-catenin is the cytolink protein connecting actin to the adherens junction; in the inset, dark brown β-catenin immunostaining (arrowhead) mimics the staining pattern of actin. suggesting colocalization of actin and β-catenin.

adherens, an actin belt that links adjacent cells into an unbroken sheet. Thus, the entire surface of the lamellar epidermis resembles a 'chainmail vest' of conjoined cells. The AJs and their connected actin network attach the apical and basolateral membranes of each highly polarized LBEC [35] and HDs, and the IF cytosketon attach to the lamellar BM that in turn is connected to the collagenous elements of the SADP (Fig. 4.14).

Cadherins are core AJ components and operate as homophilic adhesion receptors facilitating cell–cell recognition and adhesion. Cadherins have a cytoplasmic tail that interacts with the catenins, a defined set of proteins in the cytoplasm; β-catenin bound to α-catenin forms the cadherin/catenin complex. The binding of β-catenin to cadherin is crucial for full adhesive function, and this is largely dependent on its ability to bridge the cadherin with the actin-binding protein, α-catenin. This makes β-catenin an excellent candidate to mediate signal-induced changes in cadherin adhesive contacts, and therefore cell–cell adhesion. Several signaling proteins can directly bind to β-catenin, such as the epidermal growth factor (EGF) receptor or tyrosine phosphatases [32]. As cadherin–catenin clusters aggregate, they connect with actin, and actin is remodeled to propagate the AJ. Multiple actin networks associate with cadherin–catenin clusters at mature AJs to hold them in place and stabilize not only the cell but also the cell to its neighbors via 'the lamellar unbroken chainmail sheet.' Intense actin and β-catenin immunostaining staining (Fig. 4.15) occurs along the plicated, basolateral and apical boundaries of LBECs, presumably in conjunction with ultrastructural AJs (Fig. 4.13), thus providing essential adhesion, high elasticity, and resilience to this region.

Transmission electron microscopy studies of the plicated basilateral regions of LBECs show the plasma membranes of adjacent cells in close contact with mildly electron-dense plaques on opposing sides, surrounded by fine actin-like fibrillar material. The entire intercalated region is assumed to be a zone of near-continuous AJs (Fig. 4.13).

Adherens junctions are crucial for the initiation and maintenance of LBEC intercellular adhesion. Although their ultrastructure suggests that AJs form stable structures, they are in fact highly dynamic complexes. In the absence of AJs, the formation of other cell–cell adhesion structures is dramatically reduced [36].

β-Catenin is the central player in the canonical Wnt signaling pathway, and is one of the fundamental pathways that control cell processes involved not only in development but also in many disease states, including epithelial diseases such as cancer (e.g., proliferation, differentiation, polarity, motility). The core activity of the Wnt pathway is regulation of the production and stability of β-catenin in cells, including LBECs (see Chapter 15). This is important because β-catenin is a dual-function protein that: (i) serves to stabilize the cell morphology as a component of the AJ where, together with α-cadherin and vinculin, it couples the intracellular domain of E-cadherin to actin filaments (see Fig. 4.6), and (ii) mediates canonical Wnt signaling by binding to and activating members of the T-cell factor (TCF) transcriptional factor family, thus regulating the expression of specific genes involved in cell processes important in cell fate determination (as noted at the start of the paragraph). Thus, it is tempting to speculate that the function of β-catenin in AJs relates to the coordination of morphogenetic movements with cell fate determination. This proposal is corroborated by the results of a multitude of studies showing a close reciprocal relationship between intercellular adhesion and Wnt signaling [32].

If AJs are perturbed, the actin cytoskeleton follows suit, thus illustrating the linked relationship between the two. The AJs have a crucial role in maintaining the mechanical stability of keratinocytes as demonstrated by deletion of two different AJ proteins, α-catenin and E-cadherin (see Fig. 4.5). Mice carrying an epidermal-specific deletion of α-catenin have impaired intercellular adhesion, defective AJs, and epidermal detachment. Impaired intercellular adhesion and hair loss follows the deletion of E-cadherin [37].

Several enzymes produced by epithelial cells in health and disease can disrupt AJs. Metalloproteases, as well as the ADAMTS family (see Chapter 15) cleave the extracellular and transmembrane domains of E-cadherin, disrupting adhesive contacts [38, 39]. The enzymes of apoptosis-calpain and caspase-3-also target the cytosolic domains of E-cadherin, effectively abolishing its linkage with one or more catenins, and thus with the actin cytoskeleton.

Epithelial cells disassemble and reassemble their AJs to maintain the dynamics of the epithelial monolayer. In some situations, however, such as during an epithelial-to-mesenchymal transition, cells lose their adhesive contacts completely [32]. Actin filament functions are regulated by cellular signaling pathways such as those involving Rho GTPases and p38MAPK, which are important signaling molecules in their own right [40]. Reports from human pemphigus vulgaris studies show that a loss of keratinocyte adhesion was accompanied by profound changes in the actin cytoskeleton, notably displacement of the zonula adherens [40].

Hemidesmosomes

The LBECs are attached to their underlying BM by specialized structures known as hemidesmosomes (HDs). Located exclusively along the basal plasma membrane of LBECs, the HDs connect cytoskeletal IFs to the lamella densa of the BM (Figs 4.7 and 4.10). In addition to their adhesive role, HDs also participate in signal transduction [41]. There are three classes of proteins within the HD complex: (i) the intracytoplasmic plaque proteins plectin and bullous pemphigoid antigen I (BP230) that link the HD to the cytoplasmic keratin IFs; (ii) transmembrane proteins including integrin $\alpha_6\beta_4$; and (iii) the bullous pemphigoid antigen 2 (BP180 or type XVII collagen) which are cell receptors connecting the cell interior to the dermis and the BM-associated protein Ln 332 [41]. Assembled together, these molecules form the classical type I HD. Type I HDs are reported in stratified epithelium such as the skin in most species (including the horse), as well as the equine hoof [42, 43]. Plectin and BP230 form the cytoplasmic plaque mediating the attachment of IFs to the HD and therefore the basal plasma membrane of the LBEC.

Emphasizing the importance of plectin to HD integrity is the case of a Quarterhorse foal born with an inherited plectin defect. The foal developed the clinical signs of laminitis within hours of it first standing [44]. The examination of lamellar samples using TEM showed small, deformed HDs sparsely populating the lamellar BM, as well as clumps of densely staining, tonofilament material, free in the epidermal basal cell cytoplasm and condensed around the nucleus. Subsequent IHC studies showed plectin to be absent in all hoof lamellae and skin samples. Thus, a defect in a single molecule of the LBEC HD adhesion complex prevented functional HD assembly and resulted in lamellar dysfunction. It is immaterial whether HD disintegration results from an inherited gene 'knockout' or a metabolic or septic crisis in adulthood; dermoepidermal separation within the hoof lamellae – the 'signature lesion' of laminitis – will still occur [44].

Integrins are transmembrane proteins made up of an α and β subunit which associate noncovalently to participate in cell adhesion as well as signal transduction. Integrin $\alpha_6\beta_4$ is essential for HD assembly, and no HDs form in the presence $\alpha_6\beta_4$ antibody [45]. The intracellular tail of the β_4 subunit is crucial for interaction of the integrin with other HD components. The extracellular domain of the integrin $\alpha_6\beta_4$ is important for cell adhesion through association with Ln 332, the primary component of the anchoring filaments which span the lamella lucida of the BM (see Fig. 4.7) [46]. The intracellular component of β_4 is critically important in regulation of HDs; there are several sites on this part of the protein that can result in dissolution of the entire HD if phosphorylated by the different kinases involved in numerous cell signaling pathways, including growth factor signaling. This mechanism is important in the dysadhesion of basal epithelial cells for normal processes such as wound healing, but has also been found to be important in the dysadhesion of cells in disease states, such as epithelial cancers. Thus, dysregulation of the β_4 integrin, either by phosphorylation of the protein or by decreased expression of the integrin (as discussed further below), may play an important role in LBEC dysadhesion in laminitis.

Emphasizing the importance of the basement membrane protein Ln 332 to lamellar dermoepidermal integrity are Belgian foals born with an autosomal, recessive mutation within the gene encoding the gamma 2 chain of Ln 332. The mutation results in an absence of the anchoring filament Ln 332 protein, due to a premature termination codon [47]. The absence of Ln 332 results in a widespread dermoepidermal separation in skin and digital lamellae, and hoof exunguilation.

BEC adhesion to the underlying BM mediated by HDs is considered stable and robust, although appropriate signaling can cause BECs to dissociate from the BM and migrate over it during, for example, wound healing. Dissociation involves HD disassembly and matrix remodeling. Free of the basement membrane zone (BMZ), the BECs move directionally over a provisional matrix to re-establish intact, BM-bounded, epidermal structures. Upon wound coverage, the BMZ is reassembled and HDs are reformed [48].

During HD disassembly, the $\gamma 2$ subunit of Ln 332 can be enzymatically cleaved by members of the metalloprotease (MMP) family, including membrane-type 1 (MT1)-MMP, -MMP-2, -MMP-3, -MMP-12, -MMP-13, -MMP-19, and -MMP-20 [49]. Cleavage products of Ln 332, in particular the 27 kDa fragment (γ2SA), are biologically active in their own right and can mediate cell migration. The serine protease plasmin, a product of plasminogen degradation by tissue-type plasminogen activator (t-PA), not only binds the G domain of the laminin 3 subunit but also cleaves the molecule to release a fragment believed to stimulate cell migration. Inappropriate BEC migration due to the cleavage of Ln 332 was proposed as a pathophysiologic mechanism for laminitis, although, despite extensive studies, no Ln 332 cleavage products were detected during laminitis induction [50]. Despite enzymatic cleavage of Ln 332 occurring in other species, the equine molecule appears resistant, at least in the laminitis scenario.

Ultrastructural examination of normal LBECs shows HDs arranged along the BMZ, clustered in zones. Normal horses have (mean $\pm$ SEM) 4.64 $\pm$ 0.15 HDs per µm of plasmalemma (cell membrane), that occupy 28.6 $\pm$ 0.6% of the plasmalemma surface area [43]. Although four HD proteins span the plasmalemma (the 180 kDa-bullous pemphigoid antigen [termed BP180 or type XVII collagen], the two subunits of the $\alpha_6\beta_4$ integrin and a tetraspanin protein termed CD151), it is BP180 and the $\alpha_6\beta_4$ integrin that interact with the anchoring filaments (Ln 332) in the BMZ. Association of the $\alpha_6\beta_4$ integrin with the keratin cytoskeleton, rather than actin, makes this heterodimer unique among the integrin family [51]. This interaction is facilitated by the long 1000-amino acid cytoplasmic tail of the β_4 integrin subunit which binds not only BP180 but also the 230 kDa bullous pemphigoid antigen (BP230 or BPAG1e) and plectin. The latter two proteins are plakin family members that mediate the indirect but critical linkage of keratin to $\alpha_6\beta_4$ integrin (see Fig. 4.7).

The LBECs are spindle-shaped with their long axes arranged proximodistally in line with the similar orientation of the collagenous fibers of the SADP. When the plane of section is transverse, at 90° to the dorsal hoof wall, the lamellae have a characteristic well-described appearance [52]. In sections stained with hematoxylin and eosin (H&E) or PAS, most of the nuclei of lamellar basal cells are oval and situated at the apical pole of the cell (The apical pole is furthest from the BM; see Fig. 4.4). The long axis of the basal cell nucleus is oriented at right-angles to the KA of the SEL. The median width of an SEL is 25 µm (range: 21.5–28.5 µm) and the median length is 142 µm (range: 107–173 µm) [14]. PAS-stained sections locate the glycoprotein constituents of the BM, and stain the BM magenta. The BM of normal lamellae penetrates deeply into the crypt between pairs of SELs, and clearly outlines the tapered tip of each SDL (see Fig. 4.3). The proximity of the SDL tip to the KA of the PEL is, therefore, readily appreciated; it is always a distance equivalent to the length of one or two BECs. The club-shaped tips of SELs, as outlined by the BM, are always rounded and never tapered or pointed.

Masson's trichrome stain clearly shows the nature of the connective tissue of the PDLs and SDLs (Fig. 4.16). The SDL

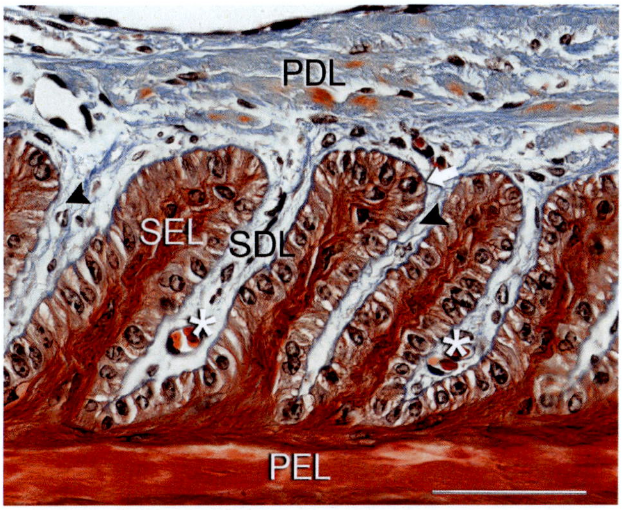

Figure 4.16 Transverse section photomicrograph of normal hoof primary dermal lamella (PDL), secondary dermal (SDL), primary epidermal lamella (PEL), and secondary epidermal lamellae (SEL) stained with Masson's trichrome. Blue-staining connective tissue fibers fill the PDL and extend to the very tip of every tapered SDL. Filamentous fibers merge into the dermal side of the blue lamellar basement membrane (arrows). Fine, thin-walled capillaries (asterisk), the diameter of one or two erythrocytes, are located within SDLs.

connective tissue consists of very fine, blue-staining fibers which fill and extend to the very tip of every tapered SDL. The fibers merge into the dermal side of the clearly delineated, blue lamellar BM. Staining the connective tissue with the Masson's trichrome stain emphasizes how much narrower the SDLs are compared to their adjacent SELs. Nevertheless, fine, thin-walled capillaries, the diameter of one or two erythrocytes, are located within the filamentous connective tissue of most of the wafer-thin SDLs. Masson's trichrome-stained sections are superior to PAS and H&E for showing the density and orientation of the SDL connective tissue.

A less familiar view, obtained when the plane of section of mid-wall lamellae is longitudinal (proximal to distal), is oriented along the long axis of the BECs and PBCs, and shows that the cells are spindle-shaped [53]. The anatomy of lamellar suspensory function is more clearly illustrated in this view/section, as the intermediate filaments of the LBEC cytoskeleton are oriented on the same axis as the collagen elements in the adjacent SDL (Fig. 4.1) [54].

In addition to the intracellular cytoskeleton, other molecules participate in equipping the lamellae to withstand the strains imposed on the SADP; this includes a lamellar ECM rich in polysulfated proteoglycans [55], shock-absorbing proteins that are usually associated with articular cartilage in joints.

A secreted enzyme, ADAMTS-4, regulates the turnover of these large proteoglycan molecules in the ECM and is located in the lamellae [55]. The main substrates of ADAMTS-4 in peripheral tissues are aggrecan and versican [56], both of which assemble massive and highly charged, anionic macromolecular complexes in the ECM that create an osmotic gradient drawing water into the tissue. The resultant hydrated gel likely helps the lamellae withstand compression and deformation, and also provides additional protection.

Lamellar Metabolism

The LBECs are metabolically active and consume energy to maintain their fundamental role of maintaining the SADP. An early insight into the nature of LBEC energy metabolism was the discovery that an absence of glucose from the culture medium that normally maintains lamellar explants intact for up to eight days caused rapid epidermal/dermal separation at the BMZ [57]. A subsequent ultrastructural investigation showed that glucose deprivation caused shrinkage and disappearance of HDs and detachment of the LBEC cytoskeleton from the HD intracellular dense plaque; the detached cytoskeleton condensed around the cell nucleus, which became round instead of oval in shape [58]. Glucose deprivation may cause HD disassembly directly by disrupting the energy-dependent phosphorylation that is vital for HD assembly and maintenance [41, 59]. Thus, glucose-deprived lamellar explants presumably separate under tension because of weak attachment of the $\alpha_6\beta_4$ integrins in the disintegrating HDs to the Ln 332-anchoring filaments in the BM. Defective $\alpha_6\beta_4$ expression, as occurs in human blistering skin disorders [60], and targeted removal of the β_4 gene in experimental mice also results in a loss of HDs and widespread dermoepidermal separation [61].

Because of the widespread realization that hyperinsulinemia was associated with an endocrinological form of laminitis [62–64], it was anticipated that LBEC glucose flux would be controlled by insulin, and that insulin receptors (IRs) or the insulin-responsive glucose transporter 4 (GLUT4), similar to the situation in muscle tissue, would also be present within the LBEC cytoplasm or at the cell surface. The argument was that insulin resistance within LBECs would result in glucose deficiency, lamellar damage and separation, as mimicked by *in vitro* glucose deprivation. However, LBECs stain weakly for GLUT4 (O.S. Wattle and C.C. Pollitt, unpublished data) and IRs stain strongly positive – but not in LBECs; only the endothelium of adjacent lamellar blood vessels were positive for IRs [65]. In addition, glucose uptake by lamellar explants in culture is not responsive to insulin [66]. Thus, glucose uptake by LBECs appears to be independent of insulin.

However, insulin can affect the lamellae. Receptors for the powerful cell mitogen/growth factor insulin-like growth factor-1 (IGF-1) are present on the LBEC [65, 67] and, presumably, respond to IGF-1 for controlled growth, remodeling, and repair. However, lamellar IGF-1 receptors are also activated by insulin, and this may trigger the inappropriate LBEC proliferative response observed in horses dosed with supraphysiological concentrations of insulin. These hyperinsulinemic horses also rapidly develop longer, thinner SELs and the clinical signs of laminitis. Among the SEL basal cells are numerous mitotic figures, and many cells stain positive for the proliferative immunohistochemical marker TPX2 [14, 67, 68]. Thus, a key aspect of lamellar homeostasis is likely revealed. Normal SELs must have an optimum width and length that is tightly maintained to keep the DP (via the SADP) suspended in its optimum position within the hoof capsule; LBEC proliferation is absent in this scenario. When hyperinsulinemia triggers cellular changes in the LBEC – including a change to a more proliferative cell phenotype that is likely associated with disruption of cytoskeletal regulation – this aberrant cell signaling likely leads to weakened, attenuated SELs, allowing a downward displacement of the distal phalanx (as observed in endocrinopathic laminitis).

GLUT1, the most abundant immunostaining glucose transporter in hoof lamellae (Fig. 4.17), is located predominantly in LBECs [69]; this pattern is similar to that described in human and rodent skin epidermis [70]. Strong GLUT1 mRNA expression in coronary band and lamellar tissue supports the immunostaining results [66]. The immunostaining of GLUT1 is absent in equine skeletal muscle, again confirmed by weak mRNA expression [66]. Presumably, LBECs continuously take up glucose from adjacent extracellular fluid (ECF) that is delivered into the ECF via lamellar blood vessels. In this way, the lamellae resemble brain tissue that depend on GLUT1 for glucose uptake independent of insulin. In the brain, glucose is the

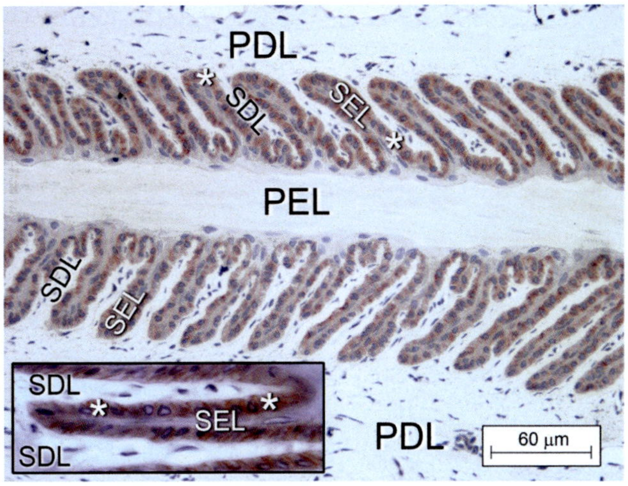

Figure 4.17 Photomicrographs of lamellar sections immunostained for GLUT-1. Only LBECs are positive (asterisks). The inset shows a higher magnification of the SEL. Inset reproduced with permission from Ref. [69]; © Elsevier.

sole substrate utilized for energy metabolism as it is the only substrate that is transported across the blood–brain barrier at a sufficient rate. In the cytoplasm of cells, glucose is converted to pyruvate and lactate [71].

Since human skin accounts for approximately 15% of the total glucose uptake under basal conditions [72], it is not surprising that an animal such as the horse, with a hoof lamellar surface area estimated to be around 0.8 m^2 per hoof [8], metabolizes considerable amounts of glucose.

Differences between arterial and venous blood reflect the metabolic processes in the tissues drained by veins. Measurements of glucose concentrations in simultaneously taken blood samples from the superficial temporal artery, the jugular vein, and a digital vein at the level of the pastern of one of the front legs of six Standardbred horses showed how much glucose was consumed per foot (O.S. Wattle and C.C. Pollitt, unpublished data). The difference between glucose concentrations in the digital veins and the artery showed that a foot in horses at rest had a glucose consumption that exceeded that of the head. One foot (1% of the body weight) consumed almost 15% of the arterial glucose delivered. In contrast, the head consumed just 8%. In comparison, the human brain consumes 20% of the glucose delivered, which is remarkable as the brain represents only 2% of the body weight [71]. Since the foot has no tissue with any glycogen storage capacity, it is reasonable to believe that the glucose consumption reflects anaerobic glycolysis, and perhaps some oxidation through the citric acid cycle. Lactate concentrations were also higher in blood from the digital veins than the jugular vein indicating that, at physiological glucose concentrations at rest, a large part of the glucose taken up is metabolized to lactate. A high glucose consumption is required since the glycolytic yield of ATP is low compared to that of oxidative phosphorylation.

The metabolism of the skin and its appendages is believed to depend mostly on anaerobic metabolism, especially in the epidermal basal layers that lack stored glycogen [73]. This appears to be the case in the epidermal lamellae of horses, as digital venous blood contains higher lactate concentrations than either arterial or jugular venous blood [69]. In addition, cryosections of LBECs are biochemically reactive for lactate dehydrogenase (LDH), suggesting that they mainly rely on glycolytically (anaerobic) generated ATP [69].

Lactate is no longer considered a waste product of anaerobic metabolism [74], but instead is a central player in cellular metabolism as a source of energy. The LBECs contain mitochondria (Figs 4.12 and 4.13) [75] and stain for reduced nicotinamide adenine dinucleotide (NADH), similar to type 1 oxidative muscle fibers [69]. However, in common with mitochondria in human skin BECs, the mitochondria are relatively small, contain few cristae, and have an electron-lucent matrix. There is a correlation between ATP production, the number of mitochondria, and their cristae [76]. The small number of cristae in LBECs implies a reduced surface area of the inner mitochondrial membrane and, consequently, insignificant oxidative phosphorylation. The mitochondria appear ineffective for the oxidative metabolism of glucose, and thus epidermal energy metabolism is probably predominantly anaerobic in spite of the formal presence of mitochondria.

There is some transcutaneous uptake of oxygen by human skin (0.529 ± 0.265 ml O_2 m^{-2} min^{-1}), which is a negligible 0.4% contribution to the pulmonary oxygen uptake (230 ml O_2 min^{-1}) at rest. Oxygen was shown to penetrate to a depth of 0.24–0.4 mm, passing through the cornified layer to the upper dermis of the skin [77]. Considering its thickness and degree of cornification, the penetration of oxygen through the equine hoof wall is probably zero. Thus, without an intrinsic circulation of its own, the lamellar epidermis must rely on oxygen delivery from erythrocytes passing through capillaries in the adjacent dermis. Between the erythrocyte and the BEC cytoplasm is the BEC plasmalemma, the BM, the dermal ECM and the capillary endothelium, which together may render the lamellar milieu relatively hypoxic. Nevertheless, sufficient oxygen is available for BEC requirements which in life may be quite small given the apparent anaerobic, glycolytic energy-generating capacity of the lamellae.

Hypoxia-inducible factor-1α (HIF-1α) is an important protein in the regulation/induction of over 100 genes in the cellular and tissue response to hypoxia, and is a central mediator in inflammatory signaling [78]. HIF-1 maintains tissue integrity and homeostasis [79] and regulates genes involved in protecting cells and tissue from low oxygen levels (and subsequent low-energy states). Thus, glucose metabolism proteins (e.g., GLUT1), glycolysis-related proteins (e.g., phosphoglycerate kinase 1; PGK1), as well as genes involved in inflammatory signaling, are regulated by HIF-1α. Increased HIF-1α concentrations will exacerbate inflammatory signaling in epidermal tissue [80]. Equine hoof SELs have a greater HIF-1α concentration than any other equine tissue, which suggests that their environment is profoundly hypoxic [81]. Unfortunately, the high HIF-1α concentration and the crosstalk between HIF-1α and inflammatory mediators such as NF-κB (nuclear factor kappa-light-chain, an enhancer of activated B cells; HIF-1α can activate NF-κB) may render the hoof lamellae uniquely prone to the effects of circulating inflammatory mediators, and thereby explain the propensity of the lamellae to injury while other organs are spared. NF-κB is a rapid-acting, first-response, primary transcription factor in the innate immune response, and is not only activated by HIF-1α but is also a critical transcriptional activator of HIF-1α [80].

Conclusions

The lamellar epidermal basal cell, as part of the suspensory apparatus of the distal phalanx, participates in an attachment function that is critical to the core survivability of the horse. The LBEC functions and reacts in a multitude of complex ways that only now are being understood as the drive to comprehend laminitis fuels research into LBEC structure and function. The integrity of the LBEC is the hinge factor determining whether or not the distal phalanx will slip away from the hoof lamellae during the progression of clinical laminitis.

The dynamics of LBEC attachment to the BM in health and disease should be a focus of future research, not only because it is intrinsically fascinating but also because it will lead to a better understanding, prevention, and treatment of laminitis [82]. How a diverse set of disease entities can lead to catastrophic failure of the SADP through: (i) a loss of morphologic integrity of the epidermal lamellae through LBEC cytoskeletal dysregulation; (ii) dysadhesion of the LBEC from its underlying basement membrane; or (iii) more likely, both, is yet to be elucidated [83].

References

1. Bragulla, H. and Hirschberg, R.M. (2003) Horse hooves and bird feathers: Two model systems for studying the structure and development of highly adapted integumentary accessory organs – The role of the dermo-epidermal interface for the micro-architecture of complex epidermal structures. *J. Exp. Zool. Part B - Mol. Dev. Evol.*, **298B** (1), 140–151.
2. Anonymous (2012) *Nomina Anatomica Veterinaria*. Hannover: International Committee on Veterinary Gross Anatomical Nomenclature, 2012, xviii + 155 p.
3. Konig, H.E. and Liebich, H.-G. (eds) (2009) *Veterinary Anatomy of Domestic Animals*. 4th revised edition. Scattauer, Stuttgart.
4. Budras, K.D., Hirschberg, R., Hinterhofer, C., Polsterer, E., and Konig, H.E. (2009) The suspensory apparatus of the coffin bone. Part 1: The fan-shaped re-inforcement of the suspensory apparatus at the tip of the coffin bone in the horse. *Pferdeheilkunde*, **25** (2), 96–104.
5. Budras, K.D., Hinterhofer, C., Hirschberg, R., Polsterer, E., and Konig, H.E. (2009) The suspensory apparatus of the coffin bone. Part 2: Clinical relevance of the suspensory apparatus and its fan-shaped reinforcement in chronic equine laminitis with coffin bone or hoof capsule rotation. *Pferdeheilkunde*, **25** (3), 198–204.
6. Pollitt, C.C. (2010) The anatomy and physiology of the suspensory apparatus of the distal phalanx. *Vet. Clin. North Am. Equine Pract.*, **26** (1), 29–49.
7. Pollitt, C.C. and Collins, S.N. (2016) The suspensory apparatus of the distal phalanx in normal horses. *Equine Vet. J.*, **48** (4), 496–501.
8. Daradka, M. (2000) *The Equine Hoof Wall: Growth, Repair and Dimensions*. PhD thesis, University of Queensland, Brisbane.
9. Van Eps, A.W. and Pollitt, C.C. (2009) Equine laminitis model: lamellar histopathology seven days after induction with oligofructose. *Equine Vet. J.*, **41** (8), 735–740.
10. Sisson, S. and Grossman, J.D. (1953) Aesthesiology; the sense organs and skin of the horse, in *The Anatomy of the Domestic Animals*, 4th edition. W.B. Saunders, Philadelphia, pp. 879–918.
11. Pollitt, C.C. and Daradka, M. (2004) Hoof wall wound repair. *Equine Vet. J.*, **36** (3), 210–215.
12. Underwood, C., Collins, S.N., Van Eps, A.W., Allavena, R.E., Medina-Torres, C.E., and Pollitt, C.C. (2014) Ultrafiltration of equine digital lamellar tissue. *Vet. J.*, **202** (2), 314–322.
13. Carter, R.A., Engiles, J.B., Megee, S.O., Senoo, M., and Galantino-Homer, H.L. (2011) Decreased expression of p63, a regulator of epidermal stem cells, in the chronic laminitic equine hoof. *Equine Vet. J.*, **43** (5), 543–551.
14. de Laat, M.A., Patterson-Kane, J.C., Pollitt, C.C., Sillence, M.N., and McGowan, C.M. (2012) Histological and morphometric lesions in the pre-clinical, developmental phase of insulin-induced laminitis in Standardbred horses. *Vet. J.*, **195**, 305–312.
15. Senoo, M., Pinto, F., Crum, C.P., and McKeon, F. (2007) p63 is essential for the proliferative potential of stem cells in stratified epithelia. *Cell*, **129**, 523–536.
16. Daradka, M. and Pollitt, C.C. (2004) Epidermal cell proliferation in the equine hoof wall. *Equine Vet. J.*, **36** (3), 236–241.
17. Van Eps, A., Collins, S.N., and Pollitt, C.C. (2010) Supporting limb laminitis. *Vet. Clin. North Am. Equine Pract.*, **26** (2), 287–302.
18. Bolliger, C. and Geyer, H. (1992) Morphology and histochemistry of the equine hoof. *Pferdeheilkunde*, **8** (5), 269–286.
19. de Laat, M.A., Patterson-Kane, J.C., Pollitt, C.C., Sillence, M.N., and McGowan, C.M. (2013) Histological and morphometric lesions in the pre-clinical, developmental phase of insulin-induced laminitis in Standardbred horses. *Vet. J.*, **195** (3), 305–312.
20. Anthauer, K., Mulling, C., and Budras, K.D. (2005) Membrane-coating granules and the intercellular cementing substance (membrane-coating material) in the epidermis in different regions of the equine hoof. *Anat. Histol. Embryol. J. Vet. Med. Series C*, **34** (5), 298–306.
21. Leach, D.H. and Oliphant, L.W. (1983) Ultrastructure of the equine hoof wall secondary epidermal lamellae. *Am. J. Vet. Res.*, **44** (8), 1561–1570.
22. Budras, K.D., Hullinger, R.L., and Sack, W.O. (1989) Light and electron microscopy of keratinization in the laminar epidermis of the equine hoof with reference to laminitis. *Am. J. Vet. Res.*, **50** (7), 1150–1160.
23. Abrahamson, D.R. (1986) Recent studies on the structure and pathology of basement membranes. *J. Pathol.*, **149**, 257–278.

24. Carter, R.A., Shekk, V., de Laat, M.A., Pollitt, C.C., and Galantino-Homer, H.L. (2010) Novel keratins identified by quantitative proteomic analysis as the major cytoskeletal proteins of equine (*Equus caballus*) hoof lamellar tissue. *J. Anim. Sci.*, **88** (12), 3843–3855.
25. Ketema, M. and Sonnenberg, A. (2011) Nesprin-3: a versatile connector between the nucleus and the cytoskeleton. *Biochem. Soc. Trans.*, **39** (6), 1719–1724.
26. Kim, S.H. and Coulombe, P.A. (2010) Emerging role for the cytoskeleton as an organizer and regulator of translation. *Nat. Rev. Mol. Cell. Biol.*, **11** (1), 75–81.
27. Moll, R., Divo, M., and Langbein, L. (2008) The human keratins: biology and pathology. *Histochem. Cell. Biol.*, **129** (6), 705–733.
28. Lee, C. and Coulombe, P. (2009) Self-organization of keratin intermediate filaments into cross-linked networks. *J. Cell Biol.*, **186** (3), 409–421.
29. Ramms, L., Fabris, G., Windoffer, R., Schwarz, N., Springer, R., Zhou, C., *et al.* (2013) Keratins as the main component for the mechanical integrity of keratinocytes. *Proc. Natl Acad. Sci. USA*, **110** (46), 18513–18518.
30. Nekrasova, O. and Green, K.J. (2013) Desmosome assembly and dynamics. *Trends Cell Biol.*, **23** (11), 537–546.
31. Young, B., Lowe, J.S., Stevens, A., and Heath, J.W. (2006) Basic tissue types, in *Wheater's Functional Histology; A Text and Colour Atlas*, 5th edition. Elsevier, St Louis, MO, pp. 88–91.
32. D'Souza-Schorey, C. (2005) Disassembling adherens junctions: breaking up is hard to do. *Trends Cell Biol.*, **15** (1), 19–26.
33. Hartsock, A. and Nelson, W.J. (2008) Adherens and tight junctions: Structure, function and connections to the actin cytoskeleton. *Biochim. Biophys. Acta. Biomembranes*, **1778** (3), 660–669.
34. Meng, W. and Takeichi, M. (2009) Adherens junction: molecular architecture and regulation. *Cold Spring Harb. Perspect. Biol.*, **1** (6), a002899.
35. Harris, T.J.C. and Tepass, U. (2010) Adherens junctions: from molecules to morphogenesis. *Nat. Rev. Mol. Cell. Biol.*, **11** (7), 502–514.
36. Vasioukhin, V. and Fuchs, E. (2001) Actin dynamics and cell-cell adhesion in epithelia. *Curr. Opin. Cell Biol.*, **13** (1), 76–84.
37. Vasioukhin, V., Bauer, C., Degenstein, L., Wise, B., and Fuchs, E. Hyperproliferation and defects in epithelial polarity upon conditional ablation of alpha-catenin in skin. *Cell*, **104** (4), 605–617.
38. Marambaud, P., Shioi, J., Serban, G., Georgakopoulos, A., Sarner, S., Nagy, V., *et al.* (2002) Presenilin-1-dependent gamma-secretase cleavage of E-cadherin controls adherens junction disassembly. *Neurobiol. Aging*, **23** (1), S212–S213.
39. Moali, C. and Hulmes, D.J.S. (2009) Extracellular and cell surface proteases in wound healing: new players are still emerging. *Eur. J. Dermatol.*, **19** (6), 552–564.
40. Gliem, M., Heupel, W.M., Spindler, V., Harms, G.S., and Waschke, J. (2010) Actin reorganization contributes to loss of cell adhesion in pemphigus vulgaris. *Am. J. Physiol. Cell Physiol.*, **299** (3), C606–C613.
41. Borradori, L. and Sonnenberg, A. (1999) Structure and function of hemidesmosomes: more than simple adhesion complexes. *J. Invest. Dermatol.*, **112** (4), 411–418.
42. Pollitt, C.C. (1994) The basement membrane at the equine hoof dermal epidermal junction. *Equine Vet. J.*, **26** (5), 399–407.
43. French, K.R. and Pollitt, C.C. (2004) Equine laminitis: loss of hemidesmosomes in hoof secondary epidermal lamellae correlates to dose in an oligofructose induction model: an ultrastructural study. *Equine Vet. J.*, **36** (3), 230–235.
44. French, K.R. and Pollitt, C.C. (2004) Equine laminitis: congenital, hemidesmosomal plectin deficiency in a Quarter Horse foal. *Equine Vet. J.*, **36** (3), 299–303.
45. Jones, J.C., Kurpakus, M.A., Cooper, H.M., and Quaranta, V. (1991) A function for the integrin alpha 6 beta 4 in the hemidesmosome. *Cell Regul.*, **2** (6), 427–438.
46. McMillan, J.R., Akiyama, M., and Shimizu, H. (2003) Ultrastructural orientation of laminin 5 in the epidermal basement membrane: an updated model for basement membrane organization. *J. Histochem. Cytochem.*, **51**, 1299–1306.
47. Spirito, F., Charlesworth, A., Linder, K., Ortonne, J.P., Baird, J., and Meneguzzi, G. (2002) Animal models for skin blistering conditions: absence of laminin 5 causes hereditary junctional mechanobullous disease in the Belgian horse. *J. Invest. Dermatol.*, **119** (3), 684–691.
48. Raja, S.K., Garcia, M.S., and Isseroff, R.R. (2007) Wound re-epithelialization: modulating keratinocyte migration in wound healing. *Front. Biosci.*, **12**, 2249–2268.
49. Tsuruta, D., Kobayashi, H., Imanishi, H., Sugawara, K., Ishii, M., and Jones, J.C.R. (2008) Laminin-332-integrin interaction: A target for cancer therapy? *Curr. Med. Chem.*, **15** (20), 1968–1975.
50. Visser, M.B. and Pollitt, C.C. (2011) The timeline of lamellar basement membrane changes during equine laminitis development. *Equine Vet. J.*, **43** (4), 471–477.
51. Jones, J.C., Hopkinson, S.B., and Goldfinger, L.E. (1998) Structure and assembly of hemidesmosomes. *BioEssays*, **20** (6), 488–494.
52. Pollitt, C.C. (1996) Basement membrane pathology: a feature of acute equine laminitis. *Equine Vet. J.*, **28** (1), 38–46.
53. Pollitt, C.C. (2015) Lamellar histology, in *The Illustrated Horse's Foot*, 1st edition. Elsevier Health Sciences, St Louis, Missouri, pp. 125–145.
54. Pollitt, C.C. (2015) *The Illustrated Horse's Foot*. Elsevier Health Sciences, St Louis, Missouri.
55. Pawlak, E., Wang, L., Johnson, P.J., Nuovo, G., Taye, A., Belknap, J.K., *et al.* (2012) Distribution and processing of a disintegrin and metalloproteinase with thrombospondin motifs-4, aggrecan, versican, and hyaluronan in equine digital laminae. *Am. J. Vet. Res.*, **73** (7), 1035–1046.
56. Salter, R.C., Ashlin, T.G., Kwan, A.P.L., and Ramji, D.P. (2010) ADAMTS proteases: key roles in atherosclerosis? *J. Mol. Med.*, **88** (12), 1203–1211.
57. Pass, M.A., Pollitt, S., and Pollitt, C.C. (1998) Decreased glucose metabolism causes separation of hoof lamellae in vitro: a trigger for laminitis? *Equine Vet. J. Suppl.*, **26**, 133–138.
58. French, K.R. and Pollitt, C.C. (2004) Equine laminitis: glucose deprivation and MMP activation induce dermo-epidermal separation *in vitro*. *Equine Vet. J.*, **36** (3), 261–266.
59. Niessen, C.M., van der Raaji-Helmer, L.M.H., Hulsman, E.H.M., van der Neut, R., Jonkman, M.F., and Sonnenberg, A. (1996) Deficiency of the integrin beta4 subunit in junctional epidermolysis bullosa with pyloric atresia: consequences for hemidesmosome formation and adhesion properties. *J. Cell Sci.*, **109**, 1695–1706.
60. Nievers, M.G., Schaapveld, R.Q.J., and Sonnenberg, A. (1999) Biology and function of hemidesmosomes. *Matrix Biol.*, **18**, 5–17.
61. McMillan, J.R., McGrath, J.A., Tidman, M.J., and Eady, R.A. (1998) Hemidesmosomes show abnormal association with the keratin

filament network in junctional forms of epidermolysis bullosa. *J. Invest. Dermatol.*, **110** (2), 132–137.
62. Coffman, J.R. and Colles, C.M. (1983) Insulin tolerance in laminitic ponies. *Can. J. Comp. Med.*, **47** (3), 347–351.
63. McGowan, C.M. (2010) Endocrinopathic laminitis. *Vet. Clin. North Am. Equine Pract.*, **26** (2), 233–237.
64. Johnson, P.J. (2002) The equine metabolic syndrome peripheral Cushing's syndrome. *Vet. Clin. North Am. Equine Pract.*, **18** (2), 271–293.
65. Burns, T.A., Watts, M.R., Weber, P.S., McCutcheon, L.J., Geor, R.J., and Belknap, J.K. (2013) Distribution of insulin receptor and insulin-like growth factor-1 receptor in the digital laminae of mixed-breed ponies: An immunohistochemical study. *Equine Vet. J.*, **45** (3), 326–332.
66. Asplin, K.E., Curlewis, J.D., McGowan, C.M., Pollitt, C.C., and Sillence, M.N. (2011) Glucose transport in the equine hoof. *Equine Vet. J.*, **43** (2), 196–201.
67. de Laat, M.A., Pollitt, C.C., Kyaw-Tanner, M.T., McGowan, C.M., and Sillence, M.N. (2013) A potential role for lamellar insulin-like growth factor-1 receptor in the pathogenesis of hyperinsulinaemic laminitis. *Vet. J.*, **197** (2), 302–306.
68. de Laat, M.A., Van Eps, A.W., McGowan, C.M., Sillence, M.N., and Pollitt, C.C. (2011) Equine laminitis: comparative histopathology 48 hours after experimental induction with insulin or alimentary oligofructose in Standardbred horses. *J. Comp. Pathol.*, **145** (4), 399–409.
69. Wattle, O. and Pollitt, C.C. (2004) Lamellar metabolism. *Clin. Tech. Equine Pract.*, **3**, 22–33.
70. Gherzi, R., Melioli, G., de Luca, M., D'Agostino, A., Distefano, G., Guastella, M., *et al.* (1992) 'HepG2/erythroid/brain' type glucose transporter (GLUT1) is highly expressed in human epidermis: keratinocyte differentiation affects GLUT1 levels in reconstituted epidermis. *J. Cell Physiol.*, **150** (3), 463–474.
71. Nordstrom, C.H. (2010) Cerebral energy metabolism and microdialysis in neurocritical care. *Childs Nervous System*, **26** (4), 465–472.
72. Johnson, J.A. and Fusaro, R.M. (1972) The role of the skin in carbohydrate metabolism. *Adv. Metab. Disord.*, **60**, 1–55.
73. Voldstedlund, M. and Dabelsteen, E. (1997) Expression of GLUT1 in stratified squamous epithelia and oral carcinoma from humans and rats. *APMIS (Acta Pathol. Microbiol. Immunol. Scand.)*, **105** (7), 537–545.
74. Gladden, L.B. (2004) Lactate metabolism: a new paradigm for the third millennium. *J. Physiol. (London)*, **558** (1), 5–30.
75. Stump, J.E. (1967) Anatomy of the normal equine foot, including microscopic features of the laminar region. *J. Am. Vet. Med. Assoc.*, **151** (12), 1588–1598.
76. Ronquist, G., Andersson, A., Bendsoe, N., and Falck, B. (2003) Human epidermal energy metabolism is functionally anaerobic. *Exp. Dermatol.*, **12** (5), 572–579.
77. Stucker, M., Struk, A., Altmeyer, P., Herde, M., Baumgartl, H., and Lubbers, D.W. (2002) The cutaneous uptake of atmospheric oxygen contributes significantly to the oxygen supply of human dermis and epidermis. *J. Physiol. (London)*, **538** (3), 985–994.
78. Gorlach, A. and Bonello, S. (2008) The cross-talk between NF-kappa B and HIF-1: further evidence for a significant liaison. *Biochem. J.*, **412**, e17–e19. Erratum in: *Biochem. J.*, **413** (3), 571.
79. Rius, J., Guma, M., Schachtrup, C., Akassoglou, K., Zinkernagel, A.S., Nizet, V., *et al.* (2008) NF-kappa B links innate immunity to the hypoxic response through transcriptional regulation of HIF-1 alpha. *Nature*, **453** (7196), 807–809.
80. Scortegagna, M., Cataisson, C., Martin, R.J., Hicklin, D.J., Schreiber, R.D., Yuspa, S.H., *et al.* (2008) HIF-1alpha regulates epithelial inflammation by cell autonomous NF-kappaB activation and paracrine stromal remodeling. *Blood*, **111** (7), 3343–3354.
81. Pawlak, E.A., Geor, R.J., Watts, M.R., Black, S.H., Johnson, P.J., and Belknap, J.K. (2014) Regulation of hypoxia-inducible factor-1α and related genes in equine digital lamellae and in cultured keratinocytes. *Equine Vet. J.*, **46**, 203–209.
82. Katz, L.M. and Bailey, S.R. (2012) A review of recent advances and current hypotheses on the pathogenesis of acute laminitis. *Equine Vet. J.*, **44** (6), 752–761.
83. Belknap, J. and Geor, R. (2012) The present state and future of laminitis research. *Equine Vet. J.*, **44** (6), 749–751.

CHAPTER 5

Digital Biomechanics Relevant to Laminitis

Jonathan Merritt, Helen Davies and Andrew H. Parks

Introduction

This chapter discusses the forces acting on the hoof (hoof biomechanics) that may be relevant to the development or treatment of laminitis.

The underlying causes of laminitis may be divided into two categories: (i) those with a biochemical or physiological basis; and (ii) those with a direct mechanical cause.

The first category, which includes the majority of types of laminitis as described in the literature, is laminitis associated with biochemical changes in the connection between the hoof wall and the dermis that leads to injury and separation of the lamellar junction. In this case, hoof biomechanics is of interest in understanding the normal load distribution through the lamellar junction around the hoof capsule, and hence the expected pattern of loss of support when there is any disruption of that connection. Biomechanics is also important in the treatment of laminitis to show how to adjust biomechanical forces acting on the hoof wall, so that further separation of the lamellae is minimized and the remaining hoof capsule is supported in such a way as to encourage the re-connection and optimum re-orientation of the damaged lamellae. This presupposes that the initiating cause of the laminitis has been treated or otherwise ceased to damage the lamellar junction, and that local deleterious events such as inflammation and infection have been controlled.

The second category of possible causes of lamellar injury is more of a traumatic origin (and possibly not included as a classic type of laminitis), and is associated with direct mechanical tearing of the lamellar junction. Direct mechanical damage may occur to the lamellae when a firmly attached shoe is wrenched off through being caught by something in the environment (wire fence, etc.) or another limb (e.g., hind foot treading on a front shoe). Such forces may directly distort the lamellae and initiate an inflammatory reaction similar to that observed in wounds elsewhere in the body. Alternatively, mechanical damage may be cumulative due to the inappropriate loading of a distorted, weakened, or otherwise damaged hoof capsule. Distortion and tearing of the lamellae would then cause local inflammation and further damage. In this chapter, attention will be focused on the first category – that is, laminitis associated with biochemical changes in the lamellar junction.

As the lamellar junction is the connection between the horse's sensitive digit (via the dermal lamellae) and the insensitive hoof capsule (via the epidermal lamellae), any load on the hoof capsule from the ground acting upwards into the standing or moving horse, or acting downwards towards the ground from the horse must go through this region.

In Thoroughbreds, the lamellar junction is approximately 4–7 mm thick [1, 2]. It is juxtaposed between the internal surface of the hoof wall and the external surface of the distal phalanx (DP). Geometrically, it forms a complex shape which can be approximated by a partial, truncated conical shell. The dorsal region most resembles part of a cone, with the radius of curvature increasing distally, while in the palmar region the wall at the heels does not diverge distally. A lamellar, or layered microstructure exists within the junction itself [3]. Primary epidermal lamellae radiate inward in long narrow strips from the internal hoof wall. These epidermal lamellae interdigitate with matching primary dermal lamellae, which radiate outward from the sublamellar dermis covering the external surface of the DP. These interdigitating lamellae are thought to increase the surface area which can support the forces on the lamellar junction. Multiple secondary lamellae protrude from the sides of each primary lamella (up to 100 secondary lamellae per primary lamella [1]), which further increases the surface area. In Thoroughbred horses, the primary lamellae are spaced at a distance of 0.36 mm at the toe, increasing to a spacing of 0.56 mm toward the heels [1]. The lamellar junction is also well-vascularized and innervated, containing blood vessels and nerves within the dermal lamellae [4].

During the earliest stages of laminitis, which reportedly can occur before hoof pain is clinically evident, the lamellar junction becomes weakened [5]. It does not appear that unusual mechanical loads are involved in the initiation of this process, but rather that the junction becomes unable to support the loads that it normally experiences. This results in the dermal lamellae pulling away from the more robust, keratinized epidermal lamellae [5]. It is this mechanical action of pull-out separation and

Equine Laminitis, First Edition. Edited by James K. Belknap and Raymond Geor.

lamellar disintegration which appears to produce not only the initial clinical pain associated with acute laminitis [6], but also the initial displacement of the DP associated with laminitis. Thus, we are motivated to understand the normal mechanical loads which may produce lamellar separation in the diseased horse. Understanding these loads informs a discussion of the mechanical attempts to reduce them, and therefore to reduce not only the degree of displacement of the DP resulting from these forces once the lamellar junction is compromised, but also the pain associated with lamellar separation. By focusing attention on the loading of the lamellar junction, and only the mechanical phenomena of the rest of the hoof which impact lamellar separation (and subsequent displacement of the DP), an attempt is made to narrow the field of investigation to those things which will be of most assistance to the laminitic horse.

Loads Acting on the Hoof

There are three major sources of loading for any joint. The first type of load is due primarily to the body weight and acts directly through the bones of the joint where they meet (the joint reaction force). The second type of load derives from the effects of any muscles that act across the joint. The third source of loading occurs whenever the ground surface is supporting the limb. This 'ground reaction force' is a sum of all the support provided by the ground surface on that hoof as the horse stands and moves. To every action there is an equal and opposite reaction (Newton's Third Law of Motion); hence, the ground reaction force is equal and opposite to the sum of the forces acting on the ground from the horse's weight and movement (otherwise, the limb would not remain in contact with the ground). All of these forces have both magnitude and direction, and so can affect the lamellar junction in various ways depending on how large they are, how frequent they are, how fast they act, and exactly what direction they are acting in relation to the lamellar junction.

For the purposes of this discussion, the hoof segment consists of the entire distal anatomical region that would be obtained by transecting the tissues around the border of the distal interphalangeal joint all the way out to the skin surface. This definition provides a 'system boundary,' with tractable boundary conditions, for the following discussion. Loads acting on the boundary of the segment are then described as 'external' loads (even if they are internal to the rest of the body of the horse), while stresses acting within the boundary are 'internal' loads.

Three main external loads are understood to act upon the hoof segment of the limb to produce substantial loading of the lamellar junction. These external loads are the joint reaction force of the distal interphalangeal joint, the ground reaction force, and the force due to the pull of the deep digital flexor tendon [2]. These external forces are not independent of each other, but instead interact in a way which depends on the specific geometry of the hoof [7]. The middle phalanx pushes down on the DP with a force that contains contributions from body weight and from a component that partially balances the pull of the deep digital flexor tendon (DDFT). This joint force is distributed nonuniformly, as a surface traction or pressure, over the cartilage of the joint surface of the DP. The DDFT pulls in a distributed fashion over its insertion site on the caudal aspect of the DP, and also produces substantial traction from wrapping around the navicular bone [7, 8]. Hence, the pull of the DDFT creates a turning force that pushes the toe of the hoof into the ground. The strength of this push on the toe is increased when the toe is longer because this increases the length of the lever arm from the center of rotation of the joint. Finally, the ground reaction force is distributed over the solear surface of the hoof segment, primarily supported by the solear periphery of the hoof wall, but also, depending on the conformation of the foot and the character of the ground (e.g., a softer ground substance that molds into the foot will incorporate more ground surface), possibly distributed over the frog, bars, and sole of the hoof [9]. The ground reaction force can reach at least 10 kN in a forelimb during gallop in a Thoroughbred [10]. The large loads acting on the hoof cause it to deform. Toward the middle of the stance phase, the heels of the hoof deform by moving laterally and the dorsal hoof wall deforms in a palmo-solear direction [4, 11]. Additional external forces also exist, such as the forces due to the extensor tendons and collateral ligaments of the distal interphalangeal joint, the hydrostatic pressure of blood vessels, and atmospheric pressure. However their role (if any) in loading the lamellar junction has not been described in the research literature.

Two of the external forces described – the joint reaction force and the pull of the tendon of the deep digital flexor muscle – act almost exclusively on the DP, or on the DP via the navicular bone. Bone, as a material, is so stiff in comparison with the lamellar junction (reportedly approximately 100-fold more stiff [2]), that we are justified in treating the DP as completely rigid. If we make this approximation, then there is no further need to consider the individual effects of the two external forces acting on the DP. Instead, we can take their vector sum, and consider the effect of the single resultant force. In more advanced finite element models of the limb, the compliance of the bone is also modeled (e.g., Ref. [2]), so in those models this approximation is not made.

Loads Acting on the Lamellar Junction

The net external force on the DP, due to the sum of the joint reaction force and the pull of the tendon of the deep digital flexor muscle, acts primarily downward, and in a standing horse is equal and opposite to the ground reaction force. Within the hoof segment, this external downward force on the bone is balanced by an upward, internal load, which is exerted by the internal boundary of the lamellar junction. This lamellar junction load is distributed in some way across its entire conical shape (mirroring the conical shape of the hoof wall). Within the lamellar junction itself, the load takes the form of a stress field, which is

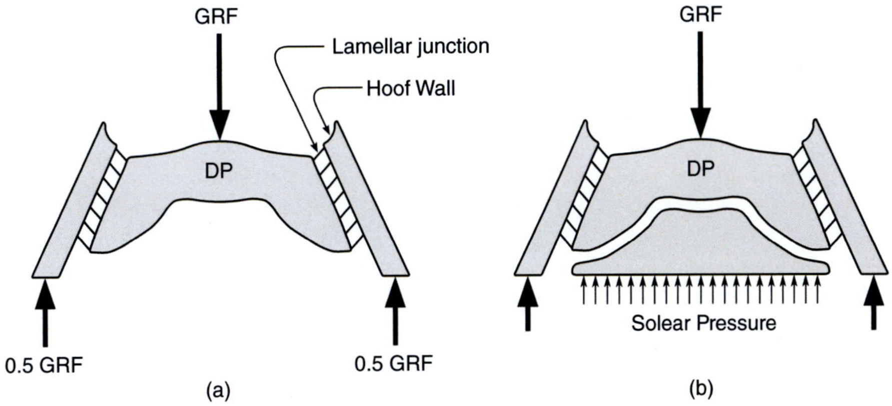

Figure 5.1 (a) Frontal plane model of the hoof. Adapted from Figure 1D of Ref. [4]; © Wiley. (b) Frontal plane model of the hoof with solear support.

mathematically rather complicated. In general, the stress is a tensor field reportedly consisting of six independent components that vary continuously throughout the volume of the lamellar junction [2]. However, although this stress field is internally complicated, we know that its net effect on the internal boundary of the junction is a force acting upward on the DP, to balance the net downward force that we previously identified. The DP may also be supported from below by forces transmitted from the solear surface of the hoof, via compression of the frog, digital cushion, and other tissues (see Fig. 5.1). If such forces are present, they reduce the total upward force that the lamellar junction must generate. Hence, increasing support from the sole may assist in reducing the force on the lamellar junction.

On the external side of the lamellar junction, its stress field acts on the internal surface of the hoof wall. The hoof wall may not be treated as rigid, since its stiffness is comparable to that of the lamellar junction [12]. Instead, another stress field is developed within the hoof wall. Via the hoof wall, the force exerted by the joint reaction force and the pull of the deep digital flexor muscle/tendon through the lamellar junction is eventually balanced by the ground reaction force. Any component of the ground reaction force which was distributed to compress the solear tissues, and support the DP from below, reduces the load applied to the hoof wall. Tensile strain predominates within the stratum medium of the toe of the normal hoof wall in midstance during simulated walking, while compression may predominate in chronically laminitic hooves [13]. Hence, loss of the connection between the hoof wall and DP due to structural failure of the lamellar junction in laminitic hooves means that the DP is no longer supported by the hoof wall as in a sling, but instead the DP is pushed down towards the sole of the hoof by the body weight. Subsequently, the toe region of the hoof wall becomes compressed by the ground reaction forces that are no longer redistributed through into the bone column. This compression of the toe may be a direct cause of the distortion seen in the hoof capsule in chronically laminitic horses.

To recap, in the hoof segment of a standing horse, we have an external downward force due to body weight, acting on the DP. This downward force is balanced by a surface traction on the internal boundary of the lamellar junction, which produces a stress field within the lamellar junction itself. The surface traction on the external boundary of the lamellar junction then acts on the hoof wall. The hoof wall, after appropriate deformations, is then acted upon by the distributed ground reaction force (Fig. 5.1a). A second load path has been described, arising from compression of the solear tissues and support of the DP from below (Fig. 5.1b). However, if the lamellar junction is not sufficiently supporting the DP within the hoof capsule, then this second load path has the potential to cause excessive compression of the solear dermis of the toe region of the DP against the sole and underlying ground surface. This position of the DP can put direct pressure on the circumflex artery at the solear margin [14], thus decreasing the normal blood supply to that region of the solear dermis and underlying bone. This concern must be kept in mind when contemplating applying sole support (e.g., with a silastic putty; see Chapter 39) during therapeutic farriery in the case with a compromised lamellar junction.

Loads Acting on the Standing and Moving Hoof

In the standing horse, all of the external and internal loads are in perfect equilibrium with each other, resulting in zero motion. In the walking horse, this equilibrium is not exact, since the forces that produce walking must exist. However, the distal limb forces that are required to produce walking are so small in comparison with the body weight of the horse that the force equilibrium is still a very good approximation [7]. Mechanically, we can say that inertial, or d'Alembert, forces are small in comparison with static forces during the stance phase in a walking horse. If we ignore the contribution of the d'Alembert forces, we perform what is referred to as a 'quasi-static' analysis. The static forces however, would necessarily be much greater during any movement when the contralateral limb is off the ground. Hence' the size of these static forces depends on what proportion of the body weight is being supported by an individual limb. Laminitic horses will strive to minimize the load on the most painful limb or limbs, and this necessarily increases the load on the other limbs (or causes the horse to lie down for long periods).

While the distribution of the ground reaction force has been widely investigated, it has not been documented experimentally how the ground reaction force is transmitted from the ground surface of the hoof capsule to the DP. As discussed above, the load may be transmitted through the wall, through the sole, or through a combination of the two. Modeling by finite element analysis suggests that the forces of weight-bearing are transmitted to the DP primarily through the hoof capsule and lamellae, and that the role of direct load transmission through the sole and underlying soft tissues to the DP is minimal. Clinical experience would tend to support this finding. Horses that have suffered marked hoof wall loss due to white line disease, such that the wall is no longer bearing significant weight, are usually markedly lame. The DP is also likely to become displaced in relation to the remaining wall, indicating significant instability. In contrast, horses that have had a large portion of their sole removed are usually relatively comfortable (at least when at rest or walking on a flat non-conformable surface), and the DP is stable in relation to the hoof capsule. The implications of the finite element analysis are that, even when a barefooted horse is standing on sand, the forces associated with weight-bearing are distributed out to the wall through the solear aspect of the hoof capsule.

Regardless of how the forces associated with weight-bearing are transmitted from the ground to the DP, the center of pressure (the center of the ground reaction force) at rest or mid-stance is close to the center of the foot, but the center of rotation of the distal interphalangeal joint (through which the forces of weight-bearing extending down the limb act) is positioned palmar to the center of pressure (see Fig. 5.2). At rest, these two opposing forces are both approximately vertically oriented, but are not aligned with each other, which generates a moment. Moments about the joint are calculated as the product of the force and the length of the moment arm. The length of the moment arm is the shortest distance between the center of rotation and the line of action of the force involved (Fig. 5.2). The moment about the distal interphalangeal joint created by the ground reaction force vector (dorsal to the center of rotation) is the extensor moment because it causes the joint to extend or dorsiflex (some models include the force with the common digital extensor tendon as part of the extensor moment). For the foot to be stable when flat on the ground, this moment must be opposed by an equal flexor moment. The flexor moment is created by tension in the DDFT. Thus, at rest the extensor moment is the product of the ground reaction force vector and the moment arm, which is the horizontal distance between the center of pressure and the center of rotation of the joint. The flexor moment is the product of tension in the DDFT and the shortest distance from the center of rotation of the joint to the deep flexor tendon, which is at the flexor surface of the navicular bone. It is not that the flexor moment causes the extensor moment, or vice versa – just that, if the foot is stationary, they must be equal and opposite. Three simple examples illustrate this principle. In a foal with a flexural deformity of the distal interphalangeal joint, the distal DDFT is under greater tension than normal. The increased tension in the tendon causes the flexor moment to increase (the flexor moment arm does not change). The flexor moment arm is the distance from the center of rotation of the joint to the flexor surface of the navicular bone. For the foot to be flat on the ground – in this case with an increased flexor moment – the extensor moment must also increase, but the weight borne by the limb has not increased. Therefore, in order for the flexor moment to increase the extensor moment arm must increase, which does happen due to the center of pressure moving to a more dorsal position. At the point when the heels come off the ground because the tension in the tendon has further increased, the center of pressure is at the toe. In this instance, an increase in tendon tension caused the center of pressure to move.

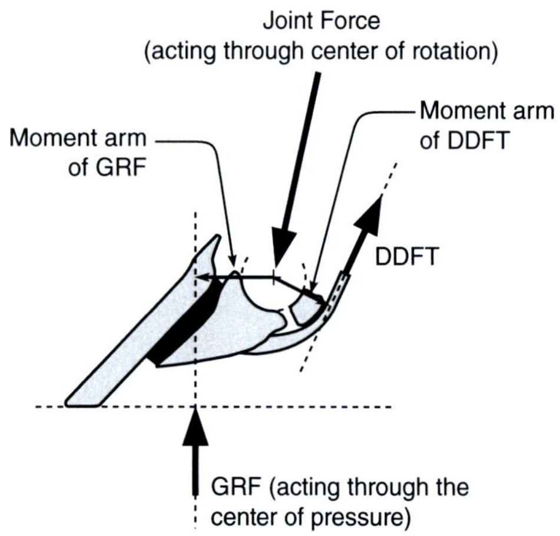

Figure 5.2 Sagittal plane model of the hoof.

However, if we consider a different scenario in which a horse is standing on the edge of a curb, such that its heels are not bearing weight, the center of pressure is moved dorsally. If the horse is to prevent excessive dorsiflexion of the distal interphalangeal joint, the flexor moment must increase and, because the flexor moment arm is fixed, this must come from an increase in tension in the DDFT. In this circumstance, a change in the center of pressure has caused a change in the tendon tension (i.e., the horse must flexe the deep digital flexor muscle to counteract the change in location of the center of pressure). In reality, the heels drop to some extent; therefore, how much of the increased tension in the tendon is caused by the heel dropping and how much is due to tension generated by the deep digital flexor tendon muscle is undetermined. Lastly, consider rupture of the distal DDFT. The flexor moment is close to zero, but the limb is still bearing weight. Therefore, in order to maintain the foot flat on the ground with both the ground reaction force and the weight being oriented vertically, the center of pressure must be directly distal to the center of rotation – that is, the center of pressure must move in a palmar direction.

When the animal walks or trots, the magnitude, direction, and center of pressure change with the phase of the stride. At the walk, the vertical component of the ground reaction force peaks twice during the stride – once during the first half and once during the second half, with a dip in the middle. The peaks are approximately two-thirds of the horse's body weight. At the trot, the vertical component of the ground reaction force peaks once approximately at mid stride with a force nearly equal to the weight of the horse. Most studies address the magnitude of the ground reaction forces and center of pressure during the stride when horses are moving at a trot. The ground reaction force vector is divided into three orthogonal components: vertical; craniocaudal; and mediolateral. Of these components, the vertical one is always positive. During the first half of the stride the craniocaudal component is negative (representing deceleration), and is positive in the second half (representing acceleration). The mediolateral component of the ground reaction force is small compared to the other two components. The center of pressure is initially positioned at the point of first contact – usually the lateral heel/quarter – before rapidly moving to the center of the foot where it remains until just before breakover. The moments about the distal interphalangeal joint are also correspondingly dynamic during the stride. During the middle of the stride, the foot is stable on the ground, the distal interphalangeal joint is passively flexed, and the center of pressure is in the center of the foot; the ground reaction force vector is vertical, and the weight of the body is acting through the center of rotation of the distal interphalangeal joint (much like it is at rest). Therefore, the lengths of both the flexor and extensor moment arms are the same as they would be at rest. Because the foot is stable on the ground, the flexor and extensor moments are equal, but both are much greater than they would be in a horse at rest because the magnitude of the ground reaction force and tension in the deep digital flexor tendon are much greater.

During the second half of the stride – after the horse's trunk passes over the foot – several events are occurring concurrently. The angle of the distal interphalangeal joint changes from flexion to extension, the magnitude of the ground reaction force progressively decreases, and the center of pressure moves towards the toe, which increases the length of the extensor moment arm. During this time the foot is still stable on the ground and therefore the flexor and extensor moments are still equal. However, the magnitudes of these moments are changing in response to the changes in weight-bearing. Just before breakover, the weight borne by the limb decreases faster than tension in the deep flexor tendon, so that the flexor moment increases relative to the extensor moment. This causes the center of pressure to move dorsally, thereby increasing the extensor moment arm, the two moments being equal all the while the foot is flat on the ground. Once the center of pressure reaches the most dorsal aspect of the foot (the toe), the extensor moment arm can no longer increase so that, in the face of a relative increase in the flexor moment (due to the force of the tension of the DDFT being relatively greater than the rapidly decreasing ground reaction force due to minimal weight-bearing as the horse reaches the end of the support phase of the stride), the heels lift off the ground. The beginning of the support phase of the stride – and to a lesser extent the end – is associated with shock waves (rapidly oscillating, high-frequency and high-magnitude vibrations). The actual effect of high-frequency vibrations on living tissues varies with the tissue and the frequency of the vibration, but in general may cause local heating, especially when there is reflection of waves at the interface of different surfaces. Localized heating may reach a level sufficient to damage tissues. Hence, there is some possibility that excessive impact vibration could increase damage to an already compromised lamellar junction. Un-shod hooves have been observed to attenuate the magnitude of impact vibrations by 67% between the hoof wall and the DP [15], which suggests that a normal lamellar junction is involved in the absorption of impact vibrations. The hoof material itself functions as a shock-absorber, while the pressure of blood in the veins of the digit increases rapidly during weight-bearing, and thus may also have a role in damping impact [16].

Models of the Hoof

The preceding discussion of loading is complicated by the difficulty of visualizing everything that has been described. We have seen that mechanical loads acting on the hoof segment consist of complicated distributed tractions from the ground reaction force, DDFT pull, and the effect of body weight acting through the distal interphalangeal joint, which all vary in a general three-dimensional manner over the surface of the segment. Within the hoof segment, the external loads generate corresponding internal stress fields, which are equally difficult to picture. To increase our level of insight, we can use some simpler mechanical models of the hoof.

None of the models described below captures all of the phenomena known to be associated with the hoof. Whether or not the model represents reality is debatable, but the response of the model itself is known precisely. This is important scientifically, because the model can be used to produce repeatable, testable predictions that then provide a basis for experimentally verifying or rejecting aspects of the model. Without a model, investigators will tend to interpret an explanation of the hoof through the filter of their own experience. A complete model provides a way to be certain that the assumptions of two different parties are precisely identical.

Finally, as in the case of this chapter, simplified models provide a way to illustrate and discuss different aspects of the problem. They afford a short-hand in which we can express ideas more easily. In the models below, attention is focused on dominant forms of loading, which are those types of load which are expected to affect the real hoof in a similar way to that in which they affect the model, despite the additional complexities of the real biological hoof. The models described below are not 'complete,' in that far more work would be required in order to make them unambiguous. However, this additional work would necessarily require the definition of mathematical equations which govern their behavior, and as such is beyond the scope of this chapter.

Frontal Plane Model: The Influence of the Ground Reaction Force

A simple model of lamellar loading (adapted from Ref. [4]) is shown in Figure 5.1a. This model is based on a frontal plane slice through the hoof segment described above. Its geometric components are the hoof wall, DP and lamellar junction. We see the angled hoof wall lying on either side of the DP; the latter is shown suspended from the hoof wall by the lamellar junction, which is adhered internally to the DP and externally to the hoof wall. The portion of the body weight borne by the limb acts downward on the DP, and the ground reaction force acts upwards on the hoof wall. Implicit in this model (though not shown in the illustration) is the idea that the hoof wall will maintain its geometry via the dorsal, conical projection of the wall that forms the toe of the hoof. Due to the fact that this supporting force from the toe is not represented, this illustration falls short of being a true 'free body diagram,' which engineers use to represent similar-force equilibria.

It is easy to see in this model that the lamellar junction will be placed primarily under tension. Just as the ropes of a hammock are placed under tension due to its occupant, the sling-like lamellar junction of this model will also experience tension (the 'occupant' of our very strong hammock is the DP). Although this model is very simple, its prediction that the lamellae should primarily experience tension has been confirmed by direct, in-vitro measurement of the strain state immediately adjacent to the lamellar junction [17].

An equilibrium of vertical forces is also evident in this model. In a static, or quasi-static situation, these forces are necessarily equal and opposite. The ground reaction force is shown acting half on the left side of the hoof wall and half on the right side. This is a short-hand representation of the fact that the ground reaction force is really distributed in some way over the hoof wall.

Of great interest in this model is the question of what would happen with support of the DP from below (depicted in Fig. 5.1b). The total ground reaction force must be equal to the fraction of the body weight borne by the limb. In this case, we have redistributed some of the ground reaction force to the solear surface of the hoof, which necessarily reduces the amount of ground reaction force borne by the hoof wall. Consequently, the tensile stress on the lamellar junction, which binds the hoof wall to the DP, is also reduced. This mechanical result – supporting the DP from below – is the one that is sought by interventions which involve some form of solear support.

As discussed above, one obvious side effect of supporting the DP via solear loading is the compression of those tissues which lie between the ground and the solear aspect of the DP. Since these tissues – which include the narrow solear dermis containing the vascular and nerve supply critical to the health of the sole – are more compliant (less stiff) than the hoof wall [2], they may experience greater deformation than the hoof wall when supporting or sharing some fraction of its load. These tissues may also be more susceptible to injury under greater compression.

A less obvious side effect of solear support, not necessarily evident from this model, is that it may alter normal hoof deformation. It is now understood that the somewhat conical shape of the hoof wall itself is likely to be at least partially responsible for causing its deformation. This likely (though not certain) conclusion is reached by knowing that hoof deformations are predicted by models of the hoof wall which only include vertical loading (e.g., Ref. [18]), and that normal heel deformation seems to occur even when the sole of the hoof does not make contact with the ground [19]. However, it is currently unclear to what extent the other, internal, structures of the hoof may play a role in determining its deformation. It is thought that both internal pressure within the hoof [20] and compression of the hoof tissues from the descending middle phalanx [21] may contribute. Experimentally, it has been observed that increasing the amount of solear support increases the deformation at the heels of the hoof [19]. The clinical significance of such modifications to the deformation of the hoof, how they relate to other things such as the return of blood from the hoof and damping of impact vibrations, are all largely unknown.

Sagittal Plane Model: The Influence of the Deep Digital Flexor Tendon

In the preceding frontal-plane model, the balance between the ground reaction force and body weight caused tension in the lamellar junction. However, that frontal plane model ignored any force exerted by the DDFT. In the model described here, we will rotate our view by 90° about a vertical axis, and examine the hoof in the sagittal plane. Bearing in mind everything we learned from the previous model, we may now also incorporate the pull of the DDFT into our mental picture.

Figure 5.2 shows a mid-sagittal view through the hoof segment. In this model, we have the same geometric features as the previous model, but viewed from a different angle: the hoof wall, the lamellar junction, and the DP. Now, only the toe region of the hoof wall is shown, and the segment of the lamellar junction which joins the hoof wall to the parietal surface of the DP is also present. In addition to the joint reaction force and the ground reaction force, we have a force due to the pull of the DDFT.

It can be seen in Figure 5.2 that the ground reaction force does not pass through the center of rotation of the distal interphalangeal joint; rather, the ground reaction force is intentionally drawn dorsal to the center of rotation, which is where it lies in the normal hoof at rest or mid stance. As described earlier in the chapter, in the later part of the stance phase (immediately prior to break-over), the point of application of the ground reaction force (center of pressure) moves towards the tip of the toe. Also illustrated is a quantity called the *moment arm* of the ground reaction force. The moment arm is the perpendicular distance between the line of force application and the center of rotation of the joint. Multiplication of this moment arm by the magnitude of the force gives the moment, or torque, that the ground reaction force exerts about the joint. In a quasi-static situation, the moment exerted by the ground reaction force must be equal to the moment exerted by the DDFT. Enforcing this equilibrium is the way that most distal forelimb models are able to compute the DDFT force [7,8]. The moment arm of the ground reaction force increases substantially just prior to break-over, as the point of application also moves to the toe, which results in an increase in the pull of the DDFT during this part of the stride [7,8,22]. The maximum force exerted by the DDFT during the stride tends to occur some time in late stance, just prior to break-over.

Whilst the above description of the DDFT force has wide agreement in the research literature, the influence of interventions that aim to reduce the DDFT pull is in dispute. As the mechanics involved are not understood well enough to draw definite conclusions, the two alternative viewpoints are presented below.

In the first alternative, attention is focused primarily on the force exerted by the DDFT, which is assumed to increase the load on the lamellar junction [23]. In our present model, we can see how an increase in the DDFT pull might increase the lamellar load. If the moment about the distal interphalangeal joint were to increase, due to a pull on the DDFT, that moment would consequently have to be supported by the lamellar junction. This moment would have to be supported in addition to the vertical load due to the body mass, thus increasing the total load. The failure to support such a moment is sometimes described as the reason that the DP can rotate as laminitis progresses [23]. If we consider only the DDFT force, then interventions to reduce the DDFT pull may be helpful as a means of reducing the lamellar junction load. Raising the heels – the most commonly used method to reduce DDFT pull – shortens the total path of the DDFT, thus reducing its pull. This also results in the point of application of the ground reaction force moving in a palmar direction, closer towards the center of rotation of the distal interphalangeal joint. This movement of the ground reaction force would reduce the torque around the joint and hence reduce the requirement for a counterbalance of tension on the DDFT, which in turn would reduce the tension on the lamellar junction emanating from the DDFT pull on the DP.

The DDFT pull is not the only concern however [2,24]. We have already seen that the body weight acts downward on the DP, loading the lamellar junction via this route. The body weight reportedly creates approximately twice the magnitude of force on the DP as that created by the DDFT pull at mid-stance [8], and thus may be of greater importance to lamellar load than that created by the pull of the DDFT. Importantly, by raising the heels, we not only reduce the pull of the DDFT but also change the direction of loading produced by the body weight. Although it seems to be a subtle point, a change in the direction of one loading component can be as important as a change in the magnitude of another [2]. Recent results using a finite element model (see below) have suggested that the benefit of reducing the pull of the DDFT by raising the heel may be entirely offset by the negative effects caused by the change in the loading direction of the body weight with a raised heel [2]. By increasing the angle of the hoof, we are likely to induce more shear loading and less tensile loading on the lamellar junction. The change in these two stress components may result in greater strain energy being absorbed by the lamellar junction, despite the force of the DDFT being reduced [2]. This increase in strain energy could make the lamellar junction more likely to fail. Tensile loading is normal in the lamellar junction and the structures and alignment of the lamellae are oriented to resist such pulls between the hoof wall and the DP. Any tensile force has to be great enough to separate the whole sequence of connections along the length of a lamella. In contrast, shear loading will tend to pull one lamella directly from its attachment to the next, and hence is much more likely to cause tearing in the lamellar junction. This may be likened to the difference between trying to pull a piece of timber apart by pulling on either end (tensile force) compared to splitting it along the line of the grain (shear force).

The practical consequence of the considerations above is that the mechanical benefits of raising or lowering the heels are currently in dispute.

It has already been mentioned that the ground reaction force moves towards the toe of the hoof during break-over. Due to the increase in moment arm of the ground reaction force, the DDFT force reaches its peak close to break-over. Some laminitis interventions aim to reduce this peak, by reducing the moment arm of the ground reaction force. Such interventions include trimming (shortening) the toes of the hoof and some types of orthopedic shoeing, in which the toe of the shoe is beveled caudally to shorten the moment arm. These interventions are less likely to suffer from the potential problems connected with raising the heels, as they address the behavior around break-over, rather than the mid-stance orientation of the hoof. However, the mechanics of these interventions would benefit from further research.

Finite Element Models: A More Complete Picture?

The two models that we have described above are quite simplistic. They take slices of the true, three-dimensional geometry of the hoof in two planes. Considering the loads in these two planes is quite useful in a conceptual understanding of dominant effects, but it lacks the detail required to make realistic predictions regarding hoof behavior. The difficulty in determining the effects of raising or lowering the heels is only a mild illustration of this problem.

More advanced models of the hoof have been constructed using an engineering technique called finite element analysis (FEA). In FEA models, the hoof is split into many small elements, with each element having a very well-defined behavior. The combined behavior of the many elements – which often number in the thousands – is then determined mathematically using a computer. The whole model can then be used to make predictions about the response of the hoof to different loads. Although further description of such models is beyond the scope of this chapter, the reader is directed to Ref. [2] as an example of a modern FEA model.

Mechanical Tearing of the Lamellae

In addition to its role in different parts of a single stride, the hoof must continue to function over longer periods of days, weeks, or months. The natural hoof wall is worn away mechanically by the ground, and grows at a replacement rate of 5–12 mm per month [25,26]. However, the placement of a shoe may interfere with the normal wear of the hoof and distort its shape.

If the shape of the hoof capsule is involved in direct mechanical tearing of the lamellar junction, then it may be associated with leverage from a longer toe during breakover. The possibility of increased leverage from a longer toe during fast gallop is supported by the finding that shod racehorses in Macau with a broken-back hoof-pastern axis are slightly more likely to win races on a grass surface, but show no difference in performance when the same horses raced on a sand surface [27]. The grains in a sand surface are likely to be more easily displaced by the toe during break-over, and hence dissipate any possible effects of a longer toe, in contrast to a turf surface where the grass roots might support the toe to some extent. This effect may be seen in the shape of the imprints made by galloping horses on these different surfaces. Shod racehorses do show a reduction in toe angle in both forelimbs during training [28] and this may lead to an increased potential for such a lever effect, especially if the lamellar junction is already weakened by other factors. A group of 11 mares that were free to exercise themselves in a large paddock showed a significant decrease in forelimb toe angle over a seven-week period when shod compared to when they were barefoot by $-1.70°$ (SEM $0.31°$; $p = 0.00004$) in the left forelimb and $-1.84°$ (SEM $0.54°$; $p = 0.0079$) in the right forelimb [29]. However, there is some evidence that in an unshod hoof there is no change in the distribution of strain at the toe when there is a change in toe angle in individual horses, even during exercise up to a 12.5 m s^{-1} gallop [30]. Hence, any potential leverage effects of a long toe may be confined to horses that are shod or that have a hoof capsule already weakened or distorted by other factors. A laminitic horse's hoof wall is likely to be weakened or distorted and hence may experience very different loads compared to a normal hoof wall. This has been demonstrated by the finding that tensile radial strain predominates within the stratum medium of the toe of the normal hoof wall during simulated walking, while compression predominates in chronically laminitic hooves [13]. Reducing the length of the toe in a laminitic horse may therefore not only reduce the leverage on the toe but also reduce the direct compression on the toe region of the hoof wall and hence assist in reducing the amount of distortion in that region of the hoof capsule.

References

1. Thomason, J.J., McClinchey, H.L., Faramarzi, B., and Jofriet, J.C. (2005) Mechanical behaviour and quantitative morphology of the equine lamellar junction. *Anat. Record Part A*, **283A**, 366–379.
2. Ramsey, G.D., Hunter, P.J., and Nash, M.P. (2011) The effect of hoof angle variations on dorsal lamellar load in the equine hoof. *Equine Vet. J.*, **43** (5), 536–542.
3. Roberts, E.D., Ochoa, R., and Haynes, P.F. (1980) Correlation of dermal-epidermal lamellar lesions of equine hoof with various disease conditions. *Vet. Pathol.*, **17**, 656–666.
4. Douglas, J.E., Biddick, T.L., Thomason, J.J., and Jofriet, J.C. (1998) Stress/strain behaviour of the equine lamellar junction. *J. Exp. Biol.*, **201**, 2287–2297.
5. Pollitt, C.C. (1996) Basement membrane pathology: a feature of acute equine laminitis. *Equine Vet. J.*, **28** (1), 38–46.
6. Pollitt, C.C. (2007) Laminitis pathophysiology, in *Equine Podiatry* (eds A.E. Floyd and R.A. Mansmann), 1st edition. Saunders Elsevier, Missouri, pp. 313–319.
7. Merritt, J.S., Davies, H.M., Burvill, C., and Pandy, M.G. (2008) Influence of muscle-tendon wrapping on calculations of joint reaction forces in the equine distal forelimb. *J. Biomed. Biotechnol.* Available from: http://www.hindawi.com/journals/bmri/2008/165730/ doi:10.1155/2008/165730.
8. Wilson, A.M., McGuigan, M.P., Fouracre, L., and MacMahon, L. (2001) The force and contact stress on the navicular bone during trot locomotion in sound horses and horses with navicular disease. *Equine Vet. J.*, **33** (2), 159–165.
9. Hood, D.M., Taylor, D., and Wagner, I.P. (2001) Effects of ground surface deformability, trimming, and shoeing on quasistatic loading patterns in horses. *Am. J. Vet. Res.*, **62**, 895–900.
10. Parsons, K.J., Pfau, T., and Wilson, A.M. (2008) High-speed gallop locomotion in the Thoroughbred racehorse. I. The effect of incline on stride parameters. *J. Exp. Biol.*, **211**, 935–944.
11. Burn, J.F. and Brockington, C. (2001) Quantification of hoof deformation using optical motion capture. *Equine Vet. J. Suppl.*, **33**, 50–53.
12. Douglas, J.E., Mittal, C., Thomason, J.J., and Jofriet, J.C. (1996) The modulus of elasticity of equine hoof wall: implications for the mechanical function of the hoof. *J. Exp. Biol.*, **199**, 1829–1836.
13. Hobbs, S.J. (2006) Measurement analysis of equine radial hoof strain and lower forelimb motion. PhD thesis, University of Central Lancashire.
14. Ritmeester, A.M., Blevins, W.E., Ferguson, D.W., and Adams, S.B. (1998) Digital perfusion, evaluated scintigraphically, and hoof wall growth in horses with chronic laminitis treated with egg bar heart bar shoeing and coronary grooving. *Equine Vet. J. Suppl.*, **26**, 111-118.
15. Willemen, M.A., Jacobs, M.W.H., and Schamhardt, H.C. (1999) *In vitro* transmission and attenuation of impact vibrations in the distal forelimb. *Equine Vet. J. Suppl.*, **30**, 245–248.
16. Ratzlaff, M.H., Shindell, R.M., and DeBowes, R.M. (1985) Changes in digital venous pressures of horses moving at the walk and trot. *Am. J. Vet. Res.*, **46** (7), 1545–1549.
17. Hobbs, S.J., Mather, J., Rolph, C., and Matuszewski, B. (2004) *In vitro* measurement of internal hoof strain. *Equine Vet. J.*, **36** (8), 683–688.

18. Newlyn, H.A., Collins, S.N., Cope, B.C., Hopegood, L., Latham, R.J., and Reilly, J.D. (1998) Finite element analysis of static loading in donkey hoof wall. *Equine Vet. J. Suppl.*, **26**, 103–110.
19. Roepstorff, L., Johnston, C., and Drevemo, S. (2001) *In vivo* and *in vitro* heel expansion in relation to shoeing and frog pressure. *Equine Vet. J. Suppl.*, **33**, 54–57.
20. Colles, C.M. (1989) A technique for assessing hoof function in the horse. *Equine Vet. J.*, **21** (1), 17–22.
21. Dyhre-Poulsen, P., Smedegaard, H.H., Roed, J., and Korsgaard, E. (1994) Equine hoof function investigated by pressure transducers inside the hoof and accelerometers mounted on the first phalanx. *Equine Vet. J.*, **26** (5), 362–366.
22. Harrison, S.M., Whitton, R.C., Kawcak, C.E., Stover, S.M., and Pandy, M.G. (2010) Relationship between muscle forces, joint loading and utilisation of elastic strain energy in equine locomotion. *J. Exp. Biol.*, **213**, 3998–4009.
23. Parks, A. and O'Grady, S.E. (2003) Chronic laminitis: current treatment strategies. *Vet. Clin. North Am. Equine Pract.*, **19**, 393–416.
24. Coffman, J.R., Johnson, J.H., Finocchio, E.J., and Guffy, M.M. (1970) Biomechanics of pedal rotation in equine laminitis. *J. Am. Vet. Med. Assoc.*, **156**, 219–221.
25. Butler, K.D. and Hintz, H.F. (1977) Effect of level of feed intake and gelatin supplementation on growth and quality of hoofs of ponies. *J. Animal Sci.*, **44**, 257–261.
26. Glade, M.J. and Salzman, R.A. (1985) Effects of toe angle on hoof growth and contraction in the horse. *J. Equine Vet. Sci.*, **5** (1), 45–50.
27. Cust, A.R., Anderson, G.A., Whitton, R.C., and Davies, H.M. (2013) Hoof conformation and performance in the racing Thoroughbred in Macau. *Austr. Vet. J.*, **91** (3), 108–112.
28. Peel, J.A., Peel, M.B., and Davies, H.M.S. (2006) The effect of gallop training on hoof angle in Thoroughbred racehorses. *Equine Vet. J. Suppl.*, **36**, 431–434.
29. Malone, S.R. and Davies, H.M.S. (2012) The effect of horse shoes on equine hoof shape, in Proceedings of the 8th International Equitation Science Conference, 18–20 July, Royal (Dick) Veterinary School, Edinburgh, p. 67.
30. Bellenzani, M.C., Merritt, J.S., Clarke, S., and Davies, H.M.S. (2012) Investigation of forelimb hoof wall strains and hoof shape in unshod horses exercised on a treadmill at various speeds and gaits. *Am. J. Vet. Res.*, **73** (11), 1735–1741.

PART 2

Pathophysiology of Laminitis

Equine Laminitis, First Edition. Edited by James K. Belknap and Raymond Geor.

CHAPTER 6
Overview

James K. Belknap

An understanding of the pathophysiology of a disease process is vital to establishing effective therapies for the clinician to use either prophylactically in animals at risk of the disease, or therapeutically in animals already suffering from the disease. The two primary requirements for determining the pathophysiologic mechanisms of a disease process are the establishment of an experimental model to effectively study the disease, and the availability of appropriate research tools to determine the pathophysiologic events that need to be targeted for effective treatment of the disease process. A greater number of advances have been made in the study of sepsis-related laminitis (including the establishment of an effective therapy) than the other types of laminitis, primarily because the most commonly used, established experimental models of laminitis for the past several decades – the carbohydrate overload models (corn starch and oligofructose models) and black walnut extract model – are models of sepsis-related laminitis.

Models of equine metabolic syndrome have only recently been introduced, with the most common model currently used being the hyperinsulinemic–euglycemic clamp in which high levels of insulin are maintained for approximately 48 h to induce laminitis. Although this model provides valuable data regarding the pathophysiologic mechanisms of endocrinopathic laminitis, there remains a need for more clinically accurate models (the insulin levels attained in the clamp model are supraphysiologic). Modeling for supporting limb laminitis has been difficult due to the need to establish a humane method of excessive weight bearing on one limb. Due to the historical lack of a model, there has been a paucity of data – and very little scientific advancement – in this type of laminitis. Recently, the use of a shoe which does not allow normal weight-bearing on one limb, and the use of a microdialysis catheter placed in the lamellar tissue for the measurement of metabolites as proxies of energy metabolism and blood flow, have provided evidence of lamellar hypoxia playing a central role in this type of laminitis.

For the first 60–70 years of the past century, research tools were primarily limited to the microscopic assessment of tissues (i.e., histology), basic radiographic imaging techniques, and fairly blunt basic techniques for assessing physiologic mechanisms such as pressures and flow rates of the respiratory and circulatory systems. Although researchers were extremely innovative with their limited choices of techniques, the lack of methods to determine mechanisms occurring at the tissue and cellular levels greatly limited progress in understanding these complex disease processes. This not only played havoc with the veterinary clinician attempting to make sense of conflicting – and commonly misinterpreted – data regarding the pathophysiology of a complex disease process such as laminitis, but also plagued physicians faced with similar disease processes in humans (e.g., sepsis). However, the past thirty years has been inundated with dramatic advancements in basic research tools to study disease processes. Some of the major advances that have had the greatest impact on the study of disease mechanisms were initially in the area of physiology/pathophysiology, but these were quickly followed by a phenomenally rapid rise in the numbers of molecular biology and protein biochemistry/proteomics research tools. It is important that, if the reader of this text does not have a scientific background, she or he should have a basic understanding of what these different fields of investigation entail, as the majority of advances made to help understand the pathophysiology of laminitis that are discussed in the following chapters involve techniques associated with these fields.

As a general rule, physiology experiments involve experimental protocols in which measurements of either systemic or local tissue events/functions are made in a live animal model or in organ/tissue baths where tissue viability is maintained during the study (e.g., the measurement of blood flow in a tissue).

Molecular biology is classically the study of the regulation of gene expression, from the level of chromosomal DNA in which genes are located (and encoded) through the production of messenger RNAs (the process of *transcription*) and proteins (the process of *translation*). *Protein biochemistry* is generally used in research to represent the study of the structure, regulation, and activity of different proteins in the body, ranging from techniques to assess the concentrations of a protein in tissues or body fluids to those used in localizing these different proteins to

Equine Laminitis, First Edition. Edited by James K. Belknap and Raymond Geor.

specific cell types. *Proteomics* is a recently introduced term that generally is used to describe the involvement of biochemistry techniques in large-scale studies of the regulation of proteins (often multiple proteins at the same time).

Many of the advances made in physiologic techniques, which showed great progress during the latter half of the twentieth century, involved improving the ability to assess physiologic processes such as blood flow, not only at the systemic level (whole body) but also at the tissue level, where events occurred in the microvasculature (small blood vessels supplying the cellular components of a tissue). Unfortunately, veterinary scientists investigating laminitis were unable to take advantage of many of the physiologic advances that allowed the in-depth assessment of local events occurring at the tissue level, due mainly to the reality that the affected tissue in laminitis is situated between two incredibly dense structures, namely the hoof wall and the distal phalanx. Thus, many of the techniques (especially on the vascular side) have not been used to their full extent in the study of laminitis due to an inability to access the tissue without disturbing its architecture. Consequently, conflicting results exist for physiologic processes such as lamellar blood flow, due to investigators being limited to rather blunt measurements (e.g., hoof warmth as an indicator of lamellar blood flow) as proxies for direct measurements.

Although all of these studies have provided valuable information to the disease, the inability to visualize the intact lamellar microvasculature leaves somewhat of a 'black box' of events actually occurring *in vivo*. Many of these questions can hopefully be answered in the future by combining advanced three-dimensional imaging techniques (e.g., magnetic resonance imaging, positron emission tomography) with physiologic techniques. One recent advance which is now providing important physiologic data in laminitis research is the insertion of a small microdialysis catheter within the lamellar tissue. This allows interstitial fluid to be obtained, providing real-time data on lamellar metabolic events such as energy levels, pH, and indicators of perfusion (via urea clearance) of the tissues.

The remarkable advances in molecular biology techniques made over the past few decades have been much more easily adapted by those investigating laminitis, due primarily to the fact that the majority of samples used are tissues, and lamellar tissue being relatively easily obtained. The primary molecular biology techniques used in laminitis research are those that detect the amount of mRNA present for a gene/protein of interest. As the detection/quantitation of mRNA of a gene of interest is generally simpler and less costly than assessment at the protein level, many investigations are still based on the mRNA concentrations of genes of interest (an increase in mRNA encoding a specific protein of interest generally indicates that more protein will also be produced). These advances, which originally were designed to assess a single mRNA/gene at a time with techniques such as polymerase chain reaction (PCR), rapidly evolved into methods such as microarrays and next-generation sequencing, which currently allow the regulation of hundreds to thousands of genes to be determined simultaneously.

The advancement of *information technology* has been crucial to advances in molecular biology, as it is essential to have computer programs to manipulate the large amounts of data now obtainable with these different techniques. These programs not only assist in the quantitation of mRNA concentrations of different genes, but also use the combined information obtained on the regulation of the different genes to determine which cell-signaling pathways (where drugs most commonly target) are likely activated (or inhibited) in the affected lamellae.

The other benchmark reached in equine molecular biology was the sequencing of the equine genome, in 2007. This information was essential for designing the reagents to be used in equine experiments, and also for the software programs used to determine which genes were differentially regulated with the mass sequencing techniques such as next-generation sequencing. In the following chapters on pathophysiology, the primary molecular biology technique used is real-time quantitative PCR (RT-qPCR or qRT-PCR). This technique has been widely used to quantitatively assess gene expression in lamellar tissue related to inflammatory signaling, metalloproteinase production, the regulation of adhesion molecules important in adherence of the lamellar epithelium to the underlying dermal lamellae, and signaling proteins important in multiple other pathways. Mass sequencing results using techniques such as microarrays and RNA Seq (a next-generation sequencing platform in which all the mRNAs present in the cell are sequenced and quantitated) have also recently been used to characterize the cell signaling that occurs in lamellar tissues in different types of laminitis.

Although some proteins produced in the cell by the translation of mRNA are immediately active with minimal post-translational modification (e.g., proinflammatory cytokines), many others may be present in the cell but inactive due to a need for post-translational events. The latter include phosphorylation, which renders the proteins active and allows them to play a role in cellular processes. Thus, it is necessary to also use protein biochemistry techniques in investigations, notably to determine the presence and concentration of the active (e.g., phosphorylated) forms of proteins of interest. Many of these investigations have been performed using antibodies that recognize the active or inactive forms of a protein, applying techniques such as *immunoblotting* to quantitate the concentrations of the protein, and qualitative techniques such as *immunohistochemistry* in which antibodies can be used to localize the presence of proteins (e.g., a phosphorylated/activated signaling protein that is important in inflammation) in tissue sections to determine the type of lamellar cells that contain proteins of interest. These techniques have recently been used to assess lamellar signaling events in experimental models of all three types of laminitis (as described in the following chapters). A technique known as *gelatin zymography* has also proved essential in determining/quantitating the concentrations of active and inactive metalloproteinases in lamellar tissues. Indeed, this technique was vital in establishing (see Chapter 15) that two matrix metalloproteinases of great interest, MMP-2 and MMP-9, were likely not playing a significant role early in the disease process as they were shown (using zymography) to be absent in their active form. In addition to being vital to studies of lamellar pathophysiology, protein biochemistry techniques (e.g., ELISAs) are critical when quantifying proteins of interest in the circulation, mainly to determine the systemic signaling events that might play a central role in the different types of laminitis. The use of protein biochemistry techniques to document insulin dysregulation in equine metabolic syndrome is perhaps the best example of an ability to use advances in biochemistry to improve the understanding of systemic events in this type of laminitis. Molecular biology and protein biochemistry techniques each also complement the use of other cutting-edge research tools currently being used in laminitis research.

In addition to advances in basic science techniques used in the laboratory, epidemiologic studies are important for increasing the understanding of laminitis. Until now, epidemiology – which is generally defined as the study of the distribution of disease, or factors determining and influencing disease in populations – has primarily been used to assess the incidence of and risk factors for laminitis in different populations of horses. Epidemiologic studies have several strengths including: (i) they are possibly more clinically relevant than experimental models due to the fact that a naturally occurring disease is being studied; (ii) they allow the study of a disease without inducing any additional pain or distress to the animals; (iii) they have methodologies for the simultaneous study of multiple factors possibly involved in the pathophysiology of the disease process; (iv) they are well suited to characterize the risk factors for diseases; and (v) they involve the methodological science of clinical trials for evaluating interventions such as preventatives, therapeutics, or procedures. The primary limitations of epidemiologic studies are the constant concerns of confounding factors, such as differences in measured or unmeasured factors (e.g., management practices) among animals that are not accounted for by the research team, and the quality of the data, for example the use of historical data or data reported by non-professionals (horse owners) as the source of medical information.

As the reader will ascertain in the chapters regarding the pathophysiology of the different types of laminitis, the incredible advances in experimental techniques now available to veterinary research workers, the establishment of experimental models for the different types of laminitis, as well as the results of epidemiologic studies, have enabled investigators to begin to establish the diverse pathophysiologic processes that occur in the different types of laminitis. Studies using different models of sepsis-related laminitis have consistently established a marked lamellar inflammation that occurs during the developmental stages of the disease process, and the derangement of different cellular processes likely to play a role in dysadhesion of the lamellar basal epithelial cell layer from the underlying dermis. Importantly, both the establishment of experimental models and the advanced experimental techniques now being used to study sepsis-related laminitis have allowed the rapid establishment of profound digital hypothermia as the first effective therapy to protect lamellar tissue from catastrophic injury in the septic equine patient. Advances in the understanding of equine metabolic syndrome have derived from advances in experimental techniques and the recent establishment of experimental models, while epidemiologic studies have also had a greater impact on understanding this type of laminitis than any other type. As described in various chapters in the text, lamellar injury/dysfunction appears to emanate more from cell signaling related to hyperinsulinemia, with minimal evidence of lamellar inflammation playing a significant role in this component of endocrinopathic laminitis. Finally, the results of recent studies of supporting limb laminitis have again pointed towards a unique cause of lamellar failure in this model compared to other types of laminitis, with investigations consistently providing evidence of decreased lamellar perfusion when using very different experimental approaches to model this disease. Clearly, the main challenge for the future will be to effectively design large-scale epidemiologic studies and, especially in the realm of endocrinopathic and supporting limb laminitis, to establish more clinically relevant animal and ex-vivo models to accurately define pathophysiologic mechanisms – and hence therapeutic targets – for the different types of laminitis.

CHAPTER 7

Experimental Models of Laminitis: Starch Overload

Susan C. Eades

Introduction

Studies conducted during the early 1970s by Harold Garner and coworkers at the University of Missouri established an experimental model for acute sepsis-related laminitis (SRL) accompanied by acute alimentary disease caused by the oral intake of large quantities of digestible carbohydrate. Garner's starch overload model, using a mixture of corn starch and wood flour, provided the first data documenting consistent responses and a course of projection to facilitate the study of laminitis in horses [1].

Animal Protocol

The preparation of horses for the starch overload model is necessary to improve the consistency of responses. Horses are stalled (to eliminate forage intake) and fed a complete pelleted ration for seven days before induction. The laminitis induction ration consists of wood flour and corn starch administered in slurry form (described as a 'starch gruel' by some authors) via a nasogastric tube. The induction dose is 17.6 g kg^{-1} of bodyweight, with the final mixture being 80% corn starch and 20% wood flour. All of the gruel (often 12–18 l total volume) can generally be administered over 25–30 min. Occasionally, horses develop signs of abdominal pain due to gastric distention; this necessitates halting the initial dosing of the gruel and administering the remainder over 1–2 h.

Clinical Signs

Laminitis generally is induced in nine out of 10 horses administered the corn starch/wood flour gruel [1]. Some variability in the progression of lameness is observed. The mean time to onset of Obel grade 3 laminitis is 40 h (range: 24–48 h); Figure 7.1 [1]. Laminitis is usually most severe in the front feet but also occurs in the hind feet. Occasionally, lameness is most severe in the hind feet. Obel grade 1 lameness, most often seen as shifting weight and lameness at a trot, can develop as early as 12 h after induction, and as late as 18 h after induction. Obel grade 2 lameness, manifested as lameness at a walk, follows Obel grade 1 lameness in 2–18 h. The animal's body temperature gradually increases so as to develop a rectal temperature of 38.9 °C between 12 and 22 h, and peaking at approximately 30–40 h after administration of the induction gruel; the heart rate usually begins to increase at approximately 12 h post gruel administration [1]. Warmth is commonly palpable in the coronary bands and dorsal hoof wall, and bounding digital pulses can sometimes be palpated either before or coincident with the onset of lameness. The limbs are frequently noted to be cold [1]. The mucous membranes can be normal, pale, or hyperemic. Ponies are not commonly used in this model because lameness takes longer to develop, and up to 30% of ponies develop severe septic shock [2].

The severity and signs of gastrointestinal injury are also variable in this model. Partial or complete anorexia commonly occurs soon after administration of the corn starch gruel. Diarrhea is the most common sign and can develop within 10 h after gruel administration. In most horses, the volume of diarrhea is mild to moderate, but in a few horses severe watery diarrhea ensues that results in severe hypovolemic shock necessitating aggressive treatment or euthanasia. Mild transient colic occurs in most horses; however, severe unrelenting abdominal pain occurs before the onset of lameness in 5–10% of horses, which may necessitate euthanasia on humane grounds.

Clinical Relevance of the Model

The starch overload (corn starch/wood flour) model of Equine Laminitis appears to more closely mimic clinical cases of laminitis that occur secondary to sepsis-related diseases (e.g., enterocolitis, large intestinal strangulation, septic metritis, pneumonia) than the BWE model of SRL. Clinical signs common to horses administered corn starch/wheat flour gruel and horses with sepsis-related diseases include increased body temperature, tachycardia, changes in mucous membrane color, and inappetence. These clinical signs commonly precede the onset of laminitis by several hours in both the experimental model and in horses with clinical disease. The starch overload model of SRL

Equine Laminitis, First Edition. Edited by James K. Belknap and Raymond Geor.

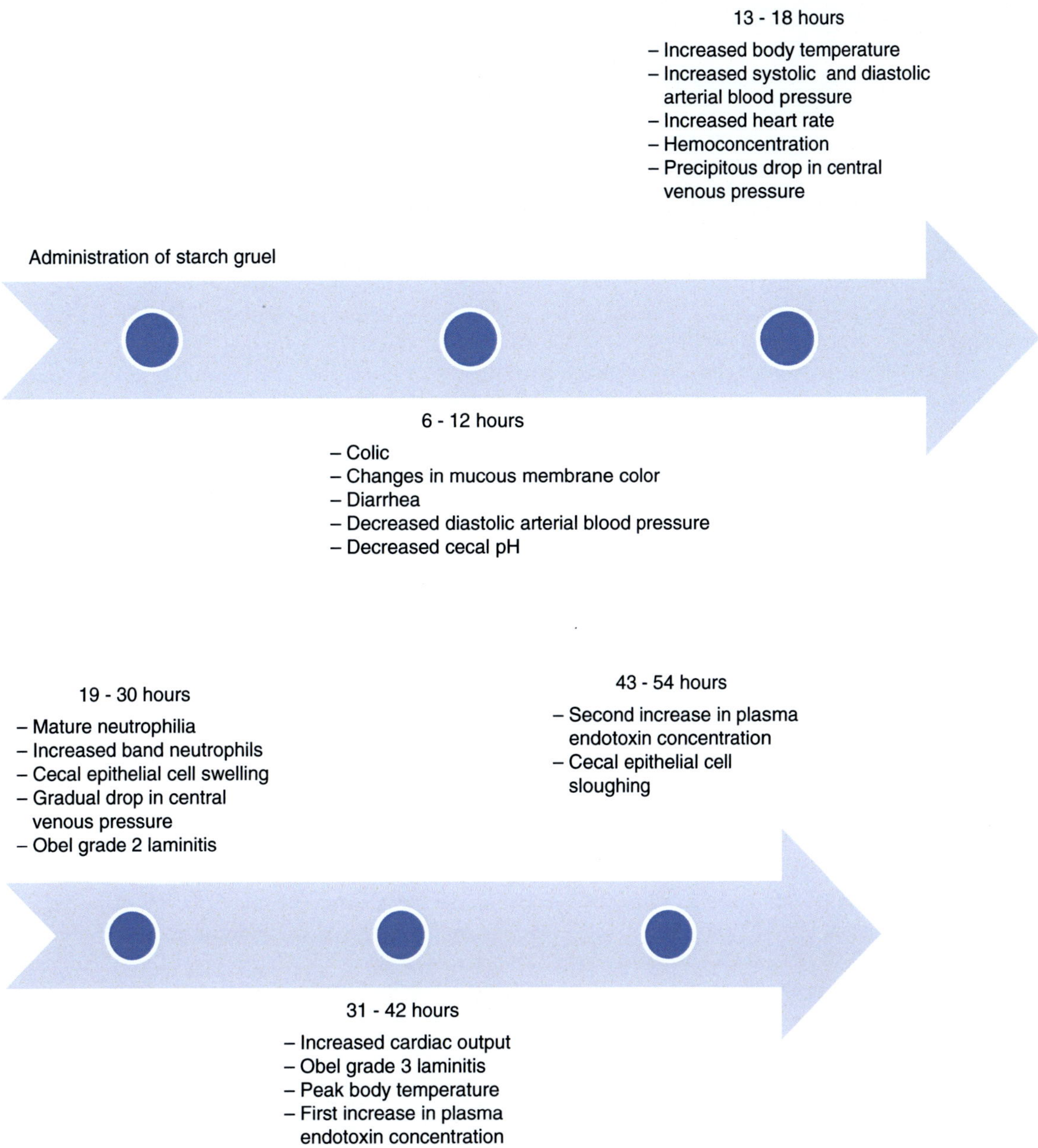

Figure 7.1 Approximate timing of events after the administration of corn starch gruel.

also induces hematologic changes (discussed in following section) similar to those which often occur in horses with these clinical diseases related to sepsis. Clinical signs of colic, diarrhea, and morphologic changes histologic changes in the large intestinal wall suggestive of colitis make the starch overload model a relevant model for the study of laminitis related to intestinal disease.

Endotoxemia has been documented in 85% of horses with laminitis induced by corn starch/wood flour gruel [3]. Endotoxemia is an important risk factor for the development of acute laminitis in horses during hospitalization for medical or surgical conditions [4]. Although endotoxemia is a common event in these diseases, whether it is directly or indirectly involved in the pathogenesis of laminitis remains unclear [5]. Although numerous models of experimental endotoxemia have been investigated, laminitis cannot be reproducibly induced by administration of endotoxin [6].

Hematologic Alterations

Although total leukocyte counts do not change significantly before and during starch overload-induced laminitis, important alterations in differential counts are observed. Segmented neutrophil counts increase at around 24 h post overload and remain increased until the onset of Obel grade 3 laminitis. Mature neutrophilia is accompanied by increased numbers of nonsegmented neutrophils. Both eosinophil and lymphocyte counts are significantly decreased after corn starch overload. Adrenalin and corticosteroid-mediated margination of mature neutrophils from the storage pool has been suggested [7]. Colitis and endotoxemia, both associated with the model, are capable of causing neutrophilia, lymphopenia, eosinopenia, and a left shift (increased numbers of non-segmented neutrophils). Blood platelet counts are decreased transiently, which may be clinically important as this may indicate to platelet aggregation.

Significant increases in packed cell volume and total protein before, during, and after Obel grade 3 laminitis have been documented [7]. Hemoconcentration is associated with an approximately 23% decrease in plasma volume [8]. Although the exact source of plasma volume loss has not been quantitated, diarrheal losses are suspected. The rapid presentation of excess soluble carbohydrate to the microbial population of the large intestine greatly increases the intraluminal production of organic acids and lactate. These particles provide the driving force – either osmotically or actively – for an additional influx of plasma water into the large intestine.

Plasma lactate concentrations increase in horses with corn starch overload, with the magnitude of such increase being greatest in horses that develop severe cardiovascular shock without developing laminitis. Horses developing Obel grade 3 laminitis have lactic acidosis that is less severe than that in horses which develop severe cardiovascular shock. Horses with less severe laminitis had only a slight increase in plasma lactate concentration [9]. Corn starch overload laminitis is accompanied by mild hyponatremia, hypokalemia, hypochloridemia, and acidosis [8, 9]. Losses of sodium, potassium, and chloride via the intestinal tract are also likely. Hyponatremia and hypovolemia are accompanied by an increase in plasma renin activity and plasma aldosterone concentration, which most likely partially compensate for the fluid and electrolyte losses by increasing intestinal and renal sodium and fluid reabsorption [8]. Anorexia developing soon after administration of the corn starch gruel probably contributes to the hypokalemia. Acidosis increases renal bicarbonate resorption and accelerates the tubular excretion of chloride to maintain electrical neutrality. Slight decreases in serum ionized calcium and phosphorus are probably not clinically important [8].

Plasma renin activity, aldosterone concentration, and hydrocortisone are all increasing when lameness and pain are most severe [8]. Plasma renin activity and aldosterone concentration are affected by serum sodium concentration, serum potassium concentration, plasma adrenocorticotropin hormone concentration, hypovolemia, sympathetic nervous system stimulation, and plasma renin activity, all of which are altered due to pain, inflammation, and diarrhea. Increased plasma renin activity could cause increases in the concentration of angiotensin, a potent vasoconstrictor that could alter tissue perfusion.

Changes in Cecal and Colonic Environment and Function

Starch overload results in enterocolitis caused by overeating soluble carbohydrate, which overwhelms the digestive capability of the small intestine. The soluble carbohydrate then enters the large intestine, where it is rapidly fermented by lactic acid-producing bacteria. The cecal pH rapidly decreases and the lactic acid concentration increases. Rapid organic acid production overwhelms the buffering capacity of the large intestine.

Highly digestible carbohydrate diets have been associated with decreases in cecal pH in horses [10]; lactic acidosis is a consistent characteristic of corn starch overload [9]. The cecal fluid pH falls from 7.18 ± 0.14 to 5.72 ± 0.13 at 8 h after corn starch overload, and to 4.14 ± 0.17 at 24 h [11]. Increases in numbers of lactic acid-producing bacteria and decreases in Gram-negative bacteria and protozoa occurs concurrent with pH changes [11]. Both, *Lactobacillus* and *Clostridial* spp. are increased significantly, while *Bacillus* spp., *Streptococcus* spp., anaerobic *Streptococcus* spp., and Enterobacteriacea are decreased [11]. High concentrations of digestible carbohydrate are conducive to the growth of *Lactobacillus* spp. which produce lactic acid. Rapid increases in cecal lactate concentrations have been documented [12]. The rapid decline in pH leads to decreased numbers of Enterobacteriacea. The release of endotoxin has been attributed to a 'die off' of these Gram-negative organisms [11]. Preliminary investigations in two horses confirmed increases in cecal fluid endotoxin concentrations after corn starch overload [12]. Sprouse *et al.* [3] monitored increases in plasma endotoxin concentrations after corn starch overload, and showed the times of such changes to vary among laminitic horses. Indeed, 13 of 20 horses administered corn starch overload developed laminitis, and increased plasma endotoxin concentrations were detected in 11 of the 13. An early peak (average 32 h after corn starch overload) and a late peak (average 38 h after) developed in five of the 11 horses [3]. No change in plasma endotoxin concentration was noted in six of the seven horses that did not develop laminitis. These reported changes in cecal and plasma endotoxin concentrations were not consistently reproducible among laboratories [13].

An electron microscopy evaluation of serial biopsies of the cecal mucosa during several hours following corn starch overload revealed pathological changes present in 50% of the sampled surface [14]. Samples collected between 3 and 7 h after starch administration appeared normal when examined microscopically, but pathological changes noted at 24–32 h after carbohydrate overload were characterized as cellular swelling and degeneration that progressed by 40–48 h to widespread cecal epithelial cell separation and some cellular sloughing. Widespread intestinal epithelial alterations observed at 72 h after corn starch administration included hydropic change and vacuolization, mitochondrial swelling and degeneration, and the unraveling of junctional complexes. Complete cell sloughing was also widespread by 72 h. Hydropic change, swollen unrecognizable organelles (including mitochondria), unraveling of junctional complexes and pyknotic nuclei were observed using transmission electron microscopy.

It has been proposed that changes in colonic and cecal fluid pH and bacterial populations could lead to ultrastructural changes, thereby altering intestinal epithelial function. Weiss and colleagues [13] determined that ponies challenged with corn starch/wheat flour gruel develop an increased intestinal permeability of a radiolabeled marker administered via a nasogastric tube. Urinary excretion of the radioisotope was increased markedly between 5—6 h after administration of the carbohydrate. Increased cecal permeability closely followed the reduction in cecal pH and increase in cecal lactate concentration, both occurring within 3 h after overload [12]. However, the permeability changes preceded the ultrastructural changes, which suggested either a more rapid damage to other intestinal segments or an altered permeability due to functional rather than structural change [14]. The effects of carbohydrate overload on intestinal permeability were diminished over the following 24 h. Intestinal permeability was not evaluated at later time points corresponding to ultrastructural changes. The incubation of cecal mucosal tissues *in vitro* with cecal contents and corn starch led to an increased paracellular permeability and permeability to a radiolabeled marker after 60–90 min. The in-vitro permeability changes correlated with a decreased pH, increased lactate concentration, and increased osmolality [15]. Although the fermentation of excess corn starch led to increased intestinal permeability, the alterations in cecal pH, lactate concentration and osmolality were not alone of sufficient magnitude to induce these changes [15].

Lactic acid is poorly absorbed by the healthy large intestine, and this results in an osmotic intestinal load causing diarrhea. Enterotoxins produced by Gram-positive lactic acid-producing bacteria are capable of damaging enterocytes. The acidity, endotoxins, and enterotoxins are capable of causing mucosal necrosis, allowing the absorption of these toxic substances capable of causing systemic inflammation and cardiovascular alterations. Secretory diarrhea resulting from pH changes and presence of inflammatory mediators worsens the acidosis and dehydration.

Cardiovascular Alterations

Typically, the animal's systolic blood pressure does not change for 16 h after induction with corn starch gruel [1]. Between 16 and 56 h, the blood pressure increases progressively and remains significantly elevated for an additional 48 h [16]. In contrast, the diastolic blood pressure decreases significantly for the first 16 h before progressively increasing between 16 and 48 h. By 40 h after corn starch overload, the systolic blood pressure reaches 139.9 ± 8.3 mmHg. The central venous pressure remains unchanged for 16 h and then decreases precipitously over the next 8 h (from 5.6 ± 1.2 mmHg to 0.75 ± 0.9 cmH_2O). The central venous pressure then decreases more slowly over the next 24–36 h. The heart rate remains normal but then begins to increase between 16 and 40 h to 73.3 ± 5.8 beats per min. Both, cardiac output and left ventricular ejection fraction are increased at the onset of Obel grade 3 lameness. The peripheral vascular resistance does not change significantly, however [16].

Increases in heart rate, systolic and diastolic blood pressures and cardiac output could result from increases in sympathetic neurotransmission or catecholamine release due to the combination of inflammatory disease, pain, and/or hypovolemia [1]. Circulatory function during and after Obel grade 3 laminitis has been characterized as hyperkinetic. A decrease in central venous pressure suggests peripheral blood pooling and a decreased circulating blood volume; simultaneous increases in packed cell volume and total protein support the movement of blood outside the vascular compartment. Increased vascular permeability due to systemic inflammatory response syndrome has been implicated. Severe decompensated cardiovascular shock can result in death, or more often may necessitate euthanasia before the onset of laminitis.

Histology

The present understanding of lamellar pathology during corn starch/wood flour-induced laminitis is limited. As histology provides only a snapshot of the lamellar changes occurring at the time of euthanasia, knowledge of the continuum of lamellar events during the disease is lacking. Early changes include secondary epidermal lamellar swelling and edema, endothelial cell swelling and deformation, red blood cell accumulation in the capillaries, and perivascular leukocyte infiltration [17]. Edema of the primary epidermal lamellae occurs within 12 h. Evaluation of the epithelium documented thinning and lengthening of the lamellar structures with flattening and displacement of the epithelial cells, redirection of the base of the secondary epidermal lamellae towards the distal phalanx, redirection of the tip of the secondary epidermal lamellae towards the hoof wall, epithelial cell swelling, vacuolization, and pyknosis beginning 24 h after carbohydrate overload [18, 19]. It has been proposed that epidermal cell vacuolization and the pyknosis and dissolution of basal cells in the presence of an intact basement membrane suggest the epidermal cell damage precedes basement membrane damage [17].

References

1. Garner, H.E., Coffman, J.R., Hahn, A.W., Hutcheson, D.P., and Tumbleson, M.E. (1975) Equine laminitis of alimentary origin: An experimental model. *Am. J. Vet. Res.*, **36**, 441–444.
2. Harkema, J.R., Robinson, N.E., and Scott, J.B. (1978) Cardiovascular, acid-base, electrolyte, and plasma volume changes in ponies developing alimentary laminitis. *Am. J. Vet. Res.*, **39**, 741–744.

3. Sprouse, R.F., Garner, H.E., and Green, E.M. (1987) Plasma endotoxin levels in horses subjected to carbohydrate-induced laminitis. *Equine Vet. J.*, **19**, 25–28.
4. Parsons, C.S., Orsini, J.A., Krafty, R., Capewell, L., and Boston, R. (2007) Risk factors for development of acute laminitis in horses during hospitalization: 73 cases (1997–2004). *J. Am. Vet. Med. Assoc.*, **230**, 885–889.
5. Belknap, J.K., Moore, J.N., and Crouser, E.C. (2009) Sepsis – From human organ failure to laminar failure. *Vet. Immunol. Immunopathol.*, **129**, 155–157.
6. Fessler, J.F., Bottoms, G.D., Coppoc, G.L., *et al.* (1989) Plasma endotoxin concentrations in experimental and clinical equine subjects. *Equine Vet. J. Suppl.*, **7**, 24–28.
7. Moore, J.N., Garner, H.E., and Coffman, J.R. (1981) Haematological changes during development of acute laminitis hypertension. *Equine Vet. J.*, **13**, 240–242.
8. Clarke, J.L., Garner, H.E., and Hatfield, D. (1982) Plasma volume, electrolyte, and endocrine changes during onset of laminitis hypertension in horses. *Am. J. Vet. Res.*, **43**, 1551–1555.
9. Garner, H.E., Hutcheson, D.P., Coffman, J.R., *et al.* (1977) Lactic acidosis: a factor associated with equine laminitis. *J. Anim. Sci.*, **45**, 1037–1041.
10. Willard, J.G., Willard, J.C., and Baker, J.P. (1977) Effect of diet on cecal pH and feeding behavior of horses. *J. Anim. Sci.*, **45**, 87–92.
11. Garner, H.E., Moore, J.N., Johnson. J.H., *et al.* (1978) Changes in the caecal flora associated with the onset of laminitis. *Equine Vet. J.*, **10**, 249–252.
12. Moore, J.N., Garner, H.E., Berg, J.N., and Sprouse, R.F. (1979) Intracecal endotoxin and lactate during the onset of equine laminitis: a preliminary report. *Am. J. Vet. Res.*, **40**, 722–723.
13. Weiss, D.J., Evanson, O.A., MacLeay, J., and Brown, D.R. (1998) Transient alteration in intestinal permeability to technetium Tc99m diethylenetraminopentaacetate during the prodromal stages of alimentary laminitis in ponies. *Am. J. Vet. Res.*, **59**, 1431–1434.
14. Krueger, A.S., Kinden, D.A., Garner, H.E., *et al.* (1986) Ultrastructural study of the equine cecum during onset of laminitis. *Am. J. Vet. Res.*, **47**, 1804–1812.
15. Weiss, D.J., Evanson, O.A., Green, B.T., and Brown, D.R. (2000) In vitro evaluation of intraluminal factors that may alter intestinal permeability in ponies with carbohydrate-induced laminitis. *Am. J. Vet. Res.*, **61**, 858–861.
16. Garner, H.E., Hahn, A.W., Salem, C., Coffman, J.R., Hutcheson, D.P., and Johnson, J.H. (1977) Cardiac output, left ventricular ejection rate, plasma volume, and heart rate changes in equine laminitis-hypertension. *Am. J. Vet. Res.*, **38**, 725–729.
17. Hood, D.M., Grosenbaugh, D.A., Mostafa, M.B., *et al.* (1993) The role of vascular mechanisms in the development of acute equine laminitis. *J. Vet. Intern. Med.*, **7**, 228–234.
18. Garner, H.E., *et al.* (1974) Clinical signs of acute alimentary laminitis correlated with cardiovascular and histopathologic alterations. *Proc. Am. Assoc. Equine Practitioners*, **20**, 61–65.
19. Morgan, S., Hood, D.M., Wagner, I.P., *et al.* (2003) Submural histopathologic changes attributable to peracute laminitis in horses. *J. Am. Vet. Res.*, **64**, 829–834.

CHAPTER 8

Experimental Models of Laminitis: Oligofructose Overload

Christopher C. Pollitt and Gabriel J. Milinovich

Introduction

Many clinical cases of laminitis result from the ingestion of excessive amounts of dietary carbohydrate, either in the form of excess cereal grain or pasture. Ingested pasture will contain variable fractions of nonstructural carbohydrate (NSC); the glucose, fructose, sucrose, and starch portions will be digested enzymatically in the stomach and small intestine, raising blood sugar levels and triggering insulin release from the pancreas. If the horse or pony is insulin-resistant, the blood insulin concentration may exceed the threshold known to cause hoof lamellar pathology and result in pasture-associated laminitis (PAL). This 'endocrinopathic' form of laminitis is the most common manifestation of the disease today, and is discussed in detail elsewhere in this book. Pasture, in addition to the sugars already mentioned, may also contain long-chain polymers of fructose called fructans that, when digested, do not appreciably raise blood sugar nor trigger the release of insulin. The fructans pass through the stomach and small intestine largely undigested [1] and reach the hindgut (the cecum and colons), where a suite of billions of microbes (the hindgut microbiome) symbiotically digest the fructans on behalf of the horse.

Laminitis Induction Models

Similarly, the ingestion of excessive quantities of uncooked cereal grain or corn (maize) may overwhelm the digestive capabilities of the stomach and small intestine and also reach the large intestine with potentially catastrophic consequences. Lameness and characteristic lamellar pathology follow the rapid microbial fermentation of the excess carbohydrate in the large intestine [2–6], resulting in a 'sepsis-related' form of laminitis. Inducing experimental laminitis by recapitulating the familiar clinical scenario of a horse or pony gorging on grain was relatively easy. In 1948, Obel dosed nine horses with rye grain and a bolus of cultured colibacilli. This induced "...violent diarrhoea, a considerable rise in temperature and pulse rate" and laminitis in eight of the nine horses [7]. In 1975, Garner led a team that established a starch overload model still used today (see Chapter 7), inducing laminitis by the nasogastric administration of a bolus dose (17.6 g kg^{-1} body weight) of 85% corn starch and 15% wood cellulose flour prepared as a gruel [8]. Eleven of 12 horses developed Obel Grade 3 laminitis within 48 h, but some developed colic and died. Although these models explained the consequences of accidental consumption of excess grain or corn by horses, the majority of horses exposed to excess carbohydrate are those consuming pasture with a high carbohydrate content over days to weeks.

Grasses and legumes make up the diet of horses in their natural state. Equids evolved and thrived eating mainly complex structural carbohydrates, in the form of cellulose, hemicellulose, and lignin, as well as NSC in the form of fructans, simple sugars, and starch. Structural carbohydrates and fructans are relatively indigestible to mammals without the aid of active hindgut fermentation by the microbiome and thus, as the ultimate hindgut fermenter, much of the equine abdomen is occupied by the cecum and colons where complex carbohydrates and fructans are fermented to absorbable end products. However, at specific times of the year and under certain environmental conditions, domestic horses and ponies can ingest excess pasture fructan. Noting a link between seasonally high pasture fructan concentration (400 g kg^{-1} dry matter) and the incidence of laminitis amongst horses and ponies grazing temperate grasses, fructan was proposed as a possible causal factor for laminitis [9].

The Fructan Laminitis Induction Model

Consequently, a laminitis induction model that utilized fructan was designed to mimic the laminitis possibly resulting from the ingestion of fructan-rich pasture [10]. Fructans are synthesized from sucrose and fructose by plants and, along with starches, constitute the predominant nonstructural plant polysaccharides. Fructan is the major storage carbohydrate of temperate (C3) plants and, in certain climatic conditions, can rapidly

Equine Laminitis, First Edition. Edited by James K. Belknap and Raymond Geor.

accumulate in grasses to attain up to 50% of the total dry matter content [11]. The van Eps and Pollitt oligofructose (OF) model used a commercially available fructan extracted from the roots of chicory (*Cichorium intybus*). OF consists of short-chain, inulin-like (β2,1-linked), fructose polymers and, dissolved in water, was administered to horses via a nasogastric tube at doses (7.5, 10 and 12.5 g kg^{-1} body weight) estimated to mimic a high consumption of fructan in temperate grasses [9]. OF administration reliably induced laminitis, with lameness occurring 24–36 h post oligofructose administration (POA). There was no excessive colonic gas production or colic, with only occasional mortality due to the rapid onset of hypovolemic, septic shock. The incidence of septic shock is greatly reduced if horses are acclimated to a soluble carbohydrate diet for three weeks prior to OF dosing. The OF induction laminitis model has proved reliable and reproducible, and may mimic field cases of laminitis when fructan concentrations are particularly high. The aim of the model was not to 'prove' that pasture fructan caused laminitis, but rather to alert the laminitis community to the dangerous possibility that fructan can contribute to laminitis and to take preventive measures accordingly.

Possible Problems with the Oligofructose Model

However, there are perceived problems with the model. The fructose molecules of OF polymers are β2,1-linked, whereas levans – the type of fructan commonly found in grass – are predominantly β2,6-linked [12], although β2,1-links also occur at polymer branch points in grasses (e.g., Timothy-grass; *Phleum pretense* [13]). However, the type of linkage may be immaterial as the fructanases of hindgut bacteria can hydrolyze either β2,1-linked or β2,6-linked fructans (e.g., *Lactobacillus paracasei* ssp. *paracasei* reportedly catalyzes the hydrolysis of β-2,6 linked fructan more rapidly than the β-2,1 linkages of inulin, although the difference is only a matter of minutes) [14].

During the OF manufacturing process, fructans extracted from chicory are enzymatically hydrolyzed to short-chain lengths with 10 degrees of polymerization (DP) or less; this is much smaller than naturally occurring fructans (30 and 50 DP) [15]. The use of a carbohydrate source with fewer DP to induce laminitis may exaggerate the proliferation response of large intestinal organisms lacking the enzymatic pathways to break down the longer fructans found in grasses [16].

The daily consumption of pasture by ponies grazing 12–17 h per day is easy to underestimate. Ponies at pasture can ingest 5% pasture dry matter (DM) of their body weight per day, considerably more than the 2–2.5% of body weight per day typically assumed. In fact, 1% of their body weight can be consumed within 3 h at pasture in autumn when pastures are particularly palatable [17]. At the higher levels of intake (2.5 and 5.2% body weight per day) from swards with an elevated NSC content, horses could have ingested between 3.5 and 7.3 kg fructan per day, respectively. These amounts are similar to and almost double the amount of OF used to induce laminitis when delivered as a single bolus.

However much fructan-rich pasture a pony may eat in a day, it does not equate to the bolus dose delivered over several minutes into the stomach of a horse to induce laminitis in the OF laminitis model. Constant grazing trickle feeds the fructan-rich fraction into the hindgut. The OF deposited in the stomach by a nasogastric tube reaches the cecum within 2 h post dosing, peaks in concentration at approximately 4 h, and takes 32 h to be completely fermented (G.J. Milinovich and C.C. Pollitt; unpublished data, 2012).

Although laminitis has yet to be induced experimentally by feeding fructan-rich pasture or a fructan-rich extract, there are anecdotal reports of clinical laminitis occurring when diets are below 10% ethanol-soluble carbohydrate (ESC) plus starch DM but high (15% DM) in NSC (K. Wilkinson, personal communication, 2015). Typically, ESC analysis excludes most of the fructan fraction, whereas the NSC includes all the simple sugars, starch, as well as fructans. The suspicion is that the hindgut fermentation of pasture fructan induces a low-grade, subclinical colitis (sepsis model) that may trigger laminitis in its own right, but may contribute to and exacerbate an already extant hyperinsulinemic form of laminitis due to the glucose absorbed from the small intestine. Fructan-rich samples of *Lolium perrenne* incubated *in vitro* with equine hindgut contents [1] produce lactate similar to the *in-vivo* dosing of OF [18]. Until specific research data are available, horse and pony owners would be well advised to avoid feeding high-NSC pasture and hays, to soak high-NSC hay to reduce the simple sugar and fructan content, or to use grazing muzzles (see Chapter 50).

Although the OF dosing regimen used experimentally does not exactly replicate laminitis by natural causes, it illuminates its pathophysiology and has led to an improved understanding and an expanded data base of knowledge. The model likely mirrors sepsis-related laminitis (versus endocrinopathic laminitis), as even dosing with low concentrations of OF (5.0 g kg^{-1}) induced laminitis without detectable changes in insulin dynamics [19]; these findings were in accord with the original OF induction studies [20]. The OF model mimics events occurring clinically in sepsis-related laminitis, and more consistently induces laminitis when compared to the traditional starch model. Since its first description in 2006, the OF model is being used increasingly by both equine and cattle laminitis research workers, as evidenced by recent publications [19, 21–24]. Indeed, the OF model is likely to be the primary model used for future sepsis-associated laminitis investigations [25].

Microbial Events in the Hindgut

Most of the consequences of OF overload occur after its arrival in the hindgut (2 h after dosing), and relate to the rapid proliferation of hindgut bacteria that use OF as a metabolic substrate. On mixing with the normally neutral caecal contents, the excess OF undergoes rapid fermentation that results in lactic acid production that lowers the caecal pH to below 5 by 6–12 h post administration [16].

To determine which organisms proliferate in the presence of OF, a novel habitat-simulating agar medium containing equine cecal fluid, agar, and OF (as the sole energy substrate) was developed [26]. Organisms with the ability to utilize oligofructose for growth were cultured from fecal samples of horses undergoing OF laminitis induction, enumerated, and identified. Most of the isolates were Gram-positive bacteria (mainly *Streptococcus bovis* and *Streptococcus equinus* [now *Streptococcus lutetiensis*]). In this model, *Escherichia coli* did not become the predominant OF-utilizing organism until after the onset of laminitis. In addition, few lactobacilli with the ability to utilize oligofructose as a growth substrate were isolated (a result which was quite different from the starch induction model [5]).

These studies relied on culture to quantify the complex changes occurring in the hindgut microbiota as laminitis developed. However, culture has serious limitations, since it is estimated that as little as 30% of the equine cecal microbiota are cultivatable [27]. Thus, modern molecular methodologies have recently been used to circumvent the limitations of culture by focusing on the unique DNA sequences in the different bacterial organisms for the small subunit rRNA genes (particularly 16S rRNA gene). Milinovich and colleagues took serial samples of gastrointestinal contents in the OF model, and analyzed them in detail using a molecular technique termed fluorescence *in-situ* hybridization (FISH), with different fluorescent probes for the unique 16S rRNA sequences of different bacterial species [28].

Initially, FISH was utilized to study changes in bacterial populations of the equine hindgut during laminitis development. This enabled changes in bacterial populations in paired cecal fluid and fecal specimens collected from five horses at 4-h intervals to be imaged and analyzed. The microbial changes were correlated with the development of histologic signs of laminitis determined by the collection and analysis of serial hoof biopsies harvested at 6-h intervals [29]. Commencing at 2 h post OF administration, there was a rapid proliferation of hindgut streptococci which peaked between 8 and 24 h. These streptococci transformed the hindgut population from predominantly Gram-negative to Gram-positive within a few hours. Thus, 60% of the total bacterial population became Gram-positive (preinduction, relative frequencies of Gram-positive bacteria were typically <10% of the total bacterial population) in all five horses before the development of lamellar histologic changes consistent with the onset of laminitis.

No other organism detected with the FISH probes used in this study (e.g., Enterobacteriaceae, *Allisonella histaminiformans*, *Enterococcus* spp., *Lactobacillus* spp., *Bacteroides fragilis*, *Mitsuokella jalaludinii*, and *Clostridium difficile*) established significant populations in the equine hindgut before onset of the disease. Interestingly, increases in Enterobacteriaceae were observed, but only after hindgut streptococci had become dominant (in all five horses) and, importantly, after the development of histologic laminitis in two of the five horses. Thus, analysis by FISH corroborated the results from the culture-based studies that showed that equine hindgut streptococcal species (EHSS) played the major role in the laminitis developmental process and that oligofructose-utilizing *E. coli* proliferated too late to be considered causative.

The DNA Fingerprint of Events in the Hindgut

When another state-of-the-art technique, DNA fingerprinting, was applied to the OF induction model, more information than could be derived from FISH alone was forthcoming [18]. Before this study, no culture-independent analysis of changes in the equine hindgut microbiome during the development of laminitis existed. Using denaturing gradient gel electrophoresis (DGGE), the DNA fingerprinting technique allows the detection of similarities and differences between samples, and can be used to monitor the changes occurring within a bacterial community over time. In the study conducted by Milinovich and colleagues, the stained gels contained columns of bands representing a unique fingerprint of the hindgut communities as they changed over the timeline of laminitis development. Selected DGGE samples were then used to design qRT-PCR assays to quantify bacterial groups of interest. The results corroborated the previous FISH and culture-based studies, and provided new insight into the laminitis development process.

In the FISH study, the EHSS population showed explosive growth until 16 h post OF administration, after which it disappeared. However, when quantified using qPCR the EHSS did not decline at 16 h but rather remained at their maximum value until the final time point 36 h post OF administration. This discrepancy was hypothesized to be due to the FISH and qPCR techniques having different targets. FISH targets the 16S rRNA in whole cells, so the signal disappears when the cell dies, whereas qPCR targets genetic material that encodes for 16S rRNA which persists in the sample long after cell death. The study concluded that, at 16 h post OF administration, the EHSS detected by qPCR but not by FISH, had undergone *en masse* lysis. This lysis of EHSS, in such high abundance before the onset of laminitis, may have released toxic cellular components that possibly contributed to laminitis pathogenesis.

The DGGE technique also showed that lactobacilli constituted only a small proportion of the total cecal microbiome during the developmental phase of laminitis. However, qPCR showed small increases in an *E. coli* subpopulation, at 16 and 24 h after OF administration, in all horses but notably after the development of pathologic changes in the foot [18].

DGGE analysis showed that other *E. coli* subpopulations, present at the time of the initial OF dosing, declined and disappeared as the EHHS population in the hindgut bloomed. Thus, endotoxin released by the lysis of *E. coli* may also contribute to the development of laminitis [30–33]. However, the attempted experimental induction of Equine Laminitis with purified endotoxin has never been successful [34–37]. Interestingly, the fact that signs of endotoxemia can be effectively controlled by drugs (e.g., polymyxin B [32,38,39] and flunixin meglumine [40,41]) but that laminitis develops regardless of their use also questions the direct role of endotoxin/ lipopolysaccharide (LPS) in laminitis. It remains difficult to directly associate genuine endotoxemia with laminitis onset. Many ill horses appear 'endotoxic,' but this is usually inferred from clinical signs rather than confirmed by endotoxin assay. As is well described in the human literature, the term 'endotoxic' or 'endotoxemia' should be replaced with the more general term 'septic' or 'sepsis,' which describes the same clinical signs being induced by multiple bacterial products from Gram-negative and Gram-positive bacteria. It is likely that multiple other bacterial products are also absorbed from the compromised hindgut in carbohydrate overload models (including the OF model) and may play an important role in laminitis pathophysiology. That said, a low concentration but significant increase in endotoxin (LPS) was detected in the systemic circulation of horses dosed with 10 g kg^{-1} OF at 8 and 12 h after dosing [42]. In the same study, increases in plasma tumor necrosis factor-alpha (TNFα), platelet p38 mitogen-activated protein kinase (MAPK) phosphorylation, plasma 5-hydroxytryptamine (5-HT) and thromboxane also occurred; these authors suggested that LPS (and/or likely other bacterial products) may contribute in the initiation of the early inflammatory changes of laminitis by activating platelets and, indirectly, leukocytes.

Conclusion

There is now rigorous evidence implicating the rapid growth and lysis of EHSS as a precipitating event in the development of alimentary overload laminitis when using the OF induction model. However, how changes in the hindgut microbiota initiate hoof lamellar basal cell cytoskeleton collapse and dysadhesion remain to be determined; the possibilities are many-fold. Caecal/colonic lymphadenopathy and eosinophilia characterized the lymph nodes of OF-dosed horses progressing to lameness without the detection of viable, translocated, gut-derived microbes in the affected lymph nodes [43]. Despite these results, it is likely that liberated cellular components of lysed EHSS and other microbes in the compromised large intestine may cross the mucosal barrier of the damaged hindgut and provoke, either locally and/or systemically, the profound systemic immune response associated with laminitis development. Thus, linking microbiotic population changes in the horse hindgut to histological and clinical evidence of laminitis has advanced the pathophysiological understanding of the disease [18].

References

1. Ince, J.C., Longland, A.C., Moore-Colyer, M.J.S., and Harris, P.A. (2014) In vitro degradation of grass fructan by equid gastrointestinal digesta. *Grass Forage Sci.*, **69** (3), 514–523.
2. Bailey, S.R., Baillon, M.L., Rycroft, A.N., Harris, P.A., and Elliott, J. (2003) Identification of equine cecal bacteria producing amines in an in vitro model of carbohydrate overload. *Appl. Environ. Microbiol.*, **69** (4), 2087–2093.
3. Elliott, J., Berhane, Y., and Bailey, S.R. (2003) Effects of monoamines formed in the cecum of horses on equine digital blood vessels and platelets. *Am. J. Vet. Res.*, **64** (9), 1124–1131.
4. Elliott, J. and Bailey, S.R. (2006) Gastrointestinal derived factors are potential triggers for the development of acute equine laminitis. *J. Nutr.*,**136** (7 Suppl.), 2103S–210-S.
5. Garner, H.E., Moore, J.N., Johnson, J.H., Clark, L., Amend, J.F., Tritschler, L.G., *et al.* (1978) Changes in the caecal flora associated with the onset of laminitis. *Equine Vet. J.*, **10** (4), 249–252.
6. Mungall, B.A., Kyaw-Tanner, M., and Pollitt, C.C. (2001) In vitro evidence for a bacterial pathogenesis of equine laminitis. *Vet. Microbiol.*, **79** (3), 209–223.
7. Obel, N. (1948) Studies of the Histopathology of Acute Laminitis. PhD Thesis, Almgvist and Wilcsells Bottrykeri Ab Uppsala, Uppsala.
8. Garner, H.E., Coffman, J.R., Hahn, A.W., Hutcheson, D.P., and Tumbleson, M.E. (1975) Equine laminitis of alimentary origin: an experimental model. *Am. J. Vet. Res.*, **36** (4 Pt.1), 441–444.
9. Longland, A.C. and Byrd, B.M. (2006) Pasture nonstructural carbohydrates and equine laminitis. *J. Nutr.*, **136**, 2099S–2102S.
10. Van Eps, A.W. and Pollitt, C.C. (2006) Equine laminitis induced with oligofructose. *Equine Vet. J.*, **38** (3), 203–208.
11. Cairns, A. and Longland, A. (eds) (1998) Sugar in grasses – an overview of sucrose and fructan accumulation in temperate grasses. International Research Conference on Equine Laminitis, Stoneleigh, Warwickshire, UK, Dodson and Horrell.
12. Sims, I.M., Pollock, C.J., and Horgan, R. (1992) Structural analysis of oligomeric fructans from excised leaves of *Lolium temulentum*. *Phytochemistry*, **31**, 2989–2992.
13. Chatterton, N.J., Harrison, P.A., Thornley, W.R., and Draper, E.A. (1990) Oligosaccharides in foliage of *Agropyron*, *Bromus*, *Dactylis*, *Festuca*, *Lolium* and *Phleum*. *New Phytologist*, **114** (2), 167–171.
14. Muller, M. and Seyfarth, W. (1997) Purification and substrate specificity of an extracellular fructanhydrolase from *Lactobacillus paracasei* ssp. *paracasei* P 4134. *New Phytologist*, **136** (1), 89–96.
15. Vijn, I. and Smeekens, S. (1999) Fructan: more than a reserve carbohydrate? *Plant Physiol.*, **120** (2), 351–360.
16. Milinovich, G.J., Klieve, A.V., Pollitt, C.C., and Trott, D.J. (2010) Microbial events in the hindgut during carbohydrate-induced equine laminitis. *Vet. Clin. North Am. Equine Pract.*, **26** (1), 79–94.
17. Longland, A.C., Barfoot, C., and Harris, P.A. (2016) Effects of grazing muzzles on intakes of dry matter and water-soluble carbohydrates by ponies grazing spring, summer and autumn swards, as well as autumn swards of different heights. *J. Equine Vet. Sci.*, **40**, 26–33.
18. Milinovich, G.J., Burrell, P.C., Pollitt, C.C., Klieve, A.V., Blackall, L.L., Ouwerkerk, D., *et al.* (2008) Microbial ecology of the equine hindgut during oligofructose-induced laminitis. *ISME J.*, **2**, 1089–1100.
19. Kalck, K.A., Frank, N., Elliott, S.B., and Boston, R.C. (2009) Effects of low-dose oligofructose treatment administered via nasogastric intubation on induction of laminitis and associated alterations in glucose and insulin dynamics in horses. *Am. J. Vet. Res.*, **70** (5), 624–632.

20. Van Eps, A.W. and Pollitt, C.C. (2006) Equine laminitis induced with oligofructose. *Equine Vet. J.*, **38** (3), 203–208.
21. Danscher, A.M., Enemark, H.L., Andersen, P.H., Aalbaek, B., and Nielsen, O.L. (2010) Polysynovitis after oligofructose overload in dairy cattle. *J. Comp. Pathol.*, **142** (2-3), 129–138.
22. Danscher, A.M., Toelboell, T.H., and Wattle, O. (2010) Biomechanics and histology of bovine claw suspensory tissue in early acute laminitis. *J. Dairy Sci.*, **93** (1), 53–62.
23. Toth, F., Frank, N., Elliott, S.B., Geor, R.J., and Boston, R.C. (2008) Effects of an intravenous endotoxin challenge on glucose and insulin dynamics in horses. *Am. J. Vet. Res.*, **69** (1), 82–88.
24. Uberti, B., Pressler, B.M., Alkabes, S.B., Chang, C.Y., Moore, G.E., Lescun, T.B., *et al.* (2010) Effect of heparin administration on urine protein excretion during the developmental stage of experimentally induced laminitis in horses. *Am. J. Vet. Res.*, **71** (12), 1462–1467.
25. Belknap, J. and Geor, R. (2012) The present state and future of laminitis research. *Equine Vet. J.*, **44** (6), 749–751.
26. Milinovich, G.J., Trott, D.J., Burrell, P.C., Van Eps, A.W., Thoefner, M.B., Blackall, L.L., *et al.* (2006) Changes in equine hindgut bacterial populations during oligofructose induced laminitis. *Environ. Microbiol.*, **8**, 885–898.
27. Mackie, R.I. and Wilkins, C.A. (1988) Enumeration of anaerobic bacterial microflora of the equine gastrointestinal tract. *Appl. Environ. Microbiol.*, **54** (9), 2155–2160.
28. Milinovich, G.J., Trott, D.J., Burrell, P.C., Croser, E.L., Al Jassim, R.A., Morton, J.M., *et al.* (2007) Fluorescence in situ hybridization analysis of hindgut bacteria associated with the development of equine laminitis. *Environ. Microbiol.*, **9** (8), 2090–2100.
29. Croser, E.L. and Pollitt, C.C. (eds) (2006) Acute laminitis: descriptive evaluation of serial hoof biopsies. 52nd Annual Convention of the American Association of Equine Practitioners, San Antonio, Texas, USA.
30. Ingle Fehr, J.E. and Baxter, G.M. (1999) The effect of oral isoxsuprine and pentoxifylline on digital and laminar blood flow in healthy horses. *Vet. Surg.*, **28** (3), 154–160.
31. Parsons, C.S., Orsini, J.A., Krafty, R., Capewell, L., and Boston, R. (2007) Risk factors for development of acute laminitis in horses during hospitalization: 73 cases (1997–2004). *J. Am. Vet. Med. Assoc.*, **230** (6), 885–889.
32. Raisbeck, M.F., Garner, H.E., and Osweiler, G.D. (1989) Effects of polymyxin B on selected features of equine carbohydrate overload. *Vet. Hum. Toxicol.*, **31** (5), 422–426.
33. Sprouse, R.F., Garner, H.E., and Green, E.M. (1987) Plasma endotoxin levels in horses subjected to carbohydrate-induced laminitis. *Equine Vet. J.*, **19** (1), 25–28.
34. Hood, D.M. (1985) Studies on the pathogenesis of equine laminitis. *Dissertation Abstracts International, B.*, **45** (9), 2835.
35. Hunt, R.J., Allen, D., and Moore, J.N. (1990) Effect of endotoxin administration on equine digital hemodynamics and Starling forces. *Am. J. Vet. Res.*, **51** (11), 1703–1707.
36. Riggs, L.M., Krunkosky, T.M., Noschka, E., Boozer, L.A., Moore, J.N., and Robertson, T.P. (2009) Comparison of characteristics and enzymatic products of leukocytes in the skin and laminar tissues of horses administered black walnut heartwood extract or lipopolysaccharide. *Am. J. Vet. Res.*, **70** (11), 1383–1390.
37. Stephens, K.A. (1984) Studies on sublethal endotoxemia in the horse. *Southwest. Vet.*, **36** (1), 27–37.
38. MacKay, R.J., Clark, C.K., Logdberg, L., *et al.* (1999) Effect of a conjugate of polymyxin B-dextran 70 in horses with experimentally induced endotoxemia. *Am. J. Vet. Res.*, **60**, 68–75.
39. Morresey, P.R. and Mackay, R.J. (2006) Endotoxin-neutralizing activity of polymyxin B in blood after IV administration in horses. *Am. J. Vet. Res.*, **67** (4), 642–647.
40. Semrad, S.D., Hardee, G.E., Hardee, M.M., and Moore, J.N. (1987) Low-dose flunixin meglumine – effects on eicosanoid production and clinical signs induced by experimental endotoxemia in horses. *Equine Vet. J.*, **19** (3), 201–206.
41. Semrad, S.D. and Moore, J.N. (1987) Effects of multiple low-doses of flunixin meglumine on repeated endotoxin challenge in the horse. *Prostaglandins Leukotrienes and Medicine*, **27** (2-3), 169–181.
42. Bailey, S.R., Adair, H.S., Reinemeyer, C.R., Morgan, S.J., Brooks, A.C., Longhofer, S.L., *et al.* (2009) Plasma concentrations of endotoxin and platelet activation in the developmental stage of oligofructose-induced laminitis. *Vet. Immunol. Immunopathol.*, **129** (3-4), 167–173.
43. Onishi, J.C., Park, J.W., Prado, J., Eades, S.C., Mirza, M.H., Fugaro, M.N., *et al.* (2012) Intestinal bacterial overgrowth includes potential pathogens in the carbohydrate overload models of equine acute laminitis. *Vet. Microbiol.*, **159** (3-4), 354–363.

CHAPTER 9

Experimental Models of Laminitis: Black Walnut Extract

John F. Peroni

Introduction

The evolution of the black walnut extract (BWE) model of laminitis, similar to the carbohydrate overload models, took place after clinical reports of laminitis surfaced regarding animals developing laminitis when bedded on wood shavings from black walnut (*Juglans nigra*) trees. The first published report of clinical cases of black walnut toxicosis was in 1978, when over 100 cases of laminitis were reported from five different farms in Connecticut and New York [1]. On these farms, a fairly high incidence of laminitis was reported, with 37% to 100% of the horses and ponies on each farm that were bedded on black walnut shavings (or a mix of black walnut with other wood) developing acute laminitis. The majority of animals exhibited distal limb edema and the classic digital signs of laminitis (hoof warmth and bounding digital pulses). Although only mild signs of laminitis were noted in most animals, more severe signs of laminitis (mainly Obel grade 2–3) were diagnosed in several animals at three of the five farms. These signs were usually apparent between 18–26 h after placing the animals on the shavings. The severity of signs appeared to differ between farms (and source of shavings). The majority of animals fully recovered with minimal treatment, but two animals were destroyed euthanized due to the severity of rotation of the distal phalanx on one farm [1]. In a later report, five of six horses exposed to a shavings mixture with 20% black walnut shavings developed transient signs of laminitis within 12–24 h, with rapid full recovery [2].

Early attempts to experimentally induce laminitis with either topical or gastric (whole or micronized in a slurry via nasogastric tube) administration of black walnut shavings were unsuccessful [1]. The first successful experimental induction was described by Minnick *et al.* in 1987, where shavings (2 g of shavings per kg body weight of horse) made from the heartwood of a branch of a black walnut tree harvested in the fall of the year were soaked in 7–8 liters of water for 12 h. The BWE was filtered to remove shavings prior to administration via a stomach tube to 10 horses. Eight horses reportedly developed Obel grade 3 or 4 laminitis within 12 h (this severity of laminitis is not typical of the model and was likely due to a more 'potent' tree than has been used in most studies, as discussed below). Two horses were 'nonresponders' (i.e., they did not develop signs of laminitis), which is not uncommon for this model. In addition to signs of laminitis, limb edema and mild sedation were (i.e. other than laminitis) observed in the 'responders.' One horse required euthanasia due to the severity of signs, whereas the other seven exhibited clinical signs but recovered fully from the laminitic episodes. Juglone was identified (via gas chromatography and mass spectrometry) in the bark and nuts, but not in the heartwood of the tree. The results of the study concluded that the aqueous extract of heartwood is 'laminogenic' to horses, but the active ingredient is not juglone. This confirmed the results of an earlier experimental study in which juglone administration did not induce laminitis [3, 4].

Protocol

Following the Minnick report, the BWE model was performed in a fairly consistent manner for approximately 20 years, with the main variability being the potency of the tree from which shavings are obtained for the study (BWE from some trees being more effective than others). It has been proposed that the extract be produced from heartwood shavings obtained from a mature black walnut tree (or branch) obtained in the fall of the year, as BWE obtained from trees harvested at other times did not consistently induce the disease. When a Black Walnut tree is felled and cut in cross-section, the outer, light-colored wood beneath the bark is termed 'sapwood,' to the inside of which is the dark purple heartwood. Once the outer sapwood is cleaned off, the heartwood can be chipped into shavings and stored in 1-kg aliquots at −20 °C. In preparation for a study, an aliquot (2 g of black walnut heartwood shavings/kg bwt) is added to 6–7 liters of water at room temperature and gently agitated for 12–24 h. The resulting dark-red color and slightly viscous solution is separated from the shavings using a cloth sheet (e.g. cheesecloth) and administered to the study subjects via a nasogastric tube.

Equine Laminitis, First Edition. Edited by James K. Belknap and Raymond Geor.

Typically, horses in the control group receive the same volume of water at room temperature.

More specifically, in preparation for an experiment, horses receive an indwelling silicone catheter positioned in the jugular vein for the collection of blood for white blood cell (WBC) counts. After performing a physical examination and obtaining the zero-time blood sample, 5 liters of BWE are administered via a nasogastric intubation to the *principal* horses. The animals' heart rate, respiratory rate, rectal temperature, digital pulses, total WBC count, and Obel grade lameness are typically monitored at 30-min intervals after dosing. Based on the results of a series of studies, it is expected that approximately 80–90% of *principal* horses will develop a 30% (or greater) decrease in WBC count by approximately 3–4 h after administration of the extract, whereas no change should occur in *control* horses given water [3, 5–7]. Often, the aforementioned decrease in WBC count is used as evidence that horses are 'responders' in the BWE model. It is expected that those principal horses that respond to the extract via a decrease in WBC count will develop Obel grade 1 laminitis (i.e., shifting of weight between the forefeet) within 8–10 h of the administration of BWE [6, 7].

Following the administration of BWE, a series of parameters are expected to change from baseline, and these are important to recognize to best follow the progression of laminitis from its prodromal phase to the onset of clinical signs. Evidence obtained using both the carbohydrate-overload and BWE models of laminitis indicate that signs of systemic inflammation precede the development of symptoms of laminitis, and represent a systemic response that may affect many body systems. The most consistent systemic response is the abrupt 30% decrease in circulating leukocytes (commonly termed 'leukopenia,' although the absolute number of total leukocytes still present may be within the normal range) at approximately 3–4 h following BWE administration [6]. The leukopenia is not due to the extravasation of neutrophils alone. In a study specifically evaluating these changes in circulating leukocytes, a significant decrease in circulating monocytes was found, as well as a shift in neutrophil population from a smaller, more mature population to a larger, immature one [8]. As a result of these studies and others, the two time points most commonly assessed using the BWE model are the onset of leukopenia (usually termed 'developmental' or prodromal time point due to the lack of clinical signs of digital pathology at that point in time) [9–12] and the onset of clinical signs of Obel grade 1 laminitis [13–15]. An earlier time point, 1.5 h post BWE administration, has also been assessed in an attempt to identify initiating events occurring in the lamellae [16].

Justification of the Black Walnut Extract Model

During the time that the majority of experimental studies using BWE were performed, only the traditional carbohydrate overload (CHO) model existed (see Chapter 7). As a result, research groups elected to induce laminitis by the administration of BWE for several reasons. First, the short time from administration of the extract to the onset of Obel grade 1 laminitis was considered an advantage over the 18–24 h required for this to occur using the CHO model [17, 18]. The development of BWE-induced laminitis was viewed as a more humane model as it is not accompanied by systemic clinical signs such as colic, diarrhea and septic shock, which are characteristic complicating factors in horses after employing CHO [17,19]. Furthermore, the model was thought of as at least as consistent, if not slightly more so, than the CHO model (e.g., same or fewer 'nonresponders') and, finally, with two consistent, distinct time points – the onset of leukopenia (usually termed the developmental or prodromal time point) and the onset of Obel grade 1 laminitis, the model rapidly became predictable and well characterized. Although the use of this model resulted in a rapid attainment of a great deal of valuable insight into sepsis-related laminitis, its use has been limited for the past decade primarily due to the fact that these animals rarely progress to lamellar failure (as is commonly observed in clinical laminitis patients). Hence, it may be less clinically relevant for studying pathophysiology and potential treatments than the CHO models.

The remainder of this chapter includes a brief overview of the various studies of laminitis pathophysiology using the BWE model. An in-depth discussion of findings using the BWE model is also provided in the separate chapters on inflammatory events, vascular events, and proteases in laminitis.

Systemic Changes

In addition to BWE-induced inflammatory events that occur in the lamellae, investigators have assessed inflammatory events in the circulation, skin, liver, lungs, and large intestine [20–22]. BWE has been reported to induce the production of reactive oxygen species (ROS) in blood (most likely due to the activation of leukocytes), and has also been found in ex-vivo experiments to increase ROS activity in equine serum [6]. As a result of the activation of the leukocytes themselves and the vascular endothelium to which leukocytes adhere (and migrate through), BWE administration leads to the extravasation of leukocytes into tissues, causing a significant decrease in the numbers of circulating monocytes together with a loss of mature neutrophils from the circulation [6]. Concentrations of both myeloperoxidase and elastase have been reported to be increased in the skin (of interest as it is also an epidermal tissue with similar cell types as lamellar tissue) of BWE-treated experimental horses [8, 20], which most likely reflects the reported influx of neutrophils into the dermal tissue of the skin at the same time points in the BWE model [16, 23]. An influx of neutrophils was also found to occur in both the lungs and liver at a developmental time point in a different study [24]. This showed not only that similar events occur in these visceral organs as occur in the lamellae, but also that similar inflammatory events occur in the visceral organs in the BWE model as are reported for organ injury in human sepsis [25]. In the lung and liver, an increase in gene expression of some of the same inflammatory molecules shown to increase in the lamellae (see below) have been reported in the BWE model at two developmental time points (1.5 h and 3–4 h; onset of leukopenia) after BWE administration, including cytokines (interleukin [IL]-1β, IL-6), chemokines (IL-8), and cyclooxygenase-2 (COX-2) [24]. Interestingly, unlike the lamellae, a significant increase in TNF-α gene expression was found in the liver and lungs at the early developmental time points [24]. Overall, the inflammatory molecule expression levels in the horse were much lower in the lungs and liver compared to those in the lamellae of the same animals, which indicates a much more fulminant inflammatory response in the lamellae than in other tissues during the early stages of laminitis. An influx of leukocytes (primarily eosinophils) into the large colon of BWE-treated horses has been reported in two studies [26, 27]. These data, when combined with a reported increase in colon wall permeability in one study [27], were interpreted as indicating that the absorption of bacterial toxins, as documented in the CHO model of laminitis, may play a role in BWE-induced laminitis. However, as the intestinal tract is also a 'target organ' of sepsis, the colon changes may merely reflect the systemic inflammatory response. Endotoxemia has never been detected in the BWE model. However, marked inflammatory changes have been documented to occur in tissues within 90 min of BWE administration [28]. This extremely short time span between ingestion and the first signs of systemic inflammation indicates that a toxic substance in the extract is absorbed in the upper gastrointestinal tract, which in turn induces the systemic inflammation; the nature of this substance is not known at present, however.

Lamellar Changes

As described in detail in various chapters of this book, the BWE model was used in many early studies of digital hemodynamics and local inflammatory events in the digital lamellae. By using an extracorporeal distal limb model to assess digital hemodynamics/Starling forces, further evidence of increased postcapillary pressure (indicating venoconstriction) occurring at the developmental stage (onset of leukopenia) was reported using the BWE model during the mid 1990s [9]. These investigations were followed many years later by *ex-vivo* studies of vasoactivity of the lamellar microvasculature in which the dysregulation of lamellar venule vasoactivity was reported [7, 29]. The BWE model was also used in the first studies documenting inflammatory events occurring in the lamellae during the developmental stages of laminitis. The initial report in 2001 used a molecular biology technique of *in-situ* hybridization to demonstrate lamellar cells expressing the pro-inflammatory cytokine IL-1β at the developmental time point (onset of leukopenia) in the BWE model [10]. Subsequent studies incorporated immunohistochemical and molecular biology techniques (e.g., RT-qPCR, differential mRNA display) to demonstrate the lamellar expression of inflammatory molecules and the influx of leukocytes at early developmental time points of the BWE model [11, 12, 16, 23]. The inflammatory events discovered in the BWE model (and later replicated in CHO models of laminitis) led to the establishment of the concept that lamellar injury occurring in cases of equine sepsis/endotoxemia most likely occurs due to a similar pathophysiology involving inflammatory mechanisms as had been reported to play a role in organ injury in human sepsis patients [25, 30]. These discoveries also assisted in delineating the different types of laminitis, and with the establishment of both BWE and CHO models as models of 'sepsis-related laminitis' [30].

BWE Versus CHO Models of Laminitis

The primary differences between the BWE and CHO models of sepsis-related laminitis are the more rapid onset of inflammatory events in the BWE model (with inflammatory events preceding the onset of lameness), and the decreased severity of lamellar injury (and reduced degree of lameness) induced. The more rapid onset of events in the BWE model may be associated with a toxin in BWE that is rapidly and directly absorbed through the small intestine into the circulation (within 90 min), whereas systemic inflammation in the CHO model only occurs after the excessive carbohydrate has reached the hindgut (cecum). It is then presumed that an injury to the mucosal lining allows the absorption of bacterial products that include endotoxin, with the first peak of detectable endotoxin being present at approximately 32 h after CHO administration [31–33]. The lack of structural failure of the lamellae in most horses treated with BWE is most likely due to the fact that there is only a transient presence of inflammatory molecules in the circulation following the administration of a single BWE bolus. In contrast, there is likely to be a much more sustained systemic inflammation due to severe injury to the large intestinal mucosa, as is documented to occur in the CHO model [17, 34].

References

1. True, R.G., Lowe, J.E., Heissen, J., *et al.* (1979) Black walnut shavings as a cause of acute laminitis. Proceedings of the Annual Convention. American Association of Equine Practitioners.
2. Uhlinger, C. (1989) Black walnut toxicosis in ten horses. *J. Am. Vet. Med. Assoc.*, **195**, 343–344.
3. Minnick, P.D., Brown, C.M., Braselton, W.E., *et al.* The induction of equine laminitis with an aqueous extract of the heartwood of black walnut (*Juglans nigra*). *Vet. Hum. Toxicol.*, **29**, 230–233.
4. True, R.G. and Lowe, J.E. (1980) Induced juglone toxicosis in ponies and horses. *Am. J. Vet. Res.*, **41**, 944–945.
5. Hurley, D.J., Hurley, K.A., Galland, K.L., *et al.* (2011) Evaluation of the ability of aqueous black walnut extracts to induce the production of reactive oxygen species. *Am. J. Vet. Res.*, **72**, 308–317.

6. Hurley, D.J., Parks, R.J., Reber, A.J., *et al.* (2006) Dynamic changes in circulating leukocytes during the induction of equine laminitis with black walnut extract. *Vet. Immunol. Immunopathol.*, **110**, 195–206.
7. Peroni, J.F., Harrison, W.E., Moore, J.N., *et al.* (2005) Black walnut extract-induced laminitis in horses is associated with heterogeneous dysfunction of the laminar microvasculature. *Equine Vet. J.*, **37**, 546–551.
8. Riggs, L.M., Franck, T., Moore, J.N., *et al.* (2007) Neutrophil myeloperoxidase measurements in plasma, laminar tissue, and skin of horses given black walnut extract. *Am. J. Vet. Res.*, **68**, 81–86.
9. Eaton, S.A., Allen, D., Eades, S.C., *et al.* (1995) Digital Starling forces and hemodynamics during early laminitis induced by an aqueous extract of black walnut (*Juglans nigra*) in horses. *Am. J. Vet. Res.*, **56**, 1338–1344.
10. Fontaine, G.L., Belknap, J.K., Allen, D., *et al.* (2001) Expression of interleukin-1beta in the digital laminae of horses in the prodromal stage of experimentally induced laminitis. *Am. J. Vet. Res.*, **62**, 714–720.
11. Waguespack, R.W., Cochran, A., and Belknap, J.K. (2004) Expression of the cyclooxygenase isoforms in the prodromal stage of black walnut-induced laminitis in horses. *Am. J. Vet. Res.*, **65**, 1724–1729.
12. Waguespack, R.W., Kemppainen, R.J., Cochran, A., *et al.* (2004) Increased expression of MAIL, a cytokine-associated nuclear protein, in the prodromal stage of black walnut-induced laminitis. *Equine Vet. J.*, **36**, 285–291.
13. Loftus, J.P., Belknap, J.K., and Black, S.J. (2006) Matrix metalloproteinase-9 in laminae of black walnut extract treated horses correlates with neutrophil abundance. *Vet. Immunol. Immunopathol.*, **113**, 267–276.
14. Belknap, J.K., Giguere, S., Pettigrew, A., *et al.* (2007) Lamellar pro-inflammatory cytokine expression patterns in laminitis at the developmental stage and at the onset of lameness: innate vs. adaptive immune response. *Equine Vet. J.*, **39**, 42–47.
15. Noschka, E., Moore, J.N., Peroni, J.F., *et al.* (2009) Thromboxane and isoprostanes as inflammatory and vasoactive mediators in black walnut heartwood extract induced equine laminitis. *Vet. Immunol. Immunopathol.*, **129**, 200–210.
16. Loftus, J.P., Black, S.J., Pettigrew, A., *et al.* (2007) Early laminar events involving endothelial activation in horses with black walnut-induced laminitis. *Am. J. Vet. Res.*, **68**, 1205–1211.
17. Pollitt, C.C. and Visser, M.B. (2010) Carbohydrate alimentary overload laminitis. *Vet. Clin. North Am. Equine Pract.*, **26**, 65–78.
18. Noschka, E., Moore, J.N., Peroni, J.F., *et al.* (2010) Evaluation of the possible role of prostaglandin F(2 alpha) in laminitis induced in horses by nasogastric administration of black walnut heartwood extract. *Am. J. Vet. Res.*, **71**, 186–193.
19. Moore, J.N., Garner, H.E., and Coffman, J.R. (1981) Haematological changes during development of acute laminitis hypertension. *Equine Vet. J.*, **13**, 240–242.
20. La Rebiere de Pouyade de G., Riggs, L.M., Moore, J.N., *et al.* (2010) Equine neutrophil elastase in plasma, laminar tissue, and skin of horses administered black walnut heartwood extract. *Vet. Immunol. Immunopathol.*, **135**, 181–187.
21. Belknap, J.K. (2010) Black walnut extract: an inflammatory model. *Vet. Clin. North Am. Equine Pract.*, **26**, 95–101.
22. Yin, C., Pettigrew, A., Loftus, J.P., *et al.* (2009) Tissue concentrations of 4-HNE in the black walnut extract model of laminitis: indication of oxidant stress in affected laminae. *Vet. Immunol. Immunopathol.*, **129**, 211–215.
23. Black, S.J., Lunn, D.P., Yin, C., *et al.* (2006) Leukocyte emigration in the early stages of laminitis. *Vet. Immunol. Immunopathol.*, **109**, 161–166.
24. Stewart, A.J., Pettigrew, A., Cochran, A.M., *et al.* (2009) Indices of inflammation in the lung and liver in the early stages of the black walnut extract model of equine laminitis. *Vet. Immunol. Immunopathol.*, **129**, 254–260.
25. Belknap, J.K., Moore, J.N., and Crouser, E.C. (2009) Sepsis – From human organ failure to laminar failure. *Vet. Immunol. Immunopathol.*, **129**, 155–157.
26. Chiavaccini, L., Hassel, D.M., Shoemaker, M.L., *et al.* (2011) Detection of calprotectin and apoptotic activity within the equine colon from horses with black walnut extract-induced laminitis. *Vet. Immunol. Immunopathol.*, **144**, 366–373.
27. McConnico, R.S., Stokes, A.M., Eades, S.C., and Moore, R.M. (2005) Investigation of the effect of black walnut extract on in-vitro ion transport and structure of equine colonic mucosa. *Am. J. Vet. Res.*, **66**, 243–247.
28. Noschka, E., Vandenplas, M.L., Hurley, D.J., *et al.* (2009) Temporal aspects of laminar gene expression during the developmental stages of equine laminitis. *Vet. Immunol. Immunopathol.*, **129**, 242–253.
29. Peroni, J.F., Moore, J.N., Noschka, E., *et al.* (2006) Predisposition for venoconstriction in the equine laminar dermis: implications in equine laminitis. *J. Appl. Physiol.*, **100**, 759–763.
30. Belknap, J.K. and Black, S.J. (2012) Sepsis-related laminitis. *Equine Vet. J.*, **44**, 738–740.
31. Garner, H.E., Moore, J.N., Johnson, J.H., *et al.* (1978) Changes in the caecal flora associated with the onset of laminitis. *Equine Vet. J.*, **10**, 249–252.
32. Garner, H.E., Coffman, J.R., Hahn, A.W., *et al.* (1975) Equine laminitis of alimentary origin: an experimental model. *Am. J. Vet. Res.*, **36**, 441–444.
33. Sprouse, R.F., Garner, H.E., and Green, E.M. (1987) Plasma endotoxin levels in horses subjected to carbohydrate induced laminitis. *Equine Vet. J.*, **19**, 25–28.
34. Faleiros, R.R., Leise, B.S., Watts, M., *et al.* (2011) Laminar chemokine mRNA concentrations in horses with carbohydrate overload-induced laminitis. *Vet. Immunol. Immunopathol.*, **144**, 45–51.

CHAPTER 10

Experimental Models of Laminitis: Hyperinsulinemia

Catherine McGowan and Janet Patterson-Kane

Introduction

Laminitis has been linked to insulin resistance and hyperinsulinemia in field studies since the 1980s [1, 2]. In ponies, cobs and certain other susceptible breeds, the term equine metabolic syndrome (EMS) has been introduced to describe the clustering of obesity, insulin resistance and laminitis, with episodes of laminitis in affected animals often associated with the grazing of carbohydrate-rich pastures [3–6]. In older horses and ponies, insulin resistance, hyperinsulinemia and laminitis may occur in association with pituitary pars intermedia dysfunction (PPID), potentially related to glucocorticoid antagonism of insulin [7,8]. Supporting the key role of hyperinsulinemia in the pathogenesis of laminitis in horses with PPID is the importance of serum insulin concentration as a prognostic indicator for survival. In one study, horses with very high serum insulin concentrations at presentation (>188 μ IU ml^{-1}) were much more likely to develop laminitis and survive less than two years after diagnosis than those with only moderate elevations or normal insulin concentrations (<62 μIU ml^{-1}) [8]. Common to both EMS and PPID appears to be disturbed glucose and insulin regulation and, most importantly, the development of insulin resistance manifesting as hyperinsulinemia. This form of laminitis, developing from hormonal influences rather than in association with proinflammatory and intestinal conditions, has been defined as 'endocrinopathic laminitis' [9].

Only relatively recently has endocrinopathic laminitis been shown to be the most common cause of laminitis in horses presenting primarily for lameness [10, 11] rather than secondary to presenting for acute severe disease and hospitalization [12]. Furthermore, until 2007, there was no experimental model of endocrinopathic laminitis. In this chapter, the hyperinsulinemic model of laminitis, possible mechanisms of laminitis development, and the histological findings in horses and ponies with hyperinsulinemic laminitis in comparison to classical descriptions of carbohydrate overload lesions will be discussed.

The Hyperinsulinemic Model of Laminitis

The hyperinsulinemic model of laminitis was developed to determine the effects of hyperinsulinemia, in the absence of cortisol manipulation, dietary modification, or hyperglycemia, on the lamellar integrity in the hooves of healthy ponies [13]. This objective was based on clinical observations that hyperinsulinemia was the hallmark of insulin resistance in the horse, that continued uncontrolled hyperinsulinemia reduced the prognosis in affected horses, and that the horse is apparently unique in that it can produce large amounts of insulin without the development of pancreatic exhaustion (as occurs in diabetes mellitus).

Laminitis was induced in 100% of normal ponies exposed to high concentrations of insulin (>1000 μIU ml^{-1}) while maintaining euglycemia of approximately 5 mmol l^{-1} (90 mg dl^{-1}) using a modified euglycemic–hyperinsulinemic clamp technique [13]. All treated ponies were healthy, young and non-obese, with no history of laminitis and no evidence of endocrine or other abnormalities on blood tests. Laminitis occurred relatively slowly (compared to models of sepsis-related laminitis) and in all four limbs, with the onset of lameness associated with laminitis (Obel grade 2) occurring by approximately 55 h. There was no evidence of gastrointestinal involvement or systemic illness throughout the experiment, and ponies remained apyrexic, as has been observed in field cases. All clinical and clinicopathological variables evaluated, including cortisol concentrations, were not significantly different from pre-infusion values throughout the clamp protocol [13]. This experiment was subsequently repeated in young athletic Standardbred ex-racehorses and the results were strikingly similar to those in the ponies, with the mean onset of Obel grade 2 laminitis of 46 h (range: 42–48 h) [14]. Although horses apparently developed laminitis more rapidly than ponies (possibly due to the effects of higher body weight on lamellar integrity), there was greater variability in the time of onset in ponies, with Obel grade 2 laminitis developing over a range of 37 to 61 h.

Equine Laminitis, First Edition. Edited by James K. Belknap and Raymond Geor.

Possible Mechanisms Involved

In both studies, laminitis was induced in horses and ponies with normal insulin sensitivity; the mean M-to-I ratios ($\times 10^{-6}$) were 3.07 ± 0.17 in horses and 3.5 ± 1.1 in ponies (where M and I are, respectively, the average rate of glucose infusion and the average serum insulin concentration during a defined period of the euglycemic–hyperinsulinemic clamp). There was also no clear indication of the development of insulin resistance at a whole-body level during the experimental protocol, with the rate of glucose infusion requiring minimal adjustments over the last half of the infusion periods. However, it is still possible that insulin infusion caused a downregulation of the insulin receptor and/or altered intracellular signaling that resulted in an altered insulin action, as has been shown in mice and humans [15]. The actions of insulin are mediated through the activation of insulin receptors on target cells. Upon binding of insulin, receptor activation involves the autophosphorylation of specific tyrosine residues on its cytoplasmic domain. These phosphotyrosine residues then serve as docking sites to recruit and activate a range of downstream proteins including the insulin receptor substrate (IRS) family proteins. These proteins regulate intracellular physiology, including the uptake and disposal of glucose and lipids, augmented by nitric oxide-mediated vasodilation. These 'metabolic' actions of insulin are mediated predominantly through the phosphoinositide 3-kinase (PI3)-kinase pathway. The MAPK pathways are also activated through IRS proteins; however, these predominantly convey 'mitogenic' signals, including an increased expression of endothelin-1 in the vasculature. Alterations in the balance of these pathways – in particular a dominance of signaling via the MAPK pathway – have been shown in murine models and human patients to be central to insulin resistance and subsequent metabolic dysfunction including dyslipidemia, vasculopathy, and coagulopathy [16]. In addition, a predominance of signaling via MAPK can result in endothelin-1-mediated vasoconstriction, an increased expression of vascular adhesion molecules and the proliferation of vascular smooth muscle cells, leading to vascular endothelial dysfunction. In studies using *ex-vivo* vascular ring models from equine digital vessels, preincubation in insulin for only 30 min resulted in a vasoconstriction response to the addition of further insulin [17]; there also was evidence of an intracellular pathway switch from PI3-kinase to MAPK dominance, with this effect being ameliorated by an inhibitor of MAPK. Similarly, lamellar arteries showed a reduced relaxation response to insulin following contraction with phenylephrine if preincubated with insulin, again reversed by a MAPK inhibitor [18]. This suggests that a form of insulin resistance associated with altered intracellular signaling can be rapidly induced under hyperinsulinemic conditions. In the hyperinsulinemic model system, horses showed downregulation of both the IGF1 receptor and insulin receptor following 48 h of insulin infusion, this being further evidence of potential insulin resistance [19].

The hyperinsulinemic model of laminitis has enabled an examination of the different mechanisms possibly involved in the development of endocrinopathic laminitis. Attention has been focused on the direct effects of insulin, including:

- Glucose deprivation
- Glucose excess
- Upregulation of matrix metalloproteases (MMPs)
- Vascular/blood flow effects
- A combination of pro-inflammatory/vascular effects

Glucose Deprivation

Glucose uptake impairment is a feature of insulin resistance; normally, insulin stimulates glucose dispersal into the tissues via insulin-dependent glucose transport proteins (especially GLUT4), particularly in muscle and adipose tissue. An underlying problem of insulin resistance is, therefore, a potential glucose deprivation of tissues causing cell death or damage. When hoof explants are incubated in the absence of glucose, or in the presence of a glucose uptake inhibitor, the layers of tissue separate rapidly, as they do when laminitis occurs [20]. Additionally, the hoof appears to utilize glucose at an exceptionally fast rate compared with most other tissues [21]. However, other studies have indicated that glucose uptake by hoof lamellae is insulin-independent – that is, glucose uptake is not dependent on or influenced by the presence of insulin [22]. When the glucose transport proteins were examined, there was a predominance of insulin-independent, type 1 glucose transport proteins (GLUT1) in lamellae [22, 23]. Together, these results provide compelling evidence that laminitis cannot be caused by the glucose deprivation that can result from insulin resistance.

Glucose Excess

The accumulation and glycation of glucose in endothelial cells (glucotoxicity) is a major pathogenic pathway in human insulin resistance. Glucotoxicity promotes the formation of advanced glycation end-products (AGEs), reducing nitric oxide production and leading to the induction of reactive oxygen species (ROS) and the promotion of endothelial expression of inflammatory mediators [24]. It was theorized that glucotoxicity may occur in the hyperinsulinemic model via insulin-mediated increased blood flow in an insulin-responsive animal. This theory was supported by the fact that tissues reliant on GLUT 1 transport proteins are more sensitive to increased blood flow and more susceptible to glycemic damage, similar to human retinal and cerebral hyperglycemic models [25]. However, the theory was not supported by research; during the prolonged euglycemic–hyperinsulinemic protocol, AGE accumulation was not evident until 48 h, there was no increase in gene expression of the equine-specific receptor for AGEs, and also no increase in ROS (protein carbonyl and malondialdehyde) [26].

Upregulation of MMPs

Matrix metalloproteinases have been studied extensively in inflammatory models of laminitis. While initial research focused on MMP2 and MMP9, it was realized that MMP9 was neutrophil-associated and not important in the developmental phase of laminitis [27]. Furthermore, Coyne *et al.* [28] found that an aggrecanase, ADAMTS4, was the most consistently proteolytic enzyme in naturally and experimentally occurring cases of non-endocrinopathic laminitis. However, in hyperinsulinemic laminitis, only minimal MMP activity was measured during the developmental and acute stages of laminitis, and only MMP9 was upregulated at later stages (48 h), correlating (as expected) with histological evidence of neutrophil infiltration [29].

Insulin Effects on Blood Flow

Insulin also has marked effects on stimulating vasodilation and blood flow in both small and large vessels via nitric oxide-mediated pathways [30]. Insulin resistance results in both reduced capillary recruitment and reduced vasodilation in animal models and in humans. Many of the effects on blood flow occur as a result of altered intracellular signaling, with a switch from primarily metabolic functions and vasodilation in health (PI3-kinase pathway) to primarily mitogenic, vasoconstrictive and proinflammatory effects (MAPK pathway) during insulin resistance [16]. In the hyperinsulinemic model, it was hypothesized that insulin-induced vasodilation may contribute to the development of laminitis. However, in separate experiments the local (intraosseous) infusion of a potent vasodilator, ATP–$MgCl_2$, did not result in any clinical or histological evidence of laminitis [31]. Another possibility is that the high insulin state results in vasoconstriction of the lamellar vasculature due to altered intracellular signaling. This was supported by the results of *ex-vivo* studies (as described above) where hyperinsulinemia induced the constriction of equine vascular rings and attenuated the lamellar arterial relaxation [17].

Histology

Studies investigating the histology of the hyperinsulinemic model of laminitis, as well as naturally occurring endocrinopathic cases, may provide important clues as to the pathogenesis of the condition. Histological descriptions of sepsis-related laminitis have typically focused on carbohydrate overload (CHO) models, spontaneous cases relating to endotoxemia and/or sepsis, or black walnut toxicosis [32–34]. The difficulty in interpreting histological lesions has been additionally complicated by the different time points examined in multiple experimental and clinical studies, the use of horses versus ponies (that are not necessarily directly comparable), and marked individual variations in the speed of progression and severity. The general impression gained from comparing CHO and hyperinsulinemia models, as detailed below, is that the lamellar structures have a limited repertoire of pathological responses to multiple etiological factors.

Elongation of the Secondary Epidermal Lamellae: A Common Early Lesion

In both CHO and hyperinsulinemia models, early histological changes include a loss of the normal perpendicular orientation of secondary epidermal lamellar nuclei relative to their basement membranes, with the nuclei becoming rounded, more central within the cytoplasm (rather than apical), more randomly oriented, and containing prominent nucleoli [35–37]. At the same time, the secondary epidermal lamellae (SEL) start to elongate, become narrower, develop tapered (rather than club-shaped) tips, and become more acutely angled to the primary epidermal lamellae (PEL) axis with irregularity of the PEL/SEL interface; they move towards each other and are often difficult to distinguish from one another. This has been seen in CHO model horses from 12 to 48 h [34] and in hyperinsulinemic horses from 6 to 48 h after initiation of the protocols (Fig. 10.1(a–c)), with changes evident before the development of clinical laminitis (personal observation). This type of elongation, tapering and more acute angulation of the SEL has also been seen in 'normal' three-year-old horses, possibly reflecting a subclinical pathology that develops from repeated cycles of mild injury [38] or underlying severe systemic disease.

There appears to be substantial between-horse variation in the rate at which the SEL elongate in the CHO model [35]. The PEL also elongate in hyperinsulinemic ponies and horses [37,39], but similar morphometric measurements have not been made for CHO models. It has been proposed that SEL elongation occurs due to the epithelial cells sliding past one another [40], but further analysis of ponies with hyperinsulinemic laminitis at approximately 50 h has indicated that the length of the cells themselves increased (i.e., they were stretched) in both forefeet and hindfeet, as did (to a lesser extent) their total number along the SEL length [39].

The Basement Membrane Focus

The most notable difference in lamellar pathology between the hyperinsulinemia and CHO models involves basement membrane (BM) lesions. In some studies of CHO laminitis, BM blebbing was evident at the tips of the SEL at 18 h and was more prominent after a further 30 h (with areas of crenation, 'blurring,' and discontinuity). This progressed rapidly as a 'de-gloving' process, with the BM forming form large vesicles at the SEL tips and then pulling away from the SEL, taking the dermal tissue and its blood supply with it [35]. This has also been seen in horses that (spontaneously) developed acute laminitis secondary to intestinal disease [32]. Interestingly, this has not been the finding of all investigators using CHO models; indeed, one group noted that the BM remained intact and attached during acute laminitis (during 4–8 h following the onset of lameness), even in horses sampled at equivalent time points [41]. Similarly, there has been minimal evidence of BM lesions in the hyperinsulinemia model; when present, the BM lesions have developed after SEL elongation. In the forefeet of ponies sampled at 55 h, there

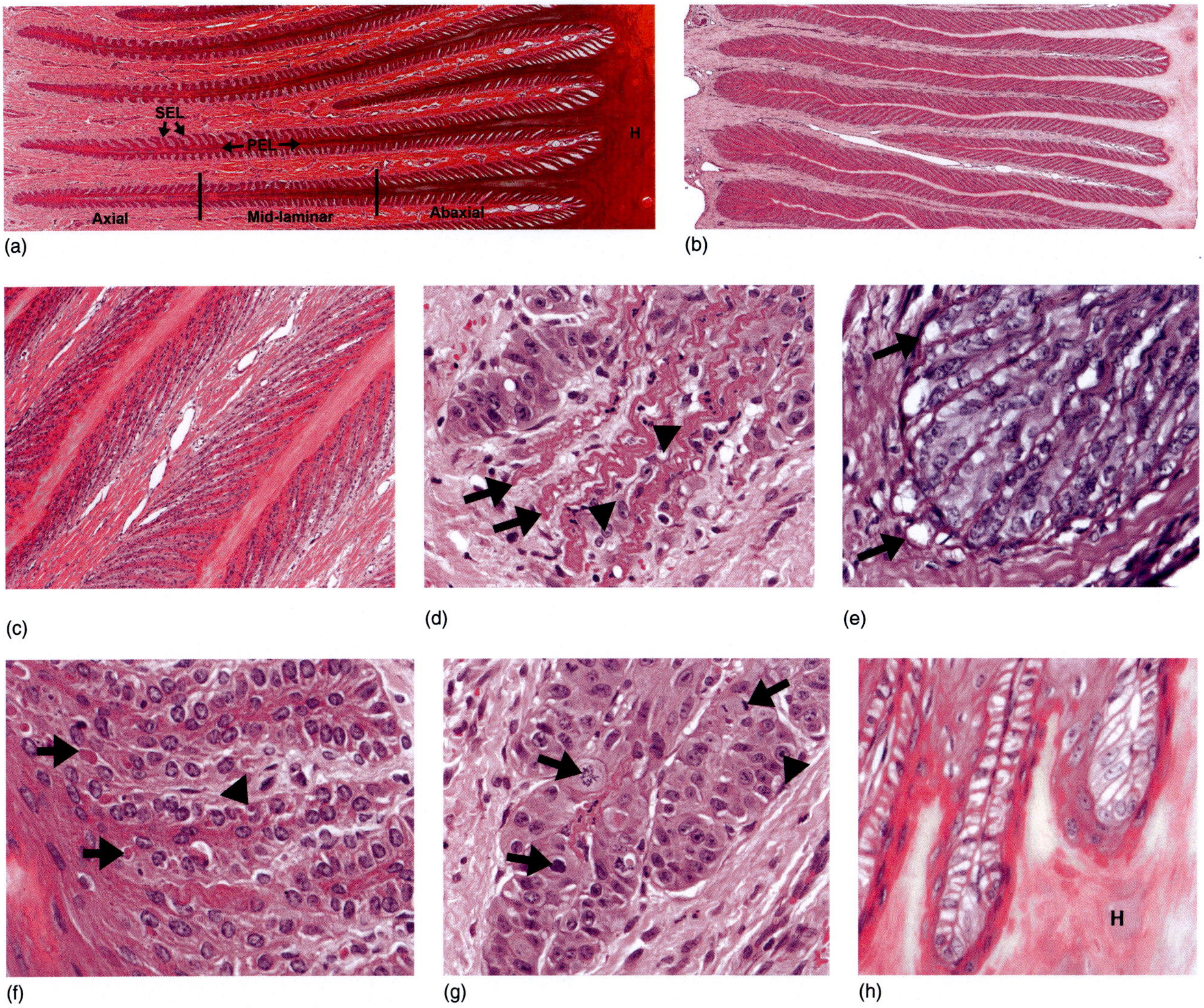

Figure 10.1 Photomicrographs of lamellae of hyperinsulinemia models. (a) Control horse, showing primary epidermal lamellae with keratinized cores (PEL), from each side of which originate large numbers of secondary epidermal lamellae (SEL). The SEL are relatively short, with club-shaped or rounded tips. The tips of the PEL are axial (closer to the third phalanx) and their bases are abaxial (i.e., they merge with the hoof horn (H)). Axial, mid-lamellar and abaxial regions are indicated. Hematoxylin and eosin (H&E) staining, original magnification × 40. (b) A hyperinsulinemic horse at 6 h, already showing marked elongation and narrowing (i.e., stretching) of the SEL; some of the SEL have tapered ends, and most are projecting at a more acute angle from their respective PEL. The elongation increased in severity from that time point up to 48 h (the last time point that was analyzed). H&E staining, original magnification × 40. (c) A hyperinsulinemic horse from another study, that was not showing clinical signs of laminitis at 48 h. The SEL, particularly in their mid-regions as shown in this image, are markedly elongated and narrowed with tapered ends. Only small numbers of apoptotic cells were noted and there was no basement membrane separation. H&E staining, original magnification × 100. Illustration courtesy of Dr Dianne McFarlane, Center for Veterinary Health Sciences, Oklahoma State University. (d) Separation and collapse of basement membrane material (arrows) from tips (axial regions) of the SEL of a hyperinsulinemic pony (with laminitis). Small numbers of neutrophils (arrowheads) are infiltrating it, this being a typical focus of the limited inflammatory response. H&E staining, original magnification ×400. (e) Blebbing (mild separation) of the basement membrane (arrows) from ends of some SEL at a PEL tip of a hyperinsulinemic horse at 24 h. Periodic acid–Schiff staining, original magnification ×400. (f) Secondary epidermal lamellae in the forefoot of a hyperinsulinemic pony (with laminitis); numerous round, hypereosinophilic apoptotic bodies are noted (arrows). Some of the apoptotic bodies have been phagocytosed by neighboring cells (arrowhead). H&E staining, original magnification × 400. (g) Cells comprising SEL at a PEL tip in the forefoot of a hyperinsulinemic pony (with laminitis); multiple mitotic figures in various phases are noted (arrows). The epidermal cells have large, variably sized nuclei containing large and often multiple nucleoli (arrowhead). H&E staining, original magnification × 400. (h) Cells adjacent to the hoof horn (H), in a hyperinsulinemic horse at 48 h that showed clinical signs of laminitis. The epidermal cells have a swollen, clear, vacuolated cytoplasm; that is, evidence of cellular injury that is reversible at this stage. Illustration courtesy of Dr Dianne McFarlane, Center for Veterinary Health Sciences, Oklahoma State University.

was a highly variable but predominantly mild and multifocal BM blebbing and separation from the most axial SEL only (at the PEL tips) in some animals [36]. In heavier Standardbred horses, however, BM lesions were first seen at 12 h and by 48 h were noted mainly in the forefeet (Fig. 10.1d,e). In some animals, these changes were limited to the most axial SEL (as in ponies), but, in others, SEL in the mid-lamellar and abaxial regions were also affected. In other words, there was a general increase in severity in horses when compared to ponies, with the involvement of greater numbers of SEL. However, BM lesions still did not approach the severity of some CHO models [35, 37]. There was a correlation in the hyperinsulinemic horses between the severity of BM lesions and a slight increase in the severity of clinical signs [37]. These findings indicate a spectrum of severity of BM separation in both models, with lesions evident after the SEL elongation phase described above.

The Role of Inflammation

In the hyperinsulinemia model, early inflammation is surprisingly limited, with neutrophils largely infiltrating into empty spaces formed by BMs that have separated from the SEL tips (Fig. 10.1d,e), and being seen around blood vessels adjacent to the PEL tips [35, 36]. Even at later stages when there has been extensive epidermal–dermal separation, the inflammation is minimal to mild, with little evidence of edema and vascular pathology, and it is largely focused on the epidermal compartment at the SEL tips [35]. In one study of the CHO model, the inflammatory cells (neutrophils and activated macrophages) were seen to have increased during the developmental phase, with more marked increases at the onset of lameness, including the infiltration of both PEL and SEL. Not all of these horses were noted to have BM pathology, and it was proposed that the inflammatory cells initiated BM damage [42]. However, other investigators identified BM changes by immunolabeling for cleaved anchoring filament proteins (from 12 h) at time points preceding the inflammatory cell infiltration [43, 44]. In general, the severity of inflammation seems to be greater in the CHO models, and, in both models, cellular infiltration follows the development of BM lesions and alterations in SEL architecture [37, 43–45]. However, the extent and severity of inflammation in both models are significantly less than would be expected in many other tissues subjected to similar levels of cellular stress and mechanical compromise, including (non-hoof) skin.

Cell Death and Proliferation

The spatial and temporal relationship between SEL stretching, cell death, and proliferation is complex [39], but the comparison of different models may again indicate how the disease develops and progresses. Apoptotic cells occur at low numbers in normal lamellar tissue [36, 39, 46]. In a study of sepsis-related laminitis using a CHO model, there were increased numbers of apoptotic (terminal deoxynucleotidyl transferase dUTP nick end labeling [TUNEL]-positive) cells at 10–18 h in the axial, mid-lamellar and abaxial regions; horses with acute naturally occurring laminitis also had elevated numbers of apoptotic cells, but those with chronic disease did not [46]. A similar increase has been reported in the hyperinsulinemia model, with apoptotic cell numbers significantly increased in the mid-lamellar and abaxial regions in all feet of ponies sampled at 50 h (Fig. 10.1f) [39]. In horses, the number of proliferating (TPX2-positive) cells was increased at 24 and 48 h without regional localization [45]. However, in ponies, the number of proliferating cells was increased in the forefeet in the axial SEL only, with remarkable increases in the sizes of nuclei and numbers of mitotic figures (Fig. 10.1g) [39]. In the hindfeet of the same ponies (that typically bear a lower proportion of the bodyweight), numbers of proliferating cells were increased in all regions, and there was a greater increase in the number of cells forming the elongated SEL [39]. It is possible that the disease is less advanced or progressive in ponies versus horses, and in the hindfeet of the ponies versus their forefeet. Vacuolar cell swelling (reversible pathology) has also been noted in both the CHO and hyperinsulinemia models (Fig. 10.1h). Thus, there appears to be a spectrum of reversible and irreversible cellular injury and death that (as would be expected) shows marked variation between individuals.

What Occurs Following the Acute Phase of Laminitis?

The classical lesions of necrosis, edema, hemorrhage, and vascular thrombosis have not been compared between different models, nor have there been comparisons of natural disease to the various laminitis models. The suspicion, however, would be that these lesions are sequelae that develop regardless of the inciting pathology – that is, they are related to the physical tearing of tissue once the lamellar tissue is sufficiently weakened [47]. In the CHO model, severe alterations in PEL and SEL microanatomy were reported seven days after laminitis induction, including fragmentation of the PEL into isolated, irregularly sized and shaped epidermal islands and columns [48]. Similar changes have been noted in naturally occurring cases of endocrinopathic laminitis [49].

Conclusions and Further Study

Research studies using the hyperinsulinemic model of laminitis in ponies and horses has shown this condition to be a disease syndrome with a clinical and histological spectrum that overlaps with other models of laminitis. With early subclinical lesions and SEL elongation evident after just 6 h of euglycemic hyperinsulinemia or 48 h of hyperglycemia [50], it is tempting to speculate that this early lesion might eventually result in hoof wall deformations and altered growth, namely laminitic rings. At the more severe end of the disease spectrum, the rapid development of irreversible mechanical destabilization and necrosis is possible. It is currently unknown exactly how hyperinsulinemia causes such rapid and profound histological changes; likewise, even the fundamental issue of whether these effects are due to direct insulin toxicity or are secondary to other mechanisms is unclear (i.e., is this rapidly induced insulin resistance or does the condition manifest as altered intracellular signaling pathways). Nonetheless, the presence of microscopic lesions has provided several theories with which to work, and further investigations of lesions seen in naturally occurring endocrinopathic laminitis are ongoing at the present authors' laboratory and other laboratories around the world.

References

1. Coffman, J.R. and Colles, C.M. (1983) Insulin tolerance in laminitic ponies. *Can. J. Comp. Med.*, **47** (3), 347–351.
2. Jeffcott, L.B., Field, J.R., McLean, J.G., *et al.* (1986) Glucose tolerance and insulin sensitivity in ponies and Standardbred horses. *Equine Vet. J.*, **18**, 97–101.
3. Treiber, K.H., Kronfeld, D.S., Hess, T.M., *et al.* (2006) Evaluation of genetic and metabolic predispositions and nutritional risk factors for pasture-associated laminitis in ponies. *J. Am. Vet. Med. Assoc.*, **228**, 1538–1545.
4. Carter, R.A., Treiber, K.H., Geor, R.J., *et al.* (2009) Prediction of incipient pasture-associated laminitis from hyperinsulinaemia, hyperleptinaemia and generalised and localised obesity in a cohort of ponies. *Equine Vet. J.*, **41**, 171–178.
5. Walsh, D.M., McGowan, C.M., McGowan, T., *et al.* (2009) Correlation of plasma insulin concentration with laminitis score in a field study of Equine Cushing's Disease and Equine Metabolic Syndrome. *J. Equine Vet. Sci.*, **29**, 87–94.
6. Frank, N., Geor, R.J., Bailey, S.R., *et al.* (2010) Equine metabolic syndrome. *J. Vet. Intern. Med.*, **24**, 467–475.
7. McGowan, C.M., Frost, R., Pfeiffer, D.U., *et al.* (2004) Serum insulin concentrations in horses with equine Cushing's syndrome: response to a cortisol inhibitor and prognostic value. *Equine Vet. J.*, **36**, 295–298.
8. McGowan, C.M. and Neiger, R. (2003) Efficacy of trilostane for the treatment of equine Cushing's syndrome. *Equine Vet. J.*, **35**, 414–418.
9. Johnson, P.J., Messer, N.T., Slight, S.H., *et al.* (2004) Endocrinopathic laminitis in the horse. *Clin. Tech. Equine Pract.*, **3**, 45–56.
10. Donaldson, M.T., Jorgensen, A.J., and Beech, J. (2004) Evaluation of suspected pituitary pars intermedia dysfunction in horses with laminitis. *J. Am. Vet. Med. Assoc.*, **224**, 1123–1127.
11. Karikoski, N.P., Horn, I., McGowan, T.W., *et al.* (2011) The prevalence of endocrinopathic laminitis among horses presented for laminitis at a first-opinion/referral equine hospital. *Domest. Anim. Endocrinol.*, **41**, 111–117.
12. Parsons, C.S., Orsini, J.A., Krafty, R., *et al.* (2007) Risk factors for development of acute laminitis in horses during hospitalization: 73 cases (1997–2004). *J. Am. Vet. Med. Assoc.*, **230**, 885–889.
13. Asplin, K.E., Sillence, M.N., Pollitt, C.C., *et al.* (2007) Induction of laminitis by prolonged hyperinsulinaemia in clinically normal ponies. *Vet. J.*, **174**, 530–535.
14. de Laat, M.A., McGowan, C.M., Sillence, M.N., *et al.* (2010) Equine laminitis: induced by 48 hours of hyperinsulinaemia in Standardbred horses. *Equine Vet. J.*, **42**, 129–135.
15. Shanik, M.H., Xu, Y., Skrha, J., *et al.* (2008) Insulin resistance and hyperinsulinemia: is hyperinsulinemia the cart or the horse? *Diabetes Care*, **Suppl. 2**, S262–S268.
16. Kim, J.A., Montagnani, M., Koh, K.K., *et al.* (2006) Reciprocal relationships between insulin resistance and endothelial dysfunction: molecular and pathophysiological mechanisms. *Circulation*, **113**, 1888–1904.
17. Venugopal, C.S., Eades, S., Holmes, E.P., *et al.* (2011) Insulin resistance in equine digital vessel rings: an in vitro model to study vascular dysfunction in equine laminitis. *Equine Vet. J.*, **43**, 744–749.
18. Wooldridge, A.A., Waguespack, R.W., Schwartz, D.D., *et al.* (2014) Vasorelaxation responses to insulin in laminar vessel rings from healthy, lean horses. *Vet J.*, **202**, 83–88.
19. de Laat, M.A., Pollitt, C.C., Kyaw-Tanner, M.T., *et al.* (2013) A potential role for lamellar insulin-like growth factor-1 receptor in the pathogenesis of hyperinsulinaemic laminitis. *Vet. J.*, **197**, 302–306.
20. Pass, M.A., Pollitt, S., and Pollitt, C.C. (1998) Decreased glucose metabolism causes separation of hoof lamellae in vitro: A trigger for laminitis? *Equine Vet. J.*, **26**, 133–138.
21. Wattle, O. and Pollitt, C.C. (2004) Lamellar metabolism. *Clin. Tech. Equine Pract.*, **13**, 22–33.
22. Asplin, K.E., Curlewis, J.D., McGowan, C.M., *et al.* (2011) Glucose transport in the equine hoof. *Equine Vet. J.*, **43**, 196–201.
23. deLaat, M.A., Clement, C.K., Pollitt, C.C., *et al.* (2013) Regulation of glucose transport during equine hyperinsulinaemia. Proceedings American College of Veterinary Internal Medicine, abstract.
24. Hartge, M.M., Unger, T., and Kintscher, U. (2007) The endothelium and vascular inflammation in diabetes. *Diabetes Vasc. Dis. Res.*, **4**, 84–8.
25. Kumagai, A.K. (1999) Glucose transport in brain and retina: implications in the management and complications of diabetes. *Diabetes Metab. Res. Rev.*, **15**, 261–273.
26. de Laat, M.A., Kyaw-Tanner, M.T., Sillence, M.N., *et al.* (2012) Advanced glycation endproducts in horses with insulin-induced laminitis. *Vet. Immunol. Immunopathol.*, **145**, 395–401.
27. Loftus, J.P., Johnson, P.J., Belknap, J.K., *et al.* (2009) Leukocyte-derived and endogenous matrix metalloproteinases in the lamellae of horses with naturally acquired and experimentally induced laminitis. *Vet. Immunol. Immunopathol.*, **129**, 221–230.
28. Coyne, M.J., Cousin, H., Loftus, J.P., *et al.* (2009) Cloning and expression of ADAM-related metalloproteases in equine laminitis. *Vet. Immunol. Immunopathol.*, **129**, 231–241.
29. de Laat, M.A., Kyaw-Tanner, M.T., Nourian, A.R., *et al.* (2011) The developmental and acute phases of insulin-induced laminitis involve minimal metalloproteinase activity. *Vet. Immunol. Immunopathol.*, **140**, 275–281.
30. Rattigan, S., Bussey, C.T., Ross, R.M., *et al.* (2007) Obesity, insulin resistance, and capillary recruitment. *Microcirculation*, **14**, 299–309.
31. de Laat, M.A., Pollitt, C.C., Walsh, D.M., *et al.* (2012) Persistent digital hyperthermia over a 48 h period does not induce laminitis in horses. *Vet. J.*, **192**, 435–440.
32. Roberts, E.D., Ochoa, R., and Haynes, P.F. (1980) Correlation of dermal-epidermal lamellar lesions of equine hoof with various disease conditions. *Vet. Pathol.*, **17**, 656–656.
33. Galey, F.D., Whiteley, H.E., Goetz, T.E., Kuenstler, A.R., Davis, C.A., and Beasley, V.R. (1991) Black walnut (*Juglans nigra*) toxicosis: a model for equine laminitis. *J. Comp. Pathol.*, **104**, 313–326.

34. Croser, E.L. and Pollitt, C.C. (2006) Acute laminitis: description evaluation of serial hoof biopsies. *AAEP Proceedings*, **52**, 542–546.
35. Pollitt, C.C. (1996) Basement membrane pathology: a feature of acute equine laminitis. *Equine Vet. J.*, **28**, 38–46.
36. Asplin, K.E., Patterson-Kane, J.C., Sillence, M.N., *et al.* (2010) Histopathology of insulin-induced laminitis in ponies. *Equine Vet. J.*, **42**, 700–706.
37. de Laat, M.A., Van Eps, A.W., McGowan, C.M., Sillence, M.N., and Pollitt, C.C. (2011) Equine laminitis: comparative histopathology 48 hours after experimental induction with insulin or alimentary oligofructose in Standardbred horses. *J. Comp. Pathol.*, **145**, 399–409.
38. Lancaster, L.S., Bowker, R.M., and Mauer, W.A. (2007) Density and morphologic features of primary epidermal lamellae in the feet of 3-year-old racing Quarter horses. *Am. J. Vet. Res.*, **68**, 11–19.
39. Karikoski, N.P., Patterson-Kane, J.C., Asplin, K.E., *et al.* (2014) Cellular changes in elongated secondary epidermal lamellae in an equine model of insulin-induced laminitis. *Am. J. Vet. Res.*, **75**, 161–168.
40. Pollitt, C.C. (2004) Equine laminitis. *Clin. Tech. Equine Pract.*, **3**, 34–44.
41. Morgan, S.J., Hood, D.M., Wagner, I.P., *et al.* (2003) Submural histopathologic changes attributable to peracute laminitis in horses. *Am. J. Vet. Res.*, **64**, 829–834.
42. Faleiros, R.R., Johnson, P.J., Nuovo, G.J., *et al.* (2011) Lamellar leukocyte accumulation in horses with carbohydrate overload-induced laminitis. *J. Vet. Intern. Med.*, **25**, 107–115.
43. Visser, M.B. and Pollitt, C.C. (2011) The timeline of lamellar basement membrane changes during equine laminitis development. *Equine Vet. J.*, **43**, 471–477.
44. Visser, M.B. and Pollitt, C.C. (2011) Lamellar leukocyte infiltration and involvement of IL-6 during oligofructose-induced equine laminitis development. *Vet. Immunol. Immunopathol.*, **144**, 120–128.
45. de Laat, M.A., Patterson-Kane, J.C., Pollitt, C.C., *et al.* (2013) Histological and morphometric lesions in the pre-clinical, developmental phase of insulin-induced laminitis in Standardbred horses. *Vet. J.*, **195**, 305–312.
46. Faleiros, R.R., Stokes, A.M., Eades, S.C., *et al.* (2004) Assessment of apoptosis in epidermal lamellar cells in clinically normal horses and those with laminitis. *Am. J. Vet. Res.*, **65**, 578–585.
47. Baxter, G.M. (1986) Equine laminitis caused by distal displacement of the distal phalanx: 12 cases (1976–1985). *J. Am. Vet. Med. Assoc.*, **189**, 326–329.
48. Van Eps, A.W. and Pollitt, C.C. (2009) Equine laminitis model: lamellar histopathology seven days after induction with oligofructose. *Equine Vet. J.*, **41**, 735–740.
49. Karikoski, N.P., McGowan, C.M., Singer, E.R., *et al.* (2015) Pathology of natural cases of equine endocrinopathic laminitis associated with hyperinsulinemia. *Vet. Pathol.*, **52**, 945–950.
50. de Laat, M.A., Sillence, M.N., McGowan, C.M., *et al.* (2012) Continuous intravenous infusion of glucose induces endogenous hyperinsulinaemia and lamellar histopathology in Standardbred horses. *Vet. J.*, **191**, 317–322.

CHAPTER 11

Hemodynamic Events in Laminitis

John F. Peroni, Susan C. Eades and Simon R. Bailey

Introduction

There is compelling evidence that the pathogenesis of Equine Laminitis includes increased post-capillary resistance, forces favorable for the formation of interstitial edema, and eventual loss of the supporting structures of the hoof. Recent evidence indicates that lamellar veins from healthy horses are predisposed to venospasm, and that intragastric administration of either black walnut extract or an overload of carbohydrate to experimentally induce laminitis selectively alters the responses of these vessels to vasoactive substances implicated in the pathogenesis of the disease.

The discovery of these pathophysiologic events raises more questions than it answers regarding the mechanism by which the integrity of lamellar attachments is lost. It has not been determined whether the increased resistance is of sufficient magnitude and duration to create ischemia or hypoxia of the lamellar tissues. The alteration of vascular resistance may result from endothelial dysfunction which may contribute to imbalances of signaling pathways that favor inflammatory events. Altered endothelial function also leads to platelet activation, causing further disruption of microvascular homeostasis. Endothelial cells and platelets both release mediators which alter the tone of the underlying vascular smooth muscle cells, potentially complicating the flow disturbances which could further reduce perfusion and oxygenation. Interstitial edema can impair the diffusion of oxygen to tissues, impair the removal of toxic byproducts of cellular metabolism, and alter cell–matrix and cell–cell signaling. Although there is clear evidence for altered vascular resistance and forces favorable for interstitial edema formation from reports using experimental models of sepsis-related laminitis (SRL), the exact contribution of any of these vascular factors to the destruction of the lamellar attachments has not been determined.

Vascular Physiology

The lamellar corium/dermis derives most of its blood supply from the branches of the terminal arterial arch, which perforates the distal phalanx. Numerous anastomoses form an arterial network beneath and between the epidermal lamellae, allowing blood to flow proximally to the coronary circumflex artery and distally to the solear circumflex artery [1]. The parallel veins join to form the terminal vein, which is joined by branches from the venous plexus to form the palmar digital vein. The majority of veins within the foot lack valves, a feature that can be exploited clinically in performing contrast radiography (venograms) or administering drugs into the foot (i.e., regional limb perfusion). The direction of flow within the veins is dependent upon weight-bearing forces [1].

In the lamellar dermal microcirculation, numerous (500 cm^{-2}) [2] arteriovenous anastomoses (AVA) connect the axial arteries to axial veins [3]. These anastomoses occur in the dermis of the coronary band, in the neurovascular structures within the dermal lamellae, and at the entrance to and along the length of the dermal lamellae [2, 4]. There are several hypotheses regarding the physiologic function of these anastomoses. One hypothesis is that, during long periods of cold exposure, the anastomoses open to allow for warming of the feet by increasing blood flow [4]. Another hypothesis is that high-pressure fluctuations that occur in the digit during galloping or jumping cause the anastomoses to open in order to diffuse the tremendous increases in pressure and may act as a 'safety valve' for the vasculature [2].

The branching of arteries results in the formation of small muscular arterioles, the function of which is to reduce blood flow coming from the larger arteries and thereby to prevent damage to the fragile capillaries that connect the arterial and venous vascular systems. Through a complex interaction with autacoids, hormones, and neurotransmitters released at sympathetic synapses, flow through the microcirculation is regulated by altering the tone of the arteriolar smooth muscle. The lamellar capillary is characterized histologically by a single layer of endothelial cells (approximately 0.25 μm), a basement membrane and, instead of a smooth muscle cell layer, envelopment by a population of pericytes or 'Rouget' cells that varies in distribution within the vascular beds [5, 6].

It is across this large surface area of the capillary bed that the majority of nutrients, cellular waste products, other solutes,

Equine Laminitis, First Edition. Edited by James K. Belknap and Raymond Geor.

water and oxygen are exchanged between the blood and the cellular constituents of the lamellae. The exchange of solutes and water usually results from simple diffusion according to solute concentration gradients and hydrostatic and osmotic pressures (i.e., Starling forces).

Research in other species has demonstrated that the distribution of blood flow in microvascular beds results from a complex interaction between endothelial and vascular smooth muscle cells of arteriolar, capillary, and venular vessel segments involving tissue metabolic demand, autacoids, hormones, and sympathetic neurotransmitters [7, 8]. Endothelial-derived substances including nitric oxide, hyperpolarizing factor, and prostacyclin cause the relaxation of vascular smooth muscle and vasodilation [7]. Endothelial cells also produce contracting agents such as endothelin-1 and angiotensin II which increase vascular tone [7]. Vascular shear stress activates endothelial nitric oxide synthase, increasing nitric oxide production which dilates vascular smooth muscle thereby increasing local blood flow [7]. The release of nitric oxide from hemoglobin in venules with reduced PO_2 also contributes to vasodilation [8]. Therefore, a number of signaling pathways responsive to metabolic and hemodynamic alterations integrate the function of smooth muscle and endothelial cells in the arteriolar, capillary, and venular segments.

The Study of Digital and Lamellar Blood Flow

The anatomy of the distal limb creates unique challenges with regards to blood flow regulation, specifically regarding venous return from the hoof capsule to the heart. It is thought that palmar digital veins may contribute to the regulation of blood flow via the maintenance of vascular tone. These veins feature a well-developed muscular layer when compared with veins in other tissues and other species [9]. In the standing horse, digital blood flow is thought to be relatively stable during minor shifts in weight-bearing [10]. In contrast, capsular blood flow reportedly decreases as weight-bearing increases during weight-shifting from one front hoof to the other [10].

Recognizing the need to measure lamellar blood flow in horses, investigators have employed several techniques including laser Doppler flowmetry, arteriography, nuclear scintigraphy, thermography, and infrared spectroscopy. Total digital arterial blood flow includes both capillary (nutrient) flow and flow through AVA. Techniques must differentiate these two forms of flow in order to discern whether reduced capillary perfusion (and therefore tissue perfusion likely leading to lamellar hypoxia) are important pathophysiologic mechanisms in laminitis. Increased total flow with shunting through AVA could be accompanied by reduced capillary perfusion and tissue hypoxia. Some of the above-mentioned techniques have been evaluated only in normal horses, whereas others have been used in experimentally induced laminitis and in horses in which drugs were administered in an attempt to alter blood flow [11–21]. The principal limitations of the aforementioned methods are associated with their use to monitor changes in blood flow in lamellar tissue beneath a relative impenetrable keratinized hoof capsule.

Some of the earliest attempts to measure digital blood flow employed nuclear scintigraphy. Hood and Kirker-Head *et al.* injected ^{99m}Te-tagged macroaggegrated albumin into the median palmar artery and immediately scanned the foot with a gamma camera, after which the radionuclide distribution and intensity were graded subjectively [20, 21]. The investigational and clinical use of nuclear scintigraphy for blood flow measurements has been extensive [22]. Distribution of the injected radionuclide is based on the size of the injected particles and the relative size of the arterioles, venules, capillaries, and AVA. Estimates of lamellar capillary size (ca. 10–20 μm) suggest that medium-sized particles (<30 μm) will pass through arterioles (ca. 30–70 μm), lodge in the capillaries, and be detected with the gamma camera, suggesting normal capillary blood flow [2, 22]. Small radionuclides (ca.10–18 μm) will pass through capillaries undetected and are more appropriate for indicator studies where venous blood is sampled and assayed for the radionuclide, allowing calculation of the blood flow based on indicator dilution principles [2, 22]. The opening of AVA (ca. 20–60 μm in diameter) allows mid-sized and small radionuclides to pass through the vasculature without gamma-camera detection, confounding estimates of nutrient flow. Because there is overlap in the size of vessel segments and variation in the size of radionuclides in aggregated preparations, it is difficult to make accurate estimates of capillary versus AVA flow with scintigraphy [2, 22]. Two studies using nuclear scintigraphy technique in traditional carbohydrate overload (CHO) models of laminitis for measuring lamellar blood flow involved either intra-arterial injection of ^{99m}Te macroaggregated albumin (MAA) [20, 21] or the intravenous injection of ^{99m}Te-diethylenetriamine pentaacetic acid (PAA) into arteries (brachiocephalic or common palmar artery) proximal to the digit [17].

Estimation of digital blood flow via thermography makes the assumption that hoof wall surface temperatures under conditions of constant ambient temperature result from changes in lamellar blood flow. Hoof surface temperature could change similarly with alterations in flow through the capillaries or AVA, so this technique provides insight into total flow but not tissue perfusion. Lamellar blood flow was evaluated in two studies using CHO models of sepsis-related laminitis. However, the two studies demonstrated conflicting results, with a decrease in hoof wall surface temperature (blood flow) in one study [23] and an increase in hoof wall surface temperature in the other [24]. Changes in either capillary perfusion or AVA flow could account for these changes. The differences in results between these studies may have been due to differences in ambient temperature, differences in the induction model and severity of disease, and the fact that hoof wall surface temperature was monitored at different times in the two studies.

More information regarding oxygen delivery via capillary perfusion is available with application of near-infrared (NIR) spectroscopy, which employs changes in light absorption at selected NIR wavelengths to detect digital hemodynamic changes [25]. The spectra investigated correspond to the absorption of cytochrome aa3 (assessment of reduction–oxidation status) and oxyhemoglobin. Using this technique, manual occlusion of the digital vessels was demonstrated to cause an increase in deoxyhemoglobin, a decrease in oxyhemoglobin, and a decrease in cytochrome aa3 typical of ischemia [25]. However, NIR spectroscopy has not been applied to the study of acute laminitis.

Doppler blood flow measurements have been used to evaluate total digital blood flow and lamellar blood flow in pharmacologic studies and investigations of endotoxemia and laminitis. Laser Doppler blood flow probes have been applied to large digital arteries for the study of total digital arterial blood flow, and have been used to measure small vessel flow in lamellar tissue by drilling multiple 8-mm holes in the hoof wall and placing a Doppler probe directly against the lamellar tissue [10–16, 19]. Laser Doppler blood flow measurements are not entirely reliable due to measurements being affected by: (i) any change in angle of the ultrasound beam in relation to the lamellar vessels being assessed; and (ii) the induction of local inflammation by tissue manipulation necessary for probe placement. These factors create a great deal of variability in flow measurements, even in normal horses [19]. This technique is also reported to be sensitive to movement artifacts that can artificially increase recorded values, and it only measures blood flow in the small area located directly under the tip of the probe. Consequently, its clinical applicability is limited, at best. Furthermore, laser Doppler perfusion probes cannot determine the relative contribution of flow through AVA and capillaries to the measurements obtained, and thus are unable to truly assess tissue capillary perfusion. Laser Doppler flowmetry has been used in studies to detect fluctuations in lamellar blood flow during the prodromal stages of black walnut extract (BWE)-induced laminitis in horses [12] and during the administration of a low dose of endotoxin (0.1 $\mu g\ kg^{-1}$ over 30 min) to normal horses [11]. In the BWE study, triphasic fluctuations in lamellar blood flow were detected, with an initial decrease followed by an increase and then a second decrease in flow near the onset of clinical signs of laminitis [12]. In the endotoxin study, although differences ($p < 0.05$) in palmar digital artery blood flow were detected using a perivascular ultrasonic flow probe, only a trend ($p > 0.05$) for a decrease in lamellar blood flow was detected with laser Doppler flowmetry [11].

Early in laminitis research, in-vivo arteriography was used to examine digital blood supply in normal horses and ponies, and horses and ponies with either experimentally induced laminitis (CHO model), or naturally induced chronic laminitis [26, 27]. This technique revealed a marked reduction in blood supply to affected hooves, including lamellar tissue, and corroborated the histopathologic identification of microthrombi in dermal veins of affected feet from three of four ponies with laminitis [18]. However, it was not possible to quantify alterations in blood flow. Furthermore, the results of studies performed by one of the present authors indicated that the contrast media used for both arteriography and venography caused the contraction of lamellar vessels *in vitro* (J. Peroni *et al*., unpublished results, 2009), most likely due to the hypertonic nature of these solutions. Rosenstein *et al.* similarly documented inconsistent but dramatic changes in equine digital arterial pressure after the intra-arterial injection of contrast media [28]. Additionally, it is difficult to use venography to accurately assess digital hemodynamics due to the fact that the tourniquet application required for venography increases venous pressure which in turn initiates compensatory hemodynamic mechanisms thereby altering blood flow measurements [29].

Lamellar Hemodynamics

The digital arteries and veins supplying the hoof have unique vasoactive properties, when compared to vessels of similar size from other tissue beds or species. Digital vessels are very sensitive to vasoconstrictor substances, particularly to norepinephrine and endothelin [30,31]. Furthermore, isolated digital veins *in vitro* are more sensitive than arteries to vasoconstrictors such as angiotensin, thromboxane, norepinephrine, serotonin, and endothelin [30]. Similarly, the results of an in-vitro study of palmar digital arteries and veins indicate that the incubation of digital veins with either acepromazine or isoxsuprine results in a greater degree of dilation than occurred when digital arteries were treated in the same manner [32]. In subsequent studies, the incubation of digital vessels with acetylcholine, prostaglandin E_2, and prostaglandin I_2 (prostacyclin) resulted in vasodilation through the endothelium-dependent actions of nitric oxide, as was demonstrated by the abolition of vasodilatory responses to the three mediators by inclusion of the nitric oxide synthase inhibitor NG-nitro-L-arginine methyl ester [32–34]. Furthermore, the palmar digital vessels were determined to be more responsive to 5-hydroxytryptamine (serotonin) than either facial or tail arteries [35].

Hemodynamic studies utilizing palmar digital veins and arteries have contributed significantly to the present understanding of digital hemodynamics. However, the results of these studies are difficult to interpret in the context of laminitis pathogenesis. In fact, profound differences in the contractile properties of large palmar digital vessels and small lamellar arteries and veins have been reported [30, 32, 36]. Studies that utilize conduit arteries (i.e., digital arteries and veins) may have very limited relevance to both the physiology and pathophysiology of laminitis. It has been established that changes in the caliber of conduit arteries and veins have little effect on vascular resistance. As a result, studies have been performed utilizing isolated small lamellar arteries and veins in order to understand the regulation of pre- and post-capillary resistance within the digits of horses [36–38].

Venoconstrictive amine compounds produced by equine hindgut bacteria during the fermentation of nonstructural carbohydrates have been identified [39]. These compounds are capable of causing digital vessel constriction (either directly or indirectly) and platelet activation displacing serotonin *in vitro* [40]. The infusion of these amines caused a reduction of digital blood flow along with increased plasma concentrations of serotonin [41]. Although these compounds have not been studied sufficiently in horses with laminitis, the fecal and plasma concentrations of these amines are increased during the first few hours after free-choice feeding of highly digestible carbohydrate feeds [42, 43]. Therefore, amines generated by hindgut bacteria could alter digital and lamellar vascular function during laminitis.

Using a technique that allowed in-vitro studies of small lamellar arteries and veins, Robertson *et al.* reported that the induction of capacitative calcium entry elicits vasoconstriction in equine lamellar veins, but not in lamellar arteries [38]. It was proposed that capacitative calcium should be considered as a potential mechanism by which selective venoconstriction occurs in horses during the development of acute laminitis [38]. In other studies, it was also shown that induction of the prodromal stages of laminitis [44, 45] resulted in a consistent and selective dysfunction of the lamellar veins, and that there may be a predisposition for venoconstriction within the vasculature of the equine digit [36]. These findings may help to explain why laminitis can result from a variety of pathological systemic conditions [36].

Impact of Hemodynamic Events in Laminitis

A central premise which was the basis for many of these studies was the notion that a common feature of laminitis is a reduction in digital perfusion, leading to ischemia of the dermal tissues within the digit. Although the presence of lamellar ischemia in the early stages of laminitis is controversial (especially in sepsis-related and endocrinopathic laminitis), disruptions of microvascular flow are likely to play a role in other events such as lamellar edema and the adhesion of platelets and leukocytes to the lamellar endothelium. Although a reduction in tissue perfusion – including lamellar perfusion – has been purported to be the result of vasospasm of arterial/arteriolar components of the tissue vasculature [21, 23, 27, 46–49], there is convincing evidence that constriction of the lamellar veins more than the arteries is responsible for the increased post-capillary resistance that occurs during development of the disease [44, 45]. While some have questioned whether the lamellar veins contain sufficient smooth muscle to significantly alter the hemodynamics of the foot, the impact of these small vessels should not be considered in isolation. Although individual lamellar veins constrict to a meager extent *in vitro* when compared to their arterial counterparts, when working in concordance within the digit their overall effects can be profound. Furthermore, lamellar veins have a relatively inelastic vascular wall, and are situated between the hoof wall and distal phalanx, resulting in a low-compliance bed [9].

The combined effects of low compliance and high sensitivity to venoconstrictive substances predispose the equine digit to increased venous and hydrostatic pressures, thereby increasing the likelihood for lamellar edema formation. Unfortunately, the microcirculation of the equine foot is poorly adapted to handling edema. For example, the main safety factors that counteract edema formation under normal circumstances are capillary permeability, precapillary-to-postcapillary resistance, and lymphatic drainage. For those tissues in which capillary permeability is low, the endothelium serves as a barrier to the movement of fluid and protein, resulting in a high gradient between capillary and tissue oncotic pressures. This situation favors the movement of fluid from the tissues into the capillary lumen. However, the results of studies performed to measure Starling forces within the equine digit have indicated that the normal equine digital capillary bed is highly permeable to fluid and macromolecules [9]. In fact, this capillary bed retains only 67% of the macromolecules within the vasculature, and thus is as 'leaky' as the capillary beds of another organ documented to have highly permeable vascular beds, namely the lung [35]. The end result is a high concentration of protein in the interstitial space, which would favor edema formation.

Under normal circumstances, far more of the resistance to blood flow in the equine digit is due to precapillary resistance (92%) than to postcapillary resistance (8%); this results in reduced capillary pressure and the hydrostatic pressure for transcapillary fluid filtration. The precapillary-to-postcapillary resistance ratio in healthy horses is comparable to that in other musculoskeletal beds in other species [9]. Allen *et al.* reported that the induction of laminitis with either the CHO or BWE model resulted in increased postcapillary resistance to flow [(9], increased tissue pressure, and a reduction in the precapillary-to-postcapillary resistance ratio [44, 45, 50, 51], all of which again favor the formation of edema within the digit.

The third factor that normally protects vascular beds from edema formation is lymphatic drainage. The lymphatic vessels of the equine digit are few in number and small in diameter; therefore, it is unlikely that the lymphatic circulation can effectively protect the foot against edema when capillary hydrostatic forces are increased [50]. It is unfortunate that the lamellar lymphatic system has not been the focus of greater scientific scrutiny. The development of modern lymphology in people may provide further insight into the role of this system in the pathophysiology of laminitis.

It is difficult to reliably and consistently document the effects of edema on the lamellar tissues. The earliest detected – but not consistently reproducible – histological changes in the lamellae after onset of lameness induced using the CHO model include the swelling of endothelial cells and mild edema formation [47]. Subsequently, lamellar capillaries become congested with erythrocytes, perivascular leukocyte infiltration occurs that then dissipates as the inflammatory cells migrate into the lamellar interstitium, and arteriolar endothelial cells become deformed as a result of cytoplasmic processes that extend into the lumen [46, 52]. Lesions detected later include microvascular thrombi, severe edema, and hemorrhage occurring within the primary dermal lamellae. The induction of laminitis also results in structural changes in the lamellae themselves, the earliest reported changes being thinning and lengthening of the lamellar structures accompanied by reduction, flattening, and displacement of epithelial cells [52]. The secondary lamellae become redirected such that lamellae nearer the base of the dermal lamellae are directed toward the distal phalanx, and those nearer the lamellar tips are directed toward the hoof wall. Morphologic alterations that have been detected later include swelling, vacuolization, nuclear swelling and/or pyknosis, and leukocytic infiltration of the secondary dermal lamellae [52].

The inability to consistently document digital edema histologically is likely due to the fact that dehydration steps in the preparation of histologic sections commonly mask any edema present in tissue sections; this fact is underlined by a study in which signs of lamellar edema (in the sublamellar dermis) were present upon magnetic resonance imaging of limbs from clinical cases of horses at risk of or with acute laminitis, whereas histologic sections of the same lamellae did not document edema [53]. The presence of lamellar edema can have several significant pathophysiologic consequences during laminitis. Small increases in tissue pressure are capable of collapsing capillary beds and significantly reducing capillary flow [44, 54]. Edema increases the diffusional barrier for oxygen, nutrients, and toxic byproducts of cellular metabolism, thereby impairing tissue function [55]. Any alteration in the flow of interstitial fluid through the tissue can alter the tethering forces at cell–matrix connections and the signaling function of cell–cell interactions [56]. Additionally, a 4% increase in extravascular water can change the composition of plasma membranes, affecting cell signaling [57]. Hence, further studies of the potential impact of edema on lamellar function/failure are required.

Alterations in endothelial cell function during the onset of acute laminitis may affect endothelium-dependent vasodilatory actions normally present in the vasculature, and therefore alter the responsiveness of the digital vasculature to vasoactive agents. The results of in-vitro studies have indicated that normal equine digital vessels have a substantial capacity for endothelial-dependent relaxation by nitric oxide (NO), a gas produced by the endothelium that normally accounts for approximately 70–85% of the maximal vascular smooth muscle relaxation induced by the vasodilator acetylcholine [30, 58]. However, it is not clear whether any endothelial dysfunction occurring in laminitis involves a dysfunction in muscarinic receptors (receptors that respond to acetylcholine) the cellular signaling processes that initiate Ca^{2+}-dependent activation of NO-synthase, or downregulation of NO-synthase, the enzyme that produces NO. Because factors that regulate endothelial cell activity – including its production of the potent vasodilator NO – are influenced by humoral factors, hypoxia, sheer stress, and nerve stimulation [8], it is possible that imbalances in the release or action of endothelial factors contribute to microvascular dysfunction in laminitis. Importantly, endothelial dysfunction is a predominant feature of ischemia–reperfusion injury [59], and inflammatory responses similar to those in laminitis occur after the reperfusion of ischemic tissues. In horses with CHO-induced laminitis, acetylcholine-mediated relaxations of digital vessels *in vitro* are reduced, suggesting that the NO-producing capacity of the digital vascular endothelium is reduced [34]. This lack of NO-mediated vasodilation would render the vessels more sensitive or vulnerable to vasoconstrictive agents [34].

Taken together, the results of studies employing CHO- and BWE-induced laminitis show that temporally related increases and decreases in digital blood flow are present in SRL. Although a variety of techniques has been used, these methods do not differentiate between capillary flow and AVA flow. Increases in total digital blood flow [12, 20, 24], decreases in total blood flow [12, 21, 23, 51], and minimal change have all been documented. However, because results using these techniques are similar for both AVA and capillaries, conclusions regarding the perfusion of lamellar tissues cannot be made [60]. It is possible that reductions in digital perfusion are transient with a low likelihood of substantial ischemia during the early stages of laminitis. With regards to the possibility of ischemia–reperfusion injury in laminitis, Loftus and colleagues failed to observe any significant increase in xanthine oxidase generation in BWE-induced laminitis, an event that would have occurred had ischemia/hypoxia been present [61]. Regardless of whether lamellar ischemia is present at the early stages of laminitis, there is little question that the lamellar microvasculature is traumatically disrupted in most cases in which displacement of the distal phalanx occurs; this would likely result in at least a furthering of lamellar epidermal hypoxia, as not only is the dermal vasculature disrupted but the distance between the lamellar epidermis and the dermal vasculature is increased by the lamellar separation.

As described in more detail elsewhere in this book (see Chapter 12), platelet activation has been observed in the early stages of CHO-induced laminitis with both platelet–platelet and platelet–neutrophil aggregates present [62]. The administration of an inhibitor of platelet activation prevented lameness in CHO-induced laminitis [63]. Activation of p38 MAP kinase in circulating platelets indicating platelet activation has also been reported in the oligofructose model of SRL [64]. Platelet activation was associated with increased plasma concentrations of endotoxin and the potent vascular smooth muscle vasoconstrictors serotonin and thromboxane [64]. These mediators could either initiate or perpetuate endothelial activation and dysfunction or systemic and local/lamellar inflammatory disease [65, 66], including the activation of endothelial leukocyte adhesion molecule expression and associated increases in leukocyte infiltration into lamellar tissues.

References

1. Kainer, R.A. (1989) Clinical anatomy of the equine foot. *Vet. Clin. North Am. Equine Pract.*, **5** (1), 1–27.
2. Pollitt, C.C. and Molyneux, G.S. (1990) A scanning electron microscopical study of the dermal microcirculation of the equine foot. *Equine Vet. J.*, **22** (2), 79–87.
3. Pollitt, C.C. (2004) Anatomy and physiology of the inner hoof wall. *Clin. Tech. Equine Pract.*, **3** (1), 3–21.
4. Molyneux, G.S., Mogg, K.C., Haller, C.J., and Pollitt, C. (1994) The structure, innervation and location of arteriovenous anastomoses in the equine foot. *Equine Vet. J.*, **26** (4), 305–312.
5. Hirschi, K.K. and D'Amore, P.A. (1996) Pericytes in the microvasculature. *Cardiovasc. Res.*, **32** (4), 687–698.
6. Khimenko, P.L., Barnard, J.W., Moore, T.M., and Taylor, A.E. (1994) Vascular permeability and epithelial transport effects on lung edema formation in ischemia and reperfusion. *J. Appl. Physiol.*, **77** (3), 1116–1121.
7. Lilly, B. (2014) We have contact: endothelial cell-smooth muscle cell interaction. *Physiology*, **29**, 234–241.
8. Sehgal, S.S. (2005) Regulation of blood flow in the microcirculation. *Microcirculation*, **12**, 33–45.
9. Allen, D., Korthuis, R.J., and Clark, S. (1988) Evaluation of Starling forces in the equine digit. *J. Appl. Physiol.*, **64** (4), 1580–1583.
10. Hunt, R.J., Brandon, C.I., and McCann, M.E. (1994) Effects of acetylpromazine, xylazine, and vertical load on digital arterial blood flow in horses. *Am. J. Vet. Res.*, **55** (3), 375–378.
11. Ingle-Fehr, J. and Baxter, G. (1998) Evaluation of digital and laminar blood flow in horses given a low dose of endotoxin. *Am. J. Vet. Res.*, **59**, 192–197.
12. Adair, H.S., Goble, D.O., Schmidhammer, J.L., and Shires, M.H. (2000) Laminar microvascular flow, measured by means of laser Doppler flowmetry, during prodromal stages of black walnut-induced laminitis in horses. *Am. J. Vet. Res.*, **61**, 862–868.
13. Adair, H.S., Goble, D.O., Shires, M.H., and Sanders, W.L. (1994) Evaluation of laser-Doppler flowmetry for measuring coronary band and laminar microcirculatory blood-flow in clinically normal horses. *Am. J. Vet. Res.*, **55**, 445–449.
14. Ingle-Fehr, J. and Baxter, G. (1999) The effect of oral isoxuprine and pentoxifylline on digital and laminar blood flow in healthy horses. *Vet. Surg.*, **28**, 154–157.
15. Adair, H., Schmidhammer, J.L., and Rivera-Walker, C. (1997) Effects of acepromazine maleate, isoxuprine hydrochloride and prazosin hydrochloride on laminar blood flow in healthy horses. *J. Equine Vet. Sci.*, **17**, 599–603.
16. Ingle-Fehr, J. and Baxter, G. (1998) Evaluation of digital and laminar blood flow in horses given a low dose of endotoxin. *Am. J. Vet. Res.*, **59**, 192–196.
17. Trout, D., Hornof, W.J., Linford, R.L., and O'Brien, T.R. (1990) Scintigraphic evaluation of digital circulation during the developmental and acute phases of equine laminitis. *Equine Vet. J.*, **22**, 416–421.
18. Weiss, D., Trent, A., and Johnston, G. (1995) Prothrombotic events in the prodromal stages of acute laminitis in horses. *Am. J. Vet. Res.*, **56**, 986–991.
19. Menzies-Gow, N. and Marr, C. (2007) Repeatability of Doppler ultrasonographic measurement of equine digital blood flow. *Vet. Radiol. Ultrasound*, **48** (3), 281–285.
20. Kirker-Head, C.A., Stephens, K.A., Toal, R.L., and Goble, D.O. (1986) Circulatory and blood gas changes accompanying the development and treatment of induced laminitis. *Equine Vet. Sci.*, **6** (6), 293–301.
21. Hood, D.M., Amoss, M.S., Hightower, D., McDonald, D.R., McGrath, F.P., McMullan, W.C., and Scrutchfield, W.L. (1978) Equine laminitis I: radioisotope analysis of the hemodynamics of the foot during acute disease. *J. Equine Med. Surg.*, **2**, 439–444.
22. Henriksen, J.H., Jensen, G.B., and Larsson, H.B. (2014) A century of indicator dilution technique. *Clin. Physiol. Funct. Imaging*, **34** (1), 1–9.
23. Hood, D.M., Wagner, I.P., and Brumbaugh, G.W. (2001) Evaluation of hoof wall surface temperature as an index of digital vascular perfusion during the prodromal and acute phases of carbohydrate-induced laminitis in horses. *Am. J. Vet. Res.*, **62**, 1167–1172.
24. Pollitt, C.C. and Davies, C.T. (1998) Equine laminitis: its development coincides with increased sublamellar blood flow. *Equine Vet. J. Suppl.*, **26**, 125–132.
25. Hinckley, K.A., Fearn, S., Howard, B.R., and Henderson, I.W. (1995) Near infrared spectroscopy of pedal haemodynamics and oxygenation in normal and laminitic horses. *Equine Vet. J.*, **27** (6), 465–470.
26. Ackerman, N., Garner, H.E., Coffman, J.R., and Clement, J.W. (1975) Angiographic appearance of the normal equine foot and alterations in chronic laminitis. *J. Am. Vet. Med. Assoc.*, **166** (1), 58–62.
27. Coffman, J.R., Johnson, J.H., Guffy, M.M., and Finocchio, E.F. (1970) Hoof circulation in equine laminitis. *J. Am. Vet. Med. Assoc.*, **156** (1), 76–83.
28. Rosenstein, D.S., Bowker, R.M., and Bartlett, P.C. (2000) Digital angiography of the feet of horses. *Am. J. Vet. Res.*, **61** (3), 255–259.
29. Johnson, P.C. (1989) The myogenic response in the microcirculation and its interaction with other control systems. *J. Hypertens. Suppl.*, **7** (4), S33–S39.
30. Baxter, G.M., Laskey, R.E., Tackett, R., and Allen, D. (1989) In vitro reactivity of digital arteries and veins to vasoconstrictive mediators in healthy horses and in horses with early laminitis. *Am. J. Vet. Res.*, **50** (4), 508–517.
31. Katz, L.M., Marr, C.M., and Elliott, J. (2003) Characterization and comparison of the responses of equine digital arteries and veins to endothelin-1. *Am. J. Vet. Res.*, **64** (11), 1438–1443.
32. Baxter, G.M., Tackett, R.L., and Moore, J.N. (1989) Reactivity of equine palmar digital arteries and veins to vasodilating agents. *Vet. Surg.*, **18** (3), 221–226.
33. Cogswell, A.M., Johnson, P.J., and Adams, H.R. (1995) Evidence for endothelium-derived relaxing factor/nitric oxide in equine digital arteries. *Am. J. Vet. Res.*, **56** (12), 1637–1641.
34. Schneider, D.A., Parks, A.H., Eades, S.C., and Tackett, R. (1999) Palmar digital vessel relaxation in healthy horses and in horses given carbohydrate. *Am. J. Vet. Res.*, **60** (2), 233–239.
35. Bailey, S.R. and Elliott, J. (1998) Plasma 5-hydroxytryptamine constricts equine digital blood vessels in vitro: implications for pathogenesis of acute laminitis. *Equine Vet. J.*, **30** (2), 124–130.

36. Peroni, J.F., Moore, J.N., Noschka, E., Grafton, M.E., Aceves-Avila, M., Lewis, S.J., *et al.* (2006) Predisposition for venoconstriction in the equine laminar dermis: implications in equine laminitis. *J. Appl. Physiol.*, **100** (3), 759–763.
37. Peroni, J.F., Harrison, W.E., Moore, J.N., Graves, J.E., Lewis, S.J., Krunkowsy, T.M., *et al.* (2005) Black walnut extract-induced laminitis in horses is associated with heterogeneous dysfunction of the laminar microvasculature. *Equine Vet. J.*, **37** (6), 546–551.
38. Robertson, T.P., Peroni, J.F., Lewis, S.J., and Moore, J.N. (2005) Effects of induction of capacitative calcium entry on equine laminar microvessels. *Am. J. Vet. Res.*, **66** (11), 1877–1880.
39. Bailey, S.R., Baillon, M.L., Rycroft, A.N., Harris, P.A., and Elliot, J. (2003) Identification of equine cecal bacteria producing amines in an in vitro model of carbohydrate overload. *Appl. Environ. Microbiol.*, **69**, 2087–2093.
40. Elliott, J., Berhane, Y., and Bailey, S.R. (2003) Effects of monoamines formed in the cecum of horses on equine digital blood vessels and platelets. *Am. J. Vet. Res.*, **64**, 1124–1131.
41. Bailey, S.R., Menzies-Gow, N.J., Marr, C.M., and Elliot, J. (2004) The effects of vasoactive amines found in the equine hindgut on digital blood flow in the normal horse. *Equine Vet. J.*, **36**, 267–272.
42. Crawford, C., Sepulveda, M.F., Elliott, J., Harris, P.A., and Bailey, S.R. (2007) Dietary fructan carbohydrate increases amine production in the equine large intestine: Implications for pasture-associated laminitis. *J. Anim. Sci.*, **85**, 2949–2958.
43. Botteon, P.T.L., Ferraz, V.P., Glória, M.B.A., Melo, M.M., Paes Leme, F.O., Faleiros, R.R., *et al.* (2008) Plasma concentrations of tryptamine, tyramine and phenylethylamine in horses under the effect of carbohydrate overload and non-steroidal anti-inflammatory compounds. *Pesq. Vet. Bras.*, **28**, 299–302.
44. Allen, D., Clark, E.S., Moore, J.N., and Prasse, K.W. (1990) Evaluation of equine distal Starling forces and haemodynamics during early laminitis. *Am. J. Vet. Res.*, **51**, 1930–1934.
45. Eaton, S., Allen, D., Eades, S.C., and Schneider, D.A. (1995) Digital Starling forces and haemodynamics during early laminitis induced by an aqueous extract of black walnut (*Juglans nigra*) in horses. *Am. J. Vet. Res.*, **56**, 321–334.
46. Hood, D. (1993) The role of vascular mechanisms in the development of acute equine laminitis. *J. Vet. Intern. Med.*, **7**, 228–234.
47. Hood, D. (1999) The pathophysiology of developmental and acute laminitis. *Vet. Clin. North Am.*, **15**, 321–334.
48. Hood, D., Amoss, M., and Grosenbaugh, D. (1990) Equine laminitis: a potential model for Raynaud's phenomenon. *Angiology*, **41**, 270–277.
49. Galey, F.D., Twardock, A.R., Goetz, T.E., Schaeffer, D.J., Hall, J.O., and Beasley, V.R. (1990) Gamma scintigraphic analysis of the distribution of perfusion of blood in the equine foot during black walnut (*Juglans nigra*)-induced laminitis. *Am. J. Vet. Res.*, **51** (4), 688–695.
50. Allen, D., Jr, Korthuis, R.J., and Clark, E.S. (1988) Capillary permeability to endogenous macromolecules in the equine digit. *Am. J. Vet. Res.*, **49** (9), 1609–1612.
51. Robinson, N.E., Scott, J.B., Dabaney, J.M., and Jones, G.A. (1976) Digital vascular responses and permeability in equine alimentary laminitis. *Am. J. Vet. Res.*, **37** (10), 1171–1176.
52. Mostafa, M.B. (1986) Studies on experimental laminitis in the horse. Thesis, Cairo University, College of Veterinary Medicine.
53. Arble, J.B., Mattoon, J.S., Drost, W.T., Weisbrode, S.E., Wassenaar, P.A., Pan, X., *et al.* (2009) Magnetic resonance imaging of the initial active stage of equine laminitis at 4.7 T. *Vet. Radiol. Ultrasound*, **50** (1), 3–12.
54. Hargens, A.R., Akeson, W.H., Mubarak, S.J., Garetto, L.P., and Akeson, W.H. (1977) Interstitial fluid pressure in muscle and compartment syndromes in man. *Microvasc. Res.*, **14**, 1–10.
55. Demling, R.H. and LaLonde, C.K. (1993) Pulmonary edema: pathophysiology, methods of measurement, and clinical importance in acute respiratory failure. *New Horiz.*, **1** (3), 371–380.
56. Miserocchi, G., Negrini, D., Passi, A., and De Luca, G. (2001) Development of lung edema: interstitial fluid dynamics and molecular structure. *Am. Physiol. Soc.*, **16** (2), 66–71.
57. Palestino, P., Calvi, C., Conforti, E., Botto, L., Fenoglio, C., and Miserocchi, G. (2002) Composition, biophysical properties, and morphometry of plasma membranes in pulmonary interstitial edema. *Am. J. Physiol. Lung Cell. Mol. Physiol.*, **282** (2), L1382–L1390.
58. Stokes, A.M., Venugopalan, C.S., Hosgood, G., Eades, S.C., and Moore, J.N. (2006) Comparison of 2 endothelin-receptor antagonists on in vitro responses of equine palmar digital arterial and venous rings to endothelin-1. *Can. J. Vet. Res.*, **70** (3), 197–205.
59. Lefer, A.M. and Lefer, D.J. (1991) Endothelial dysfunction in myocardial ischemia and reperfusion: role of oxygen derived free radicals. *Basic Res. Cardiol.*, **86** (Suppl. 2), 109–116.
60. Robinson, N.E. (1990) Digital blood flow, arteriovenous anastomoses and laminitis. *Equine Vet. J.*, **22** (6), 381–383.
61. Loftus, J.P., Belknap, K., Stankiewicz, K.M., and Black, S.J. (2007) Laminar xanthine oxidase, superoxide disumtase, and catalase activities in the prodromal state of black-walnut induced equine laminitis. *Equine Vet. J.*, **39** (1), 48–53.
62. Weiss, D.J., Trent, A.M., and Johnston, G. (1995) Prothrombotic events in the prodromal stages of acute laminitis in horses. *Am. J. Vet. Res.*, **56** (3), 986–991.
63. Weiss, D.J., Evanson, O.A., McClenahan, D., Fagliari, J.J., Dunnwiddie, C.T., and Wells, R.E. (1995) Effect of a competitive inhibitor of platelet aggregation on experimentally induced laminitis in ponies. *Am. J. Vet. Res.*, **59** (7), 814–817.
64. Bailey, S.R., Adair, H.S., Reinemeyer, C.R., Morgan, S.J., Brooks, A.C., Longhofer, S.L., *et al.* (2009) Plasma concentrations of endotoxin and platelet activation in the developmental stage of oligofructose-induced laminitis. *Vet. Immunol. Immunopathol.*, **129** (3-4), 167–173.
65. Loftus, J.P., Black, S.J., Pettigrew, A., Abrahamsen, E.J., and Belknap, J.K. (2007) Early laminar events involving endothelial activation in horses with black walnut-induced laminitis. *Am. J. Vet. Res.*, **68** (11), 1205–1211.
66. Eades, S.C., Stokes, A.M., Johnson, P.J., LeBlanc, C.J., Ganjam, V.K., Buff, P.R., *et al.* (2007) Serial alterations in digital hemodynamics and endothelin-1 immunoreactivity, platelet-neutrophil aggregation, and concentrations of nitric oxide, insulin, and glucose in blood obtained from horses following carbohydrate overload. *Am. J. Vet. Res.*, **68** (1), 87–94.

CHAPTER 12

The Role of Thrombosis and Coagulation in Equine Laminitis

Simon R. Bailey

Introduction

There is good evidence from many studies to show that platelet activation and microthrombus formation occurs in carbohydrate overload (CHO) models of sepsis-related laminitis (SRL; both starch overload and oligofructose overload models). With endocrinopathic laminitis, there is no evidence suggesting that platelet activation or microthrombus formation occurs in insulin dysregulation related to either equine metabolic syndrome (EMS) or pituitary pars intermedia dysfunction (PPID).

The role of platelet activation and coagulation abnormalities in the pathogenesis of the inflammatory/sepsis-related forms of laminitis (CHO or black walnut extract; BWE) is not clear, but possible mechanisms include the release of vasoconstrictors from platelets, activation of the vascular endothelium, and a degree of blood vessel blockage due to microthrombi. Platelet–neutrophil aggregates have been detected in the blood of horses during the developmental phase of starch overload laminitis, which is also evidence of platelets having a proinflammatory role in these forms of laminitis, enhancing the effects of bacterial toxins such as lipopolysaccharide in the circulation.

Although perhaps not critical in the disease progression, these mechanisms could certainly augment and amplify the ongoing key pathophysiological processes. Considering that antiplatelet therapies remain one of the few groups of drugs shown to be effective in reducing the severity of laminitis in experimental models, the role of coagulation and thrombosis should not be ignored in our understanding of the complex cascade of pathways leading to the development of acute laminitis.

Thrombosis and coagulation are essential events in maintaining homeostasis in the normal animal, with a primary function being a protective role in focal areas of injury allowing clots to form to decrease hemorrhage and limit the systemic effects of a focal site of disease/injury. Due to the adverse effects of excessive activation of pathways associated with thrombosis and coagulation, there are many physiologic 'checks and balances' to keep the system in hand. Unfortunately, similar to other homoeostatic mechanisms (e.g., leukocyte activation) which have evolved to protect the animal from focal injury or disease, excessive systemic activation as occurs in endotoxemia/sepsis can lead to widespread and local disruption of thrombosis and coagulation mechanisms, with deleterious consequences for the animal. Additionally, severe focal inflammation/injury as occurs in laminitis may also adversely activate events related to thrombosis and coagulation, exacerbating the ongoing injurious events in a vital tissue such as the lamellae. Both of these events are commonly occurring in SRL. In this chapter, the normal physiologic processes involved in thrombosis and coagulation (with emphasis on platelets) will first be reviewed, followed by a discussion of the possible involvement of these mechanisms in the pathophysiology of laminitis. Although attention will be focused primarily on SRL, endocrinopathic and supporting limb laminitis will also be discussed.

Overview of Thrombosis, Platelets, and Coagulation

Thrombosis is the formation of a blood clot inside a blood vessel, which may to a greater or lesser extent obstruct the flow of blood through the vasculature. The blood clot is formed by platelets (thrombocytes) and fibrin.

Platelets

Platelets are small, non-nucleated cells that circulate in the vascular system, their primary function being to initially arrest bleeding from a damaged vessel by rapidly creating a platelet plug. Platelets do not replicate by cell division but rather originate from the bone marrow, where they are shed off into the blood stream from large megakaryocytes [1]. The average lifespan of circulating platelets in the horse is estimated to between seven and nine days, similar to other species [2, 3]. The platelet surface is replete with functional receptors to facilitate platelet activation and interactions with subendothelial matrix of the

Equine Laminitis, First Edition. Edited by James K. Belknap and Raymond Geor.

vessel lumen, other blood cells, and other platelets. The platelet also contains granules that, when activated, can fuse with the platelet membrane and thereby release their contents outside the cell. The granules are categorized into the larger α-granules, the smaller dense granules (δ-granules), and lysosomes (also known as γ-granules). α-granules contain a large variety of biological active substances involved in hemostasis, including proteoglycans, adhesive glycoproteins (fibronectin, von Willebrand factor [vWF), and thrombospondin), hemostasis factors (fibrinogen, factors V, VIII, XI, and XIII, and plasminogen), protease inhibitors (α_2-macroglobulin and α_2-antitrypsin), and cellular growth factors/mitogens such as *platelet-derived growth factor* (PDGF), transforming growth factor-β (TGFβ), endothelial cell growth factor (ECGF), insulin-like growth factor (IGF), and vascular endothelial growth factor (VEGF) [4]. The dense granules mainly contain ions, such as calcium and magnesium and smaller signal molecules such as adenosine 5′-diphosphate (ADP), adenosine 5′-triphosphate (ATP) and serotonin. Lysosomes contain acid hydrolase, cathepsin and lysosomal membrane proteins [5]. A rapid and effective response from the platelets is vital. Platelets are highly sensitive towards external stimuli and can undergo a rapid activation process that is enhanced by intrinsic activation feedback loops in the form of autocrine and paracrine signaling (for a review, see Ref. [6]).

Following vessel wall injury, platelets rapidly adhere to exposed elements in the subendothelial matrix, thus initiating the first step in the hemostatic response leading to the formation of a platelet plug. This primary adhesion is mediated by the synergistic function of several receptors on the platelet surface. Collagen is the main component of the subendothelial matrix, and is also considered to play the principal role in the adhesion process of platelets to the vessel wall. In the subendothelial basement membrane, the main constituents important in platelet adhesion have been determined as collagen type I and type III [7]. The local flow conditions are also important in determining platelet behavior. Blood is always moving inside the vessels, but the conditions can vary from almost stagnant to extremely high flow rates. The velocity of blood, in relation to the stationary vessel wall, gives rise to shear forces in the moving blood. These forces will lead to a higher concentration of erythrocytes and other large blood cells in the middle of the high-velocity flow, and the platelet concentration will be highest closer to the vessel wall where the fluid velocity is lower [8, 9]. Under high-shear conditions, the initial tethering and arrest of platelets from the flowing blood to collagen is facilitated by the glycoprotein (GP) Ib-IX-V receptor [10, 11] on the platelet surface. The binding is mediated by vWF, a multimeric plasma protein that rapidly binds to exposed collagen. Long multimers of vWF can contain several binding sites for the GPIb-IX-V adhesion receptors, and upon binding GPIb-IX-V is capable of outside–in signaling (events outside the cell leading to internal cellular activation) leading to platelet activation [12, 13]. The platelet's integrin $\alpha_2\beta_1$ adhesion receptor (also known as GPIa/IIa) can bind to collagen directly. The two collagen receptors on the platelet, GPVI and $\alpha_2\beta_1$, are both essential for platelet adhesion and aggregation on collagen in flow conditions; blockade of either receptor will abolish the platelet plug-forming capabilities [14].

Once a primary layer of adhesive platelets have covered the exposed subendothelial matrix, subsequent adhesion will continue but in the form of aggregation, where platelets from flowing blood bind to adhered platelets at the wound site. The mechanism of platelet aggregation is mainly attributed to the integrin $\alpha_{II}b\beta_3$ (also known as GPIIb/IIIa) receptor. The main ligand of integrin $\alpha_{II}b\beta_3$ is fibrinogen, but the receptors also have affinity for multimeric vWF, vitronectin, fibronectin, and thrombospondin [15].

In order for the recruitment of platelets to continue during the aggregation phase, it is necessary that the activated state of the adhered and aggregated platelets can be propagated to newly arriving platelets. This propagation of activation is executed via potent autocrine and paracrine signaling pathways. Activated platelets will secrete large amounts of ADP and ATP from dense granules that in turn activate neighboring platelets via ADP- and ATP-sensitive receptors. ADP is a ligand to the receptors P2Y1 and P2Y12, located on the platelet surface [16]. The P2X1 receptor is a ligand-gated cation channel and recently was found to be a specific ATP receptor, responsible for potentiating other activation pathways [17]. Following initial platelet activation, the signal molecule thromboxane A_2 (TxA_2) is rapidly synthesized and released by platelets. Interestingly, pony platelets have been found to release significantly more thromboxane when activated than horse platelets [18]. It is not known whether this has any connection to the increased risk of acute laminitis in pony breeds compared to most horse breeds.

The target for TxA_2 is the TPa receptor. TxA_2 is a lipid signal molecule synthesized by arachidonic acid (AA) metabolism (AA metabolism/ cyclooxygenase (COX) enzymes are discussed in Chapter 31), and the synthesis can be effectively inhibited by aspirin treatment, resulting in the attenuation of platelet activation [19, 20]. Because aspirin binds irreversibly to the platelet COX enzyme, platelet thromboxane production is inhibited for many days following aspirin therapy in the horse [21].

Both, thromboxane and serotonin (released from dense granules in a calcium-dependent process) are potent vasoconstrictors, helping to reduce blood loss from the site of tissue injury. Equine digital arteries and veins possess TPa, and serotonin receptors (5-HT_1 and 5-HT_2) on their vascular smooth muscle [22, 23]. Furthermore, these digital vessels are particularly sensitive to these mediators and, in the case of serotonin, constrict at much lower concentrations compared with other peripheral blood vessels [24].

During thrombus formation, simultaneous activation of the coagulation cascade results in generation of the key coagulation enzyme thrombin. Thrombin has a dual role in hemostasis, since in addition to facilitating the fibrin network formation it also functions as an activator of two distinct platelet receptors, namely the protease-activated receptors (PARs) 1 and 4 [25–27].

Platelets also play an important proinflammatory role, in addition to their roles in hemostasis. The interaction of platelets with neutrophils promotes the recruitment of neutrophils into inflamed tissue and thus they participate in host defense [28]. This interaction of neutrophils with platelets is mainly mediated through P-selectin and β_2 and β_3 integrins (CD11b/CD18, CD41/CD61). Platelets can also interact with endothelial cells and monocytes. Adherent platelets promote the 'secondary capture' (the interaction of a freely flowing leukocyte with a rolling leukocyte or a platelet, which leads to subsequent attachment to the endothelium) of neutrophils and other leukocytes [28]. In addition, platelets secrete neutrophil and endothelial activators inducing the production of inflammatory cytokines. Thus, platelets are important amplifiers of acute inflammation.

Coagulation

Coagulation (or secondary hemostasis; the transformation of flowing blood into a stable gel) is the result of enzymatic mechanisms initiated when blood comes into contact with extravascular surfaces. The gelling of blood is accomplished when soluble fibrinogen molecules undergo enzymatic cleavage and assemble into insoluble fibrin fibers, thereby creating a fine, interconnected network to trap blood cells.

There are two separate initiation mechanisms for the enzymatic coagulation cascade, both leading to the same end point of fibrin network formation; these are the intrinsic and extrinsic pathways. The names derive from the fact that all functional components of the intrinsic pathway are bloodborne, whereas the triggering component of the extrinsic pathway, tissue factor, is not found in blood, but in extravascular tissue. These pathways are highly interconnected and also dependent on platelet surface association for proper function (for a review, see Ref. [29]).

Platelet Activation and Aggregation in Laminitis

There is good evidence from many studies to show that platelet activation and microthrombus formation occurs in the two CHO models of SRL (both starch overload and oligofructose overload models [30,31]). These models tend to result in inflammatory changes, both locally in the lamellar tissues [32] and systemically [31]. The role of thrombosis and platelet activation in the pathogenesis of this condition is not clear, but some possible mechanisms will be discussed below. Whereas neither platelet activation nor microthrombus formation are detected in EMS or PPID, it is not currently known whether thrombosis, coagulation, or platelet activation occurs to a significant extent in the early stages of pasture-associated laminitis (discussed in more detail below), largely because of the difficulties of detecting animals in the prodromal stage [34].

Platelet counts and platelet survival times have been found to be decreased during the prodromal stages of starch overload laminitis [33]. However, in an earlier larger study [35], platelet counts were only significantly decreased 8 h after the onset of lameness. Platelet counts are not the best way to determine platelet activation, and other studies have used more detailed methods of assessing platelets and have shown clear evidence of activation in the developmental and acute phases. An electron microscopy study of platelets sampled from horses undergoing CHO-induced laminitis described shape changes, increased numbers of α-granules and glycogen granules and decreased γ-granules [36]. Activation by phosphorylation of the intracellular signaling molecule, p38 MAP kinase, has been reported in platelets during the developmental phase of oligofructose-induced laminitis [31]. Peak p38 MAPK activation occurred at 12 h post induction, and Obel grade 1 laminitis started to develop between 20–30 h. Platelet activation coincided with the release of detectable but small amounts of bacterial endotoxin from the hindgut into the circulation.

Equine platelets appear to have Toll-like receptor 4 (TLR4) in their cell membrane, which binds lipopolysaccharide (LPS; endotoxin) in conjunction with LPS-binding protein and the cell surface receptor CD14 [37, 38]. Indeed, equine platelets appear to be significantly more sensitive to activation by endotoxin than leukocytes, responding at 1000-fold lower concentrations [37]. This may be one of the reasons why horses (in common with humans) are particularly sensitive to the inflammatory effects of low concentrations of endotoxin compared with most other species [39, 40]. Thus, the proinflammatory role of platelets, binding to and activating neutrophils, may be an important link in the pathogenic events in equine endotoxemia.

Consequences of Platelet Activation in Laminitis

The consequences of platelet activation in the context of the prodromal phase of laminitis are many. One of the first consequences will be the release of 5-HT from platelet-dense granules, which causes localized vasoconstriction [23]. Furthermore, arachidonic acid release from the platelet cell membrane leads to the production of thromboxane by the constitutively active COX-1 enzyme [21], leading to further vasoconstriction. A period of systemic hypertension may be observed during the development of acute CHO laminitis [35], and both serotonin and thromboxane concentrations increase in the plasma in the developmental phase [31].

In addition to serotonin being released from platelets as part of their activation process, this vasoconstrictor can also be displaced from dense granules by other monoamine compounds circulating in the plasma [41]. Compounds such as tyramine, tryptamine and β-phenylethylamine are produced by amino acid decarboxylation by lactate-producing bacteria (including streptococci and *Lactobacillus* spp.) in the equine large intestine [42]. In the CHO situation, these bacteria rapidly proliferate in the large intestine and convert fermentable carbohydrate into large quantities of lactic acid, but also produce various amines [43]. As well as being quite potent vasoconstrictors in their own right (stimulating vascular smooth muscle serotonin and adrenoreceptors) [44], these compounds are taken up by platelets by means of an active uptake process (as if they were serotonin). Serotonin is subsequently displaced

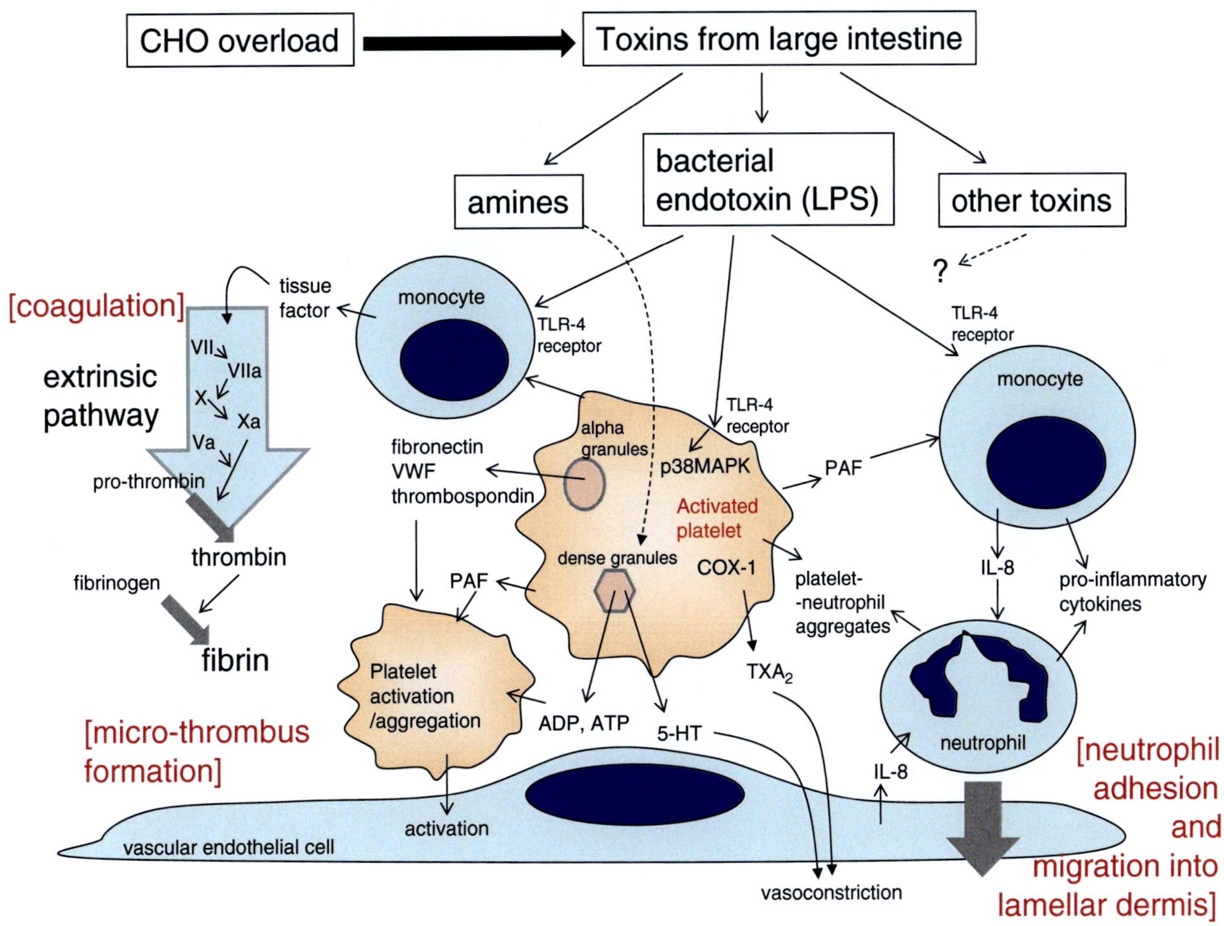

Figure 12.1 Mechanisms of platelet activation and microthrombus formation in carbohydrate overload (CHO) laminitis. Bacterial toxins from the large intestine enter the circulation and activate platelets and leukocytes. Tissue factor production (principally from monocytes) initiates the extrinsic coagulation pathway. Fibrin deposition, together with platelet aggregation, leads to the formation of microthrombi in small blood vessels. Activated platelets also cause vasoconstriction and amplify leukocyte activation, resulting in platelet–neutrophil aggregates and neutrophil adhesion to the activated vascular endothelium. The subsequent migration of neutrophils into the lamellar dermis and production of proinflammatory cytokines may be an important mechanism during the early stages of acute inflammatory laminitis. Abbreviations: ADP, adenosine diphosphate; ATP, adenosine triphosphate; COX-1, cyclooxygenase 1; 5-HT, 5-hydroxytryptamine (serotonin); IL-8, interleukin-8; LPS, lipopolysaccharide; PAF, platelet-activating factor; p38MAPK, p38 mitogen-associated protein kinase; TLR-4, toll-like receptor 4; TXA_2, thromboxane A_2.

from dense granule stores by other amines and released by the platelets [44]. These toxins appear in significant quantities in the circulation of horses in the developmental phase of starch overload laminitis [45], and also in the oligofructose overload model (S.R. Bailey, unpublished results).

Further consequences of platelet activation include aggregation and plug formation, potentially blocking blood vessels of the microcirculation, and leukocyte activation; these sequelae are discussed below. The pathways and consequences of platelet activation in acute inflammatory laminitis are outlined in Figure 12.1.

Interaction Between Platelets and Neutrophils

Platelet–neutrophil aggregates have been detected in the blood of horses during the developmental phase of starch overload laminitis, which is another indication of systemic activation of platelets. It is also evidence of platelets having a proinflammatory role in these forms of laminitis, where low levels of bacterial toxins such as LPS in the circulation may not be sufficient to cause widespread activation of leukocytes directly [31].

In one study by Eades *et al.* [46], these aggregates were only found at the 12 h time point after carbohydrate administration (samples were not assessed at the onset of clinical signs). However, in an earlier study in ponies, increased numbers of platelet–neutrophil aggregates were reported at multiple time points in the prodromal stages, together with platelet hyperaggregability [47].

Since increased numbers of platelet–neutrophil aggregates were detected free in the circulation, then not only would they be causing neutrophil activation (and subsequent proinflammatory cytokine release), but platelets adhered to the vascular endothelium would also be promoting the 'secondary capture' of neutrophils, promoting their extravasation into the tissues [28]. Given that neutrophil infiltration of the lamellar tissues (and other remote sites) appears to be an important feature of models of sepsis-related laminitis, then platelets are undoubtedly amplifying the recruitment of neutrophils to the tissues [48], in concert with the activated vascular endothelium [32].

Thrombosis in Laminitis

In the carbohydrate (starch) overload model of laminitis, multiple techniques were used to determine whether thrombosis of vessels in the lamellar corium could be demonstrated in one study [30]. In that study, radiolabeled platelets were found to accumulate distal to the coronary band at the onset of lameness. Additionally, histologic examination of the lamellar dermis from disarticulated feet demonstrated the presence of microthrombi in the dermal veins in three of the four affected animals.

However, the next question was whether these findings were simply secondary to an ongoing disease process, as the lamellar attachments were failing with extensive tissue injury likely occurring (due to distal phalanx displacement), or whether it represented an important part of the pathogenesis earlier in the disease process. Therefore, in a follow-up study, where tissues from ponies in the prodromal stages of laminitis were investigated, histologic examination of the lamellar dermis was again undertaken, and again demonstrated microthrombi in the venules of the lamellar dermis in some, but not all, affected animals [33]. Furthermore, arteriography of the disarticulated feet prior to sectioning also suggested a reduction in hoof blood supply. However, this technique would not have been able to determine whether any parts of the lamellar corium were subjected to ischemia as a result of these thrombi.

Coagulation Abnormalities in Laminitis

Despite there being some compelling evidence for platelet activation and microthrombus formation in the early stages of the models of SRL, there is little evidence for systemic activation of the coagulation system. In one comprehensive study using the starch overload model [33], there were no changes detected in prothrombin time or monocyte procoagulant activity. The activated partial thromboplastin time was only slightly altered at the onset of lameness. An earlier study by the same group had found evidence of a prolonged activated clotting time towards the onset of lameness, and also a trace of endotoxin activity in one of the ponies [30]. Therefore, systemic coagulation abnormalities, if present, are probably only seen secondary to inflammatory stimuli arising from the hindgut, and are not a major factor as they would be in severe cases of sepsis.

A more definitive study was later completed, when indices of systemic activation of coagulation, thrombin–antithrombin complexes and fibrin fragment D (D-dimers), were measured during the prodromal stages of (starch overload) laminitis in both ponies and horses [49]. Antithrombin III is an important anti-protease, which reacts as a pseudosubstrate with thrombin to form stable complexes (thrombin-antithrombin; TAT); D-dimer is a fibrin degradation product containing two crosslinked D fragments of the fibrin protein. When these factors were measured during the prodromal stages of laminitis, there were no differences between laminitic and control animals at any of the time points, with most values remaining within the normal range. This suggests that, even though there was evidence for prothrombotic events in this condition, this was not necessarily triggered by systemic activation of the coagulation or fibrinolytic systems.

In endotoxemia/sepsis in the horse, systemic activation of the coagulation system is a common finding [50]. Impairment of anticoagulant mechanisms [51] and alterations in the regulation of fibrinolysis have been documented in endotoxemic horses with gastrointestinal diseases [52]. Also accompanying endotoxemia is endothelial and leukocyte activation and vasoconstriction [53]. In CHO laminitis, inflammatory events – including platelet and leukocyte activation and increased inflammatory cytokine expression – may be associated with the small amount of endotoxin which appears to be absorbed into the systemic circulation as a result of hindgut acidosis [31].

Thrombosis and Coagulation in Supporting Limb Laminitis

Supporting limb laminitis appears to have a distinct pathophysiology from other forms of laminitis, at least until the later stages (when distal displacement of the distal phalanx occurs). In these later stages, there is evidence of secondary inflammation, enzymatic activation and vascular disruption [54]. The main hypotheses in this scenario is that the initiating factors leading to the development of acute laminitis are either a mechanical overload of the supporting digital lamellae or, more likely, a decrease in movement of the distal limb with minimal unloading of the digit, resulting in decreased lamellar blood flow [55]. In humans, alterations in blood flow resulting in stasis have been shown to lead to venous inflammation and platelet activation [56]. In horses, cyclical loading and unloading likely plays a role in promoting blood flow through the digit [55, 57]. Therefore, if there is prolonged weight-bearing on one digit with inadequate periods of unloading, a slowing of blood flow may occur with subsequent platelet activation and microthrombus formation, resulting in inadequate perfusion and ischemia of the lamellar tissue [54, 58–60]. Further studies are required to determine the importance of vascular congestion and platelet-mediated thrombosis in the pathogenesis of supporting limb laminitis. There is no evidence to date as to whether coagulation abnormalities may be associated with this form of the disease [61].

Thrombosis and Coagulation in Pasture-Associated and Endocrinopathic Laminitis

Although a significant proportion of naturally occurring laminitis cases occur at pasture, the pathophysiological pathways involved are still unclear. Although significant amounts of fructan carbohydrates may be consumed from lush pasture, and much of that will be conveyed to the hindgut, pasture laminitis does not necessarily equate with the oligofructose overload experimental model [61]. Pasture-associated laminitis most often occurs in animals with a metabolic predisposition, particularly insulin resistance/dysregulation, together with obesity or regionalized adiposity [62]. It has been confirmed that high concentrations of insulin can cause laminitis in both horses and ponies [63, 64]. However, significant evidence of microthrombi in lamellar sections from these cases has not been reported [65, 66]. It is also unlikely that systemic abnormalities of coagulation would be associated with this form of laminitis.

Antiplatelet Therapies

Despite numerous failures in many clinical trials involving novel pharmaceutical therapies for acute laminitis, one of the few groups of drugs which has been reported to show some clinical efficacy are antiplatelet drugs. In 1998, a study was conducted by Weiss and colleagues to test a synthetic analogue of the platelet fibrinogen receptor antagonist peptide (RPR110885) [67]. Ponies were pretreated with the compound before undergoing a carbohydrate overload, and none of the eight treated animals showed signs of the disease (compared with six out of eight controls). This clinical finding was supported by an attenuation of the increase in platelet–neutrophil aggregates. Therefore, platelet aggregation or activation may play important roles in this condition. However, the mechanism is not necessarily simply via the prevention of microthrombi but perhaps by targeting the intermediary role in leukocyte activation.

Another drug reported to reduce the clinical signs of laminitis was BAY TG 1000 [68]. This dihydropyridine compound, a calcium channel blocker of the same class as amlodipine and nifedipine, was proposed to enhance erythrocyte deformability; however, this class of drugs will also inhibit platelet activation and platelet thromboxane release [69]. The many different potential effects of this compound do not allow very many conclusions to be drawn about mechanisms or the role of platelets or hemodynamics.

Other therapies commonly used in the treatment of acute laminitis will also have antiplatelet effects. Dimethyl sulfoxide (DMSO) inhibits platelet activation [70], as do phosphodiesterase inhibitors such as pentoxifylline (although not at clinically relevant doses) [71]. Many nonsteroidal anti-inflammatory drugs (NSAIDs) will inhibit thromboxane production by platelets. Indeed, although flunixin and phenylbutazone do not prevent the induction of SRL by CHO [72, 73], these compounds, along with ketoprofen, have been shown to reduce the changes consistent with platelet activation occurring in this form of laminitis [36].

Heparin has also been used prophylactically for the prevention of laminitis, for example following colic surgery. Heparin is a highly sulfated glycosaminoglycan, which activates the enzyme inhibitor antithrombin III, that inactivates thrombin and other proteases involved in blood clotting. In addition to the unfractionated forms of heparin (average molecular weight about 15 kDa; range 5–40 kDa), low-molecular-weight heparins (ca. 4.5 kDa) have become available and have more predictable pharmacokinetics and anticoagulant effects. No significant beneficial effect was found when comparing the prevalence of postoperative laminitis in clinical cases of colic given unfractionated heparin, compared with postoperative colic cases not treated with heparin [74]. However, more recently, the use of low-molecular-weight heparin was reported to have a significant beneficial effect on the incidence and severity of laminitis in a large clinical study of horses undergoing colic surgery [75]. The results of heparin therapy in experimental models of laminitis have been inconclusive. Whereas, heparin was reported to reduce the severity of clinical signs in a study using the starch overload model [76], the administration of heparin did not delay the onset or decrease severity of lameness in a laminitis induction study using the oligofructose overload model [77].

Conclusions

Although it is fairly clear that coagulation deficits may occur in CHO models of SRL, there is no evidence for its occurrence or involvement in endocrinopathic laminitis, and the possible role of coagulation abnormalities in supporting limb laminitis has yet to be determined. Systemic inflammation and/or sepsis in CHO models would appear to be the cause of the observed platelet activation, coagulation abnormalities, and microthrombus formation.

These abnormalities may in theory contribute to the pathophysiology of laminitis in a number of ways. Platelet activation may lead to the release of vasoconstrictors, activation of the vascular endothelium, and the activation and adhesion of neutrophils to the luminal surface. Additionally, coagulation abnormalities and thrombosis could cause a degree of blood vessel blockage due to microthrombi. Whilst this contribution is perhaps not critical to the development of laminitis, these mechanisms could certainly augment and amplify the ongoing key pathophysiological processes as lamellar injury ensues and intensifies during later events, including displacement of the distal phalanx. Considering that antiplatelet therapies remain one of the few groups of drugs shown to be effective in reducing the severity of laminitis in experimental models, the role of coagulation and thrombosis should always be considered in the complex cascade of pathways leading to the development of acute laminitis.

References

1. Italiano, J.E. and Hartwig, J.H. (2007) Megakaryocyte development and platelet formation, in *Platelets* (ed. A.D. Michelson), Academic Press/Elsevier, Amsterdam, Boston, pp. 23–44.
2. Carter, E.I., Valli, V.E., McSherry, B.J., Milne, F.J., Robinson, G.A., and Lumsden, J.H. (1974) The kinetics of hematopoiesis in the light horse. I. The lifespan of peripheral blood cells in the normal horse. *Can. J. Comp. Med.*, **38** (3), 303–313.
3. Heyns, A.P. (1994) Thrombopoiesis and platelet kinetics, in *Haemostasis and Thrombosis* (ed. A.L. Bloom), Churchill Livingstone, Edinburgh, pp. 31–48.
4. Rendu, F. and Brohard-Bohn, B. (2002) Platelet organelles, in *Platelets in Thrombotic and Non-Thrombotic Disorders* (eds P. Gresele, C. Page, V. Fuster, and J. Vermylen), Cambridge University Press, Cambridge, UK.
5. Reed, G.L. (2007) Platelet secretion, in *Platelets* (ed. A.D. Michelson), Academic Press/Elsevier: Amsterdam, Boston, p. xlii, p. 1343.
6. Blockmans, D., Deckmyn, H., and Vermylen, J. (1995) Platelet activation. *Blood Rev.*, **9** (3), 143–156.
7. Nieswandt, B. and Watson, S.P. (2003) Platelet-collagen interaction: is GPVI the central receptor? *Blood*, **102** (2), 449–461.
8. Eskin, S.G. and McIntire, L.V. (2006) Rheology of thrombosis, in Hemostasis *and Thrombosis: Basic principles and clinical practice* (ed. R.W. Colman), Lippincott Williams & Wilkins, Philadelphia, PA, pp. 737–750.
9. Turitto, V.T. and Weiss, H.J. (1980) Red Blood Cells: Their Dual Role in Thrombus Formation. *Science*, **207** (4430), 541–543.
10. Jackson, S.P., Mistry, N., and Yuan, Y. (2000) Platelets and the injured vessel wall – 'rolling into action': focus on glycoprotein Ib/V/IX and the platelet cytoskeleton. *Trends Cardiovasc. Med.*, **10** (5), 192–197.
11. Andrews, R.K., Gardiner, E.E., Shen, Y., Whisstock, J.C., and Berndt, M.C. (2003) Glycoprotein Ib-IX-V. *Int. J. Biochem. Cell Biol.*, **35** (8), 1170–1174.
12. Schmugge, M., Rand, M.L., and Freedman, J. (2003) Platelets and von Willebrand factor. *Transfus. Apher. Sci.*, **28** (3), 269–277.
13. Broberg, M. and Nygren, H. (2001) Von Willebrand factor, a key protein in the exposure of CD62P on platelets. *Biomaterials*, **22** (17), 2403–2409.
14. Chen, J. and Lopez, J.A. (2005) Interactions of platelets with subendothelium and endothelium. *Microcirculation*, **12** (3), 235–246.
15. Plow, E.F., Pesho, M.M., and Ma, Y.-Q. (2007) Integrin alpha IIb beta 3, in *Platelets* (ed. A.D. Michelson), Academic Press/Elsevier, Amsterdam, Boston, pp. 165–178.
16. Gachet, C. (2001) ADP receptors of platelets and their inhibition. *Thromb. Haemost.*, **86** (1), 222–232.
17. Mahaut-Smith, M.P., Ennion, S.J., Rolf, M.G., and Evans, R.J. (2000) ADP is not an agonist at P2X1 receptors: evidence for separate receptors stimulated by ATP and ADP on human platelets. *Br. J. Pharmacol.*, **131** (1), 108–114.
18. McKellar, Q.A., Nolan, A.M., and Galbraith, E.A. (1990) Serum thromboxane generation by platelets in several domestic animal species. *Br. Vet. J.*, **146** (5), 398–404.
19. Davie, E.W. and Ratnoff, O.D. (1964) Waterfall sequence for intrinsic blood clotting. *Science*, **145** (3638), 1310–1312.
20. Grosser, T., Fries, S., and Fitzgerald, G.A. (2007) Thromboxane generation, in *Platelets* (ed. A.D. Michelson), Academic Press/Elsevier, Amsterdam, Boston, pp. 565–574.
21. Cambridge, H., Lees, P., Hooke, R.E., and Russell, C.S. (1991) Antithrombotic actions of aspirin in the horse. *Equine Vet. J.*, **23** (2), 123–127.
22. Bailey, S.R. (1998) A study of the vascular effects and factors regulating the concentration of 5-hydroxytryptamine in the equine digital circulation. PhD Thesis, University of London.
23. Bailey, S.R. and Elliott, J. (1998) Plasma 5-hydroxytryptamine constricts equine digital blood vessels in vitro: implications for the pathogenesis of acute laminitis. *Equine Vet. J.*, **30**, 124–130.
24. Bailey S.R. and Elliott, J. (1998) Plasma 5-hydroxytryptamine constricts equine digital blood vessels in vitro: implications for the pathogenesis of acute laminitis. *Equine Vet. J.*, **30**, 124–130.
25. Covic, L., Gresser, A.L., and Kuliopulos, A. (2000) Biphasic kinetics of activation and signaling for PAR1 and PAR4 thrombin receptors in platelets. *Biochemistry*, **39** (18), 5458–5467.
26. Kahn, M.L., Nakanishi-Matsui, M., Shapiro, M.J., Ishihara, H., and Coughlin, S.R. (1999) Protease-activated receptors 1 and 4 mediate activation of human platelets by thrombin. *J. Clin. Invest.*, **103** (6), 879–887.
27. Vretenbrant, K., Ramstrom, S., Bjerke, M., and Lindahl, T.L. (2007) Platelet activation via PAR4 is involved in the initiation of thrombin generation and in clot elasticity development. *Thromb. Haemost.*, **97** (3), 417–424.
28. Zarbock, A., Polanowska-Grabowska, R.K., and Ley K. (2007) Platelet–neutrophil-interactions: linking hemostasis and inflammation. *Blood Rev.*, **21** (2), 99–111.
29. Colman, R.W., Clowes, A.W., George, J.N., Goldhaber, S.Z., and Marder, V.J. (2006) Overview of hemostasis, in *Hemostasis and Thrombosis: Basic principles and clinical practice* (ed. R.W. Colman), Lippincott Williams & Wilkins, Philadelphia, PA, pp. 3–16.
30. Weiss, D.J., Geor, R.J., Johnston, G., and Trent, A.M. (1994) Microvascular thrombosis associated with onset of acute laminitis in ponies. *Am. J. Vet. Res.*, **55** (5), 606–612.
31. Bailey, S.R., Adair, H.S., Reinemeyer, C.R., Morgan, S.J., Brooks, A.C., Longhofer, S.L., and Elliott, J. (2009) Plasma concentrations of endotoxin and platelet activation in the developmental stage of oligofructose-induced laminitis. *Vet. Immunol. Immunopathol.*, **129**, 167–173.
32. Leise, B.S., Faleiros, R.R., Watts, M., Johnson, P.J., Black, S.J., and Belknap, J.K. (2011) Laminar inflammatory gene expression in the carbohydrate overload model of equine laminitis. *Equine Vet. J.*, **43** (1), 54–61.
33. Weiss, D.J., Trent, A.M., and Johnston, G. (1995) Prothrombotic events in the prodromal stages of acute laminitis in horses. *Am. J. Vet. Res.*, **56** (8), 986–991.
34. Bailey, S.R., Marr, C.M., and Elliott, J. (2004) Current research and theories on the pathogenesis of acute laminitis in the horse. *Vet. J.*, **167** (2), 129–142.
35. Moore, J.N., Garner, H.E., Coffman, J.R. (1981) Haematological changes during development of acute laminitis hypertension. *Equine Vet. J.*, **13** (4), 240–242.
36. Paes Leme, F.O., Wurzinger, L.J., Vasconcelos, A.C., and Alves, G.E.S. (2006) Platelet activation in equines with induced laminitis treated with ketoprophen, phenylbutazone and flunixin meglumine. *Arq. Bras. Med. Vet. Zootec.*, **58** (2), 149–157.

37. Brooks, A., Menzies-Gow, N.J., Wheeler-Jones, C., Bailey, S.R., Cunningham, F.M., and Elliott, J. (2007) Endotoxin-induced activation of equine platelets: evidence for direct activation of p38 MAPK pathways and vasoactive mediator production. *Inflamm. Res.*, **56**, 154–161.
38. Werners, A.H., Bull, S., and Fink-Gremmels, J. (2005) Endotoxaemia: a review with implications for the horse. *Equine Vet. J.*, **37** (4), 371–383.
39. King, J.N. and Gerring, E.L. (1988) Detection of endotoxin in cases of equine colic. *Vet. Rec.*, **123**, 269–271.
40. Behre, G., Schedel, I., Nentwig, B., Wormann, B., Essink, M., and Hiddemann, W. (1992) Endotoxin concentration in neutropaenic patients with suspected Gram-negative sepsis: correlation with clinical outcome and determination of anti-endotoxin core antibodies during therapy with polyclonal immunoglobulin M-enriched immunoglobulins. *Antimicrob. Agents Chemother.*, **36**, 2139–2146.
41. Bailey, S.R., Cunningham, F.M., and Elliott, J. (2000) Endotoxin and dietary amines may increase plasma 5-hydroxytryptamine in the horse. *Equine Vet. J.*, **32** (6), 497–504.
42. Bailey, S.R., Baillon, M.L., Rycroft, A.N., Harris, P.A., and Elliott, J. (2003) Identification of equine cecal bacteria producing amines in an in vitro model of carbohydrate overload. *Appl. Environ. Microbiol.*, **69** (4), 2087–2093.
43. Bailey, S.R., Rycroft, A., and Elliott, J. (2002) Production of amines in equine cecal contents in an in vitro model of carbohydrate overload. *J. Anim. Sci.*, **80** (10), 2656–2662.
44. Elliott, J., Berhane, Y., and Bailey, S.R. (2003) Effects of monoamines formed in the cecum of horses on equine digital blood vessels and platelets. *Am. J. Vet. Res.*, **64** (9), 1124–1131.
45. Botteon, P.T.L., Ferraz, V.P., Glória, M.B.A., Melo, M.M., Paes Leme, F.O., Faleiros, R.R., and Alves, G.E.S. (2008) Plasma concentrations of tryptamine, tyramine and phenylethylamine in horses under the effect of carbohydrate overload and non-steroid antinflammatory compounds. *Pesq. Vet. Bras.*, **28** (6), 299–302.
46. Eades, S.C., Stokes, A.M., Johnson, P.J., LeBlanc, C.J., Ganjam, V.K., Buff, P.R., and Moore R.M. (2007) Serial alterations in digital hemodynamics and endothelin-1 immunoreactivity, platelet-neutrophil aggregation, and concentrations of nitric oxide, insulin, and glucose in blood obtained from horses following carbohydrate overload. *Am. J. Vet. Res.*, **68** (1), 87–94.
47. Weiss, D.J., Evanson, O.A., McClenahan, D., Fagliari, J.J., and Jenkins, K. (1997) Evaluation of platelet activation and platelet-neutrophil aggregates in ponies with alimentary laminitis. *Am. J. Vet. Res.*, **58** (12), 1376–1380.
48. Faleiros, R.R., Johnson, P.J., Nuovo, G.J., Messer, N.T., Black, S.J., and Belknap, J.K. (2011) Laminar leukocyte accumulation in horses with carbohydrate overload-induced laminitis. *J. Vet. Intern. Med.*, **25** (1), 107–115.
49. Weiss, D.J., Monreal, L., Angles, A.M., and Monasterio, J. (1996) Evaluation of thrombin-antithrombin complexes and fibrin fragment D in carbohydrate-induced acute laminitis. *Res. Vet. Sci.*, **61** (2), 157–159.
50. McGovern, K.F., Lascola, K.M., Smith, S.A., Clark-Price, S.C., Wilkins, P.A., Schaeffer, D.J., and Foreman, J.H. (2013) The effects of hyperglycemia and endotoxemia on coagulation parameters in healthy adult horses. *J. Vet. Intern. Med.*, **27** (2), 347–353.
51. Dallap Schaer, B.L. and Epstein, K. (2009) Coagulopathy of the critically ill equine patient. *J. Vet. Emerg. Crit. Care (San Antonio)*, **19** (1), 53–65.
52. Collatos, C., Barton, M.H., Schleef, R., Prasse, K.W., and Moore, J.N. (1994) Regulation of equine fibrinolysis in blood and peritoneal fluid based on a study of colic cases and induced endotoxaemia. *Equine Vet. J.*, **26** (6), 474–481.
53. Menzies-Gow, N.J., Bailey, S.R., Stevens, K., Katz, L.M., Elliott, J., and Marr, C.M. (2005) Digital blood flow and plasma endothelin concentration in clinically endotoxemic horses. *Am. J. Vet. Res.*, **66**, 630–636.
54. van Eps, A., Collins, S.N., and Pollitt, C.C. (2010) Supporting limb laminitis. *Vet. Clin. North Am. Equine Pract.*, **26**, 287–302.
55. Medina-Torres, C.E., Underwood, C., Pollitt, C.C., Castro-Olivera, E.M., Hodson, M.P., Richardson, D.W., and Van Eps, A.W. (2016) The effect of weightbearing and limb load cycling on equine lamellar perfusion and energy metabolism measured using tissue microdialysis. *Equine Vet. J.*, **48** (1), 114–119.
56. Chieu, J.-J. and Chien, S. (2011) Effects of disturbed flow on vascular endothelium: pathophysiological basis and clinical perspectives. *Physiol. Rev.*, **91**, 327–387.
57. Hunt, R.J., Brandon, C.I., and McCann, M.E. (1994) Effects of acetylpromazine, xylazine, and vertical load on digital arterial blood flow in horses. *Am. J. Vet. Res.*, **55**, 375–378.
58. Hood, D.M., Grosenbaugh, D.A., Mostafa, M.B., Morgan, S.J., and Thomas, B.C. (1993) The role of vascular mechanisms in the development of acute equine laminitis. *J. Vet. Intern. Med.*, **7**, 228–234.
59. Redden, R. (2004) Preventing laminitis in the contralateral limb of horses with non-weight-bearing lameness. *Clin. Tech. Equine Pract.*, **49**, 57–63.
60. Baxter, G.M. and Morrison, S. (2008) Complications of unilateral weight bearing. *Vet. Clin. North. Am. Equine Pract.*, **24**, 621–642.
61. Katz, L.M. and Bailey, S.R. (2012) A review of recent advances and current hypotheses on the pathogenesis of acute laminitis. *Equine Vet. J.*, **44** (6), 752–761.
62. Geor, R.J. (2010) Current concepts on the pathophysiology of pasture-associated laminitis. *Vet. Clin. North. Am. Equine Pract.*, **26**, 265–276.
63. Asplin, K.E., Sillence, M.N., Pollitt, C.C., and McGowan, C.M. (2007) Induction of laminitis by prolonged hyperinsulinaemia in clinically normal ponies. *Vet. J.*, **174** (3), 530–535.
64. de Laat, M.A., McGowan, C.M., Sillence, M.N., and Pollitt, C.C. (2010) Equine laminitis: induced by 48 h hyperinsulinaemia in Standardbred horses. *Equine Vet. J.*, **42**, 129–135.
65. Asplin, K.E., Patterson-Kane, J.C., Sillence, M.N., Pollitt, C.C., and McGowan, C.M. (2010) Histopathology of insulin-induced laminitis in ponies. *Equine Vet. J.*, **42** (8), 700–706.
66. de Laat, M.A., Van Eps, A.W., McGowan, C.M., Sillence, M.N., and Pollitt, C.C. (2011) Equine laminitis: comparative histopathology 48 hours after experimental induction with insulin or alimentary oligofructose in Standardbred horses. *J. Comp. Pathol.*, **145** (4), 399–409.
67. Weiss, D.J., Evanson, O.A., McClenahan, D., Fagliari, J.J., Dunnwiddie, C.T., and Wells, R.E. (1998) Effect of a competitive inhibitor of platelet aggregation on experimentally induced laminitis in ponies. *Am. J. Vet. Res.*, **59** (7), 814–817.

68. Hood, D.M., Brumbaugh, G.W., and Wagner, I.P. (2002) Effectiveness of a unique dihydropyridine (BAYTG 1000) for prevention of laminitis in horses. *Am. J. Vet. Res.*, **62** (3), 443–447.
69. Chou, T.C., Li, C.Y., Yen, M.H., and Ding, Y.A. (1999) Antiplatelet effect of amlodipine: a possible mechanism through a nitric oxide-mediated process. *Biochem. Pharmacol.*, **58** (10), 1657–1663.
70. Lehuu, B. and Curtis-Prior, P.B. (1987) Effects of dimethyl sulphoxide (DMSO) on aggregation of human blood platelets. *J. Pharm. Pharmacol.*, **39** (1), 62–63.
71. Kornreich, B., Enyeart, M., Jesty, S.A., Nydam, D.V., and Divers, T. (2010) The effects of pentoxifylline on equine platelet aggregation. *J. Vet. Intern. Med.*, **24** (5), 1196–1202.
72. Van Eps, A. and Pollitt, C.C. (2006) Equine laminitis induced with oligofructose. *Equine Vet. J.*, **38** (3), 203–208.
73. Leme, F.O.P., Bonna, F.A.B., Marval, C.A., Xavier, S.H.N., Santos, R.L., Faleiros, R.R., and Alves, G.E.S. (2010) Histopathology of the digital laminae from horses with acute induced laminitis treated with ketoprophen, phenylbutazone, and flunixin meglumine. *Arq. Bras. Med. Vet. Zootec.*, **62** (2), 241–250.
74. Belknap, J.K. and Moore, J.N. (1989) Evaluation of heparin for prophylaxis of equine laminitis: 71 cases (1980–1986). *J. Am. Vet. Med. Assoc.*, **195** (4), 505–507.
75. de la Rebière de Pouyade, G., Grulke, S., Detilleux, J., Salciccia, A., Verwilghen, D.R., Caudron, I., Gangl, M., and Serteyn, D.D. (2009) Evaluation of low-molecular-weight heparin for the prevention of equine laminitis after colic surgery. *J. Vet. Emerg. Crit. Care (San Antonio)*, **19** (1), 113–119.
76. Hood, D.M., Stephens, K.A., and Amoss, M.S. (1982) Heparin as a preventative for equine laminitis: a preliminary report. *Am. Assoc. Equine Pract. Newsletter*, **2**, 146–149.
77. Uberti, B., Pressler, B.M., Alkabes, S.B., Chang, C.Y., Moore, G.E., Lescun, T.B., and Sojka, J.E. (2010) Effect of heparin administration on urine protein excretion during the developmental stage of experimentally induced laminitis in horses. *Am. J. Vet. Res.*, **71** (12), 1462–1467.

CHAPTER 13

Leukocytes and Inflammatory Signaling in Laminitis: Leukocytes

Rafael R. Faleiros and James K. Belknap

Introduction

The digital lamellae are a very specialized tissue that firmly connects the cornified hoof capsule to the distal phalanx (see Chapter 3). Despite an absence of hair, sweat, or sebaceous glands, the lamellar tissue is primarily derived from skin, which is modified to attend this specific function. As a component of the integumentary system, the lamellae are part of the largest organ (in weight) of the horse's body, of which the primary role is that of a physical and biological barrier.

As a biological barrier, the primary property of skin and its associated structures is to recognize pathogen-associated molecular pattern (PAMP) molecules and damage-associated molecular pattern (DAMP) molecules. Upon recognizing these molecules, cells of the epidermis and dermis send alert messages to immune tissues in the body to recruit 'the first line of defense' leukocytes and other specialized immune cells to impede body invasion by external pathogens. This dedicated response from the skin is considered to be a major part of the immune system; therefore, the term skin immune system (SIS) has been used to describe the complex milieu of immune response-associated cells present in the skin [1].

The SIS is comprised of a host of resident cells. In humans, several cell populations have been recognized as members of the SIS, including keratinocytes, Langerhans' cells, epidermal T lymphocytes, dermal T lymphocytes, mast cells, vascular endothelial cells, lymphatic endothelial cells, tissue dendritic cells, macrophages, and, possibly, fibroblasts [1]. In addition to its resident members, several cell types can be recruited to expand existing populations or to create new types of cell populations that can remain and perform their immune function in the skin. Natural killer cells, natural killer T cells, eosinophilic granulocytes, neutrophilic granulocytes, monocytes, endothelial cell precursors, dendritic cells, T lymphocytes, B lymphocytes, and basophils are examples of cells that can be recruited to the tissue depending on skin's demand resulting from events such as trauma, acute and chronic infections, neoplasia, and, immunological hypersensitivity [1]. PAMPs from infectious agents and DAMPs released during trauma and neoplasia are recognized by a host of resident cells (such as keratinocytes, dendritic cells, lymphocytes, and dermal fibroblasts) and result in the production of chemokines. The latter are small molecules that are released by cells to attract and recruit immune cells from the circulation into affected tissue. Both the resident and recruited immune cells of the SIS can trigger a cascade of events involving innate and adaptive immune responses to antigens.

In order to achieve their biological barrier targets, cell populations of SIS are involved in the innate and adaptive immunity subsystems. *Innate immunity* represents the rudimentary first line of defense and involves different cell types (e.g., neutrophils and monocytes) working together through cytokine and chemokine signaling to exterminate harmful compounds and microorganisms invading the skin. *Adaptive immunity* is the sophisticated and intelligent second line of host defense against pathogens, which also acts (mainly by dendritic cells and lymphocytes) to prepare the organism for future attacks while limiting sensitization to self-antigens [1].

Few studies have been conducted concerning the diversity of immune cell populations and subtypes in normal horse skin and lamellae, and the influence of pathologic conditions on these populations. However, most of the cells that comprise the human SIS have also been described in equine skin [2] and in equine lamellar tissue [3–5]. Studies regarding resident and recruited inflammatory cells in equine lamellar tissue in both normal and laminitic horses are reviewed in the following subsections.

A proposal for SIS cell populations in the equine digital lamellae and the indication of their main immunological subsystem are represented in Figure 13.1.

Historical Perspective of Leukocyte Evidences in Equine Laminitis

Since the first experimental models of sepsis-related laminitis were first demonstrated (see Chapters 7–9 for details of carbohydrate overload [CHO] models [oligofructose and starch

Equine Laminitis, First Edition. Edited by James K. Belknap and Raymond Geor.

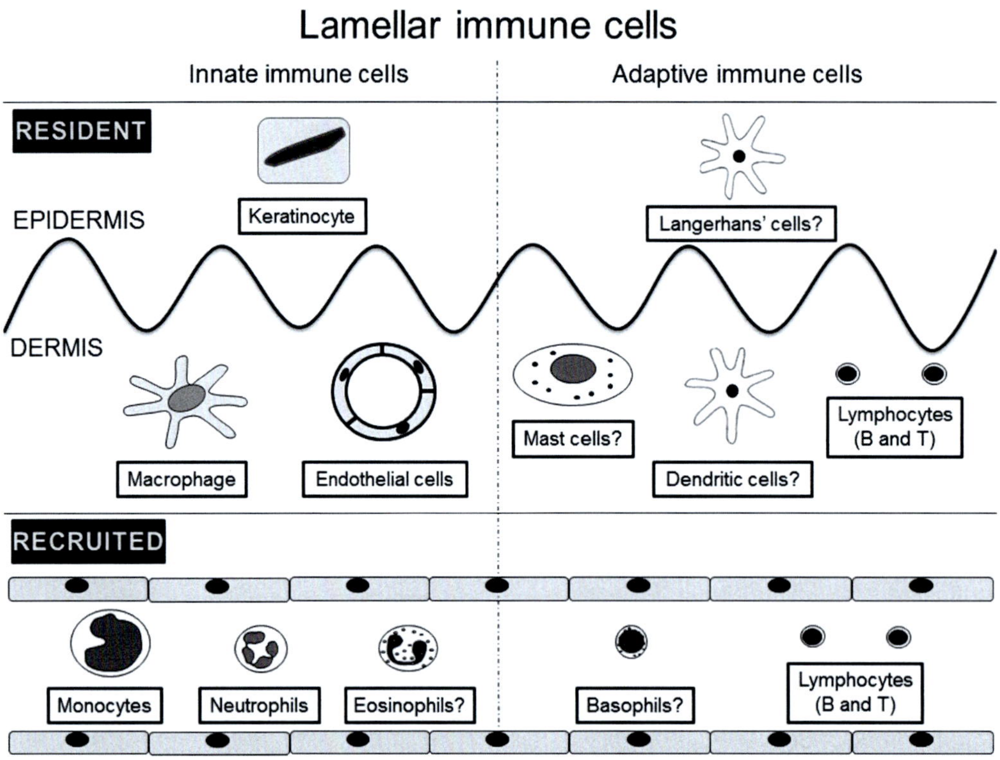

Figure 13.1 Resident and recruited cell populations that integrate the skin immune system (SIS) of the equine hoof lamellar tissue, and the indication of their subsystem (innate or adaptive). The question mark (?) designates cell types that participate in the skin immune system but have not yet been identified in equine lamellar tissue.

gruel models] [7,8] and black walnut extract (BWE) [9] Model), evidence of changes in blood leukocyte concentrations have been reported during the developmental stages of laminitis. A rapid onset of marked neutropenia has been noted in horses within 3–4 h after BWE administration [9], while neutrophilia (with increased band neutrophils) was reported as early as 16 h before Obel grade 3 laminitis occurred and remained increased through the development of Obel grade 3 laminitis in horses undergoing CHO [10]. Although demonstrating a contrasting systemic leukocyte response, these changes were considered to be related to the typical response of horses to endotoxin: an initial neutropenia followed by a rebound neutrophilia with a left shift (increase in band cells) [9]. While endotoxin has been detected in the blood of horses subjected to CHO [11,12], it does not appear to occur in those treated with BWE.

Although these early reports demonstrated systemic hematological changes after BWE or CHO treatments, there was minimal to no evidence of any infiltration of neutrophils or monocytes in the lamellar tissue. At that time, the use of basic histologic staining techniques resulted in lamellar infiltration only being consistently detected in advanced stages of the pathological process, after separation of the dermal–epidermal interface [7]. The presence of inflammatory cells in the lamellar tissue before structural failure of the dermal–epidermal interface was also not documented, even in more recent studies detailing destruction of the cellular and connective tissue (extracellular matrix [ECM] and basement membrane [BM]) components of the dermal–epidermal interface using CHO models [13,14].

Facing this absence of inflammatory clues in the early phases, leukocytes and other components of the classic inflammatory process were almost excluded as possible "players" in the developmental phase of laminitis [15]. Although extensive research was conducted, mechanisms involving inflammation and inflammatory cell function within the lamellar tissue were rarely examined [16] for approximately four decades. During that time period, a considerable amount of progress was achieved in the general understanding regarding the microvascular response, thrombus formation, glucose and insulin metabolism and the activation of enzymes that can degrade the ECM using different models of laminitis [17]. However, that effort was insufficient to identify an accurate explanation about which initial events would trigger pathologic mechanisms leading to lamellar failure.

This scenario persisted until the new millennium, when advanced laboratory techniques and improved research tools in molecular biology and protein biochemistry became available in equine applied research. One of the first reports of the exploration of molecular biology techniques in Equine Laminitis was made in 2001 [18]. Using an in-situ hybridization protocol, the expression of interleukin (IL)-1β mRNA (a key proinflammatory cytokine) was detected in lamellar tissue from horses as early as 2.5–3.5 h after enteral BWE administration.

Interestingly, most of the cells expressing IL-1β were around small lamellar venules and capillaries. These findings shed light on a local inflammatory response as a possible initiating factor, at least in BWE-induced laminitis, but also raised new relevant questions. Since it was unclear whether the cells producing IL-1β were of leukocyte origin, this report spurred further research using different cellular markers to assess the presence of leukocytes prior to the onset of advanced dermal–epidermal separation.

The first study to be published regarding lamellar leukocyte infiltration was inspired by the well-described reaction of mammalian organisms to a septic insult, the multiple organ dysfunction syndrome (MODS) that follows a systemic inflammatory response syndrome (SIRS) observed in systemic septic events such as endotoxemia [3]. Based on the knowledge that leukocyte emigration into the tissues of an affected organ is a prominent initiating factor in the inflammatory injury that leads to organ dysfunction and failure that occurs in human sepsis, it was hypothesized that systemic leukocyte events observed in laminitis models were due to a similar SIRS reaction in horses, likely leading to leukocyte infiltration (and possibly leukocyte-mediated injury) in many tissue including the lamellae and skin in the early stages of laminitis [3]. In this case, an anti-equine CD13 monoclonal antibody (a marker reported to detect the presence of in-situ monocytes and neutrophils) was used to stain lamellar tissue from horses receiving BWE [3, 19].

Results from the CD13 immunohistochemistry study indicated that a small marginal pool of $CD13^+$ cells is commonly present around the skin venules of normal horses, but not in the digital lamellar vasculature of normal horses. In horses treated with BWE, leukocyte emigration (primarily neutrophils) into the lamellar tissue was found to occur during the leukopenia phase (3–4 h after BWE administration) and was sustained through the onset of lameness [3]. These authors and others demonstrated that leukocyte emigration after BWE administration was not exclusive to the lamellar tissue, but also occurred in the skin [3], liver, lungs [20], and colon [21].

These studies inaugurated a new line of reasoning, and a new theory involving SIRS and lamellar leukocyte emigration began to be considered.

Resident Leukocyte-Derived Cells in Equine Normal Lamellae

The almost complete absence of $CD13^+$ myeloid cells in normal lamellae [3] and the lack any increase in the central myeloid leukocyte cytokine TNFα in the lamellar tissues of normal horses and horses administered BWE [22] was initially misinterpreted as indicating a lack of normal resident leukocyte-derived population of cells in the lamellae [3]. A primary reason for this misinterpretation was that it was not realized that CD13 was a poor marker for monocytes/macrophages. The use of more specific markers (i.e. CD163 and calprotectin) has more recently revealed a rich and diverse population of mononuclear inflammatory cells in the normal equine lamellar tissue [5].

In the normal horse, the majority of these mononuclear cells are macrophages expressing the CD163 receptor, which is selectively expressed on monocytes and macrophages [23]. CD163 is usually identified as a marker of the alternatively activated (M2) or 'anti-inflammatory' macrophage phenotype [24]. However, some monocytes/macrophages expressing CD163 in laminitic horses are also observed migrating from the lamellar vasculature and can also express calprotectin. As positive calprotectin staining indicates the inflammatory macrophage phenotype or classically activated (M1) phenotype [5], this finding suggests that $CD163^+$ cells can have dual roles. $CD163^+$ cells were reported to be moderately prevalent in deep/sublamellar dermis (between the digital lamellae and the distal phalanx) and lamellar regions in normal horses (Fig. 13.2). The majority of these cells in normal lamellae have a dendritic-type morphology and are primarily localized in the areolar tissue surrounding vessels and nerves in the sublamellar dermis and the interstitium of the primary and secondary dermal lamellae. Rare $CD163^+$ cells were seen in the epidermal lamellae among basal epidermal keratinocytes, suggestive of a Langerhans-type cell in the lamellar epidermis [5].

T lymphocytes ($CD3^+$) and B lymphocytes ($CD20^+$) are also present in the lamellae of normal non-laminitic horses (Fig. 13.3) [5]. The T lymphocytes occur primarily around the major vessels in the deep dermis and were infrequently seen around smaller vessels in the primary dermal lamellae [5]. Clusters of T lymphocytes resembling a lymphoid tissue can be found in the sublamellar dermis. In a similar pattern, B lymphocytes occur in the sublamellar dermis, but are rarely observed in the lamellar region [5].

Black Walnut Extract Model

As previously mentioned, leukopenia (a 30% decrease in circulating leukocyte count) is a consistent finding occurring 3–4 h following BWE administration [9, 25], and has been used as referential time point in the development of laminitis in this model [3, 25, 26]. The majority of the horses develop Obel grade 1 laminitis with this model, and those which become lame have a significant reduction in circulating leukocytes when compared to values for those that do not become lame [26].

Recruited leukocytes start to reach lamellar tissue as early as 1.5 h after BWE administration [4, 22]. Studies using a calprotectin (CP) antibody (this is a more specific marker for myeloid cells – purportedly all neutrophils and activated monocytes/macrophages – but can also stain inflamed/stressed epidermal cells) showed that CP^+ cells, either leukocytes or epithelial cells, were only rarely detected in the lamellae of normal horses. However, prominent increases in CP^+ leukocytes were detected in the lamellar regions at 1.5 h (53-fold), the onset of leukopenia (developmental time point [DTP]; 151-fold), and

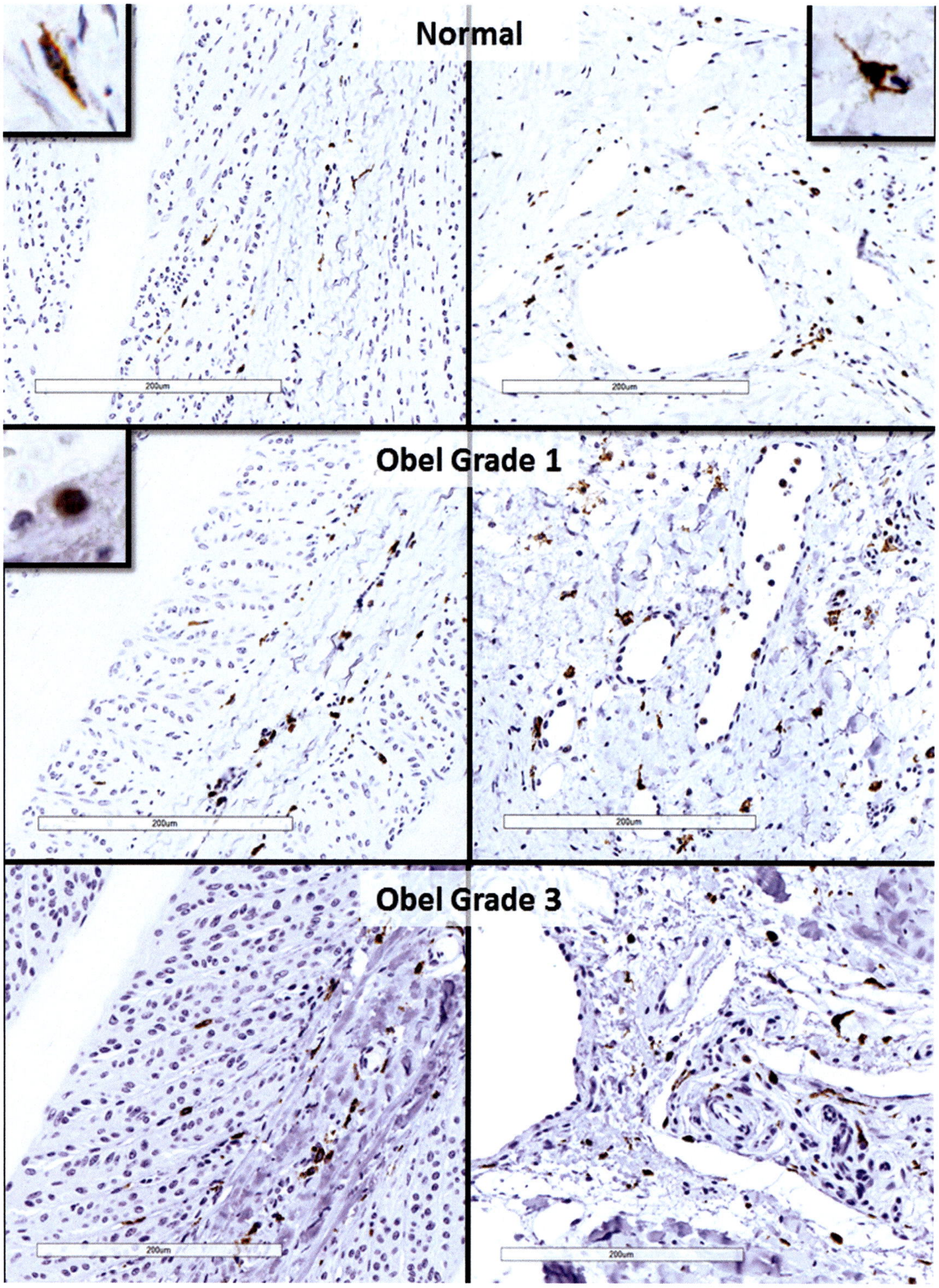

Figure 13.2 Photomicrograph of equine lamellar tissue from normal and laminitic (CHO-induced) horses at the onset of lameness (Obel grade 1) and onset of severe lameness (Obel grade 3) time points. $CD163^+$ macrophages are stained in brown. In normal horses, most of the resident cells are dendritic-shaped (right inset) and flat-shaped (upper left inset) and mainly localized in the areolar tissue surrounding vessels and nerves in the subdermis (right image) or in the interstitium of the primary and secondary dermal lamella (left image). In laminitic horses, there is intense recruitment of $CD163^+$ monocytes at the onset of lameness, which can be observed as intra- and perivascular round-shaped cells (lower left inset). Compared with normal horses, Obel grade 1 laminitic horses have threefold greater lamellar counts of $CD163^+$ cells.

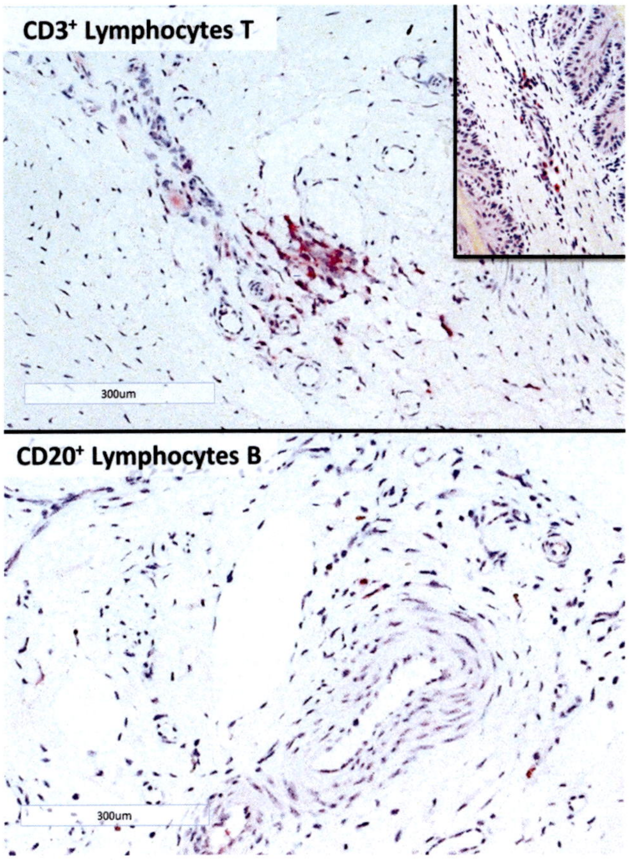

Figure 13.3 Photomicrograph of normal equine lamellar tissue showing T lymphocytes and B lymphocytes positive (red staining) for CD3 and CD20 markers, respectively. Note that both lymphocyte types occur primarily in the areolar connective tissue around the major vessels of the sublamellar dermis. As observed in the upper image, clusters of T lymphocytes resembling those found in lymphoid tissue can be identified. Additionally, T lymphocytes can be found around vessels in the lamellar primary dermal lamellae (inset).

onset of lameness (106-fold) [4], with similar emigration patterns present in the sublamellar dermis. The study results also showed that recruited leukocytes were not only confined to the perivascular space but were also able to migrate through the dense ECM of the dermal lamellae to the BM of the epidermal lamellae, starting at the DPT. However, the most relevant finding was that CP staining of the epidermal lamellae (indicating epithelial stress) occurred only at the onset of lameness (following leukocyte emigration), supporting the hypothesis that leukocyte emigration is a potential cause of lamellar epidermal damage.

Leukocytes, mainly neutrophils, are cells specialized in the production of inflammatory mediators, proteolytic enzymes and reactive oxygen species (ROS) to phagocytose and kill pathogens. These leukocyte-derived products are also believed to cause damage to normal tissue during the emigration process. Increased concentrations of ROS from systemic leukocytes [26], increased lamellar myeloperoxidase (MPO) activity [27], matrix metalloproteinase (i.e., MMP9) transcription and zymogen concentrations [28], and increased elastase concentrations [29] have all been reported in horses with BWE-induced laminitis.

Although neutrophils are reported to be the main type of myeloid cell emigrating during the developmental stages of BWE-induced laminitis [3, 4], monocytes are also participants. The total number of circulating monocytes decreases during the leukopenia phase [26], and a twofold increase in cells positive for the monocyte/macrophage marker CD163 was present compared with control horses in the secondary dermal lamellae and sublamellar dermis during the developmental phases after BWE administration [6]. However, low counts of CD163^{+} stained cells at the onset of lameness indicate that these cells may have less of a role in producing lamellar damage during BWE-induced laminitis. As lamellar damage and clinical signs of laminitis are typically less severe with BWE administration compared to CHO, it is believed that a single BWE bolus administration causes a marked but only transient systemic inflammatory response. This short lived inflammatory effect of the BWE bolus could explain the decrease in inflammatory cells counts by the onset of lameness [30], and further suggests that increased numbers of mononuclear cells may play an important role in the lamellar damage seen in other models (e.g., CHO) where a more potent and prolonged emigration of mononuclear cells is present. No changes in the numbers of lamellar B and T lymphocytes were observed in horses subjected to the BWE model [6].

CHO Models (Corn Starch and Oligofructose)

Consistent with the systemic differences in leukocyte dynamics in the CHO and BWE models (i.e., neutrophilia versus early leukopenia, respectively), lamellar leukocyte dynamics are also distinct between the two models. This difference was most evident in regards to neutrophil presence in the dermal lamellae in the two models, with large numbers of extravasating neutrophils detectable with only hematoxylin staining in the BWE model, and only rarely (if at all) observed in similar sections from CHO models. Additionally, few to no positive CD13-stained cells could be detected in lamellar tissue from horses receiving CHO (J.K. Belknap and R.R. Faleiros, unpublished data). The reason for this is now realized, in that the primary cell type which populates the lamellar tissue in the CHO model is the mononuclear cell, with an extremely limited influx of neutrophils at any time point assessed. Because the morphology of the tissue mononuclear cells appears similar to that of other lamellar dermal cells (e.g., fibroblasts) without specific stains, these cells had been missed during investigations of laminitis for multiple decades.

The developmental period of laminitis after CHO is prolonged compared to the BWE model. During the developmental period of the CHO model fever occurs typically 10–20 h after starch administration [5], but very few CP^{+} leukocytes are observed in the lamellar tissue in this developmental period in

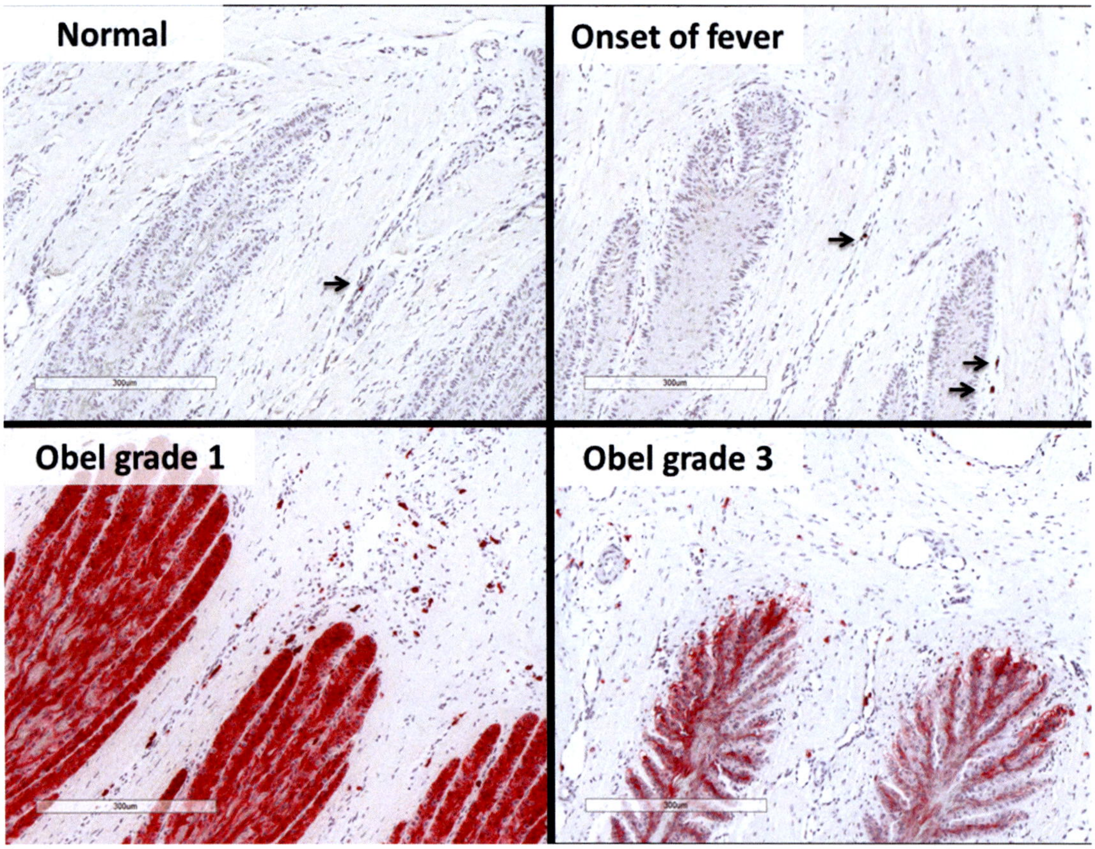

Figure 13.4 Photomicrograph of equine lamellar tissue from normal and laminitic (CHO-induced) horses at the onset of fever, onset of lameness (Obel grade 1) and onset of severe lameness (Obel grade 3) time points. The calprotectin myeloid leukocytes and epidermal positive cells are stained in red. None to rare staining is observed in normal horses, showing the absence of resident neutrophils and classically activated macrophage subpopulations in the equine lamellae. The onset of fever is coincident with the beginning of lamellar leukocyte recruitment. At the onset of lameness, diffuse and intense epidermal calprotectin expression can be easily observed together with a marked recruitment of myeloid leukocytes. When lameness progresses to Obel grade 3, leukocytes can be observed spreading into the extracellular matrix, and the architecture of epidermal lamellae is deteriorated but still shows diffuse calprotectin expression.

the CHO model compared to large numbers during the developmental period in horses receiving BWE (peak in Lamellar WBC numbers at 3–4 h post BWE administration) [5]. At the onset of lameness, the scenario is very similar to that reported in the BWE model, however, with larger numbers of CP^+ leukocytes spreading into lamellar and sublamellar dermal regions, perhaps up to 180-fold more than in normal horses [5]. At this time point, diffuse and intense CP staining is also seen in the epidermal lamellae (Fig. 13.4). Interestingly, the intensity of epidermal CP staining appears to be greater in epithelial cells adjacent to the dermal lamellae with greater numbers of CP^+ leukocytes (R.R. Faleiros and J.K. Belknap, unpublished results).

When lameness progresses to Obel grade 3 (OG3), there is a slight decrease in the number of CP^+ leukocytes and in the intensity of epidermal calprotectin staining (R.R. Faleiros and J.K. Belknap, unpublished results). At this phase, BM collapse and disintegration can easily be observed in many regions of the epidermal lamellae. Unlike the earlier time points (developmental and OG1), leukocytes can be found invading the epidermal lamellae and reaching the lamellar keratinized axis (Fig. 13.5). Thus, at the OG3 time point, the presence of recruited leukocytes in dermal lamellae appears to correlate with the intensity of epidermal damage.

$CD163^+$ macrophages and monocytes are over-represented in the starch CHO model of sepsis-related laminitis at the onset of lameness, but not at the developmental phase (see Fig. 13.2). Unlike the dendrite-type morphology of macrophages stained in the normal horse, most of the $CD163^+$ cells in horses with laminitis are round in shape. Additionally, these cells are seen to be attached to the endothelial surface in lamellar vessels and in the perivascular interstitium around vessels in lamellar and sublamellar dermis regions [5] representing newly recruited monocytes. Compared with samples obtained at the onset of lameness from the BWE model, numbers of $CD163^+$ cells were threefold greater in lamellar tissue from horses with CHO-induced laminitis [5,6].

Although described in much less detail than the traditional starch model with regards to the varying leukocyte population,

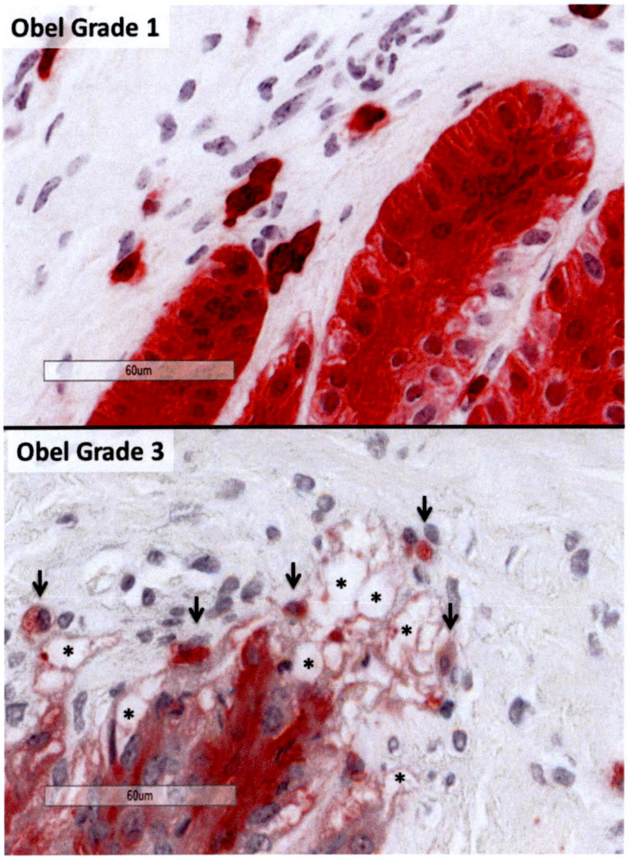

Figure 13.5 Photomicrograph of lamellar tissue from laminitic (CHO-induced) horses at the onset of lameness (Obel grade 1) and onset of severe lameness (Obel grade 3). Calprotectin expression (myeloid leukocytes and epidermal inflammation) is stained in red. At the onset of lameness, there are many leukocytes migrating towards the basal membrane. At this stage, despite intense calprotectin expression, the architecture of epidermal lamellae remains unchanged. When lameness progresses to Obel grade 3, the loss of epidermal integrity is coincident with several leukocytes (arrows) reaching the epidermal–dermal interface. Note the blank spaces (asterisks) showing detachment of epidermal cells from the basal membrane.

the oligofructose (OF) CHO model (see Chapter 8) appears to be associated with a similar pattern of leukocyte response. As occurred in starch CHO-induced laminitis, tissue leukocytes were not detected in the lamellar tissue before advanced clinical signs and interstitial and BM lesions were present when using regular histological techniques [14]. However, CP^+ leukocytes were detected in lamellar tissue at 18 h after OF administration and before epidermal CP staining and major histological BM changes were noted [31, 32].

Hyperinsulinemia Model

Recruited leukocytes have been also consistently described to be present in lamellar tissue from horses and ponies subjected to the prolonged euglycemic hyperinsulinemic clamp technique. In ponies with Obel grade 2 laminitis, in which the histological damage is not as severe as in Standardbred horses, infiltrating leukocytes have been described around sporadic areas of BM separation from epidermal basal cells [33]. In another report, induced hyperinsulinemia in Standardbred horses resulted in a diffuse infiltration of CP^+ leukocytes throughout the dermal connective tissue and around the tips of each primary epidermal lamella [32]. Occasional epidermal staining was also noted; however, staining was not as strong as in the epidermal tissue of horses receiving OF [32]. Interestingly, leukocyte infiltration in the hind feet is reported to be minor compared to the front feet [32], in contrast to the findings in horses undergoing CHO, in which leukocyte infiltration and CP epidermal staining did not differ in the front or hind feet [34].

Additionally, leukocyte oxidative burst is reportedly increased in obese hyperinsulemic horses, correlating strongly with plasma insulin levels [35]. In a recent model of equine metabolic syndrome (EMS) in which lamellae, liver, and skeletal muscle were obtained after lean and obese ponies were placed on a seven-day feeding protocol of a diet either high or low in non-structural carbohydrates, no CP^+ leukocytes were discernible in the lamellae throughout the different groups (resident $CD163^+$ macrophages were present in all samples, but did not change in number). Additionally, no change in proinflammatory cytokine or chemokine concentrations were detected in the face of significant changes in cell signaling related to growth factor activation in the lamellae of these same animals [36], suggesting that this model of EMS does not result in a significant inflammatory response.

Overall, leukocyte infiltration in the hyperinsulinemia model is reportedly less severe than in the CHO models, and actual evi dence suggests that it may be more a consequence than a cause of lamellar damage in endocrinopathic Equine Laminitis.

Potential Role of Leukocytes in the Pathophysiology of Onset Clinical Signs

Although some of the cytokines expressed in lamellar tissue after treatment with BWE or CHO are associated with an adaptive immune response [37], most of the cytokine and leukocyte responses reported to occur in lamellar tissue are much more characteristic of an innate immune response. Despite the differences in systemic leukocyte responses (e.g., neutrophilia in CHO versus neutropenia in BWE model) between the two models of sepsis-related laminitis, the magnitude of CP^+ leukocyte infiltration observed is similar. However, there does appear to be a major difference among those models at this phase, in that the predominant population of recruited cells in the CHO model is composed of monocytes whereas the majority in the BWE model are neutrophils.

It has been hypothesized that compounds in the bolus of BWE extract are quickly absorbed into circulation and act as potent PAMPs, priming leukocytes and starting a SIRS reaction [30].

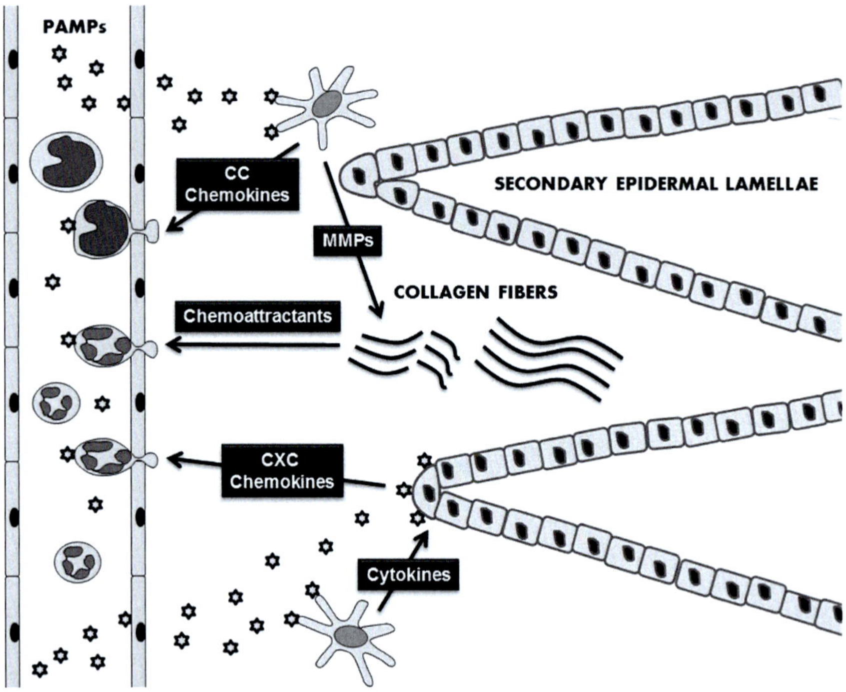

Figure 13.6 Possible role of the innate lamellar immune cell subsystem in sepsis-related laminitis. Pathogen-associated molecular patterns (PAMPs) absorbed from the primary septic focus travel in the blood to reach the lamellar tissue. Inside vessels, PAMPs activate circulating neutrophils, monocytes and lamellar endothelial cells, inducing leukocyte rolling and adhesion to the endothelium. In the tissues, PAMPs activate resident macrophages and keratinocytes. Epidermal cells secrete CXC chemokines, which attract neutrophils to the tissue. Activated macrophages can also directly recruit leukocytes secreting CC chemokines, which attract monocytes. Indirectly, macrophages secrete matrix metalloproteinases (MMPs), which break the extracellular matrix producing collagen-derived peptides that act as chemoattractants for neutrophils. In addition, macrophages release proinflammatory cytokines that can also activate the keratinocytes, inducing further chemokine release.

This mechanism can explain the intense and fast but transitory (due to the fact that only a single bolus is given) reaction caused by BWE in comparison to the reaction caused by CHO. In CHO models, increased levels of soluble carbohydrates in the cecum cause dramatic changes in the intestinal flora as well as destruction of the mucosal epithelial barrier that would lead to a possibly less intense, but progressive, sustained absorption of PAMPs [38].

By this line of reasoning, a model can easily be created to explain sepsis-related laminitis (Fig. 13.6), as in the CHO and BWE models or in clinical cases associated with causes of systemic sepsis including intestinal obstruction, colitis, enteritis, metritis, and pneumonia. Circulating PAMPs or PAMP-like substances (BWE compounds) absorbed from the gut or other primary focus reach resident cells from the SIS innate subsystem (macrophages) and from other lamellar host cells such as epithelial cells. As would be expected to occur when microorganisms and/or their microbial products invade the epidermis, these cells react by releasing destructive mediators (ROS, proteases) and produce inflammatory cytokines. Chemokines – a special type of cytokine chemotactic for leukocytes – are released from tissue macrophages and other lamellar constituents such as epithelial cells, and further recruit myeloid origin leukocytes from the blood that leave the vessels and migrate into the tissue in the direction of the source of chemokines. Recent studies have also shown that matrix metalloproteinases (MMPs) released from activated resident macrophages can degrade the ECM producing collagen-derived peptides, which can also recruit neutrophils [39]. Recruited monocytes and neutrophils invade the dermal lamellae, likely exacerbating both lamellar inflammation and tissue destruction.

Potential Role of Recruited Leukocytes in Lamellar Structural Failure

The first evidence of leukocyte-induced damage in the epidermis came from CP expression in the BWE model [4]. In this study, leukocytes leaving blood vessels, invading the interstitium and reaching the BM, could be observed before the major signs of epidermal stress/damage. Subsequently, a similar emigration of leukocytes prior to signs of epidermal stress was also observed after starch [6] and OF [31] administration, and in horses subjected to jejunal obstruction [40]. The epidermal CP expression coincident with the onset of lameness appears to link leukocyte recruitment and emigration to the detachment of epidermal cells from the BM. In corroborating these experimental findings, a recent study reported CP^+ leukocyte infiltration and epidermal CP expression preceding lamellar damage and clinical signs of laminitis in horses with naturally acquired severe gastrointestinal disorders [41].

Calprotectin/CP^+ is a heterodimer of the proteins S100A8 and S100A9 that are highly expressed in cells of myeloid origin, such as neutrophils (up to 40% of cytosolic protein content) and activated monocytes (5% of cytosolic protein content). The S100A8/9 complex can be also expressed in keratinocytes and epithelial cells, but only under inflammatory conditions [42]. By applying that knowledge and observing the temporal aspects of lamellar leukocyte invasion (see Fig. 13.4), it is easy to hypothesize that leukocytes, when migrating into the dermis, are inducing inflammation and CP expression in the epidermis.

Calprotectin expression by the epidermal cells may be involved in keratinocyte injury (and possible death) and detachment from the BM, as seen in horses with Obel Grade

3 laminitis (Fig. 13.5). Calprotectin compounds S100A8 and S100A9 have been classified as endogenous danger-associated molecular patterns (DAMPs; defined as products from injured host cells that can activate the immune system), and can directly activate Toll-like receptors (TLRs) so as to induce keratinocytes to produce several proinflammatory cytokines [42–44]. Additionally, in mouse models of arthritis, the proinflammatory and TLR activities of S100A8/A9 were found to promote severe damage mediating cartilage destruction, chondrocyte death, and osteoclastic bone resorption [42].

The question persists as to why damage progresses to more severe stages in CHO models of sepsis-related laminitis than in the BWE model. In addition to the fact that the BWE model causes only an extremely transient systemic and lamellar inflammatory response compared to the CHO model, the type of cells that predominate in the CHO models are macrophages/monocytes. These mononuclear cells are known to result in a profound proinflammatory response of a more prolonged duration compared to neutrophils, which are the predominant cell type in the BWE model [6].

Macrophage phenotype may also play a role in the difference of response between the two models (BWE versus CHO). Currently, there is a large amount of emerging information regarding phenotype and functional differences between macrophage subpopulations that involves the resident and recruited macrophages in various tissues. In tissues with abundant populations of resident macrophages associated with epithelial cells, such as intestinal mucosa [45] and pulmonary tissue [46], it is believed that the majority of resident macrophages are expressing the alternatively activated or anti-inflammatory (M2) phenotype. Like the intestinal and pulmonary macrophages, it is suspected these M2 lamellar tissue macrophages have a decreased expression of TLRs and other proinflammatory receptors, but retain phagocytic functions. When the tissue (e.g., the lamella) faces infection or inflammation, PAMPs released by invading pathogens, or DAMPs released by injured resident cells (CP from lamellar epithelial cells, for instance), not only directly activate macrophages but also induce epithelial cells to secrete cytokines and chemokines that cause a change in phenotype of the resident macrophages to a classically activated (M1) phenotype [4, 47].

The M2 phenotype mononuclear cells are basically involved in downregulating inflammation and initiating wound repair activities, including phagocytozing apoptotic neutrophils and synthesizing mediators that promote tissue remodeling and angiogenesis [47]. The M1 population orchestrates local inflammation by not only releasing destructive molecules into the tissue but also by activating other resident immune cells and recruiting neutrophils and monocytes from blood to exacerbate the macrophage-mediated tissue injury [47]. Classically activated (M1) resident macrophages and recruited monocytes have a large arsenal of mediators normally used in the destruction of invading pathogens and foreign materials, including ROS and reactive nitrogen species (RNS), proteases, and proinflammatory lipid mediators and cytokines. When these substances are generated in excessive quantities, or without control (especially remote from the infection source), normal tissue injury occurs [47].

Although markers of severe oxidative stress were not prominently increased in CHO-induced laminitis [48], it is possible that ROS released by leukocytes may cause some cellular injury or dysfunction which does not result in end-stage oxidative damage. Proteases, which have been implicated in structural failure of laminitic horses (see Chapter 15), are important products of myeloid leukocytes [49]. Neutral proteases (e.g., elastase, gelatinase, MMPs, collagenase, plasminogen activator) and acid hydrolases (e.g., proteases, lipases, cathepsins, ribonucleases, phosphatases, glycosidases) released by monocytes/macrophages can act directly on the ECM and cells, causing tissue destruction. Macrophages and monocytes have been shown to express the majority of the described MMP members, but mainly MMP-1, -2, -3, -9, -10, -14 (MT1-MMP), -17 (MT4-MMP) -19, and -25 [49]. Monocytes [50] and macrophages [51] can also express ADAMTS4 (a disintegrin and metalloprotease with thrombospondin motifs 4), a protease which was recently implicated in the progression of lamellar damage from Obel Grade 1 to Obel Grade 3 laminitis (see Chapter 15 for more in depth discussion of MMPs and ADAMTS4) [52].

MMP production depends on the stage of leukocyte maturation, but increases significantly as blood monocytes differentiate into monocyte-derived tissue macrophages [49]. Monocytes are recruited from the bloodstream into the lamellar tissue. Following endothelial transmigration, monocytes are able to cross the subendothelial BM and the interstitial matrix of collagens and fibronectin due to their production of activated MMPs [49]. Continual matrix protease activity of these recruited macrophages could result in further damage between the dermal and epidermal structures.

At present, the destructive potential of resident macrophages and recruited monocytes, combined with their prevalence at the onset of lameness (preceding major epidermal damage) in CHO-induced laminitis provides strong evidence that these cells play a fundamental role in the structural failure that occurs in laminitis. In many experimental models of SIRS and MODS, the blockade of neutrophil and monocyte recruitment and their migration to the tissues ameliorates damage to remote organs [47]. In horses, preliminary studies using a chemokine antagonist that inhibits the tissue infiltration of neutrophils demonstrated a reduction in lamellar inflammation and epidermal cell damage following OF-induced laminitis [53]. However, further studies are required to confirm the possible roles of the lamellar SIS and recruited leukocytes in lamellar pathophysiology and structural failure in Equine Laminitis.

References

1. Bos, J.D. and Luiten, R.M. (2009) Skin immune system. *Cancer Treat. Res.*, **146**, 45–62.
2. Scott, D.W. and Miller, W.H., Jr (2003) *Equine Dermatology*. Saunders, St Louis, 823 p.

3. Black, S.J., Lunn, D.P., Yin, C., *et al.* (2006) Leukocyte emigration in the early stages of laminitis. *Vet. Immunol. Immunopathol.*, **109**, 161–166.
4. Faleiros, R.R., Nuovo, G.J., and Belknap, J.K. (2009) Calprotectin in myeloid and epithelial cells of laminae from horses with black walnut extract-induced laminitis. *J. Vet. Intern. Med.*, **23**, 174–181.
5. Faleiros, R.R., Johnson, P.J., Nuovo, G.J. *et al.* (2011) Laminar leukocyte accumulation in horses with carbohydrate overload-induced laminitis. *J. Vet. Intern. Med.*, **25**, 107–115.
6. Faleiros, R.R., Nuovo, G.J., Flechtner, A.D., *et al.* (2011) Presence of mononuclear cells in normal and affected laminae from the black walnut extract model of laminitis. *Equine Vet. J.*, **43**, 45–53.
7. Garner, H.E., Coffman, J.R., Hahn, A.W., *et al.* (1975) Equine laminitis of alimentary origin: an experimental model. *Am. J. Vet. Res.*, **36**, 441–444.
8. Moore, J.N., Garner, H.E., Berg, J.N., *et al.* (1979) Intracecal endotoxin and lactate during the onset of equine laminitis: a preliminary report. *Am. J. Vet. Res.*, **40**, 722–723.
9. Galey, F.D., Whiteley, H.E., Goetz, T.E., *et al.* (1991) Black walnut (*Juglans nigra*) toxicosis: a model for equine laminitis. *J. Comp. Pathol.*, **104**, 313–326.
10. Moore, J.N., Garner, H.E., and Coffman, J.R. (1981) Haematological changes during development of acute laminitis hypertension. *Equine Vet. J.*, **13**, 240–242.
11. Sprouse, R.F., Garner, H.E., and Green, E.M. (1987) Plasma endotoxin levels in horses subjected to carbohydrate induced laminitis. *Equine Vet. J.*, **19**, 25–28.
12. Bailey, S.R., Adair, H.S., Reinemeyer, C.R., *et al.* (2009) Plasma concentrations of endotoxin and platelet activation in the developmental stage of oligofructose-induced laminitis. *Vet. Immunol. Immunopathol.*, **129**, 167–173.
13. Pollitt, C.C. (1996) Basement membrane pathology: a feature of acute equine laminitis. *Equine Vet. J.*, **28**, 38–46.
14. Croser, E.L. and Pollitt, C.C. (2006) Acute laminitis: descriptive evaluation of serial hoof biopsies, in *Proceedings of the 52nd Annual Convention of the American Association of Equine Practitioners*, San Antonio, Texas, USA.
15. Hunt, R.J. (1991) The pathophysiology of acute laminitis. *Comp. Cont. Vet. Educ.*, **13**, 401–407.
16. Weiss, D.J., Evanson, O.A., McClenahan, D., *et al.* (1997) Evaluation of platelet activation and platelet-neutrophil aggregates in ponies with alimentary laminitis. *Am. J. Vet. Res.*, **12**, 1376–1380.
17. Hood, D.M. (1999) The pathophysiology of developmental and acute laminitis. *Vet. Clin. North Am. Equine Pract.*, **15**, 321–343.
18. Fontaine, G.L., Belknap, J.K., Allen, D., *et al.* (2001) Expression of interleukin-1beta in the digital laminae of horses in the prodromal stage of experimentally induced laminitis. *Am. J. Vet. Res.*, **62**, 714–720.
19. Lunn, D.P., Holmes, M.A., Antczak, D.F., *et al.* (1998) Report of the Second Equine Leucocyte Antigen Workshop, Squaw Valley, California. *Vet. Immunol. Immunopathol.*, **62**, 101–143.
20. Stewart, A.J., Pettigrew, A., Cochran, A.M., *et al.* (2009) Indices of inflammation in the lung and liver in the early stages of the black walnut extract model of equine laminitis. *Vet. Immunol. Immunopathol.*, **129**, 254–260.
21. Chiavaccini, L., Hassel, D.M., Shoemaker, M.L., *et al.* (2011) Detection of calprotectin and apoptotic activity within the equine colon from horses with black walnut extract-induced laminitis. *Vet. Immunol. Immunopathol.*, **144**, 366–373.
22. Loftus, J.P., Black, S.J., Pettigrew, A., *et al.* (2007) Early laminar events involving endothelial activation in horses with black walnut-induced laminitis. *Am. J. Vet. Res.*, **68**, 1205–1211.
23. Fabriek, B.O., Dijkstra, C.D., and van den Berg, T.K. (2005) The macrophage scavenger receptor CD163. *Immunobiology*, **210**, 153–160.
24. Varga, G., Ehrchen, J., Tsianakas, A., *et al.* (2008) Glucocorticoids induce an activated, anti-inflammatory monocyte subset in mice that resembles myeloid-derived suppressor cells. *J. Leukoc. Biol.*, **84**, 644–650.
25. Eaton, S.A., Allen, D., Eades, S.C., *et al.* Digital Starling forces and hemodynamics during early laminitis induced by an aqueous extract of black walnut (*Juglans nigra*) in horses. *Am. J. Vet. Res.*, **56**, 1338–1344.
26. Hurley, D.J., Parks, R.J., Reber, A.J., *et al.* (2006) Dynamic changes in circulating leukocytes during the induction of equine laminitis with black walnut extract. *Vet. Immunol. Immunopathol.*, **110**, 195–206.
27. Riggs, L.M., Franck, T., Moore, J.N., *et al.* Neutrophil myeloperoxidase measurements in plasma, laminar tissue, and skin of horses given black walnut extract. *Am. J. Vet. Res.*, **68**, 81–86.
28. Loftus, J.P., Belknap, J.K., and Black, S.J. (2006) Matrix metalloproteinase-9 in laminae of black walnut extract-treated horses correlates with neutrophil abundance. *Vet. Immunol. Immunopathol.*, **113**, 267–276.
29. de la Rebière de Pouyade, G., Riggs, L.M., Moore, J.N., *et al.* Equine neutrophil elastase in plasma, laminar tissue, and skin of horses administered black walnut heartwood extract. *Vet. Immunol. Immunopathol.*, **135**, 181–187.
30. Belknap, J.K. (2010) Black walnut extract: an inflammatory model. *Vet. Clin. North Am. Equine Pract.*, **26**, 95–101.
31. Visser, M.B. and Pollitt, C.C. (2011) Lamellar leukocyte infiltration and involvement of IL-6 during oligofructose-induced equine laminitis development. *Vet. Immunol. Immunopathol.*, **144**, 120–128.
32. de Laat, M.A., Van Eps, A.W., McGowan, C.M., *et al.* (2011) Equine laminitis: comparative histopathology 48 hours after experimental induction with insulin or alimentary oligofructose in Standardbred horses. *J. Comp. Pathol.*, **145**, 399–409.
33. Nourian, A.R., Asplin, K.E., McGowan, C.M., *et al.* (2009) Equine laminitis: ultrastructural lesions detected in ponies following hyperinsulinaemia. *Equine Vet. J.*, **41**, 671–677.
34. Leise, B.S., Faleiros, R.R., Watts, M., *et al.* (2012) Hindlimb laminar inflammatory response is similar to that present in forelimbs after carbohydrate overload in horses. *Equine Vet. J.*, **44**, 633–639.
35. Holbrook, T.C., Tipton, T., and McFarlane, D. (2012) Neutrophil and cytokine dysregulation in hyperinsulinemic obese horses. *Vet. Immunol. Immunopathol.*, **145**, 283–289.
36. Burns, T.A., Watts, M.R., Weber, P.S., McCutcheon, L.J., Geor, R.J., and Belknap, J.K. (2015) Laminar inflammatory events in lean and obese ponies subjected to high carbohydrate feeding: implications for pasture-associated laminitis. *Equine Vet. J.*, **47**, 489–493.
37. Belknap, J.K., Giguère, S., Pettigrew, A., *et al.* (2007) Lamellar pro-inflammatory cytokine expression patterns in laminitis at the developmental stage and at the onset of lameness: innate vs. adaptive immune response. *Equine Vet. J.*, **39**, 42–47.

38. Garner, H.E., Coffman, J.R., Halliwell, W.H., *et al.* (1975) Clinical signs of acute alimentary laminitis correlated with cardiovascular and histopathological alterations, in Proceedings, 21st Annual Convention of the American Association of Equine Practice, pp. 61–65.
39. Gaggar, A., Jackson, P.L., Noerager, B.D., *et al.* (2008) A novel proteolytic cascade generates an extracellular matrix-derived chemoattractant in chronic neutrophilic inflammation. *J. Immunol.*, **180**, 5662–5692.
40. Laskoski, L.M., Valadão, C.C.A., Vasconcelos, R.O., *et al.* (2010) Neutrophil gelatinase-associated lipocalin and matrix metalloproteinases in laminar tissue from horses subjected to intestinal obstruction and treated with hydrocortisone *J. Equine Vet. Sci.*, **30**, 115.
41. Laskoski, L.M., Locatelli-Dittrich, R., Valadão, C.A., *et al.* (2015) Systemic leukopenia, evaluation of laminar leukocyte infiltration and laminar lesions in horses with naturally occurring colic syndrome. *Res. Vet. Sci.*, **101**, 15–21.
42. Vogl, T., Gharibyan, A.L., and Morozova-Roche, L.A. (2012) Proinflammatory S100A8 and S100A9 proteins: self-assembly into multifunctional native and amyloid complexes. *Int. J. Mol. Sci.*, **13**, 2893–2917.
43. Nurami, K., Miyakawa, R., Ueda, R., Hashimoto, H., Yamamoto, Y., Yoshida, T., and Aoki, K. (2015) Proinflammatory proteins S100A8/S100A9 activate NK cells via interaction with RAGE. *J. Immunol.*, **194**, 5539–5548.
44. Lee, Y., Jang, S., Min, J.K., *et al.* (2012) S100A8 and S100A9 are messengers in the crosstalk between epidermis and dermis modulating a psoriatic milieu in human skin. *Biochem. Biophys. Res. Commun.*, **423**, 647–653.
45. Platt, A.M. and Mowat, A.M. (2008) Mucosal macrophages and the regulation of immune responses in the intestine. *Immunol. Lett.*, **119**, 22–31.
46. Lambrecht, B.N. (2006) Alveolar macrophage in the driver's seat. *Immunity*, **24**, 366–368.
47. Laskin, D.L., Sunil, V.R., and Gardner, C.R. (2011) Macrophages and tissue injury: agents of defense or destruction? *Annu. Rev. Pharmacol. Toxicol.*, **51**, 267–288.
48. Burns, T.A., Westerman, T., Nuovo, G.J., *et al.* (2011) Role of oxidative tissue injury in the pathophysiology of experimentally induced equine laminitis: a comparison of 2 models. *J. Vet. Intern. Med.*, **25**, 540–548.
49. Webster, N.L. and Crowe, S.M. (2006) Matrix metalloproteinases, their production by monocytes and macrophages and their potential role in HIV-related diseases. *J. Leukoc. Biol.*, **80**, 1052–1066.
50. Zha, Y., Chen, Y., Xu, F., *et al.* (2010) Elevated level of ADAMTS4 in plasma and peripheral monocytes from patients with acute coronary syndrome. *Clin. Res. Cardiol.*, **99**, 781–786.
51. Salter, R.C., Arnaoutakis, K., Michael, D.R., *et al.* (2011) The expression of a disintegrin and metalloproteinase with thrombospondin motifs 4 in human macrophages is inhibited by the anti-atherogenic cytokine transforming growth factor-β and requires Smads, p38 mitogen-activated protein kinase and c-Jun. *Int. J. Biochem. Cell Biol.*, **43**, 805–811.
52. Wang, L., Pawlak, E., Johnson, P.J., *et al.* (2012) Effects of cleavage by a disintegrin and metalloproteinase with thrombospondin motifs-4 on gene expression and protein content of versican and aggrecan in the digital laminae of horses with starch gruel-induced laminitis. *Am. J. Vet. Res.*, **73**, 1047–1056.
53. Lima, L.R., Mendes, H.M.F., Soriani, F.M., *et al.* (2016) Histologic and inflammatory lamellar changes in horses with oligofructose-induced laminitis treated with a CXCR1/2 antagonist. *Pesq. Vet. Bras.*, **36**, 13–18.

CHAPTER 14

Leukocytes and Inflammatory Signaling in Laminitis: Inflammatory Signaling

Britta Leise

Introduction

Laminitis, or lamellar inflammation, was at one time thought to be an inappropriate term, as inflammation within the lamellae had not been well documented until the late 1990s. With the development of molecular biology techniques and more recent improvements in protein biochemistry specific to equine species, inflammation has been determined to be a central component in the pathophysiology of sepsis-related laminitis (SRL). Inflammation has been reported to occur early during the developmental stages of the black walnut extract (BWE) model of SRL [1–12] even before clinical signs of digital pathology or lameness are observed. In addition to the influx of leukocytes into the lamellae (see Chapter 13) [7, 13, 14], increases in numerous inflammatory mediators within the lamellar tissue have been reported in several experimental models of equine SRL [1, 9, 15, 16]. The early and aggressive inflammatory response demonstrated in the lamellae from horses undergoing experimentally induced laminitis from BWE, and carbohydrate overload (CHO) from both starch gruel (see Chapter 7) and oligofructose (OF; see Chapter 8) is similar to that of human sepsis/systemic inflammatory response syndrome (SIRS) in which an overexpression of proinflammatory mediators results in damage or complete failure of tissues/organs, such as the lamellar tissue of the horse [17].

Although inflammation occurs in causes other than SRL, the role that inflammation plays in the pathogenesis and development of supporting limb and endocrinopathic laminitis is not as well defined. Reports vary on the presence and degree of inflammation present in the lamellar tissue from these predisposing syndromes. At present, very little is known about the pathophysiology of supporting limb laminitis as the development of a humane, consistent experimental model has been difficult; however, a short-term, non-weight-bearing model has recently been developed [18]. Although causes for the development of supporting limb laminitis often have an inflammatory component to the predisposing condition, such as fractures and septic arthritis, experimentally there has been no evidence of lamellar inflammation [18]. Inconsistent results exist regarding the presence of inflammation in the lamellar tissue during the developmental and early onset of lameness periods from horses with insulin dysregulation/resistance [19, 20]. Interestingly, in recent studies using the hyperinsulinemic–euglycemic clamp model of laminitis in Standardbred horses, a 48-h period of hyperinsulinemia resulted in marked increases in lamellar concentrations of inflammatory mediators including cytokines, chemokines and cyclooxygenase-2 (COX-2) (J.K. Belknap, unpublished data). Activation of the inflammatory response systemically or in adipose tissue from obese horses has also been hypothesized to play a role in lamellar failure; however, conflicting results from several studies [19–22] question the primary role that systemic inflammation plays in the pathogenesis of the different types of endocrinopathic laminitis.

Inflammatory Signaling in Horses with Sepsis or SIRS

The pathogenesis of sepsis is complex and incompletely understood; however, dysregulation of the inflammatory response is a key factor in the development of sepsis-related tissue damage. Most inflammatory signaling present today in mammals evolved in simple organisms very early in evolution to provide a profound local inflammatory response when either a pathogenic organism invaded the organism (and needed to be destroyed by host cells [primarily immune cells]), or where tissue injury occurred (requiring clearance of the host tissue debris by host cells). The molecules present in pathogens that induce these inflammatory responses in the host are most commonly called pathogen-associated molecular patterns (PAMPs; also termed microbe-associated molecular patterns [MAMPs]), whereas the host proteins that are released by injured tissues (commonly nuclear or mitochondrial proteins) are termed *alarmins* or damage-associated molecular patterns (DAMPs) [23–25]. Both, host and pathogen proteins (DAMPs and PAMPs) bind to and activate the same host receptors, termed pattern recognition receptors (PRRs; Toll-like receptors, Nod receptors, etc.), to

Equine Laminitis, First Edition. Edited by James K. Belknap and Raymond Geor.

induce inflammatory signaling [25]. Although leukocytes are the classic cell type to recognize damage and pathogen proteins, many other cells in the body – including epithelial cells – are able to identify and respond to these proteins. The inflammatory signaling induced by the activation of PRRs varies with different cell types, but generally results in the cellular expression of inflammatory molecules (e.g., adhesion molecules, cytokines, chemokines, COX-2, all of which are discussed below).

The terms sepsis, SIRS and endotoxemia are frequently used interchangeably, as there are large overlaps in the clinical signs associated with each condition, and there are many similar cellular events that occur in all three conditions [26,27]. A localized response to infection and/or trauma can be termed *local sepsis*, and results in an inflammatory response to clear the local tissue of infection or host cellular debris. Sepsis or SIRS describes the state when the local infection/trauma is not controlled and results in the absorption of these inflammatory molecules, infectious organisms, and/or cellular debris (e.g., PAMPs and DAMPs) into the systemic circulation through the compromised tissue. The same potent inflammatory response which is vital for the resolution of a locally compromised/affected tissue now can become an uncontrolled systemic inflammatory response [26, 27]. Although organs such as the liver and lungs have evolved to clear small amounts of pathogens or their products by local tissue macrophages, these organs in sepsis can actually add to the SIRS, being activated by PAMPs and DAMPs to produce inflammatory molecules (e.g., cytokines), which enter the circulation. Thus, the host tissues in sepsis are exposed to a combined cocktail of PAMPs, DAMPs, and inflammatory molecules. The activation of PRRs and the receptors for inflammatory molecules on the host cells in the different tissues then results in a focal inflammatory response that differs in severity between different organs/tissues in different animals [27]. In humans, the most commonly affected tissues/organs include the kidneys, lungs, liver, and intestinal tract, commonly leading to organ failure. In the adult horse, the lamellar tissue is by far the tissue most prominently affected in sepsis (the kidney is likely second). Therefore, in sepsis/endotoxemia, an inflammatory response which originally evolved in simple organisms to address a focal event quickly becomes uncontrolled, resulting in an overproduction of inflammatory mediators in the systemic circulation and consequent significant tissue damage that leads to organ failure in humans and laminitis in horses.

Numerous inflammatory mediators exist and include (but are not limited to) cytokines, chemokines, COX-2, endothelial adhesion molecules, and antimicrobial proteins. Cytokines are one of the largest group of inflammatory mediators. They are small proteins secreted by various cell types and can have autocrine, paracrine, or endocrine functions [28]. Cytokines can be either proinflammatory or anti-inflammatory, which means they can have synergistic or antagonistic effects on inflammatory events occurring in the cells/tissues of the body [28]. They serve in redundant function and are often induced by a series of signaling events [28]. Chemokines are specialized cytokines that serve to recruit and attract immune cells to sites of infection and trauma. COX-2 is an enzyme important in the formation of other inflammatory mediators in the prostanoid group, including prostaglandins and thromboxane [29]. Adhesion molecule proteins are located on the surface of endothelial cells and allow for the attachment and migration of leukocytes out of the vasculature and into the tissues as the site of infection or tissue trauma. Together, these inflammatory mediators are intricately involved in both the local and systemic inflammatory response and are believed to play an important role in the development of SRL.

Inflammatory mediator production has been extensively evaluated and compared between the BWE and CHO models of SRL, and considerable temporal differences have been found to exist. Although both models involve the administration of a substance (CHO or BWE) via a nasogastric tube, systemic and local lamellar events occur much more quickly in the BWE model. Overall, CHO results in a lamellar inflammatory response that is delayed in onset [16] when compared to the early fulminant inflammatory response in the BWE model [1, 3, 4, 9]. Whereas, animals in the BWE model undergo a rapid and aggressive inflammatory response by 1.5 h following BWE administration (many hours before the onset of lameness), the majority of inflammatory genes are not significantly expressed above controls until the onset of lameness after CHO. It has been purported that the differences between the CHO model and the BWE model of SRL are similar to the differences between the two models used to induce experimental sepsis in rodents, namely the cecal ligation and puncture (CLP) and endotoxin (lipopolysaccharide; LPS) administration models [30–32]. In the BWE model, the rapid absorption of a substance which induces a profound but transient systemic inflammatory response is the likely cause of lamellar inflammation. This substance and the subsequent response are similar to the rapid and marked (but transient) systemic inflammatory reaction that follows the administration of a bolus of endotoxin in experimental animals. In the CHO model, intraluminal changes in the gastrointestinal flora and subsequent injury to the epithelium of the large intestine results in a loss of barrier function and the systemic absorption of an overwhelming amount of inflammatory 'trigger molecules' (most likely bacterial products and DAMPS from the injured intestinal cells) that takes several hours to days to occur [33]. This is similar to the CLP rodent model of sepsis, where a gradual increase in – but sustained presence of – bacterial products occurs in the circulation, resulting in a sustained inflammatory response that eventually leads to organ injury.

Numerous inflammatory mediators have been documented to be upregulated during experimental models of SRL. These include (but are not limited to) proinflammatory cytokines (interleukin (IL)-1β, IL-6, and IL-12) [1, 3, 16], neutrophilic chemokines (CXCL1, CXCL6, and CXCL8) [6, 15], monocytic chemokines (CCL2 and CCL8) [15], adhesion molecules (E-selectin and intercellular adhesion molecule-1; ICAM-1) [9,16], COX-2 [12,16,34], and antimicrobial proteins [7,10,13].

Increases in the gene expression of the proinflammatory cytokines IL-1β and IL-6 have been demonstrated in the lamellae of horses in the BWE [1,3,4], starch gruel [16], and OF [14]

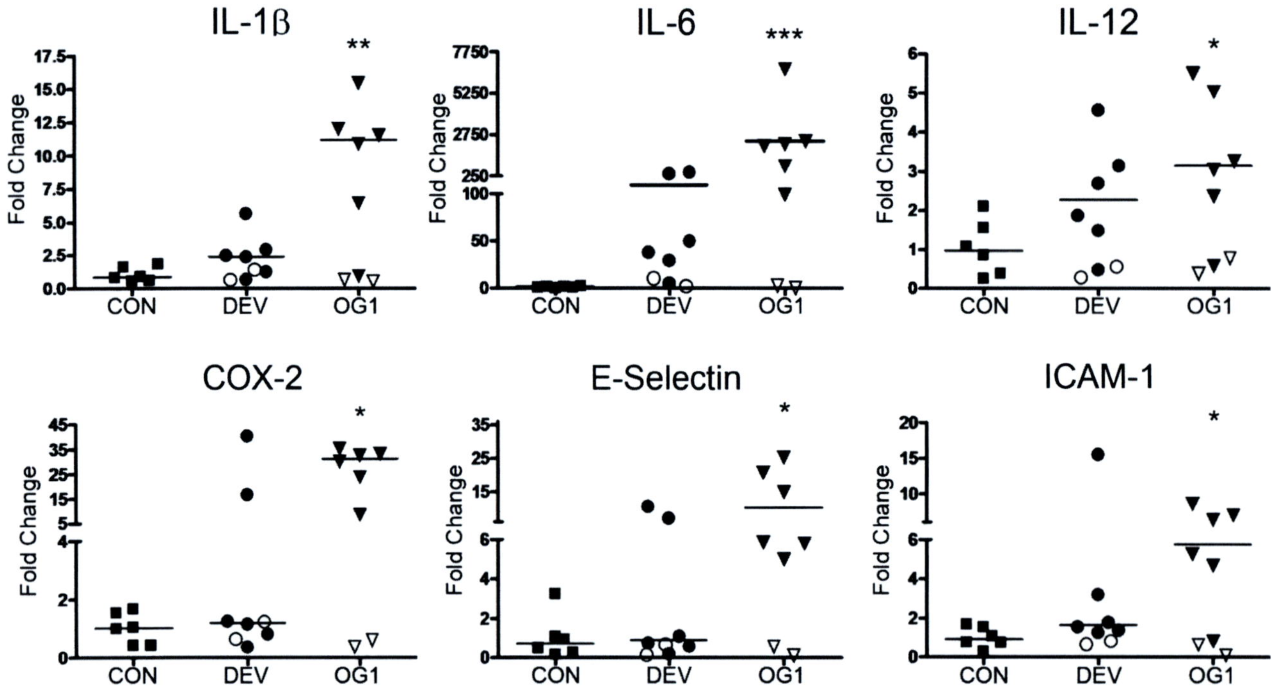

Figure 14.1 Median fold changes in lamellar mRNA concentrations after CHO in horses (development [DEV] and Obel grade 1 [OG1]). Significantly increased inflammatory mediator when compared to control (CON) horses (*P < 0.05; **P < 0.01; ***P < 0.001). Open circles indicate non-responders at the DEV time. Open triangles indicate non-responders at the OG1 time. Reproduced with permission from Ref. [16]; © Wiley.

models of sepsis-related laminitis (Fig. 14.1). Early increases in lamellar mRNA concentrations of both IL-1β and IL-6 have been reported in the BWE model, with a sustained increased in IL-6 mRNA concentration through the onset of lameness [1, 3, 9]. Lamellar mRNA concentrations of inflammatory mediators including IL-6 present at Obel grade 1 [16] begin waning by Obel grade 3 [35] after CHO. An increased gene expression of lamellar IL-6 has also been reported in the OF model as early as 12 h post administration [14]. These proinflammatory cytokines, which are an important part of the innate immune response, are also characteristic of the cytokine response reported with sepsis/SIRS in humans [36]. Increased plasma concentrations of IL-1β and IL-6 have been negatively correlated with outcome in human patients with sepsis [37]. Inflammation and metalloprotease expression and activation are closely intertwined. Whereas, the expression of MMPs and ADAMTS – molecules that can degrade important matrix molecules in the lamellae (see Chapter 15) – can be upregulated by inflammatory mediators, such as IL-1β and IL-6, MMPs (including MMP-2 and -9) can also function as negative feedback mediators by degrading cytokines [38].

Increases in mRNA concentrations of tumor necrosis factor-α (TNF-α), a prominent inflammatory cytokine present in sepsis/SIRS in humans, are not commonly found in the lamellar tissue of horses after BWE or CHO [1, 16], with only one report showing a significant difference in mRNA expression in the lamellar tissue after CHO [39]. The lack of TNF-α response in the lamellar tissue may be similar to that seen in rats after endotoxin administration, where systemic increases in TNF-α were present but local production of TNF-α in the interstitial fluid of the rat paw was not apparent [40]. Initially, the absence of a lamellar TNF-α response was purported to be due to a lack of mononuclear cells present in the lamellar tissue; however, this theory has since been disproven, as there is now strong evidence of macrophages within the primary and secondary dermis in both normal horses and those with laminitis [8, 13]. Although TNF-α is not present in lamellar tissue during the development of laminitis, increases in serum concentrations have been reported in the OF model [41]. Increases in TNF-α have also been found in the blood and peritoneal fluid of horses with acute abdominal disease [42–44], particularly in those cases at risk of developing laminitis. The source of TNF-α in the serum may not be directly related to expression within peripheral blood cells, as no change in mRNA concentrations of TNF-α was reported from peripheral blood mononuclear cells after the administration of OF to horses [45]. However, other sources of TNF-α have been documented in the BWE and CHO models of laminitis, where increased mRNA concentrations have been reported early in the developmental stages within the lung and liver after BWE administration [46] and within the liver after CHO administration [47]. Increases in systemic concentrations of TNF-α after CHO administration have also been reported, with significantly increased concentrations occurring 20 h post CHO [39]. Despite the fact that the lamellae do not demonstrate a significant

TNF-α response, it is likely that this tissue is affected by systemic increases in TNF-α in both experimental models and clinical cases of sepsis/SIRS.

Similar to other inflammatory mediators, COX-2 mRNA concentrations were not increased until the onset of Obel grade 1 lameness after CHO [16] (see Fig. 14.1) compared to increases in COX-2 expression initiated at earlier time points (both the developmental time points and onset of lameness) in horses after BWE administration [12,34]. In contrast to several other inflammatory mediators, mRNA concentrations of COX-2 remained significantly increased in Obel grade 3 horses after CHO administration when compared to controls [35]. No change in COX-1 mRNA concentrations were present at any time in either the BWE [12] or CHO [16] models; this finding is not unexpected considering that COX-1 is constitutively expressed, unlike COX-2 which is inducible in most tissues by inflammation [48]. Although increases in mRNA expression of the COX isoenzymes may not directly correlate to protein concentrations and enzyme activity [49], increases in COX-2 protein concentrations have been documented in addition to increases in mRNA concentrations in the BWE model [12, 34]. Overall, the profound and prolonged expression of COX-2 demonstrated during the acute stages of laminitis in these models suggest that therapeutic intervention inhibiting its expression (via cryotherapy) or activity (via NSAIDs) may be an important component in the prevention and treatment of horses with sepsis/SIRS.

A compensatory anti-inflammatory response is known to occur in an attempt to limit the overwhelming inflammatory response associated with sepsis/SIRS in other species [50]. This anti-inflammatory response modifies or adapts the immune status of the patient and classically involves production of the cytokine IL-10 [51, 52]. Lamellar IL-10 mRNA concentrations were reported to be decreased early in the BWE model at the 3 h developmental time, but returned to control values by the time lameness occurred [1]. A transient decrease in the expression of IL-10 was noted in the liver after BWE administration [46]. In contrast, no change in expression of IL-10 has been reported in the lamella of horses after CHO administration [16]; however, increases in IL-10 gene expression are present after CHO in both the liver and lung [47]. Compartmentalization, defined as the occurrence of varying inflammatory responses in different organs or blood compared to each other, has been described to be present during sepsis/SIRS and is believed to be a result of cellular composition of these organs [53]. Furthermore, the absence of a protective anti-inflammatory response in the lamellae versus the presence of a response in the liver and lung after CHO may in part explain why the lamellae are the site of failure and the other organs are often spared in cases of sepsis/SIRS in the horse.

The expression of adhesion molecules such as ICAM-1 and E-selectin on the luminal endothelial surface of the microvasculature of tissues plays a critical role in the activation and emigration of circulating leukocytes into target tissues in sepsis. Increases in mRNA concentrations of the leukocyte adhesion molecules E-selectin and ICAM-1 have been reported in the lamellae of horses after in both BWE [9] and CHO [16] models. In the BWE model, these adhesion molecules were markedly upregulated very early, peaking at 1.5 h after BWE administration and decreasing precipitously in expression by the onset of lameness [1, 9]. However, in the CHO model, these adhesion molecules were not increased until the onset of Obel grade 1 lameness (Fig. 14.1) [16]. Endothelial activation in the lamellae coincides with the timing of the influx of leukocytes in models of SRL, both increased endothelial leukocyte adhesion molecule expression and influx of leukocytes into the lamellar dermis occurring by the early developmental stages in the BWE model [7], and after the onset of Obel grade 1 laminitis in the starch gruel CHO overload model [13]. The delayed increases in mRNA concentrations of adhesion molecules after CHO, when compared to reports after BWE, may be explained by the delayed production of local or systemic cytokines, such as IL-1β and IL-6, which have a positive effect on the regulation of expression of these adhesion molecules [9, 54]. Furthermore, the presence of upregulated adhesion molecules during the onset of lameness may be indicative of the severity of lamellar injury in the CHO model, as a similar study comparing non-survivors of human sepsis to survivors found that a continued elevation in ICAM-1 was found more commonly in non-survivors [55].

In addition to adhesion molecules present in the endothelium, chemokines produced by numerous cell types are essential for the activation and recruitment of leukocytes into the target tissues of sepsis/SIRS. Increased lamellar mRNA concentrations of the chemokines CXCL1 [6, 15], CXCL6 [15], and CXCL8 [1, 9, 15] were present in response to CHO and BWE administration when compared to control horses. The CXC-chemokines are generally known for their neutrophil chemotaxis, but can also attract other cells, including monocytes. These CXC-chemokines were present in the lamellar tissue at both the developmental and onset of Obel grade 1 lameness periods. In contrast, mRNA concentrations for the CC-chemokines (CCL2 and CCL8), primarily known for their monocytic chemoattractant properties, were only increased at the onset of Obel grade 1 lameness horses in the CHO model [15]. The temporal differences in chemokine response between BWE and CHO models are demonstrated by a peak in CXC-chemokines by 1.5 h post BWE administration [9] and leukocyte emigration shortly thereafter [2,7]. This clustering of events in the BWE model indicates that an inflammatory molecule present in black walnut heartwood is rapidly absorbed into the circulation (most likely via the small intestine), simultaneously activating circulating leukocytes, endothelium, and other lamellar host cells. This is in contrast to the CHO model, where less of a chemokine response is present early in the developmental phase, no endothelial activation is occurring [16], and there is minimal inflammatory migration into the lamellae [13]. However, by the onset of Obel grade 1 lameness, increases in the monocytic chemokines is reflected by an increased lamellar population of monocytes/macrophages in Obel grade 1 horses [13].

Inflammatory Signaling Pathways

The determination of signaling pathways involved in lamellar inflammation requires further evaluation in order to discover novel targets for pharmaceutical intervention. One wet of signaling proteins that have been evaluated from the lamellae of horses are the signal transducing activators of transcription factors (STAT) 1 and 3 proteins of JAK-STAT signaling [56]. The STAT proteins reside in the cytoplasm of cells in a quiescent state and, once activated through phosphorylation, are translocated to the nucleus to serve as transcription factors that result in the expression of various inflammatory genes as well as those regulating cell growth and development. Both STAT1 and STAT3 have been reported to play a role in sepsis/SIRS in human and rodent models [57–61]. No significant difference in STAT1 (both tyrosine and serine) phosphorylation was present between the controls, developmental and the onset of lameness time points after BWE or CHO. As STAT1 is primarily activated by type I and type II interferons (IFNs) [62], and because there are no significant increases in mRNA concentrations of IFNα, IFNβ, or IFNγ documented at any stage in lamellar tissue from horses administered BWE or CHO [1, 16], the absence of a STAT1 response was not completely unexpected.

Lamellar STAT3 activation was present in both BWE and CHO models, with increased phosphorylation of the tyrosine and serine moieties of STAT3 at the developmental and onset of lameness time points (Fig. 14.2) [56]. Since IL-6 (one of the major activators of STAT3 [63, 64]) is greatly increased in the lamellar tissue after BWE and CHO [4, 16], lamellar STAT3 activation would be expected to occur in this tissue. However, the increase in lamellar phospho-Tyr705 concentration at the DEV time point in the CHO model (prior to reported increases in lamellar IL-6 mRNA concentration) indicates that this early activation of STAT3 may be due to either increased circulating IL-6 concentrations [64] or STAT3 activation by other signaling mechanisms (i.e., growth factor signaling [65–67]. Interestingly, increased lamellar concentrations of both IL-6 and phospho-STAT3 have also recently been found in the hyperinsulinemic–euglycemic clamp model of laminitis after 48 h of hyperinsulinemia (J.K. Belknap, unpublished data). Phosphorylation of STAT3 tyrosine and serine moieties can result in an increased expression of IL-1β, IL-6, COX-2, CXCL-8, MCP-1, ICAM1, MMP-2, and MMP-9, depending on various conditions [67–70], thereby promoting a continual inflammatory response and subsequent lamellar injury. STAT3 inhibition has had mixed effects in the rodent CLP models of sepsis, whereby the administration of STAT inhibitors reportedly decreased organ injury and mortality in one report [57]; however, liver-specific STAT3 knockout mice had increased mortality compared to wild-type mice [61]. Therefore, although current results and several compelling studies in other species have suggested that STAT3 inhibition has the potential to decrease lamellar inflammation and injury in SRL,

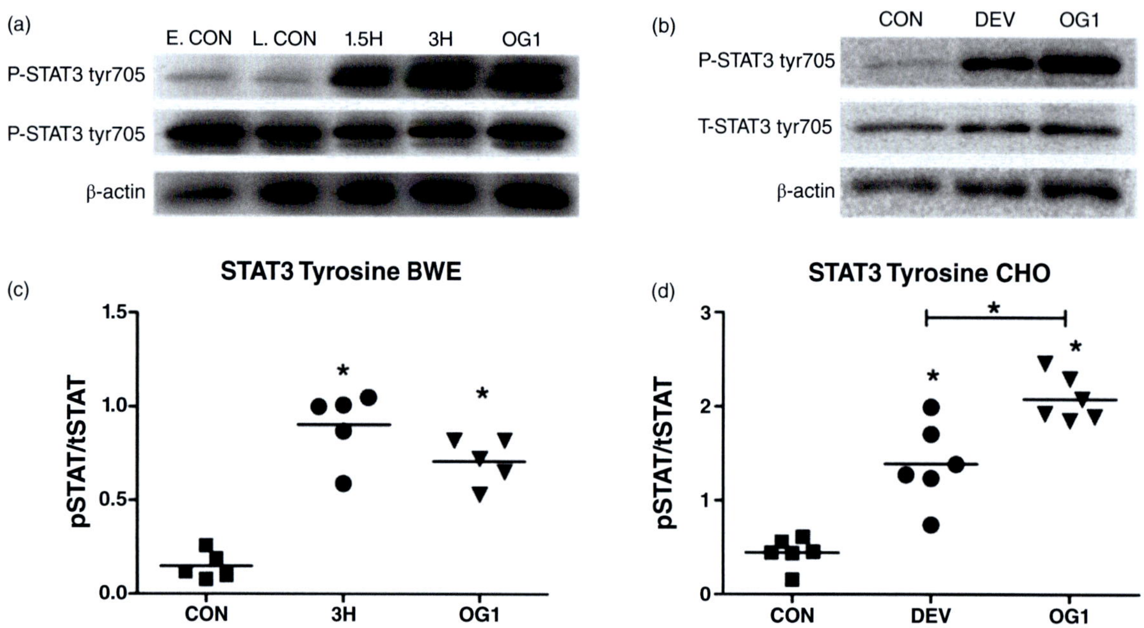

Figure 14.2 STAT3 response in the lamellar tissue of horses receiving BWE or CHO [56]. (a) Western hybridization from pooled samples from control horses (E. CON = early control; L. CON = late control), 1.5 h post BWE (1.5H), 3 h post BWE (3H), and at the onset of Obel grade 1 lameness (OG1). (b) Western hybridization from pooled samples from control horses (CON), developmental horses (DEV), and horses at onset of OG1 lameness (OG1) after CHO administration. (c) Band intensity ratios (phosphorylated STAT3/total STAT3) calculated from individual CON, 3H, and OG1 horses after BWE administration. *Increases in STAT3 ratios compared to controls at the 3H and OG1 times ($P < 0.05$). (d) Band intensity ratios (phosphorylated STAT3/total STAT3) calculated from individual CON, DEV, and OG1 horses after CHO administration. *Increases in STAT3 ratios when compared to controls at the DEV and OG1 times ($P < 0.05$). *OG1 horses also demonstrated increased STAT3 ratios when compared to DEV horses ($P < 0.05$).

further studies are required to determine if STAT3 inhibition results in a beneficial or detrimental effect during the early stages of laminitis.

Hypoxia-inducible-factor 1α (HIF-1α) is an important signaling protein that not only serves as a transcription factor for the cellular response to low tissue concentrations of oxygen, but also is involved in the inflammatory response through the NF-κB signaling pathway [71, 72]. HIF-1α-dependent signaling varies based on the mechanism involved. When hypoxia induces HIF-1α accumulation through inhibition of its degradation, genes for energy metabolism (GLUT1 and PGK1) are expressed; however, when NF-κB induces HIF-1α accumulation, genes related to inflammatory signaling (e.g., COX-2 and inducible nitric oxide synthase; iNOS) are expressed [72]. HIF-1α has been reported to play a detrimental role in models of sepsis with increases in HIF-1α concentrations resulting in the increased expression of inflammatory genes and the experimental deletion of HIF-1α improving survival [73, 74].

High concentrations of HIF-1α have been found in the normal equine parabasal lamellar epithelial cells/keratinocytes. This may be due to their relative hypoxic environment resulting from the increased distance of the parabasal keratinocytes from the vasculature of the lamellar dermis [75]. Significant increases in HIF-1α have also been reported in the lamellae of horses from both the BWE and CHO models of laminitis [75]. Additionally, two genes (COX-2 and iNOS) that can be induced by HIF-1α have been reported to be increased at similar times in both models of laminitis [75]. The lack of increased gene expression associated with hypoxia-induced HIF-1α accumulation (e.g., GLUT1), along with increased inflammatory gene expression (i.e., COX-2 and iNOS), suggests that the reported increase in HIF-1α was induced via NF-κB/inflammatory signaling and not hypoxia. However, the high concentration of HIF-1α in normal lamellar tissue, likely due to the state of relative hypoxia compared to other organs (such as liver or small intestine), may prime the lamellae for an intensified inflammatory response in cases of sepsis [75]. This may explain why the lamellar tissue appears to be uniquely prone to injury in cases of sepsis/SIRS when compared to the tissues of other organs in the horse.

Inflammatory Signaling Within the Equine Keratinocyte

Epithelial cells, particularly keratinocytes, are known to be an important part of the innate immune system through their ability to respond to bacterial ligands via PRRs [76–79]. The best characterized PRRs are the toll-like receptors (TLRs) which can recognize bacterial ligands, viral components, and various products of cellular damage. Of the ten known TLRs, the most relevant in equine endotoxemia and sepsis are TLR2 (recognizing Gram-positive related ligands), TLR4 (recognizing the Gram-negative ligand LPS), and TLR5 (recognizing bacterial flagellin from both Gram-positive and -negative sources) [80]. Equine skin keratinocytes have been reported to respond to PAMPs that are characteristic of Gram-negative bacteria (such as LPS and flagellin), and stimulation results in the expression of proinflammatory cytokines and chemokines [76]. However, a compelling question is whether or not the lamellar basal epithelial cells (LBECs; the cell layer which can dysadhere from the underlying basement membrane and dermis causing structural failure in laminitis) play an active role in lamellar inflammatory signaling (and other pathophysiologic processes) in SRL, or whether they primarily are 'victims' undergoing injury from other lamellar events (e.g., leukocyte activation). In a novel study where LBECs were isolated via laser capture microdissection and subsequently analyzed using next-generation sequencing following CHO, numerous inflammatory mediators were found to be upregulated, particularly at the onset of Obel grade 1 laminitis [81]. Increased gene expression of TLR2 and 4 was present in LBECs when compared to controls, and bioinformatics analysis revealed that the canonical pathways involving both TLR signaling and roles in pattern recognition of bacteria and viruses were activated at this time [81]. In addition to the TLRs, numerous additional inflammatory genes were differentially expressed (Table 14.1) in the LBECs, the majority of which were most prominent at the onset of Obel grade 1 lameness [81]. Many of the inflammatory molecules that were upregulated have been previously reported to be increased in SRL, and included various chemokines such as CXCL2 [MIP-2α], CCL2 [MCP-1] [10, 15, 82], CCL8 [MCP-2] [15], CCL13 [MCP-4] and CXCL6) [15], COX-2 [12, 16, 34], SOCS-3 [56], serum amyloid A [10], and beta-defensin-1 [10]. Overall, the LBECs demonstrated a strong inflammatory response, indicating that inflammatory signaling pathways are likely to play a critical role in the LBEC response during SRL. Moreover, it is clear that the LBECs are likely to be active participants in the events leading to structural failure of the lamellae.

Inflammatory Signaling in Horses with Insulin Resistance

Because insulin resistance/dysregulation occurs in horses with pituitary pars intermedia dysfunction (PPID) [83], metabolic syndrome [84, 85], and endotoxemia [86], an association between insulin resistance and laminitis is well accepted at this point in time [87]. Additionally, obesity-related systemic inflammation has been purported to play a role in tissue dysfunction in metabolic syndrome in both humans and horses. Both systemic and adipose inflammatory signaling has been studied by several research groups to determine if systemic inflammation plays a role in laminitis associated with equine metabolic syndrome. Most recently, lamellar signaling has been assessed in both a pony model mimicking pasture-associated laminitis [21] and in a hyperinsulinaemic–euglycemic clamp model developed to mimic laminitis secondary to insulin resistance [88, 89].

Table 14.1 Selected list of significantly differentially expressed inflammatory genes by the lamellar basal epithelial cells isolated via laser capture microdissection [81]. Lamellar tissue samples were collected via biopsy at three different time points: CON = control sample taken prior to CHO; DEV = developmental sample taken at 24 h post CHO; OG1 = sample taken at the onset of lameness after CHO.

CON versus DEV			
Gene ID	**Gene name**	**p-value**	**Regulation**
HRH4	histamine receptor H4	0.01384	UP
LITAF	lipopolysaccharide-induced TNF factor	0.02014	UP
CON versus OG1			
Gene ID	**Gene name**	**p-value**	**Regulation**
IL4R	interleukin 4 receptor	0.00013	UP
PTGS1	prostaglandin-endoperoxide synthase 1 (COX1)	0.00068	DOWN
PTGES	prostaglandin-E synthase	0.00244	UP
TLR2	toll-like receptor 2	0.00360	UP
BD-1	beta-defensin-1	0.00417	UP
PTGFR	prostaglandin F receptor	0.00564	UP
SOCS3	suppressor of cytokine signaling 3	0.00598	UP
C1QTNF7	C1q and tumor necrosis factor-related protein 7	0.00677	DOWN
SOD2	superoxide dismutase 2, mitochondrial	0.01138	UP
CXCL2	chemokine (C-X-C motif) ligand 2; MIP-2a	0.01543	UP
IL1RN	interleukin 1 receptor antagonist	0.01946	UP
PLA2G4A	phospholipase A2, group IVA	0.01957	UP
CCL2	chemokine (C-C motif) ligand 2; MCP-1	0.01962	UP
CASP1	caspase1; interleukin1 beta-converting enzyme	0.02133	UP
CCR2	chemokine (C-C motif) receptor 2; MCP-1 receptor	0.02309	DOWN
IL12B	interleukin 12b; IL-12 p40	0.02400	UP
TLR4	toll-like receptor 4	0.02567	UP
TNFSF12	tumor necrosis factor (ligand) superfamily, member 12	0.02628	DOWN
CXCL6	chemokine (C-X-C motif) ligand 6	0.02632	UP
SELE	E-selectin	0.02935	UP
TNFRSF13c	tumor necrosis factor receptor superfamily, member 13c	0.03033	DOWN
SPLA2	secretory phopholipase A2	0.03126	UP
PTGS2	Prostaglandin-endoperoxide synthase 2 (COX-2)	0.03191	UP
CCL8	chemokine (C-C motif) ligand 8; MCP-2	0.03455	UP
SAA1	serum amyloid A1	0.03895	UP
CCL13	chemokine (C-C motif) ligand 13 (MCP-4)	0.03948	UP
OG1 versus DEV			
Gene ID	**Gene name**	**p-value**	**Regulation**
iNOS	inducible nitric oxide synthase	0.00009	DOWN
PTGES	prostaglandin E synthase	0.00291	UP
TLR2	toll-like receptor 2	0.00389	UP
PTGFR	prostaglandin F receptor	0.00429	UP
BD-1	beta-defensin-1	0.00644	UP
C1QTNF7	C1q and tumor necrosis factor related protein 7	0.01107	DOWN
CASP1	caspase1; interleukin1 beta-converting enzyme	0.01287	UP
IL1R1	interleukin-1 receptor antagonist	0.01288	UP
CSF3	colony stimulating factor 3 (granulocyte)	0.01759	DOWN
LITAF	lipopolysaccharide-induced TNF factor	0.02018	DOWN
SOD2	superoxide dismutase 2, mitochondrial	0.02046	UP
IL-6	interleukin-6	0.02774	UP
SOCS3	suppressor of cytokine signaling 3	0.03521	UP
CCL13	chemokine (C-C motif) ligand 13 (MCP-4)	0.03576	UP
SPLA2	secretory phopholipase A2	0.03864	UP
TLR4	toll-like receptor 4	0.04020	UP
CD14	CD14 molecule	0.04172	UP
PTGS2	prostaglandin-endoperoxide synthase 2 (COX2)	0.04633	UP
CCL2	chemokine (C-C motif) ligand 2 (MCP-1)	0.04951	UP

Although the mechanisms involved in laminitis resulting from insulin administration is relatively unknown, it has been hypothesized that the activation of proinflammatory chemokines and cytokines, alterations of glucose metabolism in the lamellae, growth factor signaling, and disturbances in vascular function may all play a role [88–90].

Although obesity is considered by some to be a risk factor for endocrinopathic laminitis, the increased body weight of obesity itself is not a cause of laminitis [84]. It is much more likely that factors associated with obesity, such as insulin resistance and systemic inflammation, play a role in the development of laminitis in these horses. Adipose tissue is well described to be a producer of inflammatory mediators (including leptin, adiponecin, TNFα, IL-1β, IL-6, monocyte chemoattractant protein 1 [MCP-1] and plasminogen activator-inhibitor-1) which can act both locally and remotely throughout the body [84]. In addition to inflammatory mediators produced by adipose tissue, increases in circulating free fatty acids can also contribute to insulin resistance and are known to be proinflammatory through signaling via TLRs (e.g., TLR4) [84]. Increased TNFα and IL-1β mRNA concentrations have been reported in an obese cohort of horses [91], and found to be a risk factor for insulin resistance. However, in a study evaluating inflammatory markers (TNF, IL-1β, IL-6, and serum amyloid A [SAA]) in obese light breed horses, only plasma SAA concentrations correlated with insulin and body condition scores [92]. Additionally, when obese horses were fed diets high in carbohydrates, there were minimal changes in markers of lamellar inflammation, where only an increase in COX-2 gene expression was noted [21].

Conflicting reports do exist and the role of inflammation in insulin-resistant animals prone to laminitis remains unclear. For example, one study involving laminitis-prone ponies on pasture reported an increase in serum TNFα concentrations, suggesting that inflammation may play a role in the development of laminitis in these ponies [22]. Increases in lamellar protein expression of TLR4 and TNFα, but not IL-6, have also been reported to occur at the onset of Obel grade 2 lameness in an experimental model of prolonged euglycemic hyperinsulinemia [19]. However, recent studies have indicated an increase in inflammatory cytokine and chemokine expression in the same model, where increased lamellar mRNA concentrations of the cytokines IL-1β and IL-6, the chemokines IL-8 and MCP-1, the leukocyte adhesion molecule E-selectin, and COX-2 were all increased after a 48-h period of hyperinsulinemia (J.K. Belknap, unpublished data). An increase in the protein expression of TLR4 and SOCS3 from both visceral adipose tissue and skeletal muscle has also been demonstrated in a group of insulin-resistant horses [20]. Additionally, euglycemic insulin administration to horses for a period of 6 h resulted in an increase in plasma concentrations of IL-6 and TNFα [93]. In contrast to these findings, a different study evaluating circulating inflammatory markers in pasture ponies predisposed to laminitis found no significant differences in any of the proinflammatory markers between previous laminitic ponies versus phenotypic matched controls; however, levels of adiponectin, an anti-inflammatory marker adipokine, were found to be lower in previously laminitic ponies [94]. In the horse, increased mRNA concentrations of the proinflammatory cytokines IL-1β and IL-6 have been reported in the nuchal crest compared to other fat depots [95]. Although the nuchal crest of obese horses can become particularly thickened (this phenotype is considered to increase the risk of laminitis and/or insulin resistance), there was no difference in proinflammatory cytokine gene expression in the nuchal crest between horses that were insulin-resistant and those that were insulin-sensitive [95]. Further findings questioning the role of systemic inflammation in insulin-resistant horses were reported in a study of leukocyte responses in hyperinsulinemic obese horses, where IL-1β and IL-6 were reported to have decreased endogenous gene expression (in unstimulated leukocytes) and a similar cytokine response following immune stimulation when compared to leukocytes from control animals [96]. Overall it appears that systemic inflammation has a variable/questionable role in the pathogenesis of metabolic/endocrinopathic laminitis.

Anti-Inflammatory Therapies for Prophylaxis and Treatment of Laminitis

As successful treatment regimes for laminitis remain elusive, the majority of therapies are directed towards prevention in high-risk cases (e.g., clinical cases of sepsis) with a goal of either limiting or blocking the suspected mechanisms involved. Thus, anti-inflammatory agents have remained the cornerstones of the prevention and treatment of laminitis. Non-steroidal anti-inflammatory drugs (NSAIDs) are by far the most common therapies used in the treatment and prevention of laminitis (see Chapter 31). As significant increases in COX-2 have been documented at the onset of lameness in experimental models [12, 16, 34] of laminitis, the inhibition of COX-2 enzymes has been thought to be important in limiting the inflammatory response within the lamellae. Hence, the assessment of both non-selective and COX-2-selective NSAIDs in laminitis models is important. A recent study aimed at assessing the use of flunixin as monotherapy in a model of SRL demonstrated minimal lamellar protection [97]. With regards to the use of COX-2 selective NSAIDs (e.g., firocoxib) in laminitis, it will be important to determine if the negative vascular effects observed in some humans treated with coxibs (any NSAID used to treat pain and inflammation by inhibiting COX-2 more than COX-1), such as increased thrombus formation or vasoconstriction, would adversely affect patients with laminitis [29].

Digital hypothermia or cryotherapy has been used to successfully ameliorate experimentally induced laminitis when applied during the developmental period, immediately prior to administration of a CHO, and when not initiated until the onset of lameness [98–101]. In clinical cases of colitis the prophylactic application of digital cryotherapy also been reported to reduce the incidence of laminitis [102]. The suggested mechanisms for

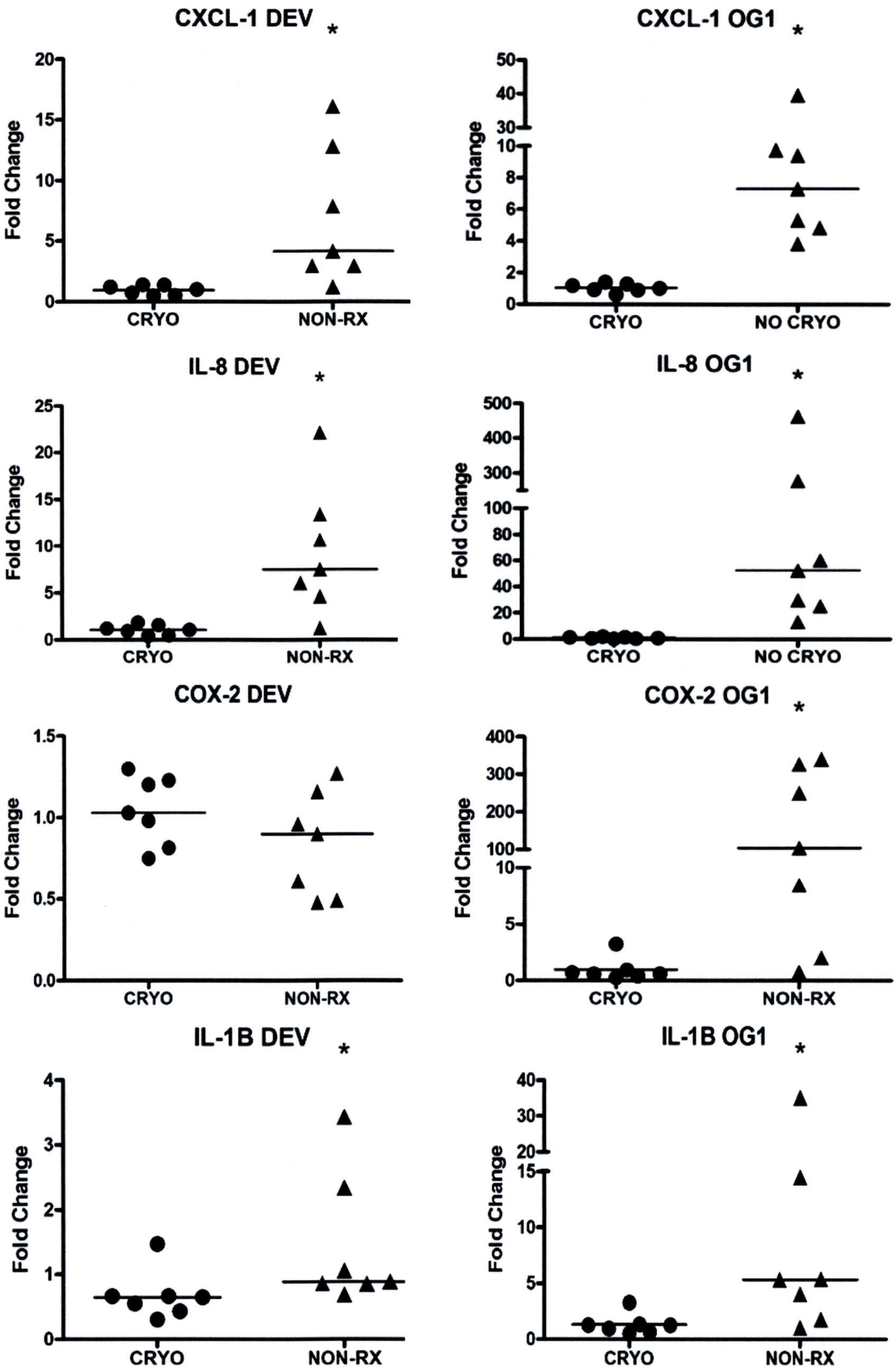

Figure 14.3 Digital hypothermia effect on lamellar inflammatory response after oligofructose administration [103]. Lamellar tissue mRNA expression for chemokines (CXCL1 and IL-8), cytokine (IL-1β) and COX-2. Digital hypothermia (cryotherapy) was associated with a significant (*P < 0.05) decrease in expression in the developmental (DEV) and onset of Obel grade 1 lameness (OG1) groups.

the prevention of laminitis using cryotherapy are thought to be related to decreasing both metabolism and inflammation in the foot [100]. Continuous cryotherapy has been found experimentally to reduce upregulation of the enzyme MMP-2 [100] and to decrease the expression of numerous proinflammatory mediators in the early stages of laminitis after OF administration [103]. Significant decreases in the mRNA concentrations of cytokines IL-1β and IL-6, chemokines CXCL1, CXCL8 and MCP-2, and COX-2 were present in the lamellae from feet treated with cryotherapy compared to normothermic controls (Fig. 14.3) [103]. In addition to the decreased lamellar expression of these inflammatory mediators, there was also a significant downregulation in the adhesion molecules ICAM-1 and E-selectin after cryotherapy (Fig. 14.3) [103].

Other treatments that have been used for their purported anti-inflammatory effects include pentoxifylline, lidocaine, and dimethyl sulfoxide (DMSO). Pentoxifylline is a non-selective phosphodiesterase inhibitor that was initially used with the hope of improving blood flow through the deformation of red blood cells; however, increases in blood flow have not been demonstrated in the horse [104]. Nonetheless, pentoxifylline has been reported to reduce cytokine production in equine whole blood after endotoxin stimulation *in vitro* [105], and to decrease the endotoxin-induced *ex vivo* production of TNFα in the horse [106]. It has also been reported to inhibit LPS-induced MMP-2 and MMP-9 activities in the horse [107]. Hence, despite the inability of pentoxifylline to alter blood flow, its possible anti-inflammatory effects can be used in the prevention and treatment of laminitis.

The use of lidocaine as an intravenous constant-rate infusion has anecdotally been helpful in the management of pain in more severe laminitic cases, and also has purported anti-inflammatory effects [108]. However, when critically evaluated in horses in the BWE model of SRL, no anti-inflammatory benefits were observed [109]. No differences were found in total leukocyte count, lamellar CD13-positive cell counts, or lamellar mRNA concentrations of IL-1β, IL-6 or IL-8 between lidocaine-treated and saline-treated animals administered BWE [109].

As the mechanisms of inflammation continue to be elucidated, and related signaling cascades revealed, the continued development of novel anti-inflammatory therapies for the treatment of laminitis can be explored.

References

1. Belknap, J.K., Giguere, S., Pettigrew, A., Cochran, A.M., Van Eps, A.W., and Pollitt, C.C. (2007) Lamellar pro-inflammatory cytokine expression patterns in laminitis at the developmental stage and at the onset of lameness: innate vs. adaptive immune response. *Equine Vet. J.*, **39**, 42–47.
2. Black, S.J., Lunn, D.P., Yin, C., Hwang, M., Lenz, S.D., and Belknap, J.K. (2006) Leukocyte emigration in the early stages of laminitis. *Vet. Immunol. Immunopathol.*, **109**, 161–166.
3. Fontaine, G.L., Belknap, J.K., Allen, D., Moore, J.N., and Kroll, D.L. (2001) Expression of interleukin-1beta in the digital laminae of horses in the prodromal stage of experimentally induced laminitis. *Am. J. Vet. Res.*, **62**, 714–720.
4. Waguespack, R.W., Kemppainen, R.J., Cochran, A., Lin, H.C., and Belknap, J.K. (2004) Increased expression of MAIL, a cytokine-associated nuclear protein, in the prodromal stage of black walnut-induced laminitis. *Equine Vet. J.*, **36**, 285–291.
5. Belknap, J.K. (2010) Black walnut extract: an inflammatory model. *Vet. Clin. North Am. Equine Pract.*, **26**, 95–101.
6. Faleiros, R.R., Leise, B.B., Westerman, T., Yin, C., Nuovo, G.J., and Belknap, J.K. (2009) In vivo and in vitro evidence of the involvement of CXCL1, a keratinocyte-derived chemokine, in equine laminitis. *J. Vet. Intern. Med.*, **23**, 1086–1096.
7. Faleiros, R.R., Nuovo, G.J., and Belknap, J.K. (2009) Calprotectin in myeloid and epithelial cells of laminae from horses with black walnut extract-induced laminitis. *J. Vet. Intern. Med.*, **23**, 174–181.
8. Faleiros, R.R., Nuovo, G.J., Flechtner, A.D., and Belknap, J.K. (2011) Presence of mononuclear cells in normal and affected laminae from the black walnut extract model of laminitis. *Equine Vet. J.*, **43** (1), 45–53.
9. Loftus, J.P., Black, S.J., Pettigrew, A., Abrahamsen, E.J., and Belknap, J.K. (2007) Early laminar events involving endothelial activation in horses with black walnut-induced laminitis. *Am. J. Vet. Res.*, **68**, 1205–1211.
10. Noschka, E., Vandenplas, M.L., Hurley, D.J., and Moore, J.N. (2009) Temporal aspects of laminar gene expression during the developmental stages of equine laminitis. *Vet. Immunol. Immunopathol.*, **129**, 242–253.
11. Riggs, L.M., Franck, T., Moore, J.N., Krunkosky, T.M., Hurley, D.J., Peroni, J.F., de la Rebiere, G., and Serteyn, D.A. (2007) Neutrophil myeloperoxidase measurements in plasma, laminar tissue, and skin of horses given black walnut extract. *Am. J. Vet. Res.*, **68**, 81–86.
12. Blikslager, A.T., Yin, C., Cochran, A.M., Wooten, J.G., Pettigrew, A., and Belknap, J.K. (2006) Cyclooxygenase expression in the early stages of equine laminitis: a cytologic study. *J. Vet. Intern. Med.*, **20**, 1191–1196.
13. Faleiros, R.R., Johnson, P.J., Nuovo, G.J., Messer, N.T., Black, S.J., and Belknap, J.K. (2011) Laminar leukocyte accumulation in horses with carbohydrate overload-induced laminitis. *J. Vet. Intern. Med.*, **25**, 107–115.
14. Visser, M.B. and Pollitt, C.C. (2011) Lamellar leukocyte infiltration and involvement of IL-6 during oligofructose-induced equine laminitis development. *Vet. Immunol. Immunopathol.*, **144**, 120–128.
15. Faleiros, R.R., Leise, B.S., Watts, M., Johnson, P.J., Black, S.J., and Belknap, J.K. (2011) Laminar chemokine mRNA concentrations in horses with carbohydrate overload-induced laminitis. *Vet. Immunol. Immunopathol.*, **144**, 45–51.
16. Leise, B.S., Faleiros, R.R., Watts, M., Johnson, P.J., Black, S.J., and Belknap, J.K. (2011) Laminar inflammatory gene expression in the carbohydrate overload model of equine laminitis. *Equine Vet. J.*, **43**, 54–61.
17. Belknap, J.K., Moore, J.N., and Crouser, E.C. (2009) Sepsis – From human organ failure to laminar failure. *Vet. Immunol. Immunopathol.*, **129**, 155–157.
18. Belknap, J. (2013) Supporting limb laminitis, in *American College of Veterinary Surgeons Symposium*, October, San Antonio, TX.

19. de Laat, M.A., Clement, C.K., McGowan, C.M., Sillence, M.N., Pollitt, C.C., and Lacombe, V.A. (2014) Toll-like receptor and pro-inflammatory cytokine expression during prolonged hyper-insulinaemia in horses: implications for laminitis. *Vet. Immunol. Immunopathol.*, **157**, 78–86.
20. Waller, A.P., Huettner, L., Kohler, K., and Lacombe, V.A. (2012) Novel link between inflammation and impaired glucose transport during equine insulin resistance. *Vet. Immunol. Immunopathol.*, **149**, 208–215.
21. Burns, T.A., Watts, M.R., Weber, P.S., McCutcheon, L.J., Geor, R.J., and Belknap, J.K. (2015) Laminar inflammatory events in lean and obese ponies subjected to high carbohydrate feeding: Implications for pasture-associated laminitis. *Equine Vet. J.*, **47** (4), 489–493.
22. Treiber, K., Carter, R., Gay, L., Williams, C., and Geor, R. (2009) Inflammatory and redox status of ponies with a history of pasture-associated laminitis. *Vet. Immunol. Immunopathol.*, **129**, 216–220.
23. Bianchi, M.E. (2007) DAMPs, PAMPs and alarmins: all we need to know about danger. *J. Leukoc. Biol.*, **81**, 1–5.
24. Xiang, M. and Fan, J. (2010) Pattern recognition receptor-dependent mechanisms of acute lung injury. *Mol. Med.*, **16**, 69–82.
25. Hirsiger, S., Simmen, H.P., Werner, C.M., Wanner, G.A., and Rittirsch, D. (2012) Danger signals activating the immune response after trauma. *Mediators Inflamm.*, **2012**, 315941.
26. Bone, R.C., Balk, R.A., Cerra, F.B., Dellinger, R.P., Fein, A.M., Knaus, W.A., Schein, R.M., and Sibbald, W.J. (1992) Definitions for sepsis and organ failure and guidelines for the use of innovative therapies in sepsis. ACCP/SCCM Consensus Conference Committee. American College of Chest Physicians/Society of Critical Care Medicine. *Chest*, **101**, 1644–1655.
27. Hotchkiss, R.S. and Karl, I.E. (2003) The pathophysiology and treatment of sepsis. *N. Engl. J. Med.*, **348**, 138–150.
28. Zhang, J.M. and An, J. (2007) Cytokines, inflammation, and pain. *Int. Anesthesiol. Clin.*, **45**, 27–37.
29. Mitchell, J.A. and Warner, T.D. (2006) COX isoforms in the cardiovascular system: understanding the activities of non-steroidal anti-inflammatory drugs. *Nat. Rev. Drug Discov.*, **5**, 75–86.
30. Villa, P., Sartor, G., Angelini, M., Sironi, M., Conni, M., Gnocchi, P., Isetta, A.M., Grau, G., Buurman, W., van Tits, L.J., *et al.* (1995) Pattern of cytokines and pharmacomodulation in sepsis induced by cecal ligation and puncture compared with that induced by endotoxin. *Clin. Diagn. Lab. Immunol.*, **2**, 549–553.
31. Remick, D.G., Newcomb, D.E., Bolgos, G.L., and Call, D.R. (2000) Comparison of the mortality and inflammatory response of two models of sepsis: lipopolysaccharide vs. cecal ligation and puncture. *Shock*, **13**, 110–116.
32. Poli-de-Figueiredo, L.F., Garrido, A.G., Nakagawa, N., and Sannomiya, P. (2008) Experimental models of sepsis and their clinical relevance. *Shock*, **30** (Suppl. 1), 53–59.
33. Sprouse, R.F., Garner, H.E., and Green, E.M. (1987) Plasma endotoxin levels in horses subjected to carbohydrate-induced laminitis. *Equine Vet. J.*, **19**, 25–28.
34. Waguespack, R.W., Cochran, A., and Belknap, J.K. (2004) Expression of the cyclooxygenase isoforms in the prodromal stage of black walnut-induced laminitis in horses. *Am. J. Vet. Res.*, **65**, 1724–1729.
35. Belknap, J.K., Eades, S.C., Johnson, P.J., and Black, S.J. (2011) Laminar inflammatory mediator expression in the CHO model: developmental stage to Obel grade 3 laminitis. *J. Equine Vet. Sci.*, **31**, 564–565.
36. Cohen, J. (2002) The immunopathogenesis of sepsis. *Nature*, **420**, 885–891.
37. Song, M. and Kellum, J.A. (2005) Interleukin-6. *Crit. Care Med.*, **33**, S463–S465.
38. Clutterbuck, A.L., Harris, P., Allaway, D., and Mobasheri, A. (2010) Matrix metalloproteinases in inflammatory pathologies of the horse. *Vet J.*, **183** (1), 27–38.
39. Kwon, S., Moore, J.N., Robertson, T.P., Hurley, D.J., Wagner, B., and Vandenplas, M.L. (2013) Disparate effects of LPS infusion and carbohydrate overload on inflammatory gene expression in equine laminae. *Vet. Immunol. Immunopathol.*, **155**, 1–8.
40. Nedrebo, T., Reed, R.K., Jonsson, R., Berg, A., and Wiig, H. (2004) Differential cytokine response in interstitial fluid in skin and serum during experimental inflammation in rats. *J. Physiol.*, **556**, 193–202.
41. Bailey, S.R., Adair, H.S., Reinemeyer, C.R., Morgan, S.J., Brooks, A.C., Longhofer, S.L., and Elliott, J. (2009) Plasma concentrations of endotoxin and platelet activation in the developmental stage of oligofructose-induced laminitis. *Vet. Immunol. Immunopathol.*, **129**, 167–173.
42. Barton, M.H. and Collatos, C. (1999) Tumor necrosis factor and interleukin-6 activity and endotoxin concentration in peritoneal fluid and blood of horses with acute abdominal disease. *J. Vet. Intern. Med.*, **13**, 457–464.
43. Morris, D.D., Moore, J.N., and Crowe, N. (1991) Serum tumor necrosis factor activity in horses with colic attributable to gastrointestinal tract disease. *Am. J. Vet. Res.*, **52**, 1565–1569.
44. Kyaw, W.O., Uhlig, A., Koller, G., Sack, U., and Schusser, G.F. (2008) Free hemoglobin and tumor necrosis factor-alpha in the blood of horses with colic or acute colitis. *Berl. Munch. Tierarztl. Wochenschr.*, **121**, 440–445.
45. Tadros, L., Frank, N., and Horohov, D.W. (2009) Inflammatory cytokine blood messenger RNA expression during the development of oligofructose-induced laminitis in horses, in *2nd American Association of Equine Practitioners: Equine Laminitis Research Workshop*, West Palm Beach, FL.
46. Stewart, A.J., Pettigrew, A., Cochran, A.M., and Belknap, J.K. (2009) Indices of inflammation in the lung and liver in the early stages of the black walnut extract model of equine laminitis. *Vet. Immunol. Immunopathol.*, **129**, 254–260.
47. Leise, B.S., Watts, M., Johnson, P.J., Black, S.J., and Belknap, J.K. (2011) Inflammatory gene expression in the liver, lung and kidney in the carbohydrate overload model of equine laminitis. *J. Equine Vet. Sci.*, **31**, 566–567.
48. Tsatsanis, C., Androulidaki, A., Venihaki, M., and Margioris, A.N. (2006) Signalling networks regulating cyclooxygenase-2. *Int. J. Biochem. Cell Biol.*, **38**, 1654–1661.
49. Wilson, J.E., Chandrasekharan, N.V., Westover, K.D., Eager, K.B., and Simmons, D.L. (2004) Determination of expression of cyclooxygenase-1 and -2 isozymes in canine tissues and their differential sensitivity to nonsteroidal anti-inflammatory drugs. *Am. J. Vet. Res.*, **65**, 810–818.
50. Adib-Conquy, M. and Cavaillon, J.M. (2009) Compensatory anti-inflammatory response syndrome. *Thromb. Haemost.*, **101**, 36–47.
51. Scumpia, P.O. and Moldawer, L.L. (2005) Biology of interleukin-10 and its regulatory roles in sepsis syndromes. *Crit. Care Med.*, **33**, S468–S471.

52. Miller, A.C., Rashid, R.M., and Elamin, E.M. (2007) The 'T' in trauma: the helper T-cell response and the role of immunomodulation in trauma and burn patients. *J. Trauma*, **63**, 1407–1417.
53. Cavaillon, J.M. and Annane, D. (2006) Compartmentalization of the inflammatory response in sepsis and SIRS. *J. Endotoxin Res.*, **12**, 151–170.
54. Stratowa, C. and Audette, M. (1995) Transcriptional regulation of the human intercellular adhesion molecule-1 gene: a short overview. *Immunobiology*, **193**, 293–304.
55. Hein, O.V., Misterek, K., Tessmann, J.P., van Dossow, V., Krimphove, M., and Spies, C. (2005) Time course of endothelial damage in septic shock: prediction of outcome. *Crit. Care*, **9**, R323–R330.
56. Leise, B.S., Watts, M., Tanhoff, E., Johnson, P.J., Black, S.J., and Belknap, J.K. (2012) Laminar regulation of STAT1 and STAT3 in black walnut extract and carbohydrate overload induced models of laminitis. *J. Vet. Intern. Med.*, **26**, 996–1004.
57. Hui, L., Yao, Y., Wang, S., Yu, Y., Dong, N., Li, H., and Sheng, Z. (2009) Inhibition of Janus kinase 2 and signal transduction and activator of transcription 3 protect against cecal ligation and puncture-induced multiple organ damage and mortality. *J. Trauma*, **66**, 859–865.
58. Matsukawa, A. (2007) STAT proteins in innate immunity during sepsis: lessons from gene knockout mice. *Acta Med. Okayama*, **61**, 239–245.
59. Scott, M.J., Godshall, C.J., and Cheadle, W.G. (2002) Jaks, STATs, Cytokines, and Sepsis. *Clin. Diagn. Lab. Immunol.*, **9**, 1153–1159.
60. Andrejko, K.M., Chen, J., and Deutschman, C.S. (1998) Intrahepatic STAT-3 activation and acute phase gene expression predict outcome after CLP sepsis in the rat. *Am. J. Physiol.*, **275**, G1423–G1429.
61. Sakamori, R., Takehara, T., Ohnishi, C., Tatsumi, T., Ohkawa, K., Takeda, K., Akira, S., and Hayashi, N. (2007) Signal transducer and activator of transcription 3 signaling within hepatocytes attenuates systemic inflammatory response and lethality in septic mice. *Hepatology*, **46**, 1564–1573.
62. Brierley, M.M. and Fish, E.N. (2005) Stats: multifaceted regulators of transcription. *J. Interferon Cytokine Res.*, **25**, 733–744.
63. Horvath, C.M. (2000) STAT proteins and transcriptional responses to extracellular signals. *Trends Biochem. Sci.*, **25**, 496–502.
64. Heinrich, P.C., Behrmann, I., Haan, S., Hermanns, H.M., Muller-Newen, G., and Schaper, F. (2003) Principles of interleukin (IL)-6-type cytokine signalling and its regulation. *Biochem. J.*, **374**, 1–20.
65. Schindler, C. and Strehlow, I. (2000) Cytokines and STAT signaling. *Adv. Pharmacol.*, **47**, 113–174.
66. Decker, T. and Kovarik, P. (1999) Transcription factor activity of STAT proteins: structural requirements and regulation by phosphorylation and interacting proteins. *Cell. Mol. Life Sci.*, **55**, 1535–1546.
67. Vij, N., Sharma, A., Thakkar, M., Sinha, S., and Mohan, R.R. (2008) PDGF-driven proliferation, migration, and IL8 chemokine secretion in human corneal fibroblasts involve JAK2-STAT3 signaling pathway. *Mol. Vis.*, **14**, 1020–1027.
68. Yu, H., Pardoll, D., and Jove, R. (2009) STATs in cancer inflammation and immunity: a leading role for STAT3. *Nat. Rev. Cancer*, **9**, 798–809.
69. Carey, R., Jurickova, I., Ballard, E., Bonkowski, E., Han, X., Xu, H., and Denson, L.A. (2008) Activation of an IL-6:STAT3-dependent transcriptome in pediatric-onset inflammatory bowel disease. *Inflamm. Bowel Dis.*, **14**, 446–457.
70. Grivennikov, S.I. and Karin, M. (2010) Dangerous liaisons: STAT3 and NF-kappaB collaboration and crosstalk in cancer. *Cytokine Growth Factor Rev.*, **21**, 11–19.
71. Rius, J., Guma, M., Schachtrup, C., Akassoglou, K., Zinkernagel, A.S., Nizet, V., Johnson, R.S., Haddad, G.G., and Karin, M. (2008) NF-kappaB links innate immunity to the hypoxic response through transcriptional regulation of HIF-1alpha. *Nature*, **453**, 807–811.
72. Jantsch, J., Wiese, M., Schodel, J., Castiglione, K., Glasner, J., Kolbe, S., Mole, D., Schleicher, U., Eckardt, K.U., Hensel, M., Lang, R., Bogdan, C., Schnare, M., and Willam, C. (2011) Toll-like receptor activation and hypoxia use distinct signaling pathways to stabilize hypoxia-inducible factor 1alpha (HIF1A) and result in differential HIF1A-dependent gene expression. *J. Leukoc. Biol.*, **90**, 551–562.
73. Cramer, T., Yamanishi, Y., Clausen, B.E., Forster, I., Pawlinski, R., Mackman, N., Haase, V.H., Jaenisch, R., Corr, M., Nizet, V., Firestein, G.S., Gerber, H.P., Ferrara, N., and Johnson, R.S. (2003) HIF-1alpha is essential for myeloid cell-mediated inflammation. *Cell*, **112**, 645–657.
74. Peyssonnaux, C., Cejudo-Martin, P., Doedens, A., Zinkernagel, A.S., Johnson, R.S., and Nizet, V. (2007) Cutting edge: Essential role of hypoxia inducible factor-1alpha in development of lipopolysaccharide-induced sepsis. *J. Immunol.*, **178**, 7516–7519.
75. Pawlak, E.A., Geor, R.J., Watts, M.R., Black, S.J., Johnson, P.J., and Belknap, J.K. (2014) Regulation of hypoxia-inducible factor-1alpha and related genes in equine digital lamellae and in cultured keratinocytes. *Equine Vet. J.*, **46**, 203–209.
76. Leise, B.S., Yin, C., Pettigrew, A., and Belknap, J.K. (2010) Proinflammatory cytokine responses of cultured equine keratinocytes to bacterial pathogen-associated molecular pattern motifs. *Equine Vet. J.*, **42**, 294–303.
77. Lebre, M.C., van der Aar, A.M., van Baarsen, L., van Capel, T.M., Schuitemaker, J.H., Kapsenberg, M.L., and de Jong, E.C. (2007) Human keratinocytes express functional Toll-like receptor 3, 4, 5, and 9. *J. Invest. Dermatol.*, **127**, 331–341.
78. Miller, L.S. and Modlin, R.L. (2007) Toll-like receptors in the skin. *Semin. Immunopathol.*, **29**, 15–26.
79. Song, P.I., Park, Y.M., Abraham, T., Harten, B., Zivony, A., Neparidze, N., Armstrong, C.A., and Ansel, J.C. (2002) Human keratinocytes express functional CD14 and toll-like receptor 4. *J. Invest. Dermatol.*, **119**, 424–432.
80. Werners, A.H. and Bryant, C.E. (2012) Pattern recognition receptors in equine endotoxaemia and sepsis. *Equine Vet. J.*, **44**, 490–498.
81. Leise, B.S., Watts, M.R., Roy, S., Yilmaz, A.S., Alder, H., and Belknap, J.K. (2015) Use of laser capture microdissection for the assessment of equine lamellar basal epithelial cell signalling in the early stages of laminitis. *Equine Vet. J.*, **47** (4), 478–488.
82. Budak, M.T., Orsini, J.A., Pollitt, C.C., and Rubinstein, N.A. (2009) Gene expression in the lamellar dermis-epidermis during the developmental phase of carbohydrate overload-induced laminitis in the horse. *Vet. Immunol. Immunopathol.*, **131**, 86–96.
83. Garcia, M.C. and Beech, J. (1986) Equine intravenous glucose tolerance test: glucose and insulin responses of healthy horses fed grain or hay and of horses with pituitary adenoma. *Am. J. Vet. Res.*, **47**, 570–572.
84. Geor, R. and Frank, N. (2009) Metabolic syndrome – From human organ disease to laminar failure in equids. *Vet. Immunol. Immunopathol.*, **129**, 151–154.

85. Geor, R.J. and Harris, P. (2009) Dietary management of obesity and insulin resistance: countering risk for laminitis. *Vet. Clin. North Am. Equine Pract.*, **25**, 51–65, vi.
86. Toth, F., Frank, N., Elliott, S.B., Geor, R.J., and Boston, R.C. (2008) Effects of an intravenous endotoxin challenge on glucose and insulin dynamics in horses. *Am. J. Vet. Res.*, **69**, 82–88.
87. Coffman, J.R. and Colles, C.M. (1983) Insulin tolerance in laminitis ponies. *Can. J. Comp. Med.*, **47**, 347–351.
88. Asplin, K.E., Sillence, M.N., Pollitt, C.C., and McGowan, C.M. (2007) Induction of laminitis by prolonged hyperinsulinaemia in clinically normal ponies. *Vet. J.*, **174**, 530–535.
89. de Laat, M.A., McGowan, C.M., Sillence, M.N., and Pollitt, C.C. (2010) Equine laminitis: induced by 48 h hyperinsulinaemia in Standardbred horses. *Equine Vet. J.*, **42**, 129–135.
90. de Laat, M.A., McGowan, C.M., Sillence, M.N., and Pollitt, C.C. (2010) Hyperinsulinemic laminitis. *Vet. Clin. North Am. Equine Pract.*, **26**, 257–264.
91. Vick, M.M., Adams, A.A., Murphy, B.A., Sessions, D.R., Horohov, D.W., Cook, R.F., Shelton, B.J., and Fitzgerald, B.P. (2007) Relationships among inflammatory cytokines, obesity, and insulin sensitivity in the horse. *J. Anim. Sci.*, **85**, 1144–1155.
92. Suagee, J.K., Corl, B.A., Crisman, M.V., Pleasant, R.S., Thatcher, C.D., and Geor, R.J. (2013) Relationships between body condition score and plasma inflammatory cytokines, insulin, and lipids in a mixed population of light-breed horses. *J. Vet. Intern. Med.*, **27**, 157–163.
93. Suagee, J.K., Corl, B.A., Crisman, M.V., Hulver, M.W., McCutcheon, L.J., and Geor, R.J. (2011) Effects of acute hyperinsulinemia on inflammatory proteins in horses. *Vet. Immunol. Immunopathol.*, **142**, 141–146.
94. Wray, H., Elliott, J., Bailey, S.R., Harris, P.A., and Menzies-Gow, N.J. (2012) Plasma concentrations of inflammatory markers in previously laminitic ponies. *Equine Vet. J.*, **45** (5), 546–551.
95. Burns, T.A., Geor, R.J., Mudge, M.C., McCutcheon, L.J., Hinchcliff, K.W., and Belknap, J.K. (2010) Proinflammatory cytokine and chemokine gene expression profiles in subcutaneous and visceral adipose tissue depots of insulin-resistant and insulin-sensitive light breed horses. *J. Vet. Intern. Med.*, **24**, 932–939.
96. Holbrook, T.C., Tipton, T., and McFarlane, D. (2012) Neutrophil and cytokine dysregulation in hyperinsulinemic obese horses. *Vet. Immunol. Immunopathol.*, **145**, 283–289.
97. Pase Leme, F., Bonna, F., De Marval, C., Xavier, S., Santos, R., Falerios, R., and Alves, G. (2010) Histopathologia das laminas do casco de equinos com laminite aguda induzida e tratados com ketoprofeno, fenibutazona e flunixin meglumine. *Arq. Bras. Med. Vet. Zootec.*, **62**, 241–250.
98. Van Eps, A.W. (2010) Therapeutic hypothermia (cryotherapy) to prevent and treat acute laminitis. *Vet. Clin. North Am. Equine Pract.*, **26**, 125–133.
99. Van Eps, A.W. (2010) Acute laminitis: medical and supportive therapy. *Vet. Clin. North Am. Equine Pract.*, **26**, 103–114.
100. Van Eps, A.W. and Pollitt, C.C. (2004) Equine laminitis: cryotherapy reduces the severity of the acute lesion. *Equine Vet. J.*, **36**, 255–260.
101. Van Eps, A.W., Pollitt, C.C., Underwood, C., Medina-Torres, C.E., Goodwin, W.A., and Belknap, J.K. (2014) Continuous digital hypothermia initiated after the onset of lameness prevents lamellar failure in the oligofructose laminitis model. *Equine Vet. J.*, **46**, 625–630.
102. Kullmann, A., Holcombe, S.J., Hurcombe, S.D., Roessner, H.A., Hauptman, J.G., Geor, R.J., and Belknap, J. (2014) Prophylactic digital cryotherapy is associated with decreased incidence of laminitis in horses diagnosed with colitis. *Equine Vet. J.*, **46**, 554–559.
103. Van Eps, A.W., Leise, B.S., Watts, M., Pollitt, C.C., and Belknap, J.K. (2012) Digital hypothermia inhibits early lamellar inflammatory signalling in the oligofructose laminitis model. *Equine Vet. J.*, **44** (2), 230–237.
104. Ingle-Fehr, J.E. and Baxter, G.M. (1999) The effect of oral isoxsuprine and pentoxifylline on digital and laminar blood flow in healthy horses. *Vet. Surg.*, **28**, 154–160.
105. Barton, M.H. and Moore, J.N. (1994) Pentoxifylline inhibits mediator synthesis in an equine in vitro whole blood model of endotoxemia. *Circ. Shock*, **44**, 216–220.
106. Barton, M.H., Ferguson, D., Davis, P.J., and Moore, J.N. (1997) The effects of pentoxifylline infusion on plasma 6-keto-prostaglandin F1 alpha and ex vivo endotoxin-induced tumour necrosis factor activity in horses. *J. Vet. Pharmacol. Ther.*, **20**, 487–492.
107. Fugler, L.A., Eades, S.C., Moore, R.M., Koch, C.E., and Keowen, M.L. (2013) Plasma matrix metalloproteinase activity in horses after intravenous infusion of lipopolysaccharide and treatment with matrix metalloproteinase inhibitors. *Am. J. Vet. Res.*, **74**, 473–480.
108. Belknap, J.K. (2005) Review of the pathophysiology of the developmental stages of equine laminitis, in Proceedings American Association of Equine Practitioners, pp. 383–388.
109. Williams, J.M., Lin, Y.J., Loftus, J.P., Faleiros, R.R., Peroni, J.F., Hubbell, J.A., Ravis, W.R., and Belknap, J.K. (2010) Effect of intravenous lidocaine administration on laminar inflammation in the black walnut extract model of laminitis. *Equine Vet. J.*, **42**, 261–269.

CHAPTER 15

Role of Proteases in Laminitis

Samuel J. Black, Le Wang, Erica Pawlak, Fengqiu Zhang, John Loftus and Dominique Alfandari

Metalloproteinases and the Extracellular Matrix

In this chapter, evidence is first presented of extracellular matrix (ECM) damage in the digital lamellae of laminitic horses, and possible contributions of matrix metalloproteinases (MMPs) and ADAMTS-4 (a disintegrin and metalloproteinase with thrombospondin motifs-4) to this pathology are subsequently addressed. The MMPs and ADAMTS-4 are proteolytic enzymes that contain a zinc (Zn)-binding motif in their catalytic site and require associated Zn^+ for their catalytic activity. Metalloproteinases are capable of degrading protein components of the ECM (the material that is produced by and surrounds the cellular components of tissues). In addition to providing a scaffolding for the cellular components of tissues, the ECM joins epidermal and dermal layers of tissues such as equine digital lamellae (as described below) and skin, and enables tissues to resist stretch and compression forces [1, 2]. Protein components of the ECM include fibrous structural proteins (e.g., collagens, fibrillins, laminins, elastin, and fibronectin), low-molecular-weight leucine-rich proteoglycans which bind collagens and affect fibril formation, and large polysulfated proteoglycans which bind to the large polysaccharide hyaluronan forming a macromolecular complex that attracts and retains water in the tissue, preserving its space-filling properties and resisting compression forces. The ECM also contains regulatory proteins including: (i) adaptors and modulators of cell and matrix interactions (e.g., galectins, thrombospondins, tenascins, osteospondin, vitronectin, the CNN family of proteins and secreted protein acidic and rich in cysteine); (ii) cytokines and growth factors which bind to the matrix; and (iii) proteases including MMPs and their inhibitors which are secreted into the matrix and respectively mediate and regulate remodeling of the ECM (e.g., to facilitate growth and tissue repair).

Matrix metalloproteinases are divided into several groups depending on their substrates and functions, namely collagenases, gelatinases, stromelysins, membrane-type (MT) MMPs, matrilysin, enamelysin, and metalloelastase, all of which are discussed below in the context of laminitis. Given the capacity of MMPs to disassemble tissues, they require close regulation, which is applied at both transcriptional and post-translational levels. MMPs are secreted as latent forms, which acquire catalytic activity only after the proteolytic removal of a regulatory propeptide, which masks their active site. However, removal of the regulatory propeptide does not ensure that an MMP will be active because Tissue Inhibitors of Metalloproteinases (TIMPs) can inactivate processed MMPs and, in some instances, prevent activation of a latent (zymogen) MMP. There are four tissue inhibitors of metalloproteinases (TIMP-1, -2, -3, and -4), which vary in their specificity for distinct metalloproteinases.

Unlike MMPs, ADAMTS-4 is secreted as an active enzyme, its regulatory propeptide being removed during its transport out of the cell. ADAMTS-4 cleaves large polysulfated proteoglycans, thus degrading molecular complexes that retain water in tissues and therefore compromising the resistance of target tissues to compression forces. TIMPS also regulate ADAMTS-4 activity, with TIMP-3 having the highest inhibitory activity against this metalloproteinase.

Structural Elements of the Digital Lamellar Extracellular Matrix

The equine digital lamellae connect the outer surface of the distal phalanx to the inner hoof wall and suspend the horse's axial skeleton within the hoof capsule. In healthy horses, the two-layer (dermis and epidermis) tissue supports the vertical load of the horse, resists force applied to the distal phalanx by the deep digital flexor tendon, accommodates compression and stretch deformation created by flexing and tilting of the hoof capsule around the distal phalanx under different loading conditions, and absorbs a portion of the concussive shock imposed when the hoof strikes a solid surface. These biomechanical properties of the lamellae are functions of the structural lamellar constituents.

The lamellae are composed of 500–600 vertical folds of keratinized epidermal tissue – the primary epidermal lamellae – which are contiguous with the inner hoof wall, and interdigitated folds of connective tissue – the primary dermal lamellae – which

Equine Laminitis, First Edition. Edited by James K. Belknap and Raymond Geor.

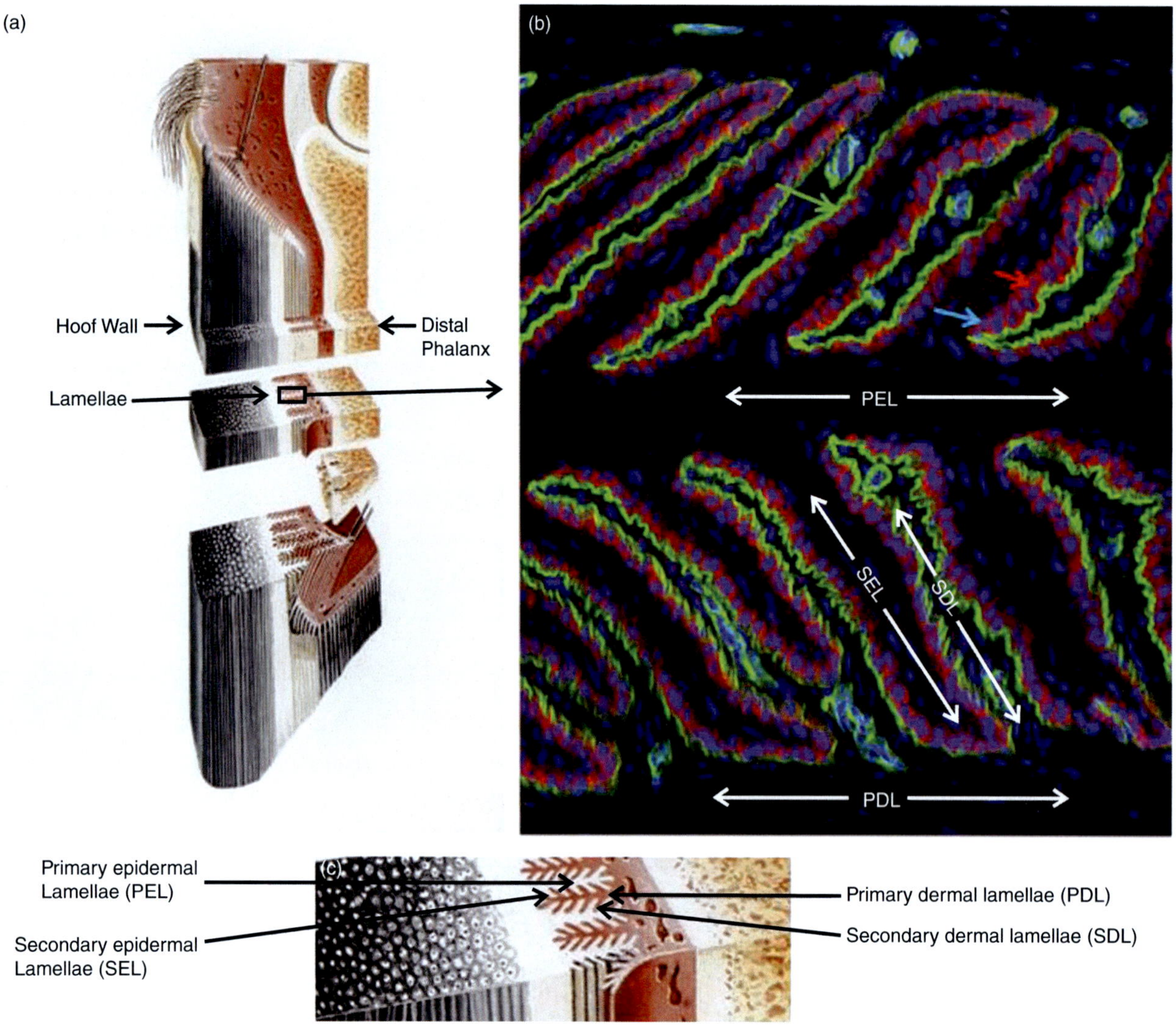

Figure 15.1 (a–c) The equine digital lamellae. (b) Cryosection of OCT-embedded lamellae from a healthy horse stained with antibodies specific for pan laminin (green), versican (red), and with the intercalating DNA stain DAPI (blue). PEL, primary epidermal lamellae; SEL, secondary epidermal lamellae; PDL, primary dermal lamellae; SDL, secondary dermal lamellae. Panels (a) and (c) reproduced with permission of John McDougall and Chris Pollitt.

are contiguous with the distal phalanx [3] (Fig. 15.1a and c). Each fold of primary epidermal and dermal lamellae has numerous interdigitated folds of secondary lamellae (shown in cross-section in Fig. 15.1b and illustrated in Fig. 15.1c) that results in a greatly expanded contact area for purposes of attachment. The secondary epidermal and dermal lamellae join at a basement membrane [4], a fibrous meshwork of collagens, laminins, entactins and various proteoglycans (the basement membrane [BM] is shown as a green [pan-laminin] stained material in a cross-section of lamellae in Fig. 15.1b). The BM lies between and is attached to the lamellar basal epithelial cells (LBECs), which sit at the boundary of the secondary epidermal lamellae. It is also attached to the connective tissue of the dermal lamellae, ensuring integrity of the two-layer tissue. The LBECs are readily identified in a cross-section of lamellae by the presence of the proteoglycan versican in their cytoplasm [5] (Fig. 15.1b, red arrow), and by alignment of their nuclei (Fig. 15.1b, blue arrow/blue nuclei) with the BM.

The LBECs are attached to the BM by protein structures called *hemidesmosomes*, which are attached via linker proteins on the cytoplasmic side of the plasma membrane to cytokeratins of the cytoskeleton (stained red in Fig. 15.2a; see Chapter 4 for more detail). LBEC are also attached to each other and to abutting parabasal keratinocytes of the secondary epidermal lamellae by plasma membrane structures called desmosomes, which are also present on the plasma membrane of parabasal keratinocytes throughout the secondary and primary epidermal lamellae and attach the parabasal keratinocytes to each other. Desmosomes are also bound via linking proteins on the cytoplasmic side of the plasma membrane to cytokeratins, which form a cable network extending through the cellular components of the epidermal lamellae to the inner hoof wall (see Chapter 4 for more detail).

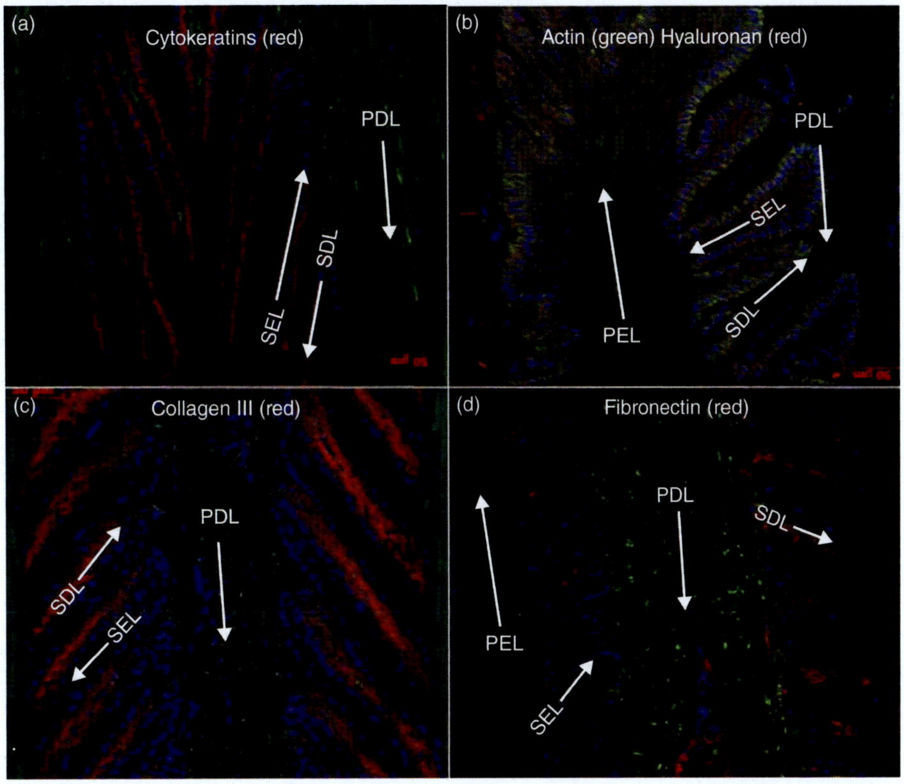

Figure 15.2 Components of the lamellar extracellular matrix and cytoskeleton. Cryosections of OCT-embedded lamellae from a healthy horse stained with antibodies specific for: (a) cytokeratins (red); (b) actin (colloidin FITC, green) hyaluronan (red); (c) collagen III (red); (d) fibronectin (red) and the intercalating DNA stain DAPI (blue). PEL, primary epidermal lamellae; SEL, secondary epidermal lamellae; PDL, primary dermal lamellae; SDL, secondary dermal lamellae. The antibody reagents do not penetrate the dense fibrous matrix of the PDL, which consequently is not stained, though it does autofluoresce green.

In addition, LBECs and other keratinocytes are attached to each other at their lateral junctions by adherens junctions. Adherens junctions are composed of E-cadherin and associated proteins. The extracellular domains of E-cadherens on neighboring cells self-associate, and their intracellular domains are bound to cellular actin by linking proteins, thus forming an actin cortical fiber network that runs through the basal epithelial cell layer and adjoining parabasal keratinocytes (stained green with the actin-binding compound phalloidin in Fig. 15.2b), contributing further structural strength to the tissue. The hemidesmosomes, desmosomes and adherens junctions, and their associated cytoskeletal elements, have been extensively studied, and well-constructed diagrams of their structure are presented in Chapter 4.

In addition to its attachment to the LBECs by hemidesmosomes, the BM is also attached to the ECM, its fibers being laced to extracellular collagen fibers of the dermal ECM (e.g., collagens I, III, and V; Fig. 15.2c). These fibers of the BM and ECM are bound to each other and to proteoglycans in the ECM of the secondary and primary dermal lamellae by adaptor proteins and fibronectin (Fig. 15.2d). Fibronectin also binds to fibrin and to the extracellular components of integrins, a family of proteins that span the plasma membranes of cells (including LBECs) and which are attached intracellularly to cytoskeletal components, thus coupling the ECM to intracellular structural elements. Collagen cables composed of Type I collagen fibers in the ECM of the primary dermal lamellae insert directly onto the outer cortex of the distal phalanx through the lamellar corium [6], thus providing a cohesive cabling system that extends from the distal phalanx to the inner hoof wall via the cellular and ECM components of the dermal and epidermal lamellae. Thus, force applied to the distal phalanx by the deep digital flexor tendon is transmitted through the cable network of the ECM of the dermal lamellar to the BM, and through LBEC BM attachments to the cytoskeletons of LBECs, parabasal epithelial cells, and fully cornified keratinocytes of the hoof capsule. This force is countered in healthy lamellae by the tensile properties of these ECM and cytoskeleton components in the lamellar epithelial cells, as well as recoil properties of elastin fibers in the dermal ECM.

Destabilization of the Lamellar Epidermal–Dermal Junction in Laminitic Horses

The junction of the epidermal and dermal lamellae (i.e., the LBEC and BM attachment, and/or the BM and dermal ECM attachment) is compromised in a variety of systemic disease conditions, including retained fetal membranes/septic

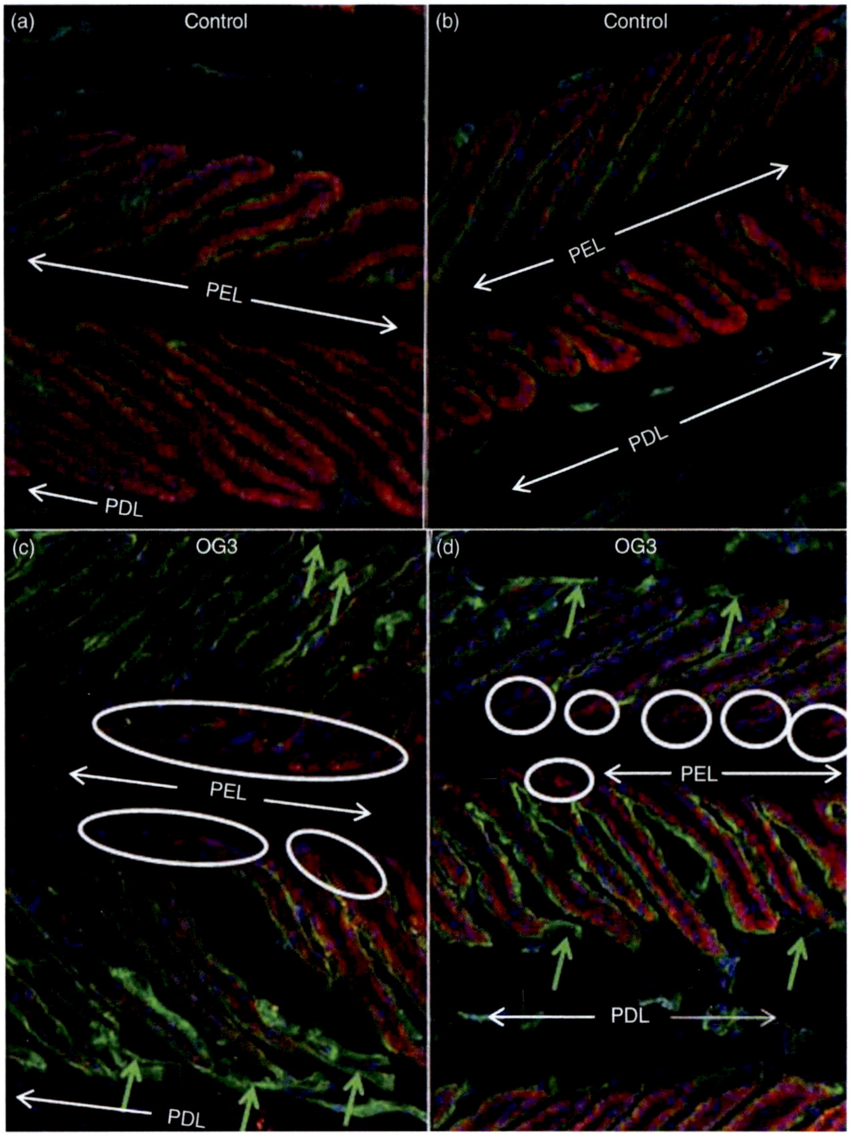

Figure 15.3 Impact of laminitis on basement membrane (BM) and basal epithelial cell attachment. Immunofluorescent images of thin cryosections of unfixed, OCT-embedded lamellae from two healthy horses (a,b) and two horses at OG3 lameness from starch-induced laminitis (c,d). The BM is stained green with anti-pan laminin, versican is stained red with specific antibody, and nuclei are stained blue with DAPI. PEL, primary epidermal lamellae; SEL, secondary epidermal lamellae; PDL, primary dermal lamellae; SDL, secondary dermal lamellae. Yellow arrows indicate the BM being pulled away from the tips of the SEL. White ovals indicate islands of lamellar basal epithelial cells detached from the BM.

metritis, Gram-negative pleuropneumonia, black walnut heartwood toxemia (occurring in horses bedded on black walnut shavings), strangulating intestinal obstruction, enterocolitis, and abnormal hindgut fermentation [7]. It is also compromised in horses experimentally administered a gastric bolus of carbohydrate (using the traditional corn starch/wood flour [here termed 'starch'] model [8] or oligofructose (OF) model [9]), or with hyperinsulinemia [10, 11] induced by intravenous infusion of insulin combined with a euglycemic clamp. These methods are respectively models of enterocolitis/related laminitis and endocrinopathic laminitis. As a result of laminitis-associated junctional instability, regional separation of the epidermal and dermal layers of the digital lamellae occurs to varying degrees and results in displacement (rotation and sinking) of the distal phalanx within the hoof capsule, accompanied by pain and lameness. The disease stages/groups used in the studies discussed here are primarily based on the Obel scale [12], with Obel grade 1 (OG1) designating lameness that is noticeable at the trot only (with minimal architectural changes present in the lamellae on histologic examination), and OG3 designating lameness even at a walk that renders the animal reluctant to move (with prominent architectural changes present in the lamellae on histologic examination).

The LBECs normally line the boundary of the secondary epidermal lamellae. In cross-sections of lamellae from healthy horses, these cells (which are stained red with anti-versican; Fig. 15.3a and b) sit perpendicular to, and are attached to, the BM (stained green with anti-laminin) [5]. However, in cross-sections of lamellae from horses with starch-induced laminitis presenting with OG3 lameness, the BM is observed to be pulled free of the tips of some secondary epidermal lamellae and to remain attached to (and appears to be streaming into) the primary dermal lamellae (Fig. 15.3c and d; indicated by green arrows), which is consistent with immunohistochemical

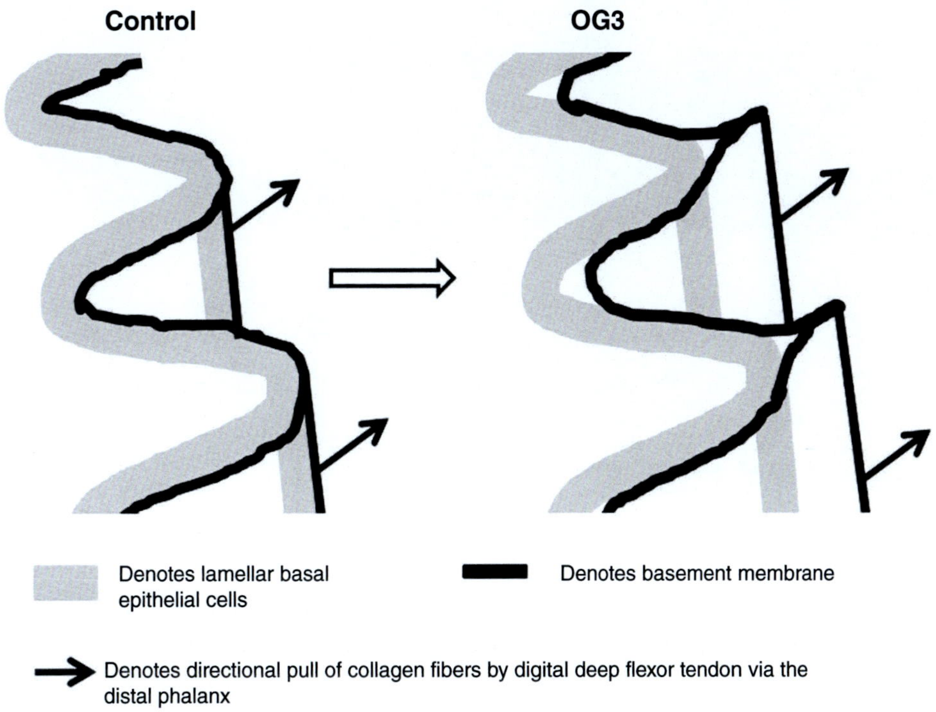

Figure 15.4 Diagram of basement membrane and lamellar basal epithelial cell interactions in healthy horses (Control) and horses with starch-induced laminitis (OG3).

observations obtained by other investigators in earlier studies [4,13]. Furthermore, in some regions of the tissue, basal epithelial cells (stained red with anti-versican) are observed to be detached from the BM and to lie marooned on the edge of the primary epidermal lamellae (Fig. 15.3c and d, indicated by white ovals).

To account for these observations, it is hypothesized that, in laminitic horses, the ambient force from the distal phalanx applied indirectly to the sheet of the lamellar BM causes directional creep of the BM on underlying LBECs in the direction of the distal phalanx (see Fig. 15.4). This would require one (or, more likely, both) of the following events to occur: (i) remodeling/disruption of hemidesmosomes (see Chapter 4), which tether LBECs to the BM; and (ii) degradation/disruption of matrix components of the BM (and underlying dermis) to which the hemidesmosomes attach. In support of this involvement of dysregulation of hemidesmosomes in lamellar pathology in laminitis, experimental studies have shown a diminished number of intact hemidesmosomes per unit area of BM in laminitic as compared to healthy horses [14], and a laminitis-associated physiologic remodeling of the cells resulting in diminished gene and protein expression of the central hemidesmosome component integrin β_4, possibly as a result of suppression of the canonical Wnt signaling pathway (discussed at end of this chapter) [15]. There is also immunohistological evidence for the reduced presence of integrin α_6, which also is a component of the hemidesmosome, as well as reduced presence and colocalization of BP180 and laminin 5, which also play a role in the attachment of hemidesmosomes to the BM [16]. This suggests that degradative processes may combine with physiologic remodeling of the LBECs to dismantle epithelial cell and BM structures critical for LBEC attachment to the BM.

Lamellar Dermal Pathology in Laminitic Horses

Pathological remodeling of digital lamellae in horses with starch-induced laminitis also manifests as the development of multifocal gaps in the ECM of the secondary dermal lamellae. In healthy horses, the secondary dermal lamellae contain fibroblasts and myeloid cells 'cocooned' in an ECM composed of elastin (P. Johnson, personal communication), collagen I, collagen III (Fig. 15.5, stained red), fibronectin, proteoglycans bearing chondroitin and keratan sulfate glycosaminoglycans [1], and most likely other elements. However, in the digital lamellae of horses that develop OG3 lameness after receiving a gastric bolus of starch gruel, multifocal gaps open in the secondary dermal lamellae. These gaps, which are observed in cross-sections of cryopreserved tissue that has not been subjected to fixation and dehydration, are devoid of collagen I, collagen III (Fig. 15.4b, dashed arrows), proteoglycans, glycosaminoglycans and fibronectin [1], and indeed appear to be entirely devoid of ECM as determined by hematoxylin and eosin staining of

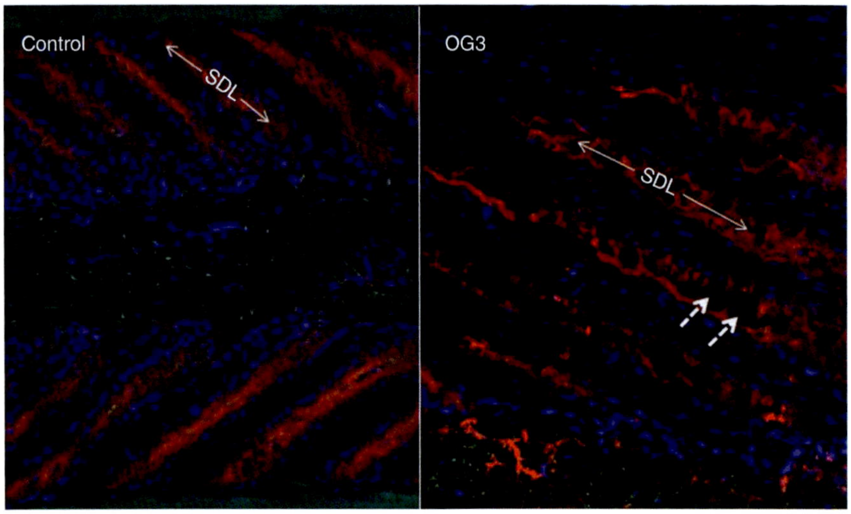

Figure 15.5 Development of multifocal gaps in secondary dermal lamellae (SDL). Immunofluorescent images of cryosections of unfixed OCT-embedded lamellae from a healthy horse (Control) and a horse with starch-induced laminitis (OG3). Sections were stained with anti-collagen III (red) and DAPI nuclear stain (blue). Dashed arrows indicate multifocal gaps.

thin sections of optimal cutting temperature compound (OCT)-embedded flash-frozen lamellae from healthy and laminitic horses (Fig. 15.6). The gaps are not observed in sections of paraffin-embedded and sucrose-permeated lamellae (data not shown), and presumably collapse during these processing steps. The development of the multifocal gaps in the dermal ECM of horses with starch-induced laminitis may result from the degradation of ECM components in affected regions by collagenases and other proteases, and from the subsequent tearing of destabilized ECM under ambient forces applied to the dermal ECM by attachments to the distal phalanx. It is also possible that the detachment of cellular elements of the dermal ECM from abutting matrix (e.g., as a result of physiological changes in these cells) contributes to destabilization of the ECM, but this has not been reported.

Lamellar Basement Membrane/Dermal Matrix injury and the Role of Proteases in Laminitis: An Overview

Molecular and biochemical analyses of metalloproteinase activity in laminitic lamellae are presented in detail in the remainder of the chapter; however, a basic overview of these studies is provided here for readers who are not well-versed in this area of science and its methodology. The interest in metalloproteases evolved from earlier studies in which the presence of two gelatinases, MMP-2 and MMP-9, were detected that are capable of degrading several components of the BM and lamellar dermis in digital lamellae. As discussed below, an examination of the regulation of these two proteases has shown that they are unlikely to play a central role in initiating lamellar structural

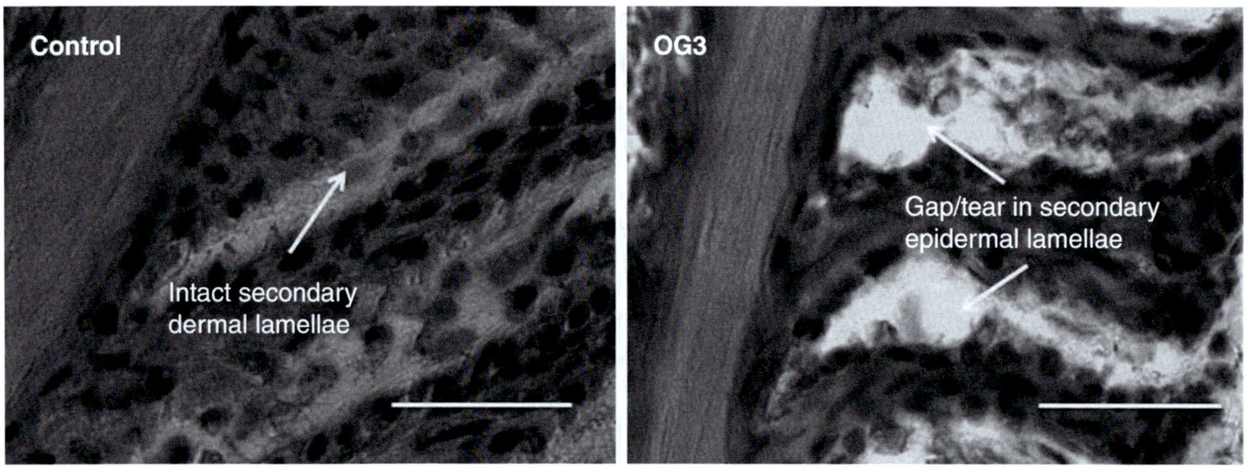

Figure 15.6 Complete loss of extracellular matrix elements in regions of secondary dermal lamellae at OG3 lameness. Grayscale image of hematoxylin and eosin-stained thin section of frozen unfixed OCT-embedded lamellae from a representative healthy horse (Control) and a representative horse with starch-induced laminitis at OG3 lameness (OG3). Original magnification ×40. Scale bars = 50 μm.

breakdown, because they are either not present or not present in active form during the acute stages of experimental or clinical laminitis when BM damage has been detected. However, two other MMPs classified as collagenases, MMP-1 and MMP-13, as well as a disintegrin and metalloproteinase with thrombospondin motifs-4 (ADAMTS-4), which cleaves large polysulfated proteoglycans, are currently of great interest due to increased lamellar expression in models of sepsis-related and endocrinopathic laminitis (see below). These metalloproteinases have been localized to the LBEC layer, consistent with release into the underlying BM and dermis where they might help remodel the ECM to accommodate hoof growth. Interestingly, increased MMP-13 activity and concentration in laminitic lamellae coincides with histologic evidence of extensive degradation of the secondary dermal lamellae (see Fig. 15.5), indicating a possible role for this collagenase in structural breakdown of the dermal matrix and therefore the 'suspensory apparatus of the distal phalanx (SADP)' (see Chapter 4). However, the involvement of these MMPs in lamellar pathology has been tempered by a recent study in which the administration of a broad-spectrum protease inhibitor, marimastat (which should inhibit MMPs-1 and -13) only slightly diminished signs of lamellar injury/failure (see below). ADAMTS-4 continues to be of interest due not only to its consistently reported increase in lamellar concentration in experimental and clinical cases of sepsis-related laminitis, but also to its increase in a model of endocrinopathic laminitis in which obese ponies were fed a high-nonstructural carbohydrate (NSC) diet for seven days (see below). Substrates for ADAMTS-4 are not detected in the lamellar ECM but are detected in LBECs (versican and aggrecan) and parabasal epithelial cells (aggrecan). Despite being a member of the water-trapping, large-polysulfated family of proteoglycans, versican in LBECs does not have associated sulfated glycosaminoglycan and consequently does not play a structural role. Rather, it is thought to be required for maintenance of the epithelial cell phenotype. On the other hand, LBEC aggrecan is richly decorated with sulfated glycosaminoglycans, and consequently might trap water in the cells so as to protect them against compression damage and sustaining keratin hydration during the cornification of parabasal epithelial cells. ADAMTS-4 cleavage products of aggrecan do not increase in concentration in the lamellae of horses with experimental and clinical laminitis, though an increased laminitis-associated cleavage of versican is well documented as discussed later in the text. This is accompanied by a greatly decreased versican gene expression that results in a loss of versican from the tissues. Although versican loss would be expected to cause epithelial cell dedifferentiation (termed 'epithelial to mesenchymal transition'; EMT), this does not occur because of a laminitis-induced shut-down in the expression of genes encoding positive regulators of the canonical Wnt signaling pathway in LBECs (discussed below); rather, a functional canonical Wnt signaling pathway is required for EMT. Despite the absence of full EMT, a decreased expression of versican and a decreased expression of the canonical Wnt signaling pathway in LBECs of laminitic lamellae is accompanied by the decreased gene and protein expression of β-catenin and integrin β_4, which are required components of attachment structures that mediate LBEC–LBEC attachment and LBEC–BM attachment, thus destabilizing the dermal–epidermal junction.

The Contribution of Metalloproteinases to the Molecular Pathology of Laminitis

Matrix metalloproteinases (MMP), which are degradative enzymes that cleave ECM proteins (as discussed above), have been a focus of interest in lamellar pathophysiology for over a decade following reports of:

- The detection of MMP-2 and MMP-9 in the digital lamellae of healthy horses [17].
- Increased levels of MMP-2 and MMP-9 in explant medium from cultured lamellae of laminitic compared to healthy horses [18].
- Increased levels of pro-MMP-9 (the enzymatically inactive pro-form of the enzyme) in the serum of horses with starch-induced laminitis compared to healthy horses [17].
- Histological evidence of ECM degradation in the lamellae of horses with starch-induced laminitis [4].
- Increased levels of collagen IV fragments in the serum of horses with naturally acquired laminitis compared to healthy horses [19]. However, the results of more recent studies have called into question the contribution of MMP-2 and MMP-9 to the loss of lamellar integrity in laminitis.

Gelatinases Revisited

Matrix metalloproteinase 2 (MMP-2) and MMP-9 belong to a subgroup of MMPs called gelatinases. They are secreted as inactive pro-enzymes/zymogens (pro-MMP-2 and pro-MMP-9), and are activated by the proteolytic removal of a regulatory pro-peptide after secretion [20]. MMP-2 and MMP-9 cleave collagens Type I and III, BM Type IV collagen, and also cleave denatured collagen. Gelatinases are identified by gelatin-zymography, a technique in which tissue extracts are subjected to sodium dodecylsulfate–polyacrylamide gel electrophoresis (SDS-PAGE) under nonreducing conditions in gels that contain gelatin, after which SDS is replaced by the non-ionic surfactant Triton X-100; this allows renaturation of the gelatinases, which degrade any neighboring gelatin, when present. Any remaining gelatin is revealed by reaction with a protein-staining dye (e.g., Coomassie blue). Regions of the gel where gelatinases are prevalent appear as protein-free clear bands against a dark, protein-rich, Coomassie-stained, background (Fig. 15.6).

Although pro-MMP-2 and pro-MMP-9 are inactive in native conformation, they acquire gelatinolytic activity during SDS-denaturation and renaturation as a result of conformational change that exposes their catalytic sites. A summary is provided in Figure 15.7 of gelatin zymographic analyses performed using extracts of lamellae from healthy horses (control), horses

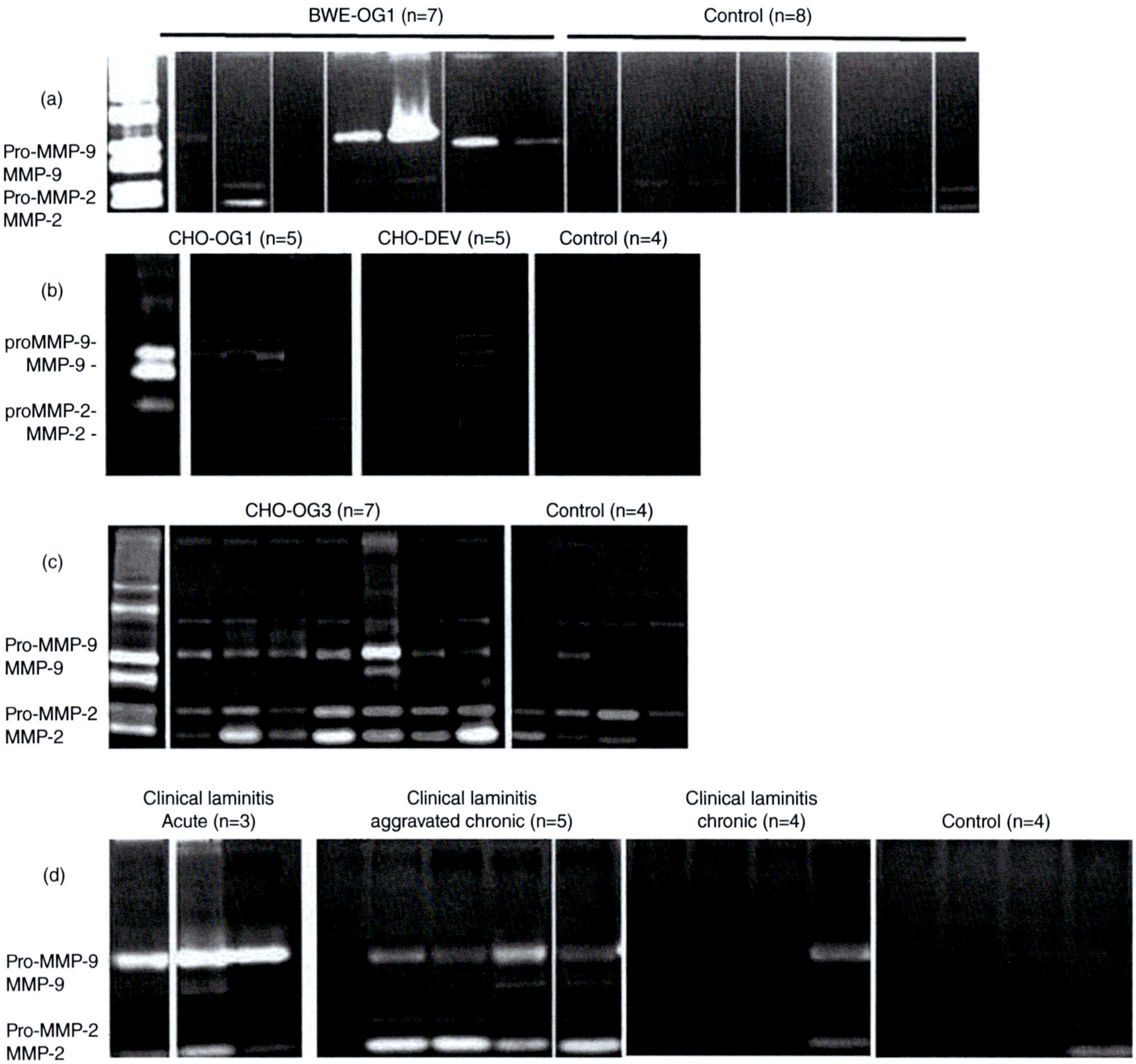

Figure 15.7 Expression of gelatinases in 0.5% NP-40 extracts of lamellae from horses with experimentally induced and naturally acquired laminitis determined by gelatin zymography after SDS–PAGE: 10 μg protein per track. Separate groups of control horses were used for studies reported in each panel. Gelatinase activity in extracts of lamellae from: Panel A: healthy horses (Control) and horses with black walnut extract (BWE)-induced laminitis. Panel B: healthy horses (Control) and horses with starch-induced laminitis presenting fever (DEV). Panel C: healthy horses (Control) and horses with starch-induced laminitis presenting OG3 lameness (OG3). Panel D: healthy horses and horses that acquired laminitis in the clinic (clinical laminitis acute), or acquired laminitis in the field and were euthanized after relapse (clinical laminitis aggravated), or at the request of the owner but not because of relapse (clinical laminitis chronic).

with black walnut extract-induced laminitis (BWE; panel A), horses with starch-induced laminitis (one of the carbohydrate overload [CHO] models of sepsis-related laminitis; panels B and C), horses that acquired laminitis in a referral hospital and were euthanized with severe lameness (Clinical laminitis acute; panel D), and horses that acquired laminitis in the field and were euthanized either after relapse (clinical laminitis aggravated; panel D), or as a result of another disease (clinical laminitis chronic; panel D). Each lane in gels recorded in Figure 15.7 contains lamellar extract from an individual horse, and all lanes were loaded with the same amount (10 μg) of lamellar protein. Although these images, together with densitometric analyses of the gelatinolytic bands, have been published [21,22], the composite zymographic images presented here facilitate an integrated analysis of gelatinase activity in extracts of lamellae from horses with laminitis of diverse etiology.

Pro-MMP-9 and MMP-9

The data presented in Figure 15.6 show that the lamellae of almost all healthy donors (n = 20) contain little or no pro-MMP-9. However, the zymogen is present in the lamellae of a high proportion of horses presenting with OG1 lameness after gastric administration of BWE, all horses presenting with starch-induced OG3 lameness laminitis, and in almost all horses with naturally acquired laminitis. In BWE-treated horses, lamellar pro-MMP-9 correlates positively and significantly with the number of neutrophils in the lamellae [21, 23], while, in horses with starch-induced and naturally acquired laminitis, it correlates positively and significantly with the content of myeloperoxidase in the tissue [22], which is also an indicator of inflammatory leukocytes. Importantly, irrespective of the pro-MMP-9 content of lamellae, little or no MMP-9 (i.e., the active form of the enzyme) is detected in the lamellae of any clinical equine case presenting for laminitis (Fig. 15.7). Thus, the pro-MMP-9 present in lamellar extracts may have been extracted from intact tissue leukocytes or, if free in the tissue at the time of harvest, was protected from pro-peptide removal (and therefore activation) by the absence of processing extracellular proteases or by inactivation of tissue proteases by tissue inhibitors of metalloproteinases (TIMPs) [24–26]. Because of its retained pro-peptide, it can be concluded that pro-MMP-9 does not contribute directly to lamellar ECM degradation; however, it cannot be concluded that this is operationally irrelevant. If released without associated TIMP, pro-MMP-9 would bind TIMPs in the ECM and hence diminish the endogenous anti-protease activity of the ECM, possibly elevating the activity of other endogenously processed (e.g., inhibitory pro-peptide-cleaved) metalloproteinases.

Pro-MMP-2, MMP-2, MT1-MMP (MMP-14), and TIMPs

Little or no pro-MMP-2 or MMP-2 is detected in the lamellae of healthy horses, or of horses presenting OG1 lameness after induction with BWE, or of horses that develop fever and OG1 lameness in the traditional CHO (starch-induction) model (Fig. 15.7). However, concentrations of MMP-2 are significantly increased in the lamellae of horses with starch-induced laminitis exhibiting OG3 lameness, and in clinical cases with aggravated chronic laminitis (Fig. 15.7) [22]. The increase in pro-MMP-2 and/or MMP-2 in the lamellae of severely lame horses did not correlate with the concentration of myeloperoxidase in extracts of lamellae, or the number of neutrophils counted in thin sections of the tissue [22], which suggested that the MMP is produced by cells other than inflammatory leukocytes. Removal of the regulatory peptide from pro-MMP-2 requires the formation of a complex with TIMP-2 and membrane type 1-MMP [27] (MT1-MMP, also called MMP-14), which cleaves the MMP-2 regulatory pro-peptide causing the release of active MMP-2. Both, MMP-2 and MMP-14 have been localized to lamellar basal epithelial cells by immunostaining of lamellae from horses with OF-induced laminitis [28, 29], which places these metalloproteinases at the site of lamellar junctional failure and identifies them as a possible factor in lamellar failure. However, based on the timing of MMP-2 increases in the lamellae relative to changes in the lamellar architecture (in the OF model of sepsis-related laminitis), it was concluded that the MMP-2/MT1–MMP complex may not play a major role in initiating lamellar BM damage [30].

Elevated MMP-2 in the lamellae of horses with aggravated chronic laminitis (Fig. 15.7, panel D) is accompanied in some instances by a high expression of TIMPs, as shown using a different zymographic technique termed *reverse zymography* (Fig. 15.8). In this procedure, the polyacrylamide gel is impregnated with both gelatin and pro-MMP-9; the tissue extract is then electrophoresed in this milieu in the presence of SDS. Upon subsequent removal of SDS and the resulting renaturation and activation of pro-MMP-9, gelatin is cleaved throughout the gel except in regions that also contain renatured, and hence inhibitory, TIMPs. The TIMPs are therefore visualized as a dark Coomassie-stained (gelatin-rich) band on a clear (gelatinolysed) background (Fig. 15.8). The results shown in Figure 15.8 indicate that TIMP protein expression is lower in the

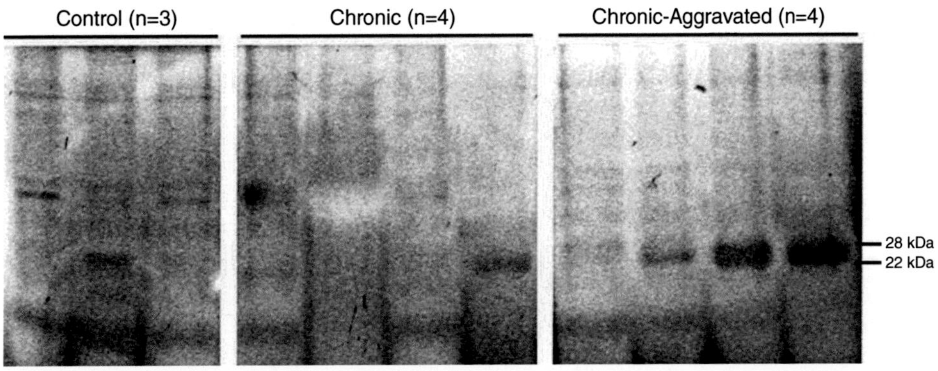

Figure 15.8 Expression of tissue inhibitors of metalloproteinases (TIMPs) in extracts of lamellae from healthy horses and horses with chronic and aggravated chronic laminitis. Reverse zymography of lamellar extracts (in 0.5% NP40) was performed in 14% polyacrylamide gels impregnated with equine neutrophil-derived pro-MMP-9. TIMPs (preventing SDS-activated pro-MMP-9 from degrading gelatin) are located in the dark bands on a clear background following Coomassie blue staining.

lamellae of healthy horses and in horses with chronic laminitis that are not currently lame, compared to most lame horses with chronic laminitis (chronic-aggravated).

To date, four tissue inhibitors of metalloproteinases have been identified, namely TIMP-1, -2, -3, and -4, which range in molecular weight from 21 kDa to 28 kDa. Of these, TIMP-1 and TIMP-2 have been partially characterized in the horse [31]. The TIMPs form non-covalent 1:1 complexes with MMP and inhibit MMP activity. Based on analyses in mouse and human systems [32, 33], it is known that TIMP-1 and TIMP-2 can inhibit secreted but not membrane-type MMPs (MT-MMPs); TIMP-1 can also bind pro-MMP-9, while TIMP-2 and TIMP-4 can bind pro-MMP-2. Thus, an increase in the extracellular content of pro-MMPs can diminish the concentration of free TIMP-1, -2, and -4 in the ECM, and consequently increase the activity of MMPs resident in the ECM. TIMP-3 has broad MMP-inhibitory activity; it inhibits MMP-1, -2, -3, -9, -13 and the MT-MMPs, while TIMP-2 is recognized as the main inhibitor of MMP-2. It is not known whether all species of TIMP are represented in the 22–28 kDa band shown in Fig. 15.8, or the relative expression of each of these proteins. However, TIMP-1 and TIMP-3 gene expression is significantly elevated in horses with starch-induced laminitis and with naturally occurring laminitis [34], while TIMP-2 gene expression is significantly suppressed in the lamellae of these horses [34] (which is also the case in the lamellae of horses with OF-induced laminitis) [28]. Thus, it is likely that the elevated presence of TIMPs in the lamellae of horses with chronic aggravated laminitis (Fig. 15.8) results from the elevated expression of TIMP-1 and TIMP-3.

Although levels of MMP-2 are increased in the lamellae of horses with CHO-induced laminitis (Fig. 15.7), the results of various unpublished studies using native zymography have suggested that MMP-2 activity is not increased. Native zymography is performed in the absence of SDS and detects processed gelatinases that lack bound TIMPs. Native gelatinase activity in extracts of lamellae from horses with starch-induced laminitis presenting OG3 lameness, and also in extracts of lamellae from horses with clinical aggravated chronic laminitis, was found to be weak and similar to that in extracts from healthy horses. This finding is supported by *in-situ* native zymography, which was performed by preparing a gelatin overlay of thin sections of cryopreserved lamellae from healthy horses and horses with wheat flour-induced laminitis; native gelatinolytic activity was absent from the sections [17]. Thus, based on both native zymography of lamellar extracts and *in-situ* gelatinolytic assays of lamellar slices, it seems unlikely that there is an accumulation of TIMP-free (and therefore active) MMP-2 in the laminitic lamellae.

Despite the above considerations, it cannot be concluded that MMP-2 plays no role in lamellar pathology. A fine balance is required between TIMPs and MMPs to ensure normal tissue growth and repair, and hence a subtle increase in active MMP-2 over regulatory TIMPs may tip the balance towards ECM damage. On the other hand, there is no compelling evidence that MMP-2 is solely, or at all, responsible for the degradation of lamellar ECM in laminitic horses. Additionally, since levels of MMP-2 vary greatly among affected horses, there is a possibility that other MMPs contribute to lamellar degradation. This reasoning led the present authors, and others, to evaluate the expression of other metalloproteinases in lamellae of laminitic horses. Consequently, gene and in many cases protein expression analyses have been completed for collagenases I and III (MMP-1, MMP-13), stromelysin I (MMP-3), membrane-type MMPs (MMP-14, MMP-15, MMP-16), a disintegrin and metalloproteinase family members (ADAM-10 and ADAM-17), and a disintegrin and metalloproteinase with thrombospondin motifs family members (ADAMTS-1, ADAMTS-4, and ADAMTS-5). Attempts to analyze neutrophil collagenase (MMP-8), macrophage metalloelastase (MMP-12), and MMP-25 (a membrane-type MMP that inactivates alpha-1-proteinase inhibitor) were unsuccessful because full-length candidate genes have not been published in the equine genome data base, thereby precluding primer design.

Collagenase I and III

MMP-1 and MMP-13 (also called collagenase I and collagenase III) are secreted as pro-enzymes which, like pro-MMP-2 and pro-MMP-9, are activated by the extracellular proteolytic removal of their regulatory pro-peptides [20]. Expression of genes encoding these enzymes is significantly increased in lamellae of horses with starch-induced laminitis compared to those of healthy horses [1] (Table 15.1). Only MMP-1 gene

Table 15.1 Changes in collagenase gene expression in the lamellae of laminitic horses.

	Primer sequence (F = forward 5′; R = reverse 5′)	Fold increase (RT-qPCR) in gene expression* in lamellae of laminitic horses presenting with: OG1 lameness	OG3 lameness
MMP-1	F- ATAACTACGATTCGGGGAGAAG-3′ R-TCTATGGGAAACCTCATAAGCA-3′	38 ($p = 0.01$; $n = 8$)	87 ($p = 0.01$; $n = 5$)
MMP-13	F-GTCCCTGATGTGGGTGAATAC-3′ R-ACATCAGACCAAACTTTGAAGG-3′	1.4 ($p = 0.67$; $n = 8$)	120 ($p = 0.01$; $n = 5$)

*Methods for RNA extraction from lamellae, generation of cDNA, performance of RT-qPCR and analysis of gene expression relative to that in lamellae of healthy horses by the $_{\Delta\Delta}$CT method using GAPDH as a reference gene have been described [1]. Primers span an intron and had high efficiency and specificity

expression was increased at OG1 lameness, while increased MMP-13 gene expression was apparent at OG3 lameness but not OG1 lameness (Table 15.1). An analysis of protein extracts (0.5% NP-40 with protease inhibitors) of lamellae from healthy and laminitic horses using SDS–PAGE and Western blotting showed that polypeptides corresponding to 52 kDa pro-MMP-1, 61 kDa pro-MMP-13 and 48 kDa MMP-13 protein are substantially and significantly (respectively fourfold, $p = 0.0001$; 12-fold, $p = 0.01$; sixfold, $p < 0.05$) increased in extracts of the lamellae of horses with OG3 lameness in a CHO (starch) model [1].

The presence of MMP-1 and MMP-13 protein in lamellar extracts has also been confirmed by proteomic analysis of lamellar extracts (H. Galantino-Homer *et al.*, unpublished results). Importantly, the expression of MMP-13 in lamellae of healthy and laminitic horses has also been localized to LBECs by immunofluorescent staining, and is absent from other cells [1], indicating that the enzyme plays a role in lamellar junctional homeostasis as well as in pathologic processes elicited by dietary starch overload. MMP-1 protein expression has not yet been localized by immunofluorescent staining due to a lack of appropriate reagents; however, the reported induction of both MMP-1 and MMP-13 transcripts in LBECs of the lamellae of horses with starch-induced laminitis as determined by laser capture microscopy, RNA extraction and gene expression analysis, makes it is likely that both MMP-1 and MMP-13 are produced by the basal epithelial cells [35].

MMP-1 and MMP-13 degrade collagens I and III, which are structural fibers of the dermal ECM. In addition, MMP-13 degrades fibronectin (which attaches ECM components to each other and to integrins expressed by cells within the ECM) and has a broad activity against other ECM components that include components of the BM [20]. Extensive remodeling of the ECM of the secondary dermal lamellae in horses with laminitis, which manifests as multifocal gaps lacking collagen I, collagen III (Fig. 15.5), fibronectin, and proteoglycans [1] correlates with increased lamellar MMP-13 activity. However, although the increased presence of MMP-13 in the lamellae is coincident with tissue damage, this does not necessarily signify a causal relationship. Thus, it is important to determine whether MMP-13 cleavage fragments of triple-helical fibrillar collagens and fibronectin accumulate in the lamellae of laminitic horses and, eventually, to establish methods to selectively inactivate MMP-13 in lamellae. In this regard, Christopher Pollitt and colleagues (notably Claire Underwood) of the Australian Equine Laminitis Research Unit, School of Veterinary Science, University of Queensland, Australia, have delivered marimastat, which is a broad-spectrum MMP inhibitor, into the lamellar blood supply by repeated regional limb perfusion through the lateral palmar digital vein in order to determine the contribution of lamellar MMPs to OF-overload induced laminitis (C. Pollitt, personal communication). An (*in-vitro*) MMP-inhibitory concentration of marimastat was detected in a lamellar ultrafiltrate collected via an ultrafiltration probe placed in the perfused foot. Control lamellae received saline without marimastat by regional limb perfusion. All horses administered a gastric OF overload developed laminitis. Although lamellae perfused with marimastat developed somewhat lesser signs of histopathology than those receiving saline, the effect was slight. The results of this study suggest against a major contribution of marimastat-perfusion-sensitive MMP to the development of laminitis. However, this conclusion has been tempered by a lack of information on the distribution of the marimastat within lamellar tissue, particularly whether or not it accumulates in the secondary dermal lamellae around the BM.

Membrane-Type MMPs

MMP-14, MMP-15, MMP-16, and MMP-25, which are also referred to respectively as membrane-type 1 MMP (MT1-MMP), MT2-MMP, MT3-MMP and MT6-MMP, are transported to the outer cell membrane as active forms, their regulatory pro-peptide being removed during intracellular transport. The expression of genes encoding MMPs-14, -15, and -16 is detected in the lamellae of healthy horses, indicating a role in normal tissue homeostasis [1]. However, levels of expression were not observed to differ between healthy horses and horses presenting with OG1 or OG3 lameness after starch induction, suggesting against a role in lamellar pathology in this form of laminitis [1]. In contrast, other investigators have reported a significant increase in MT1-MMP gene expression in the lamellae of horses with OF-induced laminitis and, as mentioned earlier, expression of the MT1-MMP protein was localized to LBECs by immunohistochemistry [29]. Further investigations are required to resolve these differences in the starch and OF models of sepsis-related laminitis.

A Disintegrin and Metalloproteinase Domain Containing Protein-10 and -17 (ADAM-10, ADAM-17)

The ADAMs are a large family of trans-membrane MMPs from which the regulatory/inhibitory pro-peptide is removed during transport to the cell surface. They function mainly to cleave membrane proteins at the cell surface, being dubbed the 'shedases.' Each ADAM can cleave many different substrates, and there is a good deal of substrate redundancy among family members. Notable substrates of ADAM-10 and ADAM-17 include tumor necrosis factor-alpha and its receptor; hence, these ADAMs play an important role in the induction and regulation of inflammation. Genes encoding ADAM-10 and ADAM-17 are expressed in the lamellae of healthy horses. However, despite the reported contribution of inflammation to CHO-induced laminitis [36–38], ADAM-10 and ADAM-17 expression is not upregulated in the lamellae of horses presenting with BWE-induced, starch-induced, or naturally acquired laminitis relative to that in the lamellae of healthy horses [34].

A Disintegrin and Metalloproteinase with Thrombospondin Motifs-4 (ADAMTS-4)

Expression of the gene encoding ADAMTS-4 is highly upregulated in the lamellae of horses with BWE- and CHO-induced

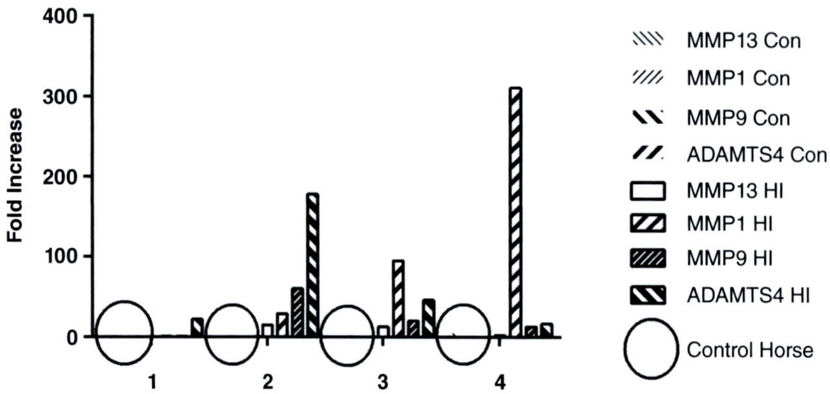

Figure 15.9 Comparative analysis using RT-qPCR of expressed genes encoding metalloproteinases in lamellae of healthy horses (Con, $n = 4$) and horses receiving sustained induction of hyperinsulinemia for 48 h (HI, $n = 4$). Con denotes control horses, which are circled because MMP expression was minimal; HI denotes hyperinsulinemic horses. The first HI horses did not become lame, whereas the other three HI horses developed OG2 lameness. Lamellar samples were supplied by Dr Susan C. Eades, Louisiana State University School of Veterinary Medicine.

laminitis (including starch [34, 35,39] and OF-induced laminitis [30]), and in the lamellae of horses with acute laminitis acquired in the clinic [34]. The expression of genes encoding ADAMTS-1 and ADAMTS-5 is also upregulated in some laminitic horses, but to a lesser degree than that of ADAMTS-4 [34]. In addition to gene expression, it has been shown that ADAMTS-4 protein and enzyme activity are significantly increased in the lamellae of horses with starch-induced laminitis [39], coincident with the increase of MMP-1 and MMP-13 gene and protein expression [1]. In contrast, the expression of genes encoding ADAMTS-4, MMP-1 and MMP-13 was not significantly (statistically) increased in the lamellae of horses with hyperinsulinemia/euglycemia-induced laminitis [40] at the 48-h time point relative to their expression in the lamellae of healthy horses (Fig. 15.9; S.J. Black *et al.*, unpublished results), consistent with studies reported by de Laat *et al.* [40]. However, these findings do not necessarily exclude a role for the metalloproteinases in insulin-induced laminitis. In this regard, expression of the metalloproteinases was minimal in the lamellae of healthy horses, but variably and often substantially increased in the lamellae of horses administered insulin (Fig. 15.9). Despite the absence of a statistically significant increase in metalloproteinase gene expression in lamellae of horses with hyperinsulinemia-induced laminitis determined by ANOVA, 'mclust discriminant analysis' of these and matching data from horses with CHO-induced laminitis indicates that increased expression of a metalloproteinase gene cluster which includes MMP-1, MMP-9, MMP-13 and ADAMTS-4, is a signature of both hyperinsulinemia- and starch-induced laminitis (J. Mayfield, F. Zhang, and S.J. Black, unpublished results). Furthermore, the use of next-generation sequencing (RNA-Seq) as an unbiased screening tool in an equine metabolic syndrome study to identify lamellar genes that are differentially expressed between ponies of two different phenotypes (obese, lean) and diets (low- and high-non-structural carbohydrate diet for seven days) resulted in the discovery that genes encoding ADAMTS-4, MMP-1 and MMP-13 underwent increased expression in ponies challenged with a high-carbohydrate diet for seven days, which also resulted in increased circulating insulin levels (J.K. Belknap, T.A. Burns, R. Geor and A.S. Yilmaz, unpublished data).

ADAMTS family members are secreted as active enzymes, their regulatory pro-peptide being removed by a furin within the endosomal system during transport out of the cell [41]. In the equine digital lamellae, ADAMTS-4 is found within lamellar basal epithelial cells [5], and is mainly present as a 51 kDa protein with minor amounts of 61 kDa and 42 kDa species [5] (Fig. 15.10), all of which bear a catalytic site neoepitope, FASLSRF, that is exposed on ADAMTS-4 only after removal of the regulatory pro-peptide [42]. The 61 kDa and 51 kDa ADAMTS-4 polypeptides are observed when extracts of lamellae are made in NP-40 extraction buffer containing protease inhibitors (Fig. 15.10), or by direct extraction in SDS-sample buffer which denatures all proteins (not shown). This latter test excludes the possibility of post-extraction enzymatic processing. In mice and humans, processed ADAMTS-4 bearing the FASLSRF neoepitope has a molecular weight of between 68 kDa and 75 kDa [43], and a portion of the material undergoes autoproteolysis to generate 61 kDa, 51 kDa, and 40 kDa polypeptides [43–46] that putatively correspond to the 61 kDa, 51 kDa, and 42 kDa forms present in the equine digital lamellae [5] (Fig. 15.10). A complete absence of the 68 kDa to 75 kDa ADAMTS-4 from extracts of equine lamellae suggests highly efficient autoproteolysis, which presumably occurs in the endosomal system of basal epithelial cells after proteolytic removal of the ADAMTS-4 regulatory pro-peptide.

ADAMTS-4 degrades large polysulfated proteoglycans, namely aggrecan, versican, neurocan, and brevican [47, 48]. Aggrecan and versican are expressed by chondrocytes in cartilage, with aggrecan predominating. Versican is also expressed by many other cell types, including muscle cells that are associated with blood vessels and epidermal epithelial cells in skin. In contrast, neurocan and brevican are largely expressed by

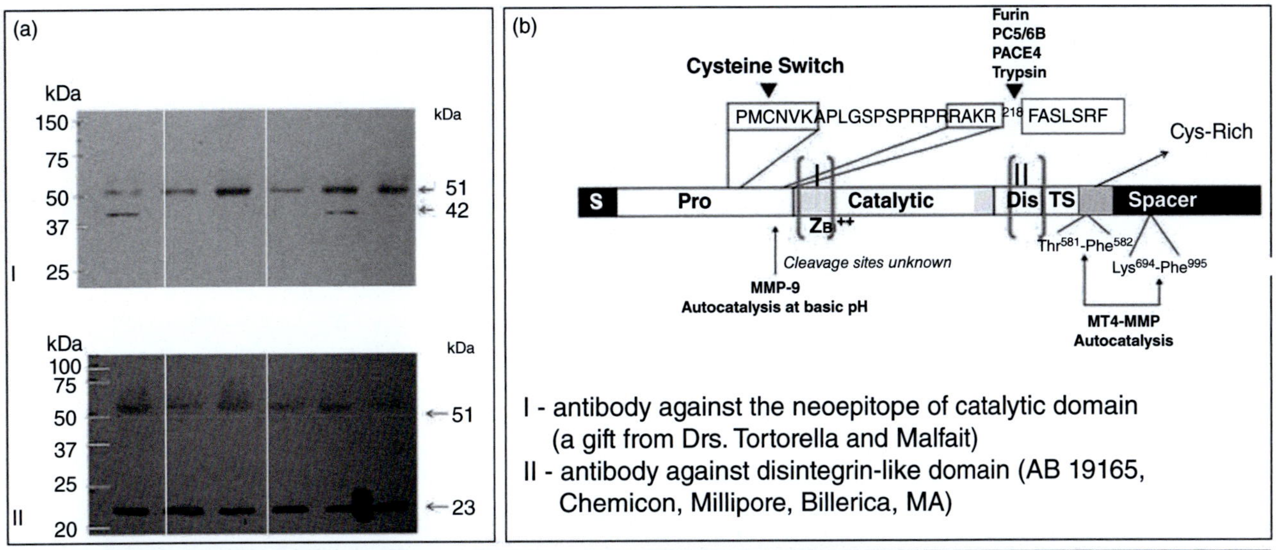

(c)

Domain (MW) Antibody	Prodomain (22)	Catalytic (24)	Dis (9)	TS (6)	Cys-rich (12)	Spacer (17)	Total MW (kDa)
I		√	√	√	√	-√-	61
		√	√	√	√		51
		√	√	√	-√-		42
II		√	√	√	√		51
			√	√	-√-		23

Figure 15.10 Expression of truncated ADAMTS-4 in equine lamellae. (a) Western blot analysis of lysates (0.5% NP-40 + protease inhibitors) of lamellae from six healthy horses using: (I) antibody specific for a catalytic site neoepitope (FASLSRF) exposed upon removal of the ADAMTS-4 propeptide domain; (II) antibody specific for a disintegrin domain epitope (Chemicon, MA). (b) Diagram showing domain structure of ADAMTS-4 and location of epitopes detected by antibodies used in panel (a). (c) Assignment of ADAMTS-4 domains to polypeptides. √, domain present; -√-, fragment of the domain present.

respectively, neuronal cells and astrocytes within the central nervous system. Aggrecan and versican play important roles in articular cartilage and tendons. The proteoglycans, which are decorated with keratan and chondroitin sulfate glycosaminoglycan side chains, are secreted into the ECM, where they attach via a binding site in their N-terminal domain and an associated linker protein, to hyaluronan, forming huge, highly charged complexes [49–51]. The proteoglycans also attach to other components of the ECM via their C-terminal, lectin-like domain. In addition, anionic groups on their glycosaminoglycan side chains carry with them positively charged counter ions, such as Na^+, creating an osmotic gradient and drawing water into the tissue. In combination with hyaluronan, the proteoglycans form hydrated gels that endow tissues with resistance to compression deformation and also serve as boundary lubricants [52, 53]. Aggrecan and versican also have signaling properties that affect cell proliferation, differentiation, adhesion, and intercellular communication and hence also have non-mechanical roles in regulating cell function [54–58].

Because hydrated large polysulfated proteoglycans prevent compression deformation of tissues such as articular cartilage, it seemed reasonable that they might play a similar role in lamellae. However, unexpectedly, versican (see Figs 15.1 and 15.2) was found by immunofluorescent staining of thin sections of frozen OCT-embedded lamellae to be selectively expressed by basal epithelial cells in the equine digital lamellae of both healthy and laminitic horses, and to be absent from the ECM. Aggrecan was selectively expressed in basal epithelial cells and parabasal keratinocytes [5,39], but was also absent from the ECM. In addition, whereas aggrecan was heavily glycosylated and required overnight extraction with 4 M guanidine-hydrochloride buffer to become soluble in extraction buffer after homogenization of lamellae, versican was minimally glycosylated and readily extracted into physiological buffer or mild detergent solutions

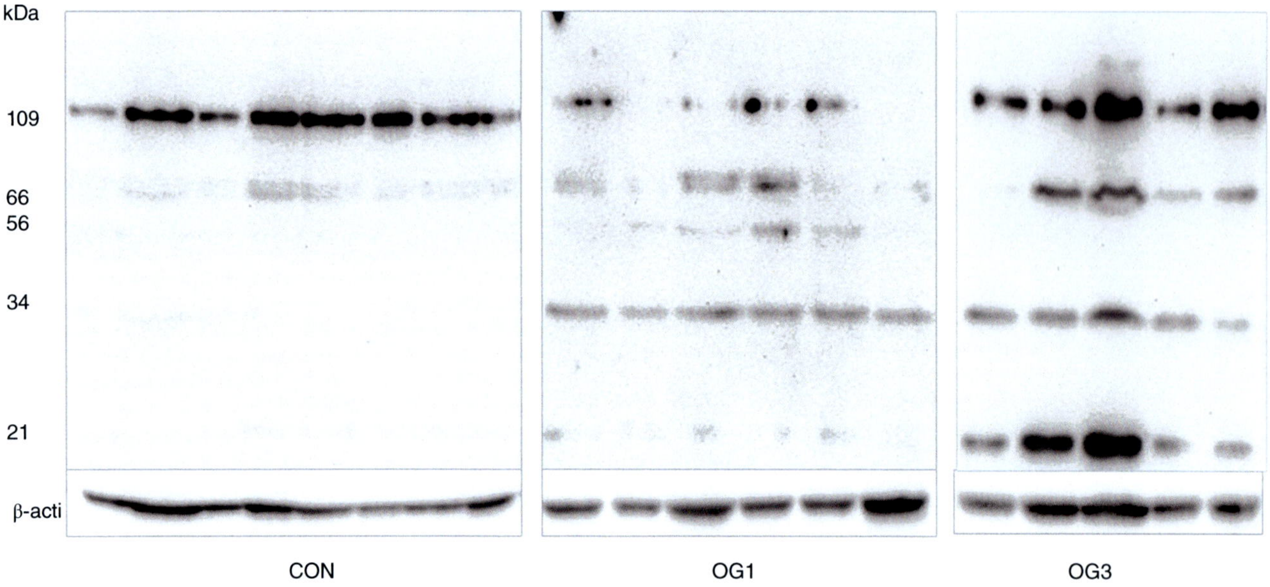

Figure 15.11 Polypeptides bearing the ADAMTS-4 versican cleavage neoepitope NIVSFE in lamellar extracts from healthy horses (CON) and horses with starch-induced laminitis presenting OG1 or OG3 lameness. Extracts of lamellae were subjected to SDS–PAGE in 10% polyacrylamide gels. Tracks were loaded with 10 μg protein from individual extracts. Western blotting was performed using antibody specific for the NIVSFE cleavage epitope (Abcam ab 28671). Beta actin was used as a load control and detected by specific antibody (Abcam ab 8226).

by homogenization [5]. Thus, while aggrecan may contribute to water retention in epidermal keratinocytes and resistance to compression forces as a result of associated glycosaminoglycans, this cannot be the role of lamellar versican which for the most part lacks glycosaminoglycans.

Like its substrates, ADAMTS-4 was also found to be present within LEBCs in the digital lamellae of healthy and laminitic horses [5,39]. In addition, a portion of lamellar aggrecan and versican had ADAMTS-4 cleavage neoepitopes, determined by SDS–PAGE and Western blot analysis, which attested to processing of the proteoglycans by the ADAMTS-4 [5]. Full-length ADAMTS-4 is known to bind to the pericellular matrix and ECM. However, removal of the ADAMTS-4 C terminal spacer domain both increases catalytic activity [43] and allows the enzyme to detach from the ECM [45]. In addition, the truncated ADAMTS-4 gains activity against multiple new cleavage sites on the aggrecan core protein and develops new activity against carboxymethylated transferrin, as well as two small leucine-rich proteoglycans (SLRPs) fibromodulin and decorin, indicative of broad proteolytic activity [45]. Interestingly, the four primary SLRPs (fibromodulin, decorin, biglycan, and lumican) were all found to be downregulated in laser microscope-dissected LBEC in the starch model of sepsis-related laminitis [35]. As SLRPs are very important in ECM fibril organization and stability, a decrease in these proteins due to possible degradation and decreased expression may play a role in the structural breakdown on the lamellar dermal ECM at OG3 lameness (as discussed above). The 51 kDa form of ADAMTS-4, which is prevalent in the lamellae of healthy horses and increased in lamellae of horses with acute laminitis [39], is expected to diffuse into and degrade the ECM if secreted from LBECs. However, extracellular 51 kDa ADAMTS-4 would be unlikely to be detected in lamellar ECM by immunofluorescent staining of OCT-embedded thin sections because it would wash away during staining. Hence, the localization of ADAMTS-4 within LBECs and its apparent absence from the ECM [5] does not exclude its secretion and extracellular activity.

Although ADAMTS-4 expression (both gene and 51 kDa truncated protein) is increased in the lamellae of horses with acute laminitis, this is not accompanied by an increase in fragments of aggrecan bearing ADAMTS-4 cleavage neoepitopes relative to those present in the lamellae of healthy horses [39]. Thus, it is unlikely that the cleavage of aggrecan is increased in the lamellae of laminitic horses. In contrast, cleavage of versican is greatly increased in the laminitic tissue, particularly cleavage of the V0/V2 isoforms which results in greatly increased concentrations of low-molecular-weight cleavage products bearing the ADAMTS-4 NIVSFE [59] cleavage neoepitope [39] (Fig. 15.11). Only a single ADAMTS-4 cleavage site on V0/V2 versican yields the NIVSFE epitope, and although cleavage fragments can vary in size depending on glycosylation [59], the dominant fragment size is approximately 68 kDa [5,59] in human tissue, and larger polypeptides have not been reported. Therefore, the ~112 kDa NIVSFE$^+$ fragment shown in Figure 15.10 in extracts of equine lamellae is unexpected and unexplained. In addition, the NIVSFE$^+$ polypeptides of ~34 kDa and ~21 kDa are also unexpected and have not been reported previously. However, quantification of these polypeptides by G-Box analysis and Pearson product moment correlation coefficient analyses performed on pairs of expressed Western blot bands indicated positive correlations (n = 19) for 68 kDa versus 34 kDa (r = 0.47, p <0.05), 68 kDa versus 21 kDa (r = 0.79, p <0.001) and 34 kDa versus 21 kDa (r = 0.73, p <0.001) NIVSFE-bearing V0/V2 versican fragments [39], consistent with their generation by the same process (i.e., by cleavage of the 68 kDa fragment), and with the possibility that there are several cleavage sites for truncated ADAMTS-4 on the N-terminal domains of V0/V2 versican isoforms. The biological significance of ADAMTS-4 cleavage fragments in laminitic lamellae, or indeed in any tissue, remains to be determined. Despite these unknowns, the results remain highly important. They are the first formal proof that metalloproteinase activity is functionally elevated in lamellae of laminitic horses and intriguingly, that this activity is a property of LBECs.

In addition to its activity against V0 and V2 isoforms of versican, ADAMTS-4 cleaves V0 and V1 isoforms yielding 66 kDa and 109 kDa fragments with a characteristic C-terminal ADAMTS-4 DPEAAE cleavage neoepitope [60]. This cleavage event is also significantly increased in the lamellae of horses with CHO-induced laminitis compared to healthy horses, and results in the accumulation of versican fragments bearing the DPEAAE cleavage epitope in the tissue [39]. Furthermore, in addition to increased cleavage of expressed versican (V0/V1/V2) isoforms, versican gene expression is suppressed, as is the generation of all versican splice variants (isoforms) [39]. Importantly, a reduced versican gene expression in the lamellae of laminitic horses is accompanied by a significantly decreased expression of versican protein in the basal epithelial cells relative to that in the lamellae of healthy horses, while aggrecan expression in these cells does not change significantly [39] (Fig. 15.11).

Degradation of Versican by ADAMTS-4 and Dysregulation of LBEC Physiology

Loss of versican gene and protein expression from the LBECs of horses that develop OG3 lameness after starch-induced laminitis (Fig. 15.12) suggests that disease progression is associated with a profound change in basal epithelial cell physiology, culminating in versican depletion from the cells. In this regard, the experimental transfer, *in vitro*, of the gene encoding versican into fibroblast cells, which do not express versican, has been shown to induce their transition to epithelial cells. This cellular transition is termed mesenchymal-to-epithelial cell transition, and is evidenced by acquisition of the epithelial cell phenotype and expression of epithelial cell differentiation antigens, namely E-cadherin, a component of adherens junctions, and integrin α_6, a component of hemidesmosomes [54,57]. Consequently, a loss of versican expression from LBECs in laminitic horses might herald a reverse transition, that is, from epithelial cells to mesenchymal cells (termed epithelial-to-mesenchymal transition [EMT], a well-studied event in epithelial cancer) and accompanying loss of cell–cell and cell–BM attachments which would destabilize

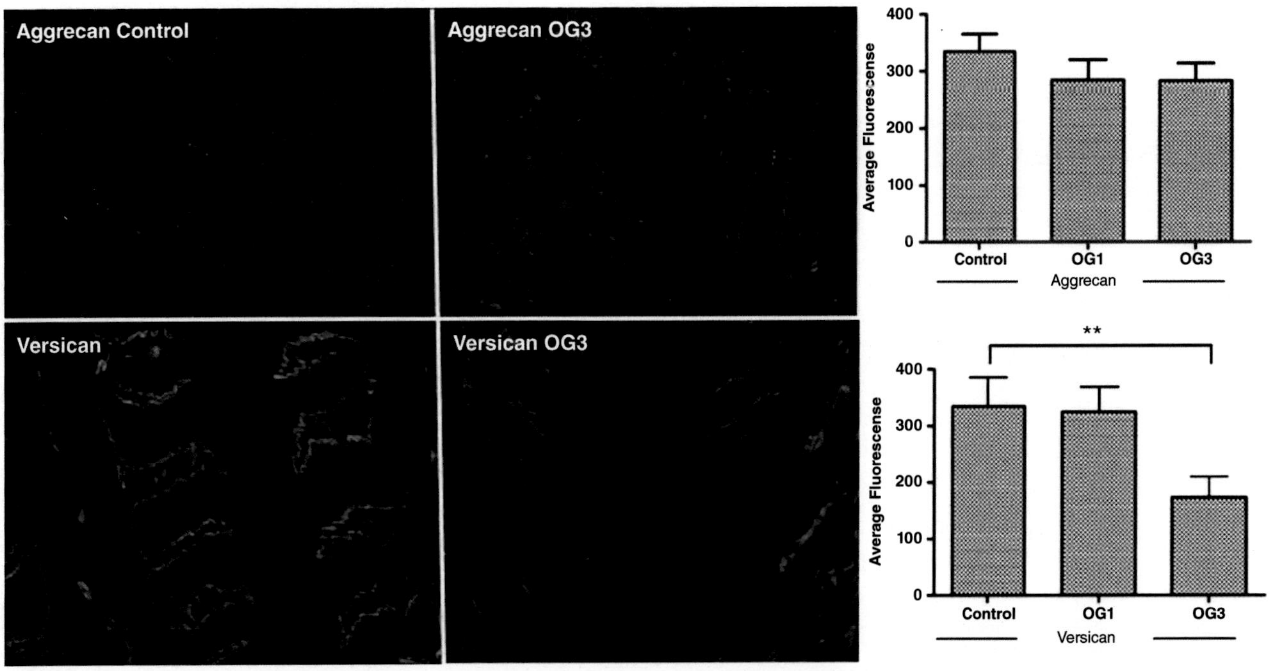

Figure 15.12 Expression of aggrecan and versican in lamellae of healthy (Control) and laminitic (OG3) horses. Thin cryosections of unfixed, OCT-embedded lamellae were stained with antibodies specific for aggrecan (red, upper panels, Abcam ab 16320), versican (red, lower panels, Santa Cruz #26706), laminin (green, lower panels, Abcam ab11575), and with DAPI (blue, all panels). To determine average fluorescence, the basal epithelial cells were traced from the base to the tip of each secondary epidermal lamellae and red stain within the region calculated. Sixty measurements were obtained from each control horse ($n = 6$) and from horses with starch-induced laminitis at OG1 ($n = 6$) and OG3 ($n = 4$) lameness. Distribution analysis of immunofluorescent data was performed using two-way ANOVA with a Duncan post-test.

the lamellar epidermal–dermal junction. However, while a suppressed expression of adherens junction and hemidesmosome attachment proteins was observed in the lamellae of horses with starch-induced laminitis compared to healthy horses, this was not a result of EMT, or because of a loss of E-cadherin or integrin α_6 gene expression [15]. The LBECs of laminitic horses retained expression of genes encoding these attachment proteins, and did not acquire expression of the mesenchymal differentiation antigen vimentin, at least up to the development of OG3 lameness [15]. Instead, the basal epithelial cells of laminitic horses developed a profound suppression of other adherens junction and hemidesmosome proteins namely, β-catenin and integrin β_4. These changes were accompanied by a suppression of the canonical Wnt signaling pathway in these cells [15] (as described below). In addition to serving as a component of the adherens junction (see Chapter 4), β-catenin is also a component of the β-catenin/T-cell factor co-transcriptional complex, which is the effector limb of the canonical Wnt signaling pathway.

The canonical Wnt signaling pathway is one of the fundamental pathways that controls multiple cellular processes including cell development, proliferation, differentiation, polarity, and motility [61, 62]. The core activity of the pathway is regulation of the concentration and stability of β-catenin in the cell. This is important because β-catenin can translocate to the nucleus where it binds to DNA-associated T-cell factor (Tcf) displacing a co-repressor and unleashing the transcriptional activity of target genes. The canonical Wnt signaling pathway regulates expression of genes encoding β-catenin itself [63], versican [64, 65], and many other proteins. In the starch model of sepsis-related laminitis, it has been shown that the regulators of canonical Wnt signaling are expressed predominantly in LBECs [15]. These include several proteins which are positive pathway regulators, namely: (i) Wnt, named after Wingless in Drosophila and integration 1 in mouse breast tumors, which is a glycoprotein that activates the pathway; (ii) its receptor, frizzled (Fz); (iii) its co-receptor, low-density lipoprotein receptor-related protein (LRP); (iv) disheveled (Dsh) which (when activated by the Wnt/FZD/LRP complex) stabilizes β-catenin by inhibiting glycogen synthase kinase 3β (GSK3β) [phosphorylation of β-catenin by GSK3β normally leads to its degradation]; (v) protein phosphatase 1 (PP1) and Protein kinase B (Akt), which also prevent β-catenin phosphorylation/degradation; and (vi) TCF, which in complex with transcriptional coactivator β-catenin induces the expression of specific target genes. There are also several negative regulators of the canonical Wnt signaling pathway which function by decreasing β-catenin concentrations by either diminishing gene expression or elevating its degradation, namely: (i) Dickkopf (DKK antagonizes Wnt signaling by binding the coreceptor LRP); (ii) components of the β-catenin degradation complex (including the scaffolding proteins Axin and *adenomatous polyposis coli* gene product [APC] which bind β-catenin); and (iii) casein kinase 1α (CK1α) and GSK3β which jointly phosphorylate bound β-catenin leading to its subsequent ubiquitination and proteasomal degradation.

In the lamellae of horses with starch overload-induced laminitis, positive regulators of the canonical Wnt signaling pathway are suppressed at the level of gene expression and, where studied, also at the level of protein expression, whereas negative regulators of the pathway are for the most part elevated relative to expression in the lamellae of healthy horses [15]. These findings, together with studies showing an increased expression of ADAMTS-4 and MMP-13 gene and protein expression in LBECs of laminitic compared to healthy horses, are summarized in Table 15.2. These data provide a time line for the expression of molecular indicators of lamellar pathology and a mechanism for destabilization of the lamellar epidermal–dermal junction in the starch-induced model of laminitis. These findings suggest that starch-induced laminitis results from a combination of: (i)

Table 15.2 Molecular indicators of lamellar pathology in starch-induced laminitis.

	Metalloproteinase expression		Canonical Wnt signaling pathway		Pathways that interact with the canonical Wnt pathway	
Stage of disease	Gene	Protein	Gene	Protein	Insulin/growth factor signaling	Integrin signaling
OG1	ADAMTS-4 ↑ MMP-1 ↑ MMP-9 ↑	*ADAMTS-4 61 kDa ↑ *ADAMTS-4 51 kDa ↑	Wnt4 ↓ Axin1 ↑ CK1α ↑	**β-catenin ↓	Akt2 ↓	Integrin β_4 ↓
OG3	ADAMTS-4 ↑ MMP-1 ↑ MMP-2 ↑ MMP-9 ↑ MMP-13 ↑	Pro-MMP-1 ↑ MMP-2 ↑ Pro-MMP-9 ↑ Pro-MMP-13 ↑ MMP-13 ↑	Wnt4 ↓ FZD4 ↓ LRP6 ↓ DSH ↓ PP1 ↓ β-catenin ↓ TCF ↓	**β–catenin ↓ GSK3β- ↑	Akt2 ↓ Integrin β_4 ↓	Integrin β_4 ↓

*Associated change: intact Versican protein significantly decreased at OG3; ADAMTS-4 cleavage fragments of V0/V1 and V0/V2 versican elevated at OG3.
**Associated change: Versican gene expression significantly decreased at OG3 (versican gene expression is regulated by the canonical Wnt signaling pathway)
↑denotes significantly increased $p < 0.05$
↓Denotes significantly decreased $p < 0.05$

dysregulation of LBEC physiology resulting in a loss of expression of adherens junction and hemidesmosome components; and (ii) degradation of dermal ECM by MMP-13 (and possibly truncated ADAMTS-4). The findings support and extend the studies of French and Pollitt, which show that failure of the lamellar junction is associated with a reduced presence of intact hemidesmosomes per unit area of BM and a reduced presence of hemidesmosome components overall [14,16].

Future Perspectives

Several questions are raised by the studies discussed above, namely: (i) what is the relationship, if any, between pathways that regulate ADAMTS-4, MMP-1 and MMP-13 gene and protein expression by LBECs; (ii) is there a relationship between the processes that regulate metalloproteinase expression by LBECs and those that regulate the canonical Wnt signaling pathway; and (iii) given that there is a strong positive correlation between loss of β-catenin and integrin β_4 gene expression [15] (Pearson's $r = 0.74$, $p = 0.0003$) in LBECs and between integrin signaling and the canonical Wnt signaling pathway [66, 67], does a loss of hemidesmosomes and integrin-signaling cause suppression of canonical Wnt signaling, or does suppression of canonical Wnt signaling and suppression of hemidesmosome-specific gene and protein expression cause suppression of hemidesmosome and integrin signaling, or are integrin and canonical Wnt signaling pathways jointly suppressed by another, as-yet undefined, change in the LBECs brought on, for example, by a 'pro-laminitis' change in the lamellar environment or in LBEC signaling pathways. These questions can be best approached *in vitro* using defined cultures of LBECs that recapitulate *in vivo* cell physiology. This technology awaits development.

Acknowledgments

The studies summarized in this chapter were funded by USDA (CSREES MAS00907; NRI CSREES 2007-01350 and 2007-35204/18313), the Morris Animal Foundation (D08EQ-054, D13EQ-004), and the American Quarter Horse Association (2012 - OGCA#112-0740), and supported by the generosity and enthusiasm of many colleagues in the field of laminitis, notably James Belknap, Philip Johnson, Hannah Galantino-Homer, Susan Eades, Ray Geor, and Christopher Pollitt.

References

1. Wang, L., Pawlak, E.A., Johnson, P.J., Belknap, J.K., Alfandari, D., and Black, S.J. (2014) Expression and activity of collagenases in the digital laminae of horses with carbohydrate overload-induced acute laminitis. *J. Vet. Intern. Med.*, **28** (1), 215–222.
2. Frantz, C., Stewart, K.M., and Weaver, V.M. (2010) The extracellular matrix at a glance. *J. Cell Sci.*, **123** (Pt 24), 4195–4200.
3. Pollitt, C.C. (2010) The anatomy and physiology of the suspensory apparatus of the distal phalanx. *Vet. Clin. North Am. Equine Pract.*, **26** (1), 29–49.
4. Pollitt, C.C. and Daradka, M. (1998) Equine laminitis basement membrane pathology: loss of type IV collagen, type VII collagen and laminin immunostaining. *Equine Vet. J. Suppl.*, **26**, 139–144.
5. Pawlak, E., Wang, L., Johnson, P.J., Nuovo, G., Taye, A., Belknap, J.K., *et al.* (2012) Distribution and processing of a disintegrin and metalloproteinase with thrombospondin motifs-4, aggrecan, versican, and hyaluronan in equine digital laminae. *Am. J. Vet. Res.*, **73** (7), 1035–1046.
6. Engiles, J.B. (2010) Pathology of the distal phalanx in equine laminitis: more than just skin deep. *Vet. Clin. North Am. Equine Pract.*, **26** (1), 155–165.
7. Eades, S.C. (2010) Overview of current laminitis research. *Vet. Clin. North Am. Equine Pract.*, **26** (1), 51–63.
8. Garner, H.E., Coffman, J.R., Hahn, A.W., Hutcheson, D.P., and Tumbleson, M.E. (1975) Equine laminitis of alimentary origin: an experimental model. *Am. J. Vet. Res.*, **36** (4 Pt.1), 441–444.
9. Van Eps, A.W. and Pollitt, C.C. (2009) Equine laminitis model: lamellar histopathology seven days after induction with oligofructose. *Equine Vet. J.*, **41** (8), 735–740.
10. Asplin, K.E., Sillence, M.N., Pollitt, C.C., and McGowan, C.M. (2007) Induction of laminitis by prolonged hyperinsulinaemia in clinically normal ponies. *Vet. J.*, **174** (3), 530–535.
11. de Laat, M.A., Van Eps, A.W., McGowan, C.M., Sillence, M.N., and Pollitt, C.C. (2011) Equine laminitis: comparative histopathology 48 hours after experimental induction with insulin or alimentary oligofructose in Standardbred horses. *J. Comp. Pathol.*, **145** (4), 399–409.
12. Obel, N. (1948) Studies on the histopathology of acute laminitis. PhD Thesis, Swedish University of Agricultural Sciences.
13. Nourian, A.R., Baldwin, G.I., Van Eps, A.W., and Pollitt, C.C. (2007) Equine laminitis: ultrastructural lesions detected 24–30 hours after induction with oligofructose. *Equine Vet. J.*, **39** (4), 360–364.
14. French, K.R. and Pollitt, C.C. (2004) Equine laminitis: loss of hemidesmosomes in hoof secondary epidermal lamellae correlates to dose in an oligofructose induction model: an ultrastructural study. *Equine Vet. J.*, **36** (3), 230–235.
15. Wang, L., Pawlak, E.A., Johnson, P.J., Belknap, J.K., Eades, S., Stack, S., *et al.* (2013) Impact of laminitis on the canonical Wnt signaling pathway in basal epithelial cells of the equine digital laminae. *PLoS ONE*, **8** (2), e56025.
16. French, K.R. and Pollitt, C.C. (2004) Equine laminitis: cleavage of laminin 5 associated with basement membrane dysadhesion. *Equine Vet. J.*, **36** (3), 242–247.
17. Mungall, B.A. and Pollitt, C.C. (1999) Zymographic analysis of equine laminitis. *Histochem. Cell Biol.*, **112** (6), 467–472.
18. Pollitt, C.C., Pass, M.A., and Pollitt, S. (1998) Batimastat (BB-94) inhibits matrix metalloproteinases of equine laminitis. *Equine Vet. J. Suppl.*, **1998** (26), 119–124.
19. Johnson, P.J., Kreeger, J.M., Keeler, M., Ganjam, V.K., and Messer, N.T. (2000) Serum markers of lamellar basement membrane degradation and lamellar histopathological changes in horses affected with laminitis. *Equine Vet. J.*, **32** (6), 462–468.
20. Visse, R. and Nagase, H. (2003) Matrix metalloproteinases and tissue inhibitors of metalloproteinases: structure, function, and biochemistry. *Circ. Res.*, **92** (8), 827–839.

21. Loftus, J.P., Belknap, J.K., and Black, S.J. (2006) Matrix metalloproteinase-9 in laminae of black walnut extract treated horses correlates with neutrophil abundance. *Vet. Immunol. Immunopathol.*, **113** (3-4), 267–276.
22. Loftus, J.P., Johnson, P.J., Belknap, J.K., Pettigrew, A., and Black, S.J. (2009) Leukocyte-derived and endogenous matrix metalloproteinases in the lamellae of horses with naturally acquired and experimentally induced laminitis. *Vet. Immunol. Immunopathol.*, **129** (3-4), 221–230.
23. Riggs, L.M., Krunkosky, T.M., Noschka, E., Boozer, L.A., Moore, J.N., Robertson, T.P., *et al.* (2009) Comparison of characteristics and enzymatic products of leukocytes in the skin and laminar tissues of horses administered black walnut heartwood extract or lipopolysaccharide. *Am. J. Vet. Res.*, **70** (11), 1383–1390.
24. Nagase, H., Visse, R., and Murphy, G. (2006) Structure and function of matrix metalloproteinases and TIMPs. *Cardiovasc. Res.*, **69** (3), 562–573.
25. Roderfeld, M., Graf, J., Giese, B., Salguero-Palacios, R., Tschuschner, A., Muller-Newen, G., *et al.* (2007) Latent MMP-9 is bound to TIMP-1 before secretion. *Biol. Chem.*, **388** (11), 1227–1234.
26. Armstrong, P.B. and Quigley, J.P. Alpha2-macroglobulin: an evolutionarily conserved arm of the innate immune system. *Dev. Comp. Immunol.*, **23** (4-5), 375–390.
27. Sato, H. and Takino, T. (2010) Coordinate action of membrane-type matrix metalloproteinase-1 (MT1-MMP) and MMP-2 enhances pericellular proteolysis and invasion. *Cancer Sci.*, **101** (4), 843–847.
28. Kyaw-Tanner, M. and Pollitt, C.C. (2004) Equine laminitis: increased transcription of matrix metalloproteinase-2 (MMP-2) occurs during the developmental phase. *Equine Vet. J.*, **36** (3), 221–225.
29. Kyaw-Tanner, M.T., Wattle, O., Van Eps, A.W., and Pollitt, C.C. (2008) Equine laminitis: membrane type matrix metalloproteinase-1 (MMP-14) is involved in acute phase onset. *Equine Vet. J.*, **40** (5), 482–487.
30. Visser, M.B. and Pollitt, C.C. (2012) The timeline of metalloprotease events during oligofructose induced equine laminitis development. *Equine Vet. J.*, **44** (1), 88–93.
31. Clutterbuck, A.L., Harris, P., Allaway, D., and Mobasheri, A. (2010) Matrix metalloproteinases in inflammatory pathologies of the horse. *Vet. J.*, **183** (1), 27–38.
32. Murphy, G. (2011) Tissue inhibitors of metalloproteinases. *Genome Biol.*, **12** (11), 233.
33. Maskos, K. and Bode, W. (2003) Structural basis of matrix metalloproteinases and tissue inhibitors of metalloproteinases. *Mol. Biotechnol.*, **25** (3), 241–266.
34. Coyne, M.J., Cousin, H., Loftus, J.P., Johnson, P.J., Belknap, J.K., Gradil, C.M., *et al.* (2009) Cloning and expression of ADAM-related metalloproteases in equine laminitis. *Vet. Immunol. Immunopathol.*, **129** (3-4), 231–241.
35. Leise, B.S., Watts, M.R., Roy, S., Yilmaz, A.S., Alder, H., and Belknap, J.K. (2015) Use of laser capture microdissection for the assessment of equine lamellar basal epithelial cell signalling in the early stages of laminitis. *Equine Vet. J.*, **47** (4), 478–488.
36. Belknap, J.K. (2010) Black walnut extract: an inflammatory model. *Vet. Clin. North Am. Equine Pract.*, **26** (1), 95–101.
37. Hensel, M., Fugler, L., Liese, B., Watts, M., Eades, S., and Belknap, J. (2011) Laminar inflammatory events and epithelial stress at Obel grade 3 lameness in the carbohydrate overload model of equine laminitis. American College of Veterinary Internal Medicine Forum, Denver, CO.
38. Leise, B.S., Faleiros, R.R., Watts, M., Johnson, P.J., Black, S.J., and Belknap, J.K. (2011) Laminar inflammatory gene expression in the carbohydrate overload model of equine laminitis. *Equine Vet. J.*, **43** (1), 54–61.
39. Wang, L., Pawlak, E., Johnson, P.J., Belknap, J.K., Alfandari, D., and Black, S.J. (2012) Effects of cleavage by a disintegrin and metalloproteinase with thrombospondin motifs-4 on gene expression and protein content of versican and aggrecan in the digital laminae of horses with starch gruel-induced laminitis. *Am. J. Vet. Res.*, **73** (7), 1047–1056.
40. de Laat, M.A., Kyaw-Tanner, M.T., Nourian, A.R., McGowan, C.M., Sillence, M.N., and Pollitt, C.C. (2011) The developmental and acute phases of insulin-induced laminitis involve minimal metalloproteinase activity. *Vet. Immunol. Immunopathol.*, **140** (3-4), 275–281.
41. Wang, P., Tortorella, M., England, K., Malfait, A.M., Thomas, G., Arner, E.C., *et al.* (2004) Proprotein convertase furin interacts with and cleaves pro-ADAMTS4 (Aggrecanase-1) in the trans-Golgi network. *J. Biol. Chem.*, **279** (15), 15434–1540.
42. Tortorella, M.D., Arner, E.C., Hills, R., Gormley, J., Fok, K., Pegg, L., *et al.* (2005) ADAMTS-4 (aggrecanase-1): N-terminal activation mechanisms. *Arch. Biochem. Biophys.*, **444** (1), 34–44.
43. Gao, G., Westling, J., Thompson, V.P., Howell, T.D., Gottschall, P.E., and Sandy, J.D. (2002) Activation of the proteolytic activity of ADAMTS4 (aggrecanase-1) by C-terminal truncation. *J. Biol. Chem.*, **277** (13), 11034–11041.
44. Miwa, H.E., Gerken, T.A., Huynh, T.D., Flory, D.M., and Hering, T.M. (2006) Mammalian expression of full-length bovine aggrecan and link protein: formation of recombinant proteoglycan aggregates and analysis of proteolytic cleavage by ADAMTS-4 and MMP-13. *Biochim. Biophys. Acta*, **1760** (3), 472–486.
45. Kashiwagi, M., Enghild, J.J., Gendron, C., Hughes, C., Caterson, B., Itoh, Y., *et al.* (2004) Altered proteolytic activities of ADAMTS-4 expressed by C-terminal processing. *J. Biol. Chem.*, **279** (11), 10109–10119.
46. Flannery, C.R., Zeng, W., Corcoran, C., Collins-Racie, L.A., Chockalingam, P.S., Hebert, T., *et al.* (2002) Autocatalytic cleavage of ADAMTS-4 (Aggrecanase-1) reveals multiple glycosaminoglycan-binding sites. *J. Biol. Chem.*, **277** (45), 42775–42780.
47. Porter, S., Clark, I.M., Kevorkian, L., and Edwards, D.R. (2005) The ADAMTS metalloproteinases. *Biochem. J.*, **386** (Pt 1), 15–27.
48. Stanton, H., Melrose, J., Little, C.B., and Fosang, A.J. (2011) Proteoglycan degradation by the ADAMTS family of proteinases. *Biochim. Biophys. Acta*, **1812** (12), 1616–1629.
49. Kiani, C., Chen, L., Wu, Y.J., Yee, A.J., and Yang, B.B. (2002) Structure and function of aggrecan. *Cell Res.*, **12** (1), 19–32.
50. Nagase, H. and Kashiwagi, M. (2003) Aggrecanases and cartilage matrix degradation. *Arthritis Res. Ther.*, **5** (2), 94–103.
51. Smith, M.M., Jacobson, E., Dart, A.J., and Little, C.B. (2013) Large proteoglycan metabolism in tendinopathy. *Br. J. Sports Med.*, **47** (9), e2.
52. Chandran, P.L. and Horkay, F. (2012) Aggrecan, an unusual polyelectrolyte: review of solution behavior and physiological implications. *Acta Biomater.*, **8** (1), 3–12.
53. Seror, J., Merkher, Y., Kampf, N., Collinson, L., Day, A.J., Maroudas, A., *et al.* (2011) Articular cartilage proteoglycans

as boundary lubricants: structure and frictional interaction of surface-attached hyaluronan and hyaluronan–aggrecan complexes. *Biomacromolecules*, **12** (10), 3432–3443.

54. Sheng, W., Wang, G., La Pierre, D.P., Wen, J., Deng, Z., Wong, C.K., *et al.* (2006) Versican mediates mesenchymal-epithelial transition. *Mol. Biol. Cell*, **17** (4), 2009–2020.
55. Ricciardelli, C., Sakko, A.J., Ween, M.P., Russell, D.L., and Horsfall, D.J. (2009) The biological role and regulation of versican levels in cancer. *Cancer Metastasis Rev.*, **28** (1-2), 233–245.
56. Kinsella, M.G., Bressler, S.L., and Wight, T.N. (2004) The regulated synthesis of versican, decorin, and biglycan: extracellular matrix proteoglycans that influence cellular phenotype. *Crit. Rev. Eukaryot. Gene Expr.*, **14** (3), 203–234.
57. Sheng, W., Dong, H., Lee, D.Y., Lu, W.Y., and Yang, B.B. (2007) Versican modulates gap junction intercellular communication. *J. Cell. Physiol.*, **211** (1), 213–219.
58. Frey, H., Schroeder, N., Manon-Jensen, T., Iozzo, R.V., and Schaefer, L. (2013) Biological interplay between proteoglycans and their innate immune receptors in inflammation. *FEBS J.*, **280** (10), 2165–2179.
59. Westling, J., Gottschall, P.E., Thompson, V.P., Cockburn, A., Perides, G., Zimmermann, D.R., *et al.* (2004) ADAMTS4 (aggrecanase-1) cleaves human brain versican V2 at Glu405-Gln406 to generate glial hyaluronate binding protein. *Biochem. J.*, **377** (Pt 3), 787–795.
60. Sandy, J.D., Westling, J., Kenagy, R.D., Iruela-Arispe, M.L., Verscharen, C., Rodriguez-Mazaneque, J.C., *et al.* (2001) Versican V1 proteolysis in human aorta in vivo occurs at the Glu441-Ala442 bond, a site that is cleaved by recombinant ADAMTS-1 and ADAMTS-4. *J. Biol. Chem.*, **276** (16), 13372–13378.
61. MacDonald, B.T., Tamai, K., and He, X. (2009) Wnt/beta-catenin signaling: components, mechanisms, and diseases. *Dev. Cell*, **17** (1), 9–26.
62. Valvezan, A.J. and Klein, P.S. (2012) GSK-3 and Wnt Signaling in neurogenesis and bipolar disorder. *Front. Mol. Neurosci.*, **5**, 1.
63. Li, Q., Dashwood, W.M., Zhong, X., Al-Fageeh, M., and Dashwood, R.H. (2004) Cloning of the rat beta-catenin gene (Ctnnb1) promoter and its functional analysis compared with the Catnb and CTNNB1 promoters. *Genomics*, **83** (2), 231–242.
64. Rahmani, M., Read, J.T., Carthy, J.M., McDonald, P.C., Wong, B.W., Esfandiarei, M., *et al.* (2005) Regulation of the versican promoter by the beta-catenin-T-cell factor complex in vascular smooth muscle cells. *J. Biol. Chem.*, **280** (13), 13019–13028.
65. Rahmani, M., Wong, B.W., Ang, L., Cheung, C.C., Carthy, J.M., Walinski, H., *et al.* (2006) Versican: signaling to transcriptional control pathways. *Can. J. Physiol. Pharmacol.*, **84** (1), 77–92.
66. Mainiero, F., Pepe, A., Wary, K.K., Spinardi, L., Mohammadi, M., Schlessinger, J., *et al.* (1995) Signal transduction by the alpha 6 beta 4 integrin: distinct beta 4 subunit sites mediate recruitment of Shc/Grb2 and association with the cytoskeleton of hemidesmosomes. *EMBO J.*, **14** (18), 4470–4481.
67. Maydan, M., McDonald, P.C., Sanghera, J., Yan, J., Rallis, C., Pinchin, S., *et al.* (2010) Integrin-linked kinase is a functional Mn^{2+}-dependent protein kinase that regulates glycogen synthase kinase-3beta (GSK-3beta) phosphorylation. *PLoS One*, **5** (8), e12356.

CHAPTER 16

Endocrine and Metabolic Dysregulation in Laminitis: Role of Pituitary Dysfunction

Philip J. Johnson

Introduction

Laminitis development in the context of underlying endocrinological disturbance has been referred to as 'endocrinopathic' laminitis, and is most commonly reported in horses affected with either or both the equine metabolic syndrome (EMS) and pituitary pars intermedia dysfunction (PPID) [1]. The link of circumstances associated with elevated corticosteroid levels (both exogenous and endogenous) to laminitis risk is well known, but a direct cause and effect relationship between corticosteroids and laminitis has been difficult to confirm. Possibly, corticosteroids cause an increased likelihood of endocrinopathic laminitis when other endocrinological predispositions are present (such as EMS and PPID). Extensive recent studies have served to highlight the role of insulin as an independent risk factor for endocrinopathic laminitis in both EMS and PPID [2,3]. Although there are some similarities between the characteristics of laminitis that result from the effects of high circulating levels of insulin when compared to laminitis resulting from sepsis-related/inflammatory causes, new information regarding the pathophysiological link between insulin and endocrinopathic laminitis suggests a unique cause for lamellar failure with this type of laminitis compared to sepsis-related or supporting limb laminitis [4–6]. An improved understanding of the role of insulin as a cause of laminitis will surely lead to better treatments and preventive strategies. The aim of the present chapter is to review the concept of endocrinopathic laminitis as a complication of PPID, as well as possible mechanisms linking exogenous corticosteroids with laminitis.

Endocrinological Factors and the Risk of Laminitis

For many years, veterinarians have recognized that laminitis sometimes develops under circumstances associated with elevated corticosteroid influence. The risk of laminitis associated with corticosteroids has been linked to both the (exogenous) administration of powerful synthetic steroid drugs including (most frequently) dexamethasone and triamcinalone [7–13], and conditions associated with heightened endogenous cortisol release (hypercortisolism resulting from stress or from PPID/equine Cushing's syndrome) [14, 15]. In direct contradiction to the recommended employment of synthetic corticosteroids for the treatment of laminitis several decades ago [16], the risk of endocrinopathic laminitis represents perhaps the most significant impediment to the broad use of synthetic corticosteroids for any disease state in modern veterinary medical practice.

An early report of elevated plasma adrenocorticotrophic hormone (ACTH) concentrations in a mature mare affected with PPID led to the conclusion that this equine condition was likely similar to pituitary-dependent Cushing's syndrome or chronic hyperadrenalocorticism in human medicine [17]. This conclusion is overly simplistic when reviewed in the light of current knowledge because ACTH-dependent hypercortisolism is currently regarded as an inconsistent finding in 'Cushingoid' (PPID-affected) horses and ponies [18–21].

Although use of the term 'equine Cushing's syndrome' has been in common use for many years, it is important to emphasize that the equine condition is distinctly different from the 'Cushing's' syndromes of human and small animal medicine, when the term 'Cushing's syndrome' is (appropriately) employed to characterize the clinical manifestations of elevated corticosteroid influence over time. A true equine 'Cushing's' syndrome resulting directly from hyperadrenalocorticism is rare in horses. Although laminitis has been described as a component of the clinical expression of pituitary-independent Cushing's in a horse with a functional adrenocortical adenoma [22], a small number of earlier reports of adrenocortical tumors in horses did not identify functionality [23–27]. Chronic hypercortisolism resulting from primary adrenocortical neoplasia is exceedingly rare in horses.

Although corticosteroid administration has been associated with a risk of laminitis, the results of extensive recent research have implicated insulin resistance (IR) and hyperinsulinemia

Equine Laminitis, First Edition. Edited by James K. Belknap and Raymond Geor.

('insulin dysregulation') as the critical endocrinopathic abnormality responsible for the development of endocrinopathic laminitis in horses affected with both PPID and EMS [28]. Laminitis occurring in association with hyperinsulinemia of any cause (including PPID) is frequently encountered in modern horses. It now appears that hyperinsulinemia *per se* may be the direct cause of endocrinopathic laminitis, rather than IR as suggested previously [28, 29].

Pituitary Pars Intermedia Dysfunction (PPID)

Significant advances pertaining to the present understanding of the pathophysiology of PPID have been made in recent years, and have led to the availability of improved diagnostic tests and therapeutic options.

Development of PPID

Endocrinopathic laminitis is an important clinical sign in horses affected with either or both EMS and PPID [29, 30]. Current thinking suggests that endocrinopathic laminitis may only develop in those PPID-affected horses that are concomitantly affected with 'insulin dysregulation' (ID, a term used recently to describe IR and hyperinsulinemia), and that endocrinopathic laminitis is much less likely to develop in those PPID-affected horses that are not concurrently affected with ID. The influence of superimposed excessive melanocortin secretion from the pars intermedia in PPID might contribute to the pathophysiological impact of pre-existing ID in terms of laminitis risk, but this possibility is speculative and deserves further investigation.

The role of chronic hypercortisolism as a direct causative factor for laminitis associated with PPID has been downplayed because post-mortem evidence of adrenocortical hyperplasia is identified in only a minority (ca. 20%) of PPID-affected horses and ponies [18–21]. However, evidence of corticosteroid influence is present to a variable degree [31] in many PPID-affected equids, and a direct or indirect effect (through inhibition of the action of insulin) should not be completely discounted [32]. Furthermore, a role for elevated cortisol production in PPID was suggested by the observation that inhibition of adrenal cortisol synthesis using the 3-beta-hydroxysteroid dehydrogenase [HSD] inhibitor trilostane resulted in improvement in the clinical signs of laminitis in PPID-affected horses [33].

Although many of the clinical manifestations of PPID result from a heightened secretion of PI-derived melanocortins over time, there have been few reports of the direct (endocrinological) effects of these important hormones throughout the body and the extent to which they affect either insulin signaling or the health of the digital lamellae in general.

The equine pituitary gland is characterized by a well-developed intermediate lobe, the pars intermedia (PI), and the principal secreting cell in the PI is the melanotrope (see Fig. 16.1). Like corticotropes in the pars ventralis (PV; also termed pars distalis) of the pituitary gland, melanotropes also synthesize the pre-pro-hormone proopiomelano(lipo)cortin (POMC; Fig. 16.1), which is then cleaved to produce multiple hormones (see below and Fig. 16.1). Whereas corticotropes

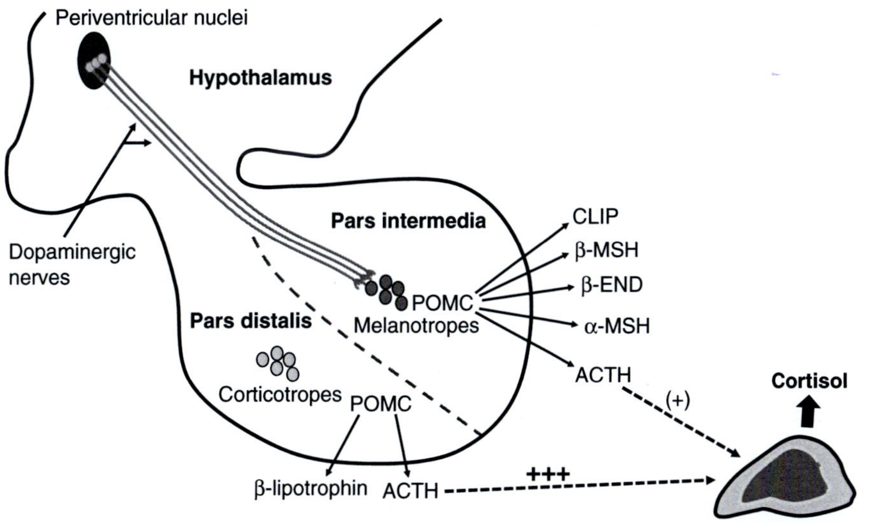

Figure 16.1 Diagrammatic representation of the equine adenohypophysis depicting the relationship between dopaminergic nerves that originate in the periventricular nuclei of the hypothalamus and melanotropes in the pars intermedia. These dopaminergic nerves are responsible for normal tonic inhibition of melanotropes. Under the influence of dopamine in the healthy state, melanotrope secretion is inhibited. Peptide hormones that constitute the secretory repertoire of melanotropes (melanocortins) include ACTH, α-MSH, β-MSH, β-END, and CLIP (see text for abbreviations), all derived from the cleavage of proopiomelanocortin (POMC). Degeneration of dopaminergic nerves and loss of tonic inhibition leads to clonal expansion of melanotropes and melanocortin hypersecretion in horses affected with PPID. In the healthy state, ACTH is primarily derived from corticotropes in the pars distalis (denoted by +++).

convert the POMC precursor to corticotropin (ACTH) and beta-lipotropin, melanotropes undertake significant further peptide cleavage and post-translational modification of POMC resulting in the following principal secretory repertoire: alpha-melanocyte-stimulating hormone (α-MSH), beta-endorphin (β-END), corticotropin-like intermediate lobe peptide (CLIP), and ACTH. As important as ACTH is for purposes of diagnosis and characterization and assessment of treatment effectiveness, PI-derived ACTH represents a significant minority (ca.2%) of the secreted output from the pituitary gland [34].

PPID results from a loss of the normal dopaminergic inhibition (and resultant proliferation [through clonal expansion] of melanotrope cells) in the PI. Secretion by melanotropes is normally tonically inhibited by dopamine released from dopaminergic nerves originating in the periventricular nucleus (a thin sheet of small neurons located in the wall of the third ventricle [not to be confused with the paraventricular nucleus]) of the hypothalamus (see Fig. 16.1). Interestingly, the periventricular nucleus does not have an effective blood–brain barrier. Released dopamine binds to dopamine D2 receptors on melanotropes and inhibits both the biosynthesis of POMC and secretion of melanocortins. It is important to emphasize that, unlike their corticotrope counterparts in the PV component of the pituitary gland, melanotropes are not inhibited by circulating corticosteroids through negative feedback inhibition.

The histological appearance of the PI obtained from PPID-affected equids is very similar to that seen in rats following PI denervation [35]. The concentration of dopamine (and its metabolites) in the PI of PPID-affected horses is markedly reduced (eightfold) and the expression of type-2 dopamine receptors in affected melanotropes is increased (consistent with a response to dopaminergic denervation) [36,37]. Furthermore, both the clinical signs of PPID and the circulating concentration of PI-derived melanocortins are significantly reduced following treatment with either dopamine or dopaminergic agonists in affected horses [38,39].

That the hormonal (melanocortin) profile of the abnormal PI is similar (i.e., melanocortin hormones are still produced in similar relative concentrations compared to each other, as occurs normally) to that of the normal PI was originally demonstrated using both biochemical [34, 37, 38, 40] and immunocytochemical [18, 37, 41] methods. Specifically, in equine PPID, the plasma concentrations of β-END, α-MSH, β-melanocyte-stimulating hormone (β-MSH), γ-melanocyte-stimulating hormone (γ-MSH), and CLIP are increased to approximately the same degree [37, 38, 42]. In contrast to the situation in human patients affected with corticotrope tumors of the PD, the plasma concentration of ACTH in many PPID-affected horses is relatively less elevated.

Using immunohistochemical methods, a reduction in the number of dopaminergic neurons in both the periventricular nuclei (cell bodies) of the hypothalamus and in the PI (nerve terminals for the same cells) was demonstrated in both aged and PPID-affected equids [43]. Loss of dopaminergic nerve fibers was greatest in those horses affected with PPID. Dopaminergic neurodegeneration in other species has been linked to oxidative stress, inflammation, neuronal accumulation of misfolded alpha-synuclein, and mitochondrial abnormalities [43].

The loss of inhibitory dopaminergic neurons in PPID-affected horses has also been attributed to the effects of oxidative stress (dopaminergic neurons are especially susceptible to oxidative stress) using immunohistochemistry for the oxidative marker 3-nitrotyrosine [43]. Oxidative stress has been associated with both obesity and an activated state of systemic inflammation, two states associated with metabolic syndrome in humans. Conflicting results are present in the equine PPID literature. Following the measurement of both systemic and PI anti-oxidant capacity in PPID-affected and age-matched controls, McFarlane *et al.* concluded that PPID is likely not a consequence of enhanced systemic oxidative stress [43]. However, in another study, Keen *et al.* showed that horses with PPID did have increased circulating markers of oxidative stress, perhaps suggesting that dopaminergic neurodegeneration could be consequent to chronic systemic oxidative stress [44].

Activation of systemic inflammatory responsiveness with advancing age is referred to as 'inflamm-aging.' When McFarlane and Holbrook evaluated systemic inflammatory responses in PPID-affected and age-matched controls [45], specifically the ratios of interleukin (IL)-6:IL-10 and tumor necrosis factor-alpha (TNF-α):IL-10 were greater in the control horses than those affected with PPID (IL-6 and TNF-α are regarded as proinflammatory cytokines and IL-10 is an anti-inflammatory cytokine). Unexpectedly, these results demonstrated that systemic inflammatory responsiveness was greater in healthy control horses than in those affected with PPID [45]. Reduced inflammatory responsiveness in PPID-affected individuals might be explained by the anti-inflammatory actions of elevated circulating melanocortin concentrations (e.g., α-MSH has an anti-inflammatory potency 23-fold that of acetaminophen [paracetamol]). If an activated state of inflammation does play a role in the development of dopaminergic neurodegeneration in horses that develop PPID, such a condition might exist earlier during the course of disease, prior to the development of the melanocortin hypersecretion that acts to inhibit inflammatory responsiveness.

Further evidence that dopaminergic neurodegeneration in horses may be similar to that reported in human patients includes the observation that an increased level of alpha-synuclein, a protein increased in affected neural tissue in Parkinson's disease, was demonstrated in the affected PI of horses [43]. Presently, a complete explanation for the accelerated development of dopaminergic neurodegeneration in horses that develop PPID is lacking and further investigation is ongoing.

Macroscopic (gross) enlargement of the pituitary gland (macroadenoma) is not evident in all cases of PPID; histological examination is needed to demonstrate small adenoma formation (microadenoma) in the PI of a minority of affected pituitary glands [18, 46]. The extent to which nonfunctional pituitary adenomas occur in horses has not been reported (non-functional pituitary adenomas represent incidental findings in approximately 25% of human autopsies [47]). However, to an increasing extent, PI adenomas are reported in young horses in which there are no clinical signs of PPID [20].

As previously noted, hypercortisolism is not uniformly or consistently identified in equine PPID. This observation may be explained by the observation that both biochemically demonstrable ACTH and ACTH immunostaining of both the normal and abnormal PI is relatively weak, and that the circulating ACTH concentration is often not greatly elevated in the face of clinical PPID [18, 38, 40–42]. Although ACTH is secreted in relatively smaller quantities compared to other melanocortins, the hypersecretion of the other melanocortins acts to potentiate the effectiveness of ACTH at the adrenal glands (e.g., the steroidogenic action of ACTH is increased sixfold in the presence of other melanocortins) [48, 49].

The overall clinical picture for PPID varies quite significantly between affected individual animals. Differences in clinical expression may be partially explained by heterogeneity in the PI-derived melanocortin repertoire being produced in a given patient, the extent to which adrenocortical stimulation is occurring, and the presence or absence of ID. It is likely that the mixture of secreted melanocortins (α-MSH, ACTH, etc.) differs significantly between affected horses (likely due to genetic variability) and over time (perhaps with a seasonal effect) [50]. Moreover, the extent to which each melanocortin is processed by post-translational modification (glycosylation, N-acetylation, etc.) before it is secreted into the circulation is likely highly variable between animals. These potentially highly variable post-translational modifications add an additional layer of heterogeneity to the composition of the (final) secreted product [37].

The net biological impact of each melanocortin is affected by these post-translational modifications. For example, although N-acetylation and carboxy-terminal proteolysis of β-END in normal horses yields a secreted product with little opioid action, these modifications are minimized in the absence of dopaminergic influence and the secreted product exerts greater opioid effectiveness [37]. Elevated levels of secreted β-END with enhanced opioid effectiveness in PPID cases may contribute to the lethargy and somnolence seen in some individuals. Therefore, PPID-associated melanocortin bioactivity differs from that associated with the same melanocortin produced in the healthy state. Thus, the endocrinological effects of PPID result from both increased circulating concentrations of melanocortins and also from the (highly variable) different biological activities of those melanocortins.

The circulating concentration of ACTH in PPID-affected horses is often higher than would be predicted from both: (i) the simple clonal expansion of the melanotrope population; and (ii) the absence of adrenocortical hyperplasia (i.e., as would be expected with ACTH stimulation). It has been shown that the bioactivity of ACTH derived from melanotropes is less than that of ACTH derived from corticotropes (see Fig. 16.1), which would lead to relatively less adrenocortical stimulation and thus less adrenal cortisol production [38]. Recently, Cordero *et al.* treated cultivated adrenal cortical cells with equimolar quantities of ACTH derived from either normal or from PPID-affected horses [51]. Interestingly, the PPID-derived ACTH was significantly less effective at stimulating cortisol release in this *in-vitro* experiment, supporting the premise that increased ACTH in PPID is less bioactive consequent to being produced by PI melanotropes.

Inhibited inflammatory responsiveness represents a very important clinical component of PPID because signs of pain associated with endocrinopathic laminitis may be inhibited (i.e., less pain than anticipated for the severity of laminitic disease). Inhibited pain expression in the face of developing laminitis may lead to severe and detrimental disruption of the digital lamellae in physically active PPID-affected individuals by virtue of the effect of uninhibited mechanical loading. Related to this concept, the common incidence of non-healing and/or recurrent corneal ulcers in PPID-affected horses may be at least partially attributed to the recent demonstration by Miller *et al.* that corneal sensitivity is reduced as a result of both age and PPID [52].

Immunosenescence and inhibited inflammatory responsiveness are also responsible for increased risk of infectious diseases in PPID-affected horses. Various opportunistic infectious conditions may be identified as a result of the immunodebilitated state of PPID-affected horses including protozoal myeloencephalitis (*Sarcocystis neurona*), dermatophilosis, dermatophytosis, subsolear abscesses, bacterial pneumonia, and urinary tract infections. Both, pneumonia and cystitis may be present at the subclinical level and are often not recognized until a post-mortem examination is conducted (PPID-associated inhibition of immune functions). Similarly, PPID-affected horses may have higher fecal egg counts when compared with healthy horses [53].

Development of Laminitis in the Context of PPID

For many years, laminitis has been widely recognized as a common clinical sign in PPID-affected individuals. Donaldson *et al.* reported that 70% of laminitis cases seen in their practice were associated with PPID (when the diagnosis was based on elevated plasma ACTH concentration) [14]. The extent to which clinically evident laminitis is reported in horses with PPID is quite variable, with reports ranging between 24% and 82%. In the author's (PJ) experience, observations suggest that subclinical laminitis may be identified by histopathological examination in many PPID-affected individuals that are examined post-mortem and in which laminitis had not been anticipated ante-mortem. However, clinically evident endocrinopathic laminitis (exhibited as pain) does not develop in a significant number of PPID-affected horses and ponies unless insulin dysregulation has been identified as a comorbidity.

Many studies pertaining to an improved understanding of the pathogenesis of endocrinopathic laminitis associated with PPID have been reported recently, especially when the role of hyperinsulinemia is taken into account. Presently, the (traditional) concept that PPID-associated laminitis results directly from elevated corticosteroid influence has been downplayed due to the facts that: (i) adrenocortical hyperplasia is an inconsistent finding; and (ii) plasma cortisol levels are highly variable with many cases of suspected PPID-associated laminitis cases having normal parameters for both.

The discovery that insulin is an independent risk factor for endocrinopathic laminitis suggests that any conditions in which IR and hyperinsulinemia are also present may be complicated by laminitis. Both IR and hyperinsulinemia are often reported in clinical cases of PPID and, when present alongside PPID, have been associated with relatively severe laminitis and an unfavorable prognosis [54]. However, modern thinking suggests that, when identified in PPID-affected equids, IR and hyperinsulinemia may represent independent comorbidities – that is, they may not be related to PPID in these animals.

Although the histopathological characteristics of the equine digital lamellae in healthy horses and in horses affected by either inflammatory or insulin-mediated laminitis have been well documented, very few studies have reported on the histopathological changes of the lamellae in equids affected by PPID. In a recent study of 16 PPID-affected animals either with ($n = 6$) or without ($n = 10$) laminitis (compared to 10 age- and breed-matched controls), Karikoski and coworkers concluded that laminitis pathology was only evident in those animals in which insulin dysregulation could also be identified [55]. The histopathological appearance of non-laminitic PPID horses was not different to that of controls. These observations further support the hypothesis that, when present in PPID-affected individuals, endocrinopathic laminitis is a result of, and a biomarker for, insulin dysregulation as comorbidity.

Insulin resistance and hyperinsulinemia ('insulin dysregulation') represent the principal endocrinological basis of EMS, currently thought to be a PPID-independent condition for which endocrinopathic laminitis is a major concern (see Chapter 18). Some EMS-affected horses may develop PPID and may therefore be at additional risk for endocrinopathic laminitis as a consequence of the additional influences of melanocortins and hypercortisolism (when present, hypercortisolism represents a significant inhibitor to the action of insulin and may serve to further reduce insulin sensitivity and worsen IR).

The effect of PI-derived melanocortin hypersecretion (independent of hypercortisolism) on insulin sensitivity is presently unknown, but may play a further role. In conclusion, endocrinopathic laminitis identified in the context of PPID could be a consequence of pre-existing/coexisting EMS or worsening insulin dysregulation as a result of the combined actions of melanocortins and hypercortisolism (if present). Many diverse etiological factors for laminitis have been proposed beyond endocrinological factors, and it is important to emphasize that PPID-affected horses should be regarded as being generally at greater risk for laminitis resulting from any cause.

References

1. Johnson, P.J., Messer, N.T., Slight, S.H., Wiedmeyer, C., Buff, P., and Ganjam, V.K. (2004) Endocrinopathic laminitis in the horse. *Clin. Tech. Equine Pract.*, **3** (1), 45–56.
2. Asplin, K.E., Sillence, M.N., Pollitt, C.C., and McGowan, C.M. (2007) Induction of laminitis by prolonged hyperinsulinaemia in clinically normal ponies. *Vet. J.*, **174** (3), 530–535.
3. Nourian, A.R., Asplin, K.E., McGowan, C.M., Sillence, M.N., and Pollitt, C.C. (2009) Equine laminitis: ultrastructural lesions detected in ponies following hyperinsulinaemia. *Equine Vet. J.*, **41** (7), 671–677.
4. de Laat, M.A., Kyaw-Tanner, M.T., Sillence, M.N., McGowan, C.M., and Pollitt, C.C. (2012) Advanced glycation endproducts in horses with insulin-induced laminitis. *Vet. Immunol. Immunopathol.*, **145** (1-2), 395–401.
5. de Laat, M.A., Pollitt, C.C., Kyaw-Tanner, M.T., McGowan, C.M., and Sillence, M.N. (2013) A potential role for lamellar insulin-like growth factor-1 receptor in the pathogenesis of hyperinsulinaemic laminitis. *Vet. J.*, **197** (2), 302–306.
6. Burns, T.A., Watts, M.R., Weber, P.S., McCutcheon, L.J., Geor, R.J., and Belknap, J.K. (2013) Distribution of insulin receptor and insulin-like growth factor-1 receptor in the digital laminae of mixed-breed ponies: an immunohistochemical study. *Equine Vet. J.*, **45** (3), 326–332.
7. Eyre, P., Elmes, P.J., and Strickland, S. (1979) Corticosteroid-potentiated vascular responses of the equine digit: a possible pharmacologic basis for laminitis. *Am. J. Vet. Res.*, **40** (1), 135–138.
8. Eyre, P. and Elmes, P.J. (1980) Corticosteroid-induced laminitis? Further observations on the isolated, perfused hoof. *Vet. Res. Commun.*, **4** (2), 139–143.
9. Johnson, P.J., Slight, S.H., Ganjam, V.K., and Kreeger, J.M. (2002) Glucocorticoids and laminitis in the horse. *Vet. Clin. North Am. Equine Pract.*, **18** (2), 219–236.
10. Johnson, P.J., Messer, N.T., Bowles, D.K., Slight, S.H., Ganjam, V.K., and Kreeger, J.M. (2004) Glucocorticoids and laminitis in horses. *Compend. Contin. Educ. Pract. Vet.*, **26** (7), 547–557.
11. Ryu, S.H., Byung, S.K., Lee, C.W., Yoon, J., and Lee, Y.L. (2004) Glucocorticoid-induced laminitis with hepatopathy in a Thoroughbred filly. *J. Vet. Sci.*, **5** (3), 271–274.
12. Cadoré, J.L. and Olive, J. (2007) Synthèse: prise en charge de la fourbure chez les équidés. (Management of laminitis in horses). *Le Nouveau Praticien Vétérinaire – Équine*, **11**, 63–64.
13. Cornelisse, C.J. and Robinson, N.E. (2013) Glucocorticoid therapy and the risk of equine laminitis. *J. Equine Vet. Educ.*, **25** (1), 39–46.
14. Donaldson, M.T., Jorgensen, A.J., and Beech, J. (2004) Evaluation of suspected pituitary pars intermedia dysfunction in horses with laminitis. *J. Am. Vet. Med. Assoc.*, **224** (7), 1123–1127.
15. Bailey, S.R. (2010) Corticosteroid-associated laminitis. *Vet. Clin. North Am. Equine Pract.*, **26** (2), 277–285.
16. Roberts, D. (1965) Treatment of equine laminitis by intra-arterial infusion of adrenocorticoid steroids. *Vet. Med. Small Animal Clin.*, **60**, 1109–1113.
17. Moore, J.N., Steiss, J., Nicholson, W.E., and Orth, D.N. (1979) A case of pituitary- adrenocorticotropin-dependent Cushing's syndrome in the horse. *Endocrinology*, **104**, 576–582.

18. Heinrichs, M., Baumgartner, W., and Capen, C. (1990) Immunocytochemical demonstration of proopiomelanocortin-derived peptides in pituitary adenomas of the pars intermedia in horses. *Vet. Pathol.*, **27**, 419–425.
19. Boujon, C.E., Bestetti, G.E., Meier, H.P., Straub, R., Junker, U., and Rossi, G.L. (1993) Equine pituitary adenoma: a functional and morphological study. *J. Comp. Pathol.*, **109** (2), 163–178.
20. Okada, T., Shimomuro, T., Oikawa, M., Nambo, Y., Kiso, Y., Morikawa, Y., Liptrap, R.M., Yamashiro, S., Little, P.B., and Sasaki, F. (1997) Immunocytochemical localization of adrenocorticotropic hormone-immunoreactive cells of the pars intermedia in Thoroughbreds. *Am. J. Vet. Res.*, **58** (8), 920–924.
21. Glover, C., Miller, L.M., and Dybdal, N.O. (2009) Extrapituitary and pituitary pathological changes in horses with pituitary pars intermedia dysfunction, a retrospective study. *J. Equine Vet. Sci.*, **29**, 146–153.
22. van der Kolk, J.H., Ijzer, J., Overgaauw, P.A., and van der Linde-Sipman, J.S. (2001) Pituitary-independent Cushing's syndrome in a horse. *Equine Vet. J.*, **33** (1), 110–112.
23. Raker, C.W. and Fegley, H. (1965) Clinico-pathologic conference. *J. Am. Vet. Med. Assoc.*, **147**, 848–860.
24. Evans, L.H., Siegel, E.T., and Hubben, K. (1968) Clinico-pathologic conference. *J. Am. Vet. Med. Assoc.*, **152**, 1778–1786.
25. Fix, A.S. and Miller, LD. (1987) Equine adrenocortical carcinoma with hypercalcemia. *Vet. Pathol.*, **24**, 190–192.
26. van der Kolk, J., Mars, M., and van der Gaag, I. (1994) Adrenocortical carcinoma in a 12-year-old mare. *Vet. Rec.*, **134** (5), 113–115.
27. Sokkar, S. and Mahmoud, A. (2003) Adrenocortical carcinoma in a donkey. *Dtsch. Tierarztl. Wochenschr.*, **110** (4), 176–177.
28. Frank, N. and Tadros, E.M. (2014) Insulin dysregulation. *Equine Vet. J.*, **46** (1), 103–112.
29. Frank, N., Geor, R.J., Bailey, S.R., Durham, A.E., and Johnson, P.J. (2010) Equine metabolic syndrome. *J. Vet. Intern. Med.*, **24** (3), 467–475.
30. Love, S. (1993) Equine Cushing's disease. *Br. Vet. J.*, **149** (2), 139–153.
31. McCue, P.M. (2002) Equine Cushing's disease. *Vet. Clin. North Am. Equine Pract.*, **18** (3), 533–543.
32. van der Kolk, J.H., Wensing, T., Kalsbeek, H.C., and Breukink, H.J. (1995) Laboratory diagnosis of equine pituitary pars intermedia adenoma. *Domest. Anim. Endocrinol.*, **12** (1), 35–39.
33. McGowan, C.M. and Neiger, R. (2003) Efficacy of trilostane for the treatment of equine Cushing's syndrome. *Equine Vet. J.*, **35** (4), 414–418.
34. Wilson, M.G., Nicholson, W.E., Holscher, M.A., Sherrell, B.J., Mount, C.D., and Orth, D.N. (1982) Proopiolipomelanocortin peptides in normal pituitary, pituitary tumor, and plasma of normal and Cushing's horses. *Endocrinology*, **110** (3), 941–954.
35. Ooki, T., Kotsu, T., and Kinutani, M. (1973) Pars intermedia of the hypophysis of rats after early postnatal lesions of the basal hypothalamus. Quantitative and qualitative observations. *Neuroendocrinology*, **11**, 22–45.
36. Levy, M. and Dybdal, N. (1997) Pituitary pars intermedia dysfunction in the horse. Part 1: Clinical signs and pathophysiology. 15th Annual Forum of the American College of Veterinary Internal Medicine, pp. 468–469.
37. Millington, W.R., Dybdal, N.O., Dawson, R., Jr, Manzini, C., and Mueller, G.P. (1988) Equine Cushing's disease: differential regulation of beta-endorphin processing in tumors of the intermediate pituitary. *Endocrinology*, **123** (3), 1598–1604.
38. Orth, D.N., Holscher, M.A., Wilson, M.G., Nicholson, W.E., Plue, R.E., and Mount, C.D. (1982) Equine Cushing's disease: plasma immunoreactive proopiolipomelanocortin peptide and cortisol levels basally and in response to diagnostic tests. *Endocrinology*, **110** (4), 1430–1441.
39. Donaldson, M.T., LaMonte, B.H., Morresey, P., Smith, G., and Beech, J. (2002) Treatment with pergolide or cyproheptadine of pituitary pars intermedia dysfunction (equine Cushing's disease). *J. Vet. Intern. Med.*, **16** (6), 742–746.
40. Pauli, B.U. and Rossi Straub, R. (1974) Interstitial cell adenoma of the hypophysis with Cushing-like symptomatology in the horse. *Vet. Pathol.*, **11** (5), 417–429.
41. Orth, D.N. and Nicholson, W.E. (1982) Bioactive and immunoreactive adrenocorticotropin in normal equine pituitary and in pituitary tumors of horses with Cushing's disease. *Endocrinology*, **111** (2), 559–563.
42. Wallace, M.A., Crisman, M.V., and Pickett, J.P. (1996) Central blindness associated with a pituitary adenoma in a horse. *Equine Pract.*, **18** (8), 8–13.
43. McFarlane, D., Dybdal, N., Donaldson, M.T., Miller, L., and Cribb, A.E. (2005) Nitration and increased alpha-synuclein expression associated with dopaminergic neurodegeneration in equine pituitary pars intermedia dysfunction. *J. Neuroendocrinol.*, **17** (2), 73–80.
44. Keen, J.A., McLaren, M., Chandler, K.J., and McGorum, B.C. (2004) Biochemical indices of vascular function, glucose metabolism and oxidative stress in horses with equine Cushing's disease. *Equine Vet. J.*, **36** (3), 226–229.
45. McFarlane, D. and Holbrook, T.C. (2008) Cytokine dysregulation in aged horses and horses with pituitary pars intermedia dysfunction. *J. Vet. Intern. Med.*, **22** (2), 436–442.
46. McFarlane, D., Miller, L.M., Craig, L.E., Dybdal, N.O., Habecker, P.L., Miller, M.A., Patterson, J.S., and Cribb, A.E. (2005) Agreement in histologic assessments of the pituitary pars intermedia in aged horses. *Am. J. Vet. Res.*, **66** (12), 2055–2059.
47. Cotran, R., Kumar, V., and Collins, T. (1999) *The Endocrine System*, 6th edition. W.B. Saunders, Philadelphia.
48. Shanker, G. and Sharma, A. (1979) Beta-endorphin stimulates corticosterone synthesis. *Biochem. Biophys. Res. Commun.*, **86** (1), 1–5.
49. Seger, M. and Bennett, H. (1986) Structure and bioactivity of the amine terminal of proopiomelanocortin. *J. Steroid Biochem.*, **25**, 703–710.
50. Haritou, S.J., Zylstra, R., Ralli, C., Turner, S., and Tortonese, D.J. (2008) Seasonal changes in circadian peripheral plasma concentrations of melatonin, serotonin, dopamine and cortisol in aged horses with Cushing's disease under natural photoperiod. *J. Neuroendocrinol.*, **20** (8), 988–996.
51. Cordero, M., Shrauner, B., and McFarlane, D. (2011) Bioactivity of plasma ACTH from PPID-affected horses compared to normal horses. *J. Vet. Intern. Med.*, **25**, 664.
52. Miller, C., Utter. M.L., and Beech, J. (2013) Evaluation of the effects of age and pituitary pars intermedia dysfunction on corneal sensitivity in horses. *Am. J. Vet. Res.*, **74** (7), 1030–1035.

53. McFarlane, D., Hale, G.M., Johnson, E.M., and Maxwell, L.K. (2010) Fecal egg counts after anthelmintic administration to aged horses and horses with pituitary pars intermedia dysfunction. *J. Am. Vet. Med. Assoc.*, **236** (3), 330–334.
54. McGowan, C.M., Frost, R., Pfeiffer, D.U., and Neiger, R. (2004) Serum insulin concentrations in horses with equine Cushing's syndrome: response to a cortisol inhibitor and prognostic value. *Equine Vet. J.*, **36** (3), 295–298.
55. Karikoski, N.P., Patterson-Kane, J.C., Singer, E.R., McFarlane, D., and McGowan, C.M. (2016) Lamellar pathology in horses with pituitary pars intermedia dysfunction. *Equine Vet. J.*, **48** (4), 472–478.

CHAPTER 17

Endocrine and Metabolic Dysregulation in Laminitis: Role of Corticosteroids

Philip J. Johnson

Introduction

As noted in Chapter 16, laminitis development in the context of underlying endocrinological disturbance has been referred to as 'endocrinopathic' laminitis, and is most commonly reported in horses affected with either or both the equine metabolic syndrome (EMS or insulin dysregulation) and pituitary pars intermedia dysfunction (PPID) [1]. That there appears to exist a risk of endocrinopathic laminitis in the context of circumstances associated with elevated corticosteroid levels (both exogenous and endogenous) is broadly accepted, but a direct cause and effect relationship between corticosteroids and laminitis has been difficult to confirm. Possibly, corticosteroids cause an increased likelihood of endocrinopathic laminitis when other endocrinological predispositions are present (such as EMS and PPID). Furthermore, extensive recent studies have served to highlight the role of insulin as an independent risk factor for endocrinopathic laminitis in both EMS and PPID [2,3]. It must be considered that, when it occurs, endocrinopathic laminitis associated with corticosteroid influence could simply be a result of aggravated insulin dysregulation in a patient with pre-existing, underlying insulin resistance. Nevertheless, both endogenous and synthetic corticosteroids are characterized by an extensively pleiotropic and diverse range of biological actions, many of which could be important in terms of endocrinopathic laminitis. The aim of this chapter is to review and discuss putative explanations regarding possible mechanisms linking corticosteroid influence to the risk of laminitis.

For many years, veterinarians have recognized that laminitis sometimes develops under circumstances associated with elevated corticosteroid influence. The risk of laminitis associated with corticosteroids has been linked to both the (exogenous) administration of powerful synthetic steroid drugs such as (especially) dexamethasone and triamcinalone [4–10], and conditions associated with heightened endogenous cortisol release (hypercortisolism resulting from stress or from PPID/equine Cushing's syndrome) [11, 12]. As previously discussed, the concept that excessive corticosteroid influence (hypercortisolism) causes endocrinopathic laminitis in PPID-affected horses has been discarded in light of the fact that pathologically enhanced cortisol influence is only identified in a minority of those patients. Moreover, newer data have shown that, when present in PPID-affected horses and ponies, endocrinopathic laminitis is more readily explained by the presence of insulin dysregulation in those cases (present as an independent comorbidity). Further explanation and discussion of insulin resistance and hyperinsulinemia ('insulin dysregulation') as a risk factor for endocrinopathic laminitis is presented in Chapter 18.

Corticosteroids as a Cause of Endocrinopathic Laminitis

Corticosteroids are powerful inhibitors of the action of insulin; endocrinopathic laminitis resulting from clinical circumstances in which corticosteroid action is increased may possibly be explained by a corticosteroid-induced loss of insulin sensitivity. Administration of the powerful synthetic corticosteroids, dexamethasone and triamcinolone, induces insulin resistance in horses [13, 14]. Although hypercortisolism may sometimes contribute to the risk of laminitis in horses affected with PPID, increased secretion of endogenous cortisol resulting from stress and the veterinary administration of synthetic corticosteroids might also be regarded as risk factors for endocrinopathic laminitis. The risk of acute laminitis represents a very important consideration before embarking on a course of corticosteroid treatment for any condition, and several incidences of corticosteroid-associated laminitis have been reported previously [8–10, 15–18].

Although iatrogenic (corticosteroid-associated) endocrinopathic laminitis is uncommon, it can cause severe laminitis necessitating euthanasia. Attempts to study the nature of laminitis that results from corticosteroid administration have generally been thwarted by the unpredictable nature of this association

Equine Laminitis, First Edition. Edited by James K. Belknap and Raymond Geor.

and the failure of corticosteroids to induce laminitis in normal horses in a predictable fashion (experimental studies performed by the present author). In another experimental study, laminitis did not develop following treatment with dexamethasone (0.08 mg kg^{-1}, administered intravenously, at 48-h intervals) over the course of 21 days [13]. Furthermore, laminitis did not occur when French *et al.* (2000) studied the effects of injected triamcinolone on pharmacokinetics and metabolism in the horse [14]. Nonetheless, the authors concluded that triamcinolone-induced laminitis may be associated with the long duration of action of this corticosteroid when higher or repeated doses are administered [14]. In 1982, Hood *et al.* reported that pretreatment with triamcinolone (15 mg, administered three times weekly for four weeks) led to significantly more severe acute laminitis in the starch grain overload model [19].

Recent studies have shown that corticosteroids drive and worsen insulin dysregulation in horses, a critical risk factor for endocrinopathic laminitis [13]. For example, Haffner *et al.* showed that dexamethasone decreases responsiveness to insulin as early as 2 h and maximally at 24 h after administration [20]. Therefore, endocrinopathic laminitis may be more likely when corticosteroid influence is elevated in (or when synthetic corticosteroids are administered to) horses with pre-existing insulin dysregulation (ID). When laminitis develops in horses affected with severe gastrointestinal disease, or other conditions in which systemic inflammation/endotoxemia is present, the influence of several laminitis-promoting pathophysiological mechanisms may be combined. For example, during the management of severe colitis, laminitis risk is likely increased by both the effect of systemic inflammation and endocrinological responses to metabolic derangement (hypercortisolism of stress along with insulin resistance/hyperinsulinemia). For this reason, the risk of laminitis should be regarded as very high whenever synthetic corticosteroids are employed as a component of the management of colitis/systemic inflammation. Nevertheless, several incidences of corticosteroid-associated acute laminitis (some severe) have been reported in horses when either risk factors for endocrinopathic laminitis of endogenous origin (obesity/IR or PPID) or sepsis-related laminitis (e.g., gastrointestinal disease and systemic inflammation) were not present as comorbidities. It might be considered that a hitherto unidentified underlying genetic predisposition to laminitis risk could be present when corticosteroid treatment results in laminitis in horses/ponies in which other underlying laminitis triggers are not identified. Because most reports of corticosteroid-associated laminitis have not included characterizations of the underlying endocrinological and metabolic profile of the affected patients prior to corticosteroid administration, it is not possible to determine whether the corticosteroid acted 'independently' of a state of underlying insulin resistance/dysregulation.

Results of epidemiological studies that have reported etiologies of laminitis suggest that corticosteroid administration is an uncommon explanation for laminitis. For example, in 1993 Hood *et al.* concluded that drug administration accounted for laminitis in 1.5% of cases (eight out of 525 horses) [21]. In another study, 8.6% of cases (three of 35 horses) were reportedly treated with a corticosteroid prior to the development of laminitis [22]. Bathe reported that corticosteroid administration represented almost 2% (four of 211 horses) of causes for laminitis [23]. In the present author's referral practice, iatrogenic corticosteroid-associated endocrinopathic laminitis has most commonly been identified when triamcinolone acetonide was used for intra-aticular steroid treatments. This risk of laminitis appears to be greater when higher total doses of the drug have been administered. In another report, only one horse out of 205 horses receiving up to 80 mg of triamcinolone acetonide developed laminitis [24]. In a well-publicized case, severe endocrinopathic laminitis developed in a valuable French dressage horse following the combination of intra-articular treatments using triamcinalone acetonide (80 mg injected into both hocks) and dexamethasone (20 mg, intramuscular), which ultimately led to significant litigation [25]. In another report, severe laminitis developed in a Thoroughbred filly that had received consecutive daily treatments with triamcinalone acetonide (20 mg per day) over the course of 10 days [8].

In conclusion, the risk of corticosteroid-induced endocrinopathic laminitis should be regarded as significantly higher when high drug doses (eight- to tenfold the recommended dose) have been administered, either during a single treatment or over the course of several days [12]. Although the risk of corticosteroid-induced laminitis is relatively lower when the drugs are used at recommended doses, some individuals may develop laminitis if pre-existing predispositions (such as IR/hyperinsulinemia, prior bouts/pre-existing laminitis, systemic inflammation) are present before the corticosteroid treatment has been started.

Linking Corticosteroid Action to Laminitis Risk

Definitive proof that corticosteroids represent an independent risk factor for the novel onset of acute laminitis is presently lacking. Moreover, a solitary pathophysiological mechanism has not been demonstrated for such an association. Importantly, the presence of pre-existing predispositions and/or risk-elevating comorbidities cannot be discounted in most reports of purported corticosteroid-induced endocrinopathic laminitis. Although corticosteroid influence throughout the body is both extensive and complex, several reasonable explanations for a putative link between corticosteroid and risk of laminitis (some with supporting experimental evidence) are presented below.

Corticosteroids and Insulin Dysregulation

Both endogenous (cortisol) and exogenous (synthetic) corticosteroids are powerful inhibitors of the action of insulin. Therefore, under conditions associated with heightened corticosteroid influence, a reduction of insulin sensitivity (worsening IR) can be anticipated [13,14]. Corticosteroids rapidly stimulate hepatic gluconeogenesis as well as insulin release from the beta-cells in pancreatic islets, leading to hyperinsulinemia. Corticosteroids also inhibit glycogen synthase kinase-3 phosphorylation in skeletal muscle, causing a reduction in insulin-stimulated glycogen synthase activity and impaired insulin sensitivity (IR) [13]. It has been shown in several studies that both dexamethasone and triamcinolone acetonide cause IR/hyperinsulinemia in horses and ponies [13, 14, 26]. A single dose of triamcinalone acetonide (0.2 mg kg^{-1}, intramuscular) led to elevated insulin levels for more than 150 h and provoked the appearance of 'growth lines' in the hoof, suggesting that the digital lamellae had been significantly affected by this treatment [14]. The administration of a low dose of dexamethasone (0.04 mg kg^{-1}, intramuscular), as used in the dexamethasone suppression test (a diagnostic test for PPID), elevates the plasma insulin concentration and the extent of this increase is significantly higher in ponies already affected with ID [26]. The extent to which insulin is increased following a dexamethasone dose is much greater at certain times of the year (when it might exceed 1000 μIU ml^{-1}) [27]. Therefore, corticosteroid influence on the plasma insulin concentration may depend on the specific drug, its dose and frequency of administration, the level of insulin sensitivity in the treated patient, and the time of year. Corticosteroid treatment may affect (weaken) the digital lamellae without necessarily causing overt signs of laminitic pain.

Corticosteroids and Glucose Availability

Adequate glucose supply to the digital lamellae is essential for normal function because the basal keratinocytes of the lamellar epithelium have a very high demand for glucose [28, 29]. When deprived of glucose (in an *ex-vivo* model), basal keratinocytes lost their attachment to the underlying basement membrane and dermo-epidermal separation (similar to that seen in laminitis) occurred [28]. Interestingly, neither insulin receptors nor insulin-responsive glucose transporter 4 (GLUT-4) are present in basal keratinocytes, which suggests that these cells acquire glucose from the circulation via other GLUTs or GLUT-like proteins. GLUT-1 is likely the principal glucose transporter for basal epidermal cells in the healthy state. In one study, GLUT-4 was not detected in lamellar tissue and glucose uptake in lamellar explants was independent of insulin [2]. Possibly, corticosteroids might increase the risk of laminitis by adversely affecting the expression, translocation, or function of hoof keratinocyte glucose transporters. The glucocorticoid actions of corticosteroids lead to an increased metabolic availability of glucose through the enhancement of gluconeogenesis, reduced tissue sensitivity to insulin, and impaired glucose tolerance.

Corticosteroids, Abnormal Glucose Homeostasis, and Risk of Endocrinopathic Laminitis

Microvascular dysfunction is a complication of abnormal glucose homeostasis in human diabetics. Glucose auto-oxidation in vascular endothelial cells leads to the production of free radicals and oxidative damage (glucotoxic endotheliopathy). Elevation of plasma levels of the following biomarkers can readily be demonstrated in human diabetic patients:

- Biomarkers of vascular dysfunction (E-selectin, thrombomodulin, vascular endothelial growth factor [VEGF] and von Willebrand factor [vWF]) [30–34].
- Biomarkers of fibrin homeostasis (tissue plasminogen activator [tPA] and plasminogen activator inhibitor [PAI] levels) [34].
- Biomarkers of oxidative stress (reduced levels of the antioxidant plasma thiols [PSHs], and increased levels of malondialdehyde [MDA], an index of lipid peroxidation) [32, 35–37].

Moreover, the levels of endothelium-derived vasoactive mediators (nitric oxide [NO] and endothelin-1 [ET-1]) are abnormal, favoring vasospasticity [34, 36]. Abnormalities in these various indices of vascular function and antioxidant status can be demonstrated prior to onset of clinical vascular disease in diabetic patients.

It has been proposed that abnormalities in glucose homeostasis, similar to those causing microvascular dysfunction in human diabetics, might also contribute to the pathogenesis of laminitis in horses with PPID. Therefore, Keen *et al.* tested the hypothesis that abnormalities in vascular function, glucose metabolism and oxidative stress (similar to those of diabetes) contribute to the development of laminitis in horses with PPID [38]. They evaluated biomarkers for glucose homeostasis (glucose, insulin and fructosamine), oxidative stress (MDA, PSH, glutathione peroxidase [GSHPx]), vascular dysfunction (vWF, VEGF, E-selectin and thrombomodulin), platelet activation (P-selectin) and fibrin homeostasis (tPA and PAI), and levels of vasoactive mediators (endothelin and nitrate/nitrite, the stable metabolites of NO) across three groups of horses designated as: (i) affected with PPID (based on the presence of hirsutism); (ii) affected with PPID (based on an absence of hirsutism but positive dexamethasone suppression test [DST] outcome); and (iii) not affected with PPID (absence of hirsutism and normal DST result). Abnormalities in systemic glucose homeostasis (increased levels of glucose and insulin) were identified in the strongly PPID-affected horses. Horses in the first two groups (likely PPID-affected) also had lower PSH levels than the control group, consistent with oxidative stress. The authors acknowledged that an accurate ante-mortem diagnosis or exclusion of PPID using the DST represented a significant limitation to the interpretation of results between groups. However, evidence of vascular dysfunction (i.e., abnormal levels of vWF, NO, ET-1, tPA, PAI) was not identified in this study [38].

Corticosteroids and Microvascular Dysregulation

As with other species, corticosteroids promote IR in horses [13]. IR-affected microvascular dysregulation in the digital lamellae could predispose to injury when other laminitis trigger factors are present. Enhanced peripheral vasoconstriction, a consequence of endothelial dysfunction, is a component of IR that might contribute to hoof lamellar microvascular dysregulation or maintenance of glucose delivery to the digital lamellae [39].

The fact that insulin receptors are present in the equine digital vasculature implies that insulin contributes to the regulation of peripheral vascular reflexes, as it does in other species. Insulin normally acts, through the vascular endothelium, to simulate both vasodilatory mechanisms (via increased nitric oxide synthase [NOS] production through the phosphatidylinositol 3-kinase [PI-3K] pathway) and vasoconstrictive mechanisms (via endothelin-1 [ET-1] release through the mitogen-activated protein kinase [MAPK] pathway) [40]. Pathways leading to activation of PI-3K are blocked in IR states (contributing to disrupted glucose disposal), at the same time as the MAPK pathways remain functional (or even overstimulated). Therefore, the ratio of NO to ET-1 is diminished and acts to promote the following pathophysiological conditions, all of which have been associated with an increased risk of laminitis: vasoconstriction; platelet activation; and leukocyte adhesion to vascular walls [41, 42].

Corticosteroids may directly affect the regulation of vascular tone in the hoof in such a way that enhanced vasoconstrictive responses could promote a risk of laminitis by reducing the availability of oxygen and/or glucose, or by promoting the development of edema (compartment syndrome) [42–44]. Corticosteroids (hydrocortisone, cortisol, dexamethasone) have been shown to markedly promote vasoconstrictive responses to epinephrine and serotonin by inhibiting their removal from the circulation [4, 5]. The treatment of horses with either dexamethasone or triamcinalone acetonide for only a few days also affects the expression of ion channels in the cell membrane of vascular smooth muscle cells (obtained from digital vessels), such that a state of relatively enhanced vasospasticity develops (corticosteroid treatment caused a decrease in voltage-dependent K+ channels (Kv) in vascular smooth muscle of vessels supplying the digital lamellae, compared to untreated animals; unpublished data from the author's laboratory). Using thermography, Cornelisse *et al.* showed that treatment with dexamethasone led to a reduction in cutaneous perfusion [45]. In that study, dexamethasone-induced reductions in skin temperature were further accentuated by the intradermal administration of phenylephrine, an alpha-1 adrenoreceptor agonist. The authors concluded that corticosteroid treatment likely also inhibits lamellar perfusion and that, during conditions characterized by hypoperfusion and/or increased catecholamines (other trigger factors for laminitis), corticosteroid treatment might further increase the risk of laminitis [45].

Corticosteroids and Apoptosis

Programmed cell death (apoptosis) in basal epidermal cells of the digital lamellae has been identified as a consistent pathological characteristic of laminitis resulting from experimental (starch, black walnut, oligofructose, and insulin) and natural causes [46]. Corticosteroids have also been shown to induce apoptosis in epithelial cells from both horses and other species. In 2010, Bailey demonstrated enhanced epithelial cell apoptosis in cultivated lamellar explants that had been treated with corticosteroids [12]. It remains to be determined whether corticosteroid-associated apoptosis might contribute to weakening of the dermo-epidermal junction and increase the risk of laminitis.

Corticosteroids and Protein Catabolism in the Integument

Pathological manifestations of corticosteroid influence in the integument have been well described in other species. A remarkably selective and localized loss of subcutaneous connective tissue at the extremities (fingers and toes) has been observed in some human cases [47]. It is not known if this variant of Cushing's syndrome in human beings is similar to events occurring in the connective tissue of the equine hoof in corticosteroid-associated laminitis. The dermo-epidermal interface of the digital lamellae of the equine hoof is uniquely subjected to persistent tensile (pull-apart) forces due to supporting the weight of the horse, so any contributing factor that might interfere with tissue maintenance at this location might increase the risk of laminitis. The structural integrity of the digital lamellae may be weakened by the effect of excessive corticosteroid influence over time. Similarly, the normal repair process is inhibited by exposure to higher than normal levels of corticosteroids. Type VII collagen is the major collagenous component of the anchoring fibrils, structures that stabilize the attachment of the lamellar basement membrane to the underlying dermis (Type VII collagen is expressed by both epidermal keratinocytes and dermal fibroblasts).

Dexamethasone has been shown to directly inhibit anchoring fibril formation, which might reduce the strength of the dermo-epidermal attachment interface and lead to an increased risk for laminitis [48]. Cortisol decreases keratinization of the bovine hoof, further supporting the contention that long-term corticosteroid influence might cause changes in the structure of the hoof that could increase the risk for laminitis from any cause [49]. Maintenance of the integrity and strength of the digital lamellae is potentially adversely affected by excessive corticosteroid effects through numerous diverse mechanisms. Corticosteroids regulate the expression of multiple genes at the dermo-epidermal junction that are likely to encode key factors in the wound repair process. Anti-inflammatory steroids, such as dexamethasone, inhibit repair processes (at least in part) by influencing the expression of various cytokines, growth factors, enzymes, and extracellular matrix molecules in both normal and wounded integument [50]. The participation of growth factors in the maintenance of dermo-epidermal integrity and tissue repair has been well established [51]. Of particular note, the biosynthesis of keratinocyte growth factor by dermal fibroblasts is markedly attenuated by dexamethasone and other corticosteroids, but not by nonsteroidal anti-inflammatory agents [52].

Corticosteroids and the Gut

Corticosteroids may predispose to laminitis by inhibiting the intestinal mucosal defense mechanisms and increasing intestinal permeability. Increased permeability of the mucosal lining of the entire gastrointestinal tract of laboratory animals has been attributed to both the action of dexamethasone and increased release of endogenous corticosteroids during times of stress [52–54]. In one study, the increased permeability was sufficient to allow luminal constituents access to the mucosal immune system [54]. There is compelling evidence that stress-associated increases in the permeability of the mucosal lining of the alimentary tract in human beings represents an important cause of morbidity [55]. Moreover, experiments using animal models have demonstrated that various types of psychological and physical stress, with consequent elevations in endogenous corticosteroids, induce dysfunction of the intestinal barrier, resulting in enhanced uptake of potentially noxious material (e.g., antigens, toxins, vasoactive amines, and other proinflammatory mediators) from the gut lumen [55].

Laminitis often arises in the face of intestinal perturbations in horses. It has been suggested that toxic factors of intestinal origin play an important role in the pathogenesis of laminitis in those cases associated with overt intestinal disease [56,57]. The starch overload method for the experimental induction of laminitis leads to both increased intestinal permeability and intestinal floral changes [57]. It is possible that conditions associated with excessive corticosteroid influence might also lead to laminitis in horses by virtue of increased intestinal permeability and the absorption of toxic factors from the intestinal lumen.

Tissue-Specific Dysregulation of Cortisol Metabolism

Corticosteroid influence in any given tissue is a consequence of both the concentration of cortisol in the circulation (derived from the adrenal cortices) and the extent to which cortisol is either degraded or amplified in the tissue. The corticosteroid-activating/-deactivating enzyme in tissues is 11β-hydroxysteroid dehydrogenase (11β-HSD), and it was reported previously that the 11β-HSD-1 isoform is present in the equine digital lamellae [58]. This specific isoform serves to convert inactive cortisone (which is always plentiful in the circulation) to the active hormone, cortisol, at the cellular level.

Moreover, it was also shown that the activity of 11β-HSD-1 was increased in lamellar tissue obtained from laminitic horses compared to controls [58]. Thus, an enhanced local tissue modulation of cortisol (cortisol amplification by 11β-HSD-1) in a manner to augment its local actions may be important. Moreover, the development of increased 11β-HSD-1 activity in the digital lamellae implies that local cortisol action is being enhanced through paracrine and autocrine mechanisms. If – as seems reasonable – corticosteroids are able to induce changes in the lamellae that predispose to laminitis, the presence of increased 11β-HSD-1 at this location could play a pivotal role.

Of particular interest in this regard is the observation that an increased corticosteroid effect interferes with the insulin-like growth factor-1 (IGF-1) system (IGF-1; IGF-1 receptor; and IGF-1 binding protein) in skin [59]. IGF-1 is a growth-promoting polypeptide that is essential for the restoration of structural integrity in wounded skin [59]. Locally enhanced cortisol production might inhibit the normal function of IGF-1 in the digital lamellae, leading to a compromise of the functional integrity of the lamellar interface. In this manner, impaired healing and weakening of the lamellar interface would be similar to the nonhealing wounds that are common problems in both experimental and clinical diabetes. The extent to which corticosteroid-mediated changes in the IGF-1 signaling system might influence insulin signaling for basal keratinocytes in the digital lamellae remains to be clarified.

Corticosteroids and Perturbations in the Canonical Wnt-Signaling Pathway

The canonical Wnt signaling pathway is a highly conserved (evolutionarily), fundamental pathway that controls cell development, proliferation, differentiation, polarity and motility [60], primarily through regulation of the production and stability of β-catenin [61]. Positive and negative regulatory components of the canonical Wnt signaling pathway are expressed in lamellar basal epithelial cells of healthy horses. Recently, Wang *et al.* reported that genes and proteins encoding multiple positive regulators of the canonical Wnt signaling pathway were decreased in the lamellae of horses affected by laminitis [62]. These authors suggested that suppression of the canonical Wnt signaling pathway, and an accompanying reduced expression of β-catenin and integrin-β_4, in lamellar basal epithelial cells causes reduced cell–cell and cell–basement membrane attachment, thus, destabilizing the lamellar dermo-epidermal junction [62]. Suppression of the canonical Wnt signaling pathway in lamellar basal epithelial cells may be a feature of laminitis irrespective of etiology. Of further note regarding the role of corticosteroids in the pathogenesis of laminitis is the observation that dexamethasone suppresses canonical Wnt signaling in some circumstances. For example, dexamethasone was reported to inhibit Wnt/β-catenin signaling in cultured human osteoblasts [63], during the development of cleft palate [64], and during adipocyte differentiation [65].

Corticosteroids, the Pancreas, and Incretins

Synthetic corticosteroids such as dexamethasone and triamcinolone are often employed as a part of the management of inflammatory and immune-mediated diseases [66]. Long-term corticosteroid influence (exogenous or endogenous) results in significant complications including insulin resistance [67]. Enhanced cortisol production in human patients (Cushing's syndrome) often results in hyperglycemia, hyperinsulinemia, and hepatic steatosis [68]. Corticosteroids normally function to offset hypoglycemia during times of acute stress and/or reduced energy intake, increasing blood glucose concentration via several mechanisms. Corticosteroids stimulate hepatic glucogenesis [69], inhibit peripheral glucose uptake [70, 71], and promote both muscle and fat breakdown to increase the availability of substrates for gluconeogenesis [72, 73]. Although long-term corticosteroid treatment may lead to abnormalities of glucose regulation, short-term treatment (<2 weeks) does not typically cause severe hyperglycemia. Short-term glucose regulation has been attributed to a corticosteroid-induced hyperinsulinemic response [74, 75]. Results of both human clinical and rodent studies documented marked elevations in glucose-stimulated insulin secretion during short-term treatment with corticosteroids [76,77]. A satisfactory explanation for the mechanism by which dexamethasone provokes a marked elevation of insulin secretion is presently lacking. In the long term, corticosteroid-enhanced hyperinsulinemia has been attributed to an increase in both pancreatic β-cell mass and function [78,79].

Two incretin hormones – glucagon-like peptide-1 (GLP-1) and glucose-dependent insulinotropic polypeptide (GIP) – are produced and secreted by gastrointestinal enteroendocrine cells in response to nutrient ingestion [80]. Specifically, GLP-1 is produced by L-cells (primarily located in the distal gastrointestinal tract), while GIP is produced by K-cells (mostly located in the duodenum and proximal jejunum). Incretins contribute to the glucose-stimulated insulin response following the ingestion of food (see Chapter 18 for further discussions of incretins). Studies in rodents have indicated that incretins promote increases in both insulin synthesis and pancreatic β-cell mass [81, 82].

In a recent study of the short-term effects of dexamethasone on glucose regulation in primates, dexamethasone caused marked increases in fasting and postprandial circulating insulin concentrations while maintaining normoglycemia in the face of marked IR (compensated IR) [83]. A short-term improvement in pancreatic β-cell function was further implied by a reduction in the pro-insulin to insulin ratio. Interestingly, treatment with dexamethasone provoked a twofold increase in postprandial GIP elevations. This response suggests that a corticosteroid-induced elevation in incretin (GIP) response to food intake may partially explain the marked postprandial hyperinsulinemia observed during treatment with synthetic corticosteroids [83].

Therefore, corticosteroids may augment the hyperinsulinemic responses to food intake, as has been linked to increased risk of endocrinopathic laminitis in horses affected with insulin dysregulation at pasture.

References

1. Johnson, P.J., Messer, N.T., Slight, S.H., Wiedmeyer, C., Buff, P., and Ganjam, V.K. (2004) Endocrinopathic laminitis in the horse. *Clin. Tech. Equine Pract.*, **3** (1), 45–56.
2. Asplin, K.E., Sillence, M.N., Pollitt, C.C., and McGowan, C.M. (2007) Induction of laminitis by prolonged hyperinsulinaemia in clinically normal ponies. *Vet. J.*, **174** (3), 530–535.
3. Nourian, A.R., Asplin, K.E., McGowan, C.M., Sillence, M.N., and Pollitt, C.C. (2009) Equine laminitis: ultrastructural lesions detected in ponies following hyperinsulinaemia. *Equine Vet. J.*, **41** (7), 671–677.
4. Eyre, P., Elmes, P.J., and Strickland, S. (1979) Corticosteroid-potentiated vascular responses of the equine digit: a possible pharmacologic basis for laminitis. *Am. J. Vet. Res.*, **40** (1), 135–138.
5. Eyre, P. and Elmes, P.J. (1980) Corticosteroid-induced laminitis? Further observations on the isolated, perfused hoof. *Vet. Res. Commun.*, **4** (2), 139–143.
6. Johnson, P.J., Slight, S.H., Ganjam, V.K., and Kreeger, J.M. (2002) Glucocorticoids and laminitis in the horse. *Vet. Clin. North Am. Equine Pract.*, **18** (2), 219–236
7. Johnson, P.J., Messer, N.T., Bowles, D.K., Slight, S.H., Ganjam, V.K., and Kreeger, J.M. (2004) Glucocorticoids and laminitis in horses. *Compend. Contin. Educ. Pract. Vet.*, **26** (7), 547–557.
8. Ryu, S.H., Byung, S.K., Lee, C.W., Yoon, J., and Lee, Y.L. (2004) Glucocorticoid-induced laminitis with hepatopathy in a Thoroughbred filly. *J. Vet. Sci.*, **5** (3), 271–274.
9. Cadoré, J.L. and Olive, J. (2007) Synthèse: prise en charge de la fourbure chez les équidés. (Management of laminitis in horses). *Le Nouveau Praticien Vétérinaire – Équine*, **11**, 63–64.
10. Cornelisse, C.J. and Robinson, N.E. (2013) Glucocorticoid therapy and the risk of equine laminitis. *J. Equine Vet. Educ.*, **25** (1), 39–46.
11. Donaldson, M.T., Jorgensen, A.J., and Beech, J. (2004) Evaluation of suspected pituitary pars intermedia dysfunction in horses with laminitis. *J. Am. Vet. Med. Assoc.*, **224** (7), 1123–1127.
12. Bailey, S.R. (2010) Corticosteroid-associated laminitis. *Vet. Clin. North Am. Equine Pract.*, **26** (2), 277–285.
13. Tiley, H.A., Geor, R.J., and McCutcheon, L.J. (2007) Effects of dexamethasone on glucose dynamics and insulin sensitivity in healthy horses. *Am. J. Vet. Res.*, **68** (7), 753–759.
14. French, K., Pollitt, C.C., and Pass, M.A. (2000) Pharmacokinetics and metabolic effects of triamcinolone acetonide and their possible relationships to glucocorticoid-induced laminitis in horses. *J. Vet. Pharmacol. Ther.*, **23** (5), 287–292.
15. Harkins, J.D., Carney, J.M., and Tobin, T. (1993) Clinical use and characteristics of the corticosteroids. *Vet. Clin. North Am. Equine Pract.*, **9**, 543–562.
16. Lawrence, R., Fessler, J.F., and Gall, C.M. (1985) Clinical forum: questions and answers. Steroid induced laminitis. *Equine Pract.*, **7**, 31–32.
17. Lose, M.P. (1980) Drug-induced laminitis in a colt. *Mod. Vet. Pract.*, **61**, 608–610.
18. Vernimb, G.D., Van Hoose, L.M., and Hennessey, P.W. (1977) Onset and duration of corticosteroid effect after injection of betasone for treating equine arthropathies. *Vet. Med. Small Anim. Clin.*, **72**, 241–244.
19. Hood, D.M., Stephens, K.A., and Amoss, M.S. (1982) The effect of exogenous steroid on the carbohydrate overload model of equine laminitis: a preliminary report. *Proc. Am. Assoc. Pract. Newsletter*, **2**, 149–151.
20. Haffner, J.C., Eiler, H., Hoffman, R.M., Fecteau, K.A., and Oliver, J.W. (2009) Effect of a single dose of dexamethasone on glucose homeostasis in healthy horses by using the combined intravenous glucose and insulin test. *J. Anim. Sci.*, **87** (1), 131–135.
21. Hood, D.M., Grosenbaugh, D.A., Mostafa, M.B., Morgan, S.J., and Thomas, B.C. (1993) The role of vascular mechanisms in the development of acute equine laminitis. *J. Vet. Intern. Med.*, **7**, 228–234.
22. Slater, M.R., Hood, D.M., and Carter, G.K. (1995) Descriptive epidemiological study of equine laminitis. *Equine Vet. J.*, **27**, 364–367.
23. Bathe, A.P. (2007) The corticosteroid laminitis story: 3. The clinician's viewpoint. *Equine Vet. J.*, **39** (1), 12–13.
24. McCluskey, M.J. and Kavenagh, P.B. (2004) Clinical use of triamcinolone acetonide in the horse (205 cases) and the incidence of

glucocorticoid-induced laminitis associated with its use. *Equine Vet. Educ.*, **16**, 86–89.

25. Dutton, H. (2007) The corticosteroid laminitis story: 1. Duty of care. *Equine Vet. J.*, **39** (1), 12–13
26. Bailey, S.R., Menzies-Gow, N.J., Harris, P.A., Habershon-Butcher, J.L., Crawford, C., Berhane, Y., Boston, R.C., and Elliott, J. (2007) Effect of dietary fructans and dexamethasone administration on the insulin response of ponies predisposed to laminitis. *J. Am. Vet. Med. Assoc.*, **231**, 1365–1373.
27. Borer, K.E., Menzies-Gow, N.J., Berhane, Y., Bailey, S.R., Harris, P.A., and Elliott, J. (2010) Seasonal influence on insulin and cortisol results from overnight dexamethasone suppression tests (DST) in normal and previously laminitic ponies (abstract). *J. Equine Vet. Sci.*, **30** (2), 103.
28. Pass, M.A., Pollitt, S., and Pollitt, C.C. (1998) Decreased glucose metabolism causes separation of hoof lamellae in vitro: a trigger for laminitis? *Equine Vet. J. Suppl.*, **26**, 133–138.
29. French, K.R. and Pollitt, C.C. (2004) Equine laminitis: glucose deprivation and MMP activation induce dermo-epidermal separation in vitro. *Equine Vet. J.*, **36**, 261–266.
30. Porta, M., Maneschi, F., White, M.C., and Kohner, E.M. (1981) Twenty-four hour variations of von Willebrand factor and factor VIII-related antigen in diabetic retinopathy. *Metabolism*, **30** (7), 695–699.
31. Greene, D.A., Sima, A.A., Stevens, M.J., Feldman, E.L., Killen, P.D., Henry, D.N., Thomas, T., Dananberg, J., and Lattimer, S.A. (1993) Aldose reductase inhibitors: an approach to the treatment of diabetic nerve damage. *Diabetes Metab. Rev.*, **9** (3), 189–217.
32. Elhadd, T.A., Khan, F., Kirk, G., McLaren, M., Newton, R.W., Greene, S.A., and Belch, J.J. (1998) Influence of puberty on endothelial dysfunction and oxidative stress in young patients with type 1 diabetes. *Diabetes Care*, **21** (11), 1990–1996.
33. McLaren, M., Elhadd, T.A., Greene, S.A., and Belch, J.J. (1999) Elevated plasma vascular endothelial cell growth factor and thrombomodulin in juvenile diabetic patients. *Clin. Appl. Thromb. Hemost.*, **5** (1), 21–24.
34. Bagg, W., Ferri, C., Desideri, G., Gamble, G., Ockelford, P., and Braatvedt, G.D. (2001) The influences of obesity and glycemic control on endothelial activation in patients with type 2 diabetes. *J. Clin. Endocrinol. Metab.*, **86** (11), 5491–5497.
35. Jennings, P.E., McLaren, M., Scott, N.A., Saniabadi, A.R., and Belch, J.J. (1991) The relationship of oxidative stress to thrombotic tendency in type 1 diabetic patients with retinopathy. *Diabetes Med.*, **8** (9), 860–865.
36. Vijayalingam, S., Parthiban, A., Shanmugasundaram, K.R., and Mohan, V. (1996) Abnormal antioxidant status in impaired glucose tolerance and non-insulin-dependent diabetes mellitus. *Diabetes Med.*, **13** (8), 715–719.
37. Giugliano, D., Ceriello, A., and Paolisso, G. (1996) Oxidative stress and diabetic vascular complications. *Diabetes Care*, **19** (3), 257–267.
38. Keen, J.A., McLaren, M., Chandler, K.J., and McGorum, B.C. (2004) Biochemical indices of vascular function, glucose metabolism and oxidative stress in horses with equine Cushing's disease. *Equine Vet. J.*, **36** (3), 226–229.
39. Caballero, A.E. (2003) Endothelial dysfunction in obesity and insulin resistance: a road to diabetes and heart disease. *Obesity Res.*, **11** (11), 1278–1289.
40. Kim, J.K., Montagnani, M., Koh, K.K., and Quon, M.J. (2006) Reciprocal relationships between insulin resistance and endothelial dysfunction: molecular and pathophysiological mechanisms. *Circulation*, **113**, 1888–1904.
41. Eades, S.C., Stokes, A.M., Johnson, P.J., LeBlanc, C.J., Ganjam, V.K., Buff, P.R., and Moore, R.M. (2007) Serial alterations in digital hemodynamics and endothelin-1 immunoreactivity, platelet-neutrophil aggregation, and concentrations of nitric oxide, insulin, and glucose in blood obtained from horses following carbohydrate overload. *Am. J. Vet. Res.*, **68** (1), 87–94.
42. Hunt, R.J. (1991) The pathophysiology of acute laminitis. *Compend. Contin. Vet. Educ.*, **13** (6), 401–407.
43. Moore, J.N. and Allen, D. (1996) The pathophysiology of acute laminitis. *Vet. Med.*, **34**, 936–939.
44. Bailey, S.R., Marr, C.M., and Elliott, J. (2004) Current research and theories on the pathogenesis of acute laminitis in the horse. *Vet. J.*, **167** (2), 129–142.
45. Cornelisse, C.J., Robinson, N.E., Berney, C.A., Eberhart, S., Hauptman, J.E., and Derksen, F.J. (2006) Thermographic study of in vivo modulation of vascular responses to phenylephrine and endothelin-1 by dexamethasone in the horse. *Equine Vet. J.*, **38**, 119–126.
46. Faleiros, R.R., Stokes, A.M., Eades, S.C., Kim, D.Y., Paulsen, D.B., and Moore, R.M. (2004) Assessment of apoptosis in epidermal lamellar cells in clinically normal horses and those with laminitis. *Am. J. Vet. Res.*, **65** (5), 578–585.
47. Groves, R.W., MacDonald, L.M., and MacDonald, D.M. (1990) Profound digital collagen atrophy: a new cutaneous presentation of adrenal-dependent Cushing's syndrome. *Br. J. Dermatol.*, **123**, 667–671.
48. Gras, M.P., Verrecchia, F., Uitto, J., and Mauviel, A. (2001) Downregulation of human type VII collagen (COL7A1) promoter activity by dexamethasone. Identification of a glucocorticoid receptor binding region. *Exp. Dermatol.*, **10** (1), 28–34.
49. Hendry, K.A., MacCallum, A.J., Knight, C.H., and Wilde, C.J. (1999) Effect of endocrine and paracrine factors on protein synthesis and cell proliferation in bovine hoof tissue culture. *J. Dairy Res.*, **66**, 23–33.
50. Beer, H.D., Fassler, R., and Werner, S. (2000) Glucocorticoid-regulated gene expression during cutaneous wound repair. *Vitam. Horm.*, **59**, 217–239.
51. Chedid, M., Hoyle, J.R., Csaky, K.G., and Rubin, J.S. (1996) Glucocorticoids inhibit keratinocyte growth factor production in primary dermal fibroblasts. *Endocrinology*, **137** (6), 2232–2237.
52. Davies, N.M., Wright, M.R., and Jamali, F. (1994) Anti-inflammatory drug-induced small intestinal permeability: the rat is a suitable model. *Pharm. Res.*, **11**, 1652–1656.
53. Kiziltaş, S., Imeryüz, N., Gürcan, T., Siva, A., Saip, S., Dumankar, A., Kalayci, C., and Ulusoy, N.B. (1998) Corticosteroid therapy augments gastroduodenal permeability to sucrose. *Am. J. Gastroenterol.*, **93**, 2420–2425.
54. Meddings, J.B. and Swain, M.G. (2000) Environmental stress-induced gastrointestinal permeability is mediated by endogenous glucocorticoids in the rat. *Gastroenterology*, **119**, 1019–1028.
55. Soderholm, J.D. and Perdue, M.H. (2001) Stress and gastrointestinal tract. II. Stress and intestinal barrier function. *Am. J. Physiol. Gastrointest. Liver Physiol.*, **280**, G7–G13.
56. Garner, H.E., Coffman, J.R., Hahn, A.W., Hutcheson, D.P., and Tumbleson, M.E. (1975) Equine laminitis of alimentary origin: an experimental model. *Am. J. Vet. Res.*, **36**, 441–444.

57. Mungall, B.A., Kyaw-Tanner, M., and Pollitt, C.C. (2001) In vitro evidence for a bacterial pathogenesis of equine laminitis. *Vet. Microbiol.*, **79**, 209–223.
58. Johnson, P.J., Ganjam, V.K., Slight, S.H., Kreeger, J.M., and Messer, N.T. (2004) Tissue-specific dysregulation of cortisol metabolism in equine laminitis. *Equine Vet. J.*, **36** (1), 41–45.
59. Bitar, M.S. (2000) Insulin and glucocorticoid-dependent suppression of the IGF-I system in diabetic wounds. *Surgery*, **127**, 687–695.
60. Johnson, M.L. and Rajamannan, N. (2006) Diseases of Wnt signaling. *Rev. Endocr. Metab. Disord.*, **7** (1-2), 41–49.
61. Villarreal, G. Jr, Chatterjee, A., Oh, S.S., Oh, D.J., Kang, M.H., and Rhee, D.J. (2014) Canonical wnt signaling regulates extracellular matrix expression in the trabecular meshwork. *Invest. Ophthalmol. Vis. Sci.*, **55** (11), 7433–7440.
62. Wang, L., Pawlak, E.A., Johnson, P.J., Belknap, J.K., Eades, S., Stack, S., Cousin, H., and Black, S.J. (2013) Impact of laminitis on the canonical Wnt signaling pathway in basal epithelial cells of the equine digital laminae. *PLoS One*, **8** (2), e56025.
63. Ohnaka, K., Tanabe, M., Kawate, H., Nawata, H., and Takayanagi, R. (2005) Glucocorticoid suppresses the canonical Wnt signal in cultured human osteoblasts. *Biochem. Biophys. Res. Commun.*, **329** (1), 177–181.
64. Hu, X., Gao, J.H., Liao, Y.J., Tang, S.J., and Lu, F. (2013) Dexamethasone alters epithelium proliferation and survival and suppresses Wnt/β-catenin signaling in developing cleft palate. *Food Chem. Toxicol.*, **56**, 67–74.
65. Naito, M., Omoteyama, K., Mikami, Y., Takahashi, T., and Takagi, M. (2012) Inhibition of Wnt/β-catenin signaling by dexamethasone promotes adipocyte differentiation in mesenchymal progenitor cells, ROB-C26. *Histochem. Cell Biol.*, **138** (6), 833–845.
66. Rosen, J. and Miner, J.N. (2005) The search for safer glucocorticoid receptor ligands. *Endocrinol. Rev.*, **26** (3), 452–464.
67. Vegiopoulos, A. and Herzig, S. (2007) Glucocorticoids, metabolism and metabolic diseases. *Mol. Cell. Endocrinol.*, **275** (1-2), 43–61.
68. Howlett, T.A., Rees, L.H., and Besser, G.M. (1985) Cushing's syndrome. *Clin. Endocrinol. Metab.*, **14** (4), 911–945.
69. McMahon, M., Gerich, J., and Rizza, R. (1988) Effects of glucocorticoids on carbohydrate metabolism. *Diabetes Metab. Rev.*, **4** (1), 17–30.
70. Weinstein, S.P., Wilson, C.M., Pritsker, A., and Cushman, S.W. (1998) Dexamethasone inhibits insulin-stimulated recruitment of GLUT4 to the cell surface in rat skeletal muscle. *Metabolism*, **47** (1), 3–6.
71. Sakoda, H., Ogihara, T., Anai, M., Funaki, M., Inukai, K., Katagiri, H., Fukushima, Y., Onishi, Y., Ono, H., Fujishiro, M., Kikuchi, M., Oka, Y., and Asano, T. (2000) Dexamethasone-induced insulin resistance in 3T3-L1 adipocytes is due to inhibition of glucose transport rather than insulin signal transduction. *Diabetes*, **49** (10), 1700–1708.
72. Divertie, G.D., Jensen, M.D., and Miles, J.M. (1991) Stimulation of lipolysis in humans by physiological hypercortisolemia. *Diabetes*, **40** (10), 1228–1232.
73. Hasselgren, P.O. (1999) Glucocorticoids and muscle catabolism. *Curr. Opin. Clin. Nutr. Metab. Care*, **2** (3), 201–205.
74. Karlsson, S., Ostlund, B., Myrsén-Axcrona, U., Sundler, F., and Ahrén, B. (2001) Beta cell adaptation to dexamethasone-induced insulin resistance in rats involves increased glucose responsiveness but not glucose effectiveness. *Pancreas*, **22** (2), 148–156.
75. Nicod, N., Giusti, V., Besse, C., and Tappy, L. (2003) Metabolic adaptations to dexamethasone-induced insulin resistance in healthy volunteers. *Obesity Res.*, **11** (5), 625–631.
76. Beard, J.C., Halter, J.B., Best, J.D., Pfeifer, M.A., and Porte, D. Jr. (1984) Dexamethasone-induced insulin resistance enhances B cell responsiveness to glucose level in normal men. *Am. J. Physiol.*, **247** (5 Pt 1), E592–E596.
77. Rafacho, A., Quallio, S., Ribeiro, D.L., Taboga, S.R., Paula, F.M., Boschero, A.C., and Bosqueiro, J.R. (2010) The adaptive compensations in endocrine pancreas from glucocorticoid-treated rats are reversible after the interruption of treatment. *Acta Physiol. (Oxf.)*, **200** (3), 223–235.
78. Ogawa, A., Johnson, J.H., Ohneda, M., McAllister, C.T., Inman, L., Alam, T., and Unger, R.H. (1992) Roles of insulin resistance and beta-cell dysfunction in dexamethasone-induced diabetes. *J. Clin. Invest.*, **90** (2), 497–504.
79. Rafacho, A., Marroquí, L., Taboga, S.R., Abrantes, J.L., Silveira, L.R., Boschero, A.C., Carneiro, E.M., Bosqueiro, J.R., Nadal, A., and Quesada, I. (2010) Glucocorticoids in vivo induce both insulin hypersecretion and enhanced glucose sensitivity of stimulus-secretion coupling in isolated rat islets. *Endocrinology*, **151** (1), 85–95.
80. Baggio, L.L. and Drucker, D.J. (2007) Biology of incretins: GLP-1 and GIP. *Gastroenterology*, **132**, 2131–2157.
81. Brubaker, P.L. and Drucker, D.J. (2004) Minireview: glucagon-like peptides regulate cell proliferation and apoptosis in the pancreas, gut, and central nervous system. *Endocrinology*, **145**, 2653–2659.
82. Kim, S.J., Winter, K., Nian, C., Tsuneoka, M., Koda, Y., and McIntosh, C.H. (2005) Glucose-dependent insulinotropic polypeptide (GIP) stimulation of pancreatic β-cell survival is dependent upon phosphatidylinositol 3-kinase (PI3K)/protein kinase B (PKB) signaling, inactivation of the forkhead transcription factor Foxo1, and down-regulation of bax expression. *J. Biol. Chem.*, **280**, 22297–22307.
83. Cummings, B.P., Bremer, A.A., Kieffer, T.J., D'Alessio, D., and Havel, P.J. (2013) Investigation of the mechanisms contributing to the compensatory increase in insulin secretion during dexamethasone-induced insulin resistance in rhesus macaques. *J. Endocrinol.*, **216** (2), 207–215.

CHAPTER 18

Metabolic Syndrome in Humans and Horses: The Relationship Between Obesity and Insulin Resistance

Teresa A. Burns and Ramiro E. Toribio

Introduction

Obesity has long been known to be associated with adverse health effects in both human and veterinary medicine [1–3]. During recent years, a clustering of risk factors associated with obesity has been identified and shown to predict the onset of cardiovascular disease and type 2 diabetes mellitus in people; this syndrome of risk factors (previously known as Syndrome X, the cardiometabolic syndrome, or insulin resistance syndrome) is now referred to as the human metabolic syndrome (HMS) [4]. The first formal definition of HMS was created by a working group of the World Health Organization in 1998 [5]; the definition adopted by this group included evidence of systemic insulin resistance and at least two additional risk factors from a list of criteria including obesity, hypertension, hypertriglyceridemia, low serum high-density lipoprotein concentration, and microalbuminuria. While seemingly inclusive, this definition has proven to be difficult to apply globally to the many diverse disease states which involve insulin resistance (such as anti-retroviral therapy for HIV/AIDS, congenital lipodystrophy, polycystic ovary syndrome, Cushing's syndrome, obesity, etc.), and exceptions to the diagnostic criteria are easily identified, particularly by individuals working in different medical specialties seeing affected patients (e.g., cardiologists, endocrinologists, gerontologists, infectious disease specialists). Consequently, the definition of metabolic syndrome in human medicine has emerged as a somewhat controversial issue [6, 7].

In 2009, a joint interim statement issued as a collaborative effort involving the International Diabetes Federation Task Force on Epidemiology and Prevention, the National Heart, Lung, and Blood Institute, the American Heart Association, the World Heart Federation, the International Atherosclerosis Society, and the International Association for the Study of Obesity suggested that the diagnosis of metabolic syndrome be made in an individual that displayed three out of the following five criteria: hypertension; hypertriglyceridemia; lowered high-density lipoprotein cholesterol; elevated fasting plasma glucose concentration; and central/truncal obesity [2]. Of these diagnostic criteria, the importance of body/adipose tissue morphometrics (waist circumference as a proxy for central/truncal obesity) was emphasized as a useful screening tool for at-risk patients, highlighting the role of adiposity in the pathogenesis and likelihood of developing complications of HMS. The latter has been shown to be associated with an increased incidence of morbidity and mortality attributed to cardiovascular disease (atherosclerotic coronary artery disease and stroke), type 2 diabetes mellitus, degenerative joint disease, and certain types of neoplasms [8–10].

Equine Metabolic Syndrome

Equine veterinary practitioners have long known from clinical experience that overweight and obese horses are prone to developing laminitis, even though the mechanisms underlying this complication remain obscure. Obesity in horses has also been associated with peripheral insulin resistance for over a decade [11, 12]. As HMS became increasingly well-described in the medical literature, parallels were drawn between the human syndrome and that noted clinically in obese horses [13]. Over time, the equine syndrome of obesity (particularly regional adiposity), peripheral insulin resistance, dyslipidemia, and increased risk of endocrinopathic laminitis was coined the 'equine metabolic syndrome' (EMS; see Chapter 23) [12, 13].

The ACVIM Consensus Statement on EMS collated and synthesized most of the available research and current best evidence regarding the condition in horses and ponies [14]. Based on available information, three primary criteria critical for the diagnosis of EMS were identified: (i) increased adiposity (generalized, regional, or both, with emphasis placed on nuchal ligament and tail head adipose tissue accumulations); (ii) peripheral insulin resistance (or insulin dysregulation [15], assessed in

Equine Laminitis, First Edition. Edited by James K. Belknap and Raymond Geor.

a variety of ways; see below and Chapter 29); and (iii) a predisposition to laminitis in the absence of risk factors for other types of the disease, such as sepsis-related laminitis (e.g., signs or history of systemic sepsis from acute pulmonary or uterine infections [16] or enterocolitis secondary to either an infectious agent or acute gross enteral carbohydrate overload [17, 18]). Additional factors that have been reportedly associated with EMS, such as hyperleptinemia [19–21], seasonally increased mean arterial blood pressure [22], and altered reproductive cyclicity in mares [23], were not included in the currently accepted diagnostic criteria. However, the possibility exists that these (and other) factors may be included in a future disease definition, pending validation studies. While the currently accepted criteria have been subjected to reasonable objective evaluation, potential flaws in their interpretation still remain (e.g., in methodology, sensitivity, etc.) that decrease their accuracy in laminitis risk prediction. Even the definition of the outcome variable, laminitis, may be ambiguous under some circumstances.

Horses with EMS are typically overweight to obese, with body condition scores ranging from 7.0 to 9.0/9.0 and clinical evidence of lamellar disease [12, 19, 24]. Whilst all breeds may be affected, most reports indicate that breed predispositions exist, with pony breeds, Morgans, American Saddlebreds, Spanish mustangs, and warmbloods over-represented [25]. There also appears to be a genetic tendency for insulin resistance in many Latin American breeds of Southern European descent (primarily Spain/Portugal), including Paso Fino, Mangalarga Marchador, and Criollo breeds (R.E. Toribio and T.A. Burns, personal communication; [26, 27]). Donkeys and hybrids also seem to be genetically predisposed to reduced insulin sensitivity [28, 29]. Within at-risk breeds, affected individuals often display pronounced regional fat deposits, particularly over the nuchal ligament and tail head. One report suggests that morphometric assessment of the neck of insulin-resistant horses (which incorporates assessment of the degree of nuchal ligament adiposity) can differentiate these horses from insulin-sensitive horses [12]. Interestingly, while the degree of insulin resistance has been shown to correlate reasonably well with body weight in horses [11, 30], not all obese horses are insulin-resistant. Conversely, some relatively lean horses may be profoundly insulin resistant, particularly if they are of a predisposed breed. Identical observations have been made in human medicine, and abnormalities in adipocyte function have been implicated in some of the more severe forms of insulin resistance (e.g., congenital lipodystrophy [31]). The underlying physiologic mechanisms that predispose some breeds of horse to EMS have not yet been elucidated, but it is a tenable hypothesis that some facet of adipocyte structure and/or function is involved, at least in part.

Unlike humans with metabolic syndrome, horses with EMS do not appear to suffer from major cardiovascular complications. While a recent report suggests that insulin-resistant ponies may be hypertensive [22], no concrete evidence of vascular disease has been demonstrated in association with EMS. However, these animals are at increased risk for the development of laminitis [19, 32]. Due to reports of an underlying inflammatory pathophysiology for: (i) severe cardiovascular complications of HMS in humans (specifically, atherosclerotic coronary artery disease); and (ii) equine sepsis-related laminitis (SRL), an inflammatory pathophysiology for EMS-associated laminitis (EMSAL) has been suggested. Although a similar role for inflammation in EMSAL as occurs in coronary artery disease and SRL has not been found (see below), recent studies have revealed a robust association between markers of EMS in ponies (namely, body condition score, plasma triglyceride concentration, and degree of insulin resistance) and the incidence of pasture-associated laminitis, which is one of the more common manifestations of endocrinopathic laminitis in horses [19, 33]. In fact, the presence of more than three clinical findings associated with EMS in one study correctly predicted the development of laminitis in 11 of 13 ponies when these animals were exposed to a high-starch pasture [33]. Anecdotal experience and survey data support the contention that EMSAL is perceived by many equine veterinarians to be the most common form of laminitis seen in their practices [34] (R.J. Geor, 2008, personal communication).

Summary of Physiology and Pathophysiology of Events Important in EMSAL

For those readers that would like only a brief overview of the physiologic mechanisms important in EMSAL, this section provides a synopsis of the in-depth discussion of these topics found in the remainder of the chapter. In the normal equid, the consumption of certain forages (and most concentrate feeds) results in the absorption of a great deal of carbohydrates in the form of sugars. There is normally a well-orchestrated physiologic response to this enteral (intestinal) exposure to carbohydrates to ensure that postprandial systemic glucose and electrolyte concentrations are rapidly and tightly regulated; while many hormones play roles, insulin is at the center of this regulation. Insulin, working primarily through insulin receptors on the surface of cells in many tissues/organs capable of taking up a great deal of glucose (primarily adipose tissue, skeletal muscle, and liver), induces the translocation of protein complexes termed glucose transporters (GLUTs; primarily GLUT-4) to the cell surface of responsive tissues which allows glucose to rapidly enter the cells; glucose is quickly processed in the cells to a form which cannot diffuse back through the GLUTs, which subsequently allows energy production in the cells. Similar to other species, insulin in the equid is secreted by β-cells within the pancreatic islets of Langerhans in response to: (i) the increase in blood glucose concentrations following absorption through the small intestinal epithelium; and (ii) the release of proteins called *incretins* from the small intestine into the bloodstream upon exposure of the intestinal lumen to ingesta that are high in sugars and starch. In the normal equid, this physiologic process not only maintains blood glucose concentrations within a physiologic range, but also allows for the storage of excess energy to be used in times of food scarcity. Throughout evolution, this adaptation likely conferred a survival advantage for those individuals able to live off stored energy when forage was sparse. In both humans and equids, the relatively constant exposure to a high-energy diet combined with the more sedentary lifestyle of modern times has resulted in a disruption of this well-orchestrated physiologic process, resulting in obesity and metabolic syndrome. In human medicine, there is well-supported evidence that adipose tissue is transformed in the setting of obesity from a tissue serving as a site of energy storage and production of regulatory molecules (e.g., adipokines, important for maintaining the body's metabolic control) to a dysregulated organ which adopts an inflammatory phenotype, releasing inflammatory mediators into the circulation and likely leading to low-grade systemic inflammation. These events, which are less well-documented in the equid, disrupt normal insulin signaling in the cells of the peripheral tissues vital to glucose regulation/uptake (e.g., liver and skeletal muscle), resulting in what is termed insulin resistance (IR) or dysregulation. Due to IR, there is a need for an increased secretion of insulin by the pancreatic β-cells to maintain normal blood glucose concentrations; this cluster of events is included in the term 'metabolic syndrome.' In the human, β-cell exhaustion frequently occurs following prolonged IR, resulting in high blood glucose concentrations and low insulin concentrations characteristic of type 2 diabetes mellitus. In the equid with metabolic syndrome, for unknown reasons, β-cell exhaustion does not occur frequently and affected horses persist in a chronic state of hyperinsulinemia (or at least a greatly exaggerated insulin response to a carbohydrate meal) and euglycemia. Whereas the cardiovascular system is most affected in humans with metabolic syndrome (resulting in sequelae such as atherosclerosis, etc.), laminitis is by far the most common complication in the equid with EMS. Although research into EMSAL is still in its infancy, recent data have suggested that lamellar dysregulation/injury in this setting is more likely due to effects of insulin on the lamellar epithelial cells (effects that are not directly related to carbohydrate substrate availability). That is, lamellar energy deprivation does not appear to be an important mechanism of injury in this type of laminitis. Additionally, lamellar inflammation – which is thought to play a central role in SRL – appears to be minimal during the development of EMSAL. Aberrant or excessive growth factor signaling in the lamellae (likely involving the activation of insulin-like growth factor-1 (IGF-1) receptors in the lamellar epithelial cells by insulin at supraphysiologic concentrations) has recently been documented in both obese ponies fed a high-energy diet and in the hyperinsulinemic–euglycemic clamp model of laminitis. This same signaling is a focus of research in epithelial disease in humans, especially in epithelial cancers, in which dysregulation of the same events affected in lamellar epithelial cells (control of cytoskeletal and cell adhesion dynamics) plays a pivotal role. Additionally, the demonstrated decrease in lamellar concentrations of the activated form of AMP-activated protein kinase (AMPK), although most commonly studied in the setting of energy metabolism, may result in the disruption of lamellar epithelial cytoskeletal dynamics proposed to occur in EMSAL.

Epidemiology of Obesity: Humans and Horses

From an epidemiologic perspective, obesity and its associated metabolic and cardiovascular consequences have emerged over the past 10–15 years as critically important disease states in human medicine worldwide, creating an increasing economic burden on the healthcare systems of developed nations worldwide [35]. In fact, in the United States and the United Kingdom, two-thirds of all adults are reported to be either overweight or obese [36–38]; accompanying this finding are increasing rates of atherothrombotic cardiovascular disease, stroke, type 2 diabetes mellitus (and all of its associated comorbidities), degenerative joint disease, and certain types of neoplastic disease [39,40]. Perhaps more alarming is the ballooning rate of obesity among young people in developed nations [41,42]; in fact, the current generation of school-age children has been suggested to have a life expectancy shorter than that of their parents, which is historically unprecedented [43]. Clearly, obesity is a major healthcare issue in human medicine, both for the wellbeing of human populations and for the prioritization of the spending of increasingly limited healthcare funding allocations. With this economic imperative, a strong research effort has been put forth over the past 10–15 years to elucidate risk factors for systemic insulin resistance and the metabolic syndrome in humans, and to characterize the role that the expanded adipose tissue itself may play in the pathogenesis of the cardiovascular and metabolic sequelae of the syndrome.

While the magnitude of the obesity epidemic in human populations is well established (and growing), far fewer studies have been performed to describe the epidemiology of obesity in equids. Additionally, most of these studies rely on owner assessments of their horses' body condition score (BCS), and as such may not accurately represent the prevalence of equine obesity. A study of 319 Scottish riding horses reported that 45% of animals were described by their owners as being 'fat' or 'very fat' [44], while another study from the UK noted that owners self-reported their horses as being 'fat' or 'very fat' only 17.7% of the time [45]. In this second study, the owners' BCS assessments were compared to those of an experienced investigator and, not surprisingly, owners tended to underscore their horses (average by owner = 3.1/5; average by investigator = 3.8/5; k = 0.04). In the United States, the prevalence of equine obesity appears to be similar to that in the UK. A study from a general equine veterinary practice population in Virginia reported that, based on the BCS of 300 horses, 1.7% were underconditioned, 47.3% were optimal, 32.3% were overweight, and 18.7% were obese [46]. The significance of these high reported prevalence rates for obesity should be stressed, since another cross-sectional study from the United States (central Ohio) investigating risk factors for hyperinsulinemia in light-breed horses reported that obesity was one of only two risk factors (along with age) that was significantly associated with hyperinsulinemia in this population [47]. Clearly, obesity is a highly prevalent condition in equids, as in humans, and associated with morbidity in both species.

Although the physiologic and pathophysiologic mechanisms associated with nutrient absorption and use/storage in the normal and obese human or equid are not entirely understood, the following is a discussion of the likely physiologic mechanisms taking place in the equid, with some of the results being extrapolated from human studies.

The Physiology of Energy Absorption and Storage

Adipose Tissue Metabolism in Health

White adipose tissue (one of two types of adipose tissue found in mammals; the other is brown adipose tissue) functions as a primary concentrated energy storage organ in animal systems, undergoing expansion or contraction in response to chronic imbalance between caloric intake and expenditure [48]. Fluctuations in adipocyte number (through proliferation and differentiation of pre-adipocytes) and volume (through alterations in the relative rates of lipid synthesis and lipolysis) are responsible for these changes, and the control of adipocyte size and number is under continuous paracrine (i.e., influence of nearby cells) and endocrine (i.e., influence of circulating hormones) control in response to dietary intake and caloric expenditure [48]. The cellular/molecular orchestration of the mechanisms governing the degree of adiposity is quite complex; one manifestation of this complexity is the variability in metabolic activity (and disease risk) associated with adipose tissue accumulation in certain regions of the body. In humans, abdominal or truncal adiposity is associated with a significantly increased risk of coronary artery disease, stroke, type 2 diabetes mellitus, and certain types of cancer [49]. Strong gender dimorphism in body fat distribution in humans (truncal in men; hips/thighs in women) suggests an important role for sex hormones in the regulation of adipose tissue deposition; in fact, the protection against cardiac disease that accompanies female gender in people is lost after the onset of menopause, which is also associated with a shift towards truncal adiposity in women [50].

In equids, a strong sexual dimorphism with respect to regional adiposity has not been described, but the concept of 'high-risk' adipose tissue depots is well-known in these species, as described above. Nuchal ligament/crest adipose tissue accumulation is associated with both insulin resistance and the risk of endocrinopathic laminitis in equids [19, 51], and these morphological changes have led to the generation of several scoring systems aimed at quantifying this location of regional adiposity and, in theory, predicting laminitis risk [12,51]. White adipose tissue, particularly when deposited in certain regions of the body, is no longer assumed to be a metabolically inert energy storage depot, but rather an endocrinologically active, dynamic tissue that plays a critical role in the regulation of intermediary metabolism of fats and carbohydrates and also contributes to systemic inflammation. Much has been learned about the endocrine roles of adipose tissue in obesity and metabolic syndrome; abdominal adipose tissue (more specifically, adipose tissue within omental and other visceral depots) appears to be more insulin-resistant, to express and secrete more adipokines and proinflammatory cytokines, and to correlate better with cardiovascular disease risk than do other adipose tissue depots in humans [52]. While horses do not appear to accumulate large deposits of omental adipose tissue routinely, omental and visceral adipose tissue have been reported to display characteristics associated with tissue insulin resistance in horses [53,54].

The association of abdominal adipose tissue with the pathogenesis of the human metabolic syndrome is clear; however, the roles of these adipose tissue depots – if any – in the equine metabolic syndrome remain to be defined. In fact, many of the metabolic and phenotypic alterations associated with insulin-resistant adipose tissue have been reported in the nuchal ligament adipose tissue of horses that were generally overweight or obese. For example, nuchal ligament adipose tissue has been reported to express interleukin (IL)-1β and IL-6 at greater levels (and leptin and adiponectin at lower levels) than other adipose tissue depots of light-breed horses, including omental, retroperitoneal, mesenteric, and tail head [55]. However, the level of expression of these factors was not associated with the degree of IR in the studied horses. Nuchal ligament adipose tissue appears to be accompanied by metabolic risk in equids, but the mechanisms by which it accumulates or how it contributes to systemic IR have not been investigated thoroughly to date.

In horses, an association has been made in several observational studies between the degree of adiposity (measured by BCS according to the method of Henneke [56], tritiated water distribution, and ultrasonographic rump fat thickness) and systemic IR [30, 57–60]. As insulin-resistant equids often display hyperinsulinemia (fasting and/or an exaggerated response to an oral or intravenous carbohydrate challenge), and hyperinsulinemia has recently been shown to precipitate laminitis experimentally, IR and subsequent hyperinsulinemia are now not only regarded as important diagnostic criteria for EMS but are also likely to be pathophysiologically linked to lamellar dysregulation/injury in EMSAL [61,62]. Further studies in ponies and small numbers of light-breed horses have shown a degree of correlation between increased size of the nuchal ligament adipose tissue (assessed via neck morphometric parameters and/or neck crest scoring) and the degree of systemic IR [12, 19]. However, the relationship between degree of adiposity and systemic IR in equids is nonlinear, with the ready identification of generally obese individuals who are quite insulin-sensitive and relatively lean individuals who are insulin-resistant (again, similar to what has been observed in HMS). This supports the theory that other factors, in addition to adipocyte size and/or metabolic activity, disturb insulin signaling in equids and potentially contribute to complications such as laminitis. There seems to be a prominent breed predisposition to this phenomenon, as breeds less commonly afflicted with EMS (e.g., Quarter Horses and Thoroughbreds) are less likely to become severely insulin-resistant with obesity; conversely, lean members of EMS-predisposed breeds, such as Morgans, Paso Finos, and American Saddlebreds, may be highly insulin-resistant [12]. While nutritional obesity may play an important role in initiating or perpetuating IR in a genetically predisposed individual, it may not be highly predictive of laminitis upon induction of obesity in all individuals, due to the above-described fact that IR and laminitis are not observed in all obese animals (and laminitis is frequently observed in otherwise lean animals). Functional assessment of the adipose tissue (in addition to an assessment of distribution) may be more relevant in this setting, as multiple adipokines (e.g., leptin, adiponectin, resistin) have been shown to have direct effects on insulin sensitivity in other species [63].

Adipose Tissue and Nutritional Obesity

Excessive dietary caloric intake leads to an expansion of white adipose tissue over time, a concept that is very familiar and easily observed clinically. Some authors have speculated that, prior to the *pathophysiologic* role that excessive adipose tissue plays in HMS (and EMS), adipose tissue likely serves a *physiologic* role, as a 'buffer' function in the normal animal by 'neutralizing' circulating free fatty acids (FFAs) by removing them from the circulation and storing them. High levels of circulating FFAs have been associated with IR and disrupted physiology in many tissues (skeletal and cardiac muscle, vascular structures, liver, endocrine pancreas, etc.) [64–67]. Perhaps less familiar is the reason(s) for continued progressive expansion of the adipose tissue when it clearly reaches the point of being nonadaptive and induces systemic complications. In other words, to a point, the accumulation of white adipose tissue can actually attenuate IR; in fact, congenital or acquired lipodystrophy in humans (associated with the absence or atrophy of white adipose tissue) results in severe systemic IR and hypertriglyceridemia [68].

In addition to possibly playing an important role in decreasing levels of circulating FFAs during times of nutrient excess, white adipose tissue serves a vital function in preserving normal metabolism during periods of nutrient scarcity (by releasing energy that was stored in adipocytes during the period of high nutrient supply). However, with the development of nutritional obesity, its phenotype can *adversely* affect metabolism. With the accumulation of intracellular triglyceride, adipocytes enlarge to the point that they are reported to outgrow their vascular supply [69], resulting in hypoxia and, ultimately, necrosis of individual adipocytes (termed 'crown cells' or 'crown-like structures' when surrounded by immune cells [70,72]). The presence of these necrotic cells is associated with leukocyte infiltration into the adipose tissue, and in other species this infiltration is highly correlated with the degree of tissue IR. The vast majority of infiltrative leukocytes in adipose tissue are macrophages, which comprise a large proportion of the stromal-vascular fraction of healthy adipose tissue. In health, most of these cells are polarized to an M2 phenotype (the so-called 'anti-inflammatory' phenotype), supporting normal tissue metabolism and suppressing inflammation [73]. In the setting of obesity, there are not only increased numbers of macrophages within the white adipose tissue, but those present have undergone a shift in polarity towards predominantly an M1, or proinflammatory, phenotype [74,75]. Carter and colleagues have reported increased IL-8, monocyte chemoattractant protein 1 (MCP-1), and plasminogen activator inhibitor-1 (PAI-1) mRNA expression in nuchal ligament white adipose tissue following the induction of nutritional obesity in Arabian geldings [76, 77]. While the number of infiltrative macrophages (assessed via CD163 immunohistochemistry) was unchanged in that study, the altered transcription profile of the adipose tissue in response to weight gain may represent an acquired shift in macrophage polarity to a proinflammatory M1 phenotype. Clearly, the adipose tissue is important and changes with obesity in horses, but the pathophysiologic role adipose tissue plays in EMS is not nearly as well characterized as it is in other species.

Dietary Components and Insulin Sensitivity

Hyperalimentation that results in increased adiposity is known to be associated with acquired systemic IR in horses [30,76,77], and if equine adipobiology is similar to what is known in other species, this is highly correlated with the degree of adipose tissue IR and leukocyte infiltration [69–71, 78]. However, even in the absence of detectable expansion of adipose tissue mass, the *composition* of the diet has been shown to have short-term effects on systemic insulin sensitivity in horses, both in adults and in young stock. For example, feeding grain-based meals high in sugar and starch was found to decrease the systemic insulin sensitivity of Thoroughbred geldings when fed over an eight-week period; obese individuals also had lower insulin sensitivity than lean animals in this study [11]. A similar study in post-foaled Thoroughbred broodmares showed higher peak plasma glucose and insulin concentrations and area under the curve (AUC) for [glucose] and [insulin] (consistent with systemic IR) in mares fed a traditional sweet feed high in sugar and starch compared to mares that consumed a feed high in fat and fiber [79]. This effect is not restricted to mature animals, as it has also been documented in young, growing horses; for example, Treiber and colleagues showed that weanling Thoroughbreds raised on pasture and supplemented with a high sugar/starch feed for approximately 200 days displayed a lower systemic insulin sensitivity than age-matched weanlings supplemented with a high-fat/-fiber feed [80]. Finally, preliminary evidence for 'metabolic programming' in equids (effects of the gestating maternal diet on postnatal insulin sensitivity in foals) has been reported. In this case, foals born to mares fed a high-starch feed during the last trimester of gestation displayed evidence of altered glucose tolerance at 80 and 160 days of age [81]. Additional information on the effects of diet on insulin sensitivity and on nutritional recommendations for the management of equine IR is available in Chapters 23 and 50.

Development of IR with Increased Adiposity: The Role of Adipokines

Recent investigations in humans and experimental rodent models has revealed the importance of aberrant insulin signaling in both the pathogenesis of the metabolic syndrome and the risk of adverse consequences in affected patients [82, 83]. Not only is basal and stimulated hyperinsulinemia considered a marker/diagnostic criterion for at-risk individuals, but insulin itself is considered to play direct and indirect roles in the pathophysiology of diseases associated with metabolic syndrome [2]. Knowledge of insulin signaling in health and mechanisms by which it becomes dysfunctional in the insulin-resistant individual is imperative for the design of rational treatment and prevention programs.

Glucose, the primary carbohydrate fuel of cellular intermediary metabolism, crosses cell membranes via facilitated diffusion through various members of a family of glucose transport proteins (GLUTs), of which 14 have been described in mammalian systems to date [84]. In the postprandial state, an elevation in plasma glucose concentration following its absorption from the gastrointestinal tract is a potent secretagogue ('inducer' of secretion) for insulin from β-cells in the islets of Langerhans of the endocrine pancreas. Upon its secretion and subsequent delivery via the systemic circulation to its target tissues (skeletal muscle, adipose tissue, liver, bone), insulin binds and activates highly specific cell-surface receptors [85]. The insulin receptor is a transmembrane heterotetrameric tyrosine kinase receptor composed of two α and two β subunits. Insulin binding to the α subunit triggers autophosphorylation of tyrosine residues on the intracellular domain of the β subunit, leading to the recruitment of cytoplasmic insulin receptor substrate (IRS) proteins [86, 87]. Although the details of several IRSs have been described (at least four), IRS-1 and IRS-2 primarily subserve the functions of signal transduction through the insulin receptor (IRS-1 is of primary importance in skeletal muscle, adipose tissue, and bone; IRS-2 is of greater importance in liver) [88]. IRSs contain multiple tyrosine and serine phosphorylation sites; in general (with a few exceptions), tyrosine phosphorylation of IRSs by activated insulin receptors results in conformational changes in the IRSs that activate and promote their function as docking proteins, recruiting additional SH-2 domain-containing molecules involved in insulin signal transduction through two main pathways [88]. Serine phosphorylation of IRSs is broadly inhibitory to their function in recruiting downstream effectors of signaling; while more than 50 canonical serine phosphorylation sites have been described on IRS-1 (the functions of all of which have not been fully characterized to date), the phosphorylation of some of these (e.g., Ser312/307) results in the retention of IRS-1 in the cytosol (in association with 14-3-3 proteins) and enhanced IRS-1 ubiquitination and degradation. In this way, serine phosphorylation of IRSs serves as an important site of negative feedback of insulin action; it is also a primary mechanism responsible for acquired insulin resistance/dysregulation in pathologic states, such as obesity and inflammation [83].

As mentioned above, IRS proteins recruit effectors of two intracellular signaling cascades that are activated by insulin binding to its receptor: (i) the mitogen-activated protein kinase (MAPK) pathway (responsible for the mitogenic and differentiation effects of insulin; does not play a significant role in glucose metabolism); and (ii) the phosphatidylinositol-3-kinase (PI3K) pathway (responsible for the increased transcellular glucose conductance observed following insulin binding). Tyrosine phosphorylation of IRS-1 and/or IRS-2 results in the recruitment of a subunit of PI3K (p85 subunit) to the plasma membrane, where its primary substrate(s) – phospholipids – are located. The phosphorylation of a specific membrane lipid, phosphatidylinositol 4,5-bisphosphate (PIP2), by PI3K (through its catalytic p110 subunit) results in the activation of a kinase, phosphatidylinositol-dependent protein kinase (PDK1). PDK1 phosphorylates PKB/Akt, a kinase that then phosphorylates the AS160 (Akt substrate of 160 kDa) protein [87, 89–92]. GLUT-4, the primary insulin-responsive glucose transporter protein in skeletal muscle, is sequestered in cytoplasmic vesicles in the absence of insulin receptor activation; AS160 is involved (likely with many other molecules) in promoting this retention. Upon phosphorylation and thus inhibition of AS160 by Akt, GLUT-4-containing vesicles translocate to and fuse with the plasma membrane, resulting in an increased cell-surface expression of GLUT-4. Plasma glucose then enters the skeletal muscle cells through GLUT-4-facilitated diffusion until these transporters are re-sequestered following cessation of the insulin signal [85]. Other GLUTs are expressed in skeletal muscle (e.g., GLUT-1, GLUT-2), but these are not insulin-responsive and their involvement in glucose transport into skeletal muscle is considered minor in comparison to that of GLUT-4 [84]. Once glucose has entered the cell, it is 'trapped' (preventing back-diffusion through GLUT-4 to the original extracellular location) via rapid phosphorylation of glucose to glucose-6-phosphate (which does not pass through GLUTs) by glucokinase/hexokinase. These are the essential steps that promote normal insulin-mediated glucose movement from the systemic circulation into the skeletal myocyte, which is primarily responsible for insulin-mediated plasma glucose disposal (the clearance of glucose from the plasma through translocation to an intracellular location) postprandially (other cell types important in insulin-mediated glucose disposal are hepatocytes and adipocytes) [85].

The Endocrine Pancreas and IR

Following the ingestion of a meal, the food components are broken down into their respective nutritional elements by salivary, gastric, pancreatic, and intestinal enzymatic activities. While an average grain meal (i.e., a 10% sweet feed preparation) for horses contains protein, lipid, and carbohydrate, the majority of said ration is carbohydrate (especially starch and simple sugars). The degradation of dietary starch and sugars to hexoses (glucose, galactose, and fructose) results in their absorption by simple and facilitated diffusion (cotransport with sodium) across the gastrointestinal tract into the portal venous blood and, ultimately, the systemic circulation. While increases in the concentration of other diet-derived substances in plasma (such as certain amino acids) can induce pancreatic insulin secretion, the postprandial increase in plasma glucose concentration is a potent (and the most physiologically important) secretagogue for insulin from the β-cells of the endocrine pancreas (located, similar to other species, in the islets of Langerhans throughout the equine pancreas). It has long been held that transport of glucose into the β-cell (primarily through passive diffusion via the GLUT-2 transporter) during times of hyperglycemia results in increased glycolysis and ATP production. An ATP-responsive potassium channel is present on the plasma membrane of the β-cell; the increased cytosolic ATP concentrations result in the channel's inhibition, inducing decreased potassium conductance out of the β-cell and the cell's relative depolarization [93,94]. This cellular depolarization leads to an increased activation of voltage-gated calcium channels on the plasma membrane and increased calcium influx into the cell, activating calcium-dependent mechanisms responsible for the fusion of insulin-containing cytoplasmic vesicles (which also contain equimolar amounts of C-peptide) with the plasma membrane. This results in insulin release into the interstitial fluid and subsequently into pancreatic venous (and then systemic) blood [95].

The results of recent studies with cultured islets suggest that this mechanism is likely not the only one responsible for insulin release, however. Two phases of insulin secretion are observed in response to an enteric glycemic load: (i) an initial, rapid phase (i.e., within the first 10 min after the administration of a glucose bolus); and (ii) a delayed, sustained phase (i.e., beginning about 15 min after the first phase) [96, 97]. The pharmacologic inhibition of the ATP-sensitive potassium channels described above significantly attenuates the initial rapid phase of insulin secretion, but has limited effects on the sustained secretion noted later. Gut-derived hormones (particularly incretins, such as glucagon-like peptide 1 [GLP-1] and glucose-dependent insulinotropic polypeptide [GIP], from the L- and K-cells of the small intestine, respectively) are likely responsible for the second phase of sustained insulin release, and have become attractive therapeutic targets for the treatment of relative insulin deficiency in humans with type II diabetes mellitus [98]. Incretins were discovered and subsequently described following the initial observation that an oral glucose load/meal would reliably elicit a two- to threefold greater insulinemic response than a similar glucose load given intravenously (thereby bypassing the gastrointestinal tract); the incretin response is severely impaired in humans with type 2 diabetes mellitus, an abnormality which can be pharmacologically reconstituted with the administration of GLP-1 analogs (e.g., exendin-4 homologues such as exenatide) or inhibitors of the enzyme that degrades incretins, dipeptidyl peptidase-4 (such as sitagliptin) [98]. The enteroinsular axis (the endocrine relationship linking local intestinal events – that is, incretin release – with alterations in pancreatic insulin secretion) has been evaluated in equids, albeit not in any great depth to date. The incretin effect has been shown to exist in horses and ponies [99], and postprandial GLP-1 plasma concentrations have been shown to be higher in breeds that are predisposed to insulin resistance/EMS [100]. Postprandial plasma insulin concentrations have been shown to be positively associated with GLP-1 concentrations in ponies, and it has been suggested that the equine enteroinsular axis contributes to insulin dysregulation in these species [101].

A primary factor likely to modify the degree of postprandial hyperinsulinemia observed in an equid consuming a meal is the composition of the meal, particularly its 'glycemic index.' The latter term is applied to human foodstuffs and is defined as the ability of a specific dose of the food in question to raise blood sugar compared to a similar quantity of white bread. This has been modified somewhat for use in equine nutrition, and the 'relative' glycemic indices of certain cereal grains have been reported (e.g., the glycemic response of the horse to a meal of corn is higher than that to one of barley) [102]. Since postprandial plasma glucose concentration is the most physiologically important secretagogue for insulin, the ability of the ingested meal to raise plasma glucose concentration would be expected to have a profound effect on the insulinemic response to that meal [103]. This is exploited therapeutically in the dietary management of horses and ponies with EMS, as attempts are made to minimize the amount of nonstructural carbohydrate in their diets [104].

The functional pancreatic β-cell mass of the individual, which has been shown to correlate to insulinemic responses to meals and to intravenous glucose challenge in experimental animals [105], is an important variable to consider when evaluating an animal's insulin response to a meal. This has not been effectively characterized in equine populations, but β-cell failure (insufficient insulin response to carbohydrate challenge) is uncommon in this species [106]. Further, β-cell mass is virtually impossible to measure accurately *in vivo* (and presents challenges *ex vivo*); it can be measured experimentally, which may shed light on the mechanisms by which equine β-cell function is preserved in the setting of prolonged hyperinsulinemia (in contrast to β-cell exhaustion/failure which leads to type 2 diabetes mellitus in humans) [107].

The relative insulin sensitivity of the most physiologically important insulin-responsive tissues (skeletal muscle, liver, and adipose tissue), which are responsible for the majority of postprandial glucose disposal, has important ramifications for the insulin secretory response. Animals that are systemically insulin-resistant show decreased glucose disposal from the plasma following a meal [14], and they display increased plasma fatty acid concentrations in both the fasting and fed states (as a result of both decreased insulin-mediated inhibition of hormone-sensitive lipase in adipose tissue and decreased inhibition of hepatic synthesis and secretion of very low-density lipoproteins [VLDLs]) [108]. Experimental glucotoxicity (structural and functional damage to pancreatic β-cells and target tissues of insulin caused by chronic hyperglycemia), lipotoxicity (cellular dysfunction resulting from the accumulation of lipid intermediates in non-adipose tissue), or both, has been shown to decrease insulin secretion from cultured islets *in vitro* over the course of several hours of glucose and lipid incubation or infusion. The mechanism for this remains to be clarified, but since the metabolic cycling of pyruvate metabolites (i.e., isocitrate–malate, citrate–malate, pyruvate–malate) during glycolysis in the β-cell is suspected to be involved in insulin secretion, the dramatic addition of metabolites to these pathways can be expected to affect their outcome (insulin secretion) [109]. Additionally, the expression and functionality of incretin receptors on β-cells has been shown to be blunted in the setting of IR; again, the mechanism for this is unclear, but this is an active area of investigation in human medicine [110]. Finally, while the pancreas is not responsible for a large amount of insulin-dependent glucose disposal within its own cells, it is insulin-responsive; insulin receptor signaling is thought to be involved in pancreatic insulin secretion, which may become dysfunctional in the setting of systemic IR (completely uncharacterized in horses and ponies) [82].

In obese humans and rodents in models of nutritional obesity, systemic IR and hyperinsulinemia are followed temporally in a majority of individuals by decreased glucose tolerance, pancreatic β-cell failure, and type 2 diabetes mellitus. In stark contrast to humans, obese horses and ponies chronically remain in what is termed a 'prediabetic' state in human medicine, characterized by hyperinsulinemic euglycemia. Few data exist describing the biology of the equine endocrine pancreas in the chronically IR animal that both explains this unique equine endocrine physiology (i.e., why β-cell exhaustion does not develop in the horse) and characterizes the animal at-risk for hyperinsulinemia-associated laminitis. In ponies subjected to a week-long enteral carbohydrate challenge, there was a trend for greater total islet surface area in pancreatic tissue from ponies fed the high-nonstructural carbohydrate (NSC) diet when compared to the ponies on the control (chopped hay) diet ($p = 0.068$); however, no difference was noted in total β-cell surface area between diet treatments ($p = 0.12$) [111]. The change in basal serum insulin concentration in these ponies was significantly greater in the high-NSC-fed animals than in controls, but this variable was not correlated with total islet surface area ($r = 0.32$; $p = 0.17$) or β-cell surface area ($r = 0.25$; $p = 0.3$). Due to the relatively modest changes in pancreatic islet surface area that accompany marked increases in serum insulin concentrations in ponies fed a high NSC diet, it is important to assess both β-cell function (insulin production) and insulin clearance mechanisms in future studies to more accurately describe the mechanism(s) of sustained hyperinsulinemia in IR equids.

Other Factors Influencing Energy Dynamics in the Horse

A number of endocrine systems for which information is lacking in equids have been implicated in energy regulation in other species [112–115]. Extensive data are available supporting a link between numerous tissues/organs (e.g., the central nervous system, the pituitary gland, the gastrointestinal tract, pancreas, adipose tissue, and bone) and metabolic functions, in particular energy homeostasis [114–116].

During the past decade, for example, it was shown that insulin promotes the release of osteocalcin (a hormone involved in bone homeostasis and metabolic regulation) by osteoblasts, which in turn enhances insulin secretion and sensitivity [114,117,118]. This has been further confirmed in animal models by manipulation of the osteocalcin gene. Mice lacking the osteocalcin gene develop hyperglycemia, IR, infertility, and increased abdominal fat [114]. Exogenous osteocalcin administration to these mice prevents the development of obesity, and the prospect of using osteocalcin to treat type 2 diabetes in people is currently being tested [114]. This endocrine energy regulatory system is known as the bone–pancreas or the bone–pancreas–testis axis [119–121], and its dysregulation is believed to contribute to the development of IR. While this example of integrative physiology is poorly described in the veterinary literature, current information legitimizes the skeleton as a tissue required for energy homeostasis. Of interest to EMS, low osteocalcin concentrations have been associated with impaired insulin secretion, obesity, metabolic syndrome, and markers of cardiovascular disease in children and adult people [122–126]. In postmenopausal woman, high osteocalcin concentrations are linked to insulin sensitivity (assessed by the homeostatic model assessment of insulin resistance [HOMA-IR]), and low osteocalcin concentrations have been associated with high glucose and hemoglobin A1C concentrations (suggesting poor short- and long-term glycemic control, respectively) and diabetes [125,127]. These observations suggest that osteocalcin, as well as other infrequently investigated factors, should be explored in horses as they may relate to energy dysregulation, insulin secretion, altered insulin signaling, and endocrinopathic laminitis.

Leptin is another endocrine factor (adipokine) that is worth mentioning in the context of adipose tissue, pancreas, bone, and the central nervous system, since this is the hormone that links the brain with energy, body condition, reproduction, and bone mass [114]. Some data on leptin have been generated in horses, ponies, and donkeys [51,128–130], mostly associating its concentrations with the BCS/adipose mass [128,129]. Although not strong, an association between leptin and the likelihood of developing laminitis has been documented [19]. In addition to its appetite-suppressing actions, leptin inhibits insulin gene expression/secretion, promotes peripheral insulin sensitivity, stimulates thermogenesis, enhances fatty acid oxidation, and reduces body fat [131,132]. Leptin resistance leads to: (i) hyperinsulinemia at the pancreatic level; and (ii) reduced insulin sensitivity in peripheral tissues [133,134]. From this information, it can be speculated that increased leptin concentrations in obese horses merely reflect adipose depots, though this finding may also be an indication of a leptin-resistant state. This intricate relationship between leptin and insulin could potentially explain metabolic abnormalities in horses with EMS and clinical evidence of laminitis.

Adiponectin is an adipokine involved with energy regulation, metabolism, and inflammation [63,135,136]. This hormone, which is secreted by adipocytes, is found in circulation in different forms. In humans, full-length adiponectin circulates as 90 kDa trimers, low-molecular-weight (LMW) hexamers of 180 kDa, and high-molecular-weight (HMW) multimers of >360 kDa [63]. The HMW form, which is subject to post-translational modifications, is considered most biologically active [63]. There is also a globular proteolytic fraction of the protein with a structure similar to that of tumor necrosis factor-alpha (TNF-α) [63]. Adiponectin increases insulin sensitivity, fatty acid oxidation, and energy consumption through activation of the peroxisome proliferator-activated receptor-α (PPAR-α), and it stimulates β-oxidation and glucose uptake via activation of a central kinase controlling cellular energy metabolism, adenosine monophosphate-activated protein kinase (AMPK) [63]. It also appears that globular adiponectin has biological actions – it promotes glucose uptake, enhances insulin sensitivity, promotes lipid oxidation, and coordinates myogenesis. HMW adiponectin seems to be protective against inflammation [136]. A number of investigations of adiponectin have been conducted in horses [137,138], and adiponectin concentrations have been shown to be associated with fat mass in humans and horses [63,136,137]. HMW adiponectin was negatively correlated with BCS and serum insulin concentrations in healthy horses [138]. Equine-specific studies on the influence of HMW and globular adiponectin on metabolic activity and cell differentiation will help to elucidate the role of this adipokine on insulin sensitivity, angiogenesis, metabolic syndrome, and laminitis.

Another system that deserves further investigation as it relates to energy homeostasis in horses is the *somatotropic axis*. Consisting of growth hormone (GH) and IGF-1, the equine somatotropic axis is likely to be integrally involved with energy metabolism, insulin sensitivity, fat accumulation/distribution, and integumentary health. It is well accepted that GH has anti-insulin properties while IGF-1 has insulin-like actions and may be a vascular protective factor [139,140]. High and low GH concentrations have been linked to HMS, while low IGF-1 seems to be a consistent finding in affected individuals. A number of studies have included the measurement of GH and IGF-1 in horses, and have associated their plasma concentrations with diet and BCS [21,141]. It is well documented in other species that GH can decrease insulin sensitivity by uncoupling PI3K signaling (a signaling pathway critical for insulin/growth factor receptor signaling; see above [142]). Increased GH and decreased IGF-1 concentrations have been associated with IR and the risk of developing metabolic syndrome [143]. It has also been suggested that low IGF-1 concentrations could be a useful marker to identify people at risk for IR and cardiovascular disease [143]. The role of the somatotropic axis in the pathogenesis of equine obesity and endocrinopathic laminitis has received little evaluation, although preliminary evidence suggests that serum IGF-1 concentrations are not increased in experimental animals subjected to a euglycemic–hyperinsulinemic clamp (under the conditions of which lamellar gene expression of insulin receptor and IGF-1 receptor [IGF-1R) is reportedly decreased) [144]. However, it is reasonable to assume that GH elevations could interfere with glucose uptake and lipid metabolism and contribute to the development of IR. Stimulation of the IGF-1R may alter numerous events relative to laminitis, including lamellar cell proliferation, cytoskeletal regulation, and cell adhesion processes, which suggests that there is a connection between this signaling system and the pathogenesis of hyperinsulinemic laminitis [144, 145]. This also supports a potential involvement of the somatotropic axis in maintaining lamellar health.

The enteroinsular axis is a poorly characterized system in the horse that likely contributes to equine metabolic disorders [113]. In general terms, this axis comprises factors from the gut that stimulate pancreatic islet cells, but specifically refers to the incretins (INtestinal seCRETion of INsulin). Of the gastrointestinal hormones, glucose-dependent insulinotropic polypeptide (GIP) and glucagon-like peptide (GLP)-1 are considered incretins, which means they promote insulin release and suppress glucagon secretion. In other species, GIP is secreted by K cells (in the proximal small intestine), and GLP-1 by L cells (from proglucagon; in the distal small intestine). Nutrients in the small intestinal lumen – carbohydrates in particular – promote incretin secretion. The incretin actions explain the increase in insulin secretion before blood glucose concentrations rise, which is considered a pre-emptive mechanism to avoid hyperglycemia and facilitate peripheral tissue glucose uptake. Incretin mimetics (e.g., GLP-1 agonists such as exenatide and liraglutide) are used in people and small animals for the treatment of type 2 diabetes mellitus. Dipeptidyl peptidase-4 (DPP-4) inactivates GIP and GLP-1. Based on this property, novel drugs (gliptins) that inhibit DPP-4 have been developed to prolong the incretin effect and reduce glycemia. These drugs have also been approved to be used alone or in combination with metformin to treat patients in which the normalization of glycemia is challenging. In addition to their actions on the endocrine pancreas, GIP and GLP-1 have a multitude of functions; notably, they inhibit gastric emptying and acid secretion, promote insulin sensitivity, influence fat metabolism, and modulate skeletal muscle metabolism and microvascular blood flow [146]. GIP enhances resistin secretion via MAPK, activates PI3K, and suppresses AMPK signaling [147]. Increased GIP concentrations have been linked to human obesity. Obese individuals have increased GIP levels and a higher response to a meal than lean individuals [148]. An impaired function of the enteroinsular axis has been linked to inadequate insulin secretion in people with type 2 diabetes mellitus. It can be speculated from this information that incretin investigation should be considered a priority to better understand equine endocrinology and metabolism, and also to elucidate the importance of the incretins in EMS. Although few investigations of incretins have been undertaken in horses [99–101], recent studies have shown that equids have a functional enteroinsular axis characterized by a positive correlation between GLP-1 and insulin concentrations [100,101]. It has been proposed that this axis may contribute to equine insulin dysregulation and the risk for laminitis in EMS [101].

The Effects of IR/Dysregulation on the Digital Lamellae

The lamellar basal epithelial cell (LBEC) integrates, through its interaction with the lamellar basement membrane (BM), the load-bearing function of the lamellae, neutralizing the downward force of gravity transmitted through the bony column of the digit and the upward ground reaction force transmitted through the hoof wall (see Chapters 4 and 5). Its importance, therefore, cannot be overstated, as the LBEC's failure to: (i) maintain its normal morphology (i.e., resist stretch, most likely through cytoskeletal homeostasis of not only the LBEC layer but also the lamellar parabasal epithelial cells); (ii) maintain attachment to the underlying BM (through adhesion complexes such as hemidesmosomes); or (iii) a combination of these two events will lead to displacement of the bony column within the hoof wall (see Chapters 4 and 19). The LBECs are highly polarized cells whose function is critically dependent on their adherence both to their neighboring epithelial cells and to the anchoring BM. In addition to this critical role, the equine LBECs appear to function similarly to other keratinocytes, responding to extracellular events by utilizing a multitude of basic signaling mechanisms, including signaling related to both inflammation and epithelial stress in SRL. Although much effort has been expended to identify a common signaling pathway by which diverse systemic disease entities can lead to laminitis/lamellar failure, it is more likely that the reason why diverse entities lead to lamellar failure is the vital function that the lamellar epithelial cells play in counteracting the great physical tension relayed through the lamellae by the lamellar dermis attached to the underlying distal phalanx (DP). Thus, any insult to the LBECs may result in a loss of function of this highly differentiated, polarized cell type (and possibly the associated parabasal epithelial cells) through dysregulation of cytoskeletal dynamics and/or BM adhesion; this would culminate in the LBEC layer stretching, followed by dysadhesion – and thus failure – of the lamellae to suspend the DP (and therefore the weight of the horse). Hence, the cause of lamellar failure in EMSAL may bear little similarity to that occurring in other types of laminitis regarding extracellular events or even cell signaling. However, lamellar failure behaves similarly in both SRL and EMSAL, resulting from the disarray of cytoskeletal and adhesion functions with subsequent stretching of the lamellae and possible dysadhesion of the LBECs from the underlying BM [17].

While Equine Laminitis has been associated with many diverse causes (including gastrointestinal tract disorders, retained placenta or metritis, severe infections, and excessive weight-bearing) [16], EMSAL is now reported to be the most common cause of laminitis, affecting primarily horses and ponies with a phenotype of obesity (especially regional adiposity) and IR when they are exposed to a high-carbohydrate diet in the form of either cereal grains and high-energy processed feeds or, most commonly, pasture forage with a high NSC content [19,33,149]. Clinical observations and the results of epidemiologic studies have indicated that the risk of EMSAL is highest when horses and ponies are grazing pastures with a high NSC content (e.g., fructans, simple sugars, and/or starch), and theories on the pathogenesis of pasture-associated EMSAL have been extrapolated from experimental models of alimentary carbohydrate overload. However, the extent to which these severe models reflect events during the development of EMSAL may be questioned. First, it is likely that the amount and rate of starch or fructan administered in a bolus via nasogastric tube for the induction of carbohydrate overload in these studies far exceeds the quantity of NSC ingested by grazing equids in a short period of time. Second, previous studies have not used animals with an EMS phenotype and thus have not addressed the interaction between diet and phenotypic factors associated with laminitis susceptibility. Subsequent studies have attempted to address these shortcomings by including an enteral carbohydrate challenge as part of the experimental model and enrolling animals considered to be at higher risk for EMSAL (e.g., ponies [61, 150, 151]).

Several cytoplasmic kinases present in the LBECs and whose activation states are affected by the concentrations of various metabolic intermediates are known to affect cytoskeletal metabolism and epithelial cell polarity *in vitro* [152, 153]. One of these kinases, AMPK, is highly regulated based on cellular energy status; increased AMPK activation (via phosphorylation) is associated with a more differentiated and polarized epithelial cell phenotype [154, 155]. It is intriguing to speculate that decreased AMPK activity (which has been recently observed in lamellar tissue of ponies challenged with an increased dietary carbohydrate load, a stimulus that has been associated with the induction of laminitis in IR equids [150]) might induce a loss of cytoskeletal polarity of the lamellar basal cell (such as has been observed *in vitro* in other epithelial cell model systems) and subsequent lamellar epithelial stretching and/or detachment from its BM. The loss of polarity of epithelial basal cells and decreased maintenance of epithelial tight junctions may lead to mechanical disruption of the lamellar interface secondary to relatively constant tension relayed through the deep digital flexor tendon.

Recent evidence of decreased lamellar AMPK phosphorylation in a model of EMSAL suggests that a decreased AMPK activity in the lamellae may be pathologic; however, it is unclear what role this enzyme plays in normal and abnormal lamellar physiology. While the net effects of AMPK activation or inhibition on the function of the equine LBEC are unknown, it is reasonable to assume that it plays a role in this highly polarized, structurally critical cell type, the cytoskeletal interactions of which are crucial to support of the weight of a horse or pony against gravity.

Insulin resistance, which has been shown to occur in obesity and in sepsis in horses, can result in hyperinsulinemia due to the stimulation of insulin production by the pancreas from a prolonged increase in blood glucose levels due to decreased glucose transport into insulin-responsive tissues (especially skeletal muscle). While IR and subsequent glucose starvation have been suggested in the past as potential mechanisms underlying lamellar failure in this state, it has recently been shown [156] that the primary glucose transporter type expressed in lamellar tissue is GLUT-1, which is neither insulin-dependent nor highly insulin-responsive. Hence, instead of glucose deprivation in the setting of IR, as might occur in insulin-dependent tissues, the lamellae may experience an *increased* glucose flux in the setting of IR (consistent with this theory, as mentioned above, AMPK phosphorylation in the lamellae has been shown to be downregulated with high-carbohydrate feeding [150]). An increased glucose flux is associated with ATP production and a decreased AMP:ATP ratio, conditions in which AMPK activity would be expected to be decreased [157]. If basal cell polarity (which is presumed to be required for correct LBEC function) is similarly dependent on AMPK function, as has been shown in other epithelial cell types *in vitro* [152], this scenario might very well result in lamellar failure (which is what is observed clinically).

It is also possible that the actin cytoskeletal reorganization events induced by AMPK activation may be *deleterious* to lamellar function in certain settings. Interesting studies conducted by a group working with alveolar epithelial cell cultures have suggested that mechanical signaling through dystroglycan (a membrane-anchored mechanoreceptor) and plectin (which binds dystroglycan and AMPK) simultaneously activates AMPK and MAPK pathways (ERK1/2) [158]. In both published and unpublished data from the Belknap laboratory, ERK1/2 was the only MAPK pathway (not p38 MAPK or SAPK) activated in the lamellae in models of laminitis, and was activated in both the carbohydrate overload (CHO) model of SRL [159] and the hyperinsulinemic–euglycemic clamp model of EMSAL (J.K. Belknap, unpublished data). This strongly suggests a pathophysiologic role for this kinase pathway in laminitis of diverse etiologies. Laminitis associated with excessive weight-bearing, which can certainly be expected to activate signaling pathways initiated by mechanoreceptors, may involve both MAPK and AMPK activation. Further investigation in this area is clearly warranted.

Hyperinsulinemia has been known to be a risk factor for the development of endocrinopathic laminitis for some time, identified by several groups independently in cross-sectional studies [12,24,33]. More recently, a direct link between insulin and laminitis has been created, with the experimental induction of laminitis via iatrogenic hyperinsulinemia in normal ponies [61] and light-breed horses [62]. Insulin is a pleiotropic hormone, the functions of which have been largely thought to be limited to the regulation of carbohydrate, lipid, and protein metabolism in times of energy surplus (i.e., during the postprandial period) [10]. However, signaling through insulin receptors has been shown to activate not only pathways that direct the fates of nutritional metabolites (through PI3K activation) but also the modulation of mitogenesis and extracellular matrix production through the activation of MAPK pathways [87]. Direct effects of insulin on LBECs, with subsequent alterations of their production of extracellular matrix (which is critically important for the integrity of the lamellar BM, known to separate from lamellar basal cells and thereby define structural failure accompanying laminitis), may play a role in endocrinopathic laminitis. However, recent studies have shown little evidence of insulin receptor expression on lamellar epidermal cells and thus have complicated the acceptance of this hypothesis [160]. Insulin signaling through insulin receptors may have a greater effect on perfusion of the lamellae, as insulin receptor expression appears to be restricted primarily to the lamellar microvasculature [160].

Prolonged exposure of endothelial cells to increased concentrations of insulin *in vitro* has been shown to alter their insulin responsiveness, inducing cellular IR over a relatively short period of time (24–48 h) [161]. Interestingly, it is shortly after this time frame, at about 48–72 h, that horses and ponies are observed to become laminitic during experimental hyperinsulinemia [61]. A rapid downregulation of the surface expression of insulin receptors has been documented on endothelial cells in response to treatment with exogenous insulin, which may partially explain the endothelial IR observed in response to hyperinsulinemia *in vivo*. Signaling through insulin receptors (through the serine phosphorylation of IRSs by Akt/PKB) also tends to be self-limiting [88]; this mechanism for IR may be more important in the lamellae, where the endothelial expression of insulin receptors appears to be increased in the setting of hyperinsulinemia [160]. An altered vascular responsiveness during IR is thought to result from decreased insulin-mediated elaboration of the potent vasodilator NO, and thus loss of its vasodilatory effects on vascular smooth muscle [162]. The attenuation of PI3K signaling downstream of insulin receptor activation results in a decreased activity of endothelial NOS (eNOS) and decreased NO production. Concurrently, while defective PI3K signaling is observed from insulin-bound insulin receptors in endothelial IR (which may be acquired over a relatively short period of time), signaling through the MAPK pathway appears to be preserved. The increased production of endothelin-1 (a potent vasoconstrictor) through this pathway, along with decreased vasodilatory effects of NO, is thought to result in inappropriate vasoconstriction, a failure to achieve flow-dependent vasodilation and, ultimately, hypertension. Local perfusion, particularly in those tissues lacking collateral circulation, may be inadequate, but it is possible that this perfusion deficit in the lamellae may activate stress kinase systems, such as MAPK and AMPK (see above). Nitric oxide also has been reported to have important anti-inflammatory and anticoagulant effects, the loss of which has been associated with the propagation of atherothrombotic lesions in humans and experimental animal models of metabolic syndrome [90]. In horses with IR, pathologic changes in vasomotor tone to a tissue with poor collateral circulation (the foot) may promote hypoxia/ischemia, both of which have been suggested to play roles in the pathogenesis of laminitis [163]. Although thrombi have also been noted in the lamellar microvasculature in experimental models of sepsis-related laminitis and naturally occurring laminitis [164], lamellar thrombi/microthrombi have not been reported in endocrinopathic laminitis (see Chapter 12). The reported decrease in lamellar AMPK activation in obese, hyperinsulinemic ponies exposed to a high NSC/high energy diet does not support ischemia as playing a central role in EMSAL [150].

Another intriguing possibility that remains purely speculative at this point is that insulin may be triggering signaling in lamellar epithelial cells through IGF-1Rs, not insulin receptors (which again, does not appear to be present at high levels on lamellar epithelial cells). Insulin has been shown to bind and activate IGF-1Rs at supraphysiologic concentrations in cell cultures (concentrations easily achievable in the average IR equid in response to a dietary carbohydrate challenge) [165], and the distribution of IGF-1Rs within the lamellae appears to be much more extensive than that of the insulin receptor [160]. While insulin receptors appear to be limited to the lamellar microvasculature, IGF-1Rs are present on lamellar epithelial cells, endothelial cells, and fibroblasts (and likely other cell types as well). Experiments using *in-vitro* skin culture systems with human keratinocytes have revealed an important role for IGF-1 in the normal maturation of epithelial cells in the skin, which progresses in an orderly fashion in the presence of IGF-1 and its receptor from basal cells to anucleate squamous cells; small interfering RNA (siRNA) knockdown of IGF-1R in this culture system results in a disordered maturation of keratinocytes and the production of histologically abnormal epidermis [166]. In the equine digital lamellae, evidence of the activation of ribosomal protein S6 (RPS6) downstream of growth factor signaling (including the IGF-1 receptor) has been documented in both ponies fed high-carbohydrate diets and in the hyperinsulinemic–euglycemic clamp models [167]; this may be a consequence of insulin activation of the IGF-1R when present at very high concentrations (as might be observed postprandially in an IR equid fed a meal containing high-NSC feedstuffs). RPS6 activation has become a recent focus of interest both in epithelial tumor formation and cytoskeletal regulation [168,169], and this signaling may play an important role in dysregulation of the lamellar epithelial cells in EMSAL. The importance of IGF-1R signaling in the lamellar epidermis – particularly its effects on the extracellular matrix and cytoskeletal/cell adhesion complex components – is currently unclear but warrants further investigation to clarify its role and identify it as a possible therapeutic target in the management of EMSAL in horses and ponies.

The Role of Systemic Inflammation in EMSAL

It appears that IR in humans is often associated with increased plasma concentrations of proinflammatory mediators (notably TNF-α, IL-1β), linking abnormal carbohydrate metabolism with chronic, low-grade inflammation [170]. This phenomenon has also been described in veterinary species, including dogs, mice, and rats, and recently, horses [171, 172]. Obesity and IR have been (loosely) positively correlated with plasma concentrations of TNF-α and IL-1β in horses [172], and several research groups have suggested (based on measurements of tissue and systemic concentrations of inflammatory mediators) that EMS represents a systemic, low-grade chronic inflammatory state [55,172,173]. The cause of laminitis in insulin-resistant horses is unknown but has been postulated to be a consequence of systemic inflammation associated with impaired insulin signaling [174]. However, this has yet to be documented conclusively in the horse, and recent evidence has suggested that equine endocrinopathic laminitis may not result in detectable lamellar inflammation [175,176].

The Role of Liver and Skeletal Muscle in Metabolic Syndrome

Liver, skeletal muscle, and adipose tissue are the primary sites of insulin's actions on carbohydrate, lipid, and protein metabolism in health. As mentioned above, skeletal muscle is the most important tissue mediating insulin-induced postprandial glucose disposal. During the development of obesity and IR, abnormal physiology in the liver and skeletal muscle contribute just as much (and perhaps more) to the initiation and persistence of systemic IR as does the obese adipose tissue. With the onset of obesity and IR, an increased efflux of FFAs from adipose tissue can result in the accumulation of lipid intermediates within hepatocytes and skeletal myocytes [64,65,177,178]. Intramyocellular and intra-hepatocellular lipid – the result of this lipid accumulation – can ultimately result in insufficiency or failure of normal function of the affected tissue; however, before this point, lipid accumulation induces cellular and tissue IR. The magnitude of ectopic lipid accumulation has been shown to correlate with systemic IR and risk outcome more tightly in humans and rodents than the degree, or even location, of adipose tissue accumulation [65,179]. When the liver develops IR, hepatic gluconeogenesis is not effectively inhibited by insulin, which results in persistent postprandial hepatic glucose production and the promotion of hyperglycemia and hyperinsulinemia. The liver is also the primary site of expression of insulin-degrading enzyme, which degrades and clears insulin from the body; during IR, hepatic insulin clearance is also impaired, which ultimately promotes persistent hyperinsulinemia and IR [180, 181]. Thus, it has become clear that, in human obesity and IR, the relative roles of skeletal muscle and hepatic IR may not be equivalent. In fact, hepatic IR appears to correlate better with systemic IR and adverse disease outcomes in people than does skeletal muscle IR [178]. Euglycemic–hyperinsulinemic clamp protocols utilizing different insulin infusion rates (a lower rate for assessing skeletal muscle IR; a higher rate for assessing hepatic IR) have been described to evaluate the differential role of these tissues, and these may have some benefit in the evaluation of equine IR (as the respective contributions of liver and skeletal muscle in this species remains unclear). Additionally, the role of ectopic lipid in the pathophysiology of equine IR remains poorly described (even though a catastrophic disease state associated with equine IR, hyperlipemia, is *defined* by ectopic lipid accumulation). The relative ease of sampling of equine skeletal muscle and liver by minimally invasive techniques, and the purported importance of these tissues to the pathophysiology of HMS, makes minimally invasive biopsy an attractive possibility for both the diagnostic evaluation of equids with EMS and for assessment of the effectiveness of treatment. Additional research is clearly warranted to further evaluate the roles of liver and skeletal muscle in the pathophysiology of IR and EMS in equids.

References

1. Must, A., Jacques, P.F., Dallal, G.E., Bajema, C.J., and Dietz, W.H. (1992) Long-term morbidity and mortality of overweight adolescents. A follow-up of the Harvard growth study of 1922 to 1935. *N. Engl. J. Med.*, **327** (19), 1350–1355.
2. Alberti, K.G., Eckel, R.H., Grundy, S.M., *et al.* (2009) Harmonizing the metabolic syndrome: A joint interim statement of the International Diabetes Federation Task Force on Epidemiology and Prevention; National Heart, Lung, and Blood Institute; American Heart Association; World Heart Federation; International Atherosclerosis Society; and International Association for the Study of Obesity. *Circulation*, **120** (16), 1640–1645.
3. Geor, R. and Frank, N. (2009) Metabolic syndrome – from human organ disease to laminar failure in equids. *Vet. Immunol. Immunopathol.*, **129** (3-4), 151–154.
4. Day, C. (2007) Metabolic syndrome, or what you will: Definitions and epidemiology. *Diabetes Vasc. Dis. Res.*, **4** (1), 32–38.
5. Alberti, K.G. and Zimmet, P.Z. (1998) Definition, diagnosis and classification of diabetes mellitus and its complications. Part 1: Diagnosis and classification of diabetes mellitus; provisional report of a WHO consultation. *Diabetes Med.*, **15** (7), 539–553.
6. Stolar, M. (2007) Metabolic syndrome: Controversial but useful. *Cleveland Clin. J. Med.*, **74** (3), 199–202, 205–208.
7. Saely, C.H., Rein, P., and Drexel, H. (2007) The metabolic syndrome and risk of cardiovascular disease and diabetes: Experiences with the new diagnostic criteria from the International Diabetes Federation. *Horm. Metab. Res.*, **39** (9), 642–650.
8. Cabarcas, S.M., Hurt, E.M., and Farrar, W.L. (2010) Defining the molecular nexus of cancer, type 2 diabetes and cardiovascular disease. *Curr. Mol. Med.*, **10** (8), 744–755.
9. Safar, M.E., Balkau, B., Lange, C., *et al.* (2013) Hypertension and vascular dynamics in men and women with metabolic syndrome. *J. Am. Coll. Cardiol.*, **61** (1), 12–19.
10. Rask-Madsen, C. and Kahn, C.R. (2012) Tissue-specific insulin signaling, metabolic syndrome, and cardiovascular disease. *Arterioscler. Thromb. Vasc. Biol.*, **32** (9), 2052–2059.
11. Hoffman, R.M., Boston, R.C., Stefanovski, D., Kronfeld, D.S., and Harris, P.A. (2003) Obesity and diet affect glucose dynamics and insulin sensitivity in thoroughbred geldings. *J. Anim. Sci.*, **81** (9), 2333–2342.
12. Frank, N., Elliott, S.B., Brandt, L.E., and Keisler, D.H. (2006) Physical characteristics, blood hormone concentrations, and plasma lipid concentrations in obese horses with insulin resistance. *J. Am. Vet. Med. Assoc.*, **228** (9), 1383–1390.
13. Johnson, P.J. (2002) The equine metabolic syndrome peripheral Cushing's syndrome. *Vet. Clin. North Am. Equine Pract.*, **18** (2), 271–293.
14. Frank, N., Geor, R.J., Bailey, S.R., Durham, A.E., and Johnson, P.J. (2010) American College of Veterinary Internal Medicine. Equine metabolic syndrome. *J. Vet. Intern. Med.*, **24** (3), 467–475.
15. Frank, N. and Tadros, E.M. (2014) Insulin dysregulation. *Equine Vet. J.*, **46** (1), 103–112.
16. Belknap, J.K., Moore, J.N., and Crouser, E.C. (2009) Sepsis – from human organ failure to laminar failure. *Vet. Immunol. Immunopathol.*, **129** (3-4), 155–157.
17. Pollitt, C.C. and Visser, M.B. (2010) Carbohydrate alimentary overload laminitis. *Vet. Clin. North Am. Equine Pract.*, **26** (1), 65–78.
18. Van Eps, A.W. and Pollitt, C.C. (2006) Equine laminitis induced with oligofructose. *Equine Vet. J.*, **38** (3), 203–208.
19. Carter, R.A., Treiber, K.H., Geor, R.J., Douglass, L., and Harris, P.A. (2009) Prediction of incipient pasture-associated laminitis from hyperinsulinaemia, hyperleptinaemia and generalised and localised obesity in a cohort of ponies. *Equine Vet. J.*, **41** (2), 171–178.
20. Kearns, C.F., McKeever, K.H., Roegner, V., Brady, S.M., and Malinowski, K. (2006) Adiponectin and leptin are related to fat mass in horses. *Vet. J.*, **172** (3), 460–465.
21. Cartmill, J.A., Thompson, D.L., Jr, Storer, W.A., Gentry, L.R., and Huff, N.K. (2003) Endocrine responses in mares and geldings with high body condition scores grouped by high vs. low resting leptin concentrations. *J. Anim. Sci.*, **81** (9), 2311–2321.
22. Bailey, S.R., Habershon-Butcher, J.L., Ransom, K.J., Elliott, J., and Menzies-Gow, N.J. (2008) Hypertension and insulin resistance in a mixed-breed population of ponies predisposed to laminitis. *Am. J. Vet. Res.*, **69** (1), 122–129.
23. Waller, C.A., Thompson, D.L., Jr, Cartmill, J.A., Storer, W.A., and Huff, N.K. (2006) Reproduction in high body condition mares with high versus low leptin concentrations. *Theriogenology*, **66** (4), 923–928.
24. Kronfeld, D.S., Treiber, K.H., Hess, T.M., *et al.* (2006) Metabolic syndrome in healthy ponies facilitates nutritional countermeasures against pasture laminitis. *J. Nutr.*, **136** (7 Suppl.), 2090S–2093S.
25. Johnson, P.J., Messer, N.T., and Ganjam, V.K. (2004) Cushing's syndromes, insulin resistance and endocrinopathic laminitis. *Equine Vet. J.*, **36** (3), 194–198.
26. Magalhaes, J.F., Lima, I.R., Lima, L.R., *et al.* (2014) Correlation study about radiographic measurements signaling laminitis in

Mangalarga Marchador mares with or without signs of overweight. *Arq. Bras. Med. Vet. Zootec.*, **66** (4), 1023–1032.
27. Faleiros, R.R., Amaral, L.A., Paz, C.F.R., and Nogueira, C.E.W. (2012) Obesidade e laminite, problemas a serem estudados na raca crioula. *Anuario Raca Crioula*, **52**, 400.
28. Mendoza, F.J., Aguilera-Aguilera, R., Gonzalez-De Cara, C.A., Toribio, R.E., Estepa, J.C., and Perez-Ecija, A. (2015) Characterization of the intravenous glucose tolerance test and the combined glucose-insulin test in donkeys. *Vet. J.*, **206** (3), 371–376.
29. Mendoza, F.J., Estepa, J.C., Gonzalez-De Cara, C.A., Aguilera-Aguilera, R., Toribio, R.E., and Perez-Ecija, A. (2015) Energy-related parameters and their association with age, gender, and morphometric measurements in healthy donkeys. *Vet. J.*, **204** (2), 201–207.
30. Carter, R.A., McCutcheon, L.J., George, L.A., Smith, T.L., Frank, N., and Geor, R.J. (2009) Effects of diet-induced weight gain on insulin sensitivity and plasma hormone and lipid concentrations in horses. *Am. J. Vet. Res.*, **70** (10), 1250–1258.
31. Wildman, R.P., Muntner, P., Reynolds, K., *et al.* (2008) The obese without cardiometabolic risk factor clustering and the normal weight with cardiometabolic risk factor clustering: Prevalence and correlates of 2 phenotypes among the US population (NHANES 1999–2004). *Arch. Intern. Med.*, **168** (15), 1617–1624.
32. Treiber, K.H., Kronfeld, D.S., and Geor, R.J. (2006) Insulin resistance in equids: Possible role in laminitis. *J. Nutr.*, **136** (7 Suppl.), 2094S–2098S.
33. Treiber, K.H., Kronfeld, D.S., Hess, T.M., Byrd, B.M., Splan, R.K., and Staniar, W.B. (2006) Evaluation of genetic and metabolic predispositions and nutritional risk factors for pasture-associated laminitis in ponies. *J. Am. Vet. Med. Assoc.*, **228** (10), 1538–1545.
34. American Association of Equine Practitioners. AAEP membership equine research study report. Available at: www.aaepfoundation.org. Updated 2009; accessed March 14, 2011.
35. Polonsky, K.S. (2012) The past 200 years in diabetes. *N. Engl. J. Med.*, **367** (14), 1332–1340.
36. Ljungvall, A. and Zimmerman, F.J. (2012) Bigger bodies: Long-term trends and disparities in obesity and body-mass index among U.S. adults, 1960–2008. *Soc. Sci. Med.*, **75** (1), 109–119.
37. Martinson, M.L. (2012) Income inequality in health at all ages: A comparison of the United States and England. *Am. J. Public Health*, **102** (11), 2049–2056.
38. Stevens, V.L., Jacobs, E.J., Sun, J., *et al.* (2012) Weight cycling and mortality in a large prospective US study. *Am. J. Epidemiol.*, **175** (8), 785–792.
39. Daviglus, M.L., Talavera, G.A., Aviles-Santa, M.L., *et al.* (2012) Prevalence of major cardiovascular risk factors and cardiovascular diseases among Hispanic/Latino individuals of diverse backgrounds in the united states. *JAMA*, **308** (17), 1775–1784.
40. Kraschnewski, J.L., Sciamanna, C.N., Stuckey, H.L., *et al.* (2013) A silent response to the obesity epidemic: Decline in US physician weight counseling. *Med. Care*, **51** (2), 186–192.
41. Robbins, J.M., Mallya, G., Polansky, M., and Schwarz, D.F. (2012) Prevalence, disparities, and trends in obesity and severe obesity among students in the Philadelphia, Pennsylvania, school district, 2006–2010. *Prev. Chronic Dis.*, **9**, E145.
42. Turchiano, M., Sweat, V., Fierman, A., and Convit, A. (2012) Obesity, metabolic syndrome, and insulin resistance in urban high school students of minority race/ethnicity. *Arch. Pediatr. Adolesc. Med.*, **166** (11), 1030–1036.
43. Bray, G.A. and Bellanger, T. (2006) Epidemiology, trends, and morbidities of obesity and the metabolic syndrome. *Endocrine*, **29** (1), 109–117.
44. Wyse, C.A., McNie, K.A., Tannahill, V.J., Murray, J.K., and Love, S. (2008) Prevalence of obesity in riding horses in Scotland. *Vet. Rec.*, **162** (18), 590–591.
45. Stephenson, H.M., Green, M.J., and Freeman, S.L. Prevalence of obesity in a population of horses in the UK. *Vet. Rec.*, **168** (5), 131.
46. Thatcher, C.D., Pleasant, R.S., Geor, R.J., and Elvinger, F. (2012) Prevalence of overconditioning in mature horses in Southwest Virginia during the summer. *J. Vet. Intern. Med.*, **26** (6), 1413–1418.
47. Muno, J., Gallatin, L., Geor, R.J., Anderson, G.A., and Hinchcliff, K.W. (2009) Seasonal variation in plasma insulin and glucose concentration in normal horses in central Ohio. Proceedings of the Forum of the American College of Veterinary Internal Medicine, Abstract #124.
48. McTernan, P.G., Anwar, A., and Kumar, S. (2005) Relationship between fat distribution and insulin resistance, in *Insulin Resistance: Insulin action and its disturbances in disease*, (eds S. Kumar and S. O'Rahilly), John Wiley & Sons, Ltd, pp. 207–235.
49. Ibrahim, M.M. (2010) Subcutaneous and visceral adipose tissue: Structural and functional differences. *Obesity Rev.*, **11** (1), 11–18.
50. Geer, E.B. and Shen, W. (2009) Gender differences in insulin resistance, body composition, and energy balance. *Gend. Med.*, **6** (Suppl. 1), 60–75.
51. Carter, R.A., Geor, R.J., Burton Staniar, W., Cubitt, T.A., and Harris, P.A. (2009) Apparent adiposity assessed by standardised scoring systems and morphometric measurements in horses and ponies. *Vet. J.*, **179** (2), 204–210.
52. Despres, J.P. and Lemieux, I. (2006) Abdominal obesity and metabolic syndrome. *Nature*, **444** (7121), 881–887.
53. Waller, A.P., Kohler, K., Burns, T.A., Mudge, M.C., Belknap, J.K., and Lacombe, V.A. (2011) Naturally occurring compensated insulin resistance selectively alters glucose transporters in visceral and subcutaneous adipose tissues without change in AS160 activation. *Biochim. Biophys. Acta*, **1812** (9), 1098–1103.
54. Burns, T.A., Geor, R.J., Mudge, M.C., McCutcheon, L.J., and Belknap, J.K. (2010) Characterization of adipose tissue macrophage infiltration in insulin-resistant and insulin-sensitive light breed horses. Proceedings of the Forum of the American College of Veterinary Internal Medicine.
55. Burns, T.A., Geor, R.J., Mudge, M.C., McCutcheon, L.J., Hinchcliff, K.W., and Belknap, J.K. (2010) Proinflammatory cytokine and chemokine gene expression profiles in subcutaneous and visceral adipose tissue depots of insulin-resistant and insulin-sensitive light breed horses. *J. Vet. Intern. Med.*, **24** (4), 932–939.
56. Henneke, D.R., Potter, G.D., Kreider, J.L., and Yeates, B.F. (1983) Relationship between condition score, physical measurements and body fat percentage in mares. *Equine Vet. J.*, **15** (4), 371–372.
57. Bamford, N.J., Potter, S.J., Harris, P.A., and Bailey, S.R. (2016) Effect of increased adiposity on insulin sensitivity and adipokine concentrations in horses and ponies fed a high fat diet, with or without a once daily high glycaemic meal. *Equine Vet. J.*, **48** (3), 368–373.
58. Selim, S., Elo, K., Jaakkola, S., *et al.* (2015) Relationships among body condition, insulin resistance and subcutaneous adipose

tissue gene expression during the grazing season in mares. *PLoS ONE*, **10** (5), e0125968.

59. Carter, R.A., McCutcheon, L.J., Valle, E., Meilahn, E.N., and Geor, R.J. (2010) Effects of exercise training on adiposity, insulin sensitivity, and plasma hormone and lipid concentrations in overweight or obese, insulin-resistant horses. *Am. J. Vet. Res.*, **71** (3), 314–321.
60. Vick, M.M., Sessions, D.R., Murphy, B.A., Kennedy, E.L., Reedy, S.E., and Fitzgerald, B.P. (2006) Obesity is associated with altered metabolic and reproductive activity in the mare: Effects of metformin on insulin sensitivity and reproductive cyclicity. *Reprod. Fertil. Dev.*, **18** (6), 609–617.
61. Asplin, K.E., Sillence, M.N., Pollitt, C.C., and McGowan, C.M. (2007) Induction of laminitis by prolonged hyperinsulinaemia in clinically normal ponies. *Vet. J.*, **174** (3), 530–535.
62. de Laat, M.A., McGowan, C.M., Sillence, M.N., and Pollitt, C.C. (2010) Equine laminitis: Induced by 48 h hyperinsulinaemia in Standardbred horses. *Equine Vet. J.*, **42** (2), 129–135.
63. Yadav, A., Kataria, M.A., Saini, V., and Yadav, A. (2013) Role of leptin and adiponectin in insulin resistance. *Clin. Chim. Acta*, **417**, 80–84.
64. Coen, P.M. and Goodpaster, B.H. (2012) Role of intramyocelluar lipids in human health. *Trends Endocrinol. Metab.*, **23** (8), 391–398.
65. Eckardt, K., Taube, A., and Eckel, J. (2011) Obesity-associated insulin resistance in skeletal muscle: Role of lipid accumulation and physical inactivity. *Rev. Endocr. Metab. Disord.*, **12** (3), 163–172.
66. Einstein, F.H., Huffman, D.M., Fishman, S., *et al.* (2010) Aging per se increases the susceptibility to free fatty acid-induced insulin resistance. *J. Gerontol. A. Biol. Sci. Med. Sci.*, **65** (8), 800–808.
67. Corcoran, M.P., Lamon-Fava, S., and Fielding, R.A. (2007) Skeletal muscle lipid deposition and insulin resistance: Effect of dietary fatty acids and exercise. *Am. J. Clin. Nutr.*, **85** (3), 662–677.
68. Petersen, K.F. and Shulman, G.I. (2006) Etiology of insulin resistance. *Am. J. Med.*, **119** (5 Suppl.1), S10–S16.
69. Lafontan, M. (2014) Adipose tissue and adipocyte dysregulation. *Diabetes Metab.*, **40** (1), 16–28.
70. Lee, B.C. and Lee, J. (2014) Cellular and molecular players in adipose tissue inflammation in the development of obesity-induced insulin resistance. *Biochim. Biophys. Acta*, **1842** (3), 446–462.
71. Revelo, X.S., Luck, H., Winer, S., and Winer, D.A. (2014) Morphological and inflammatory changes in visceral adipose tissue during obesity. *Endocr. Pathol.*, **25** (1), 93–101.
72. West, M. (2009) Dead adipocytes and metabolic dysfunction: Recent progress. *Curr. Opin. Endocrinol. Diabetes Obesity*, **16** (2), 178–182.
73. Zeyda, M., Farmer, D., Todoric, J., *et al.* (2007) Human adipose tissue macrophages are of an anti-inflammatory phenotype but capable of excessive pro-inflammatory mediator production. *Int. J. Obesity (Lond.)*, **31** (9), 1420–1428.
74. Lumeng, C.N., Deyoung, S.M., Bodzin, J.L., and Saltiel, A.R. (2007) Increased inflammatory properties of adipose tissue macrophages recruited during diet-induced obesity. *Diabetes*, **56** (1), 16–23.
75. Lumeng, C.N., Bodzin, J.L., and Saltiel, A.R. (2007) Obesity induces a phenotypic switch in adipose tissue macrophage polarization. *J. Clin. Invest.*, **117** (1), 175–184.
76. Carter, R., McCutcheon, L.J., Burns, T.A., Belknap, J.K., Frank, N., and Geor, R.J. (2008) Increased adiposity in horses is associated with decreased insulin sensitivity but unchanged inflammatory cytokine expression in subcutaneous adipose tissue. Proceedings of the Forum of the American College of Veterinary Internal Medicine.
77. Burns, T.A., Carter, R., McCutcheon, L.J., Geor, R.J., and Belknap, J.K. (2008) The relationship of infiltrative leukocytes to adipose tissue chemokine expression and insulin resistance in diet-induced obesity in horses. Proceedings of the Forum of the American College of Veterinary Internal Medicine.
78. de Luca, C. and Olefsky, J.M. (2008) Inflammation and insulin resistance. *FEBS Lett.*, **582** (1), 97–105.
79. Williams, C.A., Kronfeld, D.S., Staniar, W.B., and Harris, P.A. (2001) Plasma glucose and insulin responses of thoroughbred mares fed a meal high in starch and sugar or fat and fiber. *J. Anim. Sci.*, **79** (8), 2196–2201.
80. Treiber, K.H., Boston, R.C., Kronfeld, D.S., Staniar, W.B., and Harris, P.A. (2005) Insulin resistance and compensation in thoroughbred weanlings adapted to high-glycemic meals. *J. Anim. Sci.*, **83** (10), 2357–2364.
81. George, L.A., Staniar, W.B., Treiber, K.H., Harris, P.A., and Geor, R.J. (2009) Insulin sensitivity and glucose dynamics during preweaning foal development and in response to maternal diet composition. *Domest. Anim. Endocrinol.*, **37** (1), 23–29.
82. Wang, Q. and Jin, T. (2009) The role of insulin signaling in the development of beta-cell dysfunction and diabetes. *Islets*, **1** (2), 95–101.
83. Tanti, J.F. and Jager, J. (2009) Cellular mechanisms of insulin resistance: Role of stress-regulated serine kinases and insulin receptor substrates (IRS) serine phosphorylation. *Curr. Opin. Pharmacol.*, **9** (6), 753–762.
84. Augustin, R. (2010) The protein family of glucose transport facilitators: It's not only about glucose after all. *IUBMB Life*, **62** (5), 315–333.
85. Leto, D. and Saltiel, A.R. (2012) Regulation of glucose transport by insulin: Traffic control of GLUT4. *Nat. Rev. Mol. Cell. Biol.*, **13** (6), 383–396.
86. Saltiel, A.R. and Pessin, J.E. (2002) Insulin signaling pathways in time and space. *Trends Cell Biol.*, **12** (2), 65–71.
87. Vigneri, R., Squatrito, S., and Sciacca, L. (2010) Insulin and its analogs: Actions via insulin and IGF receptors. *Acta Diabetol.*, **47** (4), 271–278.
88. Copps, K.D. and White, M.F. (2012) Regulation of insulin sensitivity by serine/threonine phosphorylation of insulin receptor substrate proteins IRS1 and IRS2. *Diabetologia*, **55** (10), 2565–2582.
89. Avogaro, A., de Kreutzenberg, S.V., and Fadini, G.P. (2010) Insulin signaling and life span. *Pflügers Arch.*, **459** (2), 301–314.
90. Bashan, N., Kovsan, J., Kachko, I., Ovadia, H., and Rudich, A. (2009) Positive and negative regulation of insulin signaling by reactive oxygen and nitrogen species. *Physiol. Rev.*, **89** (1), 27–71.
91. Jensen, M. and De Meyts, P. (2009) Molecular mechanisms of differential intracellular signaling from the insulin receptor. *Vitam. Horm.*, **80**, 51–75.
92. Frojdo, S., Vidal, H., and Pirola, L. (2009) Alterations of insulin signaling in type 2 diabetes: A review of the current evidence from humans. *Biochim. Biophys. Acta*, **1792** (2), 83–92.
93. Aguilar-Bryan, L. and Bryan, J. (1999) Molecular biology of adenosine triphosphate-sensitive potassium channels. *Endocr. Rev.*, **20** (2), 101–135.
94. Petit, P. and Loubatieres-Mariani, M.M. (1992) Potassium channels of the insulin-secreting B cell. *Fundam. Clin. Pharmacol.*, **6** (3), 123–134.

95. Horie, M., Ishida-Takahashi, A., Ai, T., *et al.* (1997) Insulin secretion and its modulation by antiarrhythmic and sulfonylurea drugs. *Cardiovasc. Res.*, **34** (1), 69–72.
96. Henquin, J.C. (2009) Regulation of insulin secretion: A matter of phase control and amplitude modulation. *Diabetologia*, **52** (5), 739–751.
97. Henquin, J.C. (2011) The dual control of insulin secretion by glucose involves triggering and amplifying pathways in beta-cells. *Diabetes Res. Clin. Pract.*, **93** (Suppl. 1), S27–S31.
98. Nicolucci, A. and Rossi, M.C. (2008) Incretin-based therapies: A new potential treatment approach to overcome clinical inertia in type 2 diabetes. *Acta Biomed.*, **79** (3), 184–191.
99. Duhlmeier, R., Deegen, E., Fuhrmann, H., Widdel, A., and Sallmann, H.P. (2001) Glucose-dependent insulinotropic polypeptide (GIP) and the enteroinsular axis in equines (*Equus caballus*). *Comp. Biochem. Physiol. A. Mol. Integr. Physiol.*, **129** (2-3), 563–575.
100. Bamford, N.J., Baskerville, C.L., Harris, P.A., and Bailey, S.R. (2015) Postprandial glucose, insulin, and glucagon-like peptide-1 responses of different equine breeds adapted to meals containing micronized maize. *J. Anim. Sci.*, **93** (7), 3377–3383.
101. de Laat, M.A., McGree, J.M., and Sillence, M.N. (2016) Equine hyperinsulinemia: Investigation of the enteroinsular axis during insulin dysregulation. *Am. J. Physiol. Endocrinol. Metab.*, **310** (1), E61–E72.
102. Ralston, S.L. (2007) Evidence-based equine nutrition. *Vet. Clin. North Am. Equine Pract.*, **23** (2), 365–384.
103. Kasai, H., Hatakeyama, H., Ohno, M., and Takahashi, N. (2010) Exocytosis in islet beta-cells. *Adv. Exp. Med. Biol.*, **654**, 305–338.
104. Geor, R.J. and Harris, P. (2009) Dietary management of obesity and insulin resistance: Countering risk for laminitis. *Vet. Clin. North Am. Equine Pract.*, **25** (1), 51–65, vi.
105. Paulsen, S.J., Jelsing, J., Madsen, A.N., *et al.* (2010) Characterization of beta-cell mass and insulin resistance in diet-induced obese and diet-resistant rats. *Obesity (Silver Spring)*, **18** (2), 266–273.
106. Johnson, P.J., Scotty, N.C., Wiedmeyer, C., Messer, N.T., and Kreeger, J.M. (2005) Diabetes mellitus in a domesticated Spanish mustang. *J. Am. Vet. Med. Assoc.*, **226** (4), 584–588.
107. Park, S.Y. and Bell, G.I. (2009) Noninvasive monitoring of changes in pancreatic beta-cell mass by bioluminescent imaging in MIP-luc transgenic mice. *Horm. Metab. Res.*, **41** (1), 1–4.
108. Schaeffler, A., Gross, P., Buettner, R., *et al.* (2009) Fatty acid-induced induction of toll-like receptor-4/nuclear factor-kappaB pathway in adipocytes links nutritional signalling with innate immunity. *Immunology*, **126** (2), 233–245.
109. Prentki, M. and Nolan, C.J. (2006) Islet beta cell failure in type 2 diabetes. *J. Clin. Invest.*, **116** (7), 1802–1812.
110. Nichols, C.G. and Remedi, M.S. (2012) The diabetic beta-cell: Hyperstimulated vs. hyperexcited. *Diabetes Obesity Metab.*, **14** (Suppl. 3), 129–135.
111. Burns, T.A., Watts, M.R., Geor, R.J., McCutcheon, L.J., and Belknap, J.K. (2011) Evaluation of the response of the endocrine pancreas to short-term high-carbohydrate feeding in mixed breed ponies. Proceedings of the Forum of the American College of Veterinary Internal Medicine.
112. Clemens, T.L. and Karsenty, G. (2011) The osteoblast: An insulin target cell controlling glucose homeostasis. *J. Bone Miner. Res.*, **26** (4), 677–680.
113. de Graaf-Roelfsema, E. (2014) Glucose homeostasis and the enteroinsular axis in the horse: A possible role in equine metabolic syndrome. *Vet. J.*, **199** (1), 11–18.
114. Karsenty, G. and Oury, F. (2012) Biology without walls: The novel endocrinology of bone. *Annu. Rev. Physiol.*, **74**, 87–105.
115. Pi, M. and Quarles, L.I.D. (2013) Novel bone endocrine networks integrating mineral and energy metabolism. *Curr. Osteoporos. Rep.*, **11** (4), 391–399.
116. Lee, N.K. and Karsenty, G. (2008) Reciprocal regulation of bone and energy metabolism. *Trends Endocrinol. Metab.*, **19** (5), 161–166.
117. Fernandez-Real, J.M. and Ricart, W. (2011) Osteocalcin: A new link between bone and energy metabolism. Some evolutionary clues. *Curr. Opin. Clin. Nutr. Metab. Care*, **14** (4), 360–366.
118. Quarles, L.D. (2011) The bone and beyond: 'Dem bones' are made for more than walking. *Nat. Med.*, **17** (4), 428–430.
119. Karsenty, G. and Ferron, M. (2012) The contribution of bone to whole-organism physiology. *Nature*, **481** (7381), 314–320.
120. Oury, F., Ferron, M., Huizhen, W., *et al.* (2013) Osteocalcin regulates murine and human fertility through a pancreas-bone-testis axis. *J. Clin. Invest.*, **123** (6), 2421–2433.
121. Wei, J. and Karsenty, G. (2015) An overview of the metabolic functions of osteocalcin. *Rev. Endocr. Metab. Disord.*, **16** (2), 93–98.
122. Confavreux, C.B., Szulc, P., Casey, R., Varennes, A., Goudable, J., and Chapurlat, R.D. (2014) Lower serum osteocalcin is associated with more severe metabolic syndrome in elderly men from the MINOS cohort. *Eur. J. Endocrinol.*, **171** (2), 275–283.
123. Kim, G.S., Jekal, Y., Kim, H.S., Im, J.A., Park, J.Y., and Chu, S.H. (2014) Reduced serum total osteocalcin is associated with central obesity in Korean children. *Obes. Res. Clin. Pract.*, **8** (3), e201–e298.
124. Kunutsor, S.K., Apekey, T.A., and Laukkanen, J.A. (2015) Association of serum total osteocalcin with type 2 diabetes and intermediate metabolic phenotypes: Systematic review and meta-analysis of observational evidence. *Eur. J. Epidemiol.*, **30** (8), 599–614.
125. Lee, S.W., Jo, H.H., Kim, M.R., Kim, J.H., and You, Y.O. (2015) Association between osteocalcin and metabolic syndrome in postmenopausal women. *Arch. Gynecol. Obstet.*, **292** (3), 673–681.
126. Prats-Puig, A., Osiniri, I., Soriano-Rodriguez, P., *et al.* (2014) Undercarboxylated osteocalcin relates to cardiovascular risk markers in offspring of families with metabolic syndrome. *Atherosclerosis*, **233** (1), 272–277.
127. Im, J.A., Yu, B.P., Jeon, J.Y., and Kim, S.H. (2008) Relationship between osteocalcin and glucose metabolism in postmenopausal women. *Clin. Chim. Acta*, **396** (1-2), 66–69.
128. Buff, P.R., Dodds, A.C., Morrison, C.D., *et al.* (2002) Leptin in horses: Tissue localization and relationship between peripheral concentrations of leptin and body condition. *J. Anim. Sci.*, **80** (11), 2942–2948.
129. Gentry, L.R., Thompson, D.L., Jr, Gentry, G.T., Jr, Davis, K.A., Godke, R.A., and Cartmill, J.A. (2002) The relationship between body condition, leptin, and reproductive and hormonal characteristics of mares during the seasonal anovulatory period. *J. Anim. Sci.*, **80** (10), 2695–2703.
130. Diez, E., Lopez, I., Perez, C., Pineda, C., and Aguilera-Tejero, E. (2012) Plasma leptin concentration in donkeys. *Vet. Q.*, **32** (1), 13–16.

131. Marroqui, L., Gonzalez, A., Neco, P., *et al.* (2012) Role of leptin in the pancreatic beta-cell: Effects and signaling pathways. *J. Mol. Endocrinol.*, **49** (1), R9–R17.
132. Amitani, M., Asakawa, A., Amitani, H., and Inui, A. (2013) The role of leptin in the control of insulin-glucose axis. *Front. Neurosci.*, **7**, 51.
133. Gray, S.L., Donald, C., Jetha, A., Covey, S.D., and Kieffer, T.J. (2010) Hyperinsulinemia precedes insulin resistance in mice lacking pancreatic beta-cell leptin signaling. *Endocrinology*, **151** (9), 4178–4186.
134. Seufert, J. (2004) Leptin effects on pancreatic beta-cell gene expression and function. *Diabetes*, **53** (Suppl. 1), S152–S158.
135. Ebrahimi-Mamaeghani, M., Mohammadi, S., Arefhosseini, S.R., Fallah, P., and Bazi, Z. (2015) Adiponectin as a potential biomarker of vascular disease. *Vasc. Health Risk Manag.*, **11**, 55–70.
136. Tomizawa, A., Hattori, Y., Kasai, K., and Nakano, Y. (2008) Adiponectin induces NF-kappaB activation that leads to suppression of cytokine-induced NF-kappaB activation in vascular endothelial cells: Globular adiponectin vs. high molecular weight adiponectin. *Diabetes Vasc. Dis. Res.*, **5** (2), 123–127.
137. Gordon, M.E., McKeever, K.H., Betros, C.L., and Manso Filho, H.C. (2007) Plasma leptin, ghrelin and adiponectin concentrations in young fit racehorses versus mature unfit standardbreds. *Vet. J.*, **173** (1), 91–100.
138. Wooldridge, A.A., Edwards, H.G., Plaisance, E.P., *et al.* (2012) Evaluation of high-molecular weight adiponectin in horses. *Am. J. Vet. Res.*, **73** (8), 1230–1240.
139. Conti, E., Carrozza, C., Capoluongo, E., *et al.* (2004) Insulin-like growth factor-1 as a vascular protective factor. *Circulation*, **110** (15), 2260–2265.
140. Yuen, K.C. and Dunger, D.B. (2007) Therapeutic aspects of growth hormone and insulin-like growth factor-I treatment on visceral fat and insulin sensitivity in adults. *Diabetes Obesity Metab.*, **9** (1), 11–22.
141. Christensen, R.A., Malinowski, K., Massenzio, A.M., Hafs, H.D., and Scanes, C.G. (1997) Acute effects of short-term feed deprivation and refeeding on circulating concentrations of metabolites, insulin-like growth factor I, insulin-like growth factor binding proteins, somatotropin, and thyroid hormones in adult geldings. *J. Anim. Sci.*, **75** (5), 1351–1358.
142. Takano, A., Haruta, T., Iwata, M., *et al.* (2001) Growth hormone induces cellular insulin resistance by uncoupling phosphatidylinositol 3-kinase and its downstream signals in 3T3-L1 adipocytes. *Diabetes*, **50** (8), 1891–1900.
143. Sesti, G., Sciacqua, A., Cardellini, M., *et al.* (2005) Plasma concentration of IGF-I is independently associated with insulin sensitivity in subjects with different degrees of glucose tolerance. *Diabetes Care*, **28** (1), 120–125.
144. de Laat, M.A., Pollitt, C.C., Kyaw-Tanner, M.T., McGowan, C.M., and Sillence, M.N. (2013) A potential role for lamellar insulin-like growth factor-1 receptor in the pathogenesis of hyperinsulinaemic laminitis. *Vet. J.*, **197** (2), 302–306.
145. Mezi, S., Todi, L., Orsi, E., Angeloni, A., and Mancini, P. (2012) Involvement of the src-cortactin pathway in migration induced by IGF-1 and EGF in human breast cancer cells. *Int. J. Oncol.*, **41** (6), 2128–2138.
146. Abdulla, H., Phillips, B., Smith, K., Wilkinson, D., Atherton, P.J., and Idris, I. (2014) Physiological mechanisms of action of incretin and insulin in regulating skeletal muscle metabolism. *Curr. Diabetes Rev.*, **10** (5), 327–335.
147. Seino, Y., Fukushima, M., and Yabe, D. (2010) GIP and GLP-1, the two incretin hormones: Similarities and differences. *J. Diabetes Investig.*, **1** (1-2), 8–23.
148. Vilsboll, T., Krarup, T., Sonne, J., *et al.* (2003) Incretin secretion in relation to meal size and body weight in healthy subjects and people with type 1 and type 2 diabetes mellitus. *J. Clin. Endocrinol. Metab.*, **88** (6), 2706–2713.
149. USDA-NAHMS (2000) Lameness and laminitis in US horses. United States Department of Agriculture National Animal Health Monitoring System, April (#N318.0400).
150. Burns, T.A., Watts, M.R., Weber, P.S., McCutcheon, L.J., Geor, R.J., and Belknap, J.K. (2014) Effect of dietary nonstructural carbohydrate content on activation of 5'-adenosine monophosphate-activated protein kinase in liver, skeletal muscle, and digital laminae of lean and obese ponies. *J. Vet. Intern. Med.*, **28** (4), 1280–1288.
151. de Laat, M.A., Kyaw-Tanner, M.T., Nourian, A.R., McGowan, C.M., Sillence, M.N., and Pollitt, C.C. (2011) The developmental and acute phases of insulin-induced laminitis involve minimal metalloproteinase activity. *Vet. Immunol. Immunopathol.*, **140** (3-4), 275–281.
152. Zhang, L., Li, J., Young, L.H., and Caplan, M.J. (2006) AMP-activated protein kinase regulates the assembly of epithelial tight junctions. *Proc. Natl Acad. Sci. USA*, **103** (46), 17272–17277.
153. Miranda, L., Carpentier, S., Platek, A., *et al.* (2010) AMP-activated protein kinase induces actin cytoskeleton reorganization in epithelial cells. *Biochem. Biophys. Res. Commun.*, **396** (3), 656–661.
154. Lee, J.H., Koh, H., Kim, M., *et al.* (2007) Energy-dependent regulation of cell structure by AMP-activated protein kinase. *Nature*, **447** (7147), 1017–1020.
155. Jansen, M., Ten Klooster, J.P., Offerhaus, G.J., and Clevers, H. (2009) LKB1 and AMPK family signaling: The intimate link between cell polarity and energy metabolism. *Physiol. Rev.*, **89** (3), 777–798.
156. Asplin, K.E., Curlewis, J.D., McGowan, C.M., Pollitt, C.C., and Sillence, M.N. (2011) Glucose transport in the equine hoof. *Equine Vet. J.*, **43** (2), 196–201.
157. Hardie, D.G. (2011) AMP-activated protein kinase: An energy sensor that regulates all aspects of cell function. *Genes Dev.*, **25** (18), 1895–1908.
158. Takawira, D., Budinger, G.R., Hopkinson, S.B., and Jones, J.C. (2011) A dystroglycan/plectin scaffold mediates mechanical pathway bifurcation in lung epithelial cells. *J. Biol. Chem.*, **286** (8), 6301–6310.
159. Gardner, A.K., Kelly, C.S., Van Eps, A.W., Burns, T.A., Watts, M.R., and Belknap, J.K. (2015) Mitogen-activated kinase pathway activation in epidermal lamellae in the acute stages of carbohydrate overload laminitis models and the effect of regional deep hypothermia on signalling pathways. *Equine Vet. J.*, doi: 10.1111/evj.12488.
160. Burns, T.A., Watts, M.R., Weber, P.S., McCutcheon, L.J., Geor, R.J., and Belknap JK. (2013) Distribution of insulin receptor and insulin-like growth factor-1 receptor in the digital laminae of mixed-breed ponies: An immunohistochemical study. *Equine Vet. J.*, **45** (3), 326–332.

161. Schulman, I.H. and Zhou, M.S. (2009) Vascular insulin resistance: A potential link between cardiovascular and metabolic diseases. *Curr. Hypertens. Rep.*, **11** (1), 48–55.
162. Muniyappa, R. and Yavuz, S. (2013) Metabolic actions of angiotensin II and insulin: A microvascular endothelial balancing act. *Mol. Cell. Endocrinol.*, **378** (1-2), 59–69.
163. Robertson, T.P., Bailey, S.R., and Peroni, J.F. (2009) Equine laminitis: A journey to the dark side of venous. *Vet. Immunol. Immunopathol.*, **129** (3-4), 164–166.
164. Noschka, E., Moore, J.N., Peroni, J.F., Lewis, S.J., Morrow, J.D., and Robertson, T.P. (2009) Thromboxane and isoprostanes as inflammatory and vasoactive mediators in black walnut heartwood extract induced equine laminitis. *Vet. Immunol. Immunopathol.*, **129** (3-4), 200–210.
165. Varewijck, A.J. and Janssen, J.A. (2012) Insulin and its analogues and their affinities for the IGF1 receptor. *Endocr. Relat. Cancer*, **19** (5), F63–F75.
166. Sadagurski, M., Yakar, S., Weingarten, G., *et al.* (2006) Insulin-like growth factor 1 receptor signaling regulates skin development and inhibits skin keratinocyte differentiation. *Mol. Cell. Biol.*, **26** (7), 2675–2687.
167. Lane, H., Watts, M., Geor, R., Burns, T., McCutcheon, L., and Belknap, J. (2013) Laminar growth factor-related signaling in a model of equine metabolic syndrome (EMS) associated laminitis. Proceedings of the 7th International Equine Conference on Laminitis and Diseases of the Foot: West Palm Beach, FL. Poster presentation.
168. Chaisuparat, R., Rojanawatsirivej, S., and Yodsanga, S. (2013) Ribosomal protein S6 phosphorylation is associated with epithelial dysplasia and squamous cell carcinoma of the oral cavity. *Pathol. Oncol. Res.*, **19** (2), 189–193.
169. Mok, K.W., Chen, H., Lee, W.M., and Cheng, C.Y. (2015) rpS6 regulates blood-testis barrier dynamics through Arp3-mediated actin microfilament organization in rat Sertoli cells: An in-vitro study. *Endocrinology*, **156** (5), 1900–1913.
170. Yudkin, J.S., Stehouwer, C.D., Emeis, J.J., and Coppack, S.W. (1999) C-reactive protein in healthy subjects: Associations with obesity, insulin resistance, and endothelial dysfunction: A potential role for cytokines originating from adipose tissue? *Arterioscler. Thromb. Vasc. Biol.*, **19** (4), 972–978.
171. Vick, M.M., Murphy, B.A., Sessions, D.R., *et al.* (2008) Effects of systemic inflammation on insulin sensitivity in horses and inflammatory cytokine expression in adipose tissue. *Am. J. Vet. Res.*, **69** (1), 130–139.
172. Vick, M.M., Adams, A.A., Murphy, B.A., *et al.* (2007) Relationships among inflammatory cytokines, obesity, and insulin sensitivity in the horse. *J. Anim. Sci.*, **85** (5), 1144–1155.
173. Treiber, K., Carter, R., Gay, L., Williams, C., and Geor, R. (2009) Inflammatory and redox status of ponies with a history of pasture-associated laminitis. *Vet. Immunol. Immunopathol.*, **129** (3-4), 216–220.
174. Johnson, P.J., Wiedmeyer, C.E., LaCarrubba, A., Ganjam, V.K., and Messer, N.T., IV (2010) Laminitis and the equine metabolic syndrome. *Vet. Clin. North Am. Equine Pract.*, **26** (2), 239–255.
175. Burns, T.A., Watts, M.R., Weber, P.S., McCutcheon, L.J., Geor, R.J., and Belknap, J.K. (2015) Laminar inflammatory events in lean and obese ponies subjected to high carbohydrate feeding: Implications for pasture-associated laminitis. *Equine Vet. J.*, **47** (4), 489–493.
176. de Laat, M.A., Clement, C.K., McGowan, C.M., Sillence, M.N., Pollitt, C.C., and Lacombe, V.A. (2014) Toll-like receptor and pro-inflammatory cytokine expression during prolonged hyperinsulinaemia in horses: Implications for laminitis. *Vet. Immunol. Immunopathol.*, **157** (1-2), 78–86.
177. Bosma, M., Kersten, S., Hesselink, M.K., and Schrauwen, P. (2012) Re-evaluating lipotoxic triggers in skeletal muscle: Relating intramyocellular lipid metabolism to insulin sensitivity. *Prog. Lipid Res.*, **51** (1), 36–49.
178. Meshkani, R. and Adeli, K. (2009) Hepatic insulin resistance, metabolic syndrome and cardiovascular disease. *Clin. Biochem.*, **42** (13-14), 1331–1346.
179. Lara-Castro, C. and Garvey, W.T. (2008) Intracellular lipid accumulation in liver and muscle and the insulin resistance syndrome. *Endocrinol. Metab. Clin. North Am.*, **37** (4), 841–856.
180. Valera Mora, M.E., Scarfone, A., Calvani, M., Greco, A.V., and Mingrone, G. (2003) Insulin clearance in obesity. *J. Am. Coll. Nutr.*, **22** (6), 487–493.
181. Fernandez-Gamba, A., Leal, M.C., Morelli, L., and Castano, E.M. (2009) Insulin-degrading enzyme: Structure–function relationship and its possible roles in health and disease. *Curr. Pharm. Des.*, **15** (31), 3644–3655.

CHAPTER 19

Dysregulation of the Lamellar Basal Epithelial Cell in Laminitis: Role of the Cytoskeleton and Cell Junctions

Christopher C. Pollitt

Introduction

Changes in the lamellar basal epithelial cell (LBEC), observed in lamellar tissues from experimental and clinical cases of laminitis, suggest that primal laminitis pathophysiology rests with this cell type. The LBEC participates in suspending the distal phalanx (DP) from the stratum internum of the hoof capsule and has tightly regulated attachments to its basement membrane and its lamellar cell neighbors. The integrity of the LBEC and its adhesive properties is critical in determining whether or not the DP will descend into the hoof capsule and lead to clinical laminitis. The LBEC, which is robust and trouble-free in the healthy horse, may be the weak link in the hierarchy of tissues constituting the suspensory apparatus of the distal phalanx (SADP; see Chapter 4), an intact 'chain' counteracting tremendous physical forces that will fail should one 'link' give way.

The first way that LBEC impairment can lead to DP descent is for LBECs to dis-attach from their underlying basement membrane (BM). This well-documented mechanism [1–4] has been best demonstrated with both experimental models (e.g., alimentary carbohydrate overload models; see Chapters 7 and 8) and clinical cases of sepsis-related laminitis (see Chapter 22). The second way that LBEC impairment can likely lead to DP descent is a more recent finding in studies of endocrinopathic laminitis, in which LBECs – and also secondary lamellae – appear to weaken and stretch [5–8].This reportedly leads to attenuation and lengthening of the secondary epidermal lamellae (SEL) without wholesale dis-attachment from the BM but with the same net result – the DP pathologically descends towards the solear dermis. This newly documented mechanism was first associated with hyperinsulinemic laminitis. The LBEC changes overlap between the two mechanisms but, for descriptive purpose, the mechanisms are valid.

The Dysregulated Lamellar Basal Epithelial Cell

Lamellar biopsies taken from horses developing oligofructose (OF)-induced laminitis (the sepsis-related laminitis model) at 12, 18, 24, 30, 36 and 48 h after dosing show, in transverse sections, the timeline of LBEC changes as laminitis lesions develop [3,9]. The earliest change attributable to laminitis is loss of shape and normal arrangement of the lamellar basal and parabasal cells. Many LBEC nuclei become rounded, instead of oval, and attain an abnormal position in the cytoplasm of the cell (Fig. 19.1), relocating from the apex to the base of the cell, close to the BM. Some affected cells retain an oval-shaped nucleus, but the long axis of the nucleus is reoriented parallel to the BM instead of at right-angles to it.

The examination of SELs using transmission electron microscopy (TEM) (Fig. 19.2) at these early stages shows abnormal cell orientation and dislocation of the cytoskeleton, suggesting a sudden inability of the cell to maintain correct shape and tone. Junctions between adjacent cells are likely compromised as cells appear to be sliding over one another and are no longer in stable relationships.

Three important questions regarding the LBEC are: (i) why does the nucleus change shape and position, (ii) why do LBECs change shape, and (iii) why is this significant for laminitis? An initial loss of cell–cell and cell–BM attachments would untether the cytoskeleton, likely destabilizing the LBEC nucleus and causing it to change its shape and position. More profound loss of cell–cell and cell–BM attachments likely further destabilizes the lamellar epidermal–dermal junction, compromising the SADP's ability to counteract the distracting forces of the horse's weight through the DP attachments; this allows the DP to descend in the hoof capsule. The timeline of the lamellar histologic changes

Equine Laminitis, First Edition. Edited by James K. Belknap and Raymond Geor.

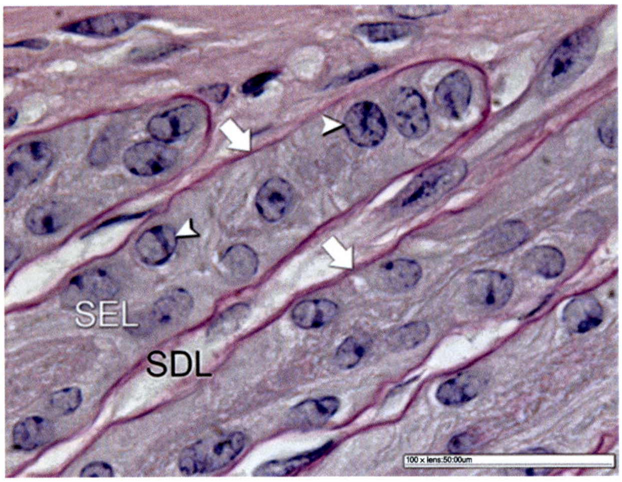

Figure 19.1 Early time point light micrograph of sepsis-related laminitis associated with colitis after carbohydrate overload (oligofructose) in an adult Standardbred (transverse section). Most lamellar basal epithelial cell (LBEC) nuclei (arrowheads) are round, suggesting a perturbation to the LBEC cytoskeleton. Some nuclei remain oval in shape but abnormally oriented in the LBEC cytoplasm; parallel to the basement membrane instead of at right-angles to it. The basement membrane (arrows) is still firmly attached to the perimeter of secondary epidermal lamellae (SEL) suggesting that, despite changes to the cytoskeleton, extensive disruption of hemidesmosomes is yet to occur. However, SELs are narrower than normal and have a stretched attenuated appearance. Periodic acid–Schiff (PAS) staining. Scale bar = 50 μm.

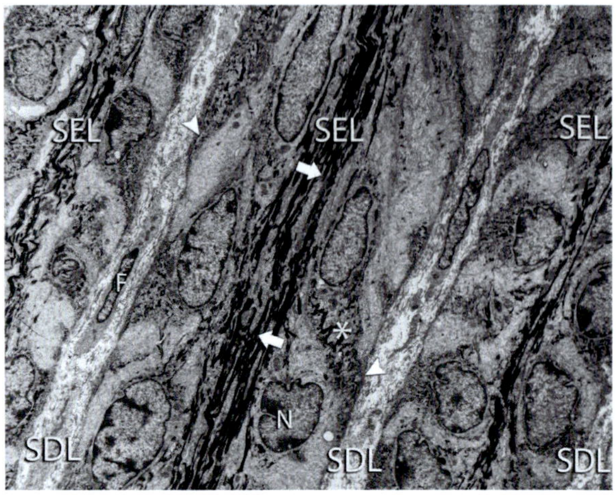

Figure 19.2 Early time point transmission electron micrograph of sepsis-related laminitis associated with colitis after carbohydrate overload (wheat grain starch) in an adult Standardbred (transverse section). There are three secondary epidermal lamellae (SEL), each characterized by central columns of dark-staining desmosomes and tonofilaments within distorted, stretched parabasal cells (arrows). Between the SELs are secondary dermal lamellae (SDLs) containing cells, most likely fibroblasts (F), and bundles of collagen fibrils. The SELs are still bound by an intact basement membrane (arrowheads). Many of the nuclei (N) of the LBECs are round instead of the usual oval shape; those that are still oval are aligned parallel to their basement membrane (BM) instead of at right-angles to it. The basal cell tonofilament cytoskeleton (*) is also misaligned; angled obliquely to the BM instead of the usual 90 degrees. This orientation suggests that the cells are being sheared; the basal cytoskeleton, attached to the BM by hemidesmosomes, appears to be moving differently than the apical cytoskeleton attached to parabasal cells by desmosomes.

in the carbohydrate overload (CHO) model of laminitis, as the histopathology progresses from mild to severe, has been well described and will not be repeated here [1, 3, 10–12]. Laminitis histopathology associated with hyperinsulinemia (HI) has also been described at various time points [5–8, 13–15].

Common to these studies were changes in the dimensions of the SEL, which became longer and narrower [6–8]. HI-induced laminitis in ponies resulted in a doubling of SEL length in some lamellar regions, an increased number of LBEC nuclei per SEL (ca. 12%), and a decreased number of LBECs per micrometer of SEL (ca. 70%). These changes led Karikoski, Patterson-Kane and colleagues to conclude that cell stretching was responsible for the SEL narrowing and elongation [8]. The LBECs were also either proliferating or undergoing apoptosis in significantly increased numbers (Fig. 19.3).

Normally, the intermediate filament (IF) cytoskeleton is 'prosurvival', and protects against apoptosis [16]. Conversely, it participates in apoptosis when damaged. Several IF proteins bind to, and are direct substrates for caspases (the enzymes important in apoptosis). Caspase-mediated cleavage of IFs promotes the timely completion of apoptosis in cultured cells. Apoptosis among SEL keratinocytes is a feature of acute laminitis when induced by CHO, black walnut extract [17], and hyperinsulinemia [6, 8, 17]. Apoptosis and SEL narrowing and stretching occur as early as 6 h post initiation of experimental HI [6] and 12 h post administration of a CHO bolus [9], suggesting

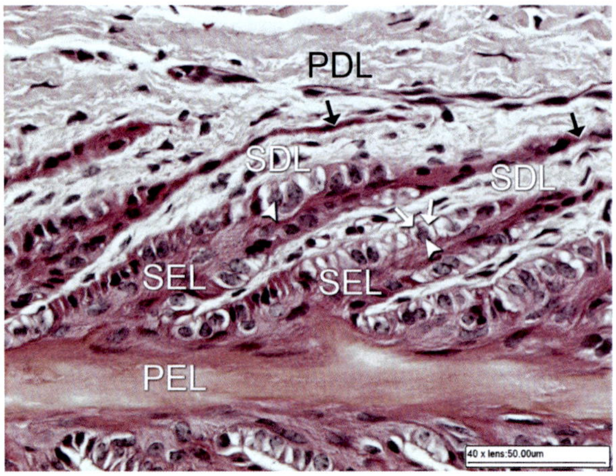

Figure 19.3 Photomicrograph of histopathology induced by 48-h hyperinsulemia in an adult Standardbred (transverse section). Most lamellar epidermal basal cells (LEBCs) have a large area of clear cytoplasm (white arrows) beside the nucleus (arrowheads), bordering the lateral walls of the cells. The keratin intermediate filament cytoskeleton is an eosinophilic band between the nucleus and the basal plasma membrane, suggesting that some hemidesmosomes are still intact. The tips of many SELs are extremely attenuated, stretched into fine threads (black arrows). The LBEC nuclei in the stretched tips are dark and condensed, consistent with apoptosis. PEL, primary epidermal lamella; PDL, primary dermal lamella. H&E staining. Scale bar = 50 μm.

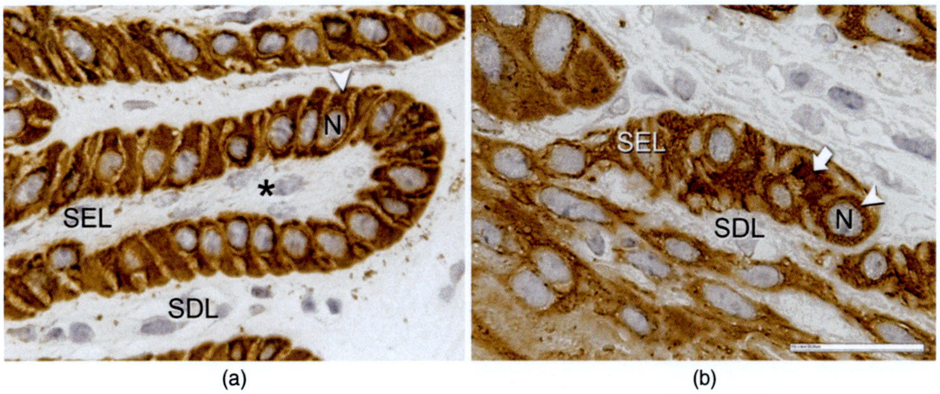

Figure 19.4 Cytokeratin 14 (K14) immunostaining of normal control (a) and laminitis (oligofructose model) -affected (b) LBECs in transverse section. The dark brown positive K14 immunostaining (arrowheads) is exclusive to LBECs; adjacent SEL parabasal cells (asterisk) contain a different cytokeratin and thus stain K14-negative. In control lamellae (a), the K14 intermediate filament (IF) cytoskeleton spans both poles of each cell suspending the oval-shaped nucleus (N) at the apical pole (the pole furthest from the basement membrane) of the basal cell. The IF cytoskeleton is tethered to the basal plasmalemma by hemidesmosomes, and to the apical and lateral plasmalemma by desmosomes (see Chapter 4). In laminitis-affected LBECs (b) the dark-immunostained K14 (arrowhead) is without plasmalemma connections, is condensed around the nucleus (N), and no longer appears to suspend the now rounded nucleus in the cytoplasm. In other LBECs, the cytoskeleton has coalesced in the center of the LBEC (arrow) and is not connected to either the basal plasmalemma or the apical and lateral plasmalemma. Lacking functional attachments between neighboring LBECs and to the basement membrane, the SELs are abnormally narrow and elongated. SEL parabasal cells are absent because they have dis-attached from LBECs and have been left behind. Scale bars = 50 μm.

an early link between cytoskeleton perturbation and apoptosis in models of both sepsis-related and endocrinopathic laminitis.

The authors of a recent report suggested that mechanical factors cause the SEL cell stretching due to unknown processes [8]. However, disruption of regulation of the LBEC cytoskeleton and associated cell adhesion complexes (see Chapter 4), including cytolinker protein depletion, attachment plaque degradation and cytoskeletal collapse, likely explain the sudden LBEC stretching and SEL lengthening. Significant decreases in cytolinker protein and gene expression and associated LBEC cytoskeletal disorganization have recently been reported in both HI- and CHO-induced laminitis [18,19].

Immunostaining for the cytokeratin CK14 of affected LBECs in both the sepsis-related and HI models of laminitis show dramatic IF disorganization [20]. As shown in Figure 19.4, IFs appear to no longer be connected to the plasma membrane but instead were clumped in the center of the cell; the nuclei were round instead of oval and surrounded by a halo of dis-attached IFs (see Fig. 19.4b).

TEMs of the same tissue show degraded desmosomes, absent adherens junctions (AJs; see Chapter 4) and extensive disassociation between LBECs (Fig. 19.5).

In CHO-induced laminitis, regulators of canonical Wnt signaling (see Chapter 15) are expressed predominantly in LBECs in the lamellar milieu. Positive regulators of genes and proteins expressed in the canonical Wnt signaling pathway are profoundly suppressed, whereas negative regulators are, for the most part, elevated [19]. Important to the LBEC actin cytoskeleton, the disruption of Wnt signaling in laminitis is associated with reduced gene and protein expression of β-catenin; in the adherens junction, binding of β-catenin to cadherin is crucial

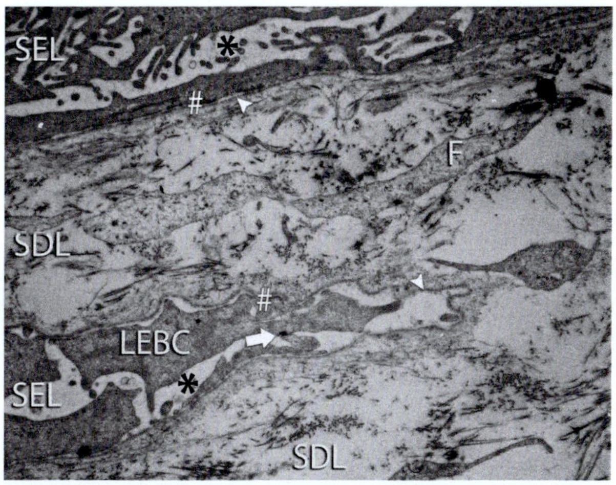

Figure 19.5 Transmission electron micrograph of sepsis-related laminitis associated with colitis after CHO (wheat grain starch) in an adult Standardbred (transverse section). There are two secondary epidermal lamellae (SEL) and two secondary dermal lamellae (SDL) containing fibroblasts (F) and bundles of collagen fibrils. The SEL basement membrane (arrowheads) is visible and close to the basal plasma membrane of lamellar epidermal basal cells (LBECs) in the upper SEL but not the lower SEL. Notably, the lateral boundaries between LBECs (*) are widely separated with few intact attachment plaques. Tonofilaments are absent from LBEC cytoplasm. A single desmosome remnant connects two LBECs (arrow). Where the basement membrane still adjoins LBECs, there are a few faded hemidesmosomes (#) but without attached tonofilaments.

for full adhesive function and, without it, basal cells disassociate from each other [21] (Fig. 19.6).

β-catenin (but not E-cadherin) progressively disappears in immunostained LBECs as CHO-mediated laminitis develops

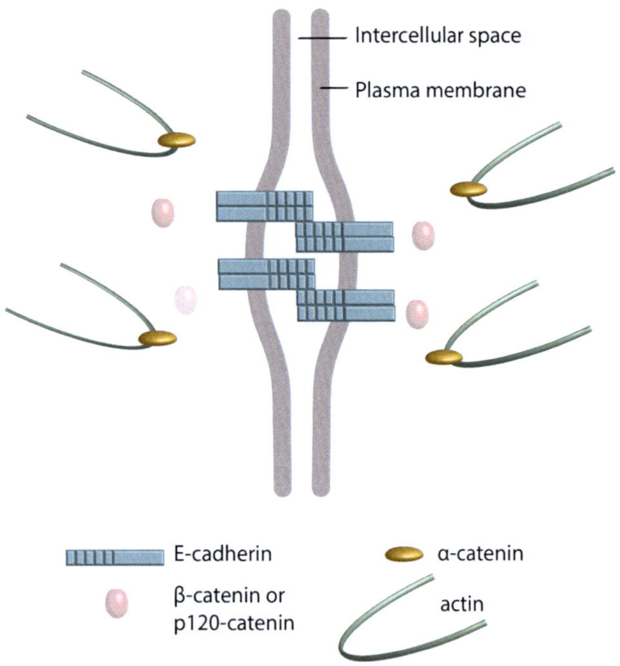

Figure 19.6 Laminitis-affected schematic adherens junction (AJ). β-catenin, the protein linking E-cadherin to the actin bearing α-catenin, disappears as laminitis progresses; this leads to the release and degradation of the actin cytoskeleton (compare to intact AJ in Fig. 4.5; see Chapter 4).

[19]; this diminution in β-catenin coincides with SEL elongation and thinning in the sections of Wang *et al.* (2013), leading to the reasonable conclusion that this event is important in the inevitable degradation of the linked actin cytoskeleton. In further support of this, sections of laminitis-affected lamellae immunostained for actin also show extensive disorganization of the LBEC actin cytoskeleton (Figs 19.7 and 19.8).

Thus, much of the laminitis-associated change in SEL architecture can likely be attributed to the LBEC actin network losing its integrity. Normally elastic (and therefore able to return to their original state after loading) SELs with degraded actin permanently yield to loading and stretch to the thin, elongated configuration characteristic of laminitis pathology. Attendant to SEL thinning and elongation are notable changes to LBEC architecture and connectivity shown by both light (Fig. 19.3) and electron microscopy (Fig. 19.9).

Furthermore, the two types of cell junction responsible for adhesion between adjacent LBECs to each other, AJs and desmosomes, interact with each other. Thus, dysfunctional AJs are associated with the disassembly of desmosomes [22].

Quantitative proteomic analysis of protein components of the desmosome in both the OF and hyperinsulinemia models of experimental laminitis detected significant decreases in the desmosomal proteins desmoplakin, plakoglobin and plakophilin when compared to sham-treated controls [18]. A loss of these desmosome cytolinker proteins untethers IFs from the cell periphery (Fig. 19.10), likely contributing to the observed nuclear rounding and IF accumulation around the nucleus (see Figs 19.1 and 19.4).

Similarly, in laminitis, the reported reduced gene and protein expression of integrin β_4 [19], the integrin in hemidesmosomes (HDs; see Chapter 4) responsible for binding the LBECs to the underlying BM (due to the integrin binding to the Ln 332 anchoring filament in the lamella densa of the BM; Fig. 19.11), also likely contributes to SEL destabilization. Without integrin β_4, Ln 332 anchoring filaments are pulled away from the LBEC basal plasma membrane, allowing the BM to be dragged downwards with the attached lamellar dermis by SADP loading (Figs. 19.12 and 19.13).

Interestingly, the vital BM matrix protein Ln 332 undergoes an epitope-revealing conformational change 12 h after OF

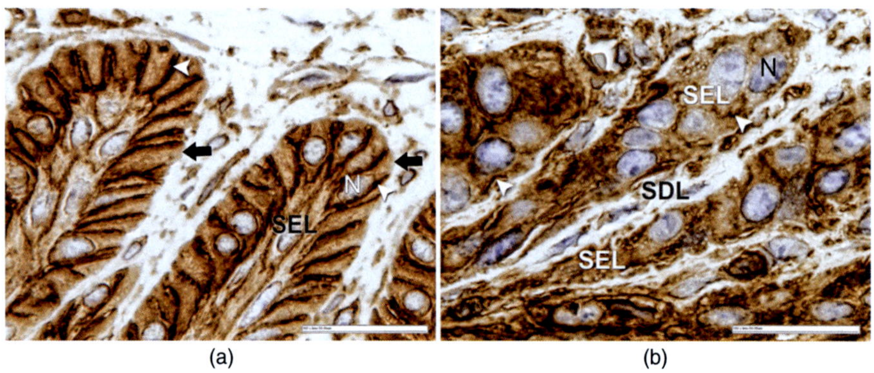

Figure 19.7 Actin immunostaining of normal control (a) and laminitis-affected (oligofructose alimentary overload) (b) lamellar basal epithelial basal cells (LBECs) in transverse section. In normal/control sections (a), actin associates with adherens junctions (the attachment plaques bridging adjacent LBECs). The dark-positive immunostaining (arrowheads) shows actin localized to the lateral and apical plasma membranes (most likely to adherens junctions) of adjacent LBECs. Staining is conspicuously absent at the basal LBEC border which lacks adherens junctions. In laminitis-affected lamellae (b), the normal pattern of actin immunostaining has been obliterated and the boundaries between adjacent LBECs can no longer be distinguished. Disintegration of the adherens junctions has dispersed actin and only remnants of organized actin remain (arrowheads). Lacking functional attachments between LBECs, the SELs are abnormally narrow and elongated. N = LBEC nucleus. Scale bar = 50 μm.

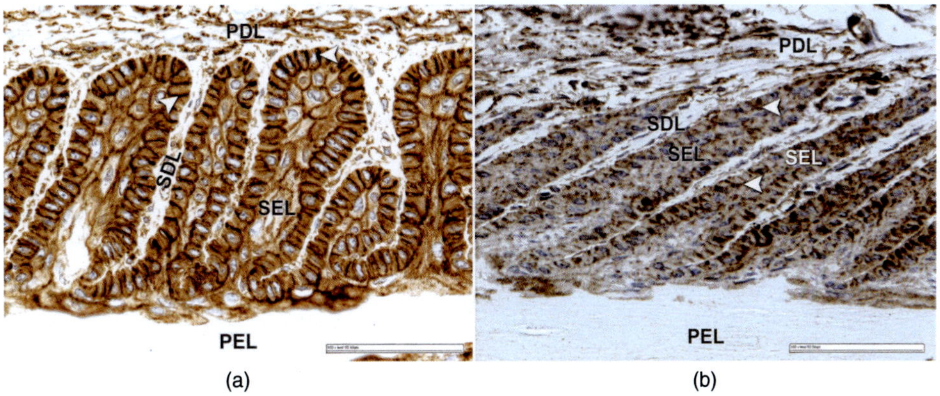

Figure 19.8 Actin immunostaining of normal control (a) and laminitis-affected (hyperinsulinemic–euglycemic clamp model) (b) lamellar basal epithelial cells (LBECs) in transverse section from Standardbred horses. Normally (a), actin associates with adherens junctions; the attachment plaques bridging adjacent LBECs. The dark immunostaining (arrowheads) shows actin localized to the zona adherens in the lateral plasma membranes of adjacent LBECs. In hyperinsulinemia laminitis-affected lamellae (b), the normal pattern of actin immunostaining has been obliterated and the boundaries between adjacent LBECs can no longer be distinguished by actin immunostaining. The disintegration of adherens junctions has dispersed actin and only remnants of organized actin remain (arrowheads). Lacking functional attachments between LBECs, the SELs are abnormally narrow and elongated. Scale bar = 50 μm.

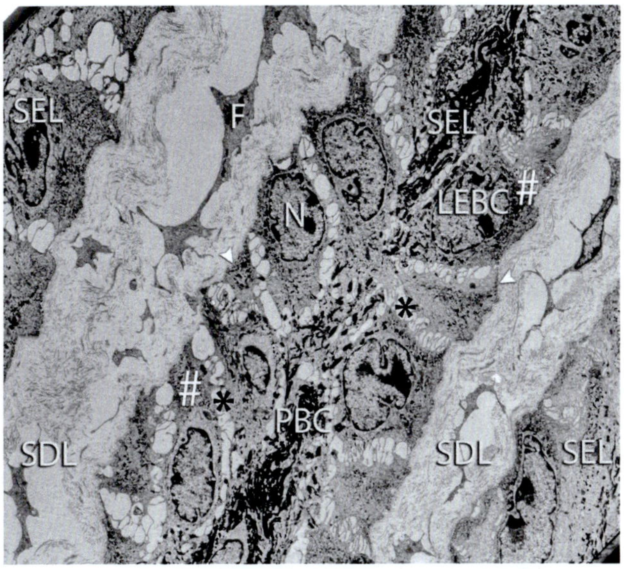

Figure 19.9 Transmission electron micrograph of sepsis-related laminitis associated with colitis after CHO (wheat grain starch) in an adult Standardbred (transverse section). There are three secondary epidermal lamellae (SEL), and between them two secondary dermal lamellae (SDL) containing fibroblasts (F) and wavy bundles of collagen fibrils. The SEL basement membrane (arrowheads) is present and still close to the basal plasma membrane of lamellar basal epithelial cells (LBECs). Some LBEC nuclei (N) are round instead of the usual oval shape, and situated abnormally close to the basement membrane. Notably, the lateral boundaries between LBECs (*) are widely separated with few intact attachment plaques; normally boundaries between the LBECs are plicated and closely joined by adherens junctions and desmosomes. The apices of LBECs, normally tightly joined to parabasal cells (PBC) by numerous desmosomes, are also widely separated. LBEC tonofilaments (#) are clumped and randomly arrayed in the cytoplasm instead of aligned between the nucleus and basement membrane. The overall impression is one of fragility; the SEL cellular cytoskeleton and the adhesion plaque array are compromised leaving the SEL exposed to mechanical stresses against which it is normally resistant.

administration to induce laminitis [3]. The three arms of the cross-shaped Ln 332 molecule are termed alpha, beta, and gamma. An antibody to a section of the gamma arm (D4B5) is unreactive until laminitis develops. The change coincided with decreased immunostaining of collagen IV, the molecular

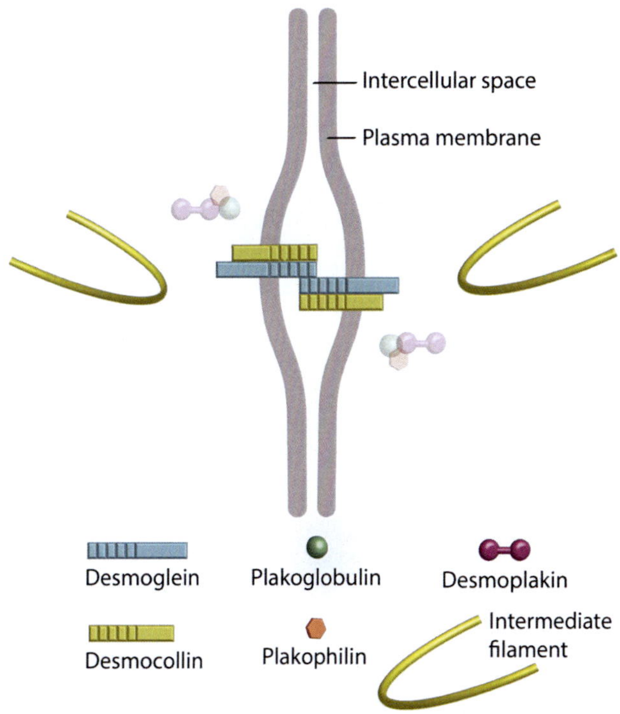

Figure 19.10 Laminitis-affected schematic desmosome (compare to intact desmosomes in Fig. 19.4; see also Chapter 4). In both the OF and hyperinsulinemia models of experimental laminitis there are decreases in the desmosomal proteins, desmoplakin (DP), plakoglobin (PG), and plakophilin (PKP). Without these cytolinker proteins, intermediate filaments (IFs) are untethered from the cell periphery contributing to nuclear rounding and IF accumulation around the nucleus.

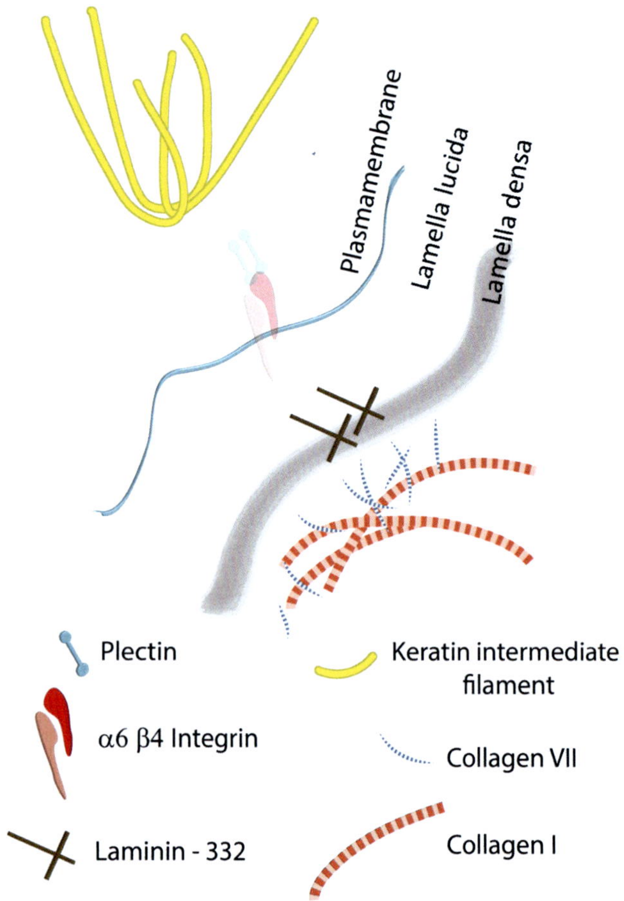

Figure 19.11 Schematic LBEC hemidesmosome affected by laminitis. As the cellular plectin concentration declines, the hemidesmosome disintegrates releasing the keratin intermediate (IF) cytoskeleton into the cytoplasm. Likewise, as the cellular concentration of β_4 integrin declines, the Ln 332 anchoring filament is released from the LBEC plasma membrane, allowing the BM to separate away. Following this the LBEC deforms and separates from the basement membrane.

backbone of the BM. Although Ln 332 was not cleaved, the change occurring to the gamma arm of the molecule may coincide with disruption of linkage to integrin β_4, thus coinciding with its downregulation via dysregulated cellular processes such as occur in the canonical Wnt pathway [19]. Changes to the BM occurred remarkably quickly, prior to the clinical signs of lameness, and much earlier than previously recognized. Changes in the stability of HD attachment at the dermo-epidermal interface, unexplained in 2011 [3] may now be linked to dysregulation of the vital HD component integrin β_4.

Thus, LBEC signaling resulting in a decreased expression of vital components of the HD, such as integrin β_4, may result in lamellar failure due to loss of adhesion of the LBECs to the underlying BM. If the LBEC effector pathways disrupted in laminitis such as the canonical Wnt pathway can be controlled by drug intervention, then loss of protein components of cell adhesion complexes including integrin β_4 of HDs and β-catenins of adherens junctions may result in protection from lamellar failure. A proposed treatment has been the use of agents that inhibit GSK3β (the kinase that causes degradation of β-catenin) and to potentially preserve the adherens junction and associated actin cytoskeleton (S. Black, personal communication). However, especially in endocrinopathic laminitis, it is likely that the stimulation of growth factor signaling cascades such as the ERK 1/2 MAPK cascade and the PI3K/Akt/mTORC1 signaling – both of which are activated by IGF-1 receptor activation by insulin (and both recently established to be activated in the lamellae in the hyperinsulinemia model of endocrinopathic laminitis; J. Belknap, personal communication) – may cause a dysregulation of LBEC adhesion and cytoskeletal signaling through the phosphorylation of HD components (e.g., integrin β_4) [23, 24] and cytoskeletal components [25]. Therefore, LBEC dysregulation of the cytoskeleton and cell adhesion complexes leading to the morphological changes (e.g., stretching) to the epidermal lamellae and disattachment from the underlying BM are likely a combination of decreased expression of vital components of the cell adhesion complexes (e.g., hemidesmosomes and adherens junctions), and direct disruption of these cellular structures through phosphorylation events.

Previously (in 1996), BM separation and degradation was described as the 'hallmark lesion' of laminitis [1], and, during the 20 years since, several studies have sought to explain why. The degree of BM separation (and hence lesion severity) graded against lameness correlated well. Likewise, increasing doses of OF used to induce laminitis via the colitis/sepsis "pathway" in Standardbred horses correlated with increasing lameness and loss of HDs from 4.64 ± 0.15 to 1.75 ± 0.01 per μm of basal plasma membrane [26, 27]. Similar HD loss was associated with experimental HI-induced laminitis in ponies [27]. The authors emphasized the fundamental importance of HDs and speculated that HD disassembly and anchoring filament failure was responsible for BM separation, cytoskeleton failure, and rounding of the basal cell nuclei. Transmission electron microscopy studies show faded HD intracytoplasmic plaques associated with absent tonofilament insertions and BM separation (Fig. 19.12).

In a timeline study of lamellar BM injury in sepsis-related laminitis (OF model), BM changes occurred at 12 h post dosing, much earlier than previously recognized and prior to clinical signs of lameness [3]. In laminitis induced by hyperinsulinemia (HI), gene and protein expression profiles similar to CHO-induced laminitis occur; positive regulators of the canonical Wnt signaling pathway are profoundly suppressed, whereas negative regulators of the pathway, are for the most part, elevated [19]. A quantitative proteomics study of HI laminitis found decreased differential protein expression for components of desmosomes (desmoplakin), hemidesmosomes (plectin), and adherens junctions (β-catenin) at 24 h and 48 h [18, 28].

Not surprisingly, the histopathologies of HI and CHO overload laminitis models have features in common (particularly with regards to SEL narrowing and elongation [7, 8]. In De Laat's (2012) Standardbred horse timeline study, the narrowing of SELs occurred throughout the developmental phase and was present

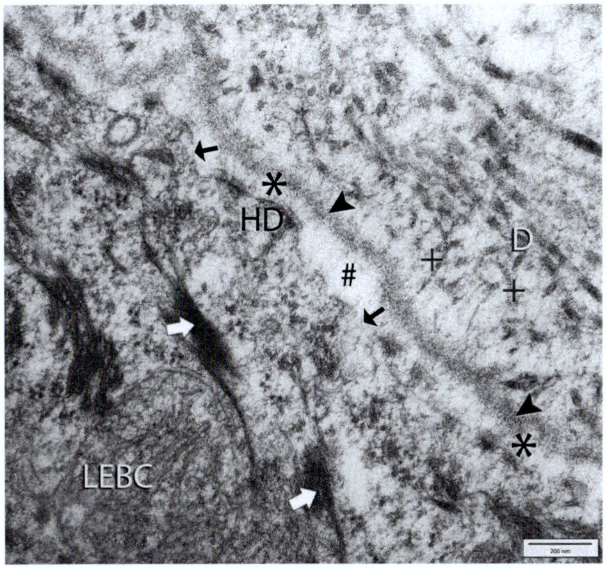

Figure 19.12 Transmission electron micrograph of sepsis-related laminitis associated with proximal enteritis in an adult Australian Stockhorse (transverse section), showing a lamellar basal epithelial cell (LBEC), its basement membrane, and the adjacent dermis (D). The lamella densa of the basement membrane (BM; arrowheads) is a gray line bordering the dermal side of the discontinuous LBEC plasma membrane (small black arrows). Cytoskeletal tonofilaments (large arrows) are clumped in the LBEC cytoplasm some distance from the BM; normally, they associate with BM hemidesmosomes (HD). A few recognizable HDs remain embedded in the plasma membrane, but most are faded remnants without linkage to tonofilaments. HD anchoring filaments span the lamella lucida where HDs are still intact (*) but are absent opposite faded HDs (#). The BM has separated from the LBEC plasma membrane opposite faded, presumably dysfunctional, HDs. The dermal side of the BM is usually characterized by anchoring fibrils and dense bundles of collagen closely associated with the lamella densa; this is largely absent in this section. Curved, banded, anchoring fibrils are present (+), but few are embedded in the lamella densa; most are free amongst the adjacent collagen fibrils. There are collagen fibrils in the dermis with the banding pattern typical of collagen I. Scale bar = 200 nm.

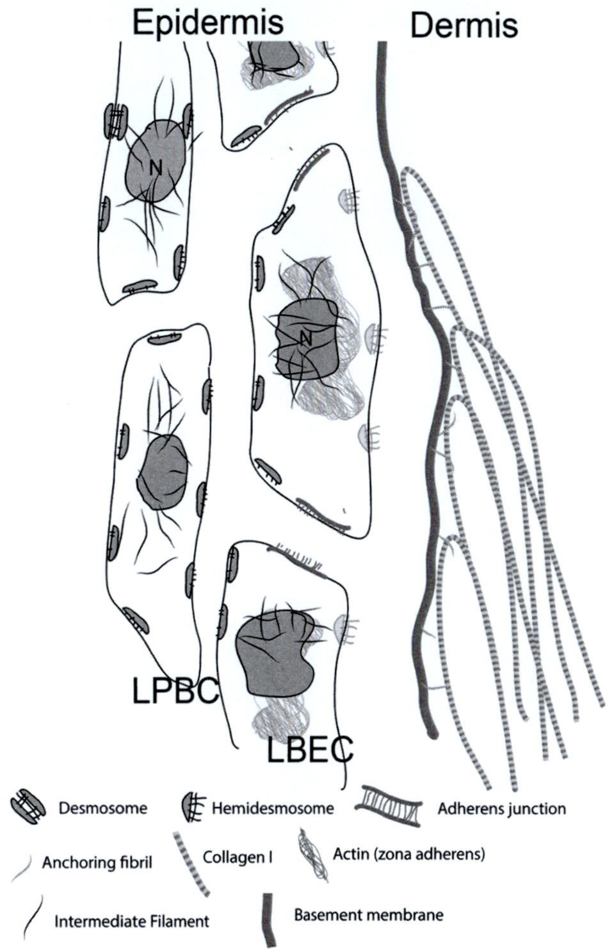

Figure 19.13 Schematic diagram of laminitis-affected cytoskeleton and cell junctions of lamellar basal epithelial cells (LBECs). Compare with normal LEBC cytoskeleton and cell junctions in Figure 4.14. Due to aberrant cell signaling, hemidesmosomes no longer attach LBECs to the basement membrane (BM); cleaved anchoring filaments release the BM and mechanical loading draws it downwards and away. Desmosomes and adherens junctions no longer connect adjacent cells as transmembrane cadherins have been lysed. Keratin intermediate filaments are free in the cytoplasm as links to hemidesmosomes and desmosomes via the cytolinkers plectin and desmoplakin have been degraded. Downregulation of β-catenin disintegrates the link between actin and the adherens junctions, causing the zona adherens to disintegrate. Without functional cell junctions and with weakened attachment to the BM, the LBECs stretch and separate from each other and the BM. LPBC, lamellar parabasal cell; N, nucleus.

between 6 h and 12 h after the onset of hyperinsulinemia [6]. SEL lengthening was concurrent with LBEC deformation and SEL narrowing, and reached significance 48 h after HI onset.

Conclusions

As depicted in Figure 19.13, the LBEC is profoundly changed as laminitis-related pathology casts its shadow over the lamellar interface. Experimental models of Equine Laminitis and studies in other species have confirmed that aberrant cell signaling results in cell junction disassembly, a loss of cell–cell and cell-matrix contacts, and a disruption in overall cell integrity. Ultimately, all of this is due to disorganization of the physical framework of the cell, the cytoskeleton [21,25].

Superimposed on the LBECs undergoing dysregulation in laminitis is an influence that all other epithelial basal cells in the body are spared, namely the distractive forces placed on these cell by weight-bearing. During laminitis induction, all epithelial basal cells in the body are likely influenced by the same circulating factors as the hoof lamellae. However, pathology develops only in LBECs. If LBECs were not subjected to mechanical stress, it is likely that much of the SEL thinning and elongation characteristic of laminitis in the standing horse would not occur. Experiments to determine if unloading during the induction/developmental phase of laminitis ameliorates laminitis pathology have not been conducted. As the LBEC – the cornerstone of the suspensory apparatus of the distal phalanx – is constantly loaded, it is understandable why LBEC dysregulation leads to a downwards dislocation of the distal phalanx, with its attendant signs of clinical laminitis.

Tissue remodeling – the acquisition of a new tissue architecture – is a feature of normal development, growth, and repair [29]. However, as laminitis develops, the LBEC is remodeling when it should not, as if it were receiving signals (e.g., wound healing) from an extraneous source. Laminitis can be associated with organ damage remote from the foot, and perhaps a spillover of wound-healing cytokines, cryptic bioactive fragments, growth factors and enzymes may reach the LBECs, via the blood, to trigger an inappropriate remodeling response. Supporting this premise, similar growth factor signaling, as has been found in epithelial cancer cells with aberrant adhesive properties, has recently been identified in lamellae from a model of metabolic syndrome and also in the traditional starch gruel model of sepsis-related laminitis (J. Belknap *et al.*, unpublished data). Thus, two seemingly disparate causes of laminitis show not only some of the same histologic changes (e.g., stretching of the secondary epidermal lamellae) but also growth factor signaling associated with the disruption of cell adhesion properties in other species. Perhaps the profound efficacy of distal limb cooling is mainly due to a diminution of the effect on the LBECs of intrinsic and extrinsic metabolic enzymes involved in laminitis development. If this were true, then laminitis severity would correlate to foot temperature. Currently, distal limb cooling is efficacious around 4.2–7.7 °C, and it would be interesting to see if lamellar pathology breaks through at incrementally higher temperatures and approaches the grade of pathology that occurs in the control, non-cooled, contralateral feet [30,31].

Recently potent pathogenic metalloproteinases have been discovered in the genome of various bacteria. *Bacteroides fragilis* secretes, from genes on a pathogenicity island, metalloproteinases that attach and cleave cellular E-cadherin and weakens cell–cell contacts *in vitro*. Interestingly, a recent investigation reported E-cadherin behaving as an adherens junction cellular receptor as well as a proteolytic target of the *B. fragilis* secretory metalloproteinases [32]. The genomes of streptococcal species, closely related to those isolated from the hindgut of horses developing oligofructose-induced laminitis (e.g., *Streptococcus equinus* ATCC700338) also secrete metalloproteinases (A. Klieve and G. Milinovich, personal communication), but their role in LBEC dysregulation and laminitis is not yet known.

While some of the participants involved in the progression of laminitis pathology are known (proteases, growth factors, other cytokines, matrix proteins and their fragments), further investigations must be conducted to unravel the multiple interactions involved.

The missing links between what the microscope shows and the observations made at the genetic and protein levels are major obstacles preventing a clear, integrated picture of the laminitis process. Fortunately, new experimental approaches are being rapidly developed that will unravel the complex network of events and enable the development of optimized therapeutic strategies.

References

1. Pollitt, C.C. (1996) Basement membrane pathology: a feature of acute equine laminitis. *Equine Vet. J.*, **28** (1), 38–46.
2. French, K.R. and Pollitt, C.C. (2004) Equine laminitis: cleavage of laminin 5 associated with basement membrane dysadhesion. *Equine Vet. J.*, **36** (3), 242–247.
3. Visser, M.B. and Pollitt, C.C. (2011) The timeline of lamellar basement membrane changes during equine laminitis development. *Equine Vet. J.*, **43** (4), 471–477.
4. Pollitt, C.C. and Daradka, M. (1998) Equine laminitis basement membrane pathology: loss of type IV collagen, type VII collagen and laminin immunostaining. *Equine Vet. J. Suppl.*, **1998** (26), 139–144.
5. Asplin, K.E., Patterson-Kane, J.C., Sillence, M.N., Pollitt, C.C., and McGowan, C.M. (2010) Histopathology of insulin-induced laminitis in ponies. *Equine Vet. J.*, **42** (8), 700–706.
6. de Laat, M.A., Patterson-Kane, J.C., Pollitt, C.C., Sillence, M.N., and McGowan, C.M. (2012) Histological and morphometric lesions in the pre-clinical, developmental phase of insulin-induced laminitis in Standardbred horses. *Vet. J.*, **195**, 305–312.
7. de Laat, M.A., Van Eps, A.W., McGowan, C.M., Sillence, M.N., and Pollitt, C.C. (2011) Equine laminitis: comparative histopathology 48 hours after experimental induction with insulin or alimentary oligofructose in Standardbred horses. *J. Comp. Pathol.*, **145** (4), 399–409.
8. Karikoski, N.P., Patterson-Kane, J.C., Asplin, K.E., McGowan, T.W., McNutt, M., Singer, E.R., *et al.* (2014) Morphological and cellular changes in secondary epidermal laminae of horses with insulin-induced laminitis. *Am. J. Vet. Res.*, **75** (2), 161–168.
9. Croser, E.L. and Pollitt, C.C. (eds) (2006) Acute laminitis: descriptive evaluation of serial hoof biopsies. 52nd Annual Convention of the American Association of Equine Practitioners, San Antonio, Texas, USA.
10. Pollitt, C.C. and Visser, M.B. (2010) Carbohydrate alimentary overload laminitis. *Vet. Clin. North Am. Equine Pract.*, **26** (1), 65–78.
11. Visser, M.B. (2009) Investigation of proteolysis of the basement membrane during the development of equine laminitis. PhD thesis, The University of Queensland, Brisbane.
12. Visser, M.B. and Pollitt, C.C. (2012) The timeline of metalloprotease events during oligofructose induced equine laminitis development. *Equine Vet. J.*, **44**, 88–93.
13. De Laat, M.A., McGowan, C.M., Sillence, M.N., and Pollitt, C.C. (2010) Equine laminitis: Induced by 48 h hyperinsulinaemia in Standardbred horses. *Equine Vet. J.*, **42**, 129–135.
14. De Laat, M.A., McGowan, C.M., Sillence, M.N., and Pollitt, C.C. (2010) Hyperinsulinemic laminitis. *Vet. Clin. North Am. Equine Pract.*, **26** (2), 257–264.
15. Karikoski, N.P., McGowan, C.M., Singer, E.R., Asplin, K.E., Tulamo, R.M., and Patterson-Kane, J.C. (2015) Pathology of natural cases of equine endocrinopathic laminitis associated with hyperinsulinemia. *Vet. Pathol.*, **52** (5), 945–956.
16. Coulombe, P.A. and Wong, P. (2004) Cytoplasmic intermediate filaments revealed as dynamic and multipurpose scaffolds. *Nat. Cell Biol.*, **6** (8), 699–706.
17. Faleiros, R.R., Stokes, A.M., Eades, S.C., Kim, D.Y., Paulsen, D.B., and Moore, R.M. (2004) Assessment of apoptosis in epidermal lamellar cells in clinically normal horses and those with laminitis. *Am. J. Vet. Res.*, **65** (5), 578–585.

18. Galantino-Homer, H.L., Johnson, P.J., Engiles, J.B., Pollitt, C.C., Linardi, R.L., Megee, S., *et al.* (2013) Loss of lamellar epidermal cytolinker and desmosomal proteins: Does it contribute to the failure of the suspensory apparatus of the distal phalanx in equine laminitis? *J. Equine Vet. Sci.*, **33** (10), 849–851.
19. Wang, L., Pawlak, E.A., Johnson, P.J., Belknap, J.K., Eades, S., Stack, S., *et al.* (2013) Impact of laminitis on the canonical wnt signaling pathway in basal epithelial cells of the equine digital laminae. *PLoS One*, **8** (2), e56025.
20. Pollitt, C.C. (2015) Laminitis, in *The Illustrated Horse's Foot*, 1st edition. Elsevier Health Sciences, St Louis, Missouri, pp. 177–222.
21. D'Souza-Schorey, C. (2015) Disassembling adherens junctions: breaking up is hard to do. *Trends Cell Biol.*, **15** (1), 19–26.
22. Gliem, M., Heupel, W.M., Spindler, V., Harms, G.S., and Waschke, J. Actin reorganization contributes to loss of cell adhesion in pemphigus vulgaris. *Am. J. Physiol. Cell Physiol.*, **299** (3), C606–C613.
23. Wilhelmsen, K., Litjens, S.H., Kuikman, I., Margadant, C., van Rheenen, J., and Sonnenberg, A. (2007) Serine phosphorylation of the integrin beta4 subunit is necessary for epidermal growth factor receptor induced hemidesmosome disruption. *Mol. Biol. Cell*, **18** (9), 3512–3522.
24. Frijns, E., Kuikman, I., Litjens, S., Raspe, M., Jalink, K., Ports, M., *et al.* (2012) Phosphorylation of threonine 1736 in the C-terminal tail of integrin beta4 contributes to hemidesmosome disassembly. *Mol. Biol. Cell*, **23** (8), 1475–1485.
25. Brosnan, R.J., Steffey, E.P., Esteller-Vico, A., Vaughan, B., and Liu, I.K. (2011) The relationship between digital perfusion pressure and hoof lamellar blood flow in isoflurane-anesthetized horses. *Res. Vet. Sci.*, **90** (1), 138–145.
26. French, K.R. and Pollitt, C.C. (2004) Equine laminitis: loss of hemidesmosomes in hoof secondary epidermal lamellae correlates to dose in an oligofructose induction model: an ultrastructural study. *Equine Vet. J.*, **36** (3), 230–235.
27. Nourian, A.R., Baldwin, G.I., Van Eps, A.W., and Pollitt, C.C. (2007) Equine laminitis: ultrastructural lesions detected 24–30 hours after induction with oligofructose. *Equine Vet. J.*, **39**, 360–364.
28. Galantino-Homer, H., Carter, R., Linardi, R., Megee, S., Engiles, J., de Laat, M., *et al.* (2011) The big picture: using quantitative proteomics to investigate laminitis pathophysiology. *J. Equine Vet. Sci.*, **31** (10), 583–584.
29. Moali, C. and Hulmes, D.J.S. (2009) Extracellular and cell surface proteases in wound healing: new players are still emerging. *Eur. J. Dermatol.*, **19** (6), 552–564.
30. Van Eps, A.W., Leise, B.S., Watts, M., Pollitt, C.C., and Belknap, J.K. (2012) Digital hypothermia inhibits early lamellar inflammatory signalling in the oligofructose laminitis model. *Equine Vet. J.*, **44** (2), 230–237.
31. Van Eps, A.W., Pollitt, C.C., Underwood, C., Medina-Torres, C.E., Goodwin, W.A., and Belknap, J.K. (2014) Continuous digital hypothermia initiated after the onset of lameness prevents lamellar failure in the oligofructose laminitis model. *Equine Vet. J.*, **46** (5), 625–630.
32. Remacle, A.G., Shiryaev, S.A., and Strongin, A.Y. (2014) Distinct interactions with cellular E-cadherin of the two virulent metalloproteinases encoded by a *Bacteroides fragilis* pathogenicity island. *PLoS One*, **9** (11), e113896.

CHAPTER 20

Structural Dynamics of Displacement of the Distal Phalanx

Andrew H. Parks

Introduction

The structural dynamics of displacement of the distal phalanx are the result of the complex interaction of biological processes and biomechanics. Three patterns of displacement of the distal phalanx are currently recognized: rotation; symmetrical distal displacement; and asymmetrical (uniaxial/unilateral) distal displacement. In most horses that develop displacement of the distal phalanx, the pattern is likely to be a combination of the three, though frequently one pattern may appear to be dominant. The structure and function of the digit have been discussed in Chapters 3 and 4; a brief review and closer examination of the attachment of the distal phalanx to the hoof capsule holds potential answers as to why these different displacements occur.

The equine hoof serves both the normal functions of skin and as an extension of the musculoskeletal system. Weight is transmitted from the distal phalanx to the hoof capsule through its soft tissue attachments, and thence to the ground. The weight of the horse is opposed by the ground reaction force (GRF) that acts through the center of pressure. The forces acting on the forelimb distal phalanx and its associated ungual cartilages during weight-bearing are therefore the weight borne by the limb acting through the center of rotation of the distal interphalangeal joint, tension in the deep digital flexor and common digital extensor tendons, and components of the ground reaction force exerted through the lamellae and the sole (this is discussed further in Chapters 3 and 5; see also Fig. 41.1a and b in Chapter 41). In the healthy horse, the GRF has been extensively studied, though it is unknown how much of the GRF is exerted through the lamellae and how much through the sole. Similarly, the force in the deep digital flexor tendon has been extensively examined in horses at rest and in motion; most models assume that there is very little tension in the common digital extensor tendon during weight-bearing by the limb. The force directed distally through the center of rotation of the distal interphalangeal joint is equal to the weight borne by the limb. How these forces change during the development of displacement of the distal phalanx (i.e., between the time of initial injury to the lamellae and the time of distal phalanx displacement) is unknown.

Movement of the distal phalanx in the sagittal plane about the distal interphalangeal joint is determined by the moments generated by the dorsopalmar position of the ground reaction force and the tension in the deep digital flexor tendon (see Fig. 41.1a). Movement of the distal phalanx in the dorsal plane is normally regulated by the mediolateral position of the ground reaction force and the collateral ligaments (see Fig. 41.1b). Why the different patterns of displacement occur is unknown. However, some statements regarding the biomechanical events associated with displacement can be made. In order for rotation of the distal phalanx about the distal interphalangeal joint to occur, the flexor moment about that joint must exceed the extensor moment. When symmetrical distal displacement occurs, the distal phalanx moves distally in the hoof capsule while the normal phalangeal axis is maintained (i.e., there is no flexion of the distal interphalangeal joint, and the dorsal aspect of the distal phalanx remains parallel to the dorsal hoof wall). In order for this to occur, the structures that support the distal phalanx within the hoof capsule must fail in such a manner that the flexor and extensor moments about the distal interphalangeal joint remain equal during the displacement process. Movement in the dorsal plane (see Fig. 41.1b) is not affected by tendons, but any change in ground reaction force in the dorsal plane to one side (i.e., medial or lateral) will create a moment that causes the distal phalanx to move slightly proximally and abaxially on that side (this is sometimes referred to as *collateromotion*) and distally and axially on the opposite side until further movement is opposed passively by the contralateral collateral ligaments and intact lamellae.

In the healthy horse, the attachments of the distal phalanx to the hoof capsule greatly exceed the stresses imposed on them by normal weight-bearing and movement; in fact, this bond is so tight that the hoof and distal phalanx are frequently considered a single biomechanical unit. Without disruption of the normal lamellar attachments of the hoof capsule to the distal phalanx in horses with laminitis, displacement would not occur. Given

Equine Laminitis, First Edition. Edited by James K. Belknap and Raymond Geor.

that it is unknown why different types of displacement occur, the potential reasons that different patterns of displacement occur can be outlined as:

- Variations in the distribution of lamellar injury.
- Variations in the distribution of forces imposed on the lamellae.
- A combination of the above.

This is complicated by the fact that there is more than one pathway by which the disease occurs (e.g., the pathologic/lamellar events associated with sepsis-associated laminitis appear to be different to that of endocrinopathic laminitis). Anecdotally, one pathway may be more likely to be associated with one type of displacement (e.g., clinicians frequently associate sepsis with symmetrical distal displacement) but again, documentation is lacking. Furthermore, there may be details about other factors such as the origin and distribution of the lamellar blood supply that may influence the outcome. It is unfortunate that no more is known about the distribution of lamellar injury, particularly during the early stages of the disease. However, one post-mortem study of horses with acute laminitis that compared magnetic resonance imaging (MRI) to radiographic imaging supports the premise that the dorsal lamellae are more at risk of separation than more palmar-located lamellae; these investigators found that MRI demonstrated an extensive separation of the dorsal lamellae but not the lamellae of the quarters or heels in animals not exhibiting displacement of the distal phalanx on digital radiography [1].

While bearing the previously mentioned uncertainties in mind, it is pertinent to review the structure of the attachment of the distal phalanx to the hoof capsule. Overall, the folding of the primary and secondary lamellae greatly increases the area of contact between the epidermis and underlying dermis, giving greater strength to the bond between the two. The strength of the normal lamellar attachment itself is dependent on the number of lamellae, the lamellar surface area, and the orientation of the lamellae around the circumference of the foot. Based on the shape of the hoof, it is clear that the macroscopic area of the parietal dermal–epidermal junction is greatest dorsally. Microscopically, the density of lamellae is greatest dorsally (which would also support a greater strength of attachment dorsally) [2]. However, the biomechanical properties of the lamellar junction do not appear to vary with either the circumferential or proximodistal location within the hoof, indicating that the strength of the attachment of the hoof per unit area is approximately the same around the circumference of the hoof [3]. Lastly, dorsally the parietal integument overlies the distal phalanx, whereas in the palmar half of the foot a significant proportion of the parietal integument (i.e., the lamellar integument) overlies the ungual cartilages. The difference in the flexibility of the underlying cartilage and the distal phalanx is likely to influence the loading pattern of the lamellae in those locations, but this point has not been investigated. It is generally considered that the lamellae suspend the distal phalanx within the hoof capsule [4, 5] and the role of the sole in directly supporting the distal phalanx is likely to be minimal in the normal horse. Clinical evidence indicates that it is possible to remove the entire sole, such that the distal phalanx is supported only by the wall, and the horse can stand relatively comfortably on a flat firm surface. However, if most of the wall is lost, such that the horse is standing on a flat firm surface bearing weight on its dorsal sole, it is likely to be much more lame. Consideration must also be given to the role the deep digital flexor tendon plays in suspending the distal phalanx within the hoof capsule. The deep digital flexor tendon does not bear weight *per se*, but it functions to lift/hold up the palmar aspect of the distal phalanx. In doing so it moves the center of pressure dorsally in relation to the center of rotation.

The nature of the forces on the ground surface of the hoof capsule have been studied in normal horses, and to a lesser extent in laminitic ponies. At rest, the weight borne by each forelimb is approximately 28% of the horse's weight. Although many studies of biomechanics of the equine foot are performed at the trot, the gait most relevant to the clinical equine patient with laminitis is the walk. At the walk, the peak force sustained by one forelimb occurring during the support phase of the stride is approximately 66% of the body weight in a healthy horse [6]. During peak loading, the center of pressure is near the center of the foot, so that the stresses associated with weight-bearing under these circumstances are approximately symmetrically distributed around the circumference of the foot. The overall magnitude of the stresses at impact and breakover are of a lesser magnitude than those during the support phase (due to the fact that the foot is not fully loaded at impact, and is already being unloaded at breakover), but both are also potentially injurious. Impact is associated with shockwaves that may both enhance injury and cause pain. At breakover, the center of pressure is at the toe, which means that, even though the overall force on the distal limb is much lower than during the support phase of the stride, breakover may be associated with a spike in load at the toe and therefore a corresponding spike in stress on the dorsal lamellae. In summary, the relative importance of the weight-bearing at rest and the events during the stride in the development of distal phalanx displacement in laminitis are undetermined. However, it is highly likely that weight-bearing at rest and during the support phase of the stride at a walk are the most important points in the development of displacement of the distal phalanx in this disease.

The following is a summary of the known biomechanical changes that are present in horses with laminitis (based on horses in which only the forelimbs are affected). It is reported that, in the acute stage of the disease, the weight borne by the forelimbs does not change, though there are changes in the frequency with which the horse shifts its weight [7]. In the chronic stage of the disease, the same authors reported a slight decrease in weight borne by the forelimbs [7]. Additionally, at least in ponies in the chronic stage of the disease, the center of pressure and force in the deep digital flexor tendon were found to be altered in another study [8]. Specifically, the ground reaction force is reportedly palmar to the center of rotation, and therefore the force in the deep digital flexor tendon is very low during the first 30% of the stride. The authors postulated that this is due to rotation of the distal phalanx with subsequent shortening of the deep digital flexor tendon; however, presumably the increased heel height in horses with rotational displacement of the distal phalanx with chronic laminitis might also contribute to this change in dynamics. An increased tension in the common digital extensor tendon in response to pain might also increase the extensor moment in relation to the flexor moment. However, these circumstances are quite different to those present in the acute stages of the disease.

To return to consideration of the different types of displacement in light of the distribution of injury versus the distribution of force on the lamellae, there may be a few clues available but they are indeed limited. With respect to the distribution of injury, the severity of regional disruption of the lamellae is relatively easy to observe once displacement has occurred, but there is no evidence about the distribution of injury prior to that and, clearly, using the former as a guide to the distribution of injury is comparable to a self-fulfilling prophesy. Examining the distribution of force as a factor in determining displacement is complicated by the fact that it changes with locomotion. That said, most laminitic horses are relatively stationary for the majority of time. Conformation and tension in the deep digital flexor tendon both have the potential to change the center of pressure and hence the distribution of force within the lamellae. For example, if the conformation of the limb places the foot significantly abaxial to the median plane of the limb, the side closest to the median plane is likely to be subject to a greater load than the opposite side. Similarly, changes in tension in the deep digital flexor tendon will alter the dorsopalmar location of the center of pressure. As previously stated, deep digital flexor tendon tension does change in horses with chronic laminitis, but it is also conceivable that a horse responds to pain in the acute phase of the disease by actively changing the tension in its deep digital flexor tendons.

Events Associated with Displacement

It seems relative easy to understand the events associated with rotation of the distal phalanx (Figs 20.1a and b). The majority of the digital lamellae are dorsal to the center of rotation of the distal phalanx, as is the center of pressure. Therefore, uniform damage to the lamellae would suggest a greater injury dorsal to the center of rotation so that the ground reaction force is no longer sufficient to oppose the moment generated by the deep digital flexor tendon, and rotation ensues.

It is widely assumed that symmetrical distal displacement (Figs 20.1c and d) results from a symmetrical loss of support of the distal phalanx around the circumference of the foot. Clinically, the depression that occurs at the coronary band appears to be symmetrical around the circumference of the foot. However, this is likely a significant oversimplification because there are more lamellae dorsal to the center of rotation than palmar to it. Therefore, it is more difficult to understand the events associated with symmetrical distal displacement because the detachment of the lamellae must occur in a manner such that the extensor moment equals the flexor moment during the process. This implies that the expected decrease in the extensor moment is matched by a decrease in the flexor moment, or that the extensor moment is maintained by support for the distal phalanx by tissues other than the lamellae. Neither is easy to comprehend. If the tension in the deep digital flexor tendon does not decrease, then either there is greater loss of lamellar support of the distal phalanx per unit area within the palmar lamellae than the dorsal lamellae, or some other structure – namely, the sole or common digital extensor tendon – are contributing to the extensor moment. Alternatively, a decrease in the flexor moment could occur because of postural accommodation or active relaxation of the tendon (the latter seems implausible because the accessory ligament of the deep digital flexor tendon would be expected to be limiting). While these are the most logical reasons for this to occur given the current understanding of the disease and digital biomechanics, none is easy to comprehend occurring and other unconsidered factors may be at play.

Asymmetrical displacement of the distal phalanx (Figs 20.1e and f) – either medial or lateral – is best explained either by a primary asymmetrical distribution of injury or an asymmetrical distribution of load. Anecdotal clinical experience suggests that this occurs most frequently on the medial side, and that it occurs most frequently in horses with outward rotation of the limb (i.e., 'toed-out' conformation). Intuitively, the latter would result in greater load on the medial side of the foot, and the increased load on the medial side would explain medial displacement under circumstances of uniform distribution of the underlying injury. However, asymmetrical distribution of the underlying injury cannot be eliminated as a cause of asymmetrical displacement.

Significance of the Pattern of Displacement

The importance of understanding the differences between the patterns is at least in part because the treatment for the various types of displacement will differ. Currently, predicting which pattern of lamellar disruption will occur before it is clinically evident is not possible. However, given that there is evidence in horses with acute laminitis that the degree of pain is indicative of the severity of lamellar injury, the deliberate manipulation of the center of pressure may provide some clues. Specifically, a horse exhibiting severe lameness due to laminitis but showing no evidence of displacement of the distal phalanx might be treated with marked heel elevation so as to move the center of pressure in a palmar direction towards the center of rotation of the distal interphalangeal joint. Then, if the lameness improves it might reasonably be inferred that the horse is predisposed to rotation of the distal phalanx. Conversely, if this maneuver makes the horse markedly worse, the animal may be predisposed to distal

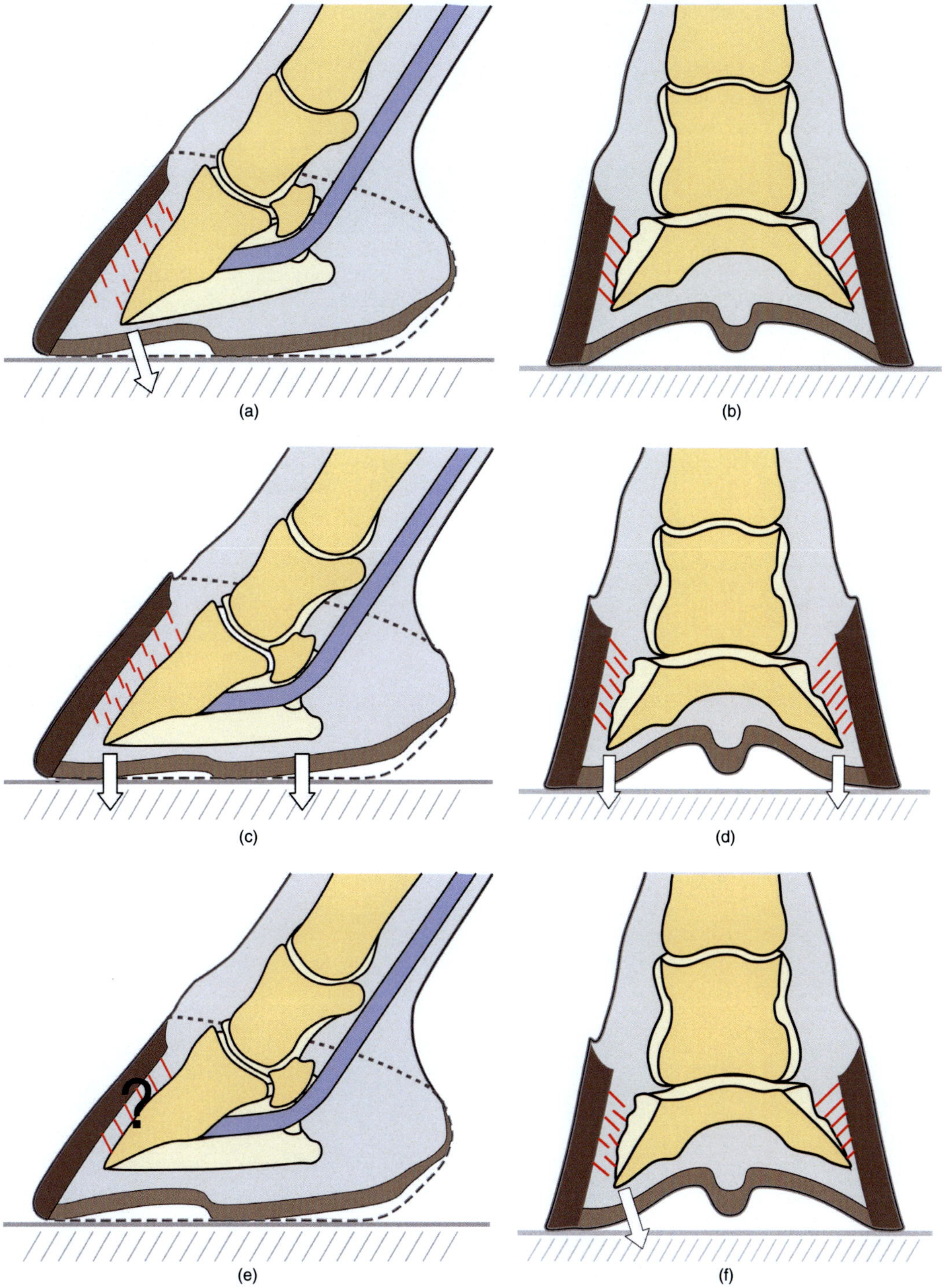

Figure 20.1 Three different patterns of displacement of the distal phalanx are recognized, but it is common, for them to occur in combination in instances of distal displacement, either symmetrical or asymmetrical, where they are commonly associated with a lesser degree of rotation. In horses with dorsal rotation, failure of the lamellae supporting the distal phalanx is greatest dorsally, while the heels may be relatively unaffected (panels a and b). In horses with symmetric distal displacement (panels c and d) disruption of the lamellae supporting the distal phalanx appears to occur around the circumference of the foot. In horses with asymmetrical distal displacement (panels e and f), lamellar failure is principally at one quarter or the other, most frequently the medial quarter; on the side that has been displaced the solear margin of the distal phalanx is displaced distally, the joint space opens ipsilaterally and is compressed contralaterally, and the hoof (wall and underlying soft tissues) appears wider than the contralateral side; it is seemingly inevitable that there is also some damage to the dorsal lamellae associated with unilateral distal displacement though the extent is variable (variability is represented by a ? in this image). Illustration courtesy of Andrew Parks, University of Georgia, Athens, GA, USA.

displacement/sinking (either symmetrically or asymmetrically) because this maneuver has increased the stress in areas where the damage is greatest. Similarly, if a horse whose conformation suggests a predisposition to asymmetrical sinking is treated by shifting the center of pressure away from the side closest to the medial plane of the limb and the lameness improves, it supports the original clinical supposition.

In a chapter such as this, reliance has been placed on the combination of basic biomechanical principles, experience, and anecdotal evidence to too great an extent due to a lack of scientific information about the specifics concerning the manner in which the effects of the disease are distributed, and about the role of the sole and the lamellae in supporting the digit within the hoof capsule. Ongoing research should provide the opportunities to fully test many of these possibilities.

References

1. Arble, J.B., Mattoon, J.S., Drost, W.T., Weisbrode, S.E, Wassenaar, P.A., Pan, X., *et al.* (2009) Magnetic resonance imaging of the initial active stage of equine laminitis at 4.7 T. *Vet. Radiol. Ultrasound*, **50** (1), 3–12.
2. Douglas, J. and Thomason, J. (2000) Shape, orientation and spacing of the primary epidermal laminae in the hooves of neonatal and adult horses (*Equus caballus*). *Cells Tiss. Org.*, **166** (3), 304–318.
3. Douglas, J., Biddick, T., Thomason, J., and Jofriet, J. (1998) Stress/strain behaviour of the equine laminar junction. *J. Exp. Biol.*, **201** (15), 2287–2297.
4. Pollitt, C.C. (1998) The anatomy and physiology of the hoof wall. *Equine Vet. Educ.*, **10** (6), 318–325.
5. Pollitt, C.C. and Collins, S.N. (2016) The suspensory apparatus of the distal phalanx in normal horses. *Equine Vet. J.*, **48** (4), 496–501.
6. Merkens, H.W. and Schamhardt, H.C. (1988) Distribution of ground reaction forces of the concurrently loaded limbs of the Dutch Warmblood horse at the normal walk. *Equine Vet. J.*, **00**, 00–00.
7. Hood, D.M., Wagner, I.P., Taylor, D.D., Brumbaugh, G.W., and Chaffin, K. (2001) Voluntary limb-load distribution in horses with acute and chronic laminitis. *Am. J. Vet. Res.*, **62** (9), 1393–1398.
8. McGuigan, M.P., Walsh, T.C., Pardoe, C.H., Day, P.S., and Wilson, A.M. (2010) Deep digital flexor tendon force and digital mechanics in normal ponies and ponies with rotation of the distal phalanx as a sequel to laminitis. *Equine Vet. J.*, **37** (2), 161–165.

PART 3

Clinical Presentation of Equine Laminitis

Equine Laminitis, First Edition. Edited by James K. Belknap and Raymond Geor.

CHAPTER 21
General Clinical Aspects of the Laminitis Case

Andrew van Eps

Introduction

There is wide variation in the history and clinical presentation of horses and ponies with laminitis. Classically, laminitis may be the primary presenting complaint or presumptive diagnosis in a horse with characteristic lameness in multiple limbs. Horses with severe laminitis may even present as being recumbent and unable to rise, with the owners, trainers, or equine health professionals suspecting other musculoskeletal or neurologic causes for the recumbency. In contrast, radiographic changes consistent with laminitis may also be found incidentally in a horse that has no history of overt lameness, making laminitis an important consideration when examining horses for pre-purchase purposes or even loss of performance.

The link between obesity and insulin resistance (IR; now commonly termed insulin dysregulation) and access to high levels of nonstructural carbohydrate in pasture has been established during recent years, and this scenario appears to account for most cases of laminitis worldwide [1–4]. Although these cases can be severe, mild chronic laminitis is most commonly the result, leading to a low-grade lameness and loss of performance in athletic horses. Laminitis still limits our ability to successfully treat horses with other predisposing causes of laminitis such as systemic illness (particularly sepsis) [5] and painful limb conditions such as fractures or synovial sepsis [6].

The recognition of (i) risk factors for the development of laminitis and (ii) the key clinical features of laminitis can facilitate early diagnosis and intervention, increasing the likelihood of successful prevention or management. A systematic and thorough approach to obtaining a history, as well as to the clinical examination, can help to identify the reasons for the development of laminitis in a particular case. This information can aid in the treatment in that particular animal, and may be of benefit when managing the problem within a herd.

Important Considerations in the Animal's History

Signalment

Laminitis is a disease of adult horses, and is generally not reported in horses aged less than one year, with the exception of congenital mechanobullous disorders that may cause similar lesions [7–9] and rarely avascular necrosis of the distal limbs in critical neonates. Laminitis may be more common in older horses due to its association with pituitary pars intermedia dysfunction (PPID), but recent epidemiological evidence has failed to demonstrate an age-based risk [10].

Pony breeds appear to be more commonly affected by chronic laminitis than horses; this is perhaps associated with a propensity towards IR and hyperinsulinemia in response to dietary carbohydrates [1]. Brood mares have a high incidence of laminitis, which may be associated with the dramatic metabolic shifts of pregnancy/lactation and also with episodic systemic inflammation associated with bouts of metritis. Breeding stallions also appear to be more susceptible, but this may be due to the tendency to keep them overconditioned (leading to IR/metabolic syndrome). Breeding stallions – particularly during the breeding season – appear to have a higher tolerance for pain, which means that they may already have quite severe digital pathology associated with laminitis before they demonstrate overt lameness.

Lameness History

It is important to carefully establish the nature, severity, and duration of lameness historically when examining the suspected laminitis case, as this information may help to differentiate laminitis from other causes of lameness and may also be of value when formulating the prognosis and treatment plan in individual cases. Classically, horses with active laminitis are described

Equine Laminitis, First Edition. Edited by James K. Belknap and Raymond Geor.

as 'stiff' or unwilling to move, and may spend more time recumbent than usual. Laminitis usually affects both forelimbs or all limbs concurrently, leading to what is described as a symmetrical 'stiff' gait, though many cases have asymmetrical signs and therefore it is not uncommon to have an owner describe lameness in a single limb or even shifting lameness in the history. Many cases of chronic laminitis are additionally complicated by hoof abscess formation, which may contribute to the episodic nature of the lameness. Owners and managers may also comment that horses are less willing to work (or even walk) over harder ground. It is important to recognize that, particularly in endocrinopathic laminitis (due to it commonly having an insidious onset), horses with laminitis-related pathology in one or multiple feet may have no history of overt lameness; this is more common if previous usage has not involved athletic/performance pursuits. Chronic lameness in a single limb, if severe and persistent enough, can cause laminitis in the contralateral limb due to excessive continuous weight-bearing (see Chapter 25) [6, 11].

History of Other Disease

Laminitis generally occurs secondary to a disease process remote from the foot; therefore, the establishment of any recent history of disease is important in the suspected laminitis case. Although endotoxin alone has not produced laminitis experimentally [12, 13], many of the diseases that are complicated by the development of acute laminitis share endotoxemia/sepsis as a common feature, and signs of endotoxemia/sepsis are a risk factor for laminitis development in hospitalized horses (i.e., sepsis-related laminitis [SRL]; see Chapter 22) [14]. Gastrointestinal disturbances such as colitis, enteritis and ingestion of excessive carbohydrate in grain or pasture, as well as pneumonia and metritis, are commonly associated with endotoxemia and are implicated in the development of acute laminitis [14–18]. In these cases, acute laminitis usually develops fairly rapidly (within 3–4 days) after the primary disease event, and can vary from mild to severe and rapidly progressive.

Bites from the *Bothrops* spp. snake have also been reported to cause acute laminitis [19]. Natural cases of acute laminitis have been associated with exposure to black walnut (*Juglans nigra*) wood shavings, generally through its use as a bedding material [20], and the ingestion of hay/pasture containing the toxic plant *Hoary alyssum* (*Berteroa incana*) [21, 22].

Changes in Management Including Exercise, Feed, and Body Condition

As most cases of laminitis occurring in the field are linked to reduced insulin sensitivity, any changes in body condition, feeding practices, and exercise levels should be determined. The ingestion of lush pasture is considered the most common cause of laminitis [23]. There is a link between laminitis and pasture accumulation of the nonstructural carbohydrate (NSC) fructan [24]. As there is evidence that NSC may vary depending on the time of day (and season), any changes in management that affect timing of access to pasture should be determined. New access to grass (within four weeks of presentation) was found to be a risk factor for laminitis in a recent study [25]. Similarly, any recent changes to other components of the diet, including hay, grain, and pelleted feeds, should be determined.

Since horses and ponies suffering from obesity and hyperinsulinemia appear to be most prone to the development of pasture-associated laminitis [26–28], and recent weight gain is an important risk factor for laminitis [25], changes in body condition and body weight should be determined where possible. Body weight is not easily determined in the field, though the use of a weight tape or similar device can provide valuable data if performed serially.

Exercise history should be examined to determine if there is an association between change in activity levels, body condition, and laminitis development, and evaluated in the light of the dietary history. In athletic horses, the performance history should be examined carefully. In some cases, progressive or sudden reductions in performance, or an unwillingness to work may be noted prior to the development of overt lameness. Similarly, in riding horses, behavioral problems during or before ridden work are sometimes noted in horses with laminitis prior to the development of overt lameness. Exercise history in the recent past, including the exercising regimen, should be determined since myositis or myopathy (including exertional rhabdomyolysis and polysaccharide storage myopathy) are important differential diagnoses in the acutely stiff horse. Although not particularly common in modern times, excessive exercise on hard surfaces can lead to laminitis (termed 'road founder') [16].

Vaccination and Medication History

The administration of exogenous corticosteroids has been empirically linked with sporadic cases of laminitis [29], although there is no proven association. The administration of larger doses of the more potent corticosteroids (triamcinolone in particular) to an 'insulin-resistant' phenotype appears to be the scenario most commonly implicated. A history of joint medication or other corticosteroid treatment should be carefully considered in the suspected laminitis case. Similarly, there are anecdotal associations between vaccination administration and laminitis, particularly if there has been an adverse vaccine reaction. In endemic areas, the vaccination status for *Neorickettsia risticii* (Potomac Horse Fever) should be considered in the history, as this disease is often associated with the development of acute laminitis [30]. It is also prudent to consider tetanus vaccination status, since this disease is an important differential diagnosis in the acutely stiff horse.

The history of nonsteroidal anti-inflammatory drug (NSAID) administration in particular should be determined because the degree of lameness in a case should be interpreted in the light of any recent administration of analgesic medication. When examining horses that have been treated aggressively with NSAIDs for several days or more, the dosage and duration of therapy is an important consideration with regards to the potential presence of (or risk of) toxic side effects, with right dorsal colitis and renal medullary necrosis being the most common and clinically significant manifestations in horses. This information may determine the need for further diagnostic tests (plasma total protein and creatinine concentration, urinalysis) or affect subsequent treatment choices, including the ongoing analgesia plan or the requirement for supportive therapy (e.g., intravenous fluids).

Shoeing and Trimming History

It is important to establish the recent shoeing and trimming history in any horse with foot-related lameness. The recent removal of shoes can cause multiple limb lameness even in normal horses if there is excessive sole contact with the ground when the animal is barefoot. Due to the insidious nature of the displacement of the distal phalanx (DP) in endocrinopathic laminitis, the first sign that the horse may exhibit is lameness from sole bruising due to exposure of a thin, compromised sole to increased ground contact with shoeing change or removal. In the chronic laminitis case, the historic effects of different shoeing and trimming techniques on the severity of lameness may be important with regards to deciding on an appropriate corrective farriery plan. Recent trimming, particularly with dressing of the dorsal wall, can also affect radiographic measurements (see Chapter 27).

Clinical Presentation of Laminitis

The clinical presentation of laminitis cases varies depending on the duration and the severity of pathology, the presence of concurrent/predisposing disease, and the systemic and behavioral responses of the individual horse to laminitis pain.

The 'Phases' of Laminitis

Laminitis is divided into developmental, acute, and chronic phases [31]. The developmental phase is not associated with any clinical signs of laminitis, although the processes ultimately leading to lamellar failure have begun. The developmental phase has been defined as the period between the initial causative insult and the first appearance of acute lameness identifiable as laminitis [31], and its duration is variable. In experimentally induced cases of carbohydrate overload (CHO), the developmental phase lasts for between 20 and 72 h, with an average duration of approximately 40 h [31–33]. A similar duration appears to generally exist in clinical cases of acute bacterial colitis. The developmental phase is commonly much shorter ($\leq$24 h) in cases of *Hoary alyssum* poisoning [22] and Potomac Horse Fever [34]. The period is also short (8–12 h) after black walnut extract (BWE) administration [35]. A longer and more variable duration may exist in association with other diseases such as pneumonia. It would be particularly advantageous from a clinical standpoint to be able to identify horses within the developmental phase, as this is likely the optimal period for therapeutic intervention. At the time of writing, there are no available biomarkers for developmental laminitis. However, several research groups are aiming to identify and evaluate serum markers of laminitis that may allow the identification of laminitis processes prior to the development of clinical signs.

The acute phase begins with the first signs of lameness and ends after 72 h, or when there is radiographic or physical evidence of displacement of the DP [31]. Acute laminitis is characterized by lameness in one or more limbs, increases in hoof temperature and digital pulse amplitude, and often an altered stance at rest [15,31,36–38]. Prior to the presence of overt lameness at the walk or trot, incessant shifting of weight in the fore and/or hind limbs may be noted. There may be pain on hoof testing, particularly in the toe region, although this response is variable. There may also be a pain response to percussion of the hoof wall.

Once horses progress to chronic laminitis, there is generally some degree of mechanical collapse of the foot [31]. This is associated with a widely varying degree of lameness and anatomical derangement [39]. Extensive acute lamellar detachment can result in downward/distal displacement ('sinking') of the pedal bone within the hoof capsule, which results in a palpable depression at the coronary band. With severe lamellar detachment, the hoof wall may separate from the integument of the coronary band; this is usually detected by hemorrhage (or serosanguineous fluid) exuding from a partial or circumferential crack in the coronary band. In severe cases, the circumferential separation and hemorrhage at the coronary band is a harbinger for catastrophic lamellar separation and exunguilation of the hoof from the underlying digit. In less severe cases, the pull of the deep flexor tendon and the proliferating epidermal lamellar tissue result in palmar and distal rotation of the pedal bone away from the dorsal hoof wall. There is a change in orientation of the dermal papillae of the coronary band associated with the changing position of the pedal bone within the hoof capsule, resulting in a modification of hoof growth. Deformed hoof growth results in visible rings in the hoof wall that converge at the toe, where the net rate of growth is the least. There may also be a concave shape to the dorsal hoof wall [40]. With more severe and progressive palmar and distal rotation of the pedal bone, a convex bulge forms in the sole overlying the DP. The pedal bone may eventually penetrate the sole.

Posture/Stance

The forelimbs are usually more severely affected than the hind limbs, and the horse loads the heels preferentially, to relieve the toes. For these reasons a characteristic 'saw horse' stance is often adopted, with the hind feet positioned forward under the body and the forefeet extended in front of the body (Fig. 21.1a) [41]. Horses with equivocal hind- and fore-limb pain due to laminitis may have a normal stance. Rarely, the hind limbs are affected more severely than the forelimbs, and, in some of these cases, there is a tendency to stand with the forefeet retracted more caudally (i.e., towards the center of gravity; Fig. 21.1b). It is always beneficial to observe the horse from a distance, preferably

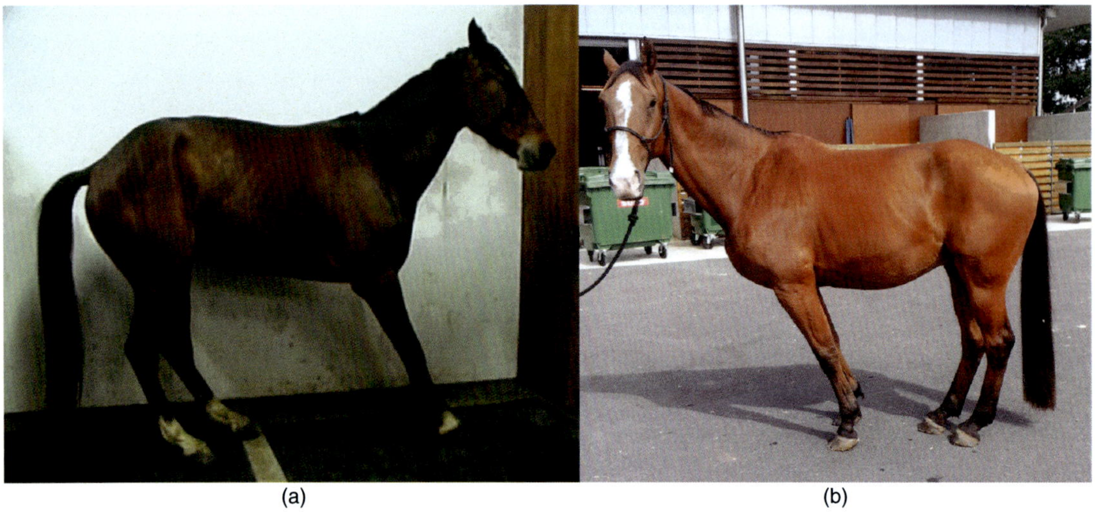

Figure 21.1 (a) Laminitis is usually worse in the front feet compared with the hind feet, and therefore horses will classically stand with the forefeet extended forwards and the hind feet either under the body or extended caudally. (b) Occasionally, laminitis is worse in the hind feet, and these horses may stand with the forefeet under the body. Horses with equivocal fore and hind foot pain may have a normal stance.

without interference from a handler, to observe posture/stance and also the rate of weight-shifting between limbs at rest.

Hoof Temperature and Digital Pulse

Increases in hoof wall surface temperature (HWST) often precede or coincide with the onset of lameness in acute laminitis cases, and increased HWST is also often evident in chronic laminitis cases experiencing a recurrent acute episode. It must be remembered that HWST is a function of ambient temperature, as well as the blood perfusion and metabolic rate of the underlying tissues of the foot [42]. The HWST rarely exceeds 35 °C, but it can fluctuate rapidly and in a cyclic fashion in normal horses across the course of a day, often with asynchrony in these fluctuations between the feet [42, 43]. In horses developing laminitis under experimental conditions, a prolonged and continuous increase in HWST precedes the development of an observable lameness that can remain throughout the acute phase. Persistently increased hoof temperature is a consistent finding in horses with acute laminitis [41]. An increase in digital pulse amplitude may precede or coincide with the onset of lameness in acute laminitis, and often persists in chronic cases. Increased digital pulse amplitude can also occur with other inflammatory conditions of the foot (hoof abscess, sole bruising, fracture, etc.) and may be present in the normal horse temporarily following travel or work on hard surfaces.

Lameness

Lameness caused by laminitis does not differ from that caused by other painful conditions of the foot, although the laminitis case most commonly presents with multiple limb lameness. The lameness is often worse in the forelimbs and is often asymmetrical. The degree of lameness can be established by careful examination at the walk in a straight line and in small circles in both directions. Horses with mild bilateral forelimb laminitis may appear normal in the straight line, though turning on a hard surface will exacerbate lameness on the inside limb in either direction. The lameness scale originally developed by Obel [37] is useful for documenting the severity of laminitis in clinical cases (Table 21.1).

Hoof testing may reveal a diffuse withdrawal response across the entire foot, or just at the toe region, or only on the medial or lateral quarter/heel region depending on the severity and type of displacement. In many cases, there is little response to hoof testing. A withdrawal reaction to the manual application of rotational force to the hoof is possibly a more reliable indicator of the presence of laminitis pain, particularly in the hind limbs.

It is important to recognize that complications of laminitis (including most commonly the development of hoof abscesses in chronic cases) may contribute to the clinical presentation of a case.

Table 21.1 The Obel grading scale used to monitor the clinical severity of laminitis [37].

Obel grade	Animal characteristics
1	At rest the horse will alternately and incessantly lift the feet. Lameness is not evident at the walk, but a short stilted gait is noted at the trot.
2	The horse moves willingly at a walk, but the gait is characteristic of laminitis. A hoof can be lifted off the ground without difficulty.
3	The horse moves very reluctantly and vigorously resists attempts to lift a forefoot.
4	The horse must be forced to move and may be recumbent.

Cardiovascular and Respiratory Signs

Laminitis can cause a sufficient pain response to modify systemic parameters, leading to increased heart and respiratory rates, sweating, and agitation. In hospitalized horses, subtle but sustained increases in heart rate (45–55 beats per minute) in particular may be noticed prior to the development of lameness and, if the heart rate is serially recorded and tracked carefully, mild tachycardia may be the first observable clinical sign of laminitis. Horses with moderate to severe acute laminitis will often have a more obviously increased resting heart rate and respiratory rate which commonly increases when the animal is standing. In both acute and chronic laminitis cases, hypertension may be noted either transiently or persistently [44–46]. Spontaneous sweating and a rectal temperature in the upper range of normal (or mild hyperthermia) may be apparent, although laminitis alone does not cause true pyrexia.

Body Condition

Since obesity and IR are causatively linked to laminitis, it is common for horses and ponies presenting with laminitis to be overweight. Increased body weight was also recently identified as a risk factor for the development of supporting-limb laminitis [6]. There is anecdotal evidence that horses with a higher body condition score (BCS) may also be more prone to iatrogenic corticosteroid-induced laminitis. However, the lack of obesity does not rule out IR; similar to human metabolic syndrome, some horses with equine metabolic syndrome and insulin dysregulation have a normal BCS. Horses with chronic laminitis, particularly if severe, will often lose body condition during the course of the disease, most likely as a result of chronic pain.

Behavioral Changes

Laminitis causes changes in behavior attributable to pain. Careful observation of the horse with laminitis at rest may reveal subtle weight shifting in the front limbs, an early clinical sign characteristic of laminitis [37, 41]. Behavioral assessment may provide additional evidence of the degree of pain in laminitis cases. In a recent study, certain behaviors (forelimb lifting and retiring towards the back of the stall) were consistently and significantly associated with laminitis pain [47]. Other behavioral changes that may be noted in response to laminitis pain include teeth grinding, sighing, groaning, self-biting, head-tossing, lip quiver, yawning, tongue extrusion, licking, sour aggression, and low head carriage. Horses with more severe pain may also spend more time recumbent. In the present author's experience, mild laminitis (even in the absence of detectable lameness) may also cause misbehavior in horses under saddle indicative of resistance to the digital pain caused by athletic work.

Integumentary Changes

In acute cases, the hooves appear normal; however, once chronic, laminitis causes progressive changes to the appearance of the hooves. Most commonly, growth rings in the hooves that diverge towards the heels (Fig. 21.2) and a dished appearance to the dorsal hoof wall are present. There is widening of the white line, visible once the foot is trimmed. In severe cases that have not undergone regular trimming, excessive distorted growth may eventually result in the development of 'slipper foot' conformation (Fig. 21.2d). In cases where there is marked symmetrical displacement of the pedal bone within the hoof capsule ('sinking'), a depression between the proximal extent of the coronary band and the pastern may be palpated. In severe cases (primarily with palmar rotation of the DP), the dorsal solear margin of the pedal bone may cause a detectable convex bulge in the sole between the tip of the frog and the white line, at times progressing to sole necrosis and perforation.

In horses with chronic laminitis, particularly if severe, skin lesions caused by pressure necrosis from prolonged recumbency (decubitus ulcers) may be evident over the *tuber coxae*, elbows, hocks, and the temporal/zygomatic region of the head.

Signs of Concurrent Disease

Since laminitis commonly occurs secondary to other disease processes remote from the foot, there are often clinical signs of concurrent disease. These may include typical signs of endotoxemia/systemic inflammatory response syndrome (SIRS; tachycardia, tachypnea, pyrexia, hypotension, depression, hyperemic mucous membranes) in the sepsis-associated laminitis case. Horses with PPID may have hirsutism, loss of muscle mass, and abnormal fat distribution (particularly bulging of the supraorbital fat pads).

Clinical Laboratory Parameters

Acute laminitis alone does not itself result in any changes in routine blood parameters, apart from the presence of a stress leukogram in moderate to severe cases. Increases in fibrinogen are indicative of inflammation associated with the primary disease or another lesion rather than the laminitis itself. Increases in serum amyloid A (SAA) occur early in experimentally induced laminitis models; the systemic inflammation present in laminitis induction models makes it difficult to determine whether the source of the elevated SAA is the injured lamellae themselves. Azotemia with concurrent hemoconcentration may be present due to dehydration. Stress due to pain in the acute or active chronic laminitis case may interfere with the results of endocrine testing for PPID and equine metabolic syndrome (EMS); horses with acute laminitis may have increased serum glucose and insulin concentrations due to stress (in the absence of EMS) [48].

Important Differential Diagnoses for Laminitis Based on Clinical Presentation

The combination of multiple limb lameness referable to the feet, increased digital pulse amplitude, increased hoof temperature, and the external hoof morphology changes often leads quickly to the presumptive diagnosis of laminitis. However, there are several important differentials in the case that is not displaying such clear clinical signs. Differential diagnoses

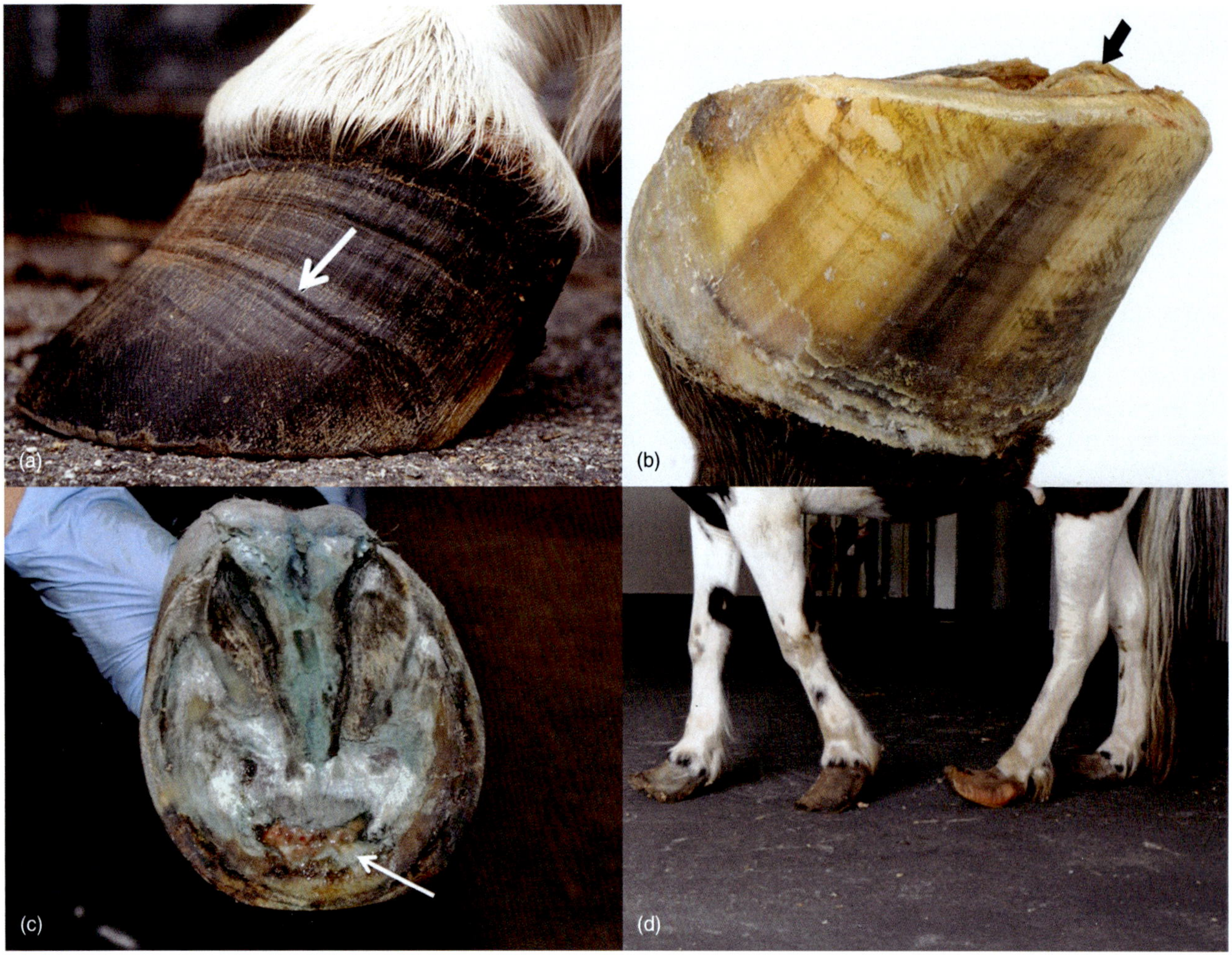

Figure 21.2 (a) Typical hoof rings that diverge towards the heels (arrow) may be noted in horses with chronic laminitis. (b, c) When there is sufficient distal displacement or rotation of the third phalanx within the hoof capsule, the sole becomes convex over the dorsal solear margin (b) and may penetrate the sole (c). (d) Due to disturbed hoof growth, the heels lengthen differentially and without trimming the feet of the chronic laminitis case may progress to the classic 'Aladdin's Slipper' appearance. The illustration in panel (b) was provided by Prof. C. Pollitt, and reproduced with his permission.

to consider in the acutely stiff horse include tetanus, myopathy, pleuritis (with pleurodynia), equine motor neuron disease, rabies, hypokalemia, and myotonia. Differential diagnoses to consider for foot-related lameness are numerous; however, hoof abscesses, fractures of the DP, navicular syndrome, white line disease, sole bruising, and seedy toe may be most important. Other conditions that may cause changes to hoof growth and conformation as well as foot pain include pemphigus foliaceus, coronitis, coronary dystrophy, selenium toxicosis, and toxicity from the ingestion of *Leucaena* sp. plants containing the toxic principle mimosine.

References

1. Geor, R.J. (2010) Current concepts on the pathophysiology of pasture-associated laminitis. *Vet. Clin. North Am. Equine Pract.*, **26**, 265–276.
2. de Laat, M.A., McGowan, C.M., Sillence, M.N., and Pollitt, C.C. (2010) Hyperinsulinemic laminitis. *Vet. Clin. North Am. Equine Pract.*, **26**, 257–264.
3. Johnson, P.J., Wiedmeyer, C.E., LaCarrubba, A., Ganjam, V.K., and Messer, N.T. (2010) Laminitis and the equine metabolic syndrome. *Vet. Clin. North Am. Equine Pract.*, **26**, 239–255.
4. Geor, R.J. (2009) Pasture-associated laminitis. *Vet. Clin. North Am. Equine Pract.*, **25**, 39–50, v–vi.
5. Kullmann, A., Holcombe, S.J., Hurcombe, S.D., Roessner, H.A., Hauptman, J.G., Geor, R.J., and Belknap, J. (2014) Prophylactic digital cryotherapy is associated with decreased incidence of laminitis in horses diagnosed with colitis. *Equine Vet. J.*, **46** (5), 554-559.
6. Virgin, J.E., Goodrich, L.R., Baxter, G.M., and Rao, S. (2011) Incidence of support limb laminitis in horses treated with half limb, full limb or transfixation pin casts: a retrospective study of 113 horses (2000–2009). *Equine Vet. J. Suppl.*, **40**, 7–11.
7. French, K.R. and Pollitt, C.C. (2004) Equine laminitis: congenital, hemidesmosomal plectin deficiency in a Quarter Horse foal. *Equine Vet. J.*, **36**, 299–303.

8. Frame, S.R., Harrington, D.D., Fessler, J., and Frame, P.F. (1988) Hereditary junctional mechanobullous disease in a foal. *J. Am. Vet. Med. Assoc.*, **193**, 1420–1424.
9. Johnson, G.C., Kohn, C.W., Johnson, C.W., Garry, F., Scott, D., and Martin, S. (1988) Ultrastructure of junctional epidermolysis bullosa in Belgian foals. *J. Comp. Pathol.*, **99**, 329–336.
10. Wylie, C.E., Collins, S.N., Verheyen, K.L., and Newton, J.R. (2013) Risk factors for equine laminitis: a case-control study conducted in veterinary-registered horses and ponies in Great Britain between 2009 and 2011. *Vet. J.*, **198**, 57–69.
11. Peloso, J.G., Cohen, N.D., Walker, M.A., Watkins, J.P., Gayle, J.M., and Moyer, W. (1996) Case-control study of risk factors for the development of laminitis in the contralateral limb in Equidae with unilateral lameness. *J. Am. Vet. Med. Assoc.*, **209**, 1746–1749.
12. Clark, E.S. and Moore, J.N. (1989) The effects of slow infusion of a low dosage of endotoxin in healthy horses. *Equine Vet. J. Suppl.*, **7**, 33–37.
13. Hunt, R.J., Allen, D., and Moore, J.N. (1990) Effect of endotoxin administration on equine digital hemodynamics and starling forces. *Am. J. Vet. Res.*, **51**, 1703–1707.
14. Parsons, C.S., Orsini, J.A., Krafty, R., Capewell, L., and Boston, R. (2007) Risk factors for development of acute laminitis in horses during hospitalization: 73 cases (1997–2004). *J. Am. Vet. Med. Assoc.*, **230**, 885–889.
15. Sloet van Oldruitenborgh Oosterbaan, M.M. (1999) Laminitis in the horse: a review. *Vet. Q.*, **21**, 121–127.
16. Hood, D.M. (1999) The pathophysiology of developmental and acute laminitis. *Vet. Clin. North Am. Equine Pract.*, **15**, 321–343.
17. Slater, M.R., Hood, D.M., and Carter, G.K. (1995) Descriptive epidemiological study of equine laminitis. *Equine Vet. J.*, **27**, 364–367.
18. Cohen, N.D., Parson, E.M., Seahorn, T.L., and Carter, G.K. (1994) Prevalence and factors associated with development of laminitis in horses with duodenitis/proximal jejunitis: 33 cases (1985–1991). *J. Am. Vet. Med. Assoc.*, **204**, 250–254.
19. Acosta de Perez, O., Teibler, P., Leiva, L., Rios, E., Sanchez Negrette, M., and Pollitt, C. (2006) Equine laminitis: bites by *Bothrops* spp. cause hoof lamellar pathology in the contralateral as well as in the bitten limb. *Toxicon*, **48**, 307–312.
20. Uhlinger, C. (1989) Black walnut toxicosis in ten horses. *J. Am. Vet. Med. Assoc.*, **195**, 343–344.
21. Geor, R.J., Becker, R.L., Kanara, E.W., Hovda, L.R., Sweeney, W.H., Winter, T.F., Rorick, J.K., Ruth, G.R., Hope, E., and Murphy, M.J. (1992) Toxicosis in horses after ingestion of hoary alyssum. *J. Am. Vet. Med. Assoc.*, **201**, 63–67.
22. Hovda, L.R. and Rose, M.L. (1993) Hoary alyssum (*Berteroa incana*) toxicity in a herd of broodmare horses. *Vet. Hum. Toxicol.*, **35**, 39–40.
23. Bailey, S.R., Marr, C.M., and Elliott, J. (2004) Current research and theories on the pathogenesis of acute laminitis in the horse. *Vet. J.*, **167**, 129–142.
24. Longland, A.C. and Byrd, B.M. (2006) Pasture nonstructural carbohydrates and equine laminitis. *J. Nutr.*, **136**, 2099S–2102S.
25. Wylie, C.E., Collins, S.N., Verheyen, K.L., and Newton, J.R. (2013) Risk factors for equine laminitis: A case-control study conducted in veterinary-registered horses and ponies in Great Britain between 2009 and 2011. *Vet. J.*, **198** (1), 57–69.
26. Vick, M.M., Adams, A.A., Murphy, B.A., Sessions, D.R., Horohov, D.W., Cook, R.F., Shelton, B.J., and Fitzgerald, B.P. (2007) Relationship between inflammatory cytokines, obesity, and insulin sensitivity in the horse. *J. Anim. Sci.*, **85** (5), 1144–1155.
27. Treiber, K.H., Kronfeld, D.S., Hess, T.M., Byrd, B.M., Splan, R.K., and Staniar, W.B. (2006) Evaluation of genetic and metabolic predispositions and nutritional risk factors for pasture-associated laminitis in ponies. *J. Am. Vet. Med. Assoc.*, **228**, 1538–1545.
28. Treiber, K.H., Kronfeld, D.S., and Geor, R.J. (2006) Insulin resistance in equids: possible role in laminitis. *J. Nutr.*, **136**, 2094S–2098S.
29. Bailey, S.R. and Elliott, J. (2007) The corticosteroid laminitis story: 2. Science of if, when and how. *Equine Vet. J.*, **39**, 7–11.
30. Bertin, F.R., Reising, A., Slovis, N.M., Constable, P.D., and Taylor, S.D. (2013) Clinical and clinicopathological factors associated with survival in 44 horses with equine neorickettsiosis (Potomac Horse Fever). *J. Vet. Intern. Med.*, **27** (6), 1528–1534.
31. Hood, D.M. (1999) Laminitis in the horse. *Vet. Clin. North Am. Equine Pract.*, **15**, 287–294, v.
32. Garner, H.E., Coffman, J.R., Hahn, A.W., Hutcheson, D.P., and Tumbleson, M.E. (1975) Equine laminitis of alimentary origin: an experimental model. *Am. J. Vet. Res.*, **36**, 441–444.
33. Pollitt, C.C. and Davies, C.T. (1998) Equine laminitis: its development coincides with increased sublamellar blood flow. *Equine Vet. J. Suppl.*, **26**, 125–132.
34. Mulville, P. (1991) Equine monocytic ehrlichiosis (Potomac horse fever): a review. *Equine Vet. J.*, **23**, 400–404.
35. Galey, F.D., Whiteley, H.E., Goetz, T.E., Kuenstler, A.R., Davis, C.A., and Beasley, V.R. (1991) Black walnut (*Juglans nigra*) toxicosis: a model for equine laminitis. *J. Comp. Pathol.*, **104**, 313–326.
36. Baxter, G.M. (1994) Acute laminitis. *Vet. Clin. North Am. Equine Pract.*, **10**, 627–642.
37. Obel, N. (1948) Studies of the Histopathology of Acute Laminitis, PhD thesis, Almgvist and Wilcsells Bottrykeri Ab Uppsala.
38. Yelle, M. (1986) Clinicians guide to equine laminitis. *Equine Vet. J.*, **18**, 156–158.
39. Hunt, R.J. (1993) A retrospective evaluation of laminitis in horses. *Equine Vet. J.*, **25**, 61–64.
40. Morgan, S.J., Grosenbaugh, D.A., and Hood, D.M. (1999) The pathophysiology of chronic laminitis. Pain and anatomic pathology. *Vet. Clin. North Am. Equine Pract.*, **15**, 395–417, vii.
41. Pollitt, C.C. (1999) Laminitis, in *Equine Medicine and Surgery*, 5th edition (eds P.T. Colahan, A.M. Merritt, J.N. Moore, and I.G. Mayhew), Mosby, St Louis, pp. 1521–1749.
42. Rosenmeier, J.G., Strathe, A.B., and Andersen, P.H. (2012) Evaluation of coronary band temperatures in healthy horses. *Am. J. Vet. Res.*, **73**, 719–723.
43. Mogg, K.C. and Pollitt, C.C. (1992) Hoof and distal limb surface temperature in the normal pony under constant and changing ambient temperatures. *Equine Vet. J.*, **24**, 134–139.
44. Navas de Solis, C., Slack, J., Boston, R.C., and Reef, V.B. (2013) Hypertensive cardiomyopathy in horses: 5 cases (1995–2011). *J. Am. Vet. Med. Assoc.*, **243**, 126–130.
45. Bailey, S.R., Habershon-Butcher, J.L., Ransom, K.J., Elliott, J., and Menzies-Gow, N.J. (2008) Hypertension and insulin resistance in a mixed-breed population of ponies predisposed to laminitis. *Am. J. Vet. Res.*, **69**, 122–129.

46. Harkema, J.R., Robinson, N.E., and Scott, J.B. (1978) Cardiovascular, acid-base, electrolyte, and plasma volume changes in ponies developing alimentary laminitis. *Am. J. Vet. Res.*, **39**, 741–744.
47. Jones, E., Vinuela-Fernandez, I., Eager, R.A., Delaney, A., Anderson, H., Patel, A., Robertson, D.C., Allchorne, A., Sirinathsinghji, E.C., Milne, E.M., MacIntyre, N., Shaw, D.J., Waran, N.K., Mayhew, J., and Fleetwood-Walker, S.M. (2007) Neuropathic changes in equine laminitis pain. *Pain*, **132**, 321–331.
48. Van Eps, A.W. and Pollitt, C.C. (2006) Equine laminitis induced with oligofructose. *Equine Vet. J.*, **38**, 203–208.

CHAPTER 22
Sepsis-Related Laminitis

Susan C. Eades

Introduction

Acute laminitis can be a devastating sequel to a wide range of causes of equine sepsis including metritis, anterior uveitis, bronchopneumonia, pleuropneumonia, and numerous causes of gastrointestinal compromise (e.g., duodenitis/proximal jejunitis, enterocolitis, surgically managed colic, grain overload). Sepsis is defined as infection with evidence of systemic inflammation [1]. Pathogens trigger sequential intracellular events in immune cells, epithelium, endothelium and neuroendocrine cells, causing the production and release of inflammatory mediators which can damage host tissues and, in severe cases, cause organ failure [1]. Laminitis may be one manifestation of host tissue damage from systemic inflammation (see Chapter 14) [2]. Unlike humans, in which a diverse array of pathogens (ranging from parasites to bacteria [both Gram-negative and Gram-positive] to viruses) can trigger sepsis-related organ damage, it is primarily sepsis related to a bacterial infection (usually with a Gram-negative component) that results in systemic inflammation and laminitis in the horse. Bacteria contain many molecules, most commonly termed pathogen-associated molecular pattern (PAMP) proteins, which can trigger a systemic inflammatory response; these include endotoxin/lipopolysaccharide (LPS), flagellin, lipoteichoic acid, lipoproteins, and peptidoglycans. Although several of these bacterial PAMPs may play a role in systemic inflammation in equine sepsis, endotoxin has received the most attention [2]. Endotoxemia, although commonly used interchangeably with the term *sepsis*, is the presence of one PAMP, endotoxin (LPS; a major structural cell wall component of Gram-negative bacteria), in the bloodstream which can stimulate similar inflammatory cascades and result in clinical signs of systemic inflammation [3]. Thus, as the term "endotoxemia" when used in the equine literature (including this text) usually refers to animals exhibiting clinical signs of sepsis (likely from the absorption of multiple bacterial PAMPs including endotoxin), the reader should realize that these animals are likely exhibiting systemic inflammation from absorption of multiple PAMPs into the systemic circulation from the originally affected organ (e.g., the colon). The major risk factor for laminitis in animals with these diseases appears to be the presence of systemic inflammation itself, as exemplified by Parsons et al. who failed to find any significant association between disease state and the development of laminitis in horses hospitalized for medical and surgical conditions, but did find the presence of endotoxemia to be an important risk factor [4]. Although the incidence of laminitis in horses with sepsis and inflammatory disease in not known, laminitis is always one of the most significant complications of these diseases. Various reviews have shown that the incidence of laminitis among cases of intestinal disease ranges from 2% to 4% [5,6], while the incidence among cases of acute diarrhea was approximately 11% [7]. Whilst diseased horses at risk of laminitis can be any age, laminitis occurs only rarely in horses aged less than one year. Most epidemiologic studies have not found any significant association between the development of acute laminitis and signalment [4,8,9]. However, in one multicenter, hospital-based study the risk for acute laminitis was found to be highest in horses aged 5–7 years or 13–31 years, in breeds other than Thoroughbreds and Quarter Horses, and in mares (compared to geldings) [10]. In addition, Hunt *et al.* [11] found the risk to be highest in stallions when compared to geldings.

Gastrointestinal tract disease is likely the most common cause of sepsis-related laminitis (SRL), and was the most common primary disease in 54% of horses that developed acute laminitis in a study conducted at seven private practices and at a university veterinary hospital [8]. More specifically, surgical colic [11], acute diarrhea [7], and duodenitis/proximal jejunitis [12] have been significantly associated with an increased risk for acute laminitis. In the present author's experience, the incidence of laminitis often seems to correlate with the severity of the primary disease (the severity of pneumonia or enterocolitis that led to systemic sepsis) or disease duration, with clinicians anecdotally associating laminitis with severe fever (e.g., >104 °F) and severe hypovolemia (e.g., packed cell volume >55%). However, there appears to be a great variability between horses regarding susceptibility to SRL, with some cases showing severe sepsis parameters and surviving without laminitis, while other sepsis cases with much more moderate clinical signs resulted in severe laminitis with complete lamellar separation. In cases of anterior enteritis (duodenitis/proximal jejunitis), horses with

Equine Laminitis, First Edition. Edited by James K. Belknap and Raymond Geor.

body weights >550 kg and those with bloody gastric reflux were reported to be more likely to have laminitis [12]. Duodenitis/proximal jejunitis, enterocolitis, surgically managed colic, interstitial pneumonia and bronchopneumonia, as well as metritis in postpartum mares, are disease states commonly associated with endotoxemia/sepsis in horses. Clinical signs common in horses with enterocolitis, duodenitis/proximal jejunitis, grain overload, surgically managed colic, bacterial bronchopneumonia/pleuritis and metritis include fever, tachycardia, injected or cyanotic mucous membranes, tachypnea, inappetence, and muscle fasciculation [3]. It has been hypothesized that these clinical signs are due to the systemic inflammatory response, which is a possible factor in the pathogenesis of laminitis [2]. Endotoxemia is a common factor leading to the systemic inflammatory response and laminitis in horses, with disease associated with Gram-negative organisms being much more commonly associated with laminitis than disease associated with Gram-positive organisms [2]. Experimentally induced endotoxemia does not cause laminitis, however, which indicates that other toxins/mediators or other local or physiologic events are necessary for the development of lamellar injury. Local inflammatory disease, pain and hypovolemia are also factors that contribute to the clinical signs in these cases, and may play a role in laminitis pathophysiology. Laminitis has a high incidence in one disease which causes enterocolitis, namely Potomac Horse Fever (PHF) [13], where the causative pathogen is a rickettsial organism with no endotoxin present. The high incidence of laminitis in PHF suggests that: (i) similar to organ injury in human sepsis, other bacterial products may be at least as important as endotoxin in causing equine sepsis and laminitis; or (ii) endotoxin (from colonic Gram-negative bacteria) is absorbed systemically in cases of PHF due to mucosal damage in the affected large intestine.

Acute laminitis is also sometimes associated with inflammatory diseases that are not accompanied by clinical signs of systemic inflammatory response. Anterior uveitis and localized sepsis (e.g., wounds, local abscessation) are sometimes accompanied by laminitis. Laminitis may also accompany acute myopathies, especially when accompanied by acute renal tubular necrosis. These cases do not always develop changes in body temperature, heart rate, respiratory rate, and mucous membrane color. The events that lead to the development of laminitis in these cases are very unclear, but possible factors include: (i) increases in the concentration of circulating inflammatory mediators that affect the lamellar tissues but are not sufficiently high to affect the autonomic control of the circulation or body temperature; (ii) sufficient pain (caused by these local diseases/events) to affect feed intake and intestinal function; or (iii) a combination of these factors. As injured and dying host cells release proteins which can bind the same receptors as bacterial products, and cause the same local and/or systemic inflammatory response (damage-associated molecular pattern molecules [DAMPs]; see Chapter 14), it is possible that diseases associated with tissue injury and cell death (e.g., myopathies, compromised bowel wall in gastrointestinal crises, tubular necrosis in kidney disease) may lead to laminitis through the systemic absorption of these products [14].

Clinical Signs

Horses with duodenitis/proximal jejunitis (also termed 'anterior enteritis') present with signs of abdominal pain which subside after gastric decompression and volume replacement. Signs of lethargy and general malaise then occur. These horses tend to have large volumes of fluid reflux (>4 liters each time decompression is attempted from a nasogastric tube) that is sometimes blood-tinged. Increases in body temperature and heart rate are common clinical signs. Mucous membranes are commonly brick red or cyanotic in color (Fig. 22.1).

Horses with enterocolitis can present with any combination of the following clinical signs, including: depression, fever, anorexia, colic, fluid reflux from nasogastric tube, septicemia

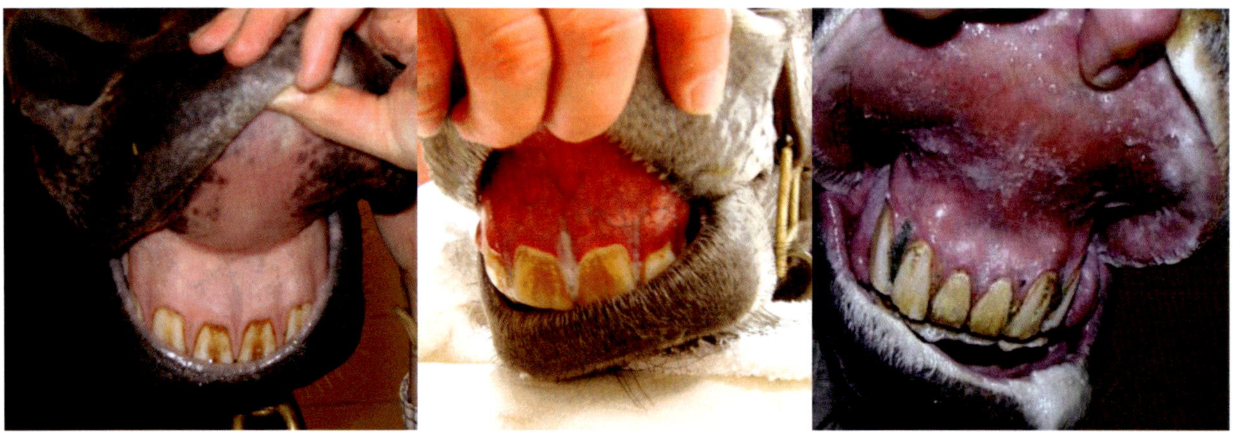

(a) (b) (c)

Figure 22.1 (a) Normal mucous membranes, and (b) mucous membranes of a horse early in sepsis (mucosal hyperemia) and (c) in late sepsis (mucosal cyanosis). Illustrations courtesy of Margaret Mudge and Eric Schroeder, Ohio State University, and Britta Leise, Louisiana State University.

with local infection/abscesses, and/or diarrhea. Fever, profound depression and anorexia, sometimes accompanied by colic, are the earliest signs. Fulminant dehydration may be obvious before diarrhea occurs. Clinical signs of sepsis/endotoxemia are common and include fever, tachycardia, tachypnea, cool extremities, weakness, and muscle fasciculations. The mucous membranes (Fig. 22.1) may be pale with perigingival hyperemia or exhibit intense hyperemia and perigingival cyanosis. Diarrhea usually occurs between 24 and 48 h after the onset of clinical signs of endotoxemia, but may not occur for several days, or at all. Grain/carbohydrate overload (i.e., the accidental exposure of an equid to excessive amounts of grain) commonly causes enterocolitis and clinical signs common to other causes of enterocolitis [15]. In grain/carbohydrate overload (CHO) cases, increases in the body temperature, heart rate and respiratory rate, hyperemic or cyanotic mucous membranes, colic, and diarrhea are common clinical signs. Nasogastric intubation may reveal significant fluid reflux. Particles of grain may be noted in the fluid reflux and feces. Abdominal auscultation and percussion may reveal reduced to absent intestinal sounds and intestinal tympany. Laminitis occurs in a high percentage of horses that have ingested excessive quantities of grain, and can be induced experimentally in approximately 90% of horses administered corn starch gruel (see Chapter 7) [16]. Changes in the intestinal microbial population and products of bacterial metabolism are likely important factors in the pathogenesis of laminitis associated with intestinal disease. In naturally occurring cases of grain overload, the amount of soluble carbohydrate necessary to induce colitis and laminitis is variable [15]. The gradual introduction of soluble carbohydrates and the concurrent feeding of high-quality forage increases the tolerance to grain feeding. Grazing of lush pasture and pasture with seed heads can be additional sources of significant ingestion of soluble carbohydrates.

The clinical signs of systemic inflammation are also prominent in postpartum mares with acute septic metritis (also termed 'retained fetal membranes') [17]. Anorexia and depression are common early clinical signs in these animals; their pulse is commonly rapid and weak, the mucous membranes are commonly affected (Fig. 22.1b), the respiratory rate is increased, body temperature is increased, and extremities may be cold. Atony of the intestinal tract can lead to reduced intestinal sounds, reduced fecal output, and colonic impaction in these metritis cases. The retention of fetal membranes and a reddish watery fetid vulvar discharge are variable in these patients.

Horses with bronchopneumonia putting the horse at risk of laminitis commonly present with clinical signs limited to an increased body temperature and inappetence early during the disease process. As pneumonia progresses, tachypnea or respiratory distress, coughing, abnormal lung sounds, nasal discharge, gurgling sounds of exudates in the trachea, exercise intolerance, and weight loss develop. Auscultation of the thorax reveals increased harsh breathing sounds dorsally, and crackles, wheezes, and dullness ventrally. Pleuropneumonia cases have additional clinical signs including a guarded and painful cough, and a stilted gait (caused by thoracic pain). Any bronchopneumonia case with a stilted gait should be closely examined to ensure that the gait is only due to thoracic pain and not the onset of laminitis.

The onset of laminitis, in association with duodenitis/proximal jejunitis, enterocolitis, surgically managed colic, bacterial bronchopneumonia/pleuritis, and metritis, generally occurs several days after onset of the primary disease and may occur as the primary disease is resolving. As discussed above, the primary disease severity does not always correlate with the incidence or severity of laminitis. Laminitis may cause an increased heart rate, an increased respiratory rate, and spontaneous sweating even after clinical signs from the primary disease have resolved. Clinical signs associated with the hoof wall surface temperature (increased wall temperature) and digital vasculature (throbbing digital artery pulses palpated at the pastern/fetlock level) sometimes precede lameness. The distal limb and hoof wall surface temperature can also be cool to the touch in horses with ongoing systemic inflammation in gastrointestinal and other sepsis-related diseases, especially when the severity of the disease leads to hypovolemia. Heat over the dorsal hoof wall associated with an increased hoof wall surface temperature may precede or occur coincident with lameness. Bounding of the digital pulse (an increase in the difference between the systolic and diastolic digital arterial pressure) is also a common sign at the onset of lameness. Sensitivity to hoof testers over the sole near the toe can precede or occur coincident with lameness.

Laminitis subsequent to septic disease can affect all four feet, the forefeet alone or, less commonly, the rear limbs alone. The increased load of the fore limbs compared with the hind limbs is thought to account for the increased occurrence of laminitis in the forelimbs. All four limbs are more commonly affected in SRL than endocrinopathic laminitis, most likely due to the increased severity of systemic disease and increased severity of insult to the lamellae. Additionally, the onset of lameness is commonly more acute and obvious in sepsis cases compared to the insidious nature of the onset of clinical signs of laminitis in endocrinopathic cases. The Obel laminitis grading system is most often used to better define the severity of lameness [18]. Grade 1 is the least severe, and states that the horse alternately and incessantly lifts the feet and that lameness is not evident at a walk but is evident at a trot as a short, stilted gait (it is not advised to trot suspected SRL cases). Minimal clinical signs may be apparent in horses at the onset of grade 1 disease. Careful observation may reveal transient periods of time where the horse shifts weight back and forth, has a slight increase in temperature at the coronary band, and has a slight increase in the digital pulse pressure. Horses that walk with a stilted gait but still will allow a foot to be lifted are classified as grade 2. Horses with Obel grade 2 laminitis can often be identified with a head-bobbing lameness when walked in a tight circle to either direction. Horses with Obel grade 3 laminitis move reluctantly and vigorously resist the lifting of a foot. The most severe classification is grade 4, noted by the horse refusing to move unless forced. A 'saw horse' stance (see Fig. 21.1), in which the horse shifts its weight to the back legs, which are moved forward under the body, is common in horses with more severe pain in the forefeet than in the hindfeet. Horses with pain equally severe in all four feet may have a normal stance. The most severe cases of laminitis often develop poor body condition and prolonged periods of recumbency with secondary pressure sores. Many severely affected horses only rise for short periods of time and demonstrate a characteristic stance of rocking or shifting their weight onto their rear feet, which is accompanied by anxiety, muscle fasciculations, and a reluctance to move.

In SRL, catastrophic failure of the lamellae is much more common than in endocrinopathic laminitis. More severe signs associate with lamellar failure in SRL include, when examining the digits, a dropped sole (loss of concavity of the sole dorsal to the apex of the frog) and/or palpation of a depression located at the level of the coronary band (see Fig. 26.5), both of which indicate rotation or distal displacement (sinking) of the distal phalanx (DP) within the hoof wall (see Chapter 6) [19]. Lateral radiographs of the digit may detect rotation and/or distal displacement of the DP within the hoof capsule (see Chapter 27). Laminitis associated with septic diseases can result in the rotation and/or distal displacement of the DP from a few hours to weeks after onset of lameness; in most cases, several days are required for rotation or distal displacement to occur. In peracute cases of SRL, serum leakage and/or bleeding from the coronary band develops within hours to a few days after the onset of lameness; this usually indicates severe lamellar damage with widespread separation of the lamellae. Mild cases may resolve without rotation or distal displacement. Once rotation or distal displacement occurs, significant lameness often persists.

Clinical Pathology

Clinical pathologic changes vary with the primary disease process leading to laminitis. There are no clinical pathologic changes specific to cases with laminitis. Hematologic abnormalities caused by enterocolitis, duodenitis/proximal jejunitis, bacterial pneumonia/pleuropneumonia, metritis, and other diseases that lead to endotoxemia/sepsis include neutropenia, leukopenia, and left shift [20, 21]. Horses with surgical intestinal disease often present with normal neutrophil and total white blood cell count; however, endotoxemia can develop after correction of intestinal strangulation leading to neutropenia and leucopenia [21]. The white blood cell count commonly rebounds after the resolution of endotoxemia-induced neutropenia, leading to neutrophilia and leukocytosis [21]. Severe dehydration associated with intestinal disease, fluid loss in diarrhea, gastric reflux, and third space fluid loss (pleuropneumonia) may result in profound hemoconcentration. All inflammatory diseases can lead to hyperfibrinogenemia; active bacterial infection leads to the most profound increases in plasma fibrinogen [21]. Protein loss due to either a compromised intestinal wall in intestinal disease or pleuropneumonia can lead to hypoproteinemia and hypoalbuminemia. Severe hypovolemia and cardiovascular shock can result in azotemia and increased hepatocellular enzyme activity. Serum lactate concentrations are elevated in horses with grain overload, colitis, and in horses with intestinal strangulation [21]. Colitis commonly results in hyponatremia, hypochloridemia, hypocalcemia, and hypokalemia. Metabolic acidosis may be present. Severe endotoxemia and sepsis can result in the activation of coagulation pathways and result in thrombocytopenia, coagulopathies, and disseminated intravascular coagulation (DIC) [22]. A high incidence of DIC associated with *Neorickettsia risticii* infection has been suggested to be linked to the high incidence of laminitis in horses with Potomac Horse Fever; however, definitive evidence of this association has not been found.

Other Diagnostic Tests

Diagnostic imaging (see Chapter 27) can be used to assess the severity of lamellar damage in horses with acute laminitis associated with septic diseases. In many circumstances, clinicians perform radiography of the distal phalanx at first sign of sepsis or, more commonly, the first sign of lamellar disease (heat in hoof, changes in digital pulse, or lameness) to determine the baseline position of the DP in relation to the hoof wall. Peritoneal fluid cytology and lactate concentration, abdominal ultrasonography, thoracic ultrasonography, thoracic radiography, transtracheal aspirate cytology and culture, abdominal radiography, exploratory celiotomy, and ocular examination are among the tests/procedures used to evaluate the primary disease process that led to systemic inflammation/sepsis and therefore SRL.

References

1. Annane, D., Bellissant, E., and Cavaillon, J.M. (2005) Septic shock. *Lancet*, **365**, 63–78.
2. Belknap, J.K., Moore, J.N., and Crouser, E.C. (2009) Sepsis – From human organ failure to laminar failure. *Vet. Immunol. Immunopathol.*, **129**, 155–157.
3. Lohmann, K.L. and Barton, M.H. (2010) Endotoxemia, in *Equine Internal Medicine* (eds S.M. Reed, W.M. Bayly, and D.C. Sellon), Saunders Elsevier, St Louis, pp. 807–823.
4. Parsons, C.S., Orsini, J.A., Krafty, R., Capewell, L., and Boston, R. (2007) Risk factors for development of acute laminitis in horses during hospitalization: 73 cases (1997–2004). *J. Am. Vet. Med. Assoc.*, **230**, 885–889.
5. Munoz, E., Arguelles, D., Areste, L., Miguel, L.S., and Prades, M. (2008) Retrospective analysis of exploratory laparotomies in 192 Andalusian and 276 horses of other breeds. *Vet. Rec.*, **162**, 303–306.
6. Rebiere, P. (2009) Evaluation of low-molecular-weight heparin for the prevention of equine laminitis after colic surgery. *J. Vet. Emerg. Crit. Care*, **19**, 113–119.

7. Cohen, N.D. and Woods, A.M. (1999) Characteristics and risk factors for failure of horses with acute diarrhea to survive: 122 cases (1990–1996). *J. Am. Vet. Med. Assoc.*, **214**, 382–390.
8. Slater, M.R., Hood, D.M., and Carter, G.K. (1995) Descriptive epidemiological study of equine laminitis. *Equine Vet. J.*, **27**, 364–367.
9. Polzer, J. and Slater, M.R. (1997) Age, breed, sex and seasonality as risk factors for equine laminitis. *Prev. Vet. Med.*, **29**, 179–184.
10. Alford, P., Geller, S., Richardson, B., Slater, M., Honnas, C., Foreman, J., Robinson, J., Messer, M., Roberts, M., Goble, D., Hood, D., and Chaffin, M. (2001) A multicenter, matched case-control study of risk factors for equine laminitis. *Prev. Vet. Med.*, **49**, 209–222.
11. Hunt, J.M., Edwards, G.B., and Clarke, K.W. (1986) Incidence, diagnosis and treatment of postoperative complications in colic cases. *Equine Vet. J.*, **18**, 264–270.
12. Cohen, N.D. (1994) Prevalence and factors associated with development of laminitis in horses with duodenitis /proximal jejunitis. 33 cases (1985–1991). *J. Am. Vet. Med. Assoc.*, **204**, 250–254.
13. Bertin, F.R., Reising, A., Slovis, N.M., Constable, P.D., and Taylor, S.D. (2013) Clinical and clinicopathological factors associated with survival in 44 horses with equine neorhickettsiosis (Potomac Horse Fever). *J. Vet. Intern. Med.*, **27**, 1528–1534.
14. Manson, J., Thiemermann, C., and Brohi, K. (2012) Trauma alarmins as activators of damage-induced inflammation. *Br. J. Surg.*, **99** (Suppl.), 12–20.
15. Atherton, R.P., McKenzie, H.C., and Furr, M.O. (2009) Acute colitis: pathophysiology and non-infectious causes. *Compend. Contin. Educ. Equine*, **October**, 366–374. Available at: http://www.vetfolio.com.
16. Garner, H.E., Coffman, J.R., Hahn, A.W., Hutcheson, D.P., and Tumbleson, M.E. (1975) Equine laminitis of alimentary origin: an experimental model. *Am. J. Vet. Res.*, **36**, 441–444.
17. Wilkins, P.A. (2009) Complications in the peri-parturient mare, in *Current Therapy in Equine Medicine*, 6th edition (eds N.E. Robinson and K.A. Sprayberry), Saunders Elsevier, St Louis, pp. 785–789.
18. Hunt, R.J. (1993) A retrospective evaluation of laminitis in horses. *Equine Vet. J.*, **25**, 61–64.
19. Baxter, G.M. (1986) Equine laminitis caused by distal displacement of the distal phalanx: 12 cases (1976–1985). *J. Am. Vet. Med. Assoc.*, **189**, 326–329.
20. Reuss, S.M. and Giguere, S. (2015) Update on bacterial pneumonia and pleuropneumonia in the adult horse. *Vet. Clin. Equine*, **31**, 105–120.
21. Lester, S.J., Mollat, W.H., and Bryant, J.E. (2015) Overview of clinical pathology and the horse. *Vet. Clin. Equine*, **31**, 247–268.
22. Divers, T.J. (2003) Prevention and treatment of thrombosis, phlebitis, and laminitis in horses with gastrointestinal diseases. *Vet. Clin. Equine*, **19**, 779–790.

CHAPTER 23

Laminitis in Equine Metabolic Syndrome

Andy E. Durham

What is Equine Metabolic Syndrome?

As metabolic syndrome has progressed to become a major threat to human health in the developed world, in association with readily available, highly caloric food and drink and a more sedentary lifestyle [1], a broadly analogous concern has developed in horses associated with more generous and relaxed feeding and management practices. In 1988, Reaven published his observation that many human patients suffering from cardiovascular disease had, at the same time, glucose intolerance, hyperinsulinemia, hypertriglyceridemia, low high-density lipoprotein (HDL)-cholesterol and hypertension [2]. Reaven considered that insulin resistance (IR) was the driving force of this syndrome. In 2002, Johnson also noted that many equine patients suffering from laminitis shared similar features, and first proposed the term equine metabolic syndrome (EMS) [3]; subsequently, working definitions have been proposed that comprise markers of obesity, insulin dysregulation, and dyslipidemia [4, 5]. Twenty-five years on from its initial description, the metabolic syndrome in humans continues to provoke debate not only regarding its pathophysiology, treatment and management, but also even regarding its fundamental definition and clinical relevance [6]. It should come as no surprise then that the much newer concept of EMS will continue to develop and evolve as new insights and research findings are presented [7].

Both human and equine metabolic syndromes are primarily created and maintained by chronically excessive caloric intake and physical inactivity with further important and related susceptibility factors also being involved. The major defining clinical consequence of EMS is laminitis, although it is possible that further pathogenic endpoints may become better recognized in the future. Thus, for the time being at least, EMS might be regarded as "…a collection of coexisting risk factors, associated with metabolic and endocrine dysregulation, that signal an increased susceptibility to laminitis." Thus far, identifiable risk factors that may alert the clinician to the presence of EMS comprise several endogenous phenotypic characteristics, along with further important interactive and influential exogenous factors (Table 23.1). Clinicopathological factors typically associated with EMS are discussed elsewhere in this book (see Chapter 29).

Identification of Animals at Risk or Exhibiting Signs of Laminitis in Association with EMS

Cases of EMS are usually first recognized and investigated following a diagnosis of laminitis. In the future, with more widespread awareness of the syndrome, more cases will hopefully be seen in a pre- or subclinical laminitic stage where risk factors are recognized and control measures are implemented before clinical disease occurs. Early recognition of EMS should therefore be encouraged by client education and preventative healthcare programs. Insulin dysregulation may represent a key pathophysiological driving force for EMS, with obesity and laminitis being the most prevalent clinical manifestations.

The recognition of clustering of common risk factors (Table 23.1), which led to the initial syndromic proposals [2, 3], is essential for the identification and differentiation of EMS from other causes of laminitis. For example, when laminitis is recurrent in a nine-year-old, obese, native pony, whilst grazing on spring pasture, that is exercised very little, and further diagnostic testing indicates insulin dysregulation and dyslipidemia, then EMS is suspected. On the other hand, supporting-limb laminitis (caused by excessive load-bearing) and sepsis-related laminitis (caused by grain engorgement, retained fetal membranes, colon torsion or acute colitis, etc.) may be less epidemiologically distinct and affect a far more diverse phenotypic range of individuals. In contrast to the laminitis patient associated with EMS, laminitis patients associated with sepsis or excessive load-bearing may be younger, leaner, fitter, of any breed, at any time of year, not grazing, and have no prior history of laminitis and no predisposing clinicopathologic features. Further discussion of recognizable factors that should lead to suspicion and/or diagnosis of EMS follows.

Equine Laminitis, First Edition. Edited by James K. Belknap and Raymond Geor.

Table 23.1 Candidate risk factors defining equine metabolic syndrome (EMS) and associated risk of laminitis.

ENDOGENOUS		
Signalment	***Clinical***	**EXOGENOUS**
Age	Obesity	Workload/activity
Breed	Previous laminitis	Diet
Gender	Hypertension	Season
	Reproductive dysfunction	

Signalment Characteristics of EMS Cases

Age

EMS is typically identified from 5–8 years of age onwards [3, 7], recognizing an apparently decreased susceptibility of young horses to laminitis [5, 8–10]. Anecdotally, many young ponies are seen to become obese during the first two to five years of life. Unfortunately, due to limited opportunities (primarily due to limited owner requests) to perform further investigations of such individuals at an early stage of obesity, the veterinarian is not summoned commonly to assess and treat the animal until after laminitis has occurred, sometimes years later. Longitudinal studies, starting in foal-hood, that describe the age of onset and development of risk factors for laminitis susceptibility later in life (e.g., obesity, insulin dysregulation) have not been published; EMS might occur – and therefore might be detectable – in young horses a long time before clinical laminitis is recognized.

The precise reason for the apparently decreased risk of laminitis in young horses is not clear, although reduced risk due to a decreased prevalence of excessive adipose deposits in an actively growing individual with higher caloric requirements, along with often higher levels of voluntary physical activity, may play a role. Age effects on insulin dysregulation *per se* have not been well described in horses; however, the findings of one study that six- to nine-month-old foals had reduced glucose tolerance compared to mature ponies [12] suggest that insulin sensitivity is not a protective mechanism that explains the reduced prevalence of laminitis in young animals.

Animals older than 15–18 years of age are also less commonly affected by EMS [3, 7], perhaps as a result of laminitis in older animals being associated with pituitary pars intermedia dysfunction (PPID) [11]. Even in the absence of PPID, decreased adiposity associated with age-related disease such as dental disorders may also be protective against EMS in older horses.

Gender

Some studies have indicated that mares and stallions may be more prone to laminitis than geldings [10, 13–15]. Any apparent gender effect could be confounded by several other factors, such as physical activity, the likelihood of the owner seeking veterinary attention, body condition, and insulin sensitivity. A decreased insulin sensitivity in females was suggested in one study of hyperlipemia in donkeys [16].

Breed/Type

It is recognized that certain 'easy-keeping' or 'good-doing' equine breeds are inherently prone to laminitis; these include Shetland, New Forest, Dartmoor, Exmoor, Welsh, Morgan, Tennessee Walking horse, Paso Fino, Arabian, Saddlebred, Spanish Mustang, and donkeys [7, 10, 13]. There may be external managemental influences to consider in the type and level of activity commonly associated with typical EMS breeds, although it is also likely that the retention of certain 'thrifty' genes is also important [17]. Several genetic traits may once have provided a survival advantage to ancestors that evolved and adapted to survive well in harsh environments where dietary energy supply was variably accessible due to seasonal drought or cold. The ration in these harsh environments would have generally been composed of low-energy density (low nonstructural carbohydrate [NSC]), high-fiber food sources. Numerous physiologic and metabolic adaptations may be inherent in these individuals, such as an increased appetite for food when available, a greater assimilative capacity (i.e., increased extraction/absorption of energy) from the ingested food, and altered metabolic/endocrine responses to the assimilated nutrients. Insulin resistance – a common feature of the EMS phenotype – is associated physiologically with the relative conservation of glucose for vital non-insulin-dependent tissues (e.g., brain, kidneys, endothelia) and the facilitation of gluconeogenesis and more readily mobilized glycogen and adipose stores. This evident evolutionary advantage that developed in a harsh and variable dietary environment no longer serves the same benefits under typical modern management systems (where food is plentiful all year round) and may, in contrast, represent a threat to health.

The recognition of particular breeds and types prone to obesity and laminitis is suggestive of genetic determination of some risk factors. Ponies have long been known to be inherently insulin-resistant when compared to horses [18–21], and a study of an inbred closed pony herd in Virginia revealed strong genetic influences on laminitis occurrence [4]; many further anecdotal reports of such exist from breeders and owners of native ponies. Complex and polygenic influences on many aspects of ingestive and exertional behaviors, digestive physiology, endocrinology and nutrient and adipose metabolism may well all play a role in EMS.

Clinical Characteristics of EMS Cases

Laminitis Characteristics in EMS Cases

When a middle-aged, obese, sedentary native pony is grazed simultaneously on the same pasture as a fit, lean, young Thoroughbred, only the former is likely to develop laminitis; this implies differing physiologic, metabolic and/or endocrine responses to the ingested nutrients. Recent studies have suggested that endocrinopathic mechanisms may be important predisposing factors in approximately 90% of clinical laminitis cases [22, 23], a figure that at first glance might seem surprisingly high. However, for far longer than the recent discussions of endocrinopathic laminitis, veterinarians and horse owners have recognized that many laminitis-prone individuals share similar characteristics such as breed, age, obesity, a rich diet, and a low workload (Table 23.1). Conversely, they would also recognize that laminitis arising in the absence of these factors is relatively unusual (i.e., less than 10% of cases!).

Thus, when considering the clinical examination and characteristics of the affected feet of animals with EMS-related laminitis, there are no special or unusual distinguishing features on which to comment as, alongside PPID, they probably constitute the regular, every-day cases that we all see [22, 23]. They may present with forelimb and/or hindlimb signs (more commonly forelimb), mild or severe pain, with acute onset signs or with mild to severe chronic anatomic foot abnormalities such as prominent and divergent hoof rings, concavity of the dorsal hoof wall, expansion of the white line and solear flattening or convexity [24, 25]. Clearly, lamellar pain and cohesive lamellar failure is not an 'all-or-nothing' event as is frequently the case in both sepsis-related and supporting-limb laminitis cases. In EMS-related laminitis, detectable anatomic changes (e.g., growth rings, expansion of white line) may be seen in the absence of a history of obvious foot pain, perhaps relating to a low-grade, chronic and insidious lamellar disease process that commonly occurs with EMS [3]. In the equine athlete with EMS-related laminitis, the lameness that the animal may exhibit the first time the veterinarian and/or farrier are summoned to perform an examination may be caused by solear pain due to bruising secondary to the insidious displacement of the distal phalanx (with no previous history of lameness during the time frame in which a gradual displacement of the phalanx must have been taking place). Due to the fact that the lameness associated with EMS is commonly mild and bilateral, affecting both forelimbs, the veterinarian needs to pay close attention to the presence of other risk factors for EMS (discussed below) and possibly be more aggressive when performing additional diagnostics such as radiographic imaging (see Chapter 27) and clinicopathologic evaluation for EMS (see Chapter 29) in animals exhibiting both digital signs (abnormalities in the hoof capsule and/or digital pain) and risk factors for EMS. It is not uncommon for these cases to first be mistaken for other causes of bilateral forelimb lameness.

Chronicity and recurrence are frequent features of EMS-related laminitis [3–5, 7]. Fundamentally, there are probably two reasons why cases of laminitis might recur: (i) damage caused by previous disease episodes makes the foot inherently more susceptible to further laminitis attacks; and (ii) the endogenous and exogenous risk factors associated with the previous laminitis episode (e.g., insulin dysregulation, obesity, excessive grazing) are still present. Indeed, a common question from the owner of a *de-novo* laminitic animal is "Will this mean that my pony will always continue to suffer from laminitis?" Intuitively, the answer is that recurrence should be expected in those cases where the fundamental causal factors are not subsequently managed and controlled effectively. It is therefore vital that laminitis cases encountered in practice are not simply treated and managed for laminitis in an insular fashion, but rather that an epidemiologic investigation is performed thoroughly so that the identification and control of significant risk factors can be instigated. This comprises investigations of historical, clinical, and clinicopathologic factors.

Obesity

Obesity has long been associated with laminitis susceptibility, and is a prominent epidemiologic feature of EMS [4,5,10,26] and human metabolic syndrome [6]. The precise links between obesity and laminitis are not fully understood, but a causal association with insulin dysregulation is a likely candidate [19,27–29].

It has been estimated that approximately half of the horses in the UK are overweight [30, 31]. Obesity is a contentious and emotive term that is surprisingly poorly recognized for what is commonly, but not invariably, an externally obvious sign. Several studies have shown that owners of many obese horses do not appear to recognize its existence in their animals [30–32]. One might surmise that this could represent 'denial' on the part of the owner – a defensive psychological response to avoid dealing with a problem that they find impossible to manage. Alternatively, it may be that many horse owners have become gradually accustomed to a slowly increasing degree of adiposity in their horses, perhaps encouraged by judges in some equestrian disciplines who actively select and reward animals carrying a certain amount of externally obvious, excessive adipose tissue. However, a further possible source of misconception is a lack of understanding about what obesity actually is.

Obesity is broadly defined in a medical context as "…excessive adiposity to an extent where health is negatively affected." Obesity is therefore primarily a functional and metabolic status, rather than simply a morphological status, and may not always directly correlate with the size of adipose deposits [33]. In contrast, in general colloquial parlance, obesity may be entirely defined according to visual preconceptions that obese individuals will represent the extreme of excess bodily condition manifesting as a severe degree of adipose coverage over the entire body. Indeed, laminitis-prone individuals are often overtly and unequivocally obese with an absence of palpable ribs, large fatty deposits behind the shoulders and tail-head, and a large firm crest in the neck. However, others may have palpable or even visible ribs leading some to describe them as 'lean,' although retaining a large cresty neck or perhaps hidden deposits of retroperitoneal fat. The point at which an individual's health becomes compromised by the presence of adipose deposits (i.e., when obesity develops) is unknown, but is likely dependent on the amount, the site, and the metabolic activity of adipose tissue in that individual, emphasizing the importance of 'regional obesity.' In human patients, there is substantial evidence indicating that fat distribution is a better predictor of cardiovascular disease than overall fat volume [34, 35]. The uneven development and disappearance of regional adipose deposits in horses and ponies

Table 23.2 Proposed working definitions of equine metabolic syndrome (EMS). Laminitis susceptibility is defined when at least three of the four listed factors are identified [4, 5].

1. **At least three of the following [4]:**
   - BCS ≥7 with localized fat deposits on neck and tailhead
   - Reverse inverse square of insulin <0.32 [mU l^{-1}]$^{-0.5}$
   - Modified insulin response to glucose >5.6 mU insulin^2/[10·l·mg glucose]
   - Triglyceride concentration >57.0 mg dl^{-1}
2. **At least three of the following [5]:**
   - BCS ≥7
   - CNS ≥4
   - Insulin >32 mU l^{-1}
   - Leptin >7.3 ng ml^{-1}

BCS, Body Condition Score; CNS, Cresty Neck Score.

is also well described [36]. Two published studies have specifically proposed clusters of risk factors defining EMS [4, 5], and both included markers of regional adiposity (Table 23.2).

Unfortunately, the definition of excessive adiposity in an individual equid when seen by a practitioner is usually based on a subjective opinion, a situation that does not facilitate the conversion of sceptical horse owners who do not believe that their animal is obese. The body mass index (body mass/height^2) has been described in horses as a possible objective index of adiposity, although it has received little attention [37]. The lack of widespread availability of weighbridges (scales) does not, in any case, encourage the use of any index relating to body mass.

The body condition score (BCS) is perhaps the most frequently used semi-objective index of obesity; however, it generally still lacks widespread acceptance and its use in practice may require tailoring for different breeds, ages, genders, and activities [21]. Any lack of clarity and user-friendliness is not aided by confusing and poorly defined descriptive terminology that is difficult to apply, requiring the user to distinguish fat deposits that feel 'spongy,' 'soft,' 'very soft,' 'patchy,' or 'bulging' [38]. Nevertheless, the BCS has been shown to correlate well with markers of IR and laminitis susceptibility [5,21,26]; indeed, in one study it was found that a BCS >6.8 was a good indication that the total body fat content exceeded 20% [39]. The 'cresty-neck score' (CNS) is a semi-objective means of describing regional obesity with respect to the apparently particular associations between neck crest fat, IR, and laminitis [5, 21] (Table 23.3). However, breed, gender, and perhaps age effects are also important in the interpretation of CNS, as in one study it was found that associations between both BCS and CNS with hyperinsulinemia were only significant for ponies and not for horses [21].

Practical and objective morphometric measures of both abdominal/trunk fat (girth:height ratio, waist:height ratio) and neck crest fat (crest height, neck circumference, neck circumference:height ratio) have been described in several studies and related to other markers of obesity, IR, and laminitis [5, 21, 26, 38]. However, these objective morphometric measures have been found to be generally less strongly correlated with body

Table 23.3 Cresty neck score. Reproduced with permission from Ref. [21]; © Elsevier.

Score	Characteristics
0	• No visual appearance of a crest • No palpable crest
1	• No visual appearance of a crest, but slight filling felt with palpation
2	• Noticeable appearance of a crest, but fat deposited fairly evenly from poll to withers • Crest easily cupped in one hand and bent from side to side
3	• Crest enlarged and thickened, so fat is deposited more heavily in middle of the neck than toward poll and withers, giving a mounded appearance. • Crest fills cupped hand and begins losing side-to-side flexibility
4	• Crest grossly enlarged and thickened, and can no longer be cupped in one hand or easily bent from side to side • Crest may have wrinkles/creases perpendicular to topline
5	• Crest is so large it permanently droops to one side

fat percentage and serum biochemical indices of IR than are the semi-objective BCS and CNS [21, 38]. Nevertheless, given the obvious attraction of objectivity, it has been suggested that certain cut-offs of morphometric measures could be used in ponies and horses to indicate overweight, obesity, and crestiness (Table 23.4). Indeed, in one large study of a particular pony herd, laminitis was predicted with reasonable accuracy in ponies with a girth:height ratio >1.30 and neck circumference:height ratio > 0.71 [5].

Fat depth measured ultrasonographically in specific areas such as the shoulder, intercostal space, rump, and retroperitoneal layer, might have potential to be used as a further objective measure of adiposity [36, 39, 40]. It was suggested that the percentage total body fat could be estimated using the formula: 8.64 + (4.7 × rump fat thickness [cm]) in horses, and 3.83 + (5.58 × rump fat thickness [cm]) in ponies [36]. In another study a slightly different formula was derived: % fat = 2.47 + (5.47 × rump fat thickness [cm]), although breeds were not specified [41].

Experience suggests that, with the exception of many PPID cases, it is rare to encounter a laminitis-prone individual where it would be unequivocally wrong to encourage further weight loss, although such cases do exist. To describe a laminitis-prone

Table 23.4 Suggested objective morphometric measurements indicative of excessive adiposity in horses and ponies [21].

Condition	Pony	Horse
Overweight	Girth:height ≥1.33	Girth:height ≥1.26
Obese	Girth:height ≥1.38	Girth:height ≥1.29
Cresty	0.5 NC:height ≥0.68	0.5 NC:height ≥0.63

0.5 NC = mid-neck circumference.

individual as 'non-obese' requires confidence that the fat deposits, which most individuals will inevitably have, are playing no direct or indirect role in the disease process.

Hypertension

Hypertension is a central feature of the metabolic syndrome in people but has received little attention in horses, perhaps due to relative inconvenience and lack of blood pressure measurements as part of a standard clinical examination of the horse. Clinical laminitis has long been recognized as a hypertensive disease, and several anti-hypertensive therapies have been advocated [42]. However, whether or not hypertension is a pathogenetic factor or simply a secondary consequence of the pain and distress associated with acute laminitis is not known. Interestingly, in one study it was found that laminitis-prone ponies had a higher mean blood pressure in the summer than non-laminitic controls, even when not clinically affected, thereby supporting hypertension as a candidate marker for laminitis-susceptibility in a striking analogy with cardiovascular-risk in the human metabolic syndrome [43]. However, other studies have not confirmed this finding [5].

Reproductive Function

Associations between IR and reproductive dysfunction are well recognized in human metabolic syndrome and polycystic ovarian syndrome [44], but are not so clearly defined in mares. Equine studies have indicated a persistence of cyclicity through the winter in obese versus lean mares, suggesting an improved reproductive function [45]. In contrast, other studies of obese and insulin-resistant mares have reported deleterious effects, including prolongation of the luteal phase and interovulatory period [46, 47]. However, no effects of exogenous insulin on cyclicity could be detected in another study [48].

Further Exogenous Factors Commonly Identified in EMS Cases

Dietary Quality and Quantity

Dietary intake is a key factor determining laminitis susceptibility, and also represents a frequently recognized final trigger event. Many EMS cases with laminitis have a long-term history of chronic caloric overprovision and a short-term history of ingestion of a high-NSC diet (usually grazing).

The chronic overprovision of dietary calories is the fundamental cause of adipose expansion which may culminate in obesity, a key risk factor for laminitis. Prediction and determination of caloric requirements is always approximate, and clearly depends on metabolic activity relating to exercise, growth, pregnancy, and lactation. It is also now recognized that there are fundamentally different energy requirements of individual animals. This is most likely due to their individual genetic makeup, but is more associated clinically with a description of their phenotype as 'easy-keepers' and 'good-doers' [49]. Metabolic efficiency is frequently used as an excuse for an inability to control obesity in laminitis-prone individuals, and it is clearly evident that weight loss is difficult to achieve in such animals. However, to suggest that obesity is absolutely resistant to dietary caloric restriction is illogical; it is simply a question of how severe the restriction needs to be. It is inconceivable that turning out an obese native-breed animal to join its feral desert-living counterparts for example, would result in long-term maintenance of its obesity! Weight loss achieved by diet and exercise is associated with improved insulin sensitivity in horses [28, 29, 40] and, by implication, a decreased risk of laminitis. There is some evidence that dietary composition may also be an important determinant of IR in that insulin responsiveness was found in one study to be lower in horses receiving high-NSC diets than high-fat and high-fiber diets [27].

Given the likely pathogenic importance of hyperinsulinemia as an acute trigger factor for laminitis [50–52], it is logical to assume that highly insulinemic diets will represent an immediate risk of laminitis. Nonstructural carbohydrates comprise simple sugars, starches and fructans, and pose the greatest insulinemic potential (although the possible insulinemic effect of other components such as amino acids in equine feeds has received little attention). Simple sugars and digestible starches clearly pose a high risk of hyperinsulinemia and form the bulk of the NSC within cereals (typically 50–70% dry matter [DM]) and leguminous pastures (typically 10–20% DM). Fructans are the major storage carbohydrate in temperate grasses and, included with simple sugars, are classified as water-soluble carbohydrate (WSC) in non-leguminous pastures, hays and silages (typically 10–20% DM). Although fructans are regarded as indigestible by the horse, the bacterial hydrolysis of fructans to fructose and glucose within the equine upper gastrointestinal tract may provide an explanation for hyperinsulinemia following fructan ingestion [53–55]. A study conducted in the UK found that serum uric acid, a metabolite of fructose, was present in slightly higher concentrations in laminitis-prone ponies compared to normal ponies during the summer [43], although this was not confirmed by a further study performed in the USA [21].

A high proportion of EMS-related laminitis cases occur in association with pasture grazing, although some might relate to cereal grain feeding or other unknown factors. The traditional explanation for this apparent link was that NSC ingested in excess of the digestible (or hydrolyzable) capacity of the upper gastrointestinal tract, led to rapid cecocolonic fermentation, dysbacteriosis, acidosis, mucosal barrier compromise, and systemic absorption of toxic 'laminogenic' trigger factors more characteristic of sepsis-related laminitis (SRL), as demonstrated by the experimental model of starch (or fructan) overload [56]. However, it is inconceivable that, under normal management conditions, NSC ingestion equivalent to the starch/fructan overload model of SRL (5–10 g NSC kg^{-1} body weight as a bolus) could occur at pasture. Although grazing ponies may eat as much as 10 g DM kg^{-1} body weight in a 3-h grazing period (P.A. Harris, personal communication), even given an extreme example of grass NSC content of 40% DM it is apparent that an intake of more than 1–2 g NSC kg^{-1} body weight per hour is implausible. Far lower rates of intake (<0.5 g NSC kg^{-1} body weight per hour) are more probably representative of realistic grazing activity. The demonstration of marked hyperinsulinemia in association with the gradual ingestion of NSC at rates much lower (<0.5 g NSC kg^{-1} body weight per hour [54, 57]) than the amount of fructan leading to sepsis strongly indicates more of an endocrinopathic link between grazing and laminitis than a link to sepsis.

Season

Laminitis has a strong seasonal incidence that has been demonstrated in several studies. The majority of non-PPID-associated laminitis cases seen in temperate climates arise in late spring/early summer [8, 13, 15], perhaps as a result of increased pasture NSC content leading to pathologic hyperinsulinemia [5]. In addition to seasonally variable NSC ingestion, there may also be seasonally differing responses to ingested NSC; however, a recent study showed that insulin responses to ingested carbohydrate in laminitis-prone ponies was higher in October/November versus May/June, contrary to expectations [55]. Significant monthly variability in resting insulin concentrations in both normal and EMS cases was also demonstrated, but this showed no distinct seasonal pattern [58]. An increased incidence of PPID-associated laminitis in the autumn has been suggested in accordance with increased pituitary secretory activity at that time in PPID cases [22]. However, it is known that pars intermedia secretory activity is also augmented in the autumn in horses without PPID [58–60]; the possible endocrinopathic consequences of this observation on EMS cases may warrant further investigation.

Workload and Activity

Many laminitis cases are relatively sedentary animals participating rarely, if at all, in organized exercise activities [10]. Enforced stable confinement is a common part of management of the acute and chronic laminitis case for the purposes of preservation of lamellar integrity and/or grazing restriction; this further adds to the lack of physical activity that typifies these animals. Conversely, it is a common anecdotal observation that fit, working ponies are generally less prone to laminitis. Perhaps the most obvious potential explanation for the apparent negative association between exercise and laminitis relates to obesity, and that the increased caloric demands of exercise mitigate against a dietary overprovision of NSC, as discussed above. However, there may be additional benefits of exercise on metabolism or even, conceivably, on lamellar cohesive strength as an adaptive response to mechanical stresses as seen in orthopedic tissues. In other species, a positive effect of exercise on insulin sensitivity is recognized independently of adiposity [61]. Several studies have also examined the effects of various exercise regimes on insulin sensitivity in horses and, although generally supportive of a beneficial effect of exercise, this has not been a consistent finding [62–65]. Whether or not such an effect exists, there are almost certainly further benefits of exercise that are likely to help reduce ongoing laminitis risk; hence, activity should be encouraged wherever lamellar integrity and comfort so allow.

Summary

The majority of cases of laminitis seen in practice are likely to share common features in respect to readily detectable endogenous and exogenous risk factors. Paramount among the controllable and reversible risk factors are overfeeding, a lack of exercise, obesity, and IR. Equine metabolic syndrome describes the clustering of these factors and, if persistent recurrence of laminitis is to be avoided, it is essential that these are identified and controlled wherever possible. However, a more ideal aspiration would be to identify and control such risk factors in young animals before the initial onset of the laminitis that they predict.

References

1. Grundy, S.M. (2008) Metabolic syndrome pandemic. *Arterioscler. Thromb. Vasc. Biol.*, **28**, 629–636.
2. Reaven, G.M. (1988) Role of IR in human disease. *Diabetes*, **37**, 1595–1607.
3. Johnson, P.J. (2002) The equine metabolic syndrome: peripheral Cushing's syndrome. *Vet. Clin. North Am. Equine Pract.*, **18**, 271–293.
4. Treiber, K.H., Kronfeld, D.S., Hess, T.M., Byrd, B.M., Splan, R.K., and Staniar, W.B. (2006) Evaluation of genetic and metabolic predispositions and nutritional risk factors for pasture-associated laminitis in ponies. *J. Am. Vet. Med. Assoc.*, **228**, 1538–1545.
5. Carter, R.A., Geor, R.J., Burton Staniar, W., Cubitt, T.A., and Harris, P.A. (2009) Prediction of incipient pasture-associated laminitis from hyperinsulinemia, hyperleptinaemia and generalised and localised obesity in a cohort of ponies. *Equine Vet. J.*, **41**, 171–178.
6. Alberti, K.G., Eckel, R.H., Grundy, S.M., Zimmet, P.Z., Cleeman, J.I., Donato, K.A., Fruchart, J.C., James, W.P., Loria, C.M., and Smith, S.C., Jr (2009) Harmonizing the metabolic syndrome. *Circulation*, **120**, 1640–1645.
7. Frank, N., Geor, R.J., Bailey, S.R., Durham, A.E., and Johnson, P.J. (2010) Equine metabolic syndrome. *J. Vet. Intern. Med.*, **24**, 467–475.
8. Peremans, K., Verschooten, F., de Moor, A., and Desmet, P. (1991) Laminitis in the pony: conservative treatment vs. dorsal hoof wall resection. *Equine Vet. J.*, **23**, 243–246.
9. Cripps, P.J. and Eustace, R.A. (1999) Factors involved in the prognosis of equine laminitis in the UK. *Equine Vet. J.*, **31**, 433–442.
10. Alford, P., Geller, S., Richrdson, B., Slater, M., Honnas, C., Foreman, J., Robinson, J., Messer, M., Roberts, M., Goble, D., Hood, D., and Chaffin, M. (2001) A multicenter, matched case-control study of risk factors for equine laminitis. *Prev. Vet. Med.*, **49**, 209–222.
11. Schott, H.C. (2006) Pituitary pars intermedia dysfunction: challenges of diagnosis and treatment. *Proc. Am. Assoc. Equine Pract.*, **52**, 60–73.

12. Murphy, D., Reid, S.W., and Love, S. (1997) The effect of age and diet on the oral glucose tolerance test in ponies. *Equine Vet. J.*, **29**, 467–470.
13. Dorn, C.R., Garner, H.E., Coffman, J.R., Hahn, A.W., and Tritschler, L.G. (1975) Castration and other factors affecting the risk of laminitis. *Cornell Vet.*, **65**, 57–64.
14. Slater, M.R., Hood, D.M., and Carter, G.K. (1995) Descriptive epidemiological study of equine laminitis. *Equine Vet. J.*, **27**, 364–367.
15. Menzies-Gow, N.J., Katz, L.M., Barker, K.J., Elliott, J., De Brauwere, M.N., Jarvis, N., Marr, C.M., and Pfeiffer, D.U. (2010) Epidemiological study of pasture-associated laminitis and concurrent risk factors in the South of England. *Vet. Rec.*, **167**, 690–694.
16. Reid, S.W. and Mohammed, H.O. (1996) Survival analysis approach to risk factors associated with hyperlipemia in donkeys. *J. Am. Vet. Med. Assoc.*, **209**, 1449–1452.
17. Neel, J.V. (1962) Diabetes mellitus: a 'thrifty' genotype rendered detrimental by 'progress'? *Am. J. Hum. Genet.*, **14**, 353–362.
18. Coffman, J.R. and Colles, C.M. (1983) Insulin tolerance in laminitic ponies. *Can. J. Comp. Med.*, **47**, 347–351.
19. Jeffcott, L.B., Field, J.R., McLean, J.G., and O'Dea, K. (1986) Glucose tolerance and insulin sensitivity in ponies and Standardbred horses. *Equine Vet. J.*, **18**, 97–101.
20. Rijnen, K.E. and van der Kolk, J.H. (2003) Determination of reference range values indicative of glucose metabolism and IR by use of glucose clamp techniques in horses and ponies. *Am. J. Vet. Res.*, **64**, 1260–1264.
21. Carter, R.A., Geor, R.J., Burton Staniar, W., Cubitt, T.A., and Harris, P.A. (2009) Apparent adiposity assessed by standardised scoring systems and morphometric measurements in horses and ponies. *Vet. J.*, **179**, 204–210.
22. Donaldson, M.T., Jorgensen, A.J., and Beech, J. (2004) Evaluation of suspected pituitary pars intermedia dysfunction in horses with laminitis. *J. Am. Vet. Med. Assoc.*, **224**, 1123–1127.
23. Karikoski, N.P., Horn, I., McGowan, T.W., and McGowan, C.M. (2011) The prevalence of endocrinopathic laminitis among horses presented for laminitis at a first opinion/referral equine hospital. *Dom. Anim. Endocr.*, **41**, 111–117.
24. Hunt, R.J. and Wharton, R.E. (2010) Clinical presentation, diagnosis, and prognosis of chronic laminitis in North America. *Vet. Clin. North Am. Equine Pract.*, **26**, 141–153.
25. Van Eps, A.W. (2010) Acute laminitis: medical and supportive therapy. *Vet. Clin. North Am. Equine Pract.*, **26**, 103–114.
26. Frank, N., Elliott, S.B., Brandt, L.E., and Keisler, D.H. (2006) Physical characteristics, blood hormone concentrations, and plasma lipid concentrations in obese horses with IR. *J. Am. Vet. Med. Assoc.*, **228**, 1383–1390.
27. Hoffman, R.M., Boston, R.C., Stefanovski, D., Kronfeld, D.S., and Harris, P.A. (2003) Obesity and diet affect glucose dynamics and insulin sensitivity in Thoroughbred geldings. *J. Anim. Sci.*, **81**, 2333–2342.
28. Freestone, J.F., Beadle, R., Shoemaker, K., Bessin, R.T., Wolfsheimer, K.J., and Church, C. (1992) Improved insulin sensitivity in hyperinsulinaemic ponies through physical conditioning and controlled feed intake. *Equine Vet. J.*, **24**, 187–190.
29. Van Weyenberg, S., Hesta, M., Buysse, J., and Janssens, G.P.J. (2008) The effect of weight loss by energy restriction on metabolic profile and glucose tolerance in ponies. *J. Anim. Physiol. Nutr.*, **92**, 538–545.
30. Wyse, C.A., McNie, K.A., Tannahil, V.J., Murray, J.K., and Love, S. (2008) Prevalence of obesity in riding horses in Scotland. *Vet. Rec.*, **162**, 590–591.
31. Stephenson, H.M., Green, M.J., and Freeman, S.L. (2011) Prevalence of obesity in a population of horses in the UK. *Vet. Rec.*, **168**, 131.
32. Ireland, J.L., Clegg, P.D., McGowan, C.M., McKane, S.A., Chandler, K.J., and Pinchbeck, G.L. (2012) Comparison of owner-reported health problems with veterinary assessment of geriatric horses in the United Kingdom. *Equine Vet. J.*, **44**, 94–100.
33. Conus, F., Rabasa-Lhoret, R., and Péronnet, F. (2007) Characteristics of metabolically obese normal-weight (MONW) subjects. *Appl. Physiol. Nutr. Metab.*, **32**, 4–12.
34. Fox, C.S., Massaro, J.M., Hoffmann, U., Pou, K.M., Maurovich-Horvat, P., Liu, C.Y., Vasan, R.S., Murabito, J.M., Meigs, J.B., Cupples, L.A., D'Agostino, R.B., Sr, and O'Donnell, C.J. (2007) Abdominal visceral and subcutaneous adipose tissue compartments: association with metabolic risk factors in the Framingham Heart Study. *Circulation*, **116**, 39–48.
35. Ibrahim, M.M. (2010) Subcutaneous and visceral adipose tissue: structural and functional differences. *Obesity Rev.*, **11**, 11–18.
36. Westervelt, R.G., Stouffer, J.R., Hintz, H.F., and Schryver, H.F. (1976) Estimating fatness in horses and ponies. *J. Anim. Sci.*, **43**, 781–785.
37. Donaldson, M., McFarlane, D., Jorgensen, A., and Beech, J. (2004) Correlation between plasma α-melanocyte-stimulating hormone concentration and body mass index in healthy horses. *Am. J. Vet. Res.*, **65**, 1469–1473.
38. Henneke, D.R., Potter, G.D., Kreider, J.L., and Yeates, B.E. (1983) Relationship between condition score, physical measurement and body fat percentage in mares. *Equine Vet. J.*, **15**, 371–372.
39. Dugdale, A.H., Grove-White, D., Curtis, G.C., Harris, P.A., and Argo, C.M. (2012) Body condition scoring as a predictor of body fat in horses and ponies. *Vet. J.*, **194**, 173–178.
40. Dugdale, A.H., Curtis, G.C., Cripps, P., Harris, P.A., and Argo, C.M. (2010) Effect of dietary restriction on body condition, composition and welfare of overweight and obese pony mares. *Equine Vet. J.*, **42**, 600–610.
41. Kane, R.A., Fisher, M., Parrett, D., and Lawrence, L.M. (1987) Estimating fatness in horses. *Proc. Equine Nutr. Physiol. Symp.*, **10**, 127–131.
42. Hinckley, K.A., Fearn, S., Howard, B.R., and Henderson, I.W. (1996) Nitric oxide donors as treatment for grass-induced acute laminitis in ponies. *Equine Vet. J.*, **28**, 17–28.
43. Bailey, S.R., Habershon-Butcher, J.L., Ransom, K.J., Elliott, J., and Menzies-Gow, N.J. (2008) Hypertension and IR in a mixed-breed population of ponies predisposed to laminitis. *Am. J. Vet. Res.*, **69**, 122–129.
44. Blank, S.K., Helm, K.D., McCartney, C.R., and Marshall, J.C. (2008) Polycystic ovary syndrome in adolescence. *Ann. N. Y. Acad. Sci.*, **1135**, 76–84.
45. Gentry, L.R., Thompson, D.L., Gentry, G.T., Davis, K.A., Godke, R.A., and Cartmill, J.A. (2002) The relationship between body condition, leptin, and reproductive and hormonal characteristics of mares during the seasonal anovulatory period. *J. Anim. Sci.*, **80**, 2695–2703.
46. Sessions, D.R., Reedy, S.E., Vick, M.M., Murphy, B.A., and Fitzgerald, B.P. (2004) Development of a model for inducing transient

insulin resistance in the mare: preliminary implications regarding the estrous cycle. *J. Anim. Sci.*, **82**, 2321–2328.

47. Vick, M.M., Sessions, D.R., Murphy, B.A., Kennedy, E.L., Reedy, S.E., and Fitzgerald, B.P. (2006) Obesity is associated with altered metabolic and reproductive activity in the mare: effects of metformin on insulin sensitivity and reproductive cyclicity. *Reprod. Fertil., Dev.*, **18**, 609–617.
48. Rambags, B.P., van Rossem, A.W., Blok, E.E., de Graaf-Roelfsema, E., Kindahl, H., van der Kolk, J.H., and Stout, T.A. (2008) Effects of exogenous insulin on luteolysis and reproductive cyclicity in the mare. *Reprod. Domest. Anim.*, **43**, 422–428.
49. National Research Council (2007) Energy, in *Nutrient Requirements of Horses*, 6th edition. National Academies Press, Washington, pp. 3–33.
50. Asplin, K.E., Sillence, M.N., Pollitt, C.C., and McGowan, C.M. (2007) Induction of laminitis by prolonged hyperinsulinaemia in clinically normal ponies. *Vet. J.*, **174**, 530–535.
51. de Laat, M.A., McGowan, C.M., Sillence, M.N., and Pollitt, C.C. (2010) Equine laminitis: induced by 48 h hyperinsulinaemia in Standardbred horses. *Equine Vet. J.*, **42**, 129–135.
52. de Laat, M.A., Sillence, M.N., McGowan, C.M., and Pollitt, C.C. (2012) Continuous intravenous infusion of glucose induces endogenous hyperinsulinaemia and lamellar histopathology in Standardbred horses. *Vet. J.*, **191**, 317–322.
53. Coenen, M., Mößeler, A., and Vervuert, I. (2006) Fermentative gases in breath indicate that inulin and starch start to be degraded by microbial fermentation in the stomach and small intestine of the horse in contrast to pectin and cellulose. *J. Nutr.*, **136**, 2108S–2110S.
54. Bailey, S.R., Menzies-Gow, N.J., Harris, P.A., Habershon-Butcher, J.L., Crawford, C., Berhane, Y., Boston, R.C., and Elliott, J. (2007) Effect of dietary fructans and dexamethasone administration on the insulin response of ponies predisposed to laminitis. *J. Am. Vet. Med. Assoc.*, **231**, 1365–1373.
55. Borer, K.E., Bailey, S.R., Menzies-Gow, N.J., Harris, P.A., and Elliott, J. (2012) Effect of feeding glucose, fructose, and inulin on blood glucose and insulin concentrations in normal ponies and those predisposed to laminitis. *J. Anim. Sci.*, **90**, 3003–3011.
56. Garner, H.E., Coffman, J.R., Hahn, A.W., Hutcheson, D.P., and Tumbleson, M.E. (1975) Equine laminitis of alimentary origin: an experimental model. *Am. J. Vet. Res.*, **36**, 441–444.
57. Frank, N., Elliott, S.B., Chameroy, K.A., Tóth, F., Chumbler, N.S., and McClamroch R. (2010) Association of season and pasture grazing with blood hormone and metabolite concentrations in horses with presumed pituitary pars intermedia dysfunction. *J. Vet. Intern. Med.*, **24**, 1167–1175.
58. Place, N.J., McGowan, C.M., Lamb, S.V., Schanbacher, B.J., McGowan, T., and Walsh, D.M. (2010) Seasonal variation in serum concentrations of selected metabolic hormones in horses. *J. Vet. Intern. Med.*, **24**, 650–654.
59. Donaldson, M.T., McDonnell, S.M., Schanbacher, B.J., Lamb, S.V., McFarlane, D., and Beech, J. (2005) Variation in plasma adrenocorticotropic hormone concentration and dexamethasone suppression test results with season, age, and sex in healthy ponies and horses. *J. Vet. Intern. Med.*, **19**, 217–222.
60. Copas, V.E. and Durham, A.E. (2012) Circannual variation in plasma adrenocorticotropic hormone concentrations in the UK in normal horses and ponies, and those with pituitary pars intermedia dysfunction. *Equine Vet. J.*, **44**, 440–443.
61. Marliss, E.B. and Vranic, M. (2002) Intense exercise has unique effects on both insulin release and its roles in glucoregulation: implications for diabetes. *Diabetes*, **51** (Suppl.1), S271–S283.
62. Powell, D.M., Reedy, D.R., Sessions, D.R., and Fitzgerald, B.P. (2002) Effect of short term exercise training on insulin sensitivity in obese and lean mares. *Equine Vet. J. Suppl.*, **34**, 81–84.
63. Graaf-Roelfsema, E., Ginneken, M.E., van Brenda, E., Winjberg, I.D., Keizer, H.A., and van der Kolk, J.H. (2006) The effect of long-term exercise on glucose metabolism and peripheral insulin sensitivity in Standardbred horses. *Equine Vet. J. Suppl.*, **36**, 221–225.
64. Carter, R.A., McCutcheon, J., Valle, E., Meilan, E.N., and Geor, R.J. (2010) Effects of exercise training on adiposity, insulin sensitivity, plasma hormone and lipid concentrations in overweight or obese, insulin-resistant horses. *Am. J. Vet. Res.*, **71**, 314–321.
65. Turner, S.P., Hess, T.M., Treiber, K., Mello, E.B., Souza, B.G., and Almeida, F.Q. (2011) Comparison of insulin sensitivity of horses adapted to different exercise intensities. *J. Equine Vet. Sci.*, **31**, 645–649.

CHAPTER 24

Laminitis in Pituitary Pars Intermedia Dysfunction

Philip J. Johnson

Introduction

Although pituitary pars intermedia dysfunction (PPID) has been recognized as a significant risk factor for endocrinopathic laminitis for many years, the role of corticosteroid (cortisol) excess as a cause of laminitis in PPID has been undermined by the realization that adrenocortical hypertrophy is an inconsistent finding in these cases. The results of more recent studies have suggested that PPID-associated laminitis may be more significantly associated with conditions of insulin resistance (IR) and hyperinsulinemia (insulin dysregulation). The extent to which chronically elevated pars intermedia-derived melanocortin secretion and hypercortisolism contribute to the risk of laminitis remains to be determined. The aim of this chapter is to provide a description of the important aspects of the history and clinical presentation of equids at risk for or exhibiting signs of laminitis in association with PPID.

Overview of the Pathophysiology of Endocrinopathic Laminitis

Laminitis is a condition of the digital lamellae at the hoof–lamellar interface (HLI) that is characterized by pain (lameness), abnormal hoof growth and appearance, and separation of the hoof from the underlying dermal connective tissue. When laminitis has occurred, the affected HLI may be permanently weakened and predisposed to further bouts of laminitis resulting from any cause. An explanation for the pathogenesis of laminitis in horses and ponies affected with PPID is the subject of extensive current investigation.

Traditionally, the development of laminitis in the context of PPID had been attributed to a direct action of cortisol (hypercortisolism). More recently, the fact that adrenocortical hypertrophy is identified in only a minority (ca.20%) of PPID-affected horses and ponies has led to some downplay for a direct corticosteroid-mediated mechanism in these cases [1]. When identified in the context of PPID, IR and hyperinsulinemia represent a significant risk factor for severe laminitis with an unfavorable prognosis [2]. Insulin resistance is the cornerstone of the equine metabolic syndrome (EMS) for which laminitis represents the principal risk [3].

Horses and ponies tend to develop 'compensated' or 'partially compensated' states of IR in which the circulating plasma concentration of insulin is elevated (hyperinsulinemia) [3]. Hyperinsulinemia represents an independent risk factor for the development of laminitis (in the absence of inflammation) [4, 5]. When subjected to a hyperinsulinemic–euglycemic clamp procedure over the course of 2–3 days (during which the blood glucose concentration was maintained in the normal range and insulin was administered to cause hyperinsulinemia), treated equids developed an acute form of laminitis [4, 6]. This observation led to the recognition that laminitis occurs in conditions associated with IR/hyperinsulinemia as a result of the direct action of heightened insulin influence over time. More recently, the insulin-mediated stimulation of insulin-like growth factor-1 (IGF-1) receptors on basal epidermal cells of the HLI has been hypothesized to promote cell proliferation and structural weakening of this important attachment zone [7]. In other studies, hyperinsulinemia caused increased vascular resistance and endothelin-1 expression in the equine digit, suggesting that abnormalities in lamellar perfusion may play a role in endocrinopathic laminitis [8].

Laminitis does not develop in every case of PPID, and it is significantly more likely in those cases of PPID that are also affected with IR/hyperinsulinemia [2]. Moreover, identification of IR/hyperinsulinemia in PPID-affected horses with laminitis has been linked to a greater clinical severity of laminitis and a more unfavorable prognosis [2]. Thus, it appears that IR/hyperinsulinemia represents the most critical risk factor for laminitis in PPID. However, the possibility that elevated cortisol and circulating pituitary-derived melanocortins also contribute to the risk of laminitis in PPID-affected equids cannot presently be discounted. For example, corticosteroid influence represents a powerful inhibitor of insulin sensitivity and promotes IR/hyperinsulinemia [9]. Melanocyte-stimulating hormone peptides exert numerous actions in the body that are incompletely understood, including aspects of cardiovascular dysfunction and impaired carbohydrate metabolism [10]. On the other hand, an increased influence of β-endorphin

Equine Laminitis, First Edition. Edited by James K. Belknap and Raymond Geor.

appears to improve peripheral insulin sensitivity in some situations [11]. The increased secretion of melanotrope-derived corticotropin-like intermediate peptide (CLIP), an insulin secretagogue [12], may further contribute to hyperinsulinemia in PPID-affected equids [13, 14], adding to the risk of endocrinopathic laminitis. Recent studies have shown that, when independent of EMS, PPID is not necessarily associated with impaired insulin sensitivity [15]. Although the pathophysiological contributions (insulin dysregulation) to laminitis risk associated with PPID and EMS are distinct from those associated with systemic inflammation and endotoxemia, it is possible that both PPID- and EMS-affected individuals are at greater risk for the development of laminitis resulting from non-endocrinological factors (e.g., gastrointestinal disease).

Laminitis

Whether it results from the activation of inflammatory processes within the digital lamellae or from endocrinopathic influences (such an hyperinsulinemia and PPID), the clinical manifestation of laminitis is broadly similar, regardless of the underlying cause.

The present author includes the following definitions:

- *Acute laminitis* is the situation in which pain resulting from activated inflammation in the digital lamellae has occurred for the first time.
- *Chronic laminitis* represents the situation in which disease of the HLI has resulted in abnormal hoof growth or deformity and may or may not be associated with pain (lameness).
- *Endocrinopathic laminitis* represents the situation in which chronic laminitis is identified in the context of underlying EMS and/or PPID [16].
- *Pasture-associated laminitis* (PAL) is the term used to describe the onset of laminitic pain when horses and ponies are allowed to graze pasture grass (usually at certain times of the year and typically resulting from the activation of underlying chronic/endocrinopathic laminitis) [17].

The point at which a new case of acute laminitis should be reclassified as 'chronic' laminitis is commonly made arbitrarily by the attending veterinarian.

For purposes of discussion, the clinical recognition of endocrinopathic laminitis will be addressed at this point. Abnormal hoof growth (discussed below) represents the most common clinical manifestation of endocrinopathic laminitis noted by laymen, veterinarians, and farriers. If present, clinical signs of digital pain (most commonly forelimb lameness) are usually identified alongside and in addition to signs of abnormal hoof growth in cases of endocrinopathic laminitis. Signs of laminitic pain (discussed below) may be precipitated by changes in management that aggravate IR (such as PAL developing at certain times of the year when horses are allowed to graze pasture grasses) and seasonally increased melanocortin secretion in the autumn months. However, digital pain also commonly first becomes evident in cases of endocrinopathic laminitis due to solear pain – commonly due to sole bruising – secondary to an insidious displacement of the distal phalanx.

Clinical Recognition of Laminitis

Abnormal Hoof Growth

Signs of chronic laminitis in cases of PPID and endocrinopathic laminitis in general that are evident upon visual inspection of the hoof are similar to chronic changes observed with other types of laminitis, and include prominent circumferential growth rings, palmar/plantar divergence of the growth rings, 'bunching-up' of growth rings at the dorsal aspect of the hoof, 'slippering' of the toe, broadening of the white line zone (especially at the toe) on solear inspection, development of 'seedy toe', solear convexity dorsal to the tip of the frog, and heel contracture (Fig. 24.1).

The normal (healthy) hoof is characterized by a white line zone (the distance between the edge of the solear horn and the inner edge of the stratum medium of the wall) that is uniformly thick along the length of the wall, and a horny/keratinized sole that is somewhat concave. In horses with chronic laminitis, conservative paring of the solear aspect of the hoof often reveals flecks of hemorrhage that result from and provide evidence of underlying laminitis. It should be emphasized that endocrinopathic laminitis is typically evident upon inspection of the hoof in the absence of any overt signs of pain or lameness. When exercised on hard ground, affected horses may develop mild bilateral forelimb lameness and the digital arterial pulses may become transiently prominent (more likely resulting from sole bruising than from lamellar injury). In endocrinopathic laminitis, bouts of acute laminitis (pain) can occur when the patient is allowed to graze pasture grass with a high sugar content, as well as during the fall when there is a seasonal elevation in the secretion of pars intermedia-derived melanocortins. Veterinary attention for horses and ponies affected with endocrinopathic laminitis (especially PPID) is often requested because the affected feet are

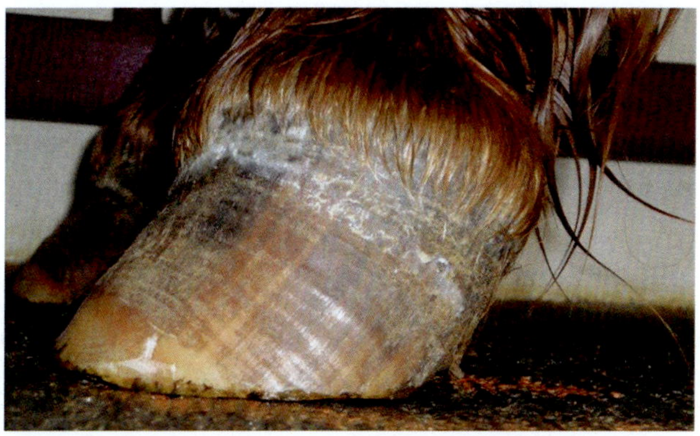

Figure 24.1 The left fore-hoof of a pony affected with pituitary pars intermedia dysfunction ('Cushing's syndrome'). Notice that the growth lines tend to diverge toward the palmar aspect. Hypertrichosis of the distal limb is also evident.

prone to develop recurrent lameness associated with sole abscessation (see Chapter 45).

Veterinary identification of abnormal hoof growth patterns characteristic for endocrinopathic (and chronic) laminitis is often an incidental finding during routine clinical examinations for unrelated (or related) reasons. Experienced farriers might also draw attention to affected feet. Critical veterinary evaluation of the hoof for growth pattern abnormalities requires that the hoof must be cleaned and scrutinized closely. An earlier recognition of endocrinopathic laminitis based on the recognition of abnormal hoof growth patterns (prior to the development of overt laminitic and/or solear pain) should lead to improved clinical outcomes. Specifically, abnormal hoof growth should warrant consideration for further diagnostics (e.g., clinical pathologic work-up for IR and PPID, radiography of the digit) and management changes intended to improve insulin sensitivity or lessen insulin responses to ingested sugar.

Pain

The clinical presentation of pain resulting from laminitis differs depending on the severity of the lamellar injury, and which foot and in how many feet it occurs. Most commonly, pain resulting from endocrinopathic laminitis is evident in both forelimbs. In severe cases of PPID-related laminitis, signs of forelimb digital pain are similar to those described for other types of laminitis (see Chapter 21) and include a reluctance to move, stiffness, or a preference for recumbency. When provoked to either walk or to stand up, affected horses exhibit uncharacteristic reluctance. When observed from a distance, affected horses often stand in one spot and stop moving around in their environment, preferring to intermittently shift weight between the forefeet. When standing, these patients tend to 'oscillate *in situ*' as they attempt to seek a comfortable stance by transferring their center of gravity toward the pelvis and shifting weight between both forelimbs. When encouraged to move, PPID horses severely affected with acute laminitis walk in a manner similar to other types of laminitis so as to avoid weight-bearing by the dorsal aspect (toe) of the forefeet, preferring to extend the forelimbs and bear greater weight at the heel. The walking movement is careful, slow, and deliberate, and the patient tends to bear increased weight in the pelvic limbs giving rise to the descriptor 'walking on eggshells.' Indications of forelimb laminitis pain are especially pronounced when the patient is required to turn sharply on a hard surface. The resulting torque within the affected hoof creates sufficient pain as to both strongly inhibit the horse's action and to cause the horse to collapse on the affected limb, quickly switching its weight to the hind quarters. As described for other types of laminitis, there may also be systemic signs that arise from the severity of pain in severe PPID-related laminitis cases such as sweating, trembling, muscle fasciculations, and rapid breathing. Importantly, many cases of endocrinopathic laminitis associated with PPID do not present with severe pain/lameness, but demonstrate mild lameness due to the insidious nature of the loss of lamellar integrity. Evidence of lameness and severity of pain may wax and wane, likely due to fluctuations in endocrine events occurring in these animals.

Other Clinical Manifestations

Although exunguilation has been reported in the context of sepsis-associated laminitis (for example, during the management of typhlocolitis) and supporting-limb laminitis, it is considered to be a rare complication of endocrinopathic laminitis, most likely due to the fact that there is rarely an acute, extensive separation of the digital lamellae with endocrinopathies, with the lamellar injury/dysregulation most commonly occurring in a gradual and insidious manner. More common hoof capsule disease entities that occur with endocrinopathic laminitis associated with PPID include diseases that occur secondarily in an abnormal lamellar/sole interface where the compromised lamellar tissue and horn exit distally (e.g., white line disease, seedy toe) and subsolear abscessation.

Clinical Recognition of Laminitis in PPID

Equine patients at risk of endocrinopathic laminitis include those affected with either or both EMS and PPID. Insulin resistance and hyperinsulinemia ('insulin dysregulation') appear to play a significant role in the pathogenesis of endocrinopathic laminitis resulting from both conditions.

Differentiating EMS from PPID

Laminitis and regional adiposity are clinical signs of EMS and PPID. Laminitis is more likely and usually more severe in those PPID-affected equids that are concurrently affected with EMS. Age of onset and the presence of clinical signs suggestive of PPID (e.g., hirsutism due to delayed or failed shedding of the winter haircoat) may enable the differentiation of PPID from EMS but, in many circumstances, endocrinological testing is necessary (see Chapter 29) to differentiate the two endocrinopathies. EMS-affected horses are typically identified in their teenage years, but IR may represent a significant risk factor for endocrinopathic laminitis in younger and older horses, including those (older) horses and ponies affected with PPID. Until recently, veterinarians' consideration of EMS was based primarily on the patient's body condition score (BCS) and the morphological distribution of subcutaneous adipose tissue. Clinical signs of EMS include 'regional adiposity,' obesity, bilateral lameness attributable to laminitis, and/or evidence of previous laminitis such as divergent growth rings on the hooves (see above). As a component of regional adiposity, the development of a thick neck ('cresty neck') resulting from the accrual of excessive subcutaneous adipose tissue has been linked to IR, and is often reported in horses and ponies affected with EMS. Other expanded repositories of subcutaneous adipose that are identified in EMS-affected horses and ponies include those areas adjacent to the base of the tail, behind the shoulders, and in the prepuce of geldings (or mammary gland in mares). It should be emphasized that EMS (IR/hyperinsulinemia) may also occur in non-obese individuals that lack the characteristic phenotype, and that it may be absent from some obese horses. Therefore, laboratory (endocrine) testing for purpose of characterizing an individual's insulin response to ingested nonstructural carbohydrates (as a standardized test or 'oral sugar test') and peripheral insulin sensitivity is recommended when either or both EMS and PPID are suspected (see Chapter 29).

Laboratory support for EMS (IR/hyperinsulinemia) currently includes testing for evidence of insulin dysregulation [3]. Clinically practical diagnostic tests for purposes of characterizing a patient's insulin sensitivity include the measurement of resting fasted plasma insulin and glucose concentrations, and dynamic insulin testing including the combined glucose and insulin test, and an oral glucose tolerance test [18]. Simple assessment of the resting fasted plasma insulin and glucose concentrations lacks sensitivity for purpose of EMS diagnosis. Recently, a two-step insulin response test was reported to provide a safe, rapid, and low-cost method to diagnose IR in horses in a clinical setting [19]. Reduced insulin sensitivity (EMS) and an increased risk for endocrinopathic laminitis have been linked to elevated levels and responses of both insulin and glucose in these tests. Methods for the diagnosis of PPID have been reviewed elsewhere, and commonly involve determination of the plasma adrenocorticotrophic hormone (ACTH) concentration and its interpretation based on seasonally adjusted reference intervals (see Chapter 29) [1, 19–23]. The plasma ACTH concentration may be reported as elevated (above a positive cut-off), not elevated (below a negative cut-off), or in an intermediate range. Specific laboratories employ different methods and cut-offs for this determination. For those horses in which an intermediate range value is reported (and for which PPID is suspected), the plasma ACTH concentration should be determined following provocation using either domperidone or thyrotropin-releasing hormone (TRH) [19, 23, 24], although the use of TRH for this purpose is currently recommended. Although many other diagnostic tests for PPID have been described previously, many of those methods lack satisfactory sensitivity and specificity. Moreover, the importance of recognizing that pars intermedia melanocortin secretion is increased during the autumn (thus affecting test result interpretation) in both healthy and in PPID-affected horses was not recognized until recently, making interpretation of some of those earlier tests difficult to impossible.

History and Clinical Signs of PPID

Recognition of the risk of endocrinopathic laminitis in the context of PPID requires that the veterinarian is cognizant of the clinical signs of PPID. It should be emphasized that endocrinopathic laminitis (abnormal hoof growth and/or pain) might be the only clinical manifestation of PPID, especially in earlier/younger cases (teenaged patients). Moreover, laminitis does not develop in every case of PPID.

Both, Morgan horses and pony breeds appear to be at greater risk for the development of PPID, but it can affect any breed. Based on more recent publications, there does not appear to be a gender predilection for PPID in horses. In many cases, the clinical manifestations (including laminitis) of PPID are reported to be more severe in the fall, compared with other times of the year. In one study, the time of onset of laminitis in PPID-affected horses was reported to occur predominantly during the month of September, possibly a result of increased pituitary melanocortin secretory output at this time of the year.

The diagnosis of PPID in older horses that have developed inappropriate hirsutism (hypertrichosis, retention of the haircoat) is often presumptively made without the use of corroborative endocrinological testing. However, it is becoming evident that PPID occurs more commonly in younger horses (and, especially, ponies) than previously believed, and that the clinical expression of the disease in these younger horses may not be so pathognomonic. Although it is most commonly diagnosed in horses and ponies aged over 18 years, PPID has been diagnosed in equids aged less than seven years of age. A diagnosis of PPID in the absence of inappropriate hirsutism can be challenging because several aspects of the clinical appearance of PPID could just as likely be attributed to other primary diseases (e.g., laminitis resulting from any cause) or the effects of advancing age.

Horses affected with PPID eventually develop a characteristic physical appearance. Veterinarians should be suspicious of PPID in mature and geriatric horses and ponies that are presented for ill-thrift, changing body condition, chronic laminitis, polyuria/polydipsia (PU/PD), and hair-coat abnormalities. Abnormalities of the hair-coat may include failure to shed out the hair coat in the spring (inappropriate hirsutism), delayed shedding, incomplete shedding, and a change (lightening) of the color of the haircoat (Fig. 24.2). PPID-affected equids tend to lose skeletal muscle mass (especially from the gluteal and epaxial musculature), and to acquire a characteristic 'regional' distribution of body fat, somewhat similar to that described for EMS. Paradoxically, some younger PPID-affected horses may be in normal or generally obese bodily condition.

As discussed briefly above, many horses that develop laminitis as a component of PPID do not exhibit significant lameness; rather, the evidence of laminitis is recognized as abnormalities in hoof structure and growth (see above). Structural and growth abnormalities of the endocrinopathic laminitis hoof may be quite severe in the absence of significant pain; expression of laminitic pain (stiffness, lameness, etc.) may be diminished as a result of the combined anti-inflammatory actions of elevated circulating melanocortins in PPID. However, PPID-associated endocrinopathic laminitis can certainly cause very severe pain and lameness in some cases.

Other clinical problems that develop as a result of PPID and that may act to draw the veterinarian's attention to this condition include abnormalities of sweating (inappropriate sweating or 'hyperhidrosis,' hypohidrosis, and anhidrosis), lethargy, infertility (mares), inappropriate lactation (galactorrhea) in

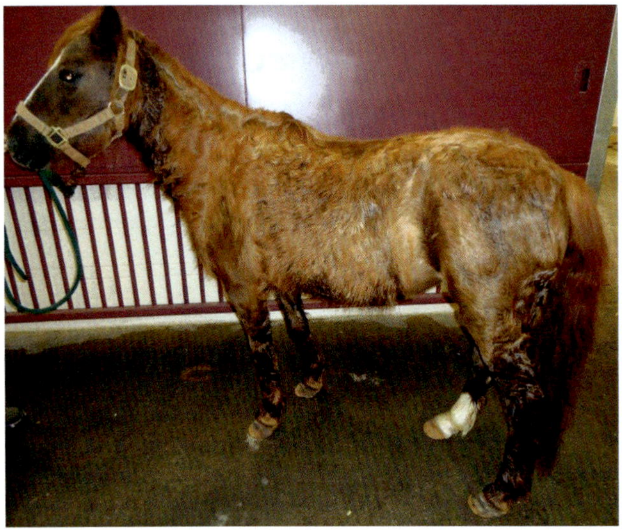

Figure 24.2 A pony affected with pituitary pars intermedia dysfunction ('Cushing's syndrome'). Notice the characteristic and pathognomonic appearance of the pony's haircoat, depicting a failure to shed out (generalized hypertrichosis).

mares, suspensory ligament degeneration, corneal ulceration, blindness, and seizures [25, 26].

The development of PPID should be considered in those teenage horses that are already being managed for EMS that begin to lose bodily condition to an unexpected degree. If baseline insulin or results of dynamic glucose/insulin studies are being undertaken on a regular basis as a part of routine wellness examinations, the development of PPID should be suspected if evidence of worsening insulin sensitivity is detected in otherwise well-managed patients (incipient PPID may or may not cause worsening IR) [15, 18].

Immune functions are reduced in horses affected with PPID because the condition is frequently identified in geriatric horses in which an age-related loss of general immune effectiveness (immunosenescence) has occurred and as a result of elevated circulating levels of the following immunosuppressive factors: alpha-melanocyte-stimulating hormone (α-MSH), β-endorphin (β-END), and cortisol [27]. Although many different infections may develop as opportunists in PPID-affected equids, some of the following are often reported: equine protozoal myeloencephalitis, chronic dermatitis, tooth root infection, bronchopneumonia, and infection of the urinary tract. Additionally, metazoan (helminth) parasites similarly become more clinically significant in immunocompromised older patients [28]. Finally, it should be noted that PPID is most commonly recognized in older horses that may coincidentally be affected by numerous other age-associated chronic diseases.

Firm clinical corroboration of the PPID diagnosis requires specific endocrinological testing.

References

1. Schott, H.C., II (2002) Pituitary pars intermedia dysfunction: equine Cushing's disease. *Vet. Clin. North Am. Equine Pract.*, **18** (2), 237–270.
2. McGowan, C.M., Frost, R., Pfeiffer, D.U., *et al.* (2004) Serum insulin concentrations in horses with equine Cushing's syndrome: response to a cortisol inhibitor and prognostic value. *Equine Vet. J.*, **36** (3), 295–298.
3. Frank, N., Geor, R.J., Bailey, S.R., Durham, A.E., and Johnson, P.J. (2010) Equine metabolic syndrome. *J. Vet. Intern. Med.*, **24** (3), 467–475.
4. Asplin, K.E., Sillence, M.N., Pollitt, C.C., and McGowan, C.M. (2007) Induction of laminitis by prolonged hyperinsulinaemia in clinically normal ponies. *Vet. J.*, **174** (3), 530–535.
5. de Laat, M.A., Sillence, M.N., McGowan, C.M., and Pollitt, C.C. (2012) Continuous intravenous infusion of glucose induces endogenous hyperinsulinaemia and lamellar histopathology in Standardbred horses. *Vet. J.*, **191** (3), 317–322.
6. Asplin, K.E., Patterson-Kane, J.C., Sillence, M.N., Pollitt, C.C., and McGowan, C.M. (2010) Histopathology of insulin-induced laminitis in ponies. *Equine Vet. J.*, **42** (8), 700–706.
7. de Laat, M.A., Pollitt, C.C., Kyaw-Tanner, M.T., McGowan, C.M., and Sillence, M.N. (2013) A potential role for lamellar insulin-like growth factor-1 receptor in the pathogenesis of hyperinsulinaemic laminitis. *Vet. J.*, **197**, 23–30.
8. Gauff, F., Patan-Zugaj, B., and Licka, T.F. (2013) Hyperinsulinaemia increases vascular resistance and endothelin-1 expression in the equine digit. *Equine Vet. J.*, **45**, 613–618.
9. Vegiopoulos, A. and Herzig, S. (2007) Glucocorticoids, metabolism and metabolic diseases. *Mol. Cell. Endocrinol.*, **275**, 43–61.
10. Humphreys, M.H. (2007) Cardiovascular and renal actions of melanocyte-stimulating hormone peptides. *Curr. Opin. Nephrol. Hypertens.*, **16** (1), 32–38.
11. Su, C.F., Chang, Y.Y., Pai, H.H., Liu, I.M., Lo, C.Y., and Cheng, J.T. (2004) Infusion of beta-endorphin improves insulin resistance in fructose-fed rats. *Horm. Metab. Res.*, **36** (8), 571–577.
12. Marshall, J.B., Kapcala, L.P., Manning, L.D., and McCullough, A.J. (1984) Effect of corticotropin-like intermediate lobe peptide on pancreatic exocrine function in isolated rat pancreatic lobules. *J. Clin. Invest.*, **74**, 1886–1889.
13. Orth, D.N., Holscher, M.A., Wilson, M.G., Nicholson, W.E., Plue, R.E., and Mount, C.D. (1982) Equine Cushing's disease: plasma immunoreactive proopiolipomelanocortin peptide and cortisol levels basally and in response to diagnostic tests. *Endocrinology*, **110**, 1430–1441.
14. Wilson, M.G., Nicholson, W.E., Holscher, M.A., Sherrell, B.J., Mount, C.D., and Orth, D.N. (1982) Proopiolipomelanocortin peptides in normal pituitary, pituitary tumor, and plasma of normal and Cushing's horses. *Endocrinology*, **110**, 941–954.
15. Mastro, L.M., Adams, A.A., and Urschel, K.L. (2015) Pituitary pars intermedia dysfunction does not necessarily impair insulin sensitivity in old horses. *Domest. Anim. Endocrinol.*, **50**, 14–25.
16. Johnson, P.J., Messer, N.T., and Ganjam, V.K. Cushing's syndromes, insulin resistance and endocrinopathic laminitis. *Equine Vet. J.*, **36** (3), 194–198.

17. Geor, R.J. (2010) Current concepts on the pathophysiology of pasture-associated laminitis. *Vet. Clin. North Am. Equine Pract.*, **26** (2), 265–276.
18. Frank, N. (2011) Equine metabolic syndrome. *Vet. Clin. North Am. Equine Pract.*, **27** (1), 73–92.
19. Bertin, F.R. and Sojka-Kritchevsky, J.E. (2013) Comparison of a 2-step insulin-response test to conventional insulin-sensitivity testing in horses. *Domest. Anim. Endocrinol.*, **44** (1), 19–25.
20. Beech, J., Boston, R., and Lindborg, S. (2011) Comparison of cortisol and ACTH responses after administration of thyrotropin releasing hormone in normal horses and those with pituitary pars intermedia dysfunction. *J. Vet. Intern. Med.*, **25** (6), 1431–1438.
21. McGowan, T.W., Pinchbeck, G.P., and McGowan, C.M. (2013) Prevalence, risk factors and clinical signs predictive for equine pituitary pars intermedia dysfunction in aged horses. *Equine Vet. J.*, **45** (1), 74–79.
22. Schreiber, C.M., Stewart, A.J., Kwessi, E., Behrend, E.N., Wright, J.C., Kemppainen, R.J., and Busch, K.A. (2012) Seasonal variation in results of diagnostic tests for pituitary pars intermedia dysfunction in older, clinically normal geldings. *J. Am. Vet. Med. Assoc.*, **241** (2), 241–248.
23. Copas, V.E. and Durham, A.E. (2012) Circannual variation in plasma adrenocorticotropic hormone concentrations in the UK in normal horses and ponies, and those with pituitary pars intermedia dysfunction. *Equine Vet. J.*, **44** (4), 440–443.
24. Beech, J., McFarlane, D., Lindborg, S., Sojka, J.E., and Boston, R.C. (2011) α-Melanocyte–stimulating hormone and adrenocorticotropin concentrations in response to thyrotropin-releasing hormone and comparison with adrenocorticotropin concentration after domperidone administration in healthy horses and horses with pituitary pars intermedia dysfunction. *J. Am. Vet. Med. Assoc.*, **238** (10), 1305–1315.
25. Hofberger, S., Gauff, F., and Licka, T. (2015) Suspensory ligament degeneration associated with pituitary pars intermedia dysfunction in horses. *Vet. J.*, **203** (3), 348–350.
26. Miller, C., Utter, M.L., and Beech, J. (2013) Evaluation of the effects of age and pituitary pars intermedia dysfunction on corneal sensitivity in horses. *Am. J. Vet. Res.*, **74** (7), 1030–1035.
27. McFarlane, D. and Holbrook, T.C. (2008) Cytokine dysregulation in aged horses and horses with pituitary pars intermedia dysfunction. *J. Vet. Intern. Med.*, **22** (2), 436–442.
28. McFarlane, D., Hale, G.M., Johnson, E.M., and Maxwell, L.K. (2010) Fecal egg counts after anthelmintic administration to aged horses and horses with pituitary pars intermedia dysfunction. *J. Am. Vet. Med. Assoc.*, **236** (3), 330–334.

CHAPTER 25

Supporting Limb Laminitis

Gary M. Baxter

Clinical Presentation

Supporting limb laminitis (SLL) is usually a sequela to the treatment of another primary condition affecting a forelimb or hind limb that results in excessive unilateral weight-bearing [1, 2]. Conditions that are most often associated with SLL include any type of complete fracture, sepsis of synovial structures, breakdown injuries, tendon lacerations, severe wounds, and unilateral neurological conditions. For example, a 16% incidence of SLL was reported in a group of 31 horses that had fracture repair or a joint arthrodesis using locking compression plates [3], and it is a known complication of fetlock arthrodesis to treat breakdown injuries. Support-limb laminitis differs from other types of laminitis because it usually occurs in only one foot, and horses that develop this complication usually do not have the systemic abnormalities that are seen with other forms of laminitis [2,4]. In addition, SLL can occur relatively spontaneously in some horses with few, if any, predictive clinical signs. The present author has seen horses show lameness in the contralateral limb long after the primary condition has resolved, only to find that the cause of lameness is chronic SLL secondary to the primary problem. Clinical signs of SLL were either not recognized or not exhibited during the initial treatment period, but became more obvious once the unilateral lameness had resolved. This subtle onset of laminitis in SLL is much rarer than the rapid, catastrophic lamellar failure that more commonly occurs once the animal exhibits signs of SLL.

Clinical Risk Factors

The primary factors believed to play a role in the development of SLL are duration and severity of lameness on the contralateral limb [4–6]. No association between specific type of lameness and the risk for laminitis in the opposite limb has been reported. However, horses that can periodically put weight on the diseased limb, thereby relieving some of the added weight-bearing on the contralateral limb, seem to be at lower risk of developing SLL than are those that refuse to bear weight on the affected limb at all [6]. Increased body weight, which often has been cited to play a role in the development of SLL, was not found to be a significant factor in a case-controlled study [5], but was found, along with duration of casting, to be significantly associated with SLL in a recent retrospective study of horses with full-limb, half-limb, and transfixation-pin casts [7]. Of the 113 horses that received casts in this study, 14 (12%) developed confirmed SLL, and horses requiring full-limb or transfixation casts were more likely to develop this complication than those requiring half-limb casts. The authors concluded that greater durations of casting and higher body weights increase the likelihood of developing this complication [7].

No study has found any association between the development of SLL and age, breed, gender, or limb (forelimb versus hind limb) affected [5, 7]. A similar lack of association of these factors with the development of traditional laminitis has also been reported [8]. A recent study reported that horses which were non-weight-bearing at presentation had a greater incidence of SLL than those that were weight-bearing (23% versus 11%), even though this difference was not statistically significant [7]. There is also the reported clinical impression that horses with healthy, robust feet are less likely to develop SLL than are those with thin soles, low heels, negative palmar angles, hoof wall defects, and other structural abnormalities [6].

Clinical Signs

Any horse with a severe unilateral lameness should be closely monitored for the development of laminitis in the other foot. Depending on the severity of the original injury, lameness may be difficult to assess in the contralateral limb; the disease can therefore go unnoticed until significant structural damage is already present. Shifting weight frequently between the injured limb and support limb, or attempts to reduce pressure and pain from the toe by rocking back on the heel of the laminitic foot may be the first clinical signs noted. A sudden apparent improvement in the severity of lameness on the injured limb may also suggest potential laminitis in the contralateral limb. Horses that

Equine Laminitis, First Edition. Edited by James K. Belknap and Raymond Geor.

suddenly begin to lie down with greater frequency or spend a greater length of time down (especially those that previously refused to lie down) should also be suspected of bilateral limb pain such as occurs with SLL. The amount of time a horse remains standing during a 24-h period can sometimes be used as a barometer of the clinical status of some horses. Although rare, some horses may not exhibit clinical signs of laminitis in the contralateral foot until the primary condition has completely resolved.

Other common findings specific for the affected limb include increased digital pulses, warmth in the affected hoof wall, and a palpable 'depression' at the coronary band [1, 4]. Most horses will also exhibit pain with hoof testers over the toe region, but this is often not possible to perform in many horses because of the severity of lameness in the opposite limb due to the primary lameness condition. Baseline digital pulses and characteristics of the coronary band should be established in all 'at-risk' horses so that subtle changes are more easily recognized. In some horses, the only detectable clinical sign prior to developing SLL is increased digital pulses. Changes in the palpable characteristics of the foot may precede radiographic changes by several days, and palpation of the coronary band has been proposed to be a more reliable early indicator of distal displacement of the third phalanx than radiography [5, 9]. As the distal phalanx 'sinks' within the hoof, the soft tissue immediately proximal to the coronary band becomes depressed, resulting in a palpable 'ridge' at the coronary band [9]. Serum or blood may ooze from the coronary band in severe cases; this is usually a very ominous clinical sign warranting a very guarded prognosis as it commonly indicates extensive lamellar failure within the digit (Fig. 25.1). The value of hoof temperature as an indicator of laminitis can be questioned, as it can fluctuate with environmental conditions, and debate exists as to whether it increases or decreases in early laminitis [10, 11]. However, it should still be considered when assessing the overall inflammatory response within the hoof.

Many of the prodromal clinical signs are subtle and difficult to interpret, especially during the early stages of disease. However, if treatment is delayed until signs are obvious, then the process is often quite advanced. For instance, waiting to begin treatment until laminitis can be definitively diagnosed clinically (increased digital pulses with pain on hoof testers over the toe) is not the correct approach. In general, preventive measures against SLL are advisable before any clinical signs are manifested. In the author's experience, horses with increased digital pulses in the contralateral limb without any other clinical or radiographic signs of supporting limb laminitis should be assumed to have SLL and treated accordingly.

Radiographic Diagnosis of SLL

Although relatively insensitive for early lamellar disease, radiography remains a useful diagnostic tool for horses with SLL. It is best used to monitor the progression of disease, rather than for an initial definitive diagnosis. Rotation is best monitored using a standard lateral view. Symmetrical distal displacement can be identified on a lateral and horizontal beam dorsopalmar/plantar view, while uniaxial/asymmetrical distal displacement can only be confirmed on the horizontal beam dorsopalmar/plantar view (the results of the lateral view can be suggestive; see Chapter 27). Dynamic contrast-enhanced computed tomography (CT) has been reported experimentally to measure lamellar blood flow and vascular permeability, but probably has yet to be used in the diagnosis of clinical cases with laminitis [12]. Nuclear scintigraphy of the foot, used to assess digital perfusion, has been reported to be predictive of clinical outcome in cases of chronic laminitis [13]. Horses refractory to treatment in that study had significantly lower dorsal lamellar scintigraphic activity and higher palmar coronary scintigraphic activity prior to treatment than did those horses that responded. Magnetic resonance imaging (MRI) may be the best imaging modality for the detection of subtle lamellar and hoof abnormalities [14], and therefore especially applicable to horses with SLL, but is not always feasible in these cases.

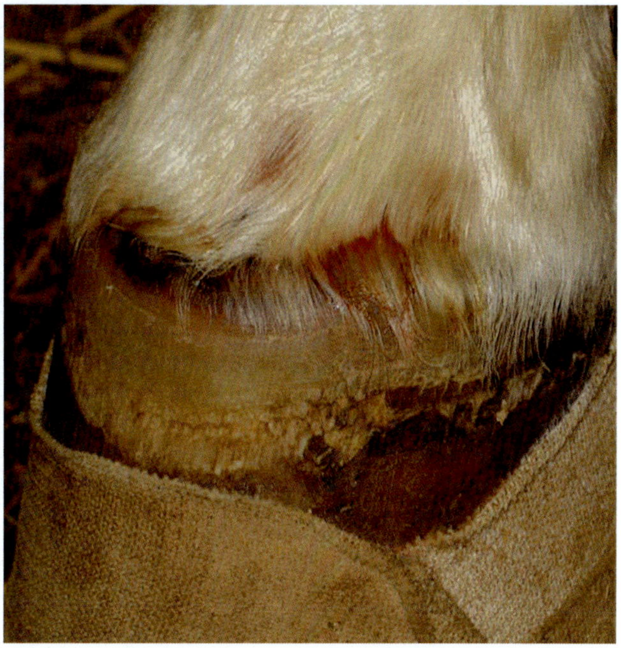

Figure 25.1 Coronary band of a horse with severe supporting limb laminitis (sinking) involving one hind foot. There is a palpable ridge along the dorsal aspect of the coronary band, bruising of the tissue, and serosanguinous discharge.

To make the best use of radiography when monitoring a horse at risk for SLL, baseline lateral and dorsopalmar/plantar views of the contralateral foot should be obtained early in the treatment period for the primary condition in the opposite limb (prior to SLL). The same radiographic technique and positioning should be used for all subsequent radiographs to permit direct comparison between the films. The soft tissue distance between

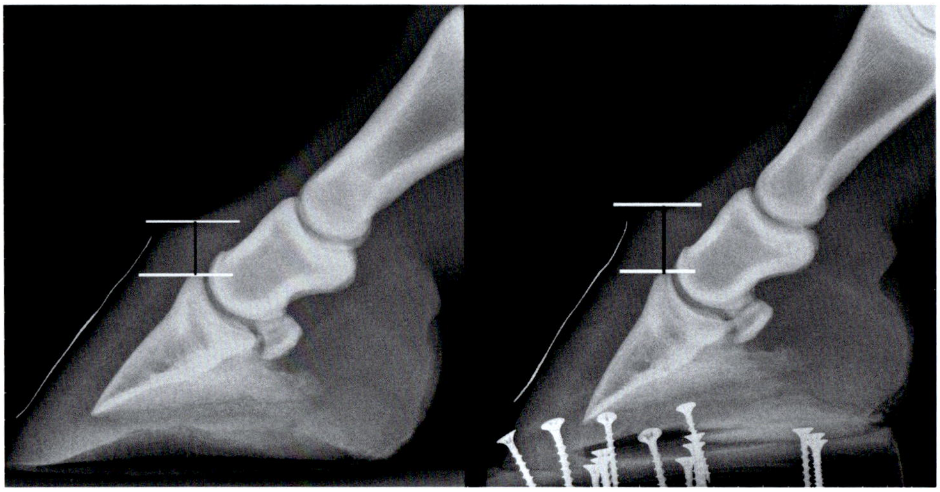

Figure 25.2 Serial radiographs of a horse with progressive distal displacement of the third phalanx. The primary injury in this horse was a second phalanx fracture in the opposite hind leg, which was in a half-limb cast. (a) Radiograph taken one day postoperatively. Few radiographic changes were present, although the 'founder distance' (black arrows) was 11 mm, which may be considered abnormal. (b) Follow-up radiograph taken six days later demonstrating that the 'founder distance' (black arrows) had increased to 18 mm. In the interim, a wooden block with a frog support had been placed in an attempt to support the foot because the horse was exhibiting clinical signs of supporting limb laminitis.

the parietal surface of the distal phalanx and the outer surface of the hoof wall (horn–lamellar zone) should be determined on baseline films and then compared to subsequent films. This thickness may vary with breed, size, and age of the horse, but in most normal horses the distance is similar at the proximal and distal aspect of the dorsal hoof wall and should be approximately 16 mm thick (range: 11–21 mm) (see Chapter 27) [15,16]. An increase in the dorsal soft tissue measurement at the distal aspect of the dorsal hoof wall compared to the proximal aspect is indicative of rotation of the distal phalanx. The dorsal soft tissue thickness has been expressed as a percentage of the palmar cortical length of the distal phalanx (distance from the tip of the distal phalanx to the midpoint of articulation between the distal phalanx and navicular bone) to allow for variations in foot size. A contralateral limb with a dorsal soft tissue thickness greater than 29% of the palmar cortical length of the distal phalanx was suggestive of SLL, despite the fact that only one of the 16 horses in the study had radiographic evidence of rotation [5].

In addition to dorsal soft tissue thickness, the distance from the proximal limit of the dorsal hoof wall (identified with a radiopaque marker) to the proximal limit of the extensor process of the distal phalanx (so-called 'founder distance' or 'coronary-extensor distance') should be measured on baseline films and compared to subsequent images (Fig. 25.2). This distance can be quite variable in normal horses, with an average distance of 4.1 mm (range: 1.8–9.7 mm) according to some, and a range of 0 to 15 mm reported by others [15, 16]. Increases in the founder distance over time are suggestive of distal displacement of the third phalanx within the hoof capsule (sinking), and this may be the only radiographic change suggestive of laminitis in some horses with SLL. In one study [17], the founder distance was determined to be the most significant radiologic prognostic measurement in cases of acute laminitis. Other radiographic signs of distal displacement include cavitation of the coronary band (Fig. 25.3), a more visible proximal aspect of the hoof wall (soft tissue line along proximal hoof wall), and a reduced distance between the apex of the distal phalanx and the solear

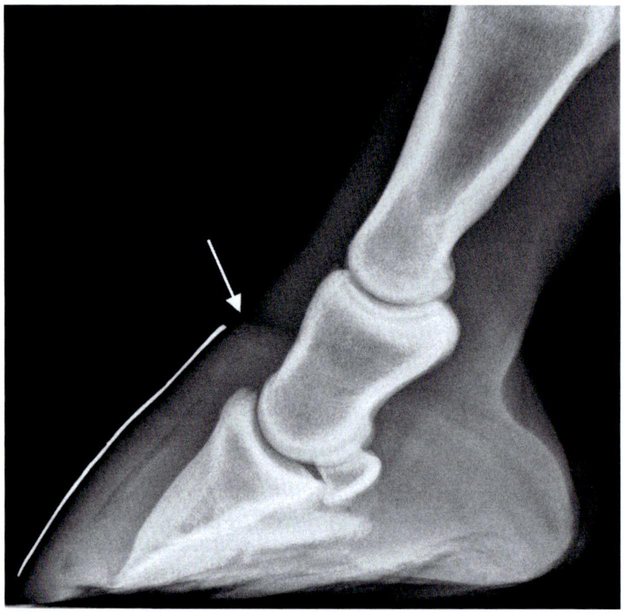

Figure 25.3 Lateral radiograph of a horse with distal displacement of the third phalanx. A distinct ridge is visualized at the coronary band (white arrow), and the sole depth distal to the solear margin of P3 is reduced. There is also mild rotation of the third phalanx.

surface (Fig. 25.3) [5,9,18]. Asymmetrical distal displacement is recognized on a dorsopalmar/plantar projection as an increased distance between the outer hoof wall and the distal phalanx, and a reduced distance between the distal phalanx and the sole on the affected side (see Chapter 27) [18]. The joint space of the distal interphalangeal joint may be increased on the affected side and narrowed on the unaffected side [18]. Many of these radiographic abnormalities can be subtle, further emphasizing the benefit of good-quality baseline radiographs of the contralateral foot in horses with a significant unilateral lameness.

Summary

Identifying animals at risk of SLL is generally more straightforward than those at risk of other types of laminitis; however, the challenge is to maintain a constant diligence regarding clinical assessment for a disease which may occur within days or not for several weeks (if at all) after the initial lameness that put the animal at risk. Even though the disease unfortunately has a poor prognosis and commonly a rapid destructive course, once diagnosed the clinician likely has a better chance of successfully intervening if close attention to the animal's clinical status results in a rapid intervention early during the course of disease. Thus, maintaining a log of both systemic clinical parameters and local parameters of the at-risk digit itself, combined with serial radiographs taken over the period of convalescence from the primary disease, is crucial to monitoring the at-risk patient.

References

1. Baxter, G.M. and Morrison, S. (2008) Complications of unilateral weight bearing. *Vet. Clin. North Am. Equine Pract.*, **24**, 621–642.
2. Eps, A., Collins, S.N., and Pollitt, C.C. (2010) Supporting limb laminitis. *Vet. Clin. Equine Pract.*, **26**, 287–302.
3. Levine, D.G. and Richardson, D.W. (2007) Clinical use of the locking compression plate (LCP) in horses: a retrospective study of 31 cases (2004–2006). *Equine Vet. J.*, **39**, 401–406.
4. Baxter, G.M. (2008) A review of SLL. *Proc. Am. Assoc. Equine Pract.*, **54**, 210–218.
5. Peloso, J.G., Cohen, N.D., Walker, M.A., *et al.* (1996) Case-control study of risk factors for the development of laminitis in the contralateral limb in Equidae with unilateral lameness. *J. Am. Vet. Med. Assoc.*, **209**, 1746–1749.
6. Redden, R.F. (2004) Preventing laminitis in the contralateral limb of horses with nonweight-bearing lameness. *Clin. Tech. Equine Pract.*, **3**, 57–63.
7. Virgin, J.E., Goodrich, L.R., Baxter, G.M., *et al.* Incidence of SLL in horses treated with a half limb, full limb, or transfixation casts: a retrospective study of 113 horses (2000–2009). *Equine Vet. J.*, **43** (Suppl. 40), 7–11.
8. Slater, M.R., Hood, D.M., and Carter, G.K. (1995) Descriptive epidemiological study of equine laminitis. *Equine Vet. J.*, **35**, 364–367.
9. Baxter, G.M. (1986) Equine laminitis caused by distal displacements of distal phalanx: 12 cases (1976–1985). *J. Am. Vet. Med. Assoc.*, **89**, 326–329.
10. Hood, D.M. (2001) Evaluation of hoof wall surface temperature as an index of digital vascular perfusion during the prodromal and acute phases of carbohydrate-induced laminitis in horses. *Am. J. Vet. Res.*, **62**, 1167–1172.
11. Pollitt, C.C. (2004) Equine laminitis. *Clin. Tech. Equine Pract.*, **3**, 34–44.
12. Kruger, E.F., Puchalski, S.M., and Pollard, R.E. (2008) Measurement of equine laminar blood flow and vascular permeability by use of dynamic contrast-enhanced computed tomography. *Am. J. Vet. Res.*, **69**, 371–377.
13. Ritmeester, A.M., Blevins, W.E., Ferguson, D.W., *et al.* (1998) Digital perfusion, evaluated scintigraphically, and hoof wall growth in horses with chronic laminitis treated with egg bar-heart bar shoeing and coronary grooving. *Equine Vet. J.*, **26**, 111–118.
14. Murray, R.C., Dyson, S.J., Schramme, M.C., *et al.* (2003) Magnetic resonance imaging of the equine digit with chronic laminitis. *Vet. Radiol. Ultrasound*, **44**, 609–617.
15. Cripps, P.J. and Eustace, R.A. (1999) Radiological measurements from the feet of normal horses with relevance to laminitis. *Equine Vet. J.*, **31**, 427–432.
16. Redden, R.F. (2003) Hoof capsule distortion: understanding the mechanisms as a basis for rational management. *Vet. Clin. North Am. Equine Pract.*, **19**, 443–462.
17. Cripps, P.J. and Eustace, R.A. (1999) Factors involved in the prognosis of equine laminitis in the UK. *Equine Vet. J.*, **31**, 433–442.
18. Parks, A.H. (2007) Patterns of displacement of the distal phalanx and it sequelae. *Proc. BEVA Congress*, **34**, 204–205.

PART 4

Diagnostic Evaluation of Equine Laminitis

Equine Laminitis, First Edition. Edited by James K. Belknap and Raymond Geor.

CHAPTER 26

Detailed Physical Examination for Laminitis

Richard A. Mansmann and Hans H. Castelijns

Introduction

Traditionally, laminitis has been described as a sudden-onset lameness with varying degrees of pain [1], with the horses exhibiting a characteristic stance of stretched-out front limbs with the hind limbs tucked under the animal for support. The lameness may be accompanied by a reluctance to move and a decreased willingness to pick up limbs due to resistance to standing on the opposite limb. Although any professional working in the equine industry has witnessed this signalment with a laminitis case, it is now realized that many horses with laminitis – mainly those suffering from endocrinopathic laminitis – do not exhibit these classic signs and commonly undergo a very insidious course for months or years with slight or no visible lameness [2]. Therefore, the aim of this chapter is to encourage equine health professionals to have a suspicion of some degree of laminitis in every soundness and pre-purchase examination, every farrier visit, and every lameness examination – and not just when a horse is 'locked to the ground.'

Currently, clinical laminitis cases are divided into three etiological categories:

- Endocrinopathic laminitis – primarily related to equine metabolic syndrome (EMS) and/or pituitary pars intermedia dysfunction (PPID; also referred to as equine Cushing's disease).
- Sepsis-related laminitis – primarily seen as a consequence of serious gastrointestinal, respiratory or uterine pathology.
- Supporting limb laminitis.

Laminitis has also been defined in three different stages [3]:

- Developmental (or prodromal) stage, where pathophysiologic events are occurring systemically (and in the digital lamellar tissue) which will lead to imminent laminitis, but no clinical signs of laminitis in the digit are present yet.
- Acute stage, where the horse shows digital signs of laminitis but no radiographic positional changes of the distal phalanx.
- Chronic stage, where radiographic evidence of positional changes of the distal phalanx is present.

Attempts have been made to develop uniformity in therapeutic farriery terms [4]; however, consensus has not yet been reached regarding the definitions, terminology, and incidence of laminitis [5]. The basis of most past discussions of the physical examination have been related to direct pain related to clinically recognized laminitis. A summary of the long revered Obel laminitis grades are:

- Grade 1: Treading, sound at walk and short-strided at trot.
- Grade 2: Short-strided at walk but feet easily picked up.
- Grade 3: Horse moves reluctantly and resists picking up feet.
- Grade 4: Horse refuses to move unless forced [6].

New, more detailed grading systems have expanded on the Obel grades. Both include more than clinical signs in their four grades (e.g., radiographic changes related to distal phalanx positioning [7, 8], venographic changes [7]), and one allowing for 250 subjective subgrades in each of the four grades [8]).

Broader definitions of laminitis such as: (i) pathophysiological forms where laminitis is some degree of failure of the soft tissue suspending the distal phalanx [2] or (ii) '...inflammation of the lamellae connecting the hoof wall to the coffin bone' [9] allows for the potential that subclinical or asymptomatic laminitis may occur where there is no pain being recognized by the horse's observers. However, as recent reports indicate that inflammation may not play the same primary role in the acute stages of endocrinopathic and supporting limb laminitis that it plays in sepsis-related laminitis (see Chapters 13, 14, 18 and 25), the inclusion of inflammation in a grading system for all types of laminitis is likely inaccurate.

The following physical examination descriptions relate to three categories of horses: (i) those with potential laminitis; (ii) those with mild lameness; and (iii) those horses with typical (more severe) painful manifestations of laminitis. The physical examination and observations of horses for laminitis is ideally part of all orthopedic evaluations, farrier observations, and preventive programs with the goal of early recognition, treatment and monitoring of potential or actual laminitis. Equine healthcare professionals such as veterinarians and farriers, along with the horses' owners, need to be looking for, recording, and monitoring changes over time:

- The horse's overall body condition and unusual stances that the animal exhibits.

Equine Laminitis, First Edition. Edited by James K. Belknap and Raymond Geor.

- Specific hoof changes to one or all four feet.
- Level of pain related to willingness to move, turn, stand or bear weight on a specific foot (including absence of pain).

When a sudden change in any of the above areas occurs, the history-taking and physical examination needs to be immediate and thorough to arrive at a diagnosis as soon as possible so that appropriate treatment can begin. As subtle changes in the above three areas begin to be noted, the healthcare professionals need to increase their intensity of history-taking, additional diagnostic testing and client education in an effort to reduce the potential for that horse developing active life-threatening acute or chronic laminitis. Each individual within a healthcare team needs to recognize the experience and sensitivity of each other – the owner, veterinarian, and farrier – each of whom need to be willing to communicate and ask questions. Potentially, the veterinarian and farrier need, if necessary, to refer to more experienced professionals in equine podiatry in a timely fashion for the sake of the horse. The owner's responsibilities will include the development of a greater vigilance and willingness to make management changes.

As it will be impossible to thoroughly describe every aspect of clinical assessment of laminitis, the reader is encouraged to investigate other general descriptions of equine foot examinations that have more depth related to hoof balance and breed-specific problems [10], farrier tools, and positioning the feet safely for examination [11], and a more detailed interaction between the physical examination and radiographs [12].

General Body Condition

The initial physical examination should begin with assessing the body condition score (BCS) of the horse and the horse's total conformation that would suggest EMS (see Chapters 16 and 22). Typically, published photographs of horses with EMS show an obese horse with fat deposits in the rump, shoulder, and dorsal neck area [13]. However, it has been suggested that this syndrome has a genetic component and recognition could begin earlier in life where the horse has become noted as an 'easy keeper' within a matter of one to three years of life. In the present authors' experience, these animals at risk of EMS may commonly be considered to be a heavy or fat horse when aged five to eight years. Subsequently, if close attention is not paid to the concerns of diet and exercise, the horse becomes obese and develops the EMS type of body conditioning. The continuum of the overweight horse can become compounded by the typical EMS horse developing PPID as it ages [14]. Developing a regular baseline examination of the 'easy keeper' type of horse at an early age may be beneficial in preventing or reducing future bouts of laminitis in these horses by noting subtle changes which may culminate in EMS. This might include recording and monitoring neck and girth circumference scores [15]. The clinician needs to bear in mind that, most likely due to the genetic component, not all horses with metabolic syndrome are obese and may only be carrying the amount of fat usually expected for their breed/activity (i.e., 'show shape').

Hoof Evaluation

During the visual and palpable external hoof evaluation, the examiner should at a minimum assess:

- The external hoof capsule.
- The coronary band.
- The solear surface (especially without a shoe in place).
- The white line (without a shoe).

The External Hoof Capsule

The initial examination from a distance should include the symmetry of the four feet. The examiner should next look at each hoof for rings that could indicate some potential stress to one, two, or all of the feet. It is important to determine if the rings are growing from the coronary band in a symmetrical fashion. If the rings are further down the hoof on one side versus the other, that might indicate that one side of the hoof is healthier than the other, the hoof is irregularly trimmed, or that there is some medial or lateral asymmetrical displacement of the distal phalanx (Fig. 26.1).

Any rings that are visible to the examiner should be discussed with the owner as to what may have occurred to cause the rings, realizing that every ring that exists on a horse's foot is not related to laminitis. A prominent ring on one foot could indicate that an individual event had occurred only in that foot (e.g., a subsolear abscess). Subtle rings in all four feet more likely indicate a systemic response to either an environmental change (e.g., a change in feed) or disease (e.g., PPID, sepsis originating from respiratory or gastrointestinal disease). Multiple rings, especially if divergent (usually being wider in the heel area than the toe area) on any or all feet, should also spark concern. This would indicate that the heel is growing faster than the toe horn, which is common in horses with chronic laminitis. Another potential cause for rings, and a long-term recognized suspect for deteriorating feet, is excessive and alternating wetness (Fig. 26.2). Feet

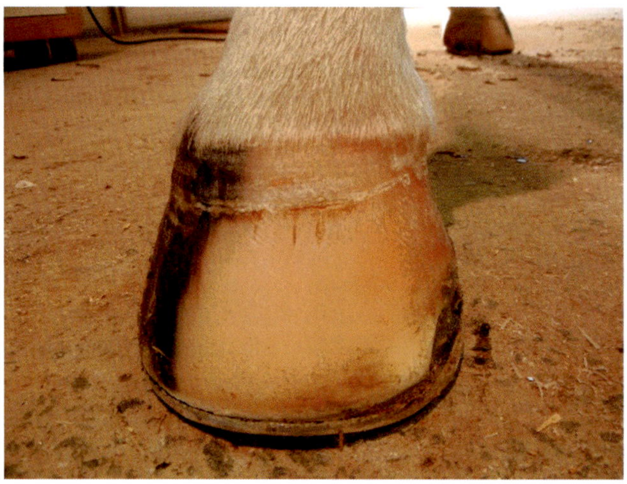

Figure 26.1 An example of a 'growth ring' showing more growth to one side of the wall than the other side. There can be several causes for this asymmetrical growth. which a dorsopalmar (plantar) radiograph can help to define.

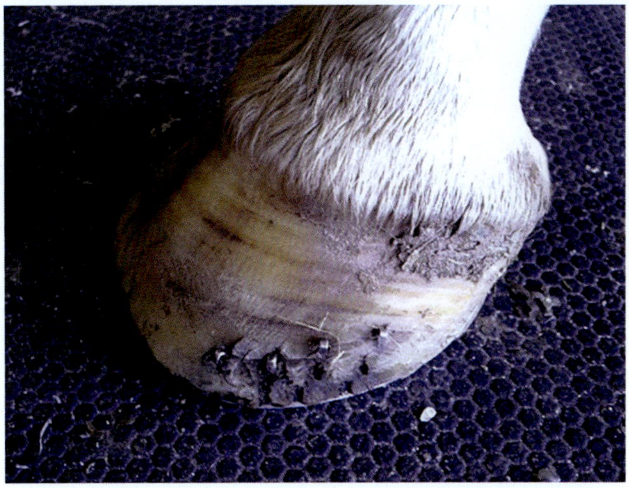

Figure 26.2 An example of a foot demonstrating the effects of excessive moisture. Note the elevated clinches, wall cracks to the nails, rings in the feet, and even some wall stretching at the toe.

with excessive moisture may have softened soles and walls with decreased strength to resist the downward pressures of the distal phalanx and the entire limb, tending to flatten, dish, and flare [16]. The added excessive moisture can increase wall separation and provide a medium for infection. This type of hoof abnormality occurs often in barefooted horses (especially brood mares) that are not on a regular trimming program.

Looking at the foot from the side, the profile of the dorsal hoof wall can be observed; if this is concave (dished) this indicates faster growth at the heels than at the toe. This condition, commonly described as 'clubfoot,' is also characterized by a broken forward phalangeal axis (phalangeal rotation). This flexion of the distal interphalangeal joint, with a high sole plane angle (commonly termed palmar or solear margin angle) of the distal phalanx, is likely to be primarily due to a strong pull of the deep digital flexor tendon (DDFT). The broken forward phalangeal axis, the strong pull of the DDFT, and the high sole plane angle tend to force the dorsodistal border of the distal phalanx into the anterior part of the sole, which may result in a remodeled dorsodistal border of the DP on radiographs (see Chapter 27) and widening of the white line at the toe. All of these findings are common to both the 'original' club foot, acquired during the foal's fast growth spurt [17], or they may be a consequence of chronic laminitis with phalangeal and capsular rotation. The sole plane angle of the distal phalanx is a result of the play of opposed forces, the DDFT pulling the distal phalanx in a palmar/plantar direction and an integral dorsal lamellar bond holding it forward. In the authors' opinion, the concave dorsal hoof wall in the developing foal is the result of a weakened dorsal lamellar bond due to laminitis and/or to an "overstrung" DDFT. It is also the authors' experience that, in a horse with mismatched front feet, severe bilateral laminitis usually results in more rotation (both capsular and phalangeal) on the straighter, club foot-type limb than on the foot with a more normal conformation. This discussion shows how important it is to obtain baseline observations and lateromedial radiographs of an individual horse's feet before clinically active laminitis occurs [18].

The Coronary Band

After the hoof examination (both visual and via palpation), a thorough inspection should be made of the coronary band. Palpating and recording an individual horse's coronary bands should become part of any orthopedic examination because there is variability in their densities among horses. Normally, the skin just above the coronet should have a mild bulge and have a somewhat firm feel on palpation and with no evidence of pain (for more detailed description, see Fig. 26.5). In the horse with distal displacement of the distal phalanx, the bulge in the coronary band may be absent or may be replaced by a 'trough' immediately above the coronary band.

The Sole

Another major area of the hoof that needs a thorough examination is the sole of each of the four feet. This is best done without the shoe (i.e., when the horse is being shod or trimmed). Certainly, the farrier is a good source of information regarding the sole as he/she has easy access to the sole during the trimming and possible shoeing procedure, and is a regular observer of this portion of the hoof. The solear surface may need to be cleaned with a hoof pick and wire brush if the white line and any wall separations are to be observed. Light rasping of the solear margin of the wall can be helpful to further expose (and therefore assist examination of) the white line. Because many laminitic horses have thin soles, the examiner should avoid using a hoof knife on the sole. The first observation of the sole is to evaluate the degree of 'flatness' or decrease in the concavity present in the a normal sole. In the more chronic laminitis case with severe positional changes of the distal phalanx, pressure from the dorsodistal aspect of the displaced distal phalanx creates a convex sole especially at the toe, which is described as a 'dropped sole.' Potentially, the flatter the sole is, the greater the risk of: (i) more serious chronic changes to the lamellar tissue and (ii) a more prominent displacement of the distal phalanx. Any evidence of widening of the lamellae within the white line is an indicator of some distal phalanx positional change relative to the dorsal hoof wall (Fig. 26.3).

It is worth noting that up to 25% of laminitic horses have changes due to the disease in their hind feet that are evident radiographically [19; M. Ertel and R.A. Mansmann, unpublished data). In cases where the hind feet are painful along with the front feet, the stance commonly adopted is that of the four limbs close together under the center of the horse's body. It has recently been determined that, in cases of laminitis, the lamellae of all four feet sustain the same initial insult from whatever systemic disease caused the lamellar injury, indicating that all four feet are always at risk and should be closely examined (realizing the increased incidence of lamellar failure is higher in the front feet) [20]. In addition to always assessing the hind limbs as potentially

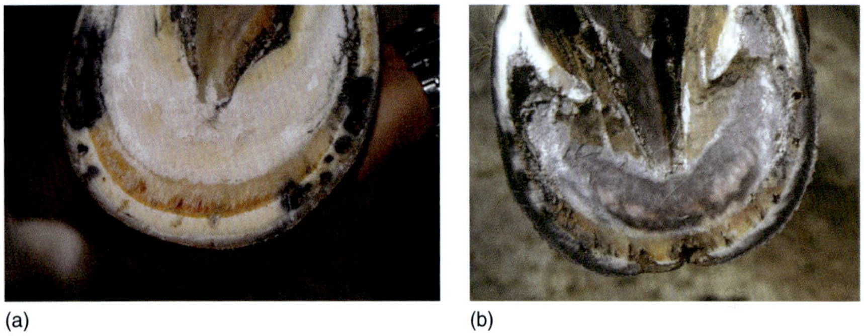

Figure 26.3 Examples of (a) mild, more acute laminitis with the reddish stretched lamellae, and (b) severe, more chronic laminitis with wider, dark lamellar stretching. In either of these visual situations, minimally lateromedial radiographs should be taken of the affected feet to evaluate the distal phalanx positioning and to aid in the trimming and/or shoeing plan.

being affected in laminitis cases, it is also important to assess for medial or lateral displacement of the distal phalanx as indicated by irregularly growing rings (see Fig. 26.1), asymmetrical (lateral or medial) coronary band depression, lateral or medial white line widening, lateral or medial sole sensitivity and/or bulging, or abnormalities in the lateral or medial hoof wall (Fig. 26.4). Dorsopalmar or dorsoplantar radiographs should be recorded if signs of asymmetric displacement are present on physical examination (see Fig. 27.8 in Chapter 27).

Lateral or medial asymmetric displacement of the distal phalanx may result from other causes than laminitis; however, the veterinarian and farrier should take this observation into account for their mechanical treatment plan.

Lameness Examination

When considering laminitis, many veterinarians and farriers think first of the horse that is 'locked to the ground' and not willing to move, or moves in a very stilted gait with its hind limbs drawn up underneath to support the painful front feet. However, in the present authors' experience, there can be many other lameness presentations that ultimately have a diagnosis of laminitis. In clinical situations where a horse is being examined for a lameness of unknown origin, the initial focus areas for examination usually includes any asymmetrical areas on the limb (e.g., foot abscess or bruise), but laminitis is not always considered by veterinarians if the animal is not demonstrating the classic signs of the disease. The present authors feel that laminitis ought to be on that primary rule-out list for any lame horse (regardless of whether the initial complaint is a unilateral lameness). If any of the following movement observations are noted, then digital pain due to laminitis should be moved up on the differential list:

- If the horse is short-strided at a walk (commonly indicating a bilateral lameness in which no characteristic head nod or limb carriage is observed due to the two sides cancelling each other).
- Also at a walk, turning the horse in hand in tight circles in each direction results in the horse's resistance to ambulate in one or both directions.
- Resistance of an animal to stand on the opposite limb when the examiner picks up one front limb.
- If, upon observation of the opposite limb when the examiner sets the originally elevated/held limb down, the opposite limb is immediately raised by the horse (indicating that there is

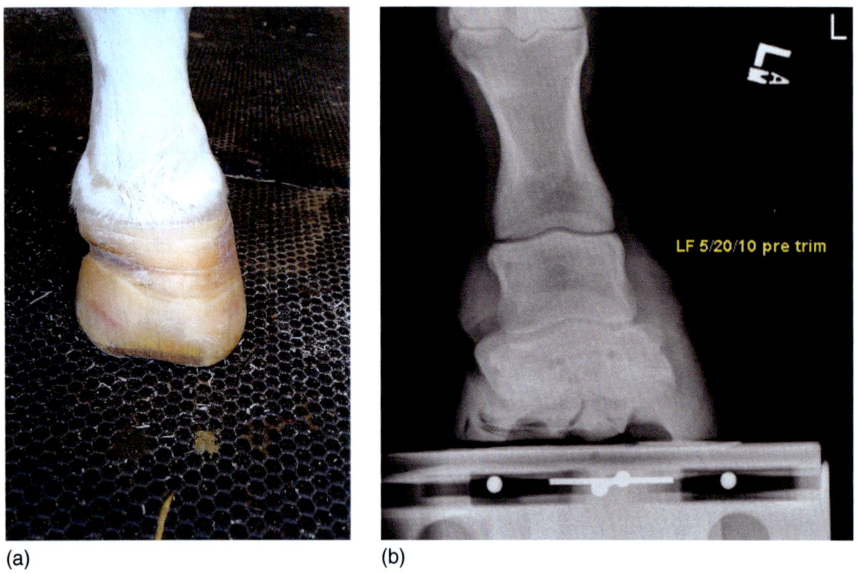

Figure 26.4 A case of sepsis-related laminitis (a sequela to a ruptured esophagus) that had significant medial asymmetrical displacement of the distal front feet phalanges about three months previously. DP radiographs were required for each trimming as the horse healed from his laminitis. The defect in the medial wall on the hoof (a) was related to the grooving and abnormal hoof that was removed around the initial bout of laminitis just distal to the coronary band. The radiograph (b) shows that the lateral wall has more growth than the medial wall.

some degree of pain when forced to bear excessive weight on that foot).

All too often, the following two scenarios are part of the complex history of horses that have an undiagnosed lameness that eventually proves to be laminitis.

A Typical Farrier Scenario

In this case, where the horse is showing some foot pain, the owner recognizes that the horse is slightly short-strided for two or three days after recent shoeings or trimmings. Subsequently, that mild short-stridedness progresses towards a mild lameness that lasts for a few more days after each shoeing or trimming. The farrier relates that he/she has done nothing different with the horse's trimming and/or shoeing. Two situations might arise in this case. First – and the best choice for the farrier, veterinarian, and owner – is that the farrier suggests a veterinary examination (including radiographs) to help explain the post-shoeing pain. Second, another farrier is introduced once a diagnosis for the post-shoeing pain is made, as the owner might feel that the first farrier should have recognized some of the previously mentioned indications of potential hoof abnormalities due to lamellar subclinical injury. This scenario demonstrates a need for good communication between the original farrier and the owner. The farrier needs to recognize subtle foot changes such as dishing and lamellar stretching, and convey that to the owner. The owner needs to convey any gait changes to the farrier, and both need to act upon the farrier's findings by involving the horse's veterinarian as soon as possible.

A Typical Veterinarian Scenario

In this case, where the horse is lame, the veterinarian is asked to examine the animal. The horse is primarily lame on one front foot, so a subsolear abscess may be the first tentative diagnosis. However, on further examination, no area of pus nor consistent area of hoof tester response can be elucidated. Next, a foot bruise may be suspected. Often there may be one of two results in this scenario. All too often, the diagnosis of progressing laminitis is delayed for several weeks due to "…let's wait and see. It's probably just a bruise," with the discomforting result of a very upset owner and a horse eventually diagnosed with advanced laminitis. The better result is that the veterinarian rechecks the horse within a few days, takes some radiographs to make the diagnosis of laminitis, and begins treatment.

Communication between the veterinarian, farrier, and owner needs to be heightened in these situations. All participants need to believe that laminitis can be an underlying cause of the presenting subtle changes, what are thought to be simple lameness. The present authors feel that a horse with this (or a similar) presentation should be rechecked within seven days if a specific diagnosis has not been made of an acute lameness. If the horse is still lame with no discrete clinical diagnosis, then, at minimum, a lateromedial radiograph of both front feet should be taken (and best to add a dorsopalmar radiograph) to rule in or out some distal phalanx positional changes.

Additional Physical Examination Considerations

These may be related to a classic acute bout of laminitis, and three important areas need to be addressed when evaluating the potentially acute laminitis case:

- Level of pain.
- Systemic effect on the vital signs.
- Foot conformation.

In the authors' experience, each of these areas has marked degrees of subtleness (or are normal) as well as degrees of severity. The examiner might assign a score from 0 being normal to 5 being very severe in each of these categories. The value of good records and a scoring system will help the examiner use the physical examination as a monitoring tool to clinically evaluate the horse in the future.

Assessing the Level of Pain

Assessment of pain level involves the consideration of several areas:

- As the examiner is approaching the horse, he/she should assess the facial expression, hair coat quality (including rubbed skin areas that may indicate bruising or presence of decubital sores), and the general demeanor of the horse. What degree of 'brightness' or 'depression' is the horse showing?
- What is the horse's stance? Is the horse laying down, and, if down, how often – and how easily – does it get up? If standing, is it in a relatively normal position or posturing abnormally, and then how long does it take to acquire a normal posture?
- Prior to touching the horse, also observe whether the horse is treading (constantly shifting weight from one foot to the opposite foot) on its front or hind feet. This occurs as the horse is trying to find a more comfortable foot on which to stand. The rate of the treading may be related to the severity of pain.
- Once the horse is haltered, the examiner should next attempt to pick up each of the four feet. The willingness or lack of willingness to pick up a foot is related to the pain in the opposite foot. How long can you hold the leg up? Is it long enough to do a reasonable foot examination, would the horse tolerate a farrier procedure, or is it impossible to pick up the foot? Even in laminitis cases where all four feet are affected, there can be a marked variation in the degree of pain in each foot.
- The level of mobility is next assessed. Is the horse willing to walk and to what degree of stiffness? What is the degree with which the horse is willing to turn in each direction (thus putting a great deal of pressure on that side of the foot/feet in the direction of the turn)? Is the horse willing to trot (this is best done on a soft surface and not to be forced on a severely affected animal)?

Systemic Effects on the Vital Signs

These include:

- The temperature, respiratory, and heart rates need to be taken. Certainly, a horse with a normal heart rate is under less stress than a horse with an elevated heart rate. The heart rate is a very good monitoring tool to evaluate the degree of pain.

Laminitis itself is not usually associated with an elevated rectal temperature; if it is elevated, other systemic problems – primarily a source of systemic sepsis – need to be suspected and diagnosed.

- Heat in the feet can be assessed by placing the palm of the hand over the dorsal wall of each hoof. The examiner may need to perform this palpation frequently alternating from one foot to another and comparing this quite subjective part of the assessment. Additionally, although it is important to compare one limb to the others for this type of clinical sign, the examiner must bear in mind that all four feet may be affected. To make the examination more objective, an infrared (laser) thermometer (available at hardware stores) may be used; in this case it is very important to aim the laser always at the same area of each foot, so as to make comparisons.
- Evaluating the digital pulses is best accomplished by pressing the fingers on the digital arteries as they pass ab-axial to each of the proximal sesamoid bones. The greater the pulse, presumably the greater the lamellar reaction/injury may be. It can be very helpful to compare one side to another (e.g., medial to lateral in the same foot), as well as one limb to another limb (both forelimbs and hindlimbs). Subjectively scoring the palpability/strength of the pulse (0 to 5/5) can be helpful as a recorded monitoring tool in future assessments.

Foot Conformation Assessment

Such assessment includes the following points:

- The coronary bands need to be thoroughly palpated and evaluated for any asymmetries or local areas of pain. If there is evidence of focal pain and possibly some swelling and heat at the coronary band, abscessation (most commonly starting near the ground/solear surface of the foot and traveling up the white line; i.e., a 'gravel') may be preparing to drain at the coronary band; this is not uncommon in chronic cases of laminitis. Obvious coronary band/wall separation without evidence of abscessation is a serious clinical sign indicating severe loss of lamellar integrity; this is more commonly associated with hemorrhage than the pus present with abscessation. A marked depression of the coronary band indicates sinking/distal displacement of the distal phalanx in the area corresponding to the depression with significant local lamellar destruction (Fig. 26.5).
- After inspecting the hoof (as described above), care must be taken with the use of hoof testers and the interpretation of their responses. Often, the examiner's digital pressure alone on the sole can cause a thinner-soled horse to respond, and immediate heavy hoof tester pressure may damage or puncture an already friable sole. It may also be a danger to the examiner! So, when hoof testers are used, begin with the slightest of pressure. Any reaction to mild pressure from hoof testers in the toe area of the sole on more than one foot is perhaps the clearest sign of an acute bout of laminitis. However, in some thicker-soled horses the hoof tester response may be minimal, thus falsely minimizing the severity of the laminitis to the examiner.
- Record any foot abnormalities that have been already described above, such as flaring, dishing, rings, any loss of sole convexity, and any abnormalities to the white line visible on the solear surface.
- Take appropriate radiographs.

Repeated monitoring of these areas of clinical assessment, along with diagnostic imaging (see Chapter 27), will have value in continuously assessing the horse's response to treatment. Additionally, the positioning of the foot and fetlock related to various levels of pain within the foot may need to be evaluated. Contracture of the deep digital flexor tendon can occur in very chronic cases. Levels of tension of the deep digital flexor tendon in the mechanical treatment can be assessed with various degrees of raising of the heels, and can be evaluated via clinical improvement (or lack thereof). The use of an instrument in the physical examination, such as the digital extension device [21],

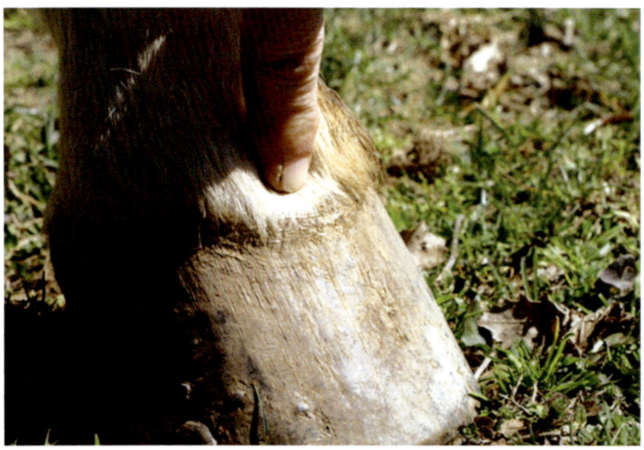

(a)

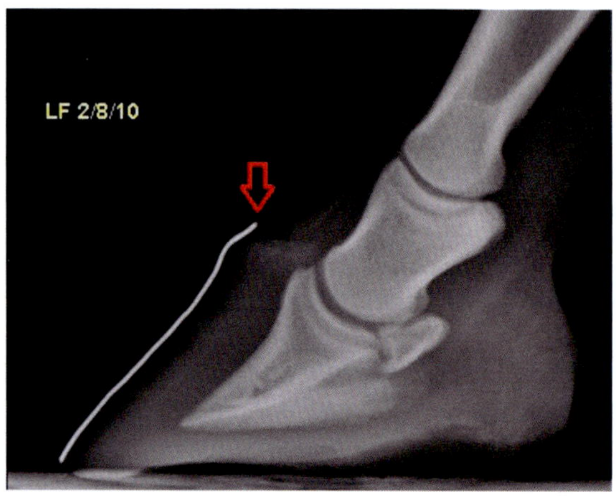

(b)

Figure 26.5 (a) Palpating the coronary band in each potential laminitic physical examination can be very helpful. Note if the palpation findings change in subsequent rechecks. Digital palpation all around the coronet is important. (b) On the lateromedial radiograph the depressed coronet (arrow) can be seen to confirm the physical examination of the coronet band. The horse with this radiograph would most likely be lame.

may be helpful in assessing the relationship of the deep digital flexor tendon to the degree of digital pain exhibited by the animal; in the present authors' opinion, this may impact the decision on whether or not to perform a deep digital flexor tenotomy.

Pre-Emptive Physical Examination and Preventive Treatment in Potential Acute Bouts of Laminitis

If general-practicing veterinarians, brood farm managers and tertiary care hospital clinicians and their staff are proactive in identifying and treating their horses at risk of septic and supporting limb laminitis, perhaps these laminitis cases which occur secondary to these other predisposing disease processes (e.g. either causes of sepsis or severe lameness in one limb) could be reduced in number or have better outcomes. The well-documented sepsis cases that are at higher risk of secondary serious laminitis are gastrointestinal medical (e.g., enterocolitis) and surgical (e.g., postoperative colon torsion) cases, pleuropneumonia, and retained placenta cases. These cases often present as emergencies, creating an immediate high level of stress for their owners and also creating a significant list of current problems and possible complications – including laminitis – that need to be communicated by the veterinarian(s) to the owner(s) or agent. The animals at risk of supporting limb laminitis are usually fairly straightforward, being those bearing minimal weight on one limb due to pain (e.g., fracture or synovial sepsis) or an inability to use the limb (e.g., radial nerve injury).

In addition to pre-emptive treatments in these cases, a thorough (possibly somewhat abbreviated due to time constraints) body and foot conformational evaluation might be helpful prior to extensive surgical and medical treatment for the above-mentioned conditions. As soon as possible, at least lateromedial radiographs of the feet should be obtained. It may be of great benefit for the veterinarian and the owner to know the baseline status of the horse's hoof conformation and distal phalanx position within the hoof prior to any clinical evidence of acute-onset laminitis. This information could help in developing a more beneficial total treatment plan, and also help with a more accurate prognosis. It could also help to defuse some of the post-septic laminitis angst that occurs even with the typical discussion about laminitis as a secondary complication to problems that have a septic or limb load component. This is particularly valuable in an animal that presents with chronic distal phalanx displacement from a previous episode of laminitis (either known or unbeknown to the owner); it can be difficult to ascertain the degree of displacement from recent or ongoing sepsis versus the amount of displacement already present if radiographs have not been taken early in the current disease process. Evidence of previous displacement not only helps to guide the treatment and prognosis of these animals, but also protects the veterinarian's practice from the possible concern by owners and trainers that these changes may have occurred at their facility. Having prior knowledge of the foot status of these septic patients will help the clinician accurately dictate the aggressiveness of preventive therapies (e.g., digital mechanics, cryotherapy, systemic medical therapy) that are discussed elsewhere in this book.

Pre-Emptive Physical Examination and Preventive Strategies in Subclinical Laminitis

Subclinical laminitis has been recognized and classified in sound cattle. The early physical signs are primarily hoof changes of deteriorating quality, sole bruising, and increasing numbers of lesions including sole ulcers, double soles, and white line disease [22]. Subclinical laminitis has also been observed in donkeys [23]. Subclinical or asymptomatic laminitis, where the horse is sound but there is evidence of hoof or radiographic change to the distal phalanx, has not been a commonly recognized form of laminitis in the equine literature. However, it is the present authors' experience that subclinical laminitis may exist quite commonly, and the initial examination to rule out laminitis should begin in horses that may be sound. Although many of the latter-twentieth century laminitis studies were focused on sepsis-related laminitis, more recent epidemiologic and clinical studies have demonstrated the importance of endocrinopathic laminitis. In the majority of equine practices, the most common type of laminitis is most likely to be of endocrinopathic origin [24,25]. This type of laminitis could commonly be described as subclinical in early stages because it can be insidious and not show clinical signs of lameness until a significant amount of positional change of the distal phalanx has occurred [26–28]. In a study examining qualitative and morphometric radiographic findings of the distal phalanx in 41 sound thoroughbred race horses that had raced twice prior to the study, radiographs were taken and repeated twice within a six-month period. Subsequently, four of the horses showed subtle radiographic signs of laminitis [29]. These signs included palmar rotation, hoof wall undulations, palmar cortical reabsorption, or distal dorsal cortical bone deposition. When the earnings records for each horse were compiled, and horses were grouped according to one or more subtle signs of laminitis, the latter horses had less earnings per race than the other sound horses. The age of these horses ranged from four to nine years, and their body condition was excellent; consequently, there was a minimal chance of these being endocrinopathic laminitic cases [29]. Interestingly, the study results indicated that other causes may exist besides endocrinopathic that can create subclinical or asymptomatic laminitis.

How Might Subclinical or Asymptomatic Laminitis Occur?

A horse with radiographic evidence of distal phalanx positional changes, with or without subtle changes to the distal phalanx, may have enough sole depth and an adequate lamellar attachment to be relatively painless. This appears to occur more frequently in the cases of endocrinopathic laminitis, where subtle, minor changes can progress and accumulate over a long period of time with: (i) progressive thinning of the dorsal sole, (ii) increased lamellar damage/thickening, and (iii) a larger positional shift of the distal phalanx in the hoof capsule. This may lead to the sudden onset of pain that is obvious to the owner and any examiner inspecting the horse, where the pain may be more from bruising due to a thin sole than from lamellar pain/instability.

Again, this proves the value of preventive foot care evaluations on an annual basis within a typical equine practice [18]. Baseline radiographs of the individual distal phalanx morphology, taken when the horse was sound, are invaluable when laminitis occurs. Slight abnormalities of original foot conformation may be recorded, making later changes due to laminitis more obvious. An example is the foot of a horse that, in its initial baseline radiographs has a negative sole plane (palmar/plantar) angle and a thinner dorsal wall distally than proximally. If, in subsequent radiographs, this horse shows a dorsal wall that is equally thick (proximally and distally) and a positive sole plane angle of the distal phalanx, this particular horse has had rotation due to laminitis. However, if no baseline radiographs were available for this horse, and only 'current' films could be assessed with no comparison against previous films, then those radiographs would most likely be considered normal.

There may be other subtle situations where a thorough overall body and foot assessment could be helpful prior to submitting the horse to specific stressors or potential laminitis triggers, such as vaccination or glucocorticoid administration. An example might be a horse that has been known to have a mild reaction to a medication or vaccination, and at this time is slightly heavier and out on spring grass. Knowing the animal's foot conformation may be helpful in making a decision of whether to treat/vaccinate the animal at that time, or not. Glucocorticoids have been related to laminitis in horses with some pre-existing foot conditions [30]. It also has been reported in a survey of 36 European Sport horse practitioners that one-third had experienced laminitis with 10 days of a normal dose of corticosteroid in a total of 22 horses. Whilst this is probably a very small percentage of the total horses treated with glucocorticoids by these practitioners, the survey further stated that the majority of the horses were overweight; 50% had to be euthanized [1]. Excessive body weight is most likely a significant contributing factor to laminitis, both from an endocrinopathic perspective and from the increased physical force sustained by the feet in the overweight animal.

Potentially, all horses – whether sound, lame, or having decreased performance – need to be considered as having subtle laminitis that could lead to a continuum that can develop into the classic Obel grades of lameness. Early diagnosis and treatment may be able to reduce these more severe grades of laminitis commonly associated with a poor outcome.

References

1. Dyson, S.J. (2011) Laminitis: Diagnosis of Laminitis, in *Diagnosis and Management of Lameness in the Horse*, 2nd edition (eds M. Ross and S.J. Dyson), Saunders Elsevier, St Louis, pp. 371–372.
2. Moore, R.M. (2010) Vision 20/20 – Conquer Laminitis by 2020. *J. Equine Vet. Sci.*, **30**, 74–76.
3. Belknap, J.K. and Parks, A. (2011) Laminitis, in *Adam's and Stashak's Lameness in Horses*, 6th edition (ed. G. Baxter), Wiley-Blackwell Publishing, Oxford, pp. 535–536.
4. O'Grady, S.E., Parks, A.H., Redden, R.F., *et al.* (2007) A glossary of therapeutic farriery terms. *Equine Vet. Educ.*, **19**, 263–271.
5. Wylie, C.E., Collins, S.N., Verheyen, K.L.P., *et al.* (2011) Frequency of equine laminitis: A systemic review with quality appraisal of published evidence. *Vet. J.*, **189**, 248–256.
6. Stashak, T.S. (1987) Lameness, in *Adam's Lameness in Horses*, 4th edition (ed. T.S. Stashak), Lea & Febiger, Philadelphia, p. 490.
7. Floyd, A.E. (2007) Grading the Laminitic Horse, in *Equine Podiatry* (eds A.E. Floyd and R.A. Mansmann), Saunders Elsevier, St Louis, pp. 320–327.
8. Redden, R.F. (1998) *Understanding Laminitis. Your Guide to Horse Health Care and Management.* The Blood-Horse, Inc., Lexington, KY, pp. 80–105.
9. Redden, R.F. (1998) *Understanding Laminitis. Your Guide to Horse Health Care and Management.* The Blood-Horse, Inc., Lexington, KY, p. 10.
10. Turner, T.A. (2006) How to subjectively and objectively examine the equine foot. *Proc. AAEP*, **52**, 531–537.
11. Moyer, W.A. and Carter, G.K. (2007) Examination of the Equine Foot, in *Equine Podiatry* (eds A.E. Floyd and R.A. Mansmann), Saunders Elsevier, St Louis, pp. 112–127.
12. Schumacher, J., Taylor, D., Schramme, M., *et al.* (2012) Localization of pain in the equine foot emphasizing the physical examination and the analgesic techniques. *Proc. AAEP*, **58**, 138–156.
13. Stewart, J. (2013) *Understanding the Horse's Feet.* The Crowood Press, Wiltshire, UK, pp. 126–136.
14. Frank, N. (2008) Endocrinopathic laminitis, obesity-associated laminitis, and pasture-associated laminitis. *Proc. AAEP*, **54**, 341–346.
15. Carter, R.A., Geor, R.J., Staniar, W.B., *et al.* (2009) Apparent adiposity assessed by standardized scoring systems and morphometric measurements in horses and ponies. *Vet. J.*, **179** (2), 204–210.
16. Emery, L., Miller, J., and Van Hoosen, N. (1977) *Horseshoeing Theory and Hoof Care.* Lea & Febiger, Philadelphia, p. 125.
17. van Heel, M.C.V., Kroekenstoel, A.M., van Dierendonck, M.C., *et al.* (2006) Uneven feet in a foal may develop as a consequence of lateral grazing behaviour induced by conformational traits. *Equine Vet. J.*, **38** (7), 646–651.
18. Mansmann, R.A., King, C., and Stewart, E. (2000) How to develop a preventive foot care program – a model. *Proc. AAEP*, **46**, 156–161.
19. Hunt, R.J. (1993) A retrospective evaluation of laminitis in horses. *Equine Vet. J.*, **25**, 61–64.
20. Leise, B.S., Faleiros, R.R., Watts, M., *et al.* (2012) Hindlimb laminar inflammatory response is similar to that present in forelimbs after carbohydrate overload in horses. *Equine Vet. J.*, **44** (6), 633–639.
21. Castelijns, H.H. (2008) How to use a digital extension device in lameness examinations. *Proc. AAEP*, **58**, 228–231.

22. Greenough, P.R. (2007) Subclinical Laminitis (SCL) (Pododermatitis Aseptica Diffusa, PAD), in *Bovine Laminitis and Lameness: A Hands-On Approach.* Greenough, PR, pp. 40–49 [electronic resource].
23. Walker, M., Taylor, T.S., Slater, M., *et al.* (1995) Radiographic appearance of the feet of mammoth donkeys and the findings of subclinical laminitis. *Vet. Radiol. Ultrasound*, **35**, 32–37.
24. Donaldson, M.T., Jorgensen, A.J., and Beech, J. (2004) Evaluation of suspected pituitary pars intermedia dysfunction in horses with laminitis. *J. Am. Vet. Med. Assoc.*, **224**, 1123–1127.
25. Karikoski, N.P., Horn, I., McGowan, T.W., *et al.* (2011) The prevalence of endocrinopathic laminitis among horses presented for laminitis at a first-opinion/referral equine hospital. *Domest. Anim. Endocrinol.*, **41**, 111–117.
26. Buckley, P., Morton, J., and Coleman, G.T. (2007) Repeated observations of naturally occurring laminitis in Pony Club horses in regional Australia. *Proc. Aust. Coll. Vet. Sci.*, **2007**, 10–11.
27. Hunt, R.J. and Wharton, R.E. (2010) Clinical Presentation, Diagnosis and Prognosis of Chronic Laminitis. *Vet. Clin. North Am. Equine Pract. Adv. Laminitis, Part I*, **26**, 141.
28. Johnson, P.J., Wiedmeyer, C.E., LaCarrubba, A., *et al.* (2010) Laminitis and the Equine Metabolic Syndrome. *Vet. Clin. North Am. Equine Pract. Adv. Laminitis, Part II*, **26**, 240.
29. Linford, R.L., O'Brien, T.R., and Trout, D.R. (1993) Qualitative and morphometric radiographic findings in the distal phalanx and digital soft tissues of sound Thoroughbred racehorses. *Am. J. Vet. Res.*, **54**, 38–51.
30. Johnson, P.J., Messer, N.T., Bowles, D.K., *et al.* (2004) Glucocorticoids and laminitis in horses. *Compendium*, **7**, 547–558.

CHAPTER 27
Diagnostic Imaging

Andrew H. Parks and James K. Belknap

Introduction

Radiographs are used to assist in the diagnosis of laminitis, to monitor the progress of the disease, to assist in determining the prognosis for a horse with the disease, and as a guide for hoof care. In order to obtain the best information from radiographs, optimal foot preparation, positioning, and radiographic exposure are essential. To make best use of the information, normal values are invaluable as a reference, and radiographs taken prior to the onset of disease (i.e., in horses known to be at risk of the disease) are even more valuable should they be available, given the degree of individual variation between normal horses.

Preparation and Positioning of the Foot

The feet should be cleaned of extraneous material as much as possible. The use of markers on the surface of the hoof capsule are useful adjuncts to aid the careful measurement of various parameters related to the hoof, and its relationship to the distal phalanx. A linear marker should be placed on the mid-dorsal hoof wall for lateral radiographs (Fig. 27.1), the proximal extent of the marker coinciding with the proximal margin of the coronary band. Both, metallic wire markers and beads of barium paste have been used for this purpose, and may enhance determining the thickness of the hoof dorsal to the distal phalanx and the position of the coronary band in relation to the extensor process of the distal phalanx. Because precise positioning of the coronary band marker is frequently not consistent between clinicians, rasping the coronary band lightly to identify the proximal extent of the firm hoof wall has been advocated [1]. With the advent of digital imaging and its enhanced ability to adjust contrast, the need for dorsal markers is not as great, and the coronary band can usually be located by following the radiodense keratinized hoof wall proximally until it intersects with the skin/periople (Figs 27.1b). However, even with digital radiographs, the location of the proximal aspect of the coronary band can still be challenging in some animals and may be more consistent if a marker is used. Additionally, many clinicians will identify the junction of the apex of the frog and the sole by trimming the dorsal extent of the frog and placing a thumbtack in the frog just behind this junction. Lastly, painting the dorsal sole (cranial to apex of frog) with barium paste provides a more accurate way to determine sole depth, both on lateral and dorsopalmar radiographs (Figs 27.3 and 27.4).

For the lateral and dorsopalmar radiographs, both feet should be positioned on blocks of equal height such that a horizontal X-ray beam intersects the hoof wall approximately 1.5 cm proximal to the ground surface of the foot (Fig. 27.2). The limb being radiographed and the contralateral limb should be bearing equal weight, and the metacarpus should be vertically aligned within 10° of vertical from a lateral–medial and dorsopalmar direction or better; even a deviation from vertical of 5° results in a significant change in mediolateral distal interphalangeal joint symmetry visible on a lateral radiograph [2]. Additionally, if the radiographic beam deviates 10° or more from perpendicular to the medial plane of the limb for a lateral radiograph, it causes an underestimation of rotation of the distal phalanx, reportedly regardless of the degree of rotation [3]. Unfortunately, it is not always possible to obtain optimally positioned radiographs because the ground is uneven or because the animal is uncomfortable standing in the appropriate position, or is even recumbent. Sedation combined with analgesia may improve a horse's ability to stand for radiographs. Many clinicians do not advocate the use of perineural analgesia solely for the purpose of taking radiographs in severely lame horses due to the concern that the horse may traumatize its lamellae or sole during the period of analgesia and exacerbate its condition. However, one of the present authors (J.B.) commonly performs perineural analgesia with lidocaine (due to its somewhat shorter duration of action versus mepivacaine), which usually only gives enough time to perform radiographs, examine the solear surfaces of the digits, and apply digital support to the feet before the animal begins to obtain sensation again. If performed, it is important that the animal be restrained from walking until sensation returns to the digit. The primary advantage, in addition to enabling a thorough examination of the sole, is that higher-quality radiographs can be obtained with minimal duress to the patient (and those taking the radiographs). It is best to keep the digit not being assessed/radiographed supported in some

Equine Laminitis, First Edition. Edited by James K. Belknap and Raymond Geor.

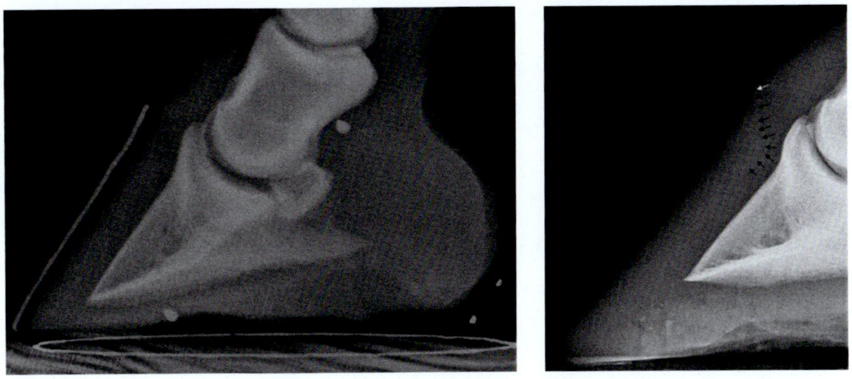

(a) (b)

Figure 27.1 (a) Linear marker on the dorsal midline ending proximally at the proximal margin of the coronary band. (b) The coronary band can also be determined by following the caudal border of the radiodense keratinized horn (black arrows) proximally until only the periople is present (white arrow).

type of temporary pad (e.g., in a SoftRide shoe) to protect it during radiographs. It is important to be ready to apply the digital support of choice to the digits once the information from the radiographs and digital examination is obtained and there is still ample analgesia present to allow each foot to be picked up and treated. As the type of digital support used may differ depending on the type of displacement of the distal phalanx found with the radiographs, the clinician would want to have the different types of support she/he uses for the different types of displacement immediately available. Radiographs obtained under suboptimal circumstances must be interpreted with caution, particularly with respect to the mediolateral symmetry of both the distal interphalangeal joint, and the distal phalanx with respect to the ground. Radiographs obtained with a horse in lateral recumbency are even more difficult to interpret. Dorsopalmar oblique radiographs (solear margin views) taken at 45° and obtained with the horse standing on a cassette box, are more important in the diagnostic work-up of a chronic laminitis case

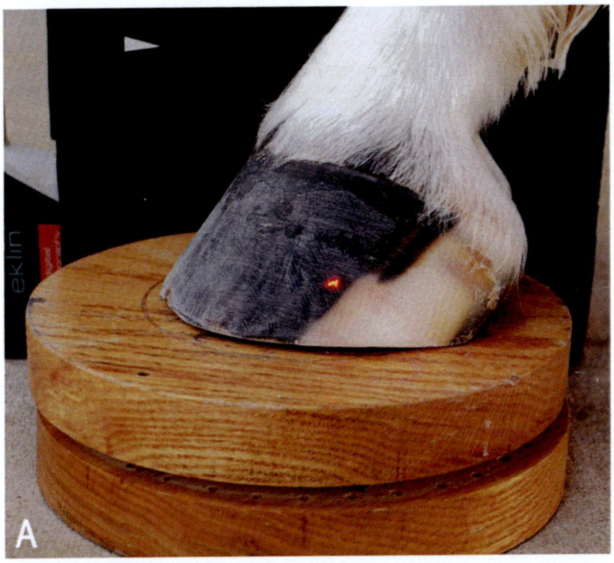

Figure 27.2 Placement of feet on blocks to allow the X-ray beam intersect the hoof wall approximately 1.5 cm proximal to the ground surface. Illustration courtesy of R. Eggleston, University of Georgia.

to allow assessment of the integrity of the solear margins of the distal phalanx; no markers should be present on the surface of the hoof capsule for this view.

Due to the increased fidelity obtained with digital radiographs, it is not only possible to measure the entire hoof thickness, but also to delineate two layers: (i) the outer hoof, a more radiodense layer which contains primarily the stratum medium of the hoof; and (ii) the inner hoof, a more radiolucent layer which contains the lamellae and the sublamellar dermis (Fig. 27.3a and b) [4,5]. As this inner layer is the more likely layer to thicken in the early stages of laminitis, its measurement may be used more in the future for assessing early laminitic changes in the hoof. Normal measurements of these two layers of the hoof wall have recently been published and are listed in Table 27.1.

General Evaluation of the Radiographs

The entire foot should be visible on the film. The density range of the radiograph should be such that soft tissue details are clearly visible. If conventional film is used, two exposures may be necessary, a 'lighter' view to evaluate the hoof capsule (soft tissue density) and its relationship to the distal phalanx, and a second 'darker' view to evaluate the morphology of the distal phalanx and the alignment of the phalanges [6].

The evaluation of radiographs of the foot made for diagnostic purposes or as a guide to treatment should be approached in a systematic manner. Which manner a clinician adopts is unlikely to matter as long as it includes the same observations. Absolute measurements of distance on a radiograph can only be made by normalizing the measurement against a marker of known length; angles may be subject to slight variation based on radiographic positioning, but are more consistent than distances.

Information Obtained from Lateral Radiographs

Measurements obtained from the lateral radiograph include several related to the keratinized horn (stratum externum and medium) of the dorsal hoof wall and sole; the clinician must

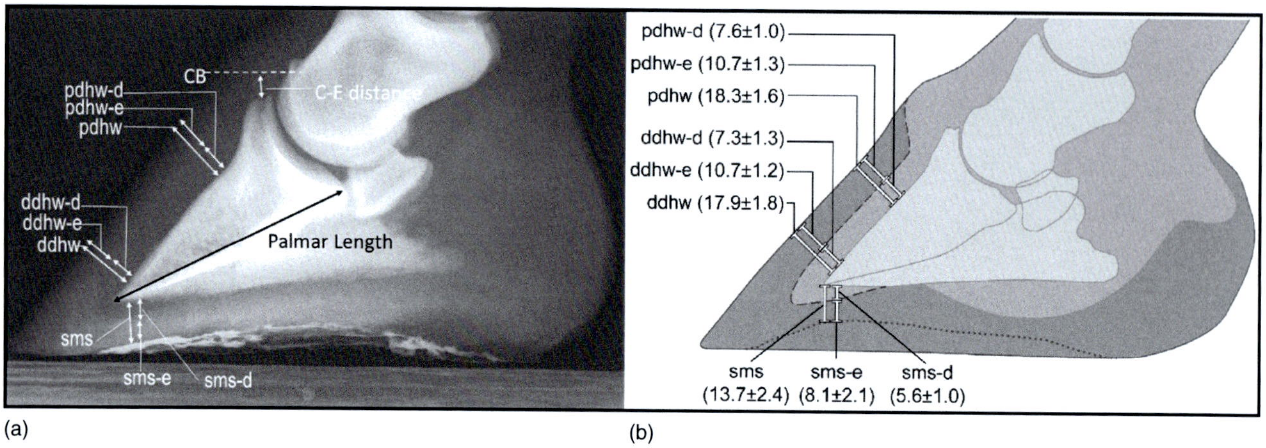

Figure 27.3 (a) Lateral radiograph with methods for quantitative assessment of displacement of the distal phalanx. (b) Average measurements obtained in light breed horses for these measurements. Reproduced with permission from Ref. [5]; © 2015, Wiley.

bear in mind that this tissue can be altered – most commonly in the horse with chronic laminitis – during trimming. Therefore, it is commonly best to obtain radiographs prior to trimming to obtain more accurate measurements, but still realizing that previous trims may be affecting the thickness of the keratinized hoof capsule. Currently, more attention is starting to be paid to the combined thickness of the lamellae and sublamellar/parietal dermis, as this tissue not only is not affected by trimming but also is the tissue which will be affected by events occurring in laminitis such as lamellar stretching and/or separation or possibly dermal edema [4, 5].

Contour of the Dorsal Surface of the Hoof Capsule

The dorsal surface of the hoof capsule is straight in normal horses and in horses that have recently become laminitic. The development of a concavity in the dorsal hoof wall – also commonly obvious by visual assessment of the hoof wall – is indicative of chronic laminitis (usually due to dorsal rotation of the distal phalanx).

Alignment of the Dorsal Surface of the Hoof Capsule in Relation to the Parietal Surface of the Distal Phalanx

Normally, the parietal surface of the distal phalanx is approximately parallel to the surface of the hoof capsule (Fig. 27.3a). When the parietal surface of the distal phalanx is less acutely angled in relation to the ground than the surface of the dorsal hoof capsule, it is indicative of dorsal rotation (Fig. 27.6). The difference between these two angles is recorded as the degree of rotation. This divergence in alignment is sometimes termed *capsular rotation* to distinguish it from phalangeal rotation. The parietal surface of the distal phalanx is normally angled 0–2° more acutely to the ground than the dorsal hoof capsule; that is, it is normal for there to be 0–2° of capsular rotation [4, 5]. Capsular rotation is always present in horses with phalangeal rotation, but can be present without phalangeal rotation (this most commonly occurs in conjunction with symmetrical distal displacement of the distal phalanx; Fig. 27.6a). In horses undergoing a first episode of laminitis with the primary displacement being rotation of the distal phalanx (versus distal displacement), capsular rotation and phalangeal rotation are always both present. With rotation of greater duration, the combination of corrective shoeing and natural repair processes may result in the alignment of the phalanges improving such that capsular rotation is present in the absence of phalangeal rotation (Fig. 27.6c).

Thickness of the Dorsal Hoof

The thickness of the hoof – that is, the entire width of the soft tissues between the dorsal surface of the hoof capsule and the dorsal (parietal) surface of the distal phalanx – is assessed proximally immediately distal to the extensor process (Fig. 27.3a, pdhw) and distally immediately proximal (approx. 5 mm) to the distal margin of the parietal surface of the distal phalanx (Fig. 27.3a, ddhw); the lines for measurement are drawn perpendicular to the parietal surface of the distal phalanx. The thickness of the hoof is the shortest distance from a given point on the parietal surface of the distal phalanx to the surface of the hoof capsule. If the thickness of the hoof has increased equally both proximally and distally, it is indicative of distal displacement of the distal phalanx. If the increase is greater distally, it is indicative of dorsal rotation of the distal phalanx (or a combination of both if the proximal measurement is greater than normal also). The measurement of the proximal dorsal hoof wall thickness has been used mostly to assess for symmetrical distal displacement (see Table 27.1); this measurement has varied from an average of 13–14 mm in ponies [1, 7], 15–16 mm in thoroughbreds [1, 8] to approximately 17–18 mm in a study of a variety of light breed horses and in Warmblood horses

Table 27.1 Normal radiographic measurement parameters.

Lateral radiograph Parameter	Breed	Mean (range or SD)	Reference
Coronary band-extensor process distance	Pony	3.1 (0–6.3)	[1]
	Pony	9.1 (± 2.2)	[7]
	WB	3.3 (–1.8–6.3)	[1]
	TB	5.2 (1.7–5.8)	[1]
	LtBr	6.9 (± 2.4)	[5]
Proximal hoof thickness (pdhw in Fig. 27.3)	Pony	13.2 (11.1–16.1)	[1]
	Pony	14.4 (± 1.5)	[7]
	WB	18 (17–19.1)	[1]
	WB	19 (± 1.4)	[11]
	WB	19.2 (± 2.1)	[4]
	TB	16.3 (13.9–19.7)	[1]
	TB	15.1 (± 0.9)	[8]
	LtBr	18.4 (± 2.4)	[4]
	LtBr	18.3 (± 1.6)	[5]
Inner hoof (pdhw-d in Fig. 27.3)	TB	5.7 (± 0.6)	[8]
	LtBr	7.0 (± 0.7)	[4]
	LtBr	7.6 (± 1.0)	[5]
Outer hoof (pdhw-e in Fig. 27.3)	TB	9.4 (± 0.6)	[8]
	LtBr	11.4 (± 2.0)	[4]
	Lt Br	10.7 (± 1.3)	[5]
Distal hoof thickness (ddhw in Fig. 27.3)	Pony	13.7 (± 1.4)	[7]
	TB	14.6 (± 1.0)	[8]
	WB	17 (± 1.7)	[11]
	WB	18.3 (± 1.8)	[4]
	LtBr	17.8 (± 2.3)	[4]
	LtBr	17.9 (± 1.8)	[5]
Inner hoof (ddhw-e in Fig. 27.3)	TB	5.5 (± 0.6)	[8]
	LtBr	6.5 (± 1.2)	[4]
	LtBr	7.3 (± 1.3)	[5]
Outer hoof (ddhw-e in Fig. 27.3)	TB	9.0 (± 0.6)	[8]
	LtBr	11.3 (± 1.9)	[4]
	LtBr	10.7 (± 1.2)	[5]
Depth of sole (sms in Fig. 27.3)	Pony	10.6 (± 2.1)	[7]
	TB	11.1 (± 1.6)	[8]
	WB	15.0 (± 2.7)	[11]
	Lt Br	13.7 (± 2.4)	[5]
Difference between DP Dorsal Cortex and Hoof Wall angles (DPDC-HW)	Pony	0.8 (0–2.0)	[1]
	Pony	–1.7 (± 1.8)	[7]
	WB	–0.4 (–4.0–2.0)	[1]
	WB	–2.8 (± 1.4)	[11]
	TB	0.4 (–1.0–2.0)	[1]
	TB	–0.5 (± 1.3)	[8]
Solear margin to ground angle (angles depicted in Figs 27.6a and b)	WB	4.0 (± 2.09)	[11]
	Pony	6.3 (± 2.6)	[7]
	LtBrP	6.1 (± 2.8)	[16]
	LtBr	5.6 (± 2.6)	[17]
Ratio of PHT: palmar length of distal cortex of DP	TB	24.9 (± 1.6)	[8]
	LtBr	26.8 (± 2.6)	[5]
	LtBr	26.7 (± 2.1)	[12]
Dorsopalmar radiograph			
Medial hoof wall thickness (mhw in Fig. 27.4)	Pony	12.3 (± 1.3)	[7]
	LtBr	19.3 (± 0.2)	[5]
Lateral hoof wall thickness (lhw in Fig. 27.4)	Pony	12.4 (± 1.4)	[7]
	LtBr	19.3 (± 0.2)	[5]
Medial sole thickness (sm in Fig. 27.4)	Pony	17.0 (± 3.0)	[7]
	WB	24.0 (± 3.8)	[11]
	LtBr	18.9 (± 4.2)	[5]
Lateral sole thickness (sl in Fig. 27.4)	Pony	18.7 (± 3.1)	[7]
	WB	26.0 (± 3.8)	[11]
	LtBr	20.7 (± 4.4)	[5]

WB, Warmblood; TB, Thoroughbred; LtBr, mixture of light breed horses; LtBrP, mixture of light breed horses and ponies.

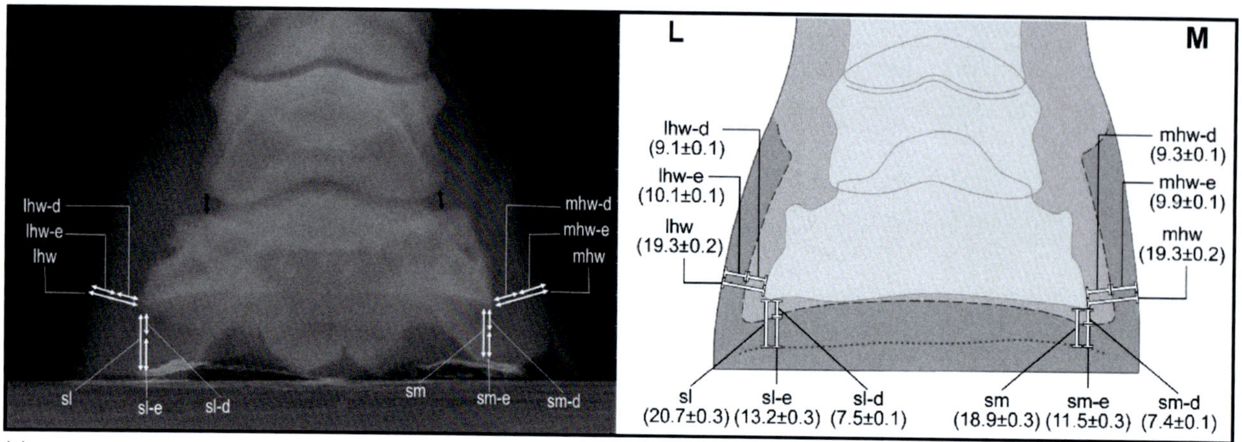

(a) (b)

Figure 27.4 (a) Dorsopalmar radiograph with methods for quantitative assessment of displacement of the distal phalanx. (b) Average measurements obtained in light breed horses for these measurements. Reproduced with permission from Ref. [5]; © 2015, Wiley.

[1,9,10], but up to 19 mm (±) has been suggested in Warmblood horses [4, 11]. Due to the variability in measurements – most likely due to different-sized feet in different animals – the ratio of the proximal dorsal hoof wall thickness to the palmar cortical length of the distal phalanx (as discussed below) has been used.

Ratio of Dorsal Hoof Wall Thickness to Palmar Cortical Length

This ratio has been assessed in multiple studies due to the impression that it is more accurate than dorsal hoof wall thickness, in that it takes into account the different sizes of horse (and therefore feet/distal phalanx). Most commonly, the

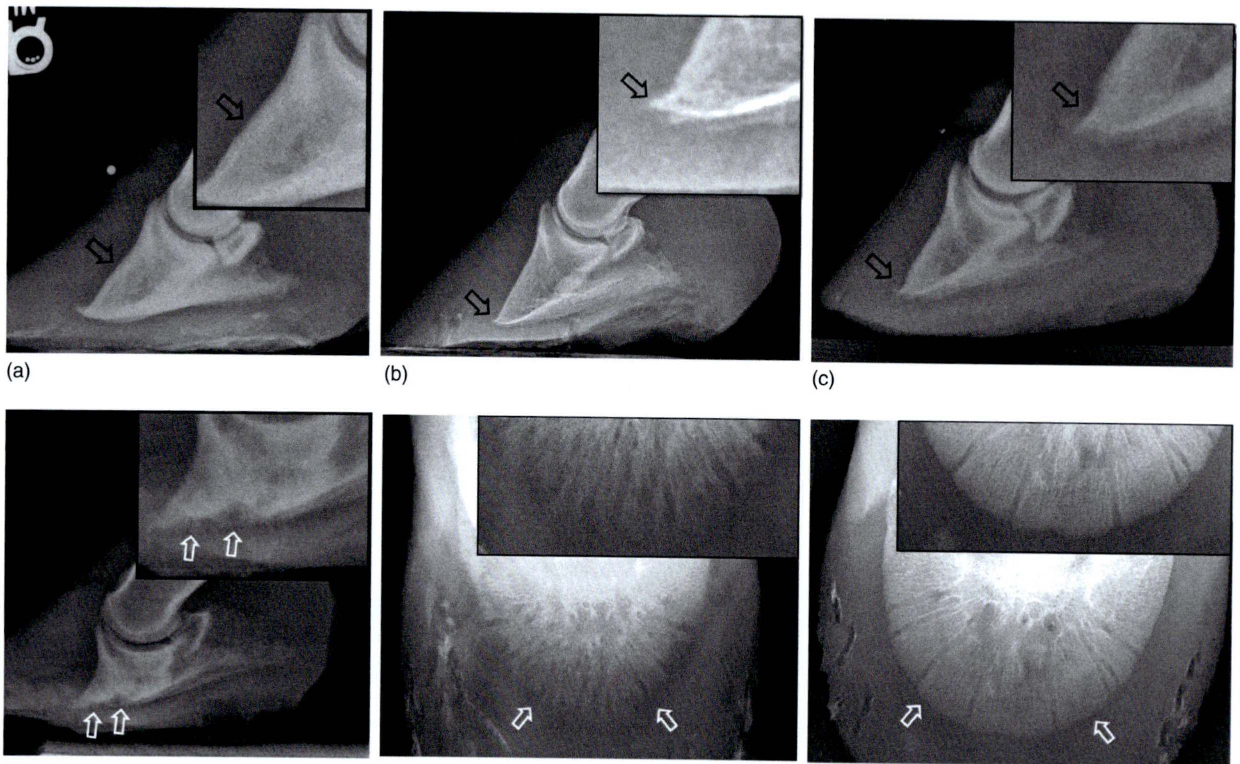

(a) (b) (c) (d) (e) (f)

Figure 27.5 Abnormalities to the distal phalanx associated with chronic laminitis on lateral radiographs include: (a) convexity of the parietal surface; (b) 'lipping' at the dorsal solear margin; (c) focal erosion of the dorsal distal margin of the distal phalanx; and (d) resorption of bone at the dorsal solear margin. Abnormalities visible on a 45° dorsopalmar oblique (solear margin) radiograph include irregularity of the dorsal solear margins in chronic laminitis (e) compared to the normal foot (f).

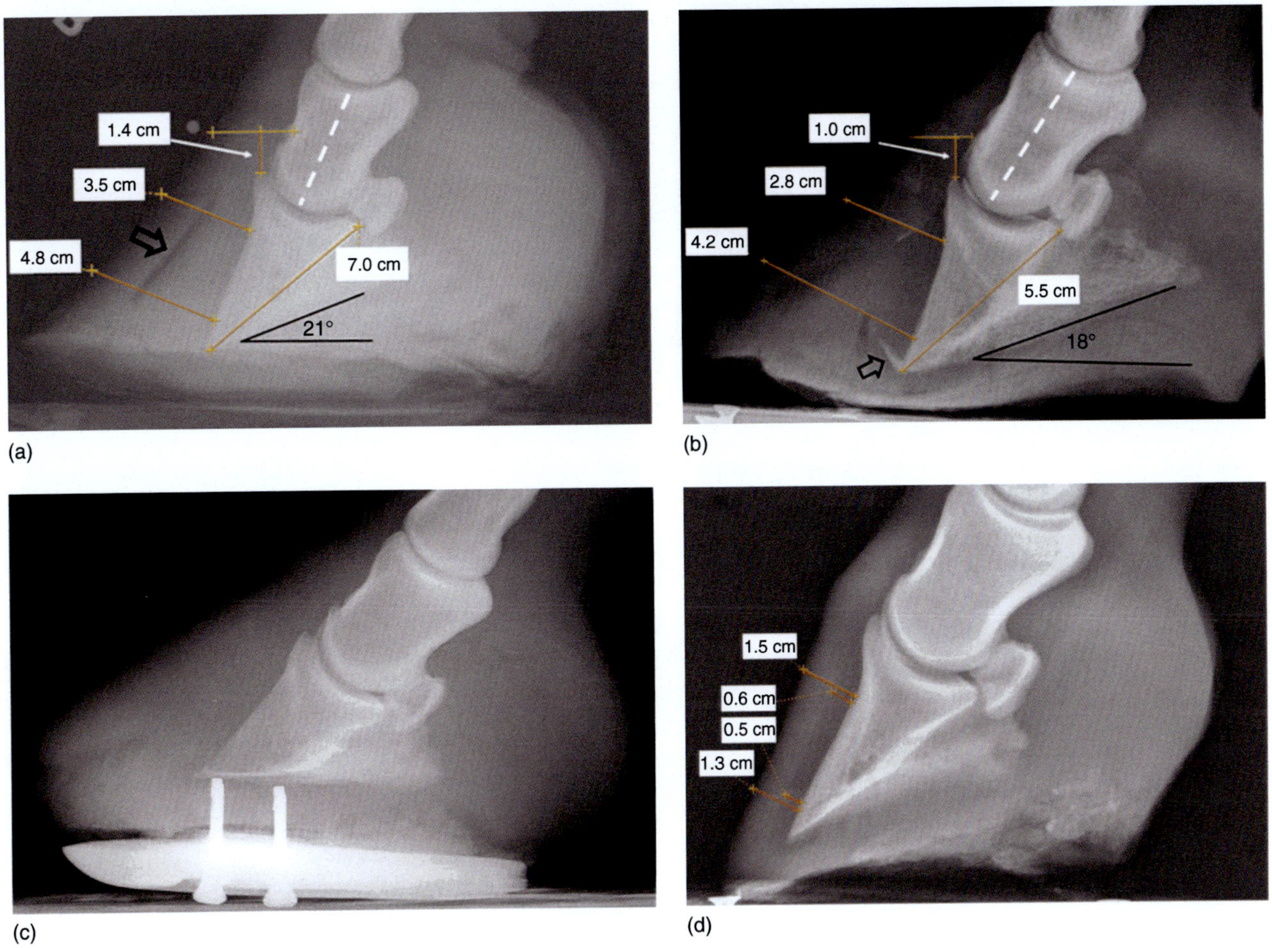

Figure 27.6 Radiographic signs of dorsal rotation including: (a) capsular rotation (with minimal phalangeal rotation [parietal surface of distal phalanx approximately parallel with axis of P2] but distal displacement/'sinking' present; (b) combined capsular and phalangeal rotation (parietal surface of distal phalanx not parallel with axis of P2; and (c) capsular rotation in a chronic case in which the phalangeal rotation has been corrected with therapeutic shoeing. Note the difference between dorsal rotation of the distal phalanx from laminitis and from a primary flexural deformity of the distal interphalangeal joint (d) in which the dorsal hoof is parallel to the parietal surface of the distal phalanx and wall measurements are not greater than normal. Dashed white lines in panels (a) and (b) represent the axis of the second phalanx (P2); the arrow in panel (a) signifies the gas line.

proximal hoof wall measurement is used in the ratio (Fig. 27.3a, pdhw). These ratios in normal animals have still varied between studies (see 27.Table 1), ranging from approximately 25% in one study of Thoroughbred race horses [8] to approximately 27% in two different studies that included a variety of breeds [9, 12]. In one of the latter studies, horses documented to have laminitis had an average (±SD) ratio of 30.6 ± 3.7%, which was significantly greater than normal [12]. However, the sensitivity and positive predictive value of using 30% as a cut-off for the diagnosis of laminitis were both poor. In the authors' opinion, any horse with a ratio of 30% or greater would be highly suggestive of distal displacement of the distal phalanx.

Hoof Capsule Thickness

The junction of the hoof capsule (Fig. 27.3a, pdhw-e) and the underlying lamellae and dermis (Fig. 27.3a, pdhw-d) is visible on digital radiographs as a change in radiodensity, the hoof capsule being more dense than the underlying dermis. An increase in thickness of the hoof is indicative of chronic laminitis (Fig. 27.6c, commonly due to lamellar wedge formation) because it does not change following the onset of laminitis until new hoof has grown distally from the coronary band [13].

Ratio of Hoof Capsule Thickness to Hoof Thickness

The reported ranges for this ratio are fairly large, from approximately 50% to 70% [1, 4, 13]. A decrease in this ratio is indicative of movement of the distal phalanx away from the surface of the hoof capsule. This ratio decreases most commonly following distal displacement or rotation, and will increase (especially on distal measurement) with chronic thickening observed with lamellar wedge formation

Coronary Band to Extensor Process (C-E) Distance

This is the vertical distance between the dorsoproximal border of the coronary band and the proximal extent of the extensor process of the distal phalanx (it has been termed the 'founder distance' [1]; see Fig. 27.3a). The founder distance will increase whenever the dorsal half of the distal phalanx moves distally. Although it is most commonly used to assess symmetrical distal displacement, the measurement is also inevitably increased in horses with acute rotation. Determining which of these is the primary cause is achieved by interpreting this in conjunction with an assessment of the alignment of the distal phalanx with the hoof capsule and the thickness of the dorsal hoof. It is not uncommon to have both symmetrical distal displacement and rotation occurring simultaneously; proximal dorsal hoof wall measurements need to be taken (immediately distal to the extensor process) in cases of rotational displacement (Fig. 27.4a) when assessing for distal displacement also.

Measurement of the C-E distance became more common after a study reporting that it was the radiographic measurement with the highest value as a predictor of outcome in laminitis cases [14]. Whereas the same authors had previously reported a normal range of C-E distance of −2 to 10 mm [1], they reported in a study of 216 laminitic horses and ponies that a C-E distance >14.0 mm had a probability of treatment success of less than 50%. Although these authors reported a mean C-E distance of 3.3–5.2 mm in different breeds of horses, a study of Warmbloods showed a value of 11 ± 3 mm) [11]. Thus, it is commonly difficult to interpret the C-E distance in an initial radiograph as the animal's normal measurement may range from −2 to 14 mm; hence, the C-E value is a more valuable tool for assessing displacement of the distal phalanx in serial radiographs (an excellent reason to take baseline radiographs prior to the onset of laminitis in horses at risk of laminitis).

Contour of the Parietal Surface of the Distal Phalanx

The parietal surface of the distal phalanx is normally straight or slightly convex and smooth. Roughening of the surface midway between the proximal and distal limits of the surface associated with a slight increase in convexity of the surface may occasionally be the only evidence of a prior episode of laminitis (Fig. 27.5a). The development of a dorsally projecting lip (Fig. 27.5b) at the junction of the parietal and solear surfaces is also indicative of remodeling, presumably caused by increased pressure on the dorsal solear margin of the bone which is usually associated with chronic laminitis. Less commonly, there is erosion of the dorsal distal margin immediately proximal to the solear margin (Fig. 27.5c), which is associated with ingrowth of dysplastic horn (associated with lamellar wedge) following the development of chronic rotation [15].

Contour of the Solear Margin of the Dorsal Aspect of the Distal Phalanx

Although somewhat variable in shape between horses, the solear margin is normally approximately straight from its dorsal margin to the palmar aspect of the palmar process (Fig. 27.3a). Following longstanding chronic laminitis, there is resorption of bone dorsally such that the dorsal portion of the solear surface of the bone is more acutely angled to the ground (Fig. 27.5d) than the palmar aspect. This makes it difficult to measure the angle that the solear margin forms with the ground.

Contour of the Solear Margins of the Palmar Processes of the Distal Phalanx

If a proper lateral radiograph is obtained with minimal obliquity, the solear margins of the two palmar processes should generally overlap with minimal disparity between the two. If there is a marked disparity between the two sides (Fig. 27.8a), this suggests asymmetrical distal displacement of the distal phalanx; the dorsopalmar (0°; Figs 27.4a and 27.8b) view is the 'gold standard' for assessing asymmetrical distal displacement (discussed below) and should be taken to fully assess the possibility of this type of displacement.

In the present authors' experience, the sole depth and solear margin angle (palmar angle) are two of the most important measurements both for case management and prognosis. In the acute case, an acute loss of sole depth appears to be a poor prognostic factor, especially in cases of symmetrical distal displacement. An increased solear margin angle in horses with either the acute or chronic laminitis indicates that pressure on the dorsal sole is increased (showing that measures must be taken to avoid solear prolapse/perforation in the acute case and subsolear bruising/abscessation in the chronic case), and also as an indicator that further injury to the dorsal lamellae may occur if the tension from the deep digital flexor tendon is not addressed (see Chapter 5).

Sole Depth

Sole depth is the proximodistal measurement from the solear margin to the ground surface of the keratinized sole; it is most commonly measured immediately caudal (ca. 5 mm) to the dorsodistal tip of the distal phalanx (Fig. 27.3a). It is important to differentiate this measurement of sole depth from the distance from the distal phalanx to the ground; the former is more important regarding the function of the sole and protection of underlying structures, while the latter is dependent on the degree of concavity of the sole.

The best way to obtain an accurate sole depth measurement is to apply a barium paste to the sole (Fig. 27.3a). A decrease in sole depth (and the distance from the distal phalanx to the ground) is expected in horses with acute dorsal rotation or symmetrical distal displacement of the distal phalanx. This is best differentiated from nonlaminitic horses with thin soles by the absence of changes associated with symmetrical distal displacement or rotational displacement, including assessments of the dorsal hoof wall and the angle of the solear margin of the distal phalanx (see below). Additionally, the thickness of the solear dermis should be normal with thin soles, but it is commonly compromised with distal phalangeal displacement (Fig. 27.7, insets). Sole depth is much more variable in horses with chronic rotation because the sole has had an opportunity

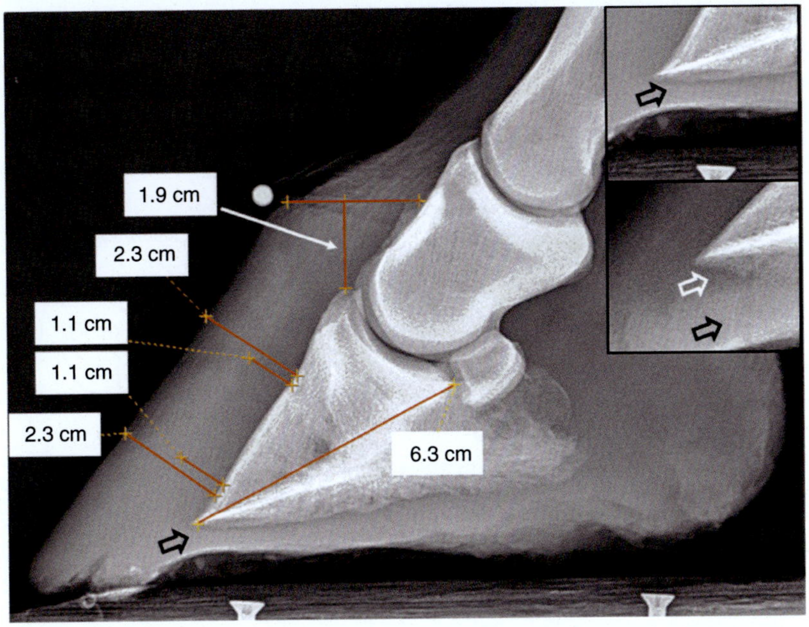

Figure 27.7 Radiographic signs of symmetrical distal displacement of the distal phalanx. Note the increased thickness (versus normal; see Fig. 27.3) but the same measurements proximally and distally for the dorsal hoof wall thickness (pdhw and ddhw in Fig. 27.3), and the thickness of the dorsal lamellar dermal/lamellar layer (pdhw-d and ddhw-d in Fig. 27.3). Also note that the solear dermal layer (sms-d in Fig. 27.3b; represented by the white arrow in the lower inset from a normal foot) is totally compressed leaving only the epidermal layer (sms-e in Fig. 27.3; black arrow on main figure and upper inset).

to regenerate, and is also one of the most variable measurements as it is commonly trimmed during routine hoof care. Average sole depth in Thoroughbred racehorses has been reported to be 1.1 cm, whereas in other studies light breeds were reported to have an average sole depth of about 1.4 cm [9], and Warmbloods 1.5 cm [11]. Interestingly, although sole depth is usually considered to be variable due to the effects of trimming, one study reported a minimal effect of trimming on sole depth measured as described above [11]. Similar to the hoof wall, the use of digital radiographs allows delineation of the solear dermis from the epidermal tissue (Figs 27.3a and b). The recent reporting of normal thicknesses for these two layers may lead to the use of dermal thickness as a more sensitive measurement when assessing for displacement in acute and possibly chronic cases [9].

Angle of the Solear Margin of the Distal Phalanx in Relation to the Ground Surface

This angle is abbreviated here to solear margin angle, but is also referred to as the palmar/plantar angle.

A decrease in the acuteness of the angle (i.e., a larger angle) formed by the solear margin of the distal phalanx and the ground is always seen in horses with acute dorsal rotation, and is sometimes termed phalangeal rotation. It must be differentiated from a flexural deformity, which is usually readily accomplished by

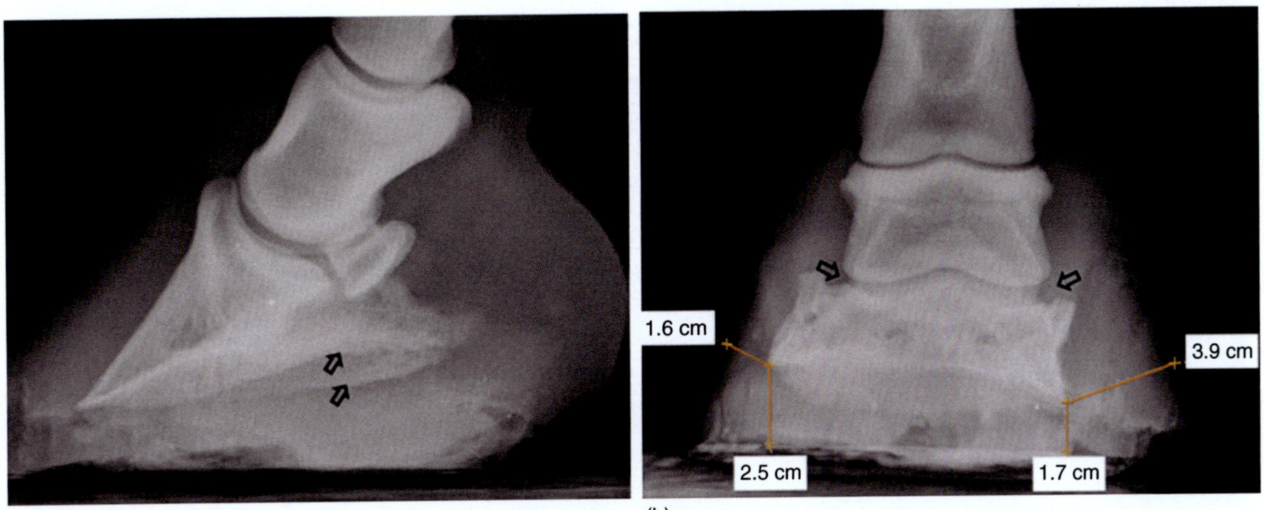

(a) (b)

Figure 27.8 (a) Radiographic signs of asymmetrical distal displacement including disparity in the solear margins of the palmar processes on lateral radiograph, and (b) on the displaced side on the dorsopalmar radiograph, decreased sole depth, increased width of the articular space of the distal interphalangeal joint, and increased hoof thickness.

taking the other radiographic signs into account (Fig. 27.6d), including a more vertical hoof wall in the horse with flexural deformity (than is observed in the normal or laminitic horse), which runs parallel to the parietal surface of the distal phalanx. In horses with chronic laminitis, this angle may vary from normal to higher than that which the horse originally developed during the early chronic phase of the disease, due to the development of a secondary flexural deformity. There is, for some reason, confusion as to which solear margin angle is considered normal, because there is considerable variabililty in this angle in normal horses (see Table 27.1). In a mixed population of sound horses the mean (SD) solear margin was 6.1 ± 2.8° [16], while in a study of horses with lameness originating from the foot excluding laminitis the solear margin angle was 5.63 ± 2.56° [17]. In another study of the effect of trimming on radiographic measurements, 40 Warmblood athletes (not lame) were trimmed by six different farriers [11]; the mean solear margin angles ranged from 4 to 4.7° before trimming, and 5.4 to 6.4° after trimming. The results of this study – which confirmed the experience of the present authors – showed that positive solear margin angles from 4–6° are not uncommon in athletes, and should not be used alone as an indication of dorsal rotation of the distal phalanx.

Phalangeal Axis

The phalangeal axis as determined on a radiograph (as distinct from the foot-pastern axis, which is determined by direct visual observation) describes the alignment of the phalanges. The normal alignment is slight dorsiflexion of the distal and proximal interphalangeal joints. Assessment of the axis on radiographs can be problematic because the axis will change depending on how much weight is borne by the limb. In horses with laminitis, the most important aspect of the axis is the angulation of the distal interphalangeal joint – more specifically, phalangeal rotation or flexion which is most commonly defined as a divergence of the dorsal surface of the distal phalanx from the axis of the first and second phalanges in a palmar/plantar direction (Fig. 27.6b). Flexion of the distal interphalangeal joint (phalangeal rotation) occurs when the flexor moment (from tension in the deep digital flexor tendon) exceeds the normal extensor moment due (from the attachments of lamellae to the distal phalanx dorsal to the center of rotation). This can occur either because the extensor moment is reduced (as in horses with laminitis due to loss of lamellar integrity; Fig. 27.6b), or the tension in the deep digital flexor tendon is increased (as in horses with flexural deformities of the distal interphalangeal joint; Fig. 27.6d).

Observations from Dorsopalmar Radiographs

The dorsopalmar radiograph is the primary view taken for determining the presence of asymmetrical distal displacement of the distal phalanx, but may also be valuable in cases of symmetrical distal displacement. Primarily, this would serve as a prognosis for the presence of lamellar changes (e.g., gas lines) on both medial and lateral aspects of the digit in this view which, combined with the same changes observed on the lateral view, would indicate a loss of the majority of the lamellae within the digit.

Symmetry of distal interphalangeal joint

The width of the distal interphalangeal joint is normally approximately equal medially and laterally (Fig. 27.4b). A marked asymmetry in the width of the joint may develop in horses that have undergone asymmetrical distal displacement; the side exhibiting an increase in the width of the joint space is the side that has displaced distally (Fig. 27.8b) [18]. However, this finding must be interpreted with caution because asymmetry in the joint space can be induced by uneven weight-bearing in the limb (an important reason to make sure that the metacarpi are vertical in a dorsopalmar direction in the standing horse while taking radiographs) [2], and is therefore best interpreted in conjunction with the thickness of the medial and lateral hoof.

Relationship Between the Articular Surface and Solear Margins of the Distal Phalanx to the Ground

Tilting of the articular surface and solear margin of the distal phalanx occur in horses with asymmetrical distal displacement, but this may also be normal for some animals. Additionally, because the solear margin of the distal phalanx is subject to remodeling, evaluating the angle of the solear margin of the distal phalanx (and also comparing the medial and lateral sole depth) is less reliable than evaluating the angle of the articular surface. Both of these measurements will also be affected by trimming; recent studies in sound horses have shown that when a skilled farrier trims a foot to perceived balance, the lateral sole depth is thicker compared to medial sole depth [11]. To differentiate between normal angulation and that which occurs with asymmetrical distal displacement, it must be interpreted in conjunction with the medial and lateral joint space and the thickness of the medial and lateral hoof (see immediately below).

Thickness of the Medial and Lateral Hoof

The medial and lateral hoof should appear approximately equal on dorsopalmar radiographs (Fig. 27.4a and b); the development of marked disparity in conjunction with an asymmetrical joint space is the best radiographic evidence for asymmetrical distal displacement (Fig. 27.8b). It should be noted that the measured width of the medial and lateral hoof walls do not represent the actual thickness of the medial and lateral wall at any point because the radiograph is a two-dimensional image of a three-dimensional object. However, it was shown in a recent study that the thickness of the hoof walls from the distomedial and distolateral aspect of the distal phalanx is much more consistent in normal horses than measurements of the medial and lateral sole depth [9].

Observations from 45° Dorsopalmar Oblique Radiographs

Evaluation of the Solear Margin

The solear margin is usually seen as a relatively smooth border interrupted by the invaginations of vascular canals with parallel sides (Fig. 27.5f), with a central indentation termed a 'crena' in many horses. The development of an irregular solear margin associated with divergence of the margins of the vascular channels as they approach the solear margin is characteristic of the aseptic form of pedal osteitis (Fig. 27.5e). Pedal osteitis is very common in horses with chronic laminitis, most likely due to chronic bruising of the dorsodistal aspect of the distal phalanx in the animal with distal phalanx displacement. However, any other chronic cause of inflammation of the distal surface of the distal phalanx (e.g., sole bruising in the thin-soled but otherwise normal foot) is also likely to cause pedal osteitis. Because of the general nature of the causes of loss of bone density, it is difficult to use this as a criterion for differentiating between septic and aseptic inflammation. Aseptic osteitis is much more common than septic osteitis of the distal phalanx; sepsis is commonly characterized by a more distinct area of lucency on dorsodistal aspect of the distal phalanx (see Fig. 45.3b and c in Chapter 45). Much less commonly, marginal fractures may develop seen as slivers of bone tangential to and separated from the solear margin.

Evaluation of Distal Phalanx Bone Density

Loss of bone density is commonly associated with inflammation of the distal phalanx or disuse of the distal limb. Late chronic laminitis is just one of the circumstances under which this may occur. Furthermore, the evaluation of bone density tends to be very subjective. The loss of bone density is a general finding observed in horses with both dorsal rotation and distal displacement.

Radiographic Changes with Different Patterns of Displacement of the Distal Phalanx

Dorsal Rotation

In horses that have recently suffered dorsal rotation, the shape and position of the wall of the hoof capsule in relation to the ground are unchanged, but the distal phalanx has rotated in a palmar direction about the distal condyles of the middle phalanx; that is, the distal interphalangeal joint is flexed (phalangeal rotation). The hallmark radiographic symptom is divergence of the parietal surface of the distal phalanx away from the hoof wall such that the distance between the surface of the dorsal hoof wall and the distal phalanx are increased, both proximally and distally, but the increase in distance is greater distally. As the extensor process rotates with the rest of the bone, the distance between the coronet and the extensor process (C-E distance) is also inevitably going to increase, though the degree to which it does is generally less than with distal displacement of the distal phalanx. Rotation also causes the distance between the dorsal solear margin of the distal phalanx and the ground to decrease and the angle of the solear margin of the distal phalanx to the ground (also termed palmar angle) to increase.

With increasing chronicity, much more variability is present in the radiographic findings than is present than in horses with recent rotation because of: (i) changes in the patterns of growth of the dorsal hoof wall; (ii) remodeling of the distal phalanx cause changes in the aforementioned parameters; and (iii) natural or farriery-enhanced attempts to achieve realignment of the distal phalanx with the hoof wall and ground. The concavity that develops in the dorsal hoof wall means that the proximal and distal aspects of the wall form different angles to the ground, so that the measurement of capsular rotation is no longer a simple single measurement; the distal wall is more acutely angled to the ground than the proximal wall. Furthermore, the tendency for the proximal hoof wall to realign with the distal phalanx, either through natural or farriery-enhanced mechanisms, causes a variable reduction in rotation of the proximal wall with time (but there is usually a residual increase in the thickness of the dorsal hoof). Resorption of bone from the dorsal distal solear margins of the distal phalanx increases the difficulty in measuring the angle the solear margin of the distal phalanx forms with the ground because the dorsal portion of the bone (where resorption has taken place) forms a different angle to the ground than the palmar aspect (Fig. 27.5d). The reason for differentiating between capsular rotation with and without phalangeal rotation is primarily because they both may occur to a similar extent in horses with early chronic rotation, but phalangeal rotation anecdotally has a better prognosis for improving (solear margin angle decreasing towards normal), over time, either naturally, with hoofcare, or with deep digital flexor tenotomy (see Chapter 43).

During the first few days to weeks after the onset of laminitis, gas densities (black arrow, Fig. 27.6a) commonly develop within the hoof before significant changes have occurred to the coronary band or white line. These early gas densities typically appear at the junction of the hoof capsule and the underlying dermis and do not extend distally to the white line or proximally to the coronary band. They are thought to represent mummification within the hoof wall where lamellar separation has occurred [19]. In the more chronically affected horse, submural or subsolear gas densities may develop later that communicate with the surface of the hoof either at the coronary band, white line, or potentially from perforation of the sole. These gas densities are likely to be associated with ongoing or previous subcapsular sepsis.

Symmetrical Distal Displacement

Early chronic symmetrical distal displacement of the distal phalanx causes an increase in the distance between the coronet and the extensor process (Fig. 27.7) and a corresponding decrease in the distance between the solear margin of the distal phalanx and the ground (Fig. 27.7). There is also an increase in the thickness of the dorsal hoof, which is the same proximally and distally (Fig. 27.7). The alignment of the phalanges does not change, nor does the angle of the solear margin of the distal phalanx. The symmetry of the distal limb on dorsopalmar radiographs is unchanged.

In late chronic distal displacement, the C-E distance may return to more normal values, but some increased thickening of the hoof commonly remains. The development of gas shadows in the hoof and the development of pedal osteitis occur in a similar manner to that seen in horses with dorsal rotation.

Asymmetrical Distal Displacement

Although indication of asymmetrical distal displacement of the distal phalanx can be visible on a lateral radiograph (as described above; see Fig. 27.8a), displacement can only be confirmed on dorsopalmar radiographs of the feet (Fig. 27.8b). The characteristic radiographic symptoms are:

- 'Tilting' of the distal phalanx distally within the hoof capsule on one side of the foot-most commonly the medial side, resulting in decreased sole thickness on the affected side compared to the unaffected side (Fig. 27.8b).
- Asymmetry of the distal interphalangeal joint such that there is an increase in joint space (arrows, Fig. 27.8b) on the side that has displaced distally and a reduction in joint space on the opposite side of the foot.
- An increase in the width of the hoof on the affected side of the foot (Fig. 27.8b).

Additionally, if there are markers at the coronary band, a greater distance between the coronary band and the palmar process may be present on the affected side; however, as the coronary band on the medial side of the foot is commonly higher than the lateral coronary band, it must be interpreted with caution. As discussed above, incorrect positioning (e.g., the horse's limb is not vertical to the ground) can lead to the artifactual appearance of a tilted distal phalanx and asymmetry of the distal interphalangeal joint (although, under these circumstances, the compressed side of the joint should be on the same side of the limb as the distal tilt of the distal phalanx in contrast to the situation in a horse with asymmetrical distal displacement). Radiographic lucencies (i.e., 'gas lines') may develop in the wall on the side of displacement, with a similar appearance to that seen dorsally with rotation. Asymmetrical distal displacement may not be detectable on lateral radiographs. However, as discussed above, if there is sufficient displacement and the positioning of the foot and radiograph technique are optimal, an asymmetry in the solear margins of the palmar processes may be quite suggestive (Fig. 27.8a).

The effect of chronic changes associated with asymmetrical distal displacement are poorly documented. However, with time, the angulation of the distal phalanx and the symmetry of the distal interphalangeal joint may return to normal. Additionally, the surface of the wall on the affected side may become irregular with new growth. Furthermore, if markers are placed at the coronary band at the widest point of the foot, the disparity in growth between the affected side and the contralateral side is evident.

The Value of Radiographs in Determining the Prognosis

Several investigators have measured various radiographic parameters with the goal of discovering cut-off values that could be useful in determining the prognosis. Stick correlated the severity of rotation with the prognosis for return to athletic function [20]. In that study, horses with less than 5.5° of rotation returned to athletic performance, whereas horses with more than 11.5° did not return to athletic performance. Hunt reviewed 202 horses with laminitis and grouped them by functional outcome for the purpose of analysis [21]. In this study, the severity of lameness did correlate with the functional outcome, but the degree of rotation did not. However, those horses that returned to athletic soundness had significantly less rotation than those that were intermittently or permanently lame. Interestingly, there was no difference in the degree of dorsal rotation between those horses that were athletically sound and those that died; the author speculated that this was because, among the horses that died, many were euthanized before significant rotation occurred. In a series of 216 horses, Eustace assigned horses to one of four groups on the basis of clinical signs and showed that the group to which a horse was assigned was more important prognostically than any radiographic parameters measured [22]. The C-E distance, when adjusted for magnification, was a useful prognostic determinant for those horses with very high or very low C-E values. Additionally, the angle of rotation was greater overall for failures than successes, but this was only statistically different in the group comprised of horses with chronic rotation.

As a single set of radiographs provides static information, serial radiographs are essential for following the progression of the disease and response to treatment. Unfortunately, radiographic studies interpreted in isolation from clinical data are of limited value. Indeed, radiographs might better be considered an adjunct to clinical findings in determining the prognosis rather than the other way around.

Radiography as a Guide to Therapeutic Trimming and Shoeing

Shoeing the feet of laminitic horses is not a 'one size and style fits all' for at least two reasons: (i) not all horses are affected by the disease in the same manner or to the same magnitude; and (ii) different clinicians/farriers with experiences with different techniques may treat the same horse with different goals or objectives in mind because objective data for one technique over another are not available. However, whatever the goal or technique to

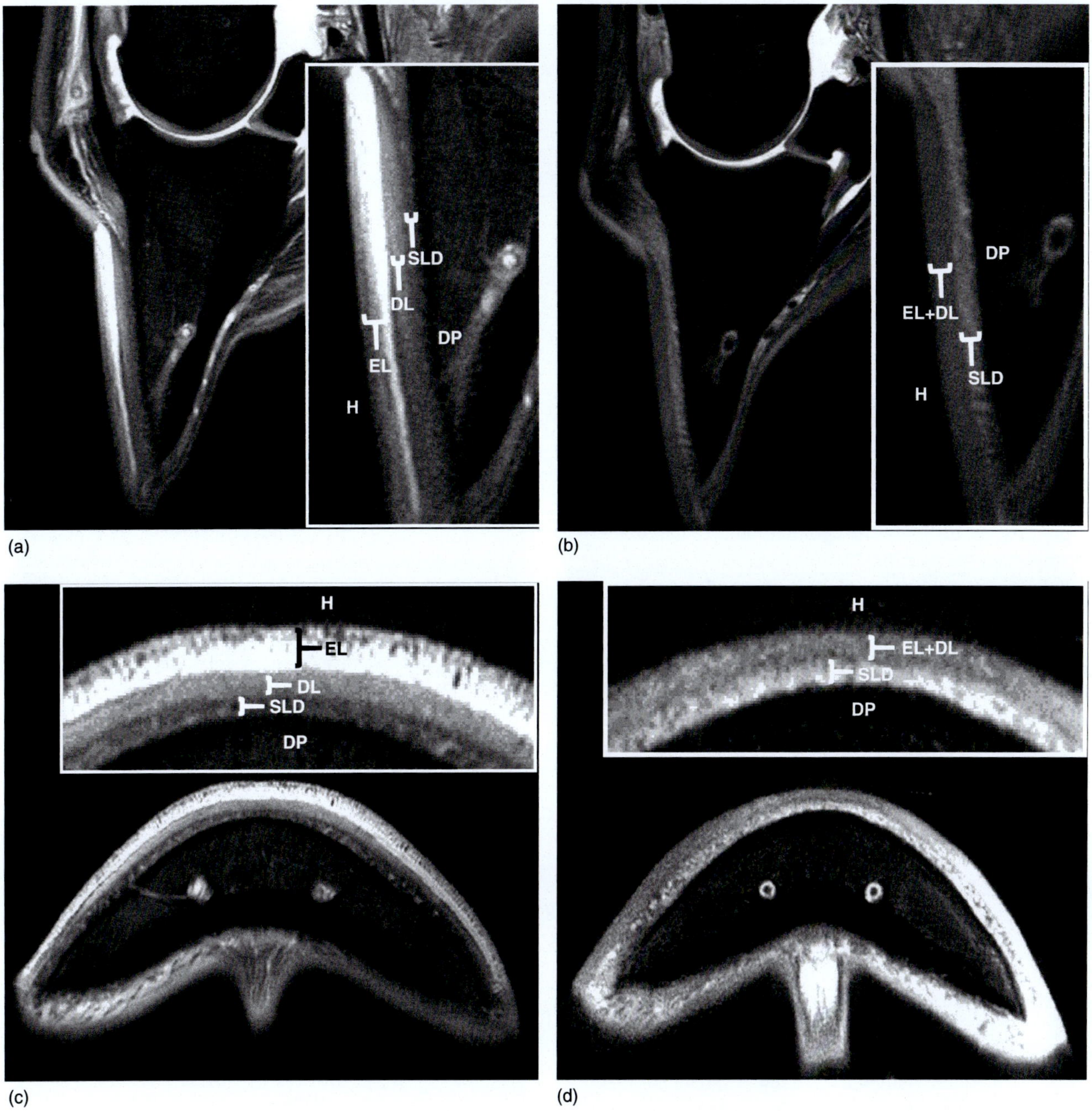

Figure 27.9 Magnetic resonance images of the affected lamellae in a clinical case with laminitis on sagittal (a) and transverse (c) views (proton density fat-suppressed), and the same views (b and d) on a normal horse. The radiographs of the affected horse appeared normal with all measurements within normal range. Note the separation of epidermal lamellae (EL) from dermal lamellae (DL) in the affected digit (panels a and c), with interdigitating EL and DL (EL+DL) forming one layer (panels b and d) in the normal digit. SLD, sublamellar dermis; DP, distal phalanx; H, cornified hoof.

be used, the external/visual landmarks of the hoof are not a consistent guideline to the position of the distal phalanx within the hoof capsule for horses with laminitis. Therefore, trimming and shoeing a laminitic horse with the benefit of radiographic guidance is required to achieve optimal and consistent results.

The lateral radiograph is most commonly used to determine how to trim the ground surface of the foot in relation to the solear margin of the distal phalanx, and the result of the trim determines the final angle of the solear margin in relation to the ground (see Chapter 38). Additionally, the lateral radiograph is used to determine the most dorsal margin of the shoe and the position of the point of breakover in relation to the distal phalanx. There is no complete agreement on what these variables should be. The present authors generally prefer a solear margin angle of between 2° and 5°. They do not place the dorsal aspect of the shoe dorsal to a point formed by the intersection of the plane of the trimmed sole and a line that represents the normal position of the surface of the dorsal wall. For the present authors, the final position for the point of breakover is usually between 0 and 1 cm dorsal to the point of intersection of the dorsal margin of the distal phalanx and the ground surface of the sole.

The depth of the sole on the lateral radiograph and the distance between the dorsal margin of the distal phalanx and the ground (sms in Fig. 27.3) is one measure of the integrity of the sole of the hoof capsule. Used in conjunction with clinical findings, it is helpful in determining whether the dorsal sole of the foot is able to bear weight (i.e. whether the dorsal part of the sole can be included when sole packing material is applied to the ground surface of the foot or whether the dorsal sole should be protected from direct pressure).

The dorsopalmar radiograph is useful in determining the position of the center of the shoe in the frontal plane in relation to the distal phalanx. For most horses, it is desirable that the shoe is directly centered under the center of the distal phalanx. However, in horses with asymmetrical distal displacement of the distal phalanx, the use of the dorsopalmar radiograph is particularly important because the distal phalanx has moved in the frontal plane so that the center of the hoof is no longer aligned with the center of the distal phalanx. Furthermore, some clinicians deliberately offset the shoe so that the shoe extends further abaxially on the least affected side of the foot (see Chapter 38).

Deep digital flexor tenotomies performed in the course of treatment may result in subluxation of the distal interphalangeal joint (see Chapter 43). The present authors consider this to be an undesirable sequel to the procedure that can be prevented or at least markedly reduced with heel elevation. Radiographic imaging during post-surgical shoeing is very helpful in determining the correct amount of heel elevation required to control the tendency of the distal interphalangeal joint to subluxate, paying particular attention that the center of the distal articular surface of the second phalanx articulates with the center of the articular surface of the distal phalanx (the distal phalanx displaces dorsally in relation to the second phalanx when subluxation occurs).

Magnetic Resonance Imaging

Although the literature is limited regarding the use of magnetic resonance imaging (MRI) in laminitis, normal measurements for MRI assessment of laminitis have recently been published [9], as have the lamellar changes using MRI been described in both acute and chronic cases of laminitis [12, 23]. The primary advantage of MRI is the enhanced visualization of the lamellae, with the ability to detect lamellar separation prior to changes in hoof wall measurements from radiographs [12]. The disadvantages are primarily the cost and the need for anesthesia – which is mainly a concern regarding causing further lamellar damage during recovery from anesthesia. MRI can be useful in diagnosing lamellar injury in animals in which the diagnosis of laminitis is not straightforward due to minimal changes on radiography and lack of support of the diagnosis upon obtaining a history and performing a clinical examination (Fig. 27.9).

Summary

Radiographs are invaluable in all steps of managing this disease. However, the information they provide is supplemental to the clinical presentation of the horse, and interpretation of radiographs in isolation of clinical findings is unlikely to be beneficial and may be misleading.

References

1. Cripps, P.J. and Eustace, R.A. (1999) Radiological measurements from the feet of normal horses with relevance to laminitis. *Equine Vet. J.*, **31** (5), 427–432.
2. Contino, E.K., Barrett, M.F., and Werpy, N.M. (2014) Effect of limb positioning on the radiographic appearance of the distal and proximal interphalangeal joint spaces of the forelimbs of horses during evaluation of dorsopalmar radiographs. *J. Am. Vet. Med. Assoc.*, **244** (10), 1186–1190.
3. Koblik, P.D., O'Brien, T.R., and Coyne, C.P. (1988) Effect of dorsopalmar projection obliquity on radiographic measurement of distal phalangeal rotation angle in horses with laminitis. *J. Am. Vet. Med. Assoc.*, **192** (3), 346–349.
4. Goulet, C., Olive, J., Rossier, Y., and Beauchamp, G. (2015) Radiographic and anatomic characteristics of dorsal hoof wall layers in nonlaminitic horses. *Vet. Radiol. Ultrasound*, **56** (6), 589–594.
5. Grundmann, I.N., Drost, W.T., Zekas, L.J., Belknap, J.K., Garabed, R.B., Weisbrode, S.E., *et al.* (2015) Quantitative assessment of the equine hoof using digital radiography and magnetic resonance imaging. *Equine Vet. J.*, **47** (5), 542–547.
6. Redden, R.F. (2003) Radiographic imaging of the equine foot. *Vet. Clin. North Am. Equine Pract.*, **19** (2), 379–92, vi.
7. Thieme, K., Ehrle, A., and Lischer, C. (2015) Radiographic measurements of the hooves of normal ponies. *Vet. J.*, **206** (3), 332–337.
8. Linford, R.L., O'Brien, T.R., and Trout, D.R. (1993) Qualitative and morphometric radiographic findings in the distal phalanx and digital soft-tissues of sound Thoroughbred racehorses. *Am. J. Vet. Res.*, **54** (1), 38–51.
9. Grundmann, I.N., Drost, W.T., Zekas, L.J., Belknap, J.K., Garabed, R.B., Weisbrode, S.E., *et al.* (2014) Quantitative assessment of the equine hoof using digital radiography and magnetic resonance imaging. *Equine Vet. J.* **47** (5), 542–547.
10. Kummer, M., Gygax, D., Lischer, C., and Auer, J. (2009) Comparison of the trimming procedure of six different farriers by quantitative evaluation of hoof radiographs. *Vet. J.*, **179** (3), 401–406.
11. Kummer, M., Geyer, H., Imboden, I., Auer, J., and Lischer, C. (2006) The effect of hoof trimming on radiographic measurements of the front feet of normal Warmblood horses. *Vet. J.*, **172** (1), 58–66.
12. Arble, J.B., Mattoon, J.S., Drost, W.T., Weisbrode, S.E., Wassenaar, P.A., Pan, X., *et al.* (2009) Magnetic resonance imaging of the initial active stage of equine laminitis at 4.7 T. *Vet. Radiol. Ultrasound*, **50** (1), 3–12.
13. Sherlock, C. and Parks, A. (2013) Radiographic and radiological assessment of laminitis. *Equine Vet. Educ.*, **25**, 524–535.
14. Cripps, P.J. and Eustace, R.A. (1999) Factors involved in the prognosis of equine laminitis in the UK. *Equine Vet. J.*, **31** (5), 433–442.

15. Collins, S.N., Van Eps, A.W., Pollitt, C.C., and Kuwano, A. (2010) The lamellar wedge. *Vet. Clin. North Am. Equine Pract.*, **26** (1), 179–195.
16. Smith, S.S., Dyson, S.J., Murray, R.C., and Weekes, J. (2004) Is there an association between distal phalanx angles and deep digital flexor tendon lesions? *Proc. Am. Assoc. Equine Pract.*, p. 1454.
17. Dyson, S.J., Tranquille, C.A., Collins, S.N., Parkin, T.D., and Murray, R.C. (2011) An investigation of the relationships between angles and shapes of the hoof capsule and the distal phalanx. *Equine Vet. J.*, **43** (3), 295–301.
18. O'Grady, S.E. and Parks, A.H. (2008) Farriery options for acute and chronic laminitis. *Proc. Am. Assoc. Equine Pract.*, **54**, 354–363.
19. van Oldruitenborgh-Oosterbaan, M.M.S. (1999) Laminitis in the horse: a review. *Vet. Q.*, **21** (4), 121–127.
20. Stick, J.A., Jann, H.W., Scott, E.A., and Robinson, N.E. (1982) Pedal bone rotation as a prognostic sign in laminitis of horses. *J. Am. Vet. Med. Assoc.*, **180** (3), 251–253.
21. Hunt, R.J. (1993) A retrospective evaluation of laminitis in horses. *Equine Vet. J.*, **25** (1), 61–64.
22. van Oldruitenborgh-Oosterbaan, M.M.S. (2011) Laminitis in the horse: a review. *Vet. Q.*, **21**, 121–127.
23. Murray, R.C., Dyson, S.J., Schramme, M.C., Branch, M., and Woods, S. (2003) Magnetic resonance imaging of the equine digit with chronic laminitis. *Vet. Radiol. Ultrasound*, **44** (6), 609–617.

CHAPTER 28

The Digital Venogram

Amy Rucker

Introduction

The digital venogram is a vascular contrast study of the foot. It was first performed in 1992, and the technique has been refined over time [1–5]. The venogram, which involves the injection of a radiopaque contrast into the palmar digital vein (as described below), is used to evaluate the integrity of the arterial and venous structures in the digital dermis of the entire foot. There are minor variations of normal feet depending on the conformation and adaptations of the distal phalanx and dermis in response to stresses associated with conformation, disease, or trauma (Fig. 28.1) [6, 7]. However, once the clinician gathers experience with venograms, these variations are easy to distinguish from the changes that occur with laminitis. Laminitis-induced dermal pathology results in venous compression and distortion of vascular structures [8]. When laminitis occurs, vascular anomalies are evident prior to measurable displacement of the distal/third phalanx, helping the veterinarian identify both the presence and severity of pathology [8]. As the distal phalanx (DP) displaces, the venogram changes become more profound.

The venogram should first be performed early during the course of the disease. Many acute laminitis patients respond favorably initially to conservative therapy that may include anti-inflammatory drugs and other pain management. Unfortunately, veterinarians are often misled by pain resolution. In the present author's view, the presence of dermal pathology may be overlooked without venograms, resulting in the horse being the horse considered 'stable' until radiographic evidence of DP displacement becomes significant later in the treatment period. Thus, what initially might have been mild pathology (diagnosed by a venogram and appropriately treated) now results in cumulative damage from a lack of resolution of dermal compression. At four to six weeks after the initial insult, the horse is no longer able to compensate and displays increasing degrees of lameness. By that time, some damage may be irreversible and the treatment becomes a race to relieve dermal compression before bone damage occurs.

The venogram demonstrates vascular and dermal integrity; venogram images aid in the assessment of severity of disease, the development of treatment strategies, and the monitoring of response to treatment [9–16]. Although the procedure is not complicated, the veterinarian should learn the technique on a sound horse to become familiar with 'normal' image patterns and to master the technique.

Procedure

Prior to removing the horse from its stall, all radiographic, farrier, and medical equipment are gathered and organized. Every attempt is made to reduce trauma to the laminitic patient by quickly and accurately completing the procedure. A vital aspect of equipment includes two foot blocks of a height that is 2 cm lower than the center of the collimator on the X-ray machine used by the clinician. This ensures that the focus of the X-ray beam is on the distal border of the DP and the solear dermis. Medical supplies necessary for venograms include: clippers; sedation (detomidine HCl); local anesthetic (mepivacaine HCl); contrast (diatrizoate meglumine and diatrizoate Na that is isotonic [some horses become painful when a hypertonic solution is used]); butterfly catheters (winged Infusion Set-21 gauge, 1.9-cm needle with 30-cm tubing); Luer-lock injection ports; 10-cm elastic tape; gauze squares; two 12-ml Luer-lock syringes; and 20 gauge X 2.5-cm needles. A tourniquet is made from a tire inner-tube (50 cm long, 2.5 cm wide). (Note: some clinicians prefer to use Esmarch tourniquets; if used, be aware that they are pliable and long, requiring extra attention to ensure that the first several wraps are secure and firm.) Two 12 ml syringes filled with contrast (24 ml total) are used for an average-sized foot. Two syringes are used because the smaller volume per syringe allows the detection of injection resistance, signaling perivascular leakage of contrast (i.e., a 'blown vein'). The volume of contrast used per foot may increase or decrease depending on the size of the foot, with the following being the general volume used depending on the greatest width of foot: 11 cm/20 ml; 12.5 cm/24 ml; 13.5 cm/30 ml and 14.5 cm/36 ml.

The horse is lightly sedated, both feet are meticulously cleaned, and regional anesthesia is performed at the level of the base of the proximal sesamoid bone (i.e., an abaxial sesamoid nerve block). Mepivicaine (3 ml) is used per site to minimize

Equine Laminitis, First Edition. Edited by James K. Belknap and Raymond Geor.

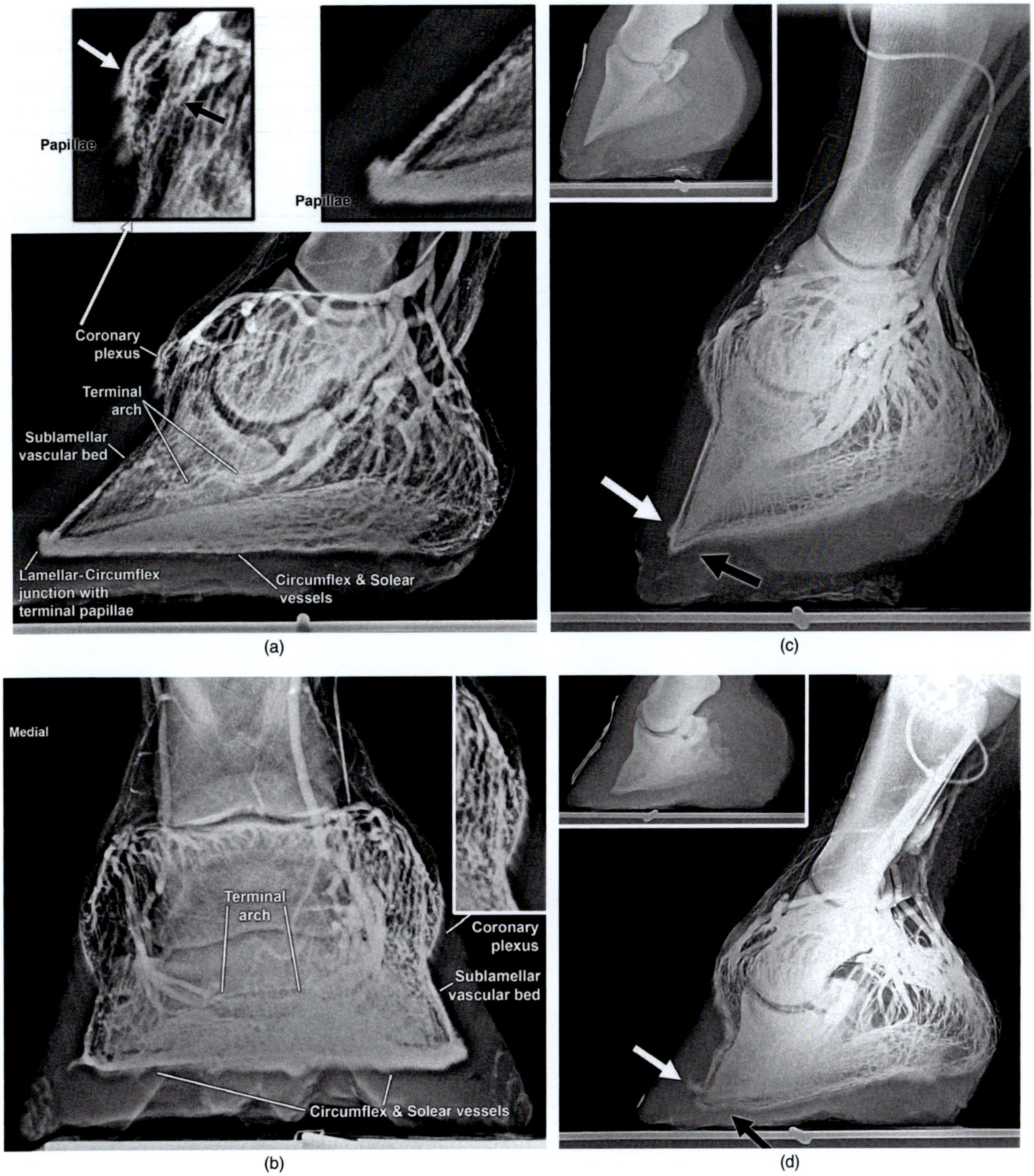

Figure 28.1 Venogram images of non-laminitic feet. (a) Lateromedial and (b) dorsopalmar views of a sound five-year-old Quarter Horse with a 0° palmar angle and 20 mm sole depth. The palmar digital arteries and veins are visualized terminating within the distal phalanx in the terminal arch. Vessels run through osseous canals and penetrate the parietal surface to anastomose with the sublamellar vascular bed, which joins proximally with the coronary plexus and distally with the circumflex vessels at the lamellar–circumflex junction. The dorsal coronary plexus (panel a, upper left inset) has a flatter caudal portion (panel a, left inset, black arrow) that parallels the distal dorsal second phalanx, and the extensor process of the DP. The more curved dorsal portion (panel a, left inset, white arrow) mirrors the coronary groove of the hoof capsule. Dermal papillae of both the coronary plexus (panel a, upper left inset) and the terminal and solear papillae (panel a, upper right inset) are parallel to the parietal surface of the DP. The lamellar–circumflex junction is of the same angle as the apex of the DP, and is located distal and peripheral to the distal margin of the DP. On the dorsopalmar view (b), the lateral coronary plexus (insert) contains more contrast and the coronary papillae are more evident (compared to the medial side). The papillae (panel b, inset) are parallel to the parietal surface of the DP. The lateral lamellar–circumflex junction is angular, while the medial papillae are reduced at the lamellar–circumflex junction. The slight reduction in contrast in the medial coronary plexus, sublamellar vascular bed, and lamellar–circumflex junction is typical of a sound horse that loads the dermis more heavily on the medial side of the foot and has mild remodeling of the distal medial border of the DP. Note that the solear and circumflex vessels and papillae are present along the entire distal border of the DP (panel b). (c) Yearling with Deep Digital Flexor Tendon contracture (inset). The SLVB is widened at the distal aspect (white arrow) and the solear papillae are compressed distal to the apex of the DP (black arrow). (d) Aged mare with club foot (inset). The SLVB is widened dorsally with remodeling of the LCJ (white arrow) and compression of the solear and CV vessels distal to the apex of the DP (black arrow). (e) Aged mare with chronic negative palmar angle (insert). The CV and solear vessels are compressed distal to the wings of the DP (black arrow.) The foot was trimmed and the venogram repeated 24 hours later (f) demonstrating that farrier techniques can alter the internal "load" and relieve dermal compression.

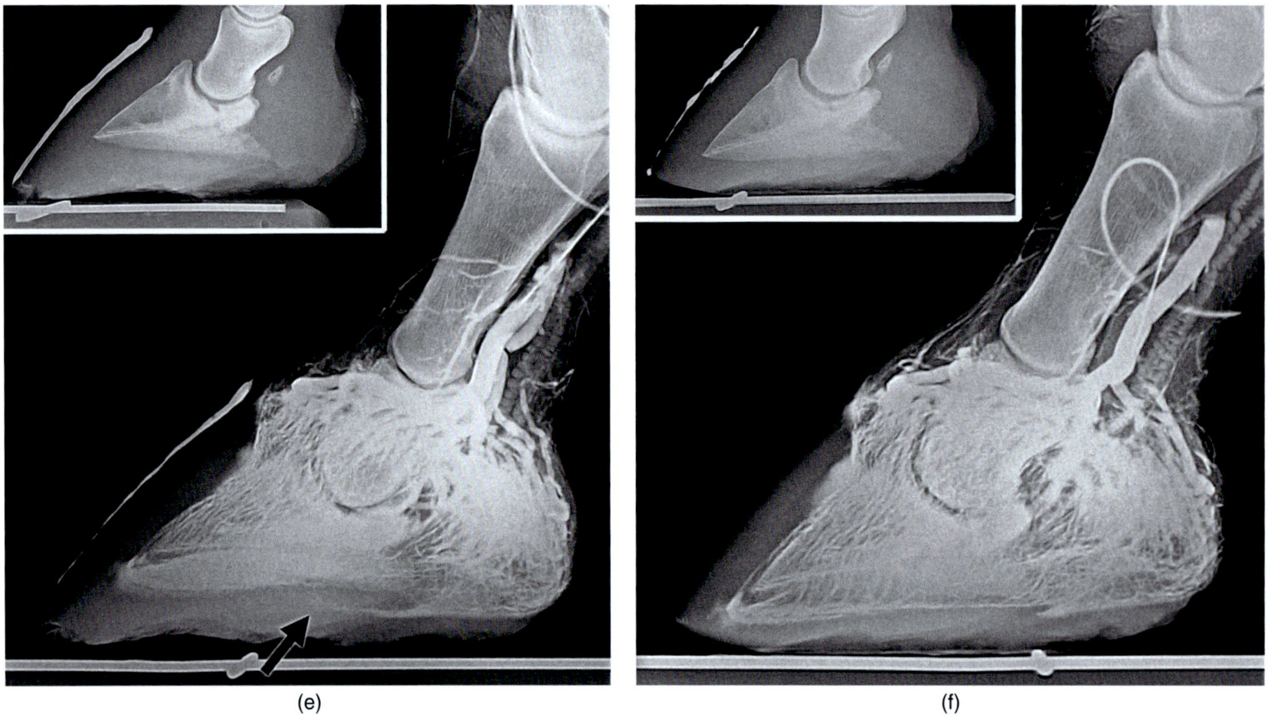

Figure 28.1 (*Continued*)

edema at the site of the tourniquet. (Note that the venogram is usually performed stall-side to minimize movement-induced lamellar injury in the blocked horse.) Hair is clipped from the medial and lateral pastern regions over the palmar digital vessels. If hair is excessive on the leg, it is also clipped from the palmar/plantar fetlock to avoid tourniquet interference.

The horse is placed on the foot blocks, making adjustments so that the horse stands with both metacarpi perpendicular to the ground (both from the lateromedial and dorsopalmar view). The feet are placed according to the conformation of the horse (i.e., base wide/toe in); this ensures that the patient stands squarely for even weight distribution. The feet are placed at the medial axial (inside) edge of the foot block to allow contact with the radiograph cassette and eliminate any image magnification. Radiopaque barium paste is applied on the dorsal hoof wall at the midline, extending from the junction with the hair (proximal coronary band) distally to assist in measurements on the lateromedial view. Baseline radiographs (dorsopalmar and lateromedial views) are taken to evaluate radiograph technique and to assist with shoeing the feet after the venograms are performed. Adjustment of the radiographic technique above that used for the baseline radiographs may be necessary to allow penetration of the contrast-filled foot (for example, depending on the radiographic machine used, the clinician may have to increase the kilovolts by 4-6, and/or milliamp seconds (mAs) by 0.05–0.1).

Immediately prior to tourniquet placement, 10 cm wide tape is wrapped twice around the widest point of the fetlock, leaving the last few centimeters of the tape free of the horse and ensuring that the distal border of the tape does not extend onto the pastern region. The tourniquet is anchored (adhered) beneath the free end of the tape, and is tightly wrapped around the fetlock, using constant tension. Care is taken not to distort the skin of the distal limb when applying the tourniquet. The tourniquet is taped in place, ending with the free end of tape on the side of the limb to be catheterized.

The veterinarian is then positioned dorsal to the foot and facing caudally. Her/his medial/inside arm is placed medial to the limb in a palmar direction. The medial hand holds the syringe for injection, and controls the limb when it is flexed. The lateral hand applies light digital pressure over the butterfly catheter and vein, and controls the hoof if the horse attempts to pick it up off the block.

The butterfly catheter is gently inserted into the lateral palmar digital vein mid-pastern. Once blood flashes back through the tubing, the needle is not advanced further. Blood should steadily drip from the catheter; if it does not, back the needle out 1 mm in case the beveled edge is against the far wall of the vessel. Once blood flows freely, the catheter is capped with an injection port.

The assistant inserts the needle of the first radiographic contrast syringe into the injection port and places the syringe of contrast into the veterinarian's inner/medial hand. The veterinarian injects the first syringe of contrast, monitoring for any extravasation of contrast by noting injection resistance with the medial hand. The outer/lateral hand monitors skin distension and temperature (perivascular contrast may be detected as a cooling of the skin adjacent to the needle). When the first syringe is empty the assistant removes it and attaches the second syringe, while being careful not to dislodge the catheter. As the

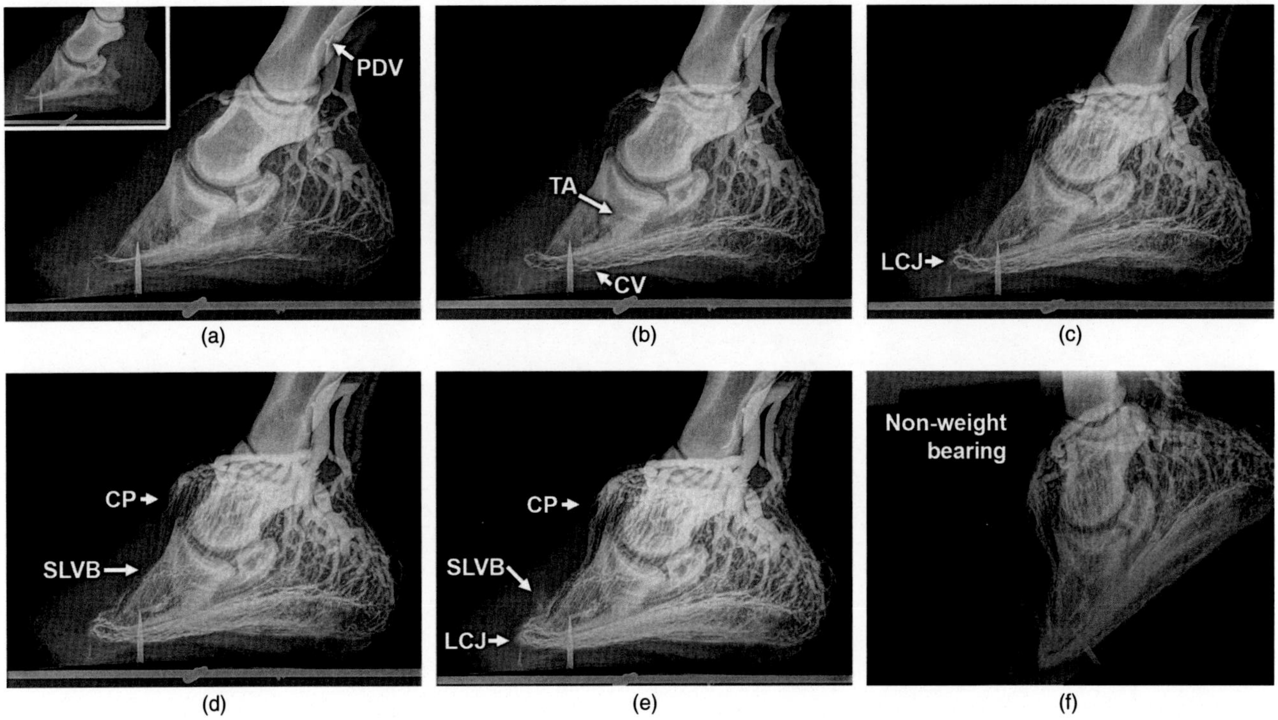

Figure 28.2 Venogram of a chronic laminitis case; the horse was relatively sound for pasture turnout and light work. These images are from a rapid sequence of radiographs taken during the injection of contrast into the palmar digital vein. This sequence demonstrates that the area with the most internal load fills last. (a) In a routine lateromedial radiograph (a, inset), the dorsal hoof wall is not parallel to the dorsal face of the DP, the distal rim of the DP has remodeled, and the sole depth is less than desirable. As contrast injected into the palmar digital vein (PDV) travels through the dorsal branch of P2 and heel, some contrast is in the terminal arch and solear dermis. (b) With continued injection, the contrast volume increases in the heel and solear dermis, and the terminal arch (TA) and solear and circumflex vessels (CV) begin to fill. (c) The coronary plexus and lamellar–circumflex junction (LCJ) then begin to fill; the PDVs are distended and the muscular-walled arteries are visible caudal to the veins. (d) Finally, contrast is present in the dorsal sublamellar vascular bed (SLVB) and coronary plexus (CP). (e) Abnormalities visible in the fully injected venogram include: discernible but short solear papillae, terminal papillae at the LCJ that are no longer parallel to the dorsal face of the DP (LCJ arrow), remodeling of the LCJ around the altered distal rim/apex of the DP, feathering of contrast into the dorsal lamellar wedge (SLVB, arrow), and narrowing and elongation of the CP arrow. (f) The non-weight-bearing venogram has a similar appearance to that in panel (e).

veterinarian injects the second syringe, she/he gently flexes the limb, releasing the tension of the deep digital flexor tendon and unloading the foot. This allows contrast to completely fill the foot. It is important to flex the limb without signaling the horse to pick up the foot. The veterinarian's medial/inside shoulder remains against the dorsal carpus as the medial arm pulls the metacarpus forward, while the lateral hand maintains the foot's position on the block. When the contrast injection is complete, the syringe and needle are removed and the injection port and catheter are quickly taped out of the way using the free end of the tourniquet tape.

Full weight-bearing lateromedial (Fig. 28.1a) and dorsopalmar (Fig. 28.1b) views are immediately taken. The veterinarian then flexes the limb and a non-weight-bearing lateromedial view is taken. Additional views may be taken if time allows, including a non-weight-bearing palmodorsal view or lateromedial images weight-bearing with the foot in different shoeing devices to aid in treatment selection (Fig. 28.2f). All images should be taken within 45 s of the injection to avoid contrast diffusion artifacts (Figs 28.3b and c). A final lateromedial view may be taken to determine if contrast has moved into pathologic areas that were compressed during the first image. When finished with radiographs, the tourniquet is removed, the catheter is removed, and both the medial and lateral palmar digital veins padded with a gauze pressure wrap for 15 min. The horse is returned to the stall to limit movement while the feet are still anesthetized.

Technique Error

If extravasation of contrast occurs during the procedure, but less than 3 ml of contrast has been injected, the tourniquet and catheter are immediately removed and digital pressure placed on the vein for 15 min. The venogram may then be performed using the opposite vein, but digital pressure is maintained on the original venipuncture site during the injection of contrast. (The assistant only removes her/his hand during radiation exposure.) Without the digital contact, the internal pressure from the added contrast will dislodge any clot and result in perivascular contrast at the original venipuncture site.

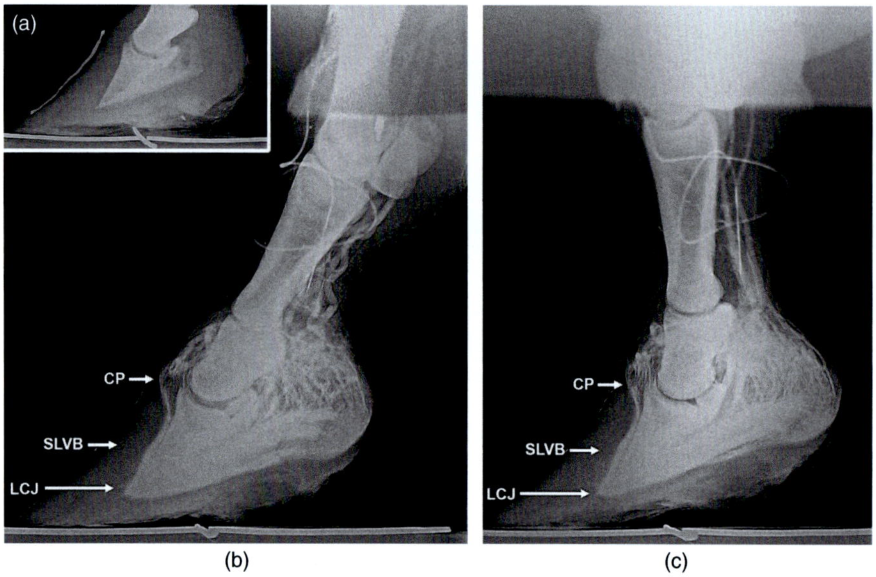

Figure 28.3 Venogram of a severely lame case of chronic laminitis case non-responsive to phenylbutazone or regional anesthesia (presented as an acute case according to the owner). An abscess was draining from the lateral coronary band bilaterally. (a, inset) The lateral radiograph confirms widening of the distal dorsal wall and remodeling of the distal apex of the DP. (b) The venogram has mild widening of the dorsal SLVB with feathering of contrast into the lamellar wedge. Contrast is present in the LCJ and CV distal to the DP. (c) There is no change in the venogram appearance when only partially bearing weight. This horse was suffering from chronic endocrinopathic laminitis unrecognized by the owner. Although the physical examination and radiographs indicated a poor prognosis, the venogram suggested the horse had a favorable prognosis for recovery. The horse made an excellent recovery with shoeing, dietary modification and treatment for endocrinopathic laminitis. The weight-bearing image demonstrates tourniquet failure. Contrast in the palmar digital veins approaches the tourniquet and is visualized proximal to the sesamoids (b). In the partial weight-bearing image (c), the palmar metacarpal arteries and veins are not within the image, however tourniquet failure would be suspected due to the palmar vascular contrast extending to the tourniquet. Both venogram images are 'fuzzy,' with loss of vessel distinction due to contrast diffusion secondary to taking the images more than 45 s after the injection of a hyperosmolar contrast diffusion.

If more than 3 ml of contrast has been injected before perivascular contrast is detected, it is not advised to switch to the other vein due to the concern that both veins may become injured ('blown'). In this scenario, radiographs are taken with no further injection of contrast to obtain any information possible while considering the inadequate contrast volume present. The venogram can be repeated in three days.

An inadequate volume of contrast reaching the foot secondary to tourniquet failure is perhaps the most common technique error. Without adequate volume, the compressed or loaded dermis does not fill. Contrast first fills the area of the foot with the least amount of load. Due to the tourniquet, contrast injected into the palmar digital vein creates a retrograde angiogram; if the tourniquet is adequate, contrast remains distal to the metacarpophalangeal joint. Veterinarians using an Esmarch tourniquet or placing the tourniquet proximal to the fetlock (many clinicians mistakenly place it in the mid-cannon bone region) commonly experience tourniquet failure. Contrast leaking proximal to the tourniquet results in inadequate contrast volume within the foot, resulting in clinicians mistakenly attributing the lack of contrast in the foot to the pathology. The hallmark of inadequate volume is that the vessels taper, gradually getting smaller and having no contrast in areas of load (Fig. 28.2b).

If contrast extends to the level of the tourniquet on venogram images, then tourniquet failure is suspected (Figs 28.3b and c). If the image area is large enough, contrast can be visualized proximal to the tourniquet. If images are time-stamped, then the clinician may compare contrast patterns and notice emptying of some vessels while contrast extends towards the fetlock in the palmar digital veins. Tourniquet failure occurs when excessive hair is not clipped from the palmar fetlock, excessive or loose tape pads the vessels beneath the tourniquet, the first wraps of the tourniquet are not tight, and when the limb is edematous. Compare the appearance of narrowed vessels secondary to inadequate contrast (Fig. 28.2) to the venogram image of distal displacement (sinker) (Fig. 28.4). The vessels are full proximal to the coronary band and in the heel, but bluntly truncated at the coronary band of the hoof capsule with minimal contrast distal to the dorsal coronet.

Interpretation

Six areas are evaluated on the venogram image (Fig. 28.1) [17–21]. The terminal arch (TA) of the palmar digital vessels is located within an osseous canal in the center of the DP. The palmar digital arteries fill retrograde from the venous injection, and are evident in the pastern due to their muscular walls. The medial and lateral vessels enter the DP between the distal impar ligament of the navicular bone and the insertion of the deep

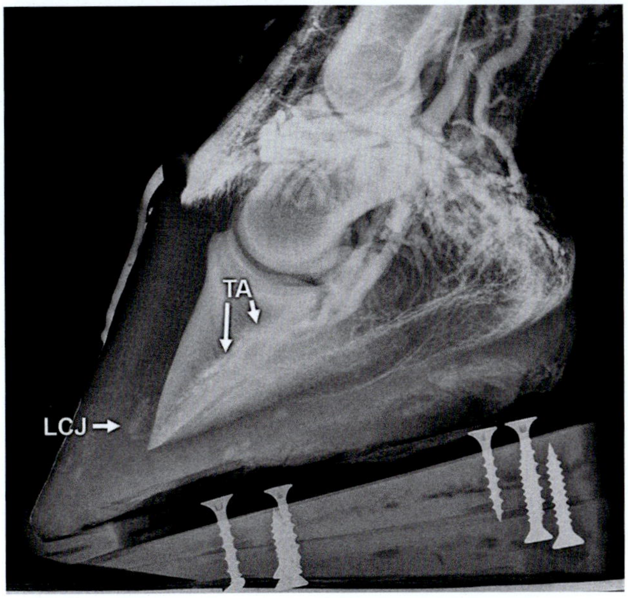

Figure 28.4 Venogram of a case of supporting limb laminitis which developed 10 days following a tendon laceration on the opposite hind limb. Although survey radiographs taken the same day have no measurable difference from those at presentation, the venogram demonstrates severe supporting limb laminitis. Vessels are bluntly truncated at the coronary band, with the exception of a small amount of contrast in the TA and heel. Contrast is absent from the CP, SLVB, CV and solear vessels. A small angle of contrast proximal and dorsal to the apex of the DP suggests displacement of the LCJ. In the pastern region a spider-web of thread-like vessels is suggestive of lymphatic distension of contrast. Post-mortem MRI confirmed changes of the lamellar dermis and identified abnormal STIR hyper-intense signaling within the DP, indicating possible bone edema/inflammation/hemorrhage. There was also an abnormal accumulation of T2 and STIR hyper-intense fluid pooling in the sole.

digital flexor tendon. Branches of the TA travel through smaller osseous canals to the parietal surface of the DP, where they anastomose with vessels of the sublamellar vascular bed (SLVB). The appearance of the TA is rarely altered, even in severe cases of laminitis. However contrast can be reduced or absent in some cases with distal displacement (sinkers) (Fig. 28.4), infarcts, and thickening of the distal aspect of the deep digital flexor tendon. Any reduction in the TA also leads to a reduction of the contribution to the lamellar bed. If the TA remains compromised, then the prognosis for survival greater than six months is guarded (Fig. 28.8). Vessels of the TA are critical for the health of the DP and the lamellar dermis.

The *heel vasculature* originates in the pastern region and supplies the digital cushion, frog, caudal/heel lamellae and coronary plexus (CP) (Figs 28.1a and 28.2a). The contrast pattern of the heel is seldom reduced in laminitis (Figs 28.2 and 28.3) [5–8], except possibly in a case of severe symmetrical distal displacement of the DP (Fig. 28.4).

Vessels of the CP originate at the level of the second phalanx (P2), proximal to the hoof capsule (Figs 28.1 and 28.2d and e). On the lateral view, the CP is proximal and dorsal to the extensor process of the DP. The rounded anterior portion reflects the concave coronary groove of the hoof capsule. Dermal coronary papillae each contain an artery and vein, and protrude into conical depressions in the coronary groove. When visible, the normal papillae are parallel to the dorsal face of the DP. The straighter posterior portion of the CP reflects the shape of distal dorsal P2 and extensor process of the DP. Contrast is not present in the center of the CP, presumably due to the pulvinus coronae [17]. On the dorsopalmar view, the medial and lateral CP can be asymmetrical due to differences in the height, shape, and internal load of the medial and lateral coronary bands (Fig. 28.1b). The appearance also varies with the dorsal-to-palmar slope of the coronary band. Occasionally, an inadequate volume of contrast creates a technique artifact (a reduction of fill within the CP and proximal SLVB) on the side opposite the catheterized vein.

When laminitis occurs, the coronary papillae become distorted (Fig. 28.5c) and may disappear. Contrast may be reduced in the distal portion of the CP and its anastomosis with the proximal dorsal SLVB (Figs 28.5a and b, 28.6a and 28.7b). As the DP displaces, the CP becomes vertically elongated and narrowed as it is compressed between the bone and proximal hoof capsule (Figs 28.2, 28.3, 28.7 and 28.8). Contrast may be reduced or absent with the vessels bluntly truncated proximal to the hoof capsule (Fig. 28.4). When chronic laminitis permanently distorts the CP, the papillae are oriented away from the face of the DP (Figs 28.5c and 28.8a) and the dorsal wall no longer grows parallel to the face of the DP (Fig. 28.7d).

The SLVB lies between the dermal/epidermal lamellar junction and the DP. In the normal foot, the SLVB is a uniform line located within 4 mm of the parietal surface of the DP (Fig. 28.1). The SLVB joins proximally with the CP, centrally with vessels contributed from the TA, and distally with the circumflex vessels (CVs) (Fig. 28.2d). The SLVB may widen and become distorted as the dermal and epidermal lamellae separate, rendering the smaller lamellar vessels more evident on the venogram image (Figs 28.5, 28.6b and 28.7). If widespread uniform lamellar separation occurs, as in symmetrical distal displacement, then the SLVB appears as a uniform rectangular 'pool' of contrast on both the lateral and dorsopalmar views (Fig. 28.5). When rotational displacement occurs, the SLVB may appear triangular. Alternatively, regardless of the type of displacement, the SLVB may be compressed and completely void of contrast (Fig. 28.4). The SLVB compression may possibly be due to any of the following: displacement of the DP trapping the dermis between the bone and hoof capsule, damage to the vessels secondary to displacement, and sublamellar edema.

In cases when the distal aspect of the DP has displaced away from the hoof capsule, a thin line of contrast may be evident at the original interface of the dermal/epidermal lamellae. In chronic cases, the line may still be apparent, but there are also 'whisps' of contrast that extend through the lamellae wedge (Figs 28.2d and e, 28.3, and 28.8a).

The CVs are located distal and peripheral to the palmar rim of the DP (Fig. 28.1). No vascular canals from the TA penetrate

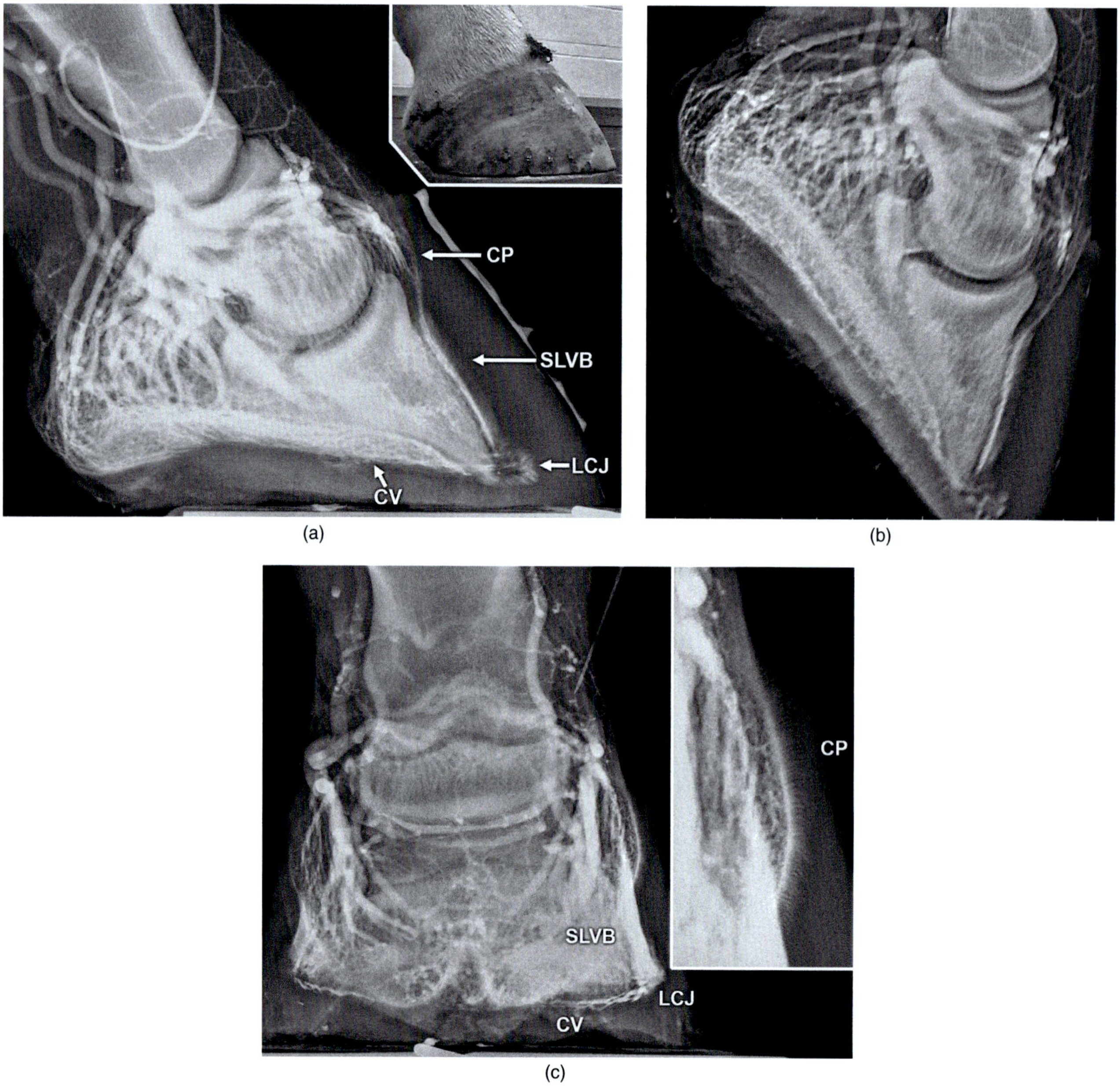

Figure 28.5 Venogram of a case of symmetrical distal displacement (five-day duration). Yellow fluid drainage is present at the dorsal coronet (inset.) In the weight-bearing image (a), the CP is narrowed and elongated, the palmar digital veins are narrowed within the DP (normal in diameter to the point they enter the canal of the terminal arch), the dorsal SLVB is uniformly widened, and the LCJ is folded and located proximal to the apex of the DP. The terminal papillae are not parallel to the dorsal face of the DP, contrast is absent distal to the apex of the DP, and there are no solear papillae in the CV. (b) The contrast pattern does not change when the foot is non-weight-bearing. (c) On the dorsopalmar view, contrast is absent from the CV at the midline, the medial and lateral SLVB are uniformly widened, and the coronary papillae of the lateral CP are oriented in a horizontal direction (inset).

the solear surface of the DP; branches from the CVs are solely responsible for maintaining the solear dermis and the solear papillae distal to the DP. This area is particularly vulnerable to compression by displacement of the DP. Of particular interest on the venogram is the lamellar–circumflex junction (LCJ) (Fig. 28.1). The LCJ mirrors the angle of the dorsodistal tip of the DP, and is the origin of the *terminal papillae* which form the white line. Both, the solear and terminal papillae are parallel to the dorsal face of the DP. On a foot with a sole depth of 20 mm, the CVs are 5 mm distal to the distal rim of the DP, and the solear papillae extend another 5 mm. (The dermis occupies 4–7 mm of space distal to the apex of the DP, and the cornified sole extends another 5–10 mm distally; Fig. 28.1a, see also Fig. 28.3b). A sound but less desirable foot may have ≤10 mm of sole depth, with the CVs only 3–4 mm distal to the DP and no solear papillae evident on the venogram. Sound horses have a large variation in the normal appearance of the CVs and sole, depending on the depth of the sole and any remodeling of the

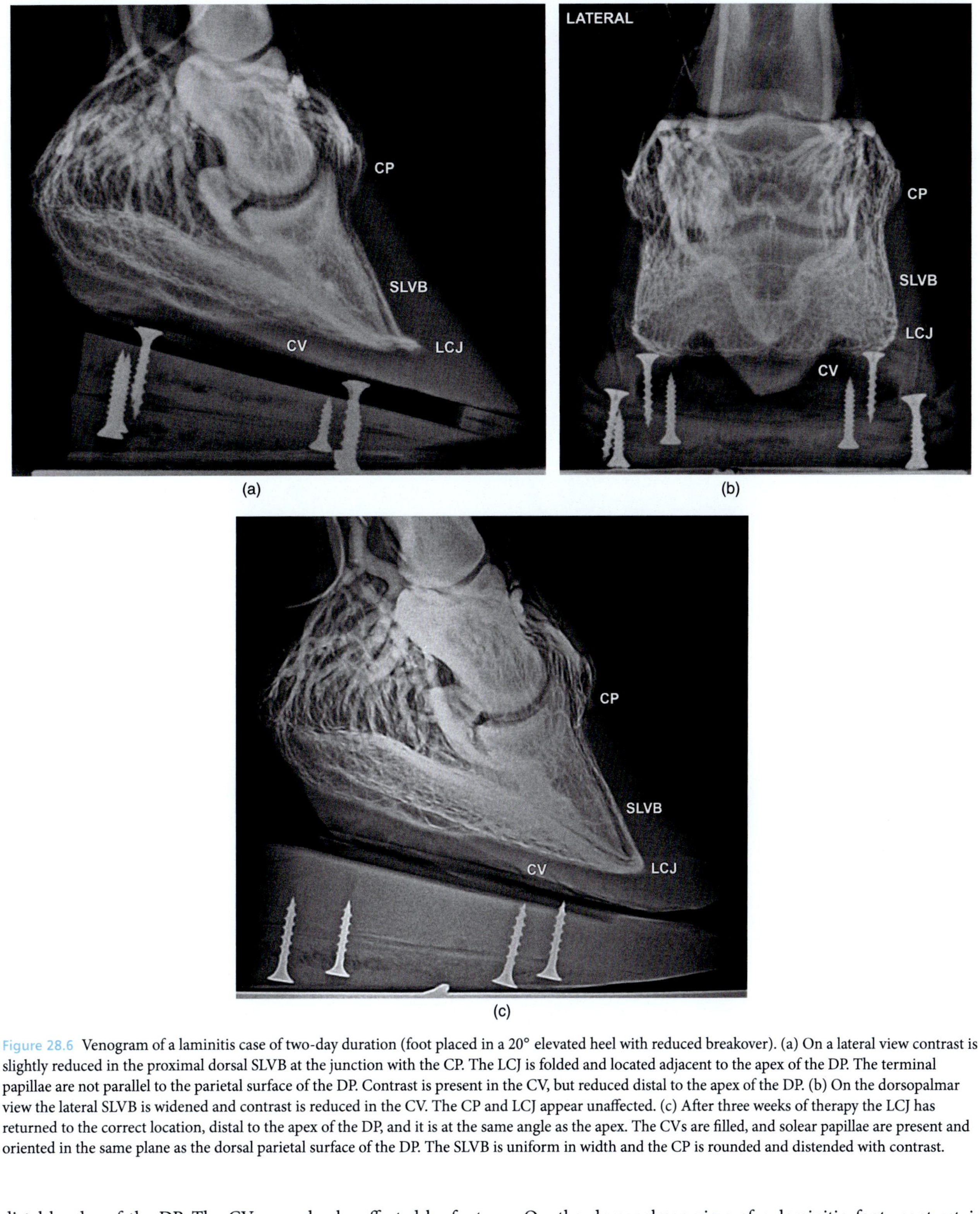

Figure 28.6 Venogram of a laminitis case of two-day duration (foot placed in a 20° elevated heel with reduced breakover). (a) On a lateral view contrast is slightly reduced in the proximal dorsal SLVB at the junction with the CP. The LCJ is folded and located adjacent to the apex of the DP. The terminal papillae are not parallel to the parietal surface of the DP. Contrast is present in the CV, but reduced distal to the apex of the DP. (b) On the dorsopalmar view the lateral SLVB is widened and contrast is reduced in the CV. The CP and LCJ appear unaffected. (c) After three weeks of therapy the LCJ has returned to the correct location, distal to the apex of the DP, and it is at the same angle as the apex. The CVs are filled, and solear papillae are present and oriented in the same plane as the dorsal parietal surface of the DP. The SLVB is uniform in width and the CP is rounded and distended with contrast.

distal border of the DP. The CV may also be affected by foot abnormalities other than laminitis; the CVs can also be compressed distal to the apex of the DP in the club foot (Figs. 28.1c and d), or distal to the wings of the DP in the negative palmar angle foot (Figs. 28.1e and f).

On the dorsopalmar view of a laminitic foot, contrast is often reduced or absent from the CVs at midline (Figs 28.5c and 28.6b). This may extend axially/abaxially depending on the degree of damage. The contrast pattern is often asymmetric due to differences in internal load within the foot. The LCJ may also

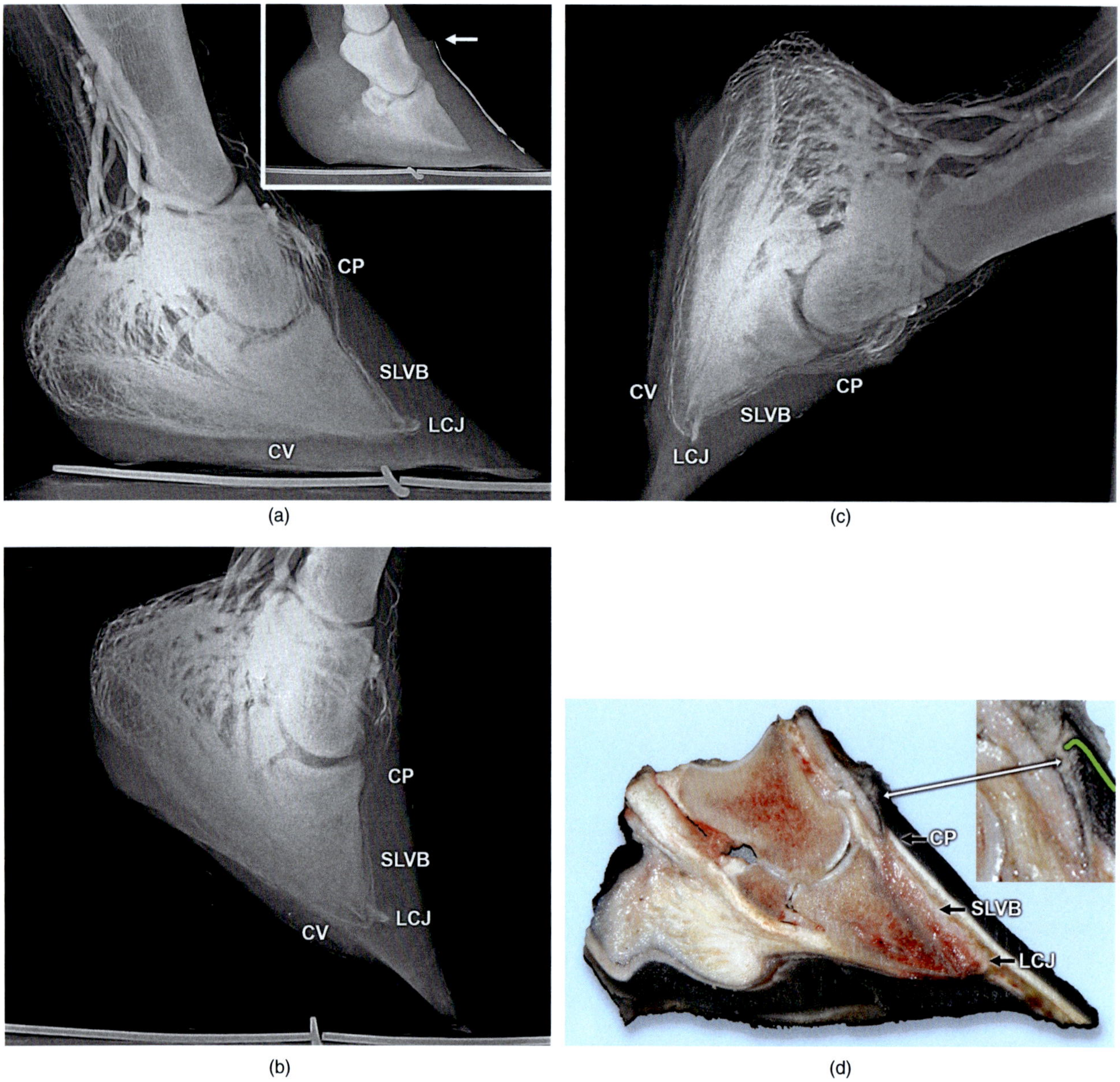

Figure 28.7 Venogram of a five-year-old Saddlebred with four-day duration of lameness following limb edema treated by an injection of dexamethasone. The lameness almost resolved (whilst feet bandaged and treated with oral antiinflammatories) and at the time of examination all four feet could easily be picked up and held. Digital pulses were unremarkable. (a) The axial border of the coronary band could be palpated, and a 'sinker halo' was evident on radiographs (arrow, inset). Note that conclusions about laminitis cannot be drawn from the increased width of the dorsal hoof wall. Note that on the lateral venogram at full weight-bearing (a), papillae are not evident at the CP or CV, the CP is elongated, the SLVB widened, the LCJ is located proximal to the apex of the DP, and the CV and solear vessels are compressed distal to the anterior half of the DP. (b) With only mild weight-bearing (toe touching), the CP is compressed and the LCJ is located proximal to the apex of the DP. Contrast has returned to the CV and solear vessels. (c) At non-weight-bearing, the majority of venous compression is eliminated, the coronary and solear papillae are not evident, the CP is elongated, and the LCJ remains folded. (d) On sagittal section at post-mortem examination two weeks later after further deterioration, tubular growth at the CP is inappropriate (in a direction perpendicular to the dorsal face of the DP), and increased width of the dorsal lamellar dermis (SLVB) and compression of the solear dermis is also apparent. The LCJ is proximal to the apex of the DP.

appear folded on the dorsopalmar view. This may be difficult to discern at midline because the vessels are overshadowed by the solear margin of the DP.

On the lateral venogram with early disease, the solear papillae are initially disoriented (no longer parallel to the dorsal surface of the DP) and then absent distal to the DP. The terminal papillae also become disoriented as the LCJ develops a folded appearance (Figs 28.5a, 28.6a, and 28.7). If disease progresses, contrast in the CVs and sole is reduced and then eliminated distal to the apex of the DP (Figs 28.6–28.8). Compression of the

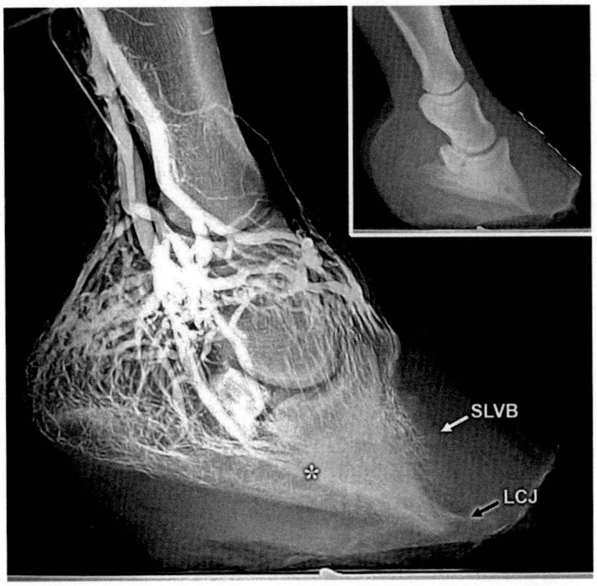

(a)

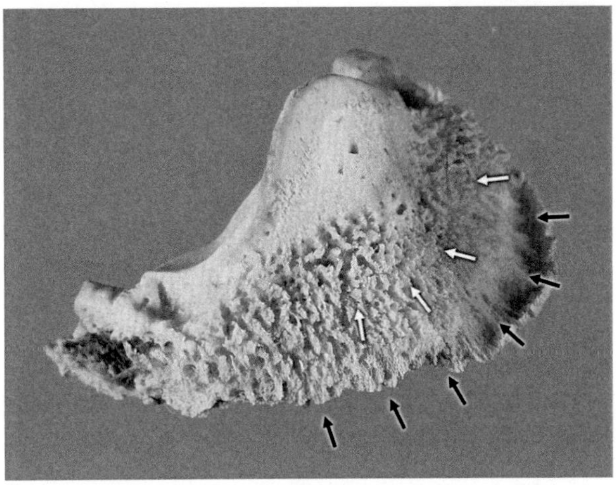

(b)

Figure 28.8 Radiograph/venogram of the DP of laminitic horse euthanized at five months after onset of symmetrical distal displacement. Increased heel growth, lack of sole growth or cornification, and deterioration of radiographic parameters indicated a need for euthanasia. (a, inset) Bone modeling included widening of the osseous canal of the terminal arch and loss of density at the distal apex with dorsal and palmar modeling. (a) The venogram demonstrates a lack of contrast in the TA (*) and CV, as well as widening of the SLVB (white arrow). The LCJ remains proximal to the remaining apex of the DP (black arrow). (b) On post-mortem examination of the DP, the distal margin of the DP has resorbed on the lateral aspect. Medially, the distal margin was 'curled' proximally with a flattened area on the parietal surface at the level of the LCJ (presumably associated with the continued growth of the terminal papillae in an inappropriate direction.) The parietal surface is irregular from bony modeling.

CVs and solear vessels may extend from the apex to the wings of the DP (Fig. 28.4). If treatment is successful, the CVs are restored on the venogram and measurable increases in sole depth begin to occur. Sole papillae again become evident on venogram (Fig. 28.6c), which is associated with improved sole growth.

In more severe cases of laminitis, the LCJ is displaced proximal to the apex of the DP (Figs 28.4, 28.5, 28.7, and 28.8); this may occur prior to radiographically measurable displacement of the DP (Fig. 28.4). The terminal papillae become oriented almost perpendicular to the dorsal face of the DP. If treatment is not successful, the papillae continue to produce epidermis but it is in an inappropriate direction. Over time, the new horn growth contributes to compression of the dermis and distal dorsal edge of the apex of the DP (Fig. 28.8).

Comparing the loaded and unloaded lateral views gives information regarding the degree of lamellar instability (Figs 28.2, 28.3, 28.5, and 28.7). Areas may have venous compression only when bearing weight in the patient with lamellar instability (Fig. 28.7). These cases may be more receptive to therapies aimed at reducing forces on the diseased tissues. The absence of contrast in both weight-bearing and non-weight-bearing views suggests that the dermal pathology is more significant (Fig. 28.5), and in the present author's experience, these cases are more difficult to treat. The extent of the void of contrast is also important; the horse which has a venogram similar to that exhibited in Figure 28.4 has a much smaller chance of survival than any of the other case examples.

The unloaded view is also helpful with chronic laminitis cases that are not responding to shoeing treatment (Fig. 28.2). Cases with lamellar instability often have compression of the sole when bearing weight, but the pattern improves when the venogram is taken when non-weight-bearing. Demonstrating the degree of instability helps to design shoeing application or indicates the need for surgical intervention.

When using venograms to monitor progress or deterioration, and to guide treatment strategies, the first four weeks of a case are particularly critical as this is the major window of opportunity to avert bone damage and halt collapse of the dermis. For a laminitic patient to return to use, they must have measurable improvement both on the venogram and in terms of sole growth within the first two to three weeks of onset. The majority of the present author's cases that return to soundness have restoration of a near-normal venogram pattern within four weeks of onset of laminitis (Fig. 28.6). (This includes cases treated conservatively with shoeing, and shoeing in conjunction with a deep digital flexor tenotomy.) Critical venographic changes indicative of a response to treatment include restoration of the CVs and solear vessels and the re-establishment of a normal orientation of the LCJ as quickly as possible (before irreversible damage occurs to the distal rim of the DP) (Fig. 28.8).

Venograms may be particularly useful when treating endocrinopathic cases of laminitis. These cases are frustrating when trying to determine progress, or differentiate the lack of progress versus an acute exacerbation of disease (Fig. 28.3). The venogram may also be useful when deciding whether to continue therapy or euthanize a laminitis patient.

The timing of additional venograms varies between cases. In a high-risk case, such as that seen with sepsis-related laminitis where the animal's condition may rapidly deteriorate, the venogram may be repeated every three days. More often, the present author repeats venograms weekly and expects measurable improvement.

As improvement will likely be slower in cases where treatment is initiated more than one week after the onset of laminitis, expectations should be lower; however, the foot must still show improvement if the animal is to survive. In this scenario, venograms would more likely be repeated on a two-weekly basis, unless the case appears to deteriorate.

Finally, in the case at risk of supporting/contralateral limb laminitis, the present author begins venograms on day 3 after the initial injury, and often repeats them weekly as cases are difficult to predict [22–24]. Venogram changes may begin mildly with compression of the solear papillae and/or circumflex and solear vessels, and then progress to distortion of the lamellar–circumflex junction. However, the initial findings may be much worse. Figure 28.4 shows a case of supporting limb laminitis 10 days after a tendon injury on the contralateral limb. The horse was euthanized and a magnetic resonance imaging scan performed (A. Rucker, J. Kramer, R. Griffin, and A. McKnight, unpublished data). Dermal pathology was confirmed as well as fluid signaling within the dermis and bone. Cases at risk of SLL are usually only monitored for clinical 'soundness' in the supporting limb, and often appear 'stable' with no measurable radiographic displacement for four to six weeks after the initial injury. At that point, there is usually recognition of rapidly progressing catastrophic supporting limb laminitis. By monitoring with serial radiographs and venograms, changes indicative of laminitis may be identified much earlier and intervention initiated prior to catastrophic breakdown of lamellar support.

Categorization of Severity of Disease Using Venograms

A laminitis case that is recognized within hours of onset of clinical signs and treated appropriately may return to use without radiographically recognizable changes of a previous disease (Fig. 28.6) (though this depends on the control of any underlying disease or risk factors). In the present author's experience, cases with mild compression of the solear vessels and mild folding of the LCJ have a good prognosis.

Cases with: (i) displacement of the apex of the DP distal to the LCJ; (ii) alterations in the CP and SLVB; and (iii) more extensive compression of the circumflex and solear vessels may respond to conservative treatment (shoeing) if presented within the first 48 h of clinical signs. However, the present author often recommends shoeing with deep digital flexor tenotomies if these cases do not respond to conservative shoeing, or if they present several days to weeks after the onset of laminitis.

In the present author's experience, treatment of distal displacement (versus rotational displacement) cases is more difficult to treat (than rotation of the DP) if the goal is return to athletic function. It is possible that, while 'sinkers' involve disruption of the dermal/epidermal lamellae (as described in detail by Pollitt and others), the most severe cases may also have a lymphatic component (Figs 28.4 and 28.5) [25,26]. Lymphatic vessels parallel the arteries and veins within the dermis of the foot. Lymphatic stasis, as well as increased pressures within the foot, could explain the compression of the vessels both within the dermis and within the terminal arch and osseous canals of the DP (as well as the lack of restoration of contrast in the non-weight-bearing images) (A. Rucker *et al.*, unpublished data). Furthermore, this increase in lymphatic pressure could contribute both to dermal pathology and also extensive bone pathology, as described by Engiles and colleagues [27,28]. This could help to explain why some sinkers are so refractory to pain control, do not respond to treatment, and have profound remodeling not just of the distal rim of the DP but also within the entire bone (Fig. 28.8).

Summary

The digital venogram documents both venous compression and dermal changes resulting from lamellar instability. It is an inexpensive, noninvasive, stall-side procedure that summarizes dermal pathology and, when combined with the history, physical examination, and radiographs, sequential venograms also aid in treatment decisions. Progress may be visualized and areas that require alternative treatment pinpointed. The majority of laminitis cases encountered by the present author have mild damage at the start of the development of clinically apparent disease. For the present author, the venogram is key to: (i) diagnosing laminitis within 24 h of the development of clinical signs; and (ii) guiding treatment. With cases that have moderate and severe damage, the venogram also guides treatment and forecasts success. Alternatively, the venogram details why treatment is not working and when euthanasia is the best treatment option.

Acknowledgments

This chapter was made possible due to collaboration on cases with the following colleagues: Dr Dick Griffin, Dr Grant Johnson, Dr Joanne Kramer DACVS, Dr Alexia McKnight DACVR, Dr Sammy Pittman, Dr. Shannon Reed DACVS, Dr Ric Redden, Dr Brad Root, Dr Roger Shaw, and Howard Wilson. As these friends will attest, any errors in the case presentations are mine alone.

References

1. Redden, R.F. (2001) A technique for performing digital venography in the standing horse. *Equine Vet. Educ.*, **3** (3), 172–178.
2. Redden, R.F. (2001) Possible therapeutic value of digital venography in two laminitic horses. *Equine Vet. Educ.*, **13** (3), 128–134.
3. Rucker, A., Redden, R.F., Arthur, E.G., *et al.* (2006) How to perform the digital venogram. Proceedings of the American Association of

Equine Practitioners, 2–6 December, San Antonio, Texas, vol. **52**, pp. 526–530.
4. Rucker, A. (2007) The digital venogram, in *Equine Podiatry* (eds A.D. Floyd and R.A. Mansmann), Saunders, St Louis, Missouri, pp. 328–346.
5. Rucker, A. and Orsini, J.A. (2014) Laminitis, in *Equine Emergencies: Treatment and Procedures*, 4th edition (eds J.A. Orsini and T.J. Divers), Elsevier-Saunders, St. Louis, Missouri, pp. 697–712.
6. Bowker, R.M. (2003) The growth and adaptive capabilities of the hoof wall and sole: functional changes in response to stress. Proceedings of the American Association of Equine Practitioners, 21–25 November, New Orleans, Louisiana, vol. **49**, pp. 146–168.
7. Bowker, R.M. (2003) Contrasting structural morphologies of 'good' and 'bad' footed horses. Proceedings of the American Association of Equine Practitioners, 21–25 November, New Orleans, Louisiana, vol. **49**, pp. 186–209.
8. Baldwin, G.I. and Pollitt, C.C. (2010) Progression of venographic changes after experimentally induced laminitis. *Vet. Clin. North Am.*, **26** (1), 135–140.
9. D'Arpe, L. and Bernardini, D. (2010) Digital venography in horses and its clinical application in Europe. *Vet. Clin. North Am.*, **26** (2), 339–359.
10. Eastman, S., Redden, R.F., and Williams, C.A. (2012) Venograms for use in laminitis treatment. *J. Equine Vet. Sci.*, **32** (11), 755–759.
11. Floyd, A.D. (2007) An approach to the treatment of the laminitic horse, in *Equine Podiatry* (eds A.D. Floyd and R.A. Mansmann), Saunders, St Louis, Missouri, pp. 347–358.
12. Hunt, R.J. and Wharton, R.E. (2010) Clinical presentation, diagnosis, and prognosis of chronic laminitis in North America. *Vet. Clin. North Am.*, **26** (1), 141–154.
13. Lyle, B.E. (2007) Venography as a tool for guiding surgery to the foot, in *Equine Podiatry* (eds A.D. Floyd and R.A. Mansmann), Saunders, St Louis, Missouri, pp. 284–293.
14. Redden, R.F. (2009) Using venograms in laminitic cases. Proceedings of Dr. Redden's In-Depth Podiatry Symposium, 16–18 January, Versailles, Kentucky, pp. 46–55.
15. Rucker, A. (2010) Clinical applications of digital venography. *J. Equine Vet. Sci.*, **30** (9), 491–503.
16. Rucker, A. (2010) Equine venography and its clinical application in North America. *Vet. Clin. North Am.*, **26** (1), 167–178.
17. Denoix, J.M. (2000) The equine foot, in *The Equine Distal Limb.* Iowa State University Press, Ames, Iowa, pp. 1–99.
18. Barone, R. (1996) *Anatomie compare des mammiferes domestiques.* Vol. 5, Angiologie. Vigot, Paris, pp. 264–271.
19. Pollitt, C.C. (1995) *Color Atlas of the Horse's Foot.* Mosby, London, pp. 10–39.
20. Pollitt, C.C. (2010) The anatomy and physiology of the suspensory apparatus of the distal phalanx. *Vet. Clin. North Am.*, **26** (1), 29–49.
21. Schummer, A., Wilkens, H., Vollmerhaus, B., *et al.* (1981) The circulatory system, the skin, and the cutaneous organs of the domestic mammals, in *The Anatomy of Domestic Animals*, Verlag Paul Parey, Berlin, pp. 540–557.
22. Orsini, J.A. (2012) Supporting limb laminitis: The four important 'whys'. *Equine Vet. J.*, **44** (6), 741–745.
23. Redden, R.F. (2004) Preventing laminitis in the contralateral limb of horses with nonweight-bearing lameness. *Clin. Tech. Equine Pract.*, **3** (1), 57–63.
24. Van Eps, A.W., Collins, S.N., and Pollitt, C.C. (2010) Supporting limb laminitis. *Vet. Clin. North Am.*, **26** (2), 287–302.
25. Walsh, D.M., Collins, S.N., Winterford, C., *et al.* (2013) The equine foot lamellar lymphatic system. *J. Equine Vet. Sci.*, **33** (13), 847–859.
26. Pollitt, C.C. and Collins, S.N. (2013) The suspensory apparatus of the distal phalanx (SADP). *J. Equine Vet. Sci.*, **33** (13), 874–876.
27. Engiles, J.B. (2010) Pathology of the distal phalanx in equine laminitis: more than just skin deep. *Vet. Clin. North Am.*, **26** (1), 155–165.
28. Engiles, J.B., Galantino-Homer, H., Boston, R.C., *et al.* (2013) Significant osteolysis in the equine distal phalanx associated with the development and progression of laminitis. Proceedings of the American Association of Equine Practitioners, 7–11 December, Nashville, Tennessee, vol. **59**, pp. 195–196.

CHAPTER 29

Endocrine and Metabolic Evaluation in Horses with Laminitis

Ramiro E. Toribio and Teresa A. Burns

Introduction

The clinical diagnosis of laminitis can be simple in horses with acute lamellar pain as well as in those with evidence of chronic lamellar disease. However, metabolic and endocrine conditions, notably pituitary pars intermedia dysfunction (PPID) and equine metabolic syndrome (EMS, obesity-associated laminitis), can lead to clinical or subclinical laminitis that may be more difficult to detect (endocrinopathic laminitis). These two conditions are associated with most cases of endocrinopathic laminitis, of which EMS accounts for the most [1]. Although there was originally a concern that hypothyroidism may play a role in endocrinopathic laminitis, a direct association between hypothyroidism and laminitis remains to be documented in the horse. However, measurements of other endocrine and metabolic factors can provide valuable information for the diagnosis, treatment, prognosis, and prevention of endocrinopathic laminitis. As there are no specific blood tests for equine lamellar disease, testing is directed toward the diagnosis of diseases known to be associated with laminitis (e.g., PPID, EMS). Hematology and serum chemistry have limited value in the diagnosis of laminitis, but they can provide valuable information on the metabolic and immune status of the animal that is prone to or currently affected by laminitis. In this chapter, attention is focused on endocrine and metabolic diagnostic methods for the evaluation of PPID, EMS, and hypothyroidism. The pathogenesis of endocrinopathic laminitis – an understanding of which is necessary for proper data interpretation – is covered elsewhere in this book.

Testing for Pituitary Pars Intermedia Dysfunction (Equine Cushing's Syndrome)

Advanced PPID can frequently be diagnosed on the basis of clinical signs alone; these cases are commonly not a diagnostic challenge (see Chapters 16 and 37 for more information on PPID). The presence of hypertrichosis (formerly referred to as hirsutism) is considered pathognomonic for PPID, especially in older horses (>15 years of age). In one study, this finding had 71% sensitivity, 95% specificity, 91% positive predictive value, and 84% negative predictive value for diagnosing the disease where a definitive diagnosis was based on post-mortem examination findings [2]. The clinical presentation of PPID in younger horses (or those in early stages of the disease) is more variable, and diagnosis of these cases is more challenging. Methods for the laboratory evaluation of PPID have included measurement of resting serum or plasma cortisol, adrenocorticotrophic hormone (ACTH), alpha-melanocyte-stimulating hormone (α-MSH), glucose, and insulin concentrations. Dynamic testing includes the ACTH stimulation test, the dexamethasone suppression test (DST), the thyrotropin-releasing hormone (TRH)-stimulation test, and the combined DST/TRH-stimulation test. Other methods that have been evaluated include the domperidone response test, salivary cortisol concentrations, and the urinary corticoid:creatinine ratio [3–5]. Before testing, it is important to know about the patient's management conditions, diet, medication history, and degree of physiologic stress (as far as it can be known) which could potentially influence the results. Another critical factor is the season, as the secretory activity of the equine pars intermedia varies throughout the year, with highest output noted during the autumn months in the northern hemisphere [6–8].

Hematology, serum biochemistry, and urinalysis can be informative regarding the immune, endocrine, and metabolic status of horses with PPID. Although many horses with PPID have normal hemograms and serum biochemistry profiles, abnormalities commonly associated with the condition include anemia, neutrophilia, lymphopenia, eosinopenia, hyperglycemia, hypertriglyceridemia (hyperlipemia), increased hepatic enzyme activities, and glucosuria [9]. Hyperglycemia is a frequent but not consistent finding in horses with PPID; it is speculated that this increase in glucose concentration is a consequence of cortisol-mediated systemic insulin resistance (IR; commonly termed insulin dysregulation [ID]). However, it is possible that other endocrine factors (e.g., ACTH, α-MSH, leptin, ghrelin,

Equine Laminitis, First Edition. Edited by James K. Belknap and Raymond Geor.

growth hormone [GH], insulin-like growth factor 1 [IGF-1]) in some way contribute to energy dysregulation in affected animals. Hypertriglyceridemia may be noted and is reportedly more frequent in ponies than in horses [5, 10]. Severe hypertriglyceridemia secondary to endocrinopathies is often associated with IR in horses and ponies, but can resolve with appropriate therapy [11].

Dexamethasone Suppression Test (DST)

The DST has historically been the most widely used method in the diagnosis of equine PPID [12–15]. The rationale behind this test is that in horses with PPID, ACTH and (subsequently) cortisol secretion are not suppressed by exogenously administered dexamethasone because ACTH in these animals is mainly produced by melanotropes of the *pars intermedia*; these cells are not subject to glucocorticoid negative feedback [12]. In healthy horses, ACTH is primarily secreted by the corticotropes of the *pars distalis*, which are suppressed by glucocorticoids.

> Protocol: Collect baseline blood sample (4–6 p.m.) and administer dexamethasone (40 μg kg^{-1}, intramuscular). Collect a second blood sample 19 h later (∼12 p.m.). In horses with an intact hypothalamic-pituitary-adrenal axis (HPAA) it is expected that serum cortisol concentrations will be below 1 μg dl^{-1} (27.6 nmol l^{-1}) after 19 h, while horses with PPID will have minimal cortisol suppression. This test is simple, inexpensive, and continues to be well accepted by equine practitioners; however, seasonally adjusted reference ranges for interpretation are not available for this test, and false-positive tests may occur if animals are tested in autumn.

Clinicians should be aware that false-positive and false-negative results occur with the DST. False positives (20–40%) are common when testing is done in the fall [8], while false-negatives may occur early in the disease process. For horses with clinical evidence of PPID and a non-diagnostic DST, it is recommended to repeat testing four to six months later, or to consider other tests. In regard to steroid-induced laminitis, while some authors have suggested an association between short-acting glucocorticoids and laminitis [16], it should be emphasized that no controlled study has demonstrated this to be the case [17]. The DST did not induce or worsen the signs of laminitis in 66 horses with evidence of PPID [12]. Many theoretical explanations exist as to why horses may develop laminitis after glucocorticoid exposure [18, 19]. It has been proposed that impaired glucose metabolism may be responsible for steroid-induced laminitis, in particular with triamcinolone [20]. Despite this lack of objective information (including the lack of an experimental model for the induction of corticosteroid-associated laminitis), disclosure of risk to clients (however small it may be) is important because using glucocorticoids in horses at risk of developing laminitis could have legal implications [21]. Of interest, a recent study evaluating medical records from a large number of horses found no association between triamcinolone administration and the risk of developing laminitis [22]. If the veterinarian or the client is worried about the DST, other methods (e.g., resting ACTH concentration, TRH-stimulation test) are available. The DST is being gradually replaced by other methods (e.g., resting ACTH concentration, TRH-stimulation test) that are more time-efficient and accurate than the DST in reaching a diagnosis of PPID (see Fig. 29.1).

Resting ACTH Concentrations

Horses with PPID have excessive secretion of POMC-derived peptides, including ACTH and α-MSH [23–28]. Resting ACTH concentration *per se* is a good screening test for the diagnosis of PPID, although the clinician should be aware that values may fall within the reference range in early disease. In one study using the DST as the 'gold standard,' resting ACTH concentrations had a sensitivity of 91% in horses and 82% in ponies, and a specificity of 100% [23]. Other publications have reported lower and higher sensitivities and specificities for this test [29–33]. Similar to cortisol, ACTH concentrations can be increased by stress and glycemia. A resting ACTH level >58 pg ml^{-1} had a sensitivity of 83% and a specificity of 79% to predict future laminitic episodes in one study in ponies [34].

In the northern hemisphere, ACTH concentrations in healthy horses are higher in the late summer and fall than in spring months [8], and, recently, seasonally adjusted reference ranges have been established for this test. In fall months (August to October), most healthy ponies and horses have ACTH concentrations below 100 pg ml^{-1} (∼22 pmol l^{-1}), while in non-fall months ACTH concentrations are <35 pg ml (∼7.7 pmol l^{-1}) [8, 35]. Different cut-off values have been reported for resting ACTH concentrations depending on the specific immunoassay used, but the consensus is that, for the period November through July, concentrations >35 pg ml^{-1} measured using the immunochemiluminescent assay are diagnostic for PPID [8, 30–33, 35]. For the period August to October (and likely the analogous months for late summer/autumn in the Southern hemisphere), an ACTH concentration >100 pg ml^{-1} is strongly indicative of PPID, while values between 50 and 100 pg ml^{-1} are considered suspicious and justify repeat evaluation three to six months later. McGowan *et al.* showed that resting ACTH and α-MSH concentrations have better sensitivity and specificity for the diagnosis of PPID during the fall when compared to other times of the year, and it has therefore been recommended that testing via these modalities should be ideally performed at this time of the year [33]. Feeding also affects baseline and stimulated ACTH concentrations – fed horses have higher resting and post-TRH stimulation ACTH concentrations than non-fed horses [36]. However, no influence of the time of the day on baseline or stimulated ACTH concentrations was found [36].

To perform this test, blood should be collected in EDTA-containing tubes (preferably plastic tubes), kept on ice for shipping, or centrifuged and the plasma separated and frozen until

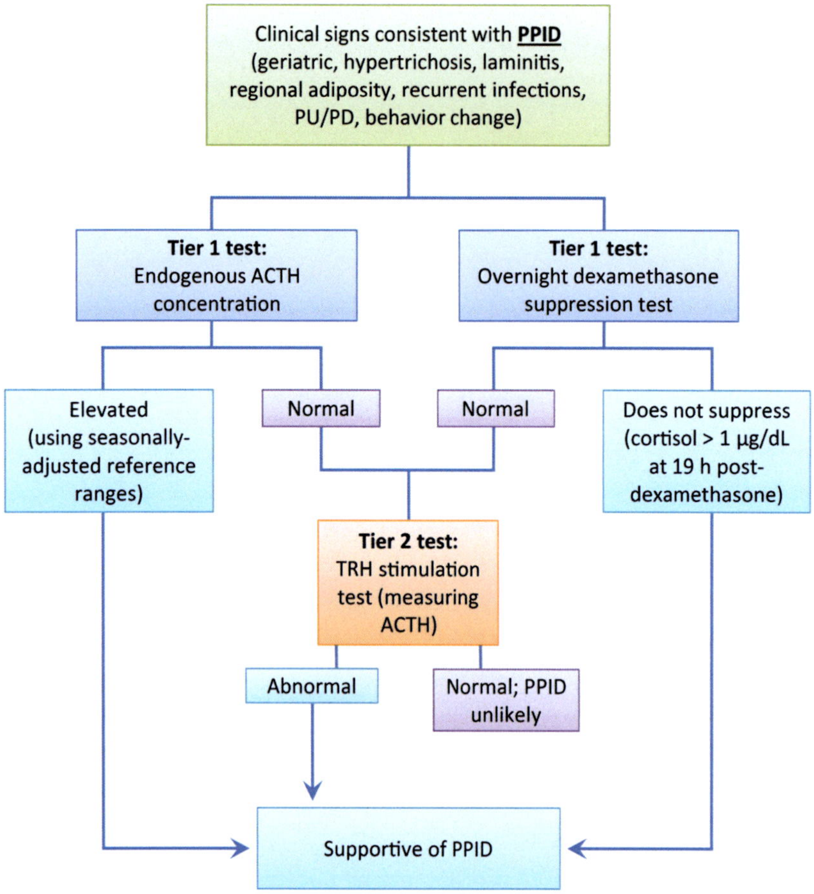

Figure 29.1 Schematic for the diagnosis of pituitary pars intermedia dysfunction (PPID) in horses.

analyzed [23,37]. When collected in plastic EDTA tubes, equine ACTH is stable for 8 h in whole blood [37, 38], and longer if the plasma is separated and frozen promptly [38]. Freezing and thawing have minimal effects on ACTH concentrations [37]. ACTH concentrations tend to be lower in samples collected in glass tubes, but this difference is minimal [37]; overall, equine ACTH is more stable than previously believed. When resting ACTH concentrations are higher than the upper reference limit (taking into consideration confounding factors [season, stress]), there does not appear to be any additional benefit of performing other more complex tests to establish a diagnosis of PPID (e.g., TRH stimulation see Fig. 29.1) [32].

TRH-Stimulation Test

The TRH-stimulation test was developed under the rationale that TRH administration to horses with PPID will result in a higher cortisol secretion when compared to healthy horses [39]. This effect of TRH appears to be indirect from the release of POMC-derived peptides (ACTH and α-MSH) by hyperplastic melanotropes in the pars intermedia [30, 32, 40, 41]. TRH increases the secretion of α-MSH and ACTH in healthy horses and horses with PPID [31,32,40], but concentrations are greater and more prolonged in horses with PPID [32]. Moreover, the percentage increase in secretion in horses with PPID is greater for α-MSH than for ACTH [32], and α-MSH concentrations remain elevated longer [32]. In healthy horses, ACTH and α-MSH release following TRH administration exhibits seasonal variation, with higher values measured in summer and fall months compared to winter months [41]. ACTH and cortisol concentrations are disassociated in horses with PPID [30], and measuring ACTH concentrations after TRH administration appears to be more diagnostically accurate than measuring post-TRH cortisol in differentiating normal horses from those with PPID [30]. For example, in horses with PPID, TRH (1 mg, intravenous) induced an approximately 10-fold increase in ACTH concentrations at 4–14 min post-administration, while in healthy horses the increase was about twofold [30–32]. The increase in cortisol concentration at 14 and 30 min was minimal in both PPID and healthy horses [30]. A similar response to what is observed with ACTH is also seen with α-MSH when measured post-TRH, but there is no evidence that α-MSH is superior to ACTH if measurements are made within 30 min of TRH administration [32]. A labeled TRH solution for equine use is not readily available to the equine practitioner; however, chemical-grade TRH powder can be purchased from a number of companies,[a,b] diluted in saline solution, filter-sterilized,

[a] TRH, Sigma-Aldrich Co., St Louis, MO.
[b] TRH, Phoenix Pharmaceutical, Burlingame, CA.

and frozen in 1 mg aliquots until used. Veterinary compounding pharmacies are also offering TRH as an injectable solution.[c]

Protocol: Collect baseline blood sample (EDTA tubes), administer TRH (1 mg, intravenous), and take additional blood samples at 10 and 30 min. In horses with PPID, it is expected that ACTH concentrations will be more than fourfold higher than baseline at 10–30 min, while cortisol concentrations will double [30]. ACTH concentrations higher than 75 pg ml^{-1} (16.5 pmol l^{-1}) at 30 min post-TRH administration suggest PPID when testing is performed from November through July [31, 32]. There is a weaker indication of PPID if the ACTH concentration is between 35 and 75 pg ml^{-1}. If samples are collected at 10 min post-TRH, ACTH values can be interpreted as follows: negative if <85 pg ml^{-1}, weak indication if 85–100 pg ml^{-1}, and strong indication if >100 pg ml^{-1}. Side effects that may be observed in horses after TRH administration include yawning, lip movements, salivation, and trembling.

The TRH-stimulation test is becoming the method of choice to diagnose PPID for equine practitioners because it provides reliable results, is of short duration, evaluates pituitary and adrenal gland function, and is without significant complications [30,32,40]. Another potential advantage of the TRH-stimulation test is that it can also be used to assess thyroid gland function [42, 43]. Hypothyroidism is often misdiagnosed in horses afflicted with PPID and EMS. In addition to sampling at 10 and 30 min for ACTH measurements, samples can be collected at 2 and 4 h to determine T3 and T4 concentrations. In this manner, a single TRH administration is used to evaluate two endocrine axes (RET/TAB). The TRH-stimulation test should not be repeated within 24 h, and compounded TRH solution stored at room temperature is effective for stimulation testing in horses [44] (see Fig. 29.1).

Resting α-MSH Concentrations

Similar to plasma ACTH, resting α-MSH concentrations follow a similar secretion pattern in healthy and PPID-affected horses throughout the year [7, 41]. Resting α-MSH concentration has the potential to become a routine diagnostic test for PPID; however, commercial assays are not readily available, and, at this point, it can be very expensive to measure. Currently, α-MSH concentrations in horses are only determined for research purposes. It is recommended to collect blood samples in EDTA-containing tubes. Normal seasonal values for plasma α-MSH in healthy and PPID horses have been published [6,7,32,40,45,46]. Reported sensitivities and specificities for resting α-MSH concentrations ≥30 pmol l^{-1} were 68% and 93%, respectively, and α-MSH >50 pmol l^{-1} were 63% and 93%, respectively [32]. In the same group of horses, at 30 min after TRH stimulation, sensitivities and specificities were 93% and 87% for α-MSH ≥30 pmol l^{-1}, and 81% and 93% for α-MSH >50 pmol l^{-1} [32]. Based on these results, the α-MSH response to TRH stimulation displays minor diagnostic advantage compared to baseline α-MSH values; this differs from the ACTH response to TRH, which has greatly improved diagnostic value over baseline ACTH concentrations.

Other Tests

The Combined DST/TRH Test

Some clinicians preferred a combination of the DST with the TRH stimulation test to obtain a more accurate diagnosis of PPID [37]. The reported sensitivity, specificity, positive predictive value, and negative predictive value for this test were 88%, 76%, 71%, and 90%, respectively [2]. This test is tedious, and there is no evidence (for the reasons previously described) that it is superior to baseline ACTH concentrations or to the TRH stimulation test.

Protocol: Collect the first blood sample, administer dexamethasone (40 μg kg^{-1}, intravenous or intramuscular; 8:00–10:00 AM) and collect second blood sample 3 h later. Administer TRH (1 mg, intravenous) and collect third sample 30 min later. A fourth blood sample is collected 24 h after dexamethasone administration, and cortisol concentration is measured in all samples. The test is considered positive if cortisol concentration is >1 μg dl^{-1} at 24 h, or the cortisol concentration increases by ≥66% at 30 min after TRH administration.

Baseline Cortisol Concentrations

Measurement of resting cortisol concentration is not recommended for diagnosis of PPID. Cortisol secretion is affected by stress, exercise, glucose concentrations, and sedatives. Additionally, resting cortisol concentrations are most often in the normal range in horses with PPID [47]. Cortisol metabolites have also been measured in the saliva and urine of horses with PPID, but values often overlap with those of healthy horses to the point that they do not reliably differentiate diseased from healthy horses [4, 5, 48].

ACTH Stimulation Test

The administration of ACTH has been evaluated in a number of studies with different results [12, 26, 27, 48–50]. In healthy horses, it is expected that cortisol concentrations will be doubled by 30–60 min after ACTH administration (0.1–0.25 μg kg^{-1} of cosyntropin, intravenous) [51], while in horses with PPID there is an exaggerated (more than fourfold) increase in cortisol [26]. This test is rarely used due to its impracticality and cost. Rather, methods such as the DST, baseline ACTH concentrations, and the TRH-stimulation test are preferred, as they are more reliable and cost-effective. The ACTH stimulation test is more useful to

[c] Protirelin (TRH), Wedgewood Pharmacy, Wedesboro, NJ.

evaluate adrenal gland function when adrenal insufficiency or exhaustion is suspected.

Resting Glucose and Insulin Concentrations

Basal glucose and insulin concentrations have been used by some clinicians as a screening test for PPID; however, hyperinsulinemia is not a reliable clinicopathologic finding in this condition [52]. Persistent hyperinsulinemia and hyperglycemia, findings consistent with IR, are occasionally documented in horses with PPID [15]. However, these abnormalities are not specific to PPID, and it remains to be determined whether insulin dysregulation in PPID is directly related to pituitary dysfunction or is an indirect consequence from increased concentrations of pro-opiomelanocortin (POMC) peptides and adrenocortical steroids. Under the premise that diabetes mellitus (DM) is defined as persistent hyperglycemia, a number of horses with PPID are also diagnosed with DM [15]. However, it is unclear how often these horses truly have type 2 DM (hyperglycemia, hyperinsulinemia, polyuria/polydipsia) or whether many of their clinical signs are the result of pituitary endocrine dysfunction [53]. A more accurate diagnosis will require evaluation of insulin sensitivity and pancreatic β-cell function. In an epidemiologic study of aged horses (>15 years old), those with evidence of PPID were more likely to be hyperinsulinemic (insulin >20 μIU ml^{-1}) when compared to aged horses without PPID; however, only 32% of the horses with PPID were hyperinsulinemic [54]. Mastro *et al.* [55] reported that insulin sensitivity measured with the euglycemic–hyperinsulinemic clamp method did not differ between groups of aged horses (mean age 25 years) with and without PPID, suggesting that PPID is not always associated with altered insulin sensitivity. On the other hand, the detection of hyperinsulinemia or other evidence of insulin dysregulation in horses with PPID may have important prognostic implications, given the association between hyperinsulinemia and laminitis [34, 56, 57]. Horses with PPID that had very high serum insulin concentrations at presentation (>188 μIU ml^{-1}) were more likely to develop laminitis and survive less than two years after diagnosis when compared to horses with normal insulin concentrations or only moderate hyperinsulinemia [58]. In a recent study, it was found that more often than not, horses with PPID and laminitis had fasting hyperinsulinemia, whereas those horses with PPID without laminitis had serum insulin concentrations in the normal range [59].

Serial measurements of serum glucose and insulin concentrations over time, therefore, may be useful to assess disease progression, response to treatment, as well as risk of endocrinopathic laminitis. Unlike ACTH or α-MSH, a seasonal pattern for insulin secretion in healthy horses is poorly defined [6, 60, 61]. One study in healthy horses in the US found increased insulin concentrations in November compared to other months, but the range was wide [60]. Another study found slightly lower concentrations in healthy ponies and horses in June, with no differences noted in horses with PPID [6]; a third study evaluating healthy horses found no differences in insulin concentrations across the year [61].

Domperidone Response Test

Domperidone is a dopamine D_2 receptor antagonist that does not cross the blood–brain barrier. Based on the understanding that the pathogenesis of PPID involves a lack of dopaminergic inhibition of the pars intermedia melanotropes, it has been proposed that, in horses with PPID, additional dopaminergic blockade could result in greater ACTH and α-MSH secretion [3, 32]. In a study of 33 horses, plasma ACTH concentrations at 8 h after domperidone administration were positively correlated to the pituitary histological PPID severity score [3]. However, not all animals classified as positive by the domperidone test and histologic evaluation had clinical signs of PPID. When using doubling in baseline ACTH concentrations at 2 and 4 h as a positive diagnosis of PPID, domperidone administration to 28 horses was less accurate than baseline ACTH ≥36 pg ml^{-1} or ACTH ≥36 pg ml^{-1} at 30 min after TRH administration to diagnose PPID [32]. Other than for research purposes, there is not a good justification to recommend this test over other available options.

Testing for Equine Metabolic Syndrome

Equine metabolic syndrome (EMS) describes a condition characterized by generalized and/or regional adiposity, laminitis, and IR/ID (see Chapters 18 and 23 for more information on EMS) [62, 63]. It is speculated that hyperinsulinemia and perhaps also a proinflammatory state lead to the development of laminitis in affected horses and ponies (see Chapter 18), although the mechanism(s) by which insulin induces lamellar pathology are currently unclear. Clinical findings (phenotype) and history can be used as indicators that a horse is suffering from EMS and endocrinopathic laminitis [34]. In one study of Welsh ponies, measurements of adiposity (body condition score [BCS], cresty neck score, neck circumference, girth:height ratio) had good sensitivity but poor specificity to predict endocrinopathic laminitis [34]. Specific blood screening (static, basal) and dynamic tests based on glucose and insulin concentrations must be performed for an accurate diagnosis of IR [63]. Screening tests rely on single determinations of glucose, with or without insulin and leptin concentrations, while dynamic tests are centered on the sequential measurement of glucose and insulin concentrations after glucose is given (oral or intravenous) alone or followed by insulin (intravenous) administration. These tests provide an overall picture of the metabolic and endocrine status of the horse at a particular time, and are helpful in assessing insulin sensitivity, disease progression, risk of laminitis, time for intervention, and response to treatment. Dynamic tests, on the other hand, evaluate: (i) how the energy endocrine system responds when challenged (insulin sensitivity, pancreatic β-cell function, and hepatic insulin extraction), (ii) give a better

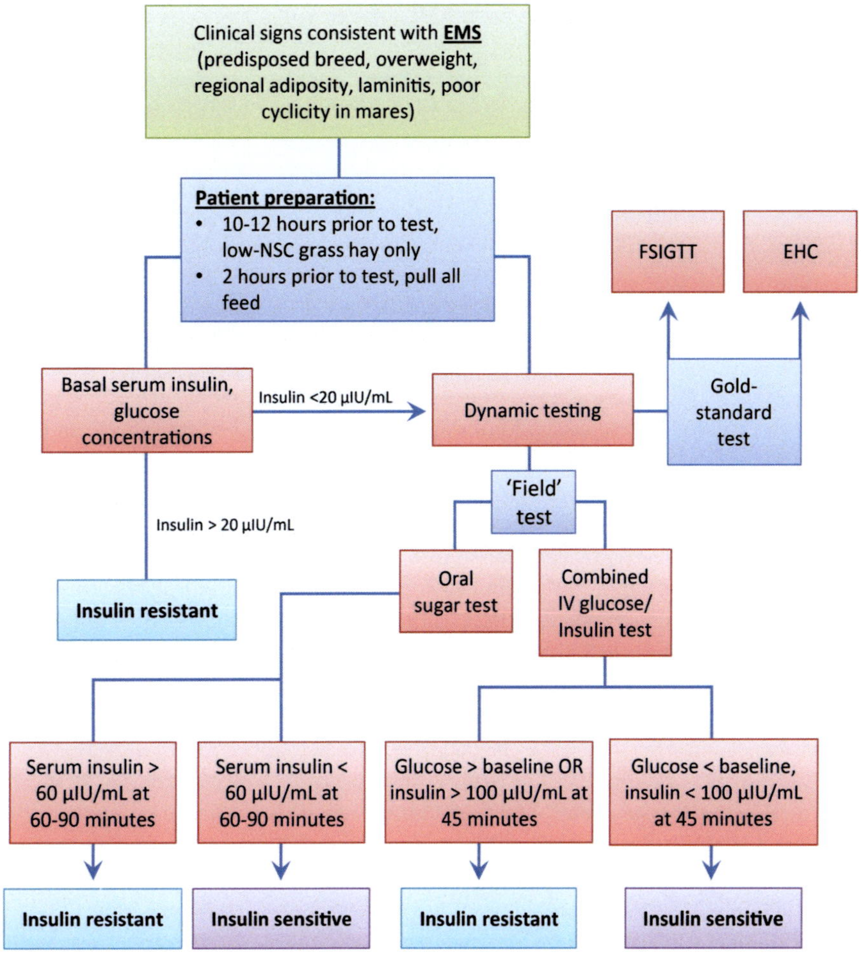

Figure 29.2 Schematic for the assessment of insulin sensitivity in horses.

assessment of glucose and insulin kinetics, (iii) are diagnostic, (iv) provide valuable information on disease progression and laminitis risk, and (v) have prognostic value. Depending on which dynamic test is chosen, they range in practicality from those requiring a few blood samples to the more complex in which frequent blood sampling is necessary to obtain valid information (see Fig. 29.2).

Screening Tests

Screening tests include fasting glucose and insulin concentrations. Additionally, leptin concentrations have also been measured in horses with EMS and laminitis [34, 64], and the measurement of high-molecular-weight (HMW) adiponectin shows promise as a biomarker for EMS and laminitic status (see Chapter 18 for further information on leptin and adiponectin in EMS) [65, 66]. Serum triglyceride concentrations and liver enzyme activity may provide information on severity of hepatic involvement and lipid mobilization. As part of the routine evaluation of IR and laminitis, it is also recommended to measure resting ACTH concentrations, especially in older horses [34,63].

Fasting/Basal Glucose and Insulin Concentrations

The measurement of basal blood glucose and insulin concentrations has been recommended as a screening test for EMS. Horses should not be provided feedstuffs rich in nonstructural carbohydrates within 6–8 h of testing in order to accurately interpret the results. Frank [63] recommends a standardized method in which the horse is fed one flake of hay overnight (after 10:00 PM), with blood collected in the morning (ideally between 7:00–10:00 AM). Blood samples must be refrigerated and sent for analysis to a laboratory running an assay validated for horses. Horses are considered to have IR/ID if the fasting glucose concentrations are >110 mg dl^{-1} (6.1 mmol l^{-1}) and insulin concentrations are >20 µIU ml^{-1} [63]. In one cohort of ponies, resting insulin concentrations >32 µIU ml^{-1} had a sensitivity and specificity to predict laminitis of 100% and 78%, respectively [34]. These cut-off values for insulin were based on measurements using the Siemens Coat-A-Count^{TM} insulin radioimmunoassay, which was well-validated for horses but is no longer commercially available. Accordingly, there is a need to develop new reference ranges and cut-off values based on alternative assays.

Additionally, it is now recognized that many EMS-affected animals that exhibit abnormally high insulin responses to dynamic challenge tests (see below) have normal basal insulin concentrations. In one study from the present authors' group, the evaluation of basal serum insulin concentration was normal (<20 μIU ml^{-1}) in all of 12 horses; according to the frequently sampled intravenous glucose tolerance test (FSIGTT) with minimal model analysis (see below), seven of these horses were actually IR [67]. Based on these results, the basal insulin concentration, while specific, has insufficient sensitivity to be used as a single screening test for IR in equids. It should also be noted that, within an individual animal, there can be marked inter-day variation in serum insulin concentrations; this is another major limitation in the use of resting insulin for diagnosis of IR.

Proxy estimates of insulin sensitivity and pancreatic β-cell function from single measurements of glucose and insulin have been used for the diagnosis of IR [57, 63, 68, 69]. Commonly used proxies have included the glucose-to-insulin ratio, the reciprocal of the square root of insulin (RISQI; $\text{insulin}^{-0.5}$), the quantitative insulin sensitivity check index (QUICKI; $1/(\log[\text{insulin}] + \log[\text{glucose}])$), the homeostatic model assessment of insulin resistance (HOMA-IR; $[\text{glucose} \times \text{insulin}]/22.5$), and the modified insulin-to-glucose ratio (MIRG; $800 - 0.3 \times [\text{insulin} - 50)^2/[\text{glucose} - 30])$ [63, 69], the latter being an estimate of pancreatic β-cell responsiveness. In two separate studies, these proxy measurements were useful for distinguishing groups of laminitis-prone and control ponies [57, 68], but they did not accurately predict any predisposition to laminitis in individual ponies. Seasonal variation in the proxy measurements of insulin sensitivity also have been observed, confounding interpretation [68] (see Fig. 29.2).

Serum Triglycerides

Increased serum triglyceride concentration was a feature of the EMS phenotype in a closed herd of Welsh ponies (97.2 ± 10.7 mg dl^{-1} for ponies with previous laminitis versus 52.3 ± 3.6 mg dl^{-1} for non-laminitic ponies) [57]. In a cohort of mixed-breed ponies, animals with the EMS phenotype had higher serum triglyceride levels in summer but not in winter [70]. Recent studies in a large cohort of horses and ponies ($n > 600$) have also shown that serum triglyceride concentrations are higher in animals with a history of laminitis and other features of EMS [71]. Therefore, serum triglyceride values may be a useful in the diagnosis of EMS.

Resting Leptin and Adiponectin Concentrations

There is interest in the diagnostic utility of the adipokines leptin and adiponectin in EMS. Increased leptin concentrations have been associated with IR and laminitis in horses and ponies [34, 64]. In one cohort of ponies, leptin concentrations >7.3 ng ml^{-1} had a sensitivity and specificity of 83% and 78%, respectively, to predict laminitis [34]. However, in recent studies, serum leptin was not useful for the identification laminitis-prone animals (although, consistent with previous studies in horses and other species, leptin concentrations were strongly correlated with the BCS) [72]. Adiponectin is involved with energy regulation, metabolism, and inflammation, and also increases insulin sensitivity, fatty acid oxidation, energy consumption, β-oxidation, and glucose uptake [73]. Full-length adiponectin (30 kDa) does not circulate as a monomer but rather as 90 kDa trimers, low-molecular-weight (LMW; 180 kDa) hexamers, and high-molecular-weight (HMW; >360 kDa) multimers [73]. The HMW form is considered the most active [73]. A proteolytic product of adiponectin known as globular adiponectin also circulates in human and rodent plasma [73,74]; globular adiponectin ameliorates hyperglycemia and hyperinsulinemia, and decreases plasma free fatty acids [74]. Adiponectin concentrations are associated with fat mass in humans and horses [65,66,73,75]. Concentrations were higher in lean compared to obese horses, and lower in EMS and laminitic animals when compared to healthy cohorts [65, 66, 75]. HMW adiponectin was negatively correlated with BCS and serum insulin concentrations in healthy horses [65]. Equine-specific studies on the influence of HMW and globular adiponectin on metabolic activity and cell differentiation will help to elucidate the role of this adipokine on insulin sensitivity, angiogenesis, metabolic syndrome, and laminitis.

Dynamic Testing

When the results of basal insulin concentrations are inconsistent, or when insulin levels are <20 μIU ml^{-1} in the face of other clinical or historical findings indicative of EMS, the dynamic evaluation of insulin sensitivity and/or glucose tolerance is recommended. These tests are also useful to assess the severity of IR, to monitor disease progression, and to evaluate response to treatment. Dynamic tests include the intravenous glucose tolerance test (IVGTT), the combined glucose–insulin test (CGIT) [63, 76], the insulin tolerance test (ITT) [77, 78], the two-step insulin tolerance test (2-ITT) [77], and the oral glucose tolerance test (OGTT)/oral sugar test (OST) [79]. Methods for the quantitative assessment of insulin sensitivity such as the euglycemic–hyperinsulinemic clamp (EHC) and minimal model analysis of a FSIGTT provide valuable information in the research setting, but they can be impractical for clinical use [63].

Intravenous Glucose Tolerance Test (IVGTT)

The IVGTT has historically been one of the most frequently used methods for the assessment of glucose tolerance in horses [63]. It requires dextrose administration and sequential blood sampling to measure blood glucose concentrations, which can be done at the stall side/on-farm using a handheld glucometer. Horses should be held off-feed for 6–8 h prior to testing. Dextrose (150–300 mg kg^{-1} body weight; 50% solution) is administered intravenously after the collection of a baseline blood sample. Additional blood samples are collected every 30 min for a total of 180 min. In insulin-sensitive horses, glucose concentrations should be back to baseline values by 150 min after dextrose administration. Horses with elevated glucose at 180 min are likely to have IR. This test can be simplified for the field use by collecting samples at 0, 150, and 180 min.

Alpha 2-adrenoreceptor agonists such as xylazine, detomidine, and romifidine should be avoided before and during dynamic testing or before taking blood samples to measure glucose and insulin concentrations as they interfere with insulin release and glucose disposal [76].

Combined Glucose–Insulin Test (CGIT)

The goal of the CGIT is to assess insulin sensitivity by determining the time when glucose concentrations return to baseline values after the combined intravenous administration of dextrose and insulin boluses. An intravenous catheter is placed the day before or just prior to testing. The horse is fasted or offered one flake of hay overnight. After collection of a baseline blood sample, dextrose (150 mg kg^{-1} body weight; 50% solution) is administered intravenously, followed immediately by an injection of regular insulin (0.1 IU kg^{-1} body weight, intravenous). Blood samples are collected at 0, 1, 5, 15, 25, 35, 45, 60, 75, 90, 105, 120, 135, and 150 min to measure glucose concentrations [63]. The insulin concentration can be measured in a sample collected 45 min after its administration. A horse is considered to have IR if the blood glucose concentration is above baseline or the insulin concentration is >100 μIU ml^{-1} at 45 min after dextrose administration [63]. This test can be performed in the field, and glucose concentrations can be measured with a hand-held glucometer. It is important to keep in mind when performing the CGIT that hypoglycemia can be a potential complication and having a dextrose solution at hand is highly recommended. A more practical and economical modification of this test protocol is to collect a baseline blood sample, administer dextrose immediately followed by insulin, and then to measure glucose and insulin concentrations at 45 min after their administration. Interpretation is as previously described. It is important to note that, in a recent study, the repeatability of glucose dynamics with the CGIT was found to be low [80].

Extrapolating the CGIT to donkeys and likely ponies can be misleading. In insulin-sensitive donkeys, the glucose curve is shifted to the right, reaching nadir at 120 minutes compared to 75 minutes for horses, and taking 240 minutes for glucose concentrations to return to baseline compared to 150 minutes for horses. Moreover, 45 minutes after insulin administration, donkeys could have glucose concentrations above baseline, which under equine reference values would categorize them as insulin-resistant. This indicates that for an equivalent glucose and insulin dose, insulin-mediated glucose uptake in donkeys is delayed, supporting differences in insulin sensitivity between equid species [81].

Insulin Response or Tolerance Test (ITT)

The ITT is a simple method to assess tissue insulin sensitivity by measuring the glucose response to a single intravenous injection of regular insulin [78,82–84]. The test also assesses the animal's response to hypoglycemia. It is important to consider factors that could influence the glucose response to insulin, including age, breed, stress, and drugs. The standard ITT that requires multiple blood samples over 180 min has been simplified to two blood samples (0 and 30 min), making it easy and useful for the practitioner [77]. The insulin doses used are variable (0.02–0.6 IU kg^{-1}; 20–600 mIU kg^{-1}) but 0.1 IU kg^{-1} [77, 78, 82–84]. In insulin-sensitive horses, glucose concentrations decrease by 50% within 30 min and return to baseline by 2 h [82–84]. In insulin-resistant animals the glucose concentrations do not decrease as expected and return to baseline sooner than in insulin-sensitive horses. A potential complication of the ITT is severe hypoglycemia. To avoid this, the clinician can proceed with two ITTs using different insulin doses a few days apart [78, 84], or employ a two-step ITT [77]. For the two ITTs, the horse is fasted, a baseline blood sample is collected, regular insulin (30 mIU kg^{-1}; 0.03 IU kg^{-1}) is administered, and a second blood sample is collected at 30 min after injection. If the glucose concentrations fall by 50% at 30 min the horse is considered to be insulin-sensitive and no further testing is required. However, if the glucose concentrations do not fall by 50% at 30 min, the second ITT should be conducted a few days later, this time using 60–100 mIU kg^{-1} (0.06–0.1 IU kg^{-1}) of regular insulin, with samples collected as before. It is important to have a glucose solution available when performing this test in case the horse develops hypoglycemia. In a study of 16 horses with EMS comparing the OST with two ITTs (30 and 60 mIU kg^{-1}), the area under the glucose curve for the OST was significantly correlated with the slope of maximal glucose reduction during the ITT ($r = -0.74$; $P = 0.001$) [84].

Two-Step Insulin Response Test (2-ITT)

In 2013, Bertin and Sojka-Kritchevsky (2013) described a two-step ITT test in which the blood glucose response to an intravenous injection of regular insulin (0.1 U kg^{-1} regular human insulin) is assessed [77]. Blood samples for measurements of glucose concentrations, which may be accomplished by use of a hand-held glucometer, are taken at baseline and 30 min after the injection of insulin. To avoid potential hypoglycemia, after the second sample the clinician can administer dextrose (150 mg kg^{-1}, intravenous) [77]. The time taken to reach a 50% reduction of glucose from baseline is calculated from the two measurements. Bertin and Sojka-Kritchevsky suggested that the two-step test provided a safe, rapid, and low-cost method for the diagnosis of IR in horses [77].

Oral Glucose Tolerance Test (OGTT)/Oral Sugar Test (OST)

The primary utility of the OGTT in equine practice has been to evaluate the small intestinal absorptive capacity, in particular in animals with protein-losing enteropathies. However, unlike in human medicine, the classical OGTT has not been widely used as a tool to assess insulin sensitivity in the horse. A modified approach, the OST, has recently been recommended as the preferred method for dynamic assessment of glucose and insulin dynamics in clinical settings [79]. The OST evaluates the enteroinsular axis (described in separate section below) as carbohydrate detection by enteric endocrine cells leads to the release of the incretins glucagon-like peptide 1 (GLP-1) and glucose-dependent insulinotropic polypeptide (GIP; also termed gastric inhibitory peptide), which stimulate pancreatic β-cell insulin secretion (see below, FSIGTT). Recent studies have shown that horses have a functional enteroinsular axis [85, 86].

The OST test involves the oral administration of corn syrup (Karo® Light[d] at a dosage of 15 ml per 100 kg body weight, equivalent to 150 mg sugar per kg bodyweight) after a short period (8–10 h) of feed withholding. Blood samples are collected at 60 and 90 min after sugar administration for the measurement of glucose and insulin concentrations (see Fig. 29.2). As discussed below, the sensitivity of the OST has recently been questioned, as it shows good specificity but lacks sensitivity when compared to the FSIGTT [67]. Using current insulin diagnostic values (>60 μIU/mL between 60–90 minutes), the OST did not perform better than basal insulin concentrations in a group of horses [67]. That being said, the OST is a useful method to quantify insulin dysregulation; it mimics physiologic conditions of glucose loads that stimulate the enteroinsular axis, which may be involved in insulin and glucose dysregulation. In addition, it is easy to perform and does not require IV catheter placement.

Protocol for the OST The test should be performed after an 8–10 h period of feed withholding. For horses kept in a stall or dry lot, this can be accomplished by leaving one flake of hay with the horse between 10:00 PM and midnight, with testing initiated at about 8:00 AM the next day. Alternatively, the horse can be fed in the morning with testing initiated after 3:00–4:00 PM on the same day. Corn syrup (Karo® Light) is administered by mouth using 60-ml catheter-tipped syringes at a dosage of 15 ml per 100 kg body weight. The current recommendation is to collect blood samples at 60 and 90 min after corn syrup administration for measurements of glucose and insulin concentrations. An insulin concentration >60 μIU ml^{-1} at either time point indicates abnormal hyperinsulinemia [63, 79]. An excessive glucose response is indicated by a glucose concentration >125 mg dl (>6.9 mmol l^{-1}) at 60 or 90 min.

An 'in-feed OGTT' has also been used to assess glucose and insulin responses in EMS suspects; this test has been used in place of the OST due in part to limited access to corn syrup in many countries [87, 88]. For this test, the animal is provided a small meal composed of dextrose powder (1 g kg^{-1} bodyweight) mixed with a small amount (ca. 450 g) of a low-glycemic feedstuff, such as hay chaff. A blood sample for measurement of insulin concentration is collected 2 h after feeding; values >85 μIU ml^{-1} are considered to be abnormal [87]. For both the OST and in-feed OGTT, owners may be concerned about adverse effects associated with the administration of sugar/glucose to insulin-resistant animals (e.g., laminitis), but the risk appears to be very small based on the present authors' experience. Additionally, investigators who have administered hundreds of OSTs to horses and ponies for epidemiologic and genetic studies of EMS have reported no new laminitic episodes immediately post-testing (Dr Jane Manfredi, personal communication); the risk appears, again, to be quite low.

[d] Karo Light Corn Syrup, ACH Food Companies, Cordova, TN.

Frequently Sampled Intravenous Glucose Tolerance Test (FSIGTT)

Minimal model analysis of the FSIGTT is considered the 'gold standard' to estimate insulin-dependent and insulin-independent glucose dynamics, although high intra-subject variation has been reported [89]. The FSIGTT has been modified and optimized to a lower glucose dose to reduce urinary glucose spilling while not affecting performance of the test [90, 91]. For the modified FSIGTT, two jugular venous catheters are placed the night prior to testing. One catheter is used for blood collection and the other for dextrose and insulin administration. Blood samples are collected 10, 5 and 1 min before 50% dextrose solution (150 mg kg^{-1}, intravenous) is rapidly administered (time 0). Blood samples are collected at 1, 2, 3, 4, 5, 6, 7, 8, 9, 10, 12, 14, 16, 19, 22, 23, 24, 25, 27, 30, 35, 40, 50, 60, 70, 80, 90, 100, 120, 150, and 180 min after 50% dextrose infusion [67]. At 20 min after dextrose infusion, regular insulin (0.02 IU kg^{-1}, intravenous) diluted in 3–5 ml of 0.9% sodium chloride solution is given. Information from the FSIGTT is analyzed through the minimal model to calculate values for the insulin sensitivity index (SI), glucose effectiveness (Sg), acute insulin response to glucose (AIRg), and disposition index (DI) [67, 69, 92, 93]. The FSIGTT is a time- consuming test that requires trained personnel and specific software to generate valid information; thus, it is mostly used for research purposes although under specific conditions it can be performed in clinical cases.

In summary, a number of screening and dynamic tests are available to assess the energy status and insulin sensitivity in obese horses or horses at risk of developing laminitis. For the general practitioner, a single measurement of glucose and insulin concentrations may provide sufficient information to implement preventive and therapeutic measures. In other instances, additional tests that depend on the administration of sugars with sequential measurements of glucose and insulin concentrations may be necessary to obtain a better assessment of the patient. At present, the OST is the dynamic field test of choice because it is easy to perform, requires few blood samples, the results are highly correlated with the FSIGTT, and the test evaluates β-cell function, glucose disposal, and the integrity of the enteroinsular axis. It is important to note that agreement between many of these tests has been questioned [67, 69, 79, 89, 92–94]. A recent study conducted in adult horses using minimal model analysis of the FSIGTT as reference, found a poor to fair agreement between basal insulin concentrations, OST, and the CGIT [67]. The authors concluded that current criteria to diagnose IR/ID using baseline insulin concentrations and the OST are highly specific, but lack sensitivity.

The Enteroinsular Axis and its Potential Role in EMS

The enteroinsular axis comprises enteroendocrine factors known as incretins (INtestinal seCRETion of INsulin) that modulate the secretion of pancreatic hormones but also have metabolic actions. The incretins, which include glucagon-like peptide 1 (GLP-1) and glucose-dependent insulinotropic polypeptide (gastric inhibitory peptide; GIP), promote insulin release and suppress glucagon secretion [95]. In other species, GIP is secreted by K cells (proximal small intestine) and GLP-1 by L cells (from proglucagon; distal small intestine) [95]. Nutrients (soluble carbohydrates, amino acids, and fatty acids) and neuroenteric activation promote incretin secretion. The incretin actions explain the rise in insulin secretion before blood glucose concentrations increase, which is considered a pre-emptive mechanism to avoid hyperglycemia and facilitate peripheral tissue glucose uptake. In addition to their insulinotropic actions, GLP-1 and GIP have a multitude of functions; they inhibit gastric emptying and acid secretion, enhance insulin sensitivity, promote fat deposition, modulate skeletal muscle metabolism, stimulate bone formation, increase microvascular blood flow, and control appetite [95, 96]. Understanding the physiology of enteroendocrine cells and the gut–pancreatic–brain axis has become a major area of research, in particular to develop therapeutic strategies that modulate incretin activity in diabetes, obesity, and hypertension [97]. From all this information, it is reasonable to assume that incretin dysregulation contributes to equine conditions related to metabolic activity, insulin secretion and sensitivity, nutrient uptake, inflammation, obesity, and satiety. There is evidence that equids have a functional enteroinsular axis [85, 86, 98]. Oral soluble carbohydrates enhanced GIP, GLP-1, and insulin secretion in horses and ponies [85, 86], and these effects were more evident for oral than intravenous glucose administration [86]. Relevant to EMS and endocrinopathic laminitis, it was also observed that many insulin-resistant ponies had a hyperresponsive enteroinsular axis to oral and intravenous glucose [86]. These findings suggest that endocrine research beyond pancreatic β-cell function is necessary and long overdue to understand pathophysiologic processes involved in energy dysregulation and its detrimental consequences to equine health.

Testing for Thyroid Function

Measurement of thyroid hormone (TH) concentrations is common in equine practice. Historically, it has been believed that many horses with weight loss, obesity, laminitis, reproductive problems, and poor performance have hypothyroidism [43]. However, it is important to mention that hypothyroidism is a rare pathological condition in the horse, and that low TH concentrations is not equivalent to hypothyroidism [43]. In fact, more often than not, TH concentrations are below the normal range in sick horses and foals (non-thyroidal illness syndrome, euthyroid sick syndrome) [43,99,100]. This could clearly lead to a misdiagnosis of hypothyroidism and unnecessary (sometimes life-long) replacement therapy.

Thyroid function can be evaluated through screening and dynamic tests. Screening tests involve the measurement of free and total forms of resting serum T3 (triiodothyroidine) and T4 (thyroxine) concentrations [43,101]. Measuring resting TH concentrations can have some merit if repeated multiple times, taking into consideration the health status, management, and ongoing treatments of the patient [43, 101]. However, resting TH concentrations may be more valuable to assess hyperthyroidism, which is also rare in the horse. Under similar management conditions, donkeys have higher TH concentrations than horses [102].

In order to determine if a horse has a hypofunctional thyroid gland, a dynamic test must be performed. Of these, the TRH-stimulation test is recommended due to its simplicity, cost, minimal side effects, and extensive validation. In addition, as mentioned above in the section on PPID, this test can serve a dual purpose by evaluating pituitary, thyroid, and adrenal gland function after a single intravenous dose of TRH.

TRH-Stimulation Test for thyroid function

The TRH-stimulation test is the best available dynamic method to assess thyroid gland function in the horse [42, 101, 103–106], and is also becoming a routine test to evaluate PPID, as described above [31, 32, 39–41]. In this test, TRH is administered intravenously (1 mg to horses or 0.5 mg to ponies and foals), with hormone measurements taken at baseline and at 2 and 4 h after TRH administration. In horses with a functional thyroid gland, serum T3 and T4 concentrations should double at 2 and 4 h after TRH administration, respectively [42, 43, 101, 103–105, 107]. A lack of response to TRH will suggest pituitary or thyroid disease. Due to the lack of commercial assays to measure equine TSH, and that diseases of the pituitary pars distalis are rare in the horse, it is reasonable to assume that low TH concentrations are the result of a hypofunctional thyroid gland. It may be speculated that horses with PPID could have secondary hypopituitarism from compression of the pars distalis by an enlarged pars intermedia.

TRH-Stimulation Test for PPID and thyroid gland function

In this case, TRH (1 mg) is administered intravenously. Blood samples are collected at baseline, at 10 and 30 min (PPID), and at 2 and 4 h (thyroid gland function). For the interpretation of results, see the previous sections.

References

1. Karikoski, N.P., Horn, I., McGowan, T.W., and McGowan, C.M. (2011) The prevalence of endocrinopathic laminitis among horses presented for laminitis at a first-opinion/referral equine hospital. *Domest. Anim. Endocrinol.*, **41** (3), 111–117.
2. Frank, N., Andrews, F.M., Sommardahl, C.S., Eiler, H., Rohrbach, B.W., and Donnell, R.L. (2006) Evaluation of the combined dexamethasone suppression/ thyrotropin-releasing hormone stimulation test for detection of pars intermedia pituitary adenomas in horses. *J. Vet. Intern. Med.*, **20** (4), 987–993.
3. Miller, M.A., Pardo, I.D, Jackson, L.P., Moore, G.E., and Sojka, J.E. (2008) Correlation of pituitary histomorphometry with adrenocorticotrophic hormone response to domperidone administration in the diagnosis of equine pituitary pars intermedia dysfunction. *Vet. Pathol.*, **45** (1), 26–38.
4. van der Kolk, J.H., Nachreiner, R.F., Schott, H.C., Refsal, K.R., and Zanella, A.J. (2001) Salivary and plasma concentration of cortisol in normal horses and horses with Cushing's disease. *Equine Vet. J.*, **33** (2), 211–213.
5. van der Kolk, J.H. and Wensing, T. (2000) Urinary concentration of corticoids in ponies with hyperlipoproteinaemia or hyperadrenocorticism. *Vet. Q.*, **22** (1), 55–57.
6. Beech, J., Boston, R.C., McFarlane, D., and Lindborg, S. (2009) Evaluation of plasma ACTH, alpha-melanocyte-stimulating hormone, and insulin concentrations during various photoperiods in clinically normal horses and ponies and those with pituitary pars intermedia dysfunction. *J. Am. Vet. Med. Assoc.*, **235** (6), 715–722.
7. Cordero, M., Brorsen, B.W., and McFarlane, D. (2012) Circadian and circannual rhythms of cortisol, ACTH, and alpha-melanocyte-stimulating hormone in healthy horses. *Domest. Anim. Endocrinol.*, **43** (4), 317–324.
8. Donaldson, M.T., McDonnell, S.M., Schanbacher, B.J., Lamb, S.V., McFarlane, D., and Beech, J. (2005) Variation in plasma adrenocorticotropic hormone concentration and dexamethasone suppression test results with season, age, and sex in healthy ponies and horses. *J. Vet. Intern. Med.*, **19** (2), 217–222.
9. McFarlane, D. and Toribio, R.E. (2010) Pituitary pars intermedia dysfunction (Equine Cushing's Disease), in *Equine Internal Medicine*, 3rd edition (eds S.M. Reed, W.M. Bayly, and D.C. Sellon), Saunders/Elsevier, St Louis, MO, pp. 1262–1270.
10. van der Kolk, J.H., Wensing, T., Kalsbeek, H.C., and Breukink, H.J. (1995) Lipid metabolism in horses with hyperadrenocorticism. *J. Am. Vet. Med. Assoc.*, **206** (7), 1010–1012.
11. Dunkel, B., Wilford, S.A., Parkinson, N.J., Ward, C., Smith, P., Grahame, L., *et al.* (2014) Severe hypertriglyceridaemia in horses and ponies with endocrine disorders. *Equine Vet. J.*, **46** (1), 118–122.
12. Dybdal, N.O., Hargreaves, K.M., Madigan, J.E., Gribble, D.H., Kennedy, P.C., and Stabenfeldt, G.H. (1994) Diagnostic testing for pituitary pars intermedia dysfunction in horses. *J. Am. Vet. Med. Assoc.*, **204** (4), 627–632.
13. Levy, M., Sojka, J.E., and Dybdal, N.O. (1999) Diagnosis and treatment of equine Cushing's disease. *Compend. Contin. Educ. Pract. Vet.*, **21**, 766–769.
14. Sojka, J.E., Johnson, M.A., and Bottoms, G.D. (1993) The effect of starting time on dexamethasone suppression test results in horses. *Domest. Anim. Endocrinol.*, **10** (1), 1–5.
15. McFarlane, D. (2011) Equine pituitary pars intermedia dysfunction. *Vet. Clin. North Am. Equine Pract.*, **27** (1), 93–113.
16. Eustace, R.A. and Redden, R.R. (1990) Iatrogenic laminitis. *Vet. Rec.*, **126** (23), 586.
17. Bailey, S.R. and Elliott, J. (2007) The corticosteroid laminitis story: 2. Science of if, when and how. *Equine Vet. J.*, **39** (1), 7–11.
18. Johnson, P.J., Slight, S.H., Ganjam, V.K., and Kreeger, J.M. (2002) Glucocorticoids and laminitis in the horse. *Vet. Clin. North Am. Equine Pract.*, **18** (2), 219–236.
19. Johnson, P.J., Ganjam, V.K., Slight, S.H., Kreeger, J.M., and Messer, N.T. (2004) Tissue-specific dysregulation of cortisol metabolism in equine laminitis. *Equine Vet. J.*, **36** (1), 41–45.
20. French, K., Pollitt, C.C., and Pass, M.A. (2000) Pharmacokinetics and metabolic effects of triamcinolone acetonide and their possible relationships to glucocorticoid-induced laminitis in horses. *J. Vet. Pharmacol. Ther.*, **23** (5), 287–292.
21. Dutton, H. (2007) The corticosteroid laminitis story: 1. Duty of care. *Equine Vet. J.*, **39** (1), 5–6.
22. Hammersley, E., Duz, M., and Marshall, J.F. (2015) Triamcinolone administration does not increase overall risk of developing laminitis. *Equine Vet. J. Suppl.*, **48**, 24.
23. Couetil, L., Paradis, M.R., and Knoll, J. (1996) Plasma adrenocorticotropin concentration in healthy horses and in horses with clinical signs of hyperadrenocorticism. *J. Vet. Intern. Med.*, **10** (1), 1–6.
24. Millington, W.R., Dybdal, N.O., Dawson, R., Jr, Manzini, C., and Mueller, G.P. (1988) Equine Cushing's disease: differential regulation of beta-endorphin processing in tumors of the intermediate pituitary. *Endocrinology*, **123** (3), 1598–1604.
25. Orth, D.N., Holscher, M.A., Wilson, M.G., Nicholson, W.E., Plue, R.E., and Mount, C.D. (1982) Equine Cushing's disease: plasma immunoreactive proopiolipomelanocortin peptide and cortisol levels basally and in response to diagnostic tests. *Endocrinology*, **110** (4), 1430–1441.
26. Sojka, J.E. and Levy, M. (1995) Evaluation of endocrine function. *Vet. Clin. North Am. Equine Pract.*, **11** (3), 415–435.
27. van der Kolk, J.H., Wensing, T., Kalsbeek, H.C., and Breukink, H.J. (1995) Laboratory diagnosis of equine pituitary pars intermedia adenoma. *Domest. Anim. Endocrinol.*, **12** (1), 35–9.
28. Wilson, M.G., Nicholson, W.E., Holscher, M.A., Sherrell, B.J., Mount, C.D., and Orth, D.N. (1982) Proopiolipomelanocortin peptides in normal pituitary, pituitary tumor, and plasma of normal and Cushing's horses. *Endocrinology*, **110** (3), 941–954.
29. Schott, H.C., Coursen, C.L., Eberhart, S.W., Nachreiner, R.J., Refsal, K.R., Ewart, S.L., *et al.* (2001) The Michigan Cushing's project. *Proceedings of the 47th Annual Convention of the American Association of Equine Practitioners*, vol. **47**, pp. 22–24.
30. Beech, J., Boston, R., and Lindborg, S. (2011) Comparison of cortisol and ACTH responses after administration of thyrotropin releasing hormone in normal horses and those with pituitary pars intermedia dysfunction. *J. Vet. Intern. Med.*, **25** (6), 1431–1438.
31. Beech, J., Boston, R., Lindborg, S., and Russell, G.E. (2007) Adrenocorticotropin concentration following administration of thyrotropin-releasing hormone in healthy horses and those with pituitary pars intermedia dysfunction and pituitary gland hyperplasia. *J. Am. Vet. Med. Assoc.*, **231** (3), 417–426.
32. Beech, J., McFarlane, D., Lindborg, S., Sojka, J.E., and Boston, R.C. (2011) Alpha-melanocyte-stimulating hormone and

adrenocorticotropin concentrations in response to thyrotropin-releasing hormone and comparison with adrenocorticotropin concentration after domperidone administration in healthy horses and horses with pituitary pars intermedia dysfunction. *J. Am. Vet. Med. Assoc.*, **238** (10), 1305–1315.

33. McGowan, T.W., Pinchbeck, G.P., and McGowan, C.M. (2013) Evaluation of basal plasma alpha-melanocyte-stimulating hormone and adrenocorticotrophic hormone concentrations for the diagnosis of pituitary pars intermedia dysfunction from a population of aged horses. *Equine Vet. J.*, **45** (1), 66–73.
34. Carter, R.A., Treiber, K.H., Geor, R.J., Douglass, L., and Harris, P.A. (2009) Prediction of incipient pasture-associated laminitis from hyperinsulinaemia, hyperleptinaemia and generalised and localised obesity in a cohort of ponies. *Equine Vet. J.*, **41** (2), 171–178.
35. Copas, V.E. and Durham, A.E. (2012) Circannual variation in plasma adrenocorticotropic hormone concentrations in the UK in normal horses and ponies, and those with pituitary pars intermedia dysfunction. *Equine Vet. J.*, **44** (4), 440–443.
36. de Diez, C.E., Lopez, I., Cortes, B., Pineda, C., Garfia, B., and Guilera-Tejero, E. (2014) Influence of feeding status, time of the day, and season on baseline adrenocorticotropic hormone and the response to thyrotropin releasing hormone-stimulation test in healthy horses. *Domest. Anim. Endocrinol.*, **48**, 77–83.
37. Perkins, G.A., Lamb, S., Erb, H.N., Schanbacher, B., Nydam, D.V., and Divers, T.J. (2002) Plasma adrenocorticotropin (ACTH) concentrations and clinical response in horses treated for equine Cushing's disease with cyproheptadine or pergolide. *Equine Vet. J.*, **34** (7), 679–685.
38. Prutton, J.S., Kass, P.H., Watson, J.L., and Pusterla, N. (2015) Pre-analytical stability of adrenocorticotrophic hormone from healthy horses in whole blood, plasma and frozen plasma samples. *Vet. J.*, **204** (1), 123–124.
39. Beech, J. and Garcia, M. (1985) Hormonal response to thyrotropin-releasing hormone in healthy horses and in horses with pituitary adenoma. *Am. J. Vet. Res.*, **46** (9), 1941–1943.
40. McFarlane, D., Beech, J., and Cribb, A. (2006) Alpha-melanocyte stimulating hormone release in response to thyrotropin releasing hormone in healthy horses, horses with pituitary pars intermedia dysfunction and equine pars intermedia explants. *Domest. Anim. Endocrinol.*, **30** (4), 276–288.
41. Funk, R.A., Stewart, A.J., Wooldridge, A.A., Kwessi, E., Kemppainen, R.J., Behrend, E.N., *et al.* (2011) Seasonal changes in plasma adrenocorticotropic hormone and alpha-melanocyte-stimulating hormone in response to thyrotropin-releasing hormone in normal, aged horses. *J. Vet. Intern. Med.*, **25** (3), 579–585.
42. Breuhaus, B.A. (2002) Thyroid-stimulating hormone in adult euthyroid and hypothyroid horses. *J. Vet. Intern. Med.*, **16** (1), 109–115.
43. Toribio, R.E. (2010) Thyroid Gland, in *Equine Internal Medicine*, 3rd edition (eds S.M. Reed, W.M. Bayly, and D.C. Sellon), Saunders/Elsevier, St Louis, MO, pp. 1252–1260.
44. Goodale, L., Frank, N., Hermida, P., and D'Oench, S. (2015) Evaluation of a thyrotropin-releasing hormone solution stored at room temperature for pituitary pars intermedia dysfunction testing in horses. *Am. J. Vet. Res.*, **76** (5), 437–444.
45. McFarlane, D., Donaldson, M.T., McDonnell, S.M., and Cribb, A.E. (2004) Effects of season and sample handling on measurement of plasma alpha-melanocyte-stimulating hormone concentrations in horses and ponies. *Am. J. Vet. Res.*, **65** (11), 1463–1468.
46. McFarlane, D., Paradis, M.R., Zimmel, D., Sykes, B., Brorsen, B.W., Sanchez, A., *et al.* (2011) The effect of geographic location, breed, and pituitary dysfunction on seasonal adrenocorticotropin and alpha-melanocyte-stimulating hormone plasma concentrations in horses. *J. Vet. Intern. Med.*, **25** (4), 872–881.
47. Boujon, C.E., Bestetti, G.E., Meier, H.P., Straub, R., Junker, U., and Rossi, G.L. (1993) Equine pituitary adenoma: a functional and morphological study. *J. Comp. Pathol.*, **109** (2), 163–178.
48. van der Kolk, J.H., Kalsbeek, H.C., Wensing, T., and Breukink, H.J. (1994) Urinary concentration of corticoids in normal horses and horses with hyperadrenocorticism. *Res. Vet. Sci.*, **56** (1), 126–128.
49. Eiler, H., Goble, D., and Oliver, J. (1979) Adrenal gland function in the horse: effects of cosyntropin (synthetic) and corticotropin (natural) stimulation. *Am. J. Vet. Res.*, **40** (5), 724–726.
50. van der Kolk, J.H., Kalsbeek, H.C., van Garderen, E., Wensing, T., and Breukink, H.J. (1993) Equine pituitary neoplasia: a clinical report of 21 cases (1990–1992). *Vet. Rec.*, **133** (24), 594–597.
51. Stewart, A.J., Behrend, E.N., Wright, J.C., Martin, L.G., Kemppainen, R.J., Busch, K.A., *et al.* (2011) Validation of a low-dose ACTH stimulation test in healthy adult horses. *J. Am. Vet. Med. Assoc.*, **239** (6), 834–841.
52. Reeves, H.J., Lees, R., and McGowan, C.M. (2001) Measurement of basal serum insulin concentration in the diagnosis of Cushing's disease in ponies. *Vet. Rec.*, **149** (15), 449–452.
53. Moses, M.E., Johnson, P.J., Messer, N.T., and Wilson, D.A. (2016) Antidiuretic response of a horse affected with pituitary pars intermedia dysfunction to desmopressin acetate. *Equine Vet. Educ.*, **25**, 111–115.
54. McGowan, T.W., Pinchbeck, G.P., and McGowan, C.M. (2013) Prevalence, risk factors and clinical signs predictive for equine pituitary pars intermedia dysfunction in aged horses. *Equine Vet. J.*, **45** (1), 74–79.
55. Mastro, L.M., Adams, A.A., and Urschel, K.L. (2015) Pituitary pars intermedia dysfunction does not necessarily impair insulin sensitivity in old horses. *Domest. Anim. Endocrinol.*, **50**, 14–25.
56. de Laat, M.A., McGowan, C.M., Sillence, M.N., and Pollitt, C.C. (2010) Hyperinsulinemic laminitis. *Vet. Clin. North Am. Equine Pract.*, **26** (2), 257–264.
57. Treiber, K.H., Kronfeld, D.S., Hess, T.M., Byrd, B.M., Splan, R.K., and Staniar, W.B. (2006) Evaluation of genetic and metabolic predispositions and nutritional risk factors for pasture-associated laminitis in ponies. *J. Am. Vet. Med. Assoc.*, **228** (10), 1538–1545.
58. McGowan, C.M., Frost, R., Pfeiffer, D.U., and Neiger, R. (2004) Serum insulin concentrations in horses with equine Cushing's syndrome: response to a cortisol inhibitor and prognostic value. *Equine Vet. J.*, **36** (3), 295–298.
59. Karikoski, N.P., Patterson-Kane, J.C., Singer, E.R., McFarlane, D., and McGowan, C.M. (2016) Lamellar pathology in horses with pituitary pars intermedia dysfunction. *Equine Vet. J.*, **48** (4), 472–478.
60. Schreiber, C.M., Stewart, A.J., Kwessi, E., Behrend, E.N., Wright, J.C., Kemppainen, R.J., *et al.* (2012) Seasonal variation in results of diagnostic tests for pituitary pars intermedia dysfunction in older, clinically normal geldings. *J. Am. Vet. Med. Assoc.*, **241** (2), 241–248.

61. Place, N.J., McGowan, C.M., Lamb, S.V., Schanbacher, B.J., McGowan, T., and Walsh, D.M. (2010) Seasonal variation in serum concentrations of selected metabolic hormones in horses. *J. Vet. Intern. Med.*, **24** (3), 650–654.
62. Frank, N., Geor, R.J., Bailey, S.R., Durham, A.E., and Johnson, P.J. (2010) Equine metabolic syndrome. *J. Vet. Intern. Med.*, **24** (3), 467–475.
63. Frank, N. (2011) Equine metabolic syndrome. *Vet. Clin. North Am. Equine Pract.*, **27** (1), 73–92.
64. Frank, N., Elliott, S.B., Brandt, L.E., and Keisler, D.H. (2006) Physical characteristics, blood hormone concentrations, and plasma lipid concentrations in obese horses with insulin resistance. *J. Am. Vet. Med. Assoc.*, **228** (9), 1383–1390.
65. Wooldridge, A.A., Edwards, H.G., Plaisance, E.P., Applegate, R., Taylor, D.R., Taintor, J., *et al.* (2012) Evaluation of high-molecular weight adiponectin in horses. *Am. J. Vet. Res.*, **73** (8), 1230–1240.
66. Wray, H., Elliott, J., Bailey, S.R., Harris, P.A., and Menzies-Gow, N.J. (2013) Plasma concentrations of inflammatory markers in previously laminitic ponies. *Equine Vet. J.*, **45** (5), 546–551.
67. Dunbar, L.K., Mielnicki, K.A., Dembek, K.A., Toribio, R.E., and Burns, T.A. (2016) Evaluation of four diagnostic tests for insulin dysregulation in adult Light-Breed horses. *J. Vet. Intern. Med.*, **30** (3), 885–891.
68. Borer, K.E., Bailey, S.R., Menzies-Gow, N.J., Harris, P.A., and Elliott, J. (2012) Use of proxy measurements of insulin sensitivity and insulin secretory response to distinguish between normal and previously laminitic ponies. *Equine Vet. J.*, **44**, 444–448.
69. Treiber, K.H., Kronfeld, D.S., Hess, T.M., Boston, R.C., and Harris, P.A. (2005) Use of proxies and reference quintiles obtained from minimal model analysis for determination of insulin sensitivity and pancreatic beta-cell responsiveness in horses. *Am. J. Vet. Res.*, **66** (12), 2114–2121.
70. Bailey, S.R., Habershon-Butcher, J.L., Ransom, K.J., Elliott, J., and Menzies-Gow, N.J. (2008) Hypertension and insulin resistance in a mixed-breed population of ponies predisposed to laminitis. *Am. J. Vet. Res.*, **69** (1), 122–129.
71. Geor, R.J., McCue, M.E., and Schultz, N. (2013) Current understanding of equine metabolic syndrome. Proceedings of the 59th Annual Convention of the American Association of Equine Practitioners, vol. **59**, pp. 297–304.
72. Schultz, N., Geor, R.J., Manfredi, J.M., and McCue, M.E. (2014) Factors associated with leptin and adiponectin concentrations in a large across breed cohort of horses and ponies. *J. Vet. Intern. Med.*, **28**, 998.
73. Yadav, A., Kataria, M.A., Saini, V., and Yadav, A. (2013) Role of leptin and adiponectin in insulin resistance. *Clin. Chim. Acta*, **417**, 80–84.
74. Chandran, M., Phillips, S.A., Ciaraldi, T., and Henry, R.R. (2003) Adiponectin: more than just another fat cell hormone? *Diabetes Care*, **26** (8), 2442–2450.
75. Kearns, C.F., McKeever, K.H., Roegner, V., Brady, S.M., and Malinowski, K. (2006) Adiponectin and leptin are related to fat mass in horses. *Vet. J.*, **172** (3), 460–465.
76. Eiler, H., Frank, N., Andrews, F.M., Oliver, J.W., and Fecteau, K.A. (2005) Physiologic assessment of blood glucose homeostasis via combined intravenous glucose and insulin testing in horses. *Am. J. Vet. Res.*, **66** (9), 1598–1604.
77. Bertin, F.R. and Sojka-Kritchevsky, J.E. (2013) Comparison of a 2-step insulin-response test to conventional insulin-sensitivity testing in horses. *Domest. Anim. Endocrinol.*, **44** (1), 19–25.
78. Frank, N. (2015) Equine metabolic syndrome, in *Current Therapy in Equine Medicine*, 7th edition (eds N.E. Robinson and K.A. Sprayberry), Elsevier, St Louis, MO, pp. 569–573.
79. Schuver, A., Frank, N., Chameroy, K.A., and Elliott, S.B. (2014) Assessment of insulin and glucose dynamics by using an oral sugar test in horses. *J. Equine Vet. Sci.*, **34**, 465–470.
80. Brojer, J., Lindase, S., Hedenskog, J., Alvarsson, K., and Nostell, K. (2013) Repeatability of the combined glucose-insulin tolerance test and the effect of a stressor before testing in horses of 2 breeds. *J. Vet. Intern. Med.*, **27** (6), 1543–1550.
81. Mendoza FJ, Aguilera-Aguilera R, Gonzalez-De Cara CA, Toribio RE, Estepa JC, Perez-Ecija A. (2015) Characterization of the intravenous glucose tolerance test and the combined glucose-insulin test in donkeys. *Vet. J.*, **206** (3), 371–376.
82. Firshman, A.M. and Valberg, S.J. (2007) Factors affecting clinical assessment of insulin sensitivity in horses. *Equine Vet. J.*, **39** (6), 567–575.
83. De La Corte, F.D., Valberg, S.J., MacLeay, J.M., Williamson, S.E., and Mickelson, J.R. (1999) Glucose uptake in horses with polysaccharide storage myopathy. *Am. J. Vet. Res.*, **60** (4), 458–462.
84. Reiche, D., Johnston, L., and Frank, N. (2013) Comparison of an oral sugar test and intravenous insulin tolerance test to characterize horses with equine metabolic syndrome. *J. Vet. Intern. Med.*, **27**, 650.
85. Bamford, N.J., Baskerville, C.L., Harris, P.A., and Bailey, S.R. (2015) Postprandial glucose, insulin, and glucagon-like peptide-1 responses of different equine breeds adapted to meals containing micronized maize. *J. Anim. Sci.*, **93** (7), 3377–3383.
86. de Laat, M.A., McGree, J.M., and Sillence, M.N. (2016) Equine hyperinsulinemia: investigation of the enteroinsular axis during insulin dysregulation. *Am. J. Physiol. Endocrinol. Metab.*, **310** (1), E61–E72.
87. Smith, S., Harris, P.A., and Menzies-Gow, N.J. (2016) Comparison of the in-feed glucose test and the oral sugar test. *Equine Vet. J.*, **48** (2), 224–227.
88. Tadros, E.M. and Frank, N. (2013) Endocrine disorders and laminitis. *Equine Vet. Educ.*, **25**, 152–162.
89. Pratt, S.E., Geor, R.J., and McCutcheon, L.J. (2005) Repeatability of 2 methods for assessment of insulin sensitivity and glucose dynamics in horses. *J. Vet. Intern. Med.*, **19** (6), 883–888.
90. Hoffman, R.M., Boston, R.C., Stefanovski, D., Kronfeld, D.S., and Harris, P.A. (2003) Obesity and diet affect glucose dynamics and insulin sensitivity in Thoroughbred geldings. *J. Anim. Sci.*, **81** (9), 2333–2342.
91. Toth, F., Frank, N., Elliott, S.B., Perdue, K., Geor, R.J., and Boston, R.C. (2009) Optimisation of the frequently sampled intravenous glucose tolerance test to reduce urinary glucose spilling in horses. *Equine Vet. J.*, **41** (9), 844–851.
92. Toth, F., Frank, N., Chameroy, K.A., and Bostont, R.C. (2009) Effects of endotoxaemia and carbohydrate overload on glucose and insulin dynamics and the development of laminitis in horses. *Equine Vet. J.*, **41** (9), 852–858.
93. Treiber, K.H., Boston, R.C., Kronfeld, D.S., Staniar, W.B., and Harris, P.A. (2005) Insulin resistance and compensation in

Thoroughbred weanlings adapted to high-glycemic meals. *J. Anim. Sci.*, **83** (10), 2357–2364.

94. Pratt-Phillips, S.E., Geor, R.J., and McCutcheon, L.J. (2015) Comparison among the euglycemic-hyperinsulinemic clamp, insulin-modified frequently sampled intravenous glucose tolerance test, and oral glucose tolerance test for assessment of insulin sensitivity in healthy Standardbreds. *Am. J. Vet. Res.*, **76** (1), 84–91.
95. Seino, Y., Fukushima, M., and Yabe, D. (2010) GIP and GLP-1, the two incretin hormones: Similarities and differences. *J. Diabetes Investig.*, **1** (1-2), 8–23.
96. Abdulla, H., Phillips, B., Smith, K., Wilkinson, D., Atherton, P.J., and Idris, I. (2014) Physiological mechanisms of action of incretin and insulin in regulating skeletal muscle metabolism. *Curr. Diabetes Rev.*, **10** (5), 327–335.
97. Ezcurra, M., Reimann, F., Gribble, F.M., and Emery, E. (2013) Molecular mechanisms of incretin hormone secretion. *Curr. Opin. Pharmacol.*, **13** (6), 922–927.
98. Duhlmeier, R., Deegen, E., Fuhrmann, H., Widdel, A., and Sallmann, H.P. (2001) Glucose-dependent insulinotropic polypeptide (GIP) and the enteroinsular axis in equines (*Equus caballus*). *Comp. Biochem. Physiol. A. Mol. Integr. Physiol.*, **129** (2-3), 563–575.
99. Himler, M., Hurcombe, S.D., Griffin, A., Barsnick, R.J., Rathgeber, R.A., MacGillivray, K.C., *et al.* (2012) Presumptive nonthyroidal illness syndrome in critically ill foals. *Equine Vet. J. Suppl.*, **41**, 43–47.
100. Hilderbran, A.C., Breuhaus, B.A., and Refsal, K.R. (2014) Nonthyroidal illness syndrome in adult horses. *J. Vet. Intern. Med.*, **28** (2), 609–617.
101. Breuhaus, B.A. (2011) Disorders of the equine thyroid gland. *Vet. Clin. North Am. Equine Pract.*, **27** (1), 115–128.
102. Mendoza, F.J., Perez-Ecija, R.A., Toribio, R.E., and Estepa, J.C. (2013) Thyroid hormone concentrations differ between donkeys and horses. *Equine Vet. J.*, **45** (2), 214–218.
103. Harris, P., Marlin, D., and Gray, J. (1992) Equine thyroid function tests: a preliminary investigation. *Br. Vet. J.*, **148** (1), 71–80.
104. Lothrop, C.D., Jr and Nolan, H.L. (1986) Equine thyroid function assessment with the thyrotropin-releasing hormone response test. *Am. J. Vet. Res.*, **47** (4), 942–944.
105. Rothschild, C.M., Hines, M.T., Breuhaus, B., Gay, J., and Sellon, D.C. (2004) Effects of trimethoprim-sulfadiazine on thyroid function of horses. *J. Vet. Intern. Med.*, **18** (3), 370–373.
106. Breuhaus, B.A. 2014) Thyroid function and dysfunction in term and premature equine neonates. *J. Vet. Intern. Med.*, **28** (4), 1301–1309.
107. Chen, C.L. and Li, W.I. (1986) Effect of thyrotropin releasing hormone (TRH) on serum levels of thyroid hormones in thoroughbred mares. *J. Equine Sci.*, **6**, 58.

PART 5

Medical Treatment of the Laminitic Patient

Equine Laminitis, First Edition. Edited by James K. Belknap and Raymond Geor.

CHAPTER 30

General Supportive Care for the Laminitis Case

Andrea E. Floyd and Debra R. Taylor

Introduction

The recovering laminitic horse has many challenges which must be overcome. The simplest change in the environment of the lame or recumbent horse may make the difference between life and death. If a human being were to find him/herself in an intensive care unit, they would realize that they were at the mercy of the doctors, caretakers, the bed they lay on, the food brought to them, and the machines that supported them. Their physical comfort and the rate of the healing process would be entirely dependent upon the aforementioned, as well as their psychological health and feeling of safety and wellbeing. This frame of mind should serve as a starting point when considering the needs of an animal that is totally dependent on a veterinarian.

The factors that are important to implement in an intensive care situation are the following:

- The intensive care stall and supportive apparatus.
- Nutrition and hydration.
- Monitoring physical wellbeing
- Pharmacological management.

The Intensive Care Stall and Supportive Apparatus

Laminitic horses have trouble rising. Normally, horses elevate their front ends before using their hind ends. Since the front feet of a laminitic horse are usually the worst affected, the animal will tend to stumble forward or sideways when trying to find their balance. Laminitic horses also have a tendency to find themselves in awkward situations when trying to lie down, and may crash into a wall or become cast once down. Stalls housing laminitic horses should be at least 15 feet (4.5 m) wide and 20 feet (6 m) long. This amount of space allows the horse to gain its bearings without crashing into a wall, and also allows a handler to get out of the way should the need arise.

It is recommended that the walls of the intensive care stall be made of wood such as $^{3}/_{4}$-inch (20 mm) plywood, covered with foam sheets (the type used under plastic house siding) and then covered with medium-gauge metal (4 × 8 ft; 1.2 × 2.5 m) sheets. Concrete block is not recommended, not only because it holds moisture – and thus mold and bacteria – but also because it has no shock absorbency should the horse crash into it on attempting to rise. Metal panels are also easy to disinfect.

Supportive rings should be placed around the stall at head height that can be used to assist the horse that has difficulty rising. The rings can be judiciously used for support of the head and tail. The rings should be well-anchored in the walls and capable of supporting the weight of the horse. The rings should be at least 2 in (50 mm; inside diameter; Fig. 30.1a).

Horses with severe hind limb lameness will benefit from a rump bar placed at the height of the tuber ischii. Rump bars allow the horse to support part of their weight on the bar and stand without placing compression on the injured hind feet (Fig. 30.1c).

An overhead rail will allow the use of a body sling to help the horse rise if necessary. Generally, these are not needed and the present author does not like to place horses in slings in order to force them to stand for long periods. If a horse does not want to stand, then it should be made comfortable on the floor and flipped over every 4 h.

A centered intravenous hook should be placed in the ceiling. Supportive intravenous fluids administered through coiled lines work well for the horse in need of hydration, but these cases require 24-h monitoring.

Video monitoring of all stalls is a good practice. Horses tend to react differently in human company than they do alone. Monitoring their activities will show true pain levels, changes in attitude, destructive behavior, and will give early warning of problems, such as colic. Bandage chewing at the level of the heel bulbs or coronary bands is a symptom of an underlying problem such as impending coronary band rupture (Fig. 30.2).

Bedding

A recumbent horse is an intensive care horse – they are truly at the veterinarian's mercy. A type of bedding should be used that fluffs (lofts) easily so as to decrease the frequency and severity of decubital ulcers. Pine sawdust that is banked against the walls

Equine Laminitis, First Edition. Edited by James K. Belknap and Raymond Geor.

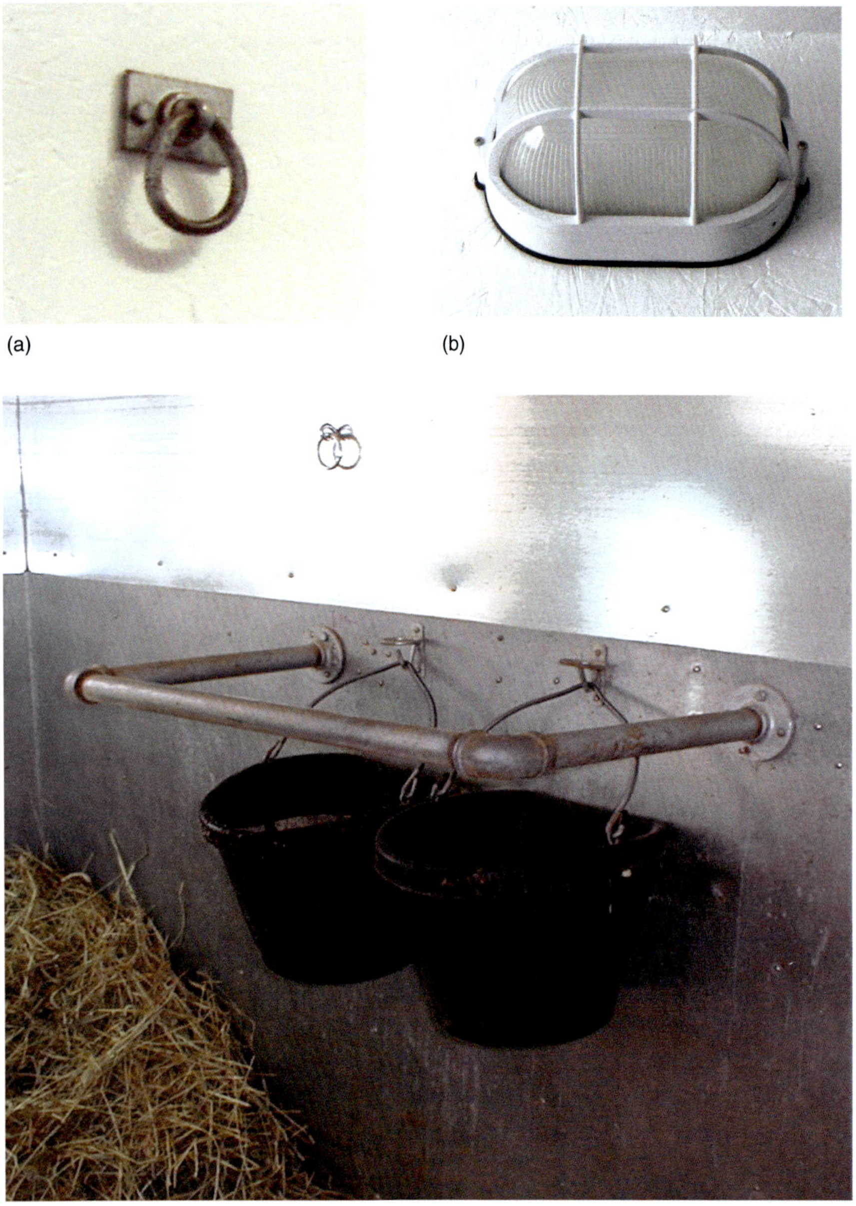

(a) (b) (c)

Figure 30.1 (a) Rings attached to the walls of the stall at head height should be strong enough to support the weight of the horse as they attempt to rise. (b) Lighting should be waterproof and placed near the ceiling around the stall to give adequate illumination for veterinary procedures and bandage changes. (c) Rump bars give the horse with hind-end laminitis the opportunity to stand while resting their injured feet.

(Fig. 30.3) and at least 10 in (25 cm) deep under the horse gives sufficient comfort and padding. This bedding should be lifted with a metal pitchfork several times a day to re-establish the softness (loft). The horse should never be allowed to 'bottom out' in the stall and thus be found lying directly on the subflooring, especially if the subflooring is concrete or asphalt. If this occurs, the depth of the bedding must be increased immediately. 'Bottoming out' is a common occurrence when recumbent horses are bedded with pine shavings rather than pine sawdust. The latter bedding is also naturally absorbent, causing urine to form a 'clump' rather than to seep under the recumbent horse. The pine oil in the bedding acts as an astringent and mild fly deterrent. Straw that is clean and bright may be used over sawdust or shavings to provide a bed with loft; however, straw has the disadvantage of attracting flies as manure and urine will cling to the straw. Fly control by spraying around the horse is essential, regardless of the bedding used. Overhead fly control misters may intoxicate the recumbent horse and should not be used. Whatever the form of bedding used, it is extremely important that the bedding be cleaned on an hourly basis. Many horses urinate and defecate without rising, and they must have all the urine and feces removed, new bedding placed behind

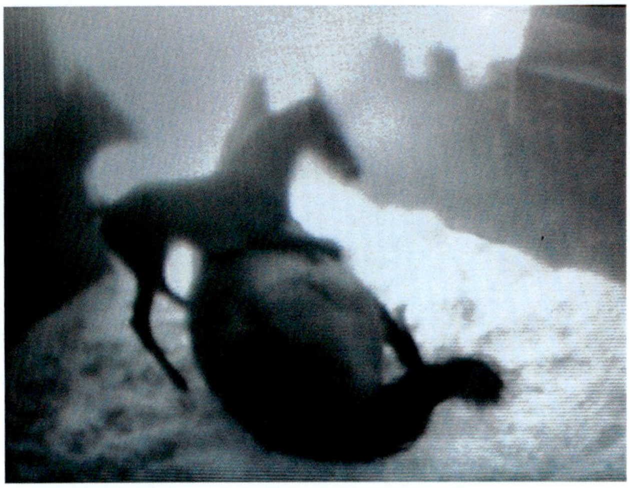

Figure 30.2 Video monitoring of stalls enables constant viewing of the horse. This video shows a recumbent mare and a playing foal.

them, and their perineal and/or scrotal and abdominal areas washed with mild soap and water and dried to prevent scalding. Prompt removal of urine will also keep the ammonia levels low and protect the respiratory environment of the recumbent horse.

Slinkies (a spandex, lightweight body cover) are used routinely by the present author on recumbent horses (Fig. 30.3). These body covers protect the skin from abrasion and help move urine and manure away from the body; they also help with fly control. Any full body covering must not trap a horse's limbs when they attempt to rise. Slinkies with short-stretch Velcro straps stay tight to the body and do not tangle around the legs. Avoid any slinky that has metal or plastic closures.

If the horse is being maintained in rubber hoof boots, cotton (human) athletic socks can be utilized as inexpensive boot

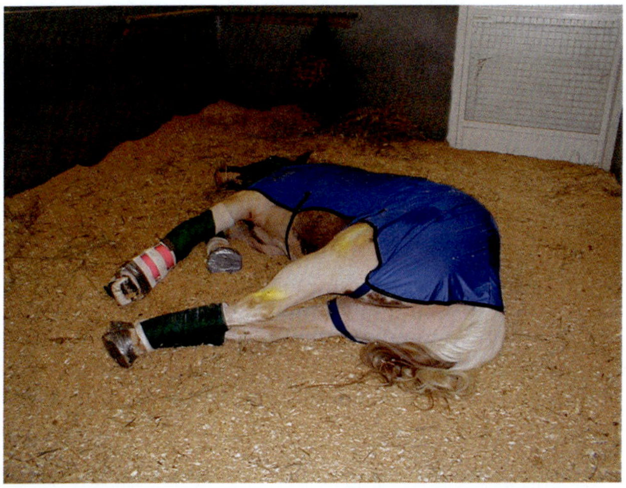

Figure 30.3 Slinky or spandex sheet used to protect recumbent horses. Spandex sheets with Velcro straps are available from Norman Equine Design, Subiaco, AR 72865.

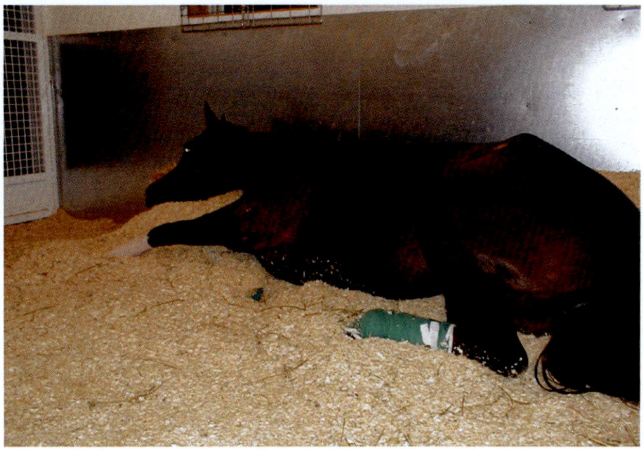

Figure 30.4 Sawdust banked around the stall allows for sternal recumbency. Note the open window and the horse's interest in the outside environment.

liners (Fig. 30.5). The socks can be pulled up the cannon bone to help protect the skin of the fetlocks (and the carpi if long socks are used) from decubitis. Note that rubber or other synthetic material hoof appliances that cover the bulbs of the heels will trap heat and moisture. Socks should be changed and the heel bulbs checked for rubs on a daily basis when utilizing hoof boots.

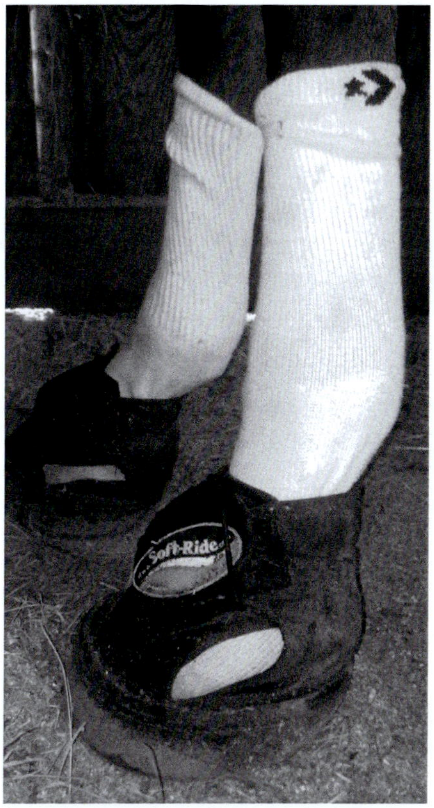

Figure 30.5 Cotton human athletic socks should be used as hoof boot liners whenever rubber or synthetic hoof boots are being used for hoof protection. Socks should be changed once or twice daily to minimize moisture and the chance of heel bulb rubbing.

Obel Grade 4 patients are predisposed to eye ulcers. An eye mask should be used during this stage of the disease to keep bedding out of the eyes.

Ventilation, Temperature, and Lighting

Horses in pain commonly have high body temperatures, and the pyrexia generally cannot be controlled through the use of nonsteroid anti-inflammatory drugs (NSAIDs), pain killers, or sedatives.

Recumbent horses absorb heat from the bedding which, combined with their sweating, will set up a strong environment for skin scalding and large decubital ulcers. Keeping the temperature as low as possible will improve the horse's attitude, stop the sweating and subsequent scalding, and make them much more comfortable. Adding air conditioning to the intensive care stall or suite of stalls will greatly enhance case outcome. Good ventilation within the air-conditioned stall is also a must. Venting away the odors of urine, manure and medicine is beneficial for everyone. It is crucial to supply a constant source of fresh air, while using a fan ventilation system that does not cause a constant wash of bedding particles. If the horse is repeatedly found wet in the stall, the bedding and the air flow should be modified. This may require a fan with a $^1/_4$ to $^1/_2$ horsepower motor. These large fans can be wall-mounted at a level of approximately 4 ft (1.1 m) above the floor, with the air stream pointed parallel to the recumbent horse. This will allow for a constant air movement without a constant wash of bedding particles. Overhead ceiling fans may also be installed. The use of air-conditioning units in intensive care stalls helps with the pain-induced pyrexia, sweating and decubital ulcer formation, and has been the present author's preferred method of dealing with the painful recumbent horse.

Having windows within the intensive care unit will provide an escape from boredom and also provide sunlight. The windows should be of sufficient strength and quality to allow disinfection, closure while the air-conditioning is running, and strong enough to withstand impact. A heavy-gauge screen mesh window guard that can be opened for cleaning is a good idea. Placing the windows low enough that a sternally recumbent horse can see out improves the horse's attitude. It is recommended that tall narrow windows be installed that allow the horse to view the outside environment, whether it is sternal or standing (Fig. 30.4).

Light fixtures placed on all the walls just below ceiling height will allow good observation of the horse from any angle, and also makes medicating and treating the horse much easier (Fig. 30.1b).

Nutrition and Hydration

Horses in extreme pain (Obel grades 3 and 4) have difficulty eating sufficient calories to maintain their body weight. Pain can increase energy expenditure by as much as 199% in humans with similar injury [1]. Horses in pain are also not able to walk to the hay, or to supplement tub or water supply. Even the originally obese horse may rapidly become cachectic. It is imperative that food is brought to the horse and water is offered every 2 h.

One way to provide a calorie-dense diet and hydration simultaneously is to soak a mixture of beet pulp, alfalfa pellets, a high-protein sweet feed or pellet (or a high-protein/high-fat, moderate nonstructural carbohydrate [NSC] feed in a horse with metabolic syndrome concerns), salt, rice bran oil, and molasses. The mixture is broken down by the added hot water to the consistency of a slurry. The mixture has more fluid and particulate than solid feed, it can be easily swallowed in the same manner as water, and the horse will readily consume it. Such a gruel can be fed to the sternal horse in a large tub. If the horse has problems getting sternal, handlers can hold the animal in a sternal position for the length of time it takes to consume the food. In a standing horse that has trouble moving, the tub can be held by a handler. There may be some questions raised about the use of a high-NSC feed (e.g., sweet feed) or molasses in an insulin-resistant horse. However, any horse with a high pain index and suffering from significant tissue damage is likely to be hypermetabolic [1]. The present author has found it near-impossible to normalize the body condition of severely affected laminitis patients without carbohydrates (in moderation) within the diet.

High-quality soft hay is placed under the sternal horse's head and around the head so that any movement will bring them into direct contact with edible forage. In the horse which is standing but unwilling to move, the present author places hay around the entire perimeter of the stall on the banks of bedding. Placing it on the banks makes it easier to reach than on the ground, and placing it around the perimeter means that the horse will always find hay within easy reach. Fresh hay should be offered several times a day, and water offered from a small (2 gallon; 9 liter) bucket every 2 h. The author recommends keeping a chart on recumbent horses that shows the hourly consumption of feed and water, the recumbent position, heart rate (standing and recumbent), and the fecal and urinary output (approximate).

Hand-sized portions of the following diet can be administered: apples, carrots, freshly cut grass, herbs, sugar-free peppermints (for insulin-resistant horses), grains, beet pulp-based treats or alfalfa pellets. Appropriate treats can be offered several times throughout the day to break up boredom and provide interaction.

Monitoring Physical Wellbeing

The basic physical examination parameters of body temperature, heart rate, respiratory rate, appetite, urinary and fecal output should be monitored twice daily. Laminitic horses rarely lose their appetite due to laminitis alone, so if inappetance is noted then other etiologies should be investigated.

Pain Assessment

The Obel Pain Scale [2] has historically been used to evaluate laminitis pain. This scale lacks sensitivity to detect the subtle day-to-day and week-to-week changes in laminitic patients. The original Obel grading system and suggested modifications to create subcategories is provided in Table 30.1. A similar system has been described for postoperative colic patients [3]. The original scale is in **bold** font, while suggested modifications are in regular font.

Heart Rate

Heart rate has been used for equine pain assessment after arthroscopic surgery [4], and is a major focus of colic assessment. The laminitic patient is no less in crisis than is the colic patient, and therefore the heart rate is a sensitive and valuable indicator of pain and overall stress level. The present author expects the heart rate to normalize if the therapeutic plan is appropriate. If the heart rate increases following treatment, then the primary treatment or supportive care is not working. A decrease in heart rate can be considered a positive prognostic indicator. The heart rate and respiratory rates should be monitored and recorded at least twice daily, and notations made as to whether the horse was standing or recumbent at the time of examination.

Limb and Pelvic Position

The most common presentation of laminitis is for the horse to be most severely affected by laminitis in the forelimbs. However, lamellar events always occurs in all four feet and therefore the hind feet should not be forgotten. Forelimb position is an important indicator of treatment appropriateness in horses with laminitis of the forelimbs. In the present author's opinion, forelimb extension of the classic laminitis stance is likely due to the horse trying to create 'slack' in the deep digital flexor tendon and muscle unit by extending the elbow (origin of deep digital flexor is on the caudal side of the humerus) and straightening the fetlock (Fig. 30.6). The present author (AF) believes that, when hoof and limb mechanical treatment applications have created loading mechanics where deep digital flexor tension is not aggravating the situation, the horse will pull its forelimbs back under its shoulder to the normal vertical position. The other reason laminitic horses will extend their forelimbs is in an attempt to unload the toe region of the foot. Either way, if the patient is not able to bring the forelimbs to a normal vertical position, the current therapy should be considered inappropriate or inadequate and change is mandated if treatment success is expected. Rather than rampaging the pharmacy for more pain medication to 'mask the pain' created by jeopardized hoof tissues, focus on abolishing the source of the pain rather than masking it. This will give the tissues an opportunity to heal.

When a horse is laminitic in the forelimbs, the weight is shifted to the hindlimbs. The hindlimb position is moved forward, the pelvis becomes tilted, and the back is arched (Fig. 30.7a). This protective stance causes muscle spasms of the back and gluteal muscles. During stride, the hindlimbs are awkward and are slapped to the ground in the anterior phase of the stride (Fig. 30.7b). Owners and veterinarians often question that the horse is neurologic or has a primary hindlimb condition. The hind feet should be closely re-evaluated for laminitis because they may have become worse than the forefeet. If the hind feet are found to be normal, increasing the comfort of the lamintic forefeet should be the primary focus to re-establish normal hindlimb stance and movement. If the hindlimb stance and stride characteristics are not normalizing over time, the forelimb treatment strategy is likely in need of change. Alternative therapies such as massage, acupuncture and chiropractics may also help to minimize and ameliorate the negative impact of forelimb pain on the muscles and joints of the back and pelvic limbs.

Stall cameras, pedometers and heart rate monitors are an ideal method to confirm the horse's activity level and track the response to various treatment protocols.

Pharmacological Management

Perfusion Enhancement

The lack of suspension of the bone within the hoof capsule allows the boney column to be pushed into the hoof capsule as the horse bears weight, and this compresses the solear dermis and stretches the lamellar dermis. Compression and stretching of the dermis physically occludes blood flow within the dermis. But tissues cannot heal without blood flow, and re-establishing blood flow is the key to 'creating a healing environment' by providing needed nutrients and oxygen. While it would be everyone's dream to have a 'silver bullet' medication to do this, no such treatment currently exists [5–7]. Even if drugs can pharmacologically reverse the increased vascular resistance that occurs during the hours after experimental laminitis induction [8], it would be quite impossible for any pharmacological agent to reverse the ongoing mechanical compression and stretching of the corium that exists in a standing horse once the suspensory apparatus has failed. Therefore, the first order of business in re-establishing perfusion in the naturally occurring disease is minimizing mechanical compression and stretching of the corium within the capsule. Therefore, *mechanics* should be considered the most important therapeutic target for addressing digital perfusion. The corium will not heal (nor will systemically administered drugs likely have access to the injured corium) as long as it is being crushed (coronary and solear corium) and/or stretched (lamellar corium). A thorough discussion of vasoactive drugs is provided in Chapter 32.

Pain and Inflammation

The present author believes that it is impossible to medicate a way out of high-scale laminitis pain. The primary focus of pain management should be to minimize the source of pain by optimizing hoof loading mechanics to unload the stresses and strains on inflamed/injured tissues so they can heal. Residual

Table 30.1 Modified Obel grading scale (the original scale is shown in bold text). The Obel scale takes into account gait and willingness to lift feet and move forward when coaxed. It is suggested that other parameters such as heart rate, respiratory rate, limb position, pelvic position and willingness to make a normal response to stimuli, be added to the current scale, similar to that previously described for postoperative colic patients [3]. This scoring system was previously published in *Care and Rehabilitation of the Equine Foot* (ed. P. Ramey), 2001.

Obel grade	Original scale	Modified scale
1	**When in the standing position the horse lifts the feet incessantly, often at intervals of but a few seconds (paddling). At a walking pace it does not show any lameness, but the trotting gait is short and stilty. When the animal is recovering, this stage is characterized by the latter symptom alone**.	All limbs are in normal vertical position at all times, rear limb stride is long and smooth, may resist or avoid sharp turns, may self-initiate trotting on straight lines or large circles. Resting heart and respiratory rates are normal if recovering, elevated if acute. i When approached by a feed bucket from behind, the horse will promptly turn around and walk briskly or trot toward the feed bucket (or spooks and trots away). ii When approached by a feed bucket from behind the horse reluctantly turns around and faces the bucket and walks slowly toward the feed. iii When approached by a feed bucket from behind the horse does not turn around, but stands in one spot and turns its head to look behind.
2	**The horse moves quite willing at a walking pace, but the gait is characteristic for laminitis. A forefoot may be lifted without difficulty**.	Forelimbs are maintained vertical at all times, rear limbs near normal position standing but are slapped or stomped to ground during anterior phase of stride when walking, horse may or may not freely initiate movement on its own but warms out of forelimb lameness upon slight coaxing to walk a short distance in straight line, decubitis is mild or healing with mostly intact skin, some hair loss may be present. Occasional shifting of weight from forelimb-to-forelimb is noted. Resting heart rate is less than 44 bpm. Respiratory rate is usually normal. i When standing, initiates straight line movement on its own, without being coaxed to interact with environment, rear limb stride is long with little evidence of slapping motion at anterior phase. ii When standing, shows no resistance when being coaxed to start walking but only initiates one step at a time to graze on its own, rear limbs have moderate slapping movement in anterior phase of stride, tail head is slightly low, noticeably awkward appearance to rear limb stride. iii When standing, shows slight resistance when coaxed to start walking for first few strides, forelimb stride length increases as horse moves, rear limbs are slapped down during anterior phase of stride, back is slightly arched and tail head is low, quite awkward appearance to rear limb stride
3	**The horse moves most reluctantly. Vigorously resists attempts to lift a forefoot.**	The forelimbs are gradually adjusted to vertical upon standing, rear limbs are variable position upon standing. At walk, forelimbs land flat or heel first (while padded), rear limbs are short-strided and quickly slapped or stomped to ground at anterior phase of stride, back is arched and tail head is low, very awkward appearing rear limb stride, decubitus with eroded skin and hair loss may be present. Frequent shifting of weight from forelimb-to-forelimb is noted. Resting heart rate is 40–60 bpm. Respiratory rate may be elevated. i When recumbent, quickly rises at the introduction of a stimulus, brings forelimbs to vertical almost immediately upon rising (rear feet may be normal position or slightly forward but behind the flank) ii When recumbent, rises with some delay at the introduction of a stimulus, brings forelimbs to vertical within 15 s (rear feet may be normal or positioned or as far forward as the flank) iii When recumbent, rises with reluctance or after a period of calculated delay at the introduction of a stimulus such as opening the stall door, brings forelimbs to vertical after 15 s or longer, maintains rear limbs markedly under the abdomen (rear feet in front of flank)
4	**At this stage the horse does not move without being forced**	Rises from recumbency with great reluctance and requires coaxing. Forelimbs are extended when standing, rear limbs well under flank, back is arched and tail head is very low, decubitus may be present with full thickness skin ulceration on hips, stifles, shoulders and/or lateral aspect of fetlocks. Horse trembles when standing. Heart rate is >56 bpm. Elevated respiratory rate is present. i While recumbent, eats in sternal recumbency, moves from lateral to sternal as soon as approached or stall door is opened ii While recumbent, eats in sternal recumbency, must be lightly patted or stimulated to elicit moving from lateral to sternal recumbency iii While recumbent, eats in lateral recumbency, must be aggressively patted or stimulated to elicit moving from lateral to sternal recumbency

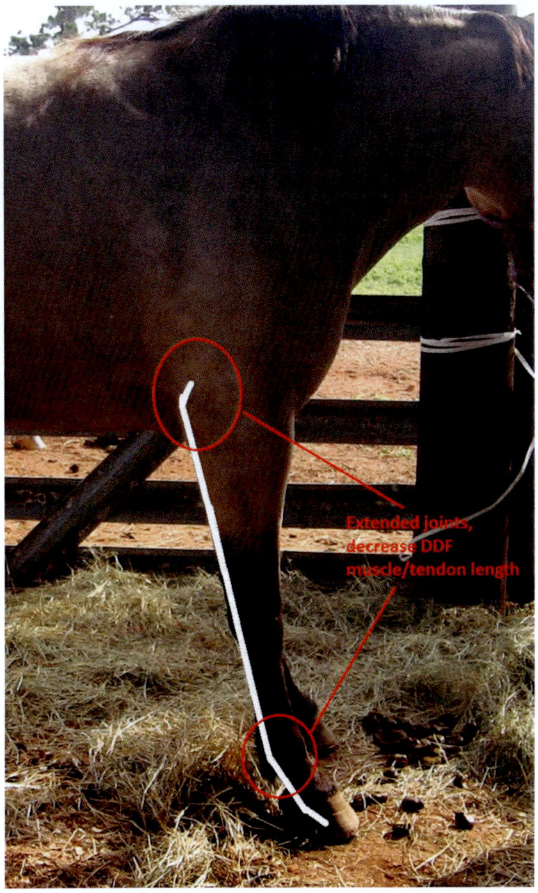

Figure 30.6 The course of the deep digital flexor (DDF) muscle and tendon as indicated by the white line on the forelimb of this horse with the classic extended stance. The origin of the DDF muscle is on the caudal aspect of the medial humeral condyle, above the elbow. Extending the elbow and the fetlock decreases the overall muscle tendon unit length (adds 'slack') by straightening its course from origin to insertion.

pain can then be addressed with medication. It is important to establish a 'baseline' pain management regimen which is familiar and knowledge is available as to how other horses have responded. New regimens should be tried gradually with caution, always comparing them to the familiar 'baseline' regimen. Switching and/or stacking medications can lead to either over- or under-medicating the case at hand, which may lead to confusion and cause the clinician to miss or ignore the big picture which is "...where is the ongoing pain originating"? Most frequently, ongoing pain is originating from loading mechanics that cause weight-bearing to be transferred to inflamed/injured dermis. A failure to address the source of pain and ameliorate it mechanically sets the horse up for 'wind-up' pain – a phenomenon where the painful stimulation of peripheral nerves at sufficient intensity to stimulate C-fibers (see Chapter 33) leads to a slow cumulative effect that progressively increases the response in the spinal neurons even to normally non-painful stimuli. Once the 'wind-up' phenomenon has started it is a challenge to break. Establishing a healing environment for the dermis through mechanics early is the best method of long-term pain management. Thorough discussions of the use of NSAIDs and other analgesic drugs are available in Chapters 31 and 33. In the present author's opinion on NSAID treatment, the laminitic horse which fails to respond positively (by improving one to three levels on the modified Obel scale) to a low-dose phenylbutazone (e.g., 4.4 mg kg^{-1} day^{-1}) should be addressed with the same diligence as the colic that fails to respond to 1.1 mg kg^{-1} of flunixin. Although it has been reported that failure of a laminitis patient to respond to phenylbutazone is a diagnostic indicator of a poor prognosis [5], in the present author's (AF) experience it means that it is essential to achieve better mechanics and instigate a deeper investigation of the true cause of the ongoing pain that is not being controlled by low-dose phenylbutazone. The results of a study conducted in 2005 suggested that there

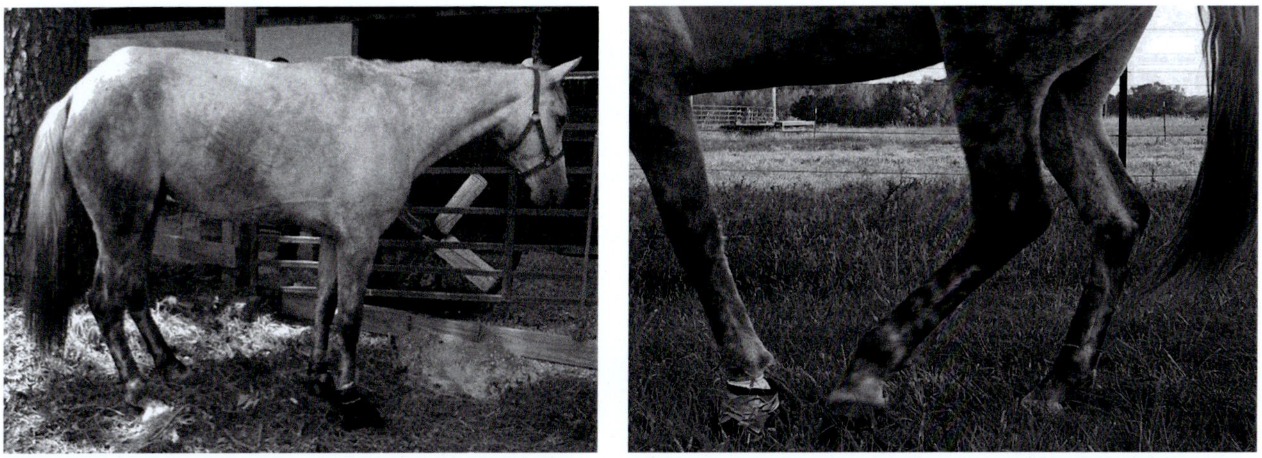

(a) (b)

Figure 30.7 (a) The pelvis of this mare with forelimb laminitis is tilted so that the tail head is low, the back is arched, and the hind limbs are forward under the flank. (b) The rear limbs of the horse in Fig. 30.6a are angled forward, well under the horse's abdomen, just before being slapped down awkwardly during the anterior phase of the stride.

was no benefit in administering phenylbutazone doses higher than 4.4 mg kg^{-1} day^{-1} for chronic lameness [15]. Finally, as various reports indicate that it takes approximately four days for analgesia to stabilize on a new phenylbutazone dose regimen, the present authors do not suggest frequent changes in phenylbutazone dosing [16]. Other options described elsewhere in this book include firocoxib (Chapter 31), gabapentin (Chapter 33), pentoxifylline (Chapters 31, 32, and 35), dimethyl sulfoxide (DMSO; Chapter 31), and cryotherapy/digital hypothermia (Chapters 34 and 35).

References

1. Graves, C., Saffle, J., Morris, S., *et al.* (2005) Caloric requirements in patients with necrotizing fasciitis. *Burns*, **31** (1), 55–59.
2. Obel, N. (1948) Studies of the Histopathology of Acute Laminitis. Thesis, Almqvist and Wilcsells Bottrykeri Ab Uppsala.
3. Pritchett, L.C., Ulibarri, C., Roberts, M.C., *et al.* (2003) Identification of potential physiological and behavioral indicators of postoperative pain in horses after exploratory celiotomy for colic. *Appl. Anim. Behav. Sci.*, **80**, 31–43.
4. Raekallio, M., Taylor, P., and Bennett, R. (1997) Preliminary investigation of pain and analgesia assessment in horses administered phenylbutazone or placebo after arthroscopic surgery. *Vet. Surg.*, **26** (2), 150–155.
5. Divers, T.J. (2010) Clinical application of current research findings toward the prevention and treatment of acute laminitis in horses with systemic inflammatory diseases: an internist's perspective. *J. Equine Vet. Sci.*, **30** (9), 517–524.
6. Moore, R.M. (2008) Evidence-based treatment for laminitis – what works? *J. Equine Vet. Sci.*, **28** (3), 176–179.
7. Moyer, W., Schumacher, J., and Schumacher, J. (2008) Are drugs effective treatment for horses with acute laminitis? *Am. Assoc. Equine Pract.*, **54**, 337–340.
8. Eades, S.C., Stokes, A.M., and Moore, R.M. (2006) Effects of an endothelin receptor antagonist and nitroglycerin on digital vascular function in horses during the prodromal stages of carbohydrate overload-induced laminitis. *Am. J. Vet. Res.*, **67** (7), 1204–1211.

CHAPTER 31

Common Therapies: Anti-Inflammatory Therapy

Thomas J. Divers

Introduction

Medical treatments that are commonly used as anti-inflammatory therapy in treating laminitis include nonsteroidal anti-inflammatory drugs (NSAIDS), cytokine inhibitors, enzyme inhibitors, inhibitors of neutrophils and platelets, antioxidants, and cryotherapy. If there is ongoing systemic inflammation, the anti-inflammatory therapy must be directed at both the 'whole horse' and the hoof. The initial steps in trying to prevent or control laminitis in horses with ongoing systemic inflammatory disease are correct treatment of the primary disease, control of the systemic inflammation, and cryotherapy of the feet. Treatments for the first two of these are based on:

- *Sepsis containment* (e.g., uterine lavage in septic metritis cases, administration of intestinal toxin absorbents and/or cathartics for grain overload, early administration of antibiotics, such as tetracycline for Potomac Horse Fever) when appropriate.
- *Cardiovascular support* (e.g., crystalloids and colloids).

Anti-inflammatory treatments that are commonly used in treating the systemic inflammation and that have evidence-based support include hyperimmune plasma, flunixin meglumine or other NSAIDS, pentoxifylline, lidocaine, and polymixin B [1–7].

Nonsteroidal Anti-Inflammatory Drug Treatments for Laminitis

Nonsteroidal anti-inflammatory drugs (NSAIDs) are cyclooxygenase (COX) inhibitors which have anti-inflammatory, analgesic, and antipyretic properties, primarily by blocking the synthesis of prostanoids (prostaglandins [PGs] and thromboxanes [TXs]). The two primary COX isoenzymes, COX-1 and COX-2, produce the same central prostaglandin PGH2 from arachidonic acid released from cell membrane phospholipids; PGH2 is then used as a substrate by different prostanoid synthase enzymes to produce specific PGs and TXs. The COX-1 enzyme has been classically considered a constitutive (constantly expressed/present) enzyme associated with the production of a variety of cytoprotective prostanoids, which are important for normal gastrointestinal, renal, vascular, and other body system physiologic functions. The COX-2 enzyme is more tightly regulated, being induced by both proinflammatory cytokines and growth factors. Because COX-2 is the primary COX enzyme involved in the production of prostaglandins involved in inflammation, pain, and fever, some have referred to the COX-2 enzyme as the 'bad COX,' and the COX-1 enzyme as the 'good COX.' Unfortunately, it is not that simple! Some selective COX-2 activity is constitutive and protective (e.g., endothelial expression associated with the homeostatic maintenance of blood vessels through the production of prostacyclin and PGE_2 in the renal medulla) and some COX-1 increases (e.g., associated with platelet production of TX) may enhance pathophysiologic processes. Additionally, inducible COX-2 activity is vital for embryonic/fetal development and wound healing. COX activity has now been further divided into COX-3 activity, which appears to have its activity centrally in the brain. In horses, the ability of NSAIDS to inhibit platelet activity is mostly limited to aspirin in systemically healthy horses only.

Prostaglandins are centrally involved in pain sensation, primarily through COX-2 and associated prostanoid synthases to produce PGI2 and PGE2 in peripheral and central nerves. The prostanoids are not only involved directly in neural signaling, but also induce a hypersensitivity to other nociceptive stimuli (e.g., bradykinin) by lowering the threshold of activation for peripheral and central sensory nerves, therefore causing a peripheral and central hyperalgesia. Thus, a great deal of the analgesia supplied by NSAIDs/COX inhibitors is by the inhibitory effects of blocking COX-2 on the nerve activation/transmission of the sensory nerves themselves, not just from decreasing tissue inflammation. An inhibition of approximately 80% of COX-2 activity is necessary to provide consistent analgesia in experimental pain models [8], and is likely to be true in clinical patients also. Therefore, when assessing the efficacy and selectivity of NSAIDs, most investigators use the concentration of the NSAID of interest which is the IC_{80} (inhibitory concentration to block 80% of activity) for COX-2 in the species of interest (there is a great deal of variability between species) [9].

Equine Laminitis, First Edition. Edited by James K. Belknap and Raymond Geor.

Table 31.1 Commonly used nonsteroidal anti-inflammatory drugs (NSAIDs) used for the treatment or prevention of laminitis.

Drug	Route/Dosage	Selectivity	Advantages	Disadvantages
Phenylbutazone	Intravenous, oral 2.2–4.4 mg kg^{-1} b.i.d.	Nonselective	Effective for musculoskeletal pain. Inexpensive	Higher incidence of gastrointestinal, renal side effects versus some other NSAIDs
Flunixin meglumine	Intravenous, oral 0.25–1.0 mg kg^{-1} b.i.d. or t.i.d.	Nonselective	High efficacy for systemic inflammation/sepsis	Moderate or higher incidence of gastrointestinal, renal side effects
Meloxicam	Oral 0.6 mg kg^{-1} SID	Nonselective	Low incidence of side effects at suggested dose	Intravenous preparation expensive in United States
Firocoxib	Intravenous, oral 0.09–0.1 mg kg^{-1} SID	COX-2-selective	Low incidence of side effects	May not effectively inhibit thromboxane, long half-life and lower plasma levels on day 1 may require dose adjustment for initial treatment

SID, once daily.

Choosing the most appropriate COX inhibitor for horses with laminitis based on current information is not always straightforward, and must be based on the stage of the disease process, concurrent diseases, pharmacokinetic and dynamic studies, safety, cost, and personal experiences (see Table 31.1). Considerations for choosing an NSAID to treat laminitis must include the relative importance of each of the following: (i) the need to inhibit ongoing systemic inflammatory mediator production (e.g., endotoxemia/sepsis); (ii) the level of concern for intestinal and renal injury from the COX inhibitor; (iii) possible administration routes (e.g., intravenous, oral, intramuscular); (iv) whether or not platelet inhibition is desirable; (v) what level of analgesia is needed (e.g., how much in pain the horse is); and (vi) expense. Although well-documented to be effective in alleviating many of the clinical signs of systemic inflammatory diseases that are commonly associated with a high risk of laminitis, NSAIDS likely have little or no efficacy in directly preventing laminitis in horses. The upregulation of COX-2 in the lamellae occurs in the prodromal stage of the black walnut extract (BWE) model of laminitis, but COX-2 increases have not been found in the lamellae during the development stage (prior to the onset of clinical signs of pain) of laminitis with the carbohydrate overload (CHO) model [10–12]. COX-2 is consistently increased in the lamellae with the onset of early clinical laminitis [13]. The clinical application of these research findings on prostanoid production in the different stages of laminitis is difficult, and the following questions should be considered:

1 Should selective or nonselective COX-2 inhibitors be used?
2 Should the NSAID treatment be focused on inflammation associated with the COX-2 isoenzyme or on vascular abnormalities (i.e., vasoconstriction which may be associated more with COX-1 isoenzymes).
3 Should attention be focused on COX-2 inhibition while at the same time providing some (albeit a lesser) degree of COX-1 inhibition?

Nonselective COX inhibitors (e.g., flunixin, phenylbutazone, and to a lesser degree ketoprofen) have been the NSAID standard of care for inhibiting inflammatory mediators and controlling laminitic pain in horses for four decades in North America.

Firocoxib, a relatively new and highly selective COX-2 inhibitor, is available as both an injectable and orally administered product for the treatment of pain and inflammation in horses. Due to its highly selective COX-2 inhibition (with minimal COX-1 inhibition), it is the least toxic of the NSAIDs [14]. Unfortunately, due to its prolonged half-life and time required for reaching steady state, the initial dose may not have the desired therapeutic effect and many veterinarians administer three times the recommended dose as the initial dose [15]. Also, due to its highly selective COX-2 inhibition, it may not inhibit TX, which can have various proinflammatory and vasoactive effects on tissue microvasculature.

Meloxicam has been used successfully in Europe for several years and is now beginning to be used in the United States (0.6 mg kg^{-1} oral, q. 24 h) [16]. Meloxicam has been termed a 'COX-2 preferential' drug due to its slightly more selective COX-2 inhibition (versus COX-1) in *in-vitro* assays [9,16]. Although meloxicam is relatively nonselective (it inhibits ca. 70% of COX-1 activity) at its IC_{80} concentration for COX-2 [9], the drug at the 0.6 mg kg^{-1} q.24 h dose is still found to have fewer deleterious gastrointestinal effects than phenylbutazone and flunixin [17]. A parenteral form of meloxicam is available, but its use is limited by the high cost. The oral product is affordable and may, due to its relatively balanced COX1–COX-2 inhibition, be an NSAID with reasonable efficacy and low toxicity for treating both systemic inflammation and laminitis [17]. Due to their enhanced safety, either firocoxib or meloxicam would be a reasonable NSAID selection for the long-term NSAID treatment of laminitis, assuming that the pain relief is acceptable and cost is affordable.

Many practitioners believe the best and most consistent NSAID for musculoskeletal pain control is the nonselective COX inhibitor phenylbutazone. In severely painful laminitic cases, it is important to administer, early during the course of the disease, a NSAID that provides an adequate degree of analgesia for both patient comfort (humane reasons) and to decrease the possible development of 'wind-up'/neuropathic pain [18]. Treatment with an appropriate dose of an NSAID that reliably provides analgesia can also be used as a prognostic guide. For example, in the present author's clinical experience, in acute laminitis caused by grain overload, affected horses can often be divided clinically into two groups: (i) those that respond within 6–24 h to 4–6 mg kg^{-1} of phenylbutazone and have a good prognosis; and (iii) those that have minimal or no noticeable response to the same treatment and have a guarded to poor prognosis.

If systemic toxemia is present (evidenced by fever, band neutrophils or toxic-appearing neutrophils) in a horse with either laminitis or is at risk of laminitis, flunixin may be a preferred NSAID because of its efficacy against several endotoxin-induced clinical signs and inflammatory mediators such as TX. Flunixin may have a greater selective effect on TX inhibition than phenylbutazone, may marginally alleviate platelet dysregulation more than ketoprofen or phenlybutazone, and may decrease the activation of nuclear factor kappa B (NFκB; a transcription protein which is rapidly activated by bacterial products and associated with several inflammatory genes) [19–21]. Additionally, even a 'low' dose of flunixin (0.25 mg kg^{-1}) can inhibit the production of TX (a vasoconstrictor increased with endotoxemia that promotes microvascular dysfunction leading to tissue inflammation), and partially alleviates clinical signs associated with endotoxemia [3].

The type of NSAID and dose used to treat laminitis and/or decrease systemic inflammation may depend on the primary disease causing the systemic inflammation. For example, horses with systemic inflammation with no intestinal disease (e.g., metritis) can be treated with either full or reduced doses of a nonselective or a more selective COX-2 inhibitor in the hope of: (i) reducing the systemic inflammatory trigger factors for laminitis; (ii) providing analgesia; and (iii) providing COX-2 inhibition within the hoof during clinical laminitis. In contrast, the use of NSAIDs to prevent or treat laminitis in horses with colitis should be more restricted due to the potential adverse effects of NSAIDs on intestinal repair and the need for parenteral administration in those cases. For horses being treated for laminitis and having significant risk of intestinal or renal injury from prolonged NSAID use, firocoxib (the most selective COX-2 inhibitor available) may be a medically sound selection. However, the one concern of using a COX-2-selective NSAID in acute laminitis is the potential for possibly creating a more 'prothrombotic' environment in the lamellar vasculature (where platelet activation has been reported) [22], by preferentially blocking endothelial PGE2 and PGI2 which inhibit platelet activation/aggregation, while sparing platelet COX-1 which is associated with thromboxane synthase and the production of this vasoactive prostanoid (TX promotes platelet adhesion and vasoconstriction). The bioavailability of all NSAIDs is generally excellent, but, in horses with severe intestinal diseases, there is a concern about absorption and the ability of the drug to reach therapeutic levels. Additionally, low albumin concentrations often present with enterocolitis in horses could disrupt the pharmacokinetics of these normally highly protein-bound drugs, thus enhancing toxicity.

When treating horses with NSAIDs, strict attention should be given to the animal's hydration status and plasma albumin concentration. It is very important to maintain normal hydration in horses/ponies being treated with NSAIDs, as dehydration enhances the drugs' toxic effects. This can be a significant problem in laminitic horses that spend large amounts of time in recumbency. Intramuscular flunixin administration is not recommended if there are alternatives, because of the relatively high incidence of clostridial myositis that follows intramuscular injections of this drug. Feeding a moderate protein/low carbohydrate feed with added corn oil and glutamine may help to protect against the intestinal and renal injury sometimes associated with NSAIDs. Omeprazole (a proton pump inhibitor; 4 mg kg oral, q. 24 h) can be given to decrease the risk of gastric ulcers. Misoprostol (a synthetic prostaglandin E1; 2–4 μg kg^{-1} oral, q. 8–12 h) is frequently administered to horses requiring high-dose NSAID therapy at the present author's hospital. This has been shown to be effective in preventing NSAID-induced intestinal injury in humans, and is an effective inhibitor of basal gastric acid secretion in horses [23]. Although combining NSAIDs may improve analgesia, it is generally not recommended because it may increase intestinal toxicity, as was demonstrated in normal horses given normal doses of both phenylbutazone and flunixin for five consecutive days [24].

Rarely, 'low-dose' aspirin (10 mg kg^{-1} given rectally or orally every two to three days) is combined with moderate doses of phenylbutazone, meloxicam, or firocoxib for the treatment of chronic laminitis, in the hope of providing both pain relief and platelet inhibition [25]. Clopidogrel might be a better choice for platelet inhibition due to the fact that aspirin and all other tested NSAIDs have little effect on equine platelet function during systemic inflammation [26].

Nonselective and both COX-2 and COX-1-selective inhibitors may all have some effect on intestinal motility. COX-2-selective inhibitors may reduce some forms of intestinal motility, while flunixin has been reported to decrease colonic motility [27, 28]. Consideration must also be given to the different pharmacodynamics of NSAIDs in ponies and donkeys when compared to horses. In mules and donkeys, the metabolism and elimination of most NSAIDs is faster, and more frequent administration of the drugs (three times per day for some NSAIDs instead of twice daily) may be required [29]. Some NSAIDs (e.g., phenylbutazone) appear to be more toxic to the intestine of ponies than the intestine of horses at similar doses; hence, firocoxib might be particularly indicated in ponies with chronic laminitis. Other highly protein-bound drugs (e.g., antibiotics) may be affected by

NSAIDs, such that higher free/active drug levels may arise when given concurrently with NSAIDs.

Enzyme Inhibition and Decreasing Inflammation

As described in detail in Chapter 15, there is little doubt that matrix metalloproteinase (MMP) enzymes (e.g., MMP-2, -9, -13) and other proteases (e.g., ADAMTS-4) are involved in the pathology and possibly the repair of lamellar tissue [30–33]. It is unclear if the enzyme activation is an initiating injury mechanism, or more likely it is secondary to an earlier inflammatory insult. It is also unclear when, how, and if this process should be interrupted. Similar to many other endogenous proteins, MMPs can have detrimental effects associated with overwhelming inflammation, but beneficial effects in the remodeling of some tissues following injury [34]. Recent studies conducted at Louisiana State University described the inhibition of MMP production by doxycycline, oxytetracycline, pentoxifylline, and flunixin meglumine in both a low-dose endotoxin model and a CHO overload laminitis model [35]. Although doxycycline, tetracycline, and pentoxifylline decreased MMP production following endotoxin, only pentoxifylline had a measurable effect on decreasing the severity of lameness in the experimental horse. Doxycycline and minocycline will inhibit MMP-13 production in interleukin (IL)-1-stimulated equine synoviocytes [36] and may improve joint lameness in some horses, but there is little evidence suggesting that these drugs are effective in preventing or treating laminitis. In the present author's experience, oxytetracycline does not appear to be effective in treating sepsis-related laminitis (SRL) based on the early treatment of Potomac horse fever (PHF) enterocolitis cases with the drug (due to efficacy of oxytetracycline as a therapeutic agent for the PHF pathogen), where yet a relatively high incidence of laminitis occurs in spite of the treatment.

Pentoxifylline is a nonselective phosphodiesterase inhibitor that has been used commonly to treat laminitis in equine practice. It has been shown to inhibit cytokine production in experimental equine toxemia when given prior to an endotoxin challenge, but had fewer effects when given intravenously after an endotoxin challenge [37]. Pentoxifylline could have numerous beneficial effects in treating endotoxemia, including cytokine and MMP reduction, but it is only commercially available for oral administration, which somewhat limits its usefulness in horses with intestinal disorders. Although pentoxifylline has not been shown to have direct anti-inflammatory effects in the lamellae itself, there is some evidence from an *ex vivo* study that it may enhance vasodilatation in equine digital veins via both endothelium-dependent and -independent pathways involving nitric oxide synthase and cyclo-oxygenase [38]. At the present author's hospital, pentoxifylline is formulated for intravenous administration (and is compounded in the intravenous form by many commercial pharmacies); it is frequently used orally (10 mg kg^{-1}, q. 12 h) or intravenously (7.5 mg kg^{-1}, q. 8–12 h) for the treatment of horses with systemic inflammation, and in both the prevention and treatment of laminitis.

Inhibiting Neutrophil and Platelet Margination and Preventing or Treating Laminitis

Although neutrophil (polymorphonucleocyte; PMN) and platelet margination onto endothelial cells in the hoof are not the initial event in either inflammatory model of laminitis, their margination is known to occur during the prodromal stage following chemokine and cytokine upregulation, and likely plays a role in the initiation of and/or progression of laminitis [39–43]. The adhesion of PMNs to lamellar endothelial cells and migration through the vascular wall into the lamellar tissue would affect vascular tone, activating endothelial cells and likely triggering/exacerbating lamellar inflammation from neutrophil-derived enzymes (e.g., elastase in addition to the downstream production of MMPs) and further increasing cytokine, chemokine, and free radical production in the lamellae. Platelet aggregation, which may precede but enhance PMN margination, would have similar effects on the endothelium in addition to release of TXA_2 and serotonin, both of which are potent vasoconstrictors. Early platelet activation may be particularly important in the CHO model of laminitis [39]. Unfortunately, drugs proven to inhibit the endothelial margination of both platelets and neutrophils are currently either not known or are not available for routine use in the horse. Available drugs which may have some effect on neutrophil and platelet margination include pentoxifylline, low-molecular-weight heparin (LMWH), clopidogrel, and corticosteroids. LMWH has been reported to decrease the incidence of laminitis in horses undergoing intestinal surgery [44]. Heparins – both unfractionated and fractionated (LMWH) – have been shown to decrease neutrophilic myeloperoxidase uptake by equine venous endothelial cells [45]. LMWH has the potential to decrease cytokines, TXB_2 activity, and neutrophil margination on the endothelium when given prior to endotoxemia. Unfortunately, the currently available LMWH drugs are cost-prohibitive for most equine cases in the United States. Lidocaine infusions have been administered to horses in an attempt to inhibit neutrophil adhesion to endothelium and inflammation, but this apparently is not the case [46, 47]. Lidocaine infusion is effective as an analgesic in horses with laminitis, and is often used in an attempt to decrease pain, decrease NSAID use, and to possibly inhibit apoptosis. Lastly, to suggest that corticosteroids could be used in the prevention of laminitis seems counterproductive, but a recent abstract reported that treatment with hydrocortisone prior to the correction of an equine small intestinal obstruction inhibited lamellar neutrophils emigration and MMP-9 activity/concentration [48]. Hydrocortisone should be further evaluated as an initial therapy for preventing laminitis in horses with systemic inflammation. A single dose of short-acting corticosteroids administered prior to clinical procedures that can result in a bolus release of laminitic trigger factors (procedures such as flushing septic metritis, correction of intestinal strangulation, etc.) may have beneficial effects and limited adverse effects; however, further studies are required before this can be recommended.

Anti-Oxidant Treatments

The role of oxidative injury in the pathogenesis of laminitis is unknown. Horses have low levels of superoxide dismutase (SOD) in the lamellae, which could make the latter susceptible to lamellar oxidative damage [49]. Evidence of lipid perioxidation has been found in both the developmental and early clinical phases of the disease only in the BWE model of SRL. When tissues from starch-overload laminitis were compared using similar techniques, no evidence was found of tissue oxidation [50]. There is no evidence-based information to suggest that dimethyl sulfoxide (DMSO) is helpful in preventing or treating the disease.

Cryotherapy

As described in detail in Chapter 34, cryotherapy is the only proven treatment for preventing laminitis in horses with CHO overload models of SRL [51, 52]. Cryotherapy has recently been reported to decrease the incidence of laminitis in hospital patients with entercolitis [53]. In an experimental study on the efficacy of cryotherapy in a CHO model of laminitis, horses stood in 1–7 °C iced water from the hoof to the mid-cannon region. This has recently become practical in the clinics with the availability of a commercial ice boot (SoftRide, Inc., Vermillion, OH, USA) which reaches the level of the distal carpus; other practical yet successful methods of cooling the hoof have been reported [54]. Currently, the present author is using commercial boots that cover the feet and distal one-third of the limb, or a 5-liter fluid bag filled with an ice slurry and duct-taped over the hoof, and further held in place by an ice slurry-filled leg boot that extends down over the coronary band (Fig. 31.1). The efficacy

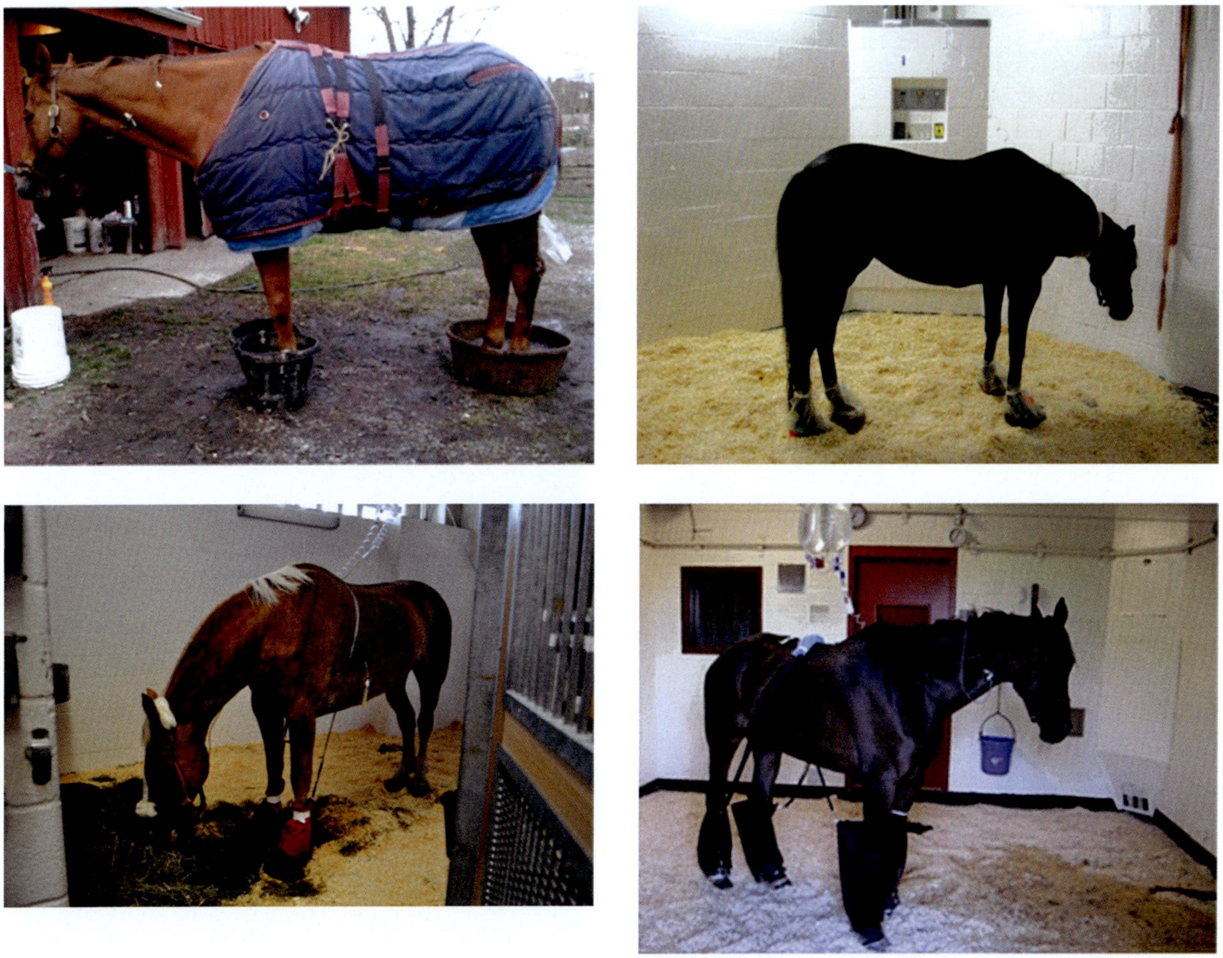

Figure 31.1 Photographs showing several methods used at the present author's practice to provide continual multiple limb cryotherapy to horses.

of cryotherapy may be related to its ability to decrease lamellar inflammation, including inhibiting adhesion molecules, COX-2 gene expression, platelet and neutrophil activation, and decreasing apoptosis. Cryotherapy would also be expected to decrease lamellar oxygen and nutrient requirements and inhibit destructive enzymes and oxidative reactions if they are present. It has been proposed that cryotherapy can prevent laminitis in some at-risk horses by decreasing the delivery of blood-borne toxins that trigger enzymatic destruction of the lamellae. Horses at high risk for developing laminitis, or horses with acute laminitis, should be place in ice boots as soon as possible. The cryotherapy should be continual and can be administered for at least three to four days. Careful attention should be paid to the coronary band to ensure that the boot is not rubbing and damaging the tissue. As a prophylaxis, icing of the feet, along with other medical therapies for systemic inflammation, should be continued for 24 h after no clinical (normal heart rate, digital pulses, and rectal temperature) or laboratory findings (no band or toxic neutrophils) suggestive of systemic inflammation have been identified.

Digital hypothermia with cryotherapy, when not initiated until the detection of lameness, has recently been shown to reduce the severity of lamellar injury and to prevent lamellar structural failure in an acute laminitis model [55]. Whereas, previous studies had investigated cryotherapy as a preventive approach to laminitis, this study also supports the use of therapeutic digital hypothermia as a treatment for acute laminitis. This is not surprising due to the likelihood that the clinical stage of laminitis is a continuation (with some differences [e.g., physical tearing of lamellae]) of many of the inflammatory, vascular, and other destructive events observed during the prodromal stage. Although no studies have yet been conducted to dictate the length of time that horses with acute clinical laminitis should be treated with cryotherapy, the present author feels that it should be continued until there is no clinical evidence of lamellar inflammation (normal digital pulses and normal hoof temperature) and until pain is easily controlled with NSAIDs.

References

1. Baskett, A., Barton, M.H., Norton, N., *et al.* (1997) Effect of pentoxifylline, flunixin meglumine, and their combination on a model of endotoxemia in horses. *Am. J. Vet. Res.*, **58**, 121–129.
2. Forbes, G., Bailey, S.R., Church, S., *et al.* (2010) Effects of hyperimmune equine plasma on clinical and cellular responses in a low-dose endotoxemia model in horses. Proceedings of the Annual Meeting of the American College of Veterinary Internal Medicine.
3. Semrad, S.D., Hardee, G.E., Hardee, M.M., *et al.* (1987) Low-dose flunixin meglumine: effects on eicosanoid production and clinical signs induced by experimental endotoxaemia in horses. *Equine Vet. J.*, **19**, 201–206.
4. Barton, M.H., Parviainen, A., and Norton, A. (2004) Polymyxin B protects horses against induced endotoxaemia *in vivo*. *Equine Vet. J.*, **36**, 397–401.
5. Spier, S.J. (1990) Use of hyperimmune plasma containing antibody to gram-negative core antigens. Proceedings, *Annual Convention of the American Association of Equine Practitioners*, vol. **35**, pp. 91–94.
6. Forbes, G., Church, S., Savage, C.J., *et al.* (2012) Effects of hyperimmune equine plasma on clinical and cellular responses in a low-dose endotoxaemia model in horses. *Res. Vet. Sci.*, **92**, 40–44.
7. Peiró, J.R., Barnabé, P.A., Cadioli, F.A., *et al.* (2010) Effects of lidocaine infusion during experimental endotoxemia in horses. *J. Vet. Intern. Med.*, **24**, 940–948.
8. Huntjens, D.R., Danhof, M.D., and Pasqua, O.E. (2005) Pharmacokinetic-pharmacodynamic correlations and biomarkers in the development of COX-2 inhibitors. *Rheumatology (Oxford)*, **44**, 846–859.
9. Beretta, C., Garavaglia, G., and Cavalli, M. (2005) COX-1 and COX-2 inhibition in horse blood by phenylbutazone, flunixin, carprofen and meloxicam: an in vitro analysis. *Pharm. Res.*, **52**, 302–306.
10. Belknap, J.K., Giguère, S., Pittigrew, A., *et al.* (2007) Lamellar pro-inflammatory cytokine expression patterns in laminitis at the developmental stage and at the onset of lameness: innate vs. adaptive immune response. *Equine Vet. J.*, **39**, 42–47.
11. Waguespack, R.W., Cochran, A., and Belknap, J.K. (2004) Expression of the cyclooxygenase isoforms in the prodromal stage of black walnut-induced laminitis in horses. *Am. J. Vet. Res.*, **65**, 1724–1729.
12. Bilkslager, A.T., Yin, C., Cochran, A.M., *et al.* (2006) Cyclooxygenase expression in the early stages of equine laminitis: a cytologic study. *J. Vet. Intern. Med.*, **20**, 11911–1196.
13. Leise, B.S., Faleiros, R.R., Watts, M., *et al.* (2011) Laminar inflammatory gene expression in the carbohydrate overload model of equine laminitis. *Equine Vet. J.*, **43**, 54–61.
14. Yamaga, T., Tsuzuki, N., Seo Jong, P., *et al.* (2012) Effects of cyclooxygenase-2 inhibitor on equine gastric mucosa. *J. Jpn. Vet. Med. Assoc.*, **65**, 597.
15. Cox, S., Villarino, N., Sommardahl, C., *et al.* (2013) Disposition of firocoxib in equine plasma after an oral loading dose and a multiple dose regimen. *Vet. J.*, **98**, 382–385.
16. Noble, G., Edwards, S., Livevaart, J., *et al.* (2012) Pharmacokinetics and safety of single and multiple oral doses of meloxicam in adult horses. *J. Vet. Intern. Med.*, **26**, 1192–1201.
17. D'Arcy-Moskwa, E., Noble, G.K., Weston, L.A., *et al.* Effects of meloxicam and phenylbutazone on equine gastric mucosal permeability. *J. Vet. Intern. Med.*, **26**, 1494–1499.
18. Driessen, B., Bauquier, S.H., and Zarucco, L. (2010) Neuropathic pain management in chronic laminitis. *Vet. Clin. North Am. Equine Pract.*, **26**, 315–337.
19. Moore, J.N., Hardee, M.M., and Hardee, G.E. (1986) Modulation of arachidonic acid metabolism in endotoxic horses: comparison of flunixin meglumine, phenylbutazone, and a selective thromboxane synthetase inhibitor. *Am. J. Vet. Res.*, **47**, 110–113.
20. Bryant, C.E., Farnfield, B.A., and Janicke, H.J. (2003) Evaluation of the ability of carprofen and flunixin meglumine to inhibit activation of nuclear factor kappa B. *Am. J. Vet. Res.*, **64**, 211–215.
21. Jackman, B.R., More, J.N., Barton, M.H., *et al.* (1994) Comparison of the effects of ketoprofen and flunixin meglumine on the *in vitro* response of equine peripheral blood monocytes to bacterial endotoxin. *Can. J. Vet. Res.*, **58**, 138–143.
22. Leme, F.O.P., Wurzinger, L.J., Vasconcelos, A.C., *et al.* (2006) Platelet activation in equine with induced laminitis and treated with ketoprofen, phenylbutazone and flunixin meglumine. *Arq. Bras. Med. Vet. Zootec.*, **2**, 149–157.

23. Sangiah, S., MacAllister, C.C., and Amouzadeh, H.R. (1989) Effects of misoprostol and omeprazole on basal gastric pH and free acid content in horses. *Res. Vet. Sci.*, **47**, 350–354.
24. Reed, S.K., Messer, N.T., Tessman, R.K., *et al.* (2006) Effects of phenylbutazone alone or in combination with flunixin meglumine on blood protein concentrations in horses. *Am. J. Vet. Res.*, **67**, 398–402.
25. Cambridge, H., Lees, P., Hooke, R.E., *et al.* (1991) Antithrombotic actions of aspirin in the horse. *Equine Vet. J.*, **23**, 123–127.
26. Watts, A.E., Ness, S.L., Divers, T.J., *et al.* (2014) Effects of clopidogrel on horses with experimentally induced endotoxemia. *Am. J. Vet. Res.*, **75**, 760–769.
27. Menozzi, A., Pozzoli, C., Poli, E., *et al.* (2009) Effects of nonselective and selective cyclooxygenase inhibitors on small intestinal motility in the horse. *Res. Vet. Sci.*, **86**, 129–135.
28. Van Hoogmoed, L.M., Snyder, R., and Harmon, F. (2000) *In vitro* investigation of the effect of prostaglandins and nonsteroidal anti-inflammatory drugs on contractile activity of the equine smooth muscle of the dorsal colon, ventral colon, and pelvic flexure. *Am. J. Vet. Res.*, **61**, 1259–1266.
29. Mealey, K.L., Matthews, N.S., Peck, K.E., *et al.* (1997) Comparative pharmacokinetics of phenylbutazone and its metabolite oxyphenbutazone in clinically normal horses and donkeys. *Am. J. Vet. Res.*, **58**, 53–55.
30. Clutterbuck, A.L., Harris, P., Allaway, D., *et al.* (2010) Matrix metalloproteinases in inflammatory pathologies of the horse. *Vet. J.*, **183**, 27–38.
31. Kyaw-Tanner, M.T., Wattle, O., van Eps, A.W., *et al.* (2008) Equine laminitis: membrane type matrix metalloproteinase-1 (MMP-14) is involved in acute phase onset. *Equine Vet. J.*, **40**, 482-487.
32. Loftus, J.P., Johnson, P.J., Belknap, J.K., *et al.* (2009) Leukocyte-derived and endogenous matrix metalloproteinases in the malellae of horses with naturally acquired and experimentally induced laminitis. *Vet. Immunol. Immunopathol.*, **129**, 221–230.
33. Visser, M.B. and Pollitt, C.C. (2012) The timeline of metalloproteinase events during oligofructose induced equine laminitis development. *Equine Vet. J.*, **44**, 88–93.
34. Clutterbuck, A.L., Asplin, K.E., Harris, P., *et al.* (2009) Targeting matrix metalloproteinases in inflammatory conditions. *Curr. Drug Targets*, **10**, 1245–1254.
35. Eades, S.C. (2009) Laminitis research: Louisiana State University. Proceedings of the Fifth International Equine Conference on Laminitis and Diseases of the Foot, November, pp. 34–35.
36. Fortier, L.A., Motta, T., Greenwald, R.A., *et al.* (2010) Synoviocytes are more sensitive than cartilage to the effects of minocycline and doxycycline on IL-1α and MMP-13-induced catabolic gene responses. *J. Orthop. Res.*, **28**, 522–528.
37. Barton, M.H., Moore, J.N., and Norton, N. (1997) Effects of pentoxifylline infusion on response of horses to *in vivo* challenge exposure with endotoxin. *Am. J. Vet. Res.*, **58**, 1300–1307.
38. Kabbesh, N., Gogny, M., Chatagnon, G., *et al.* (2012) Vasodilatory effect of pentoxifylline in isolated equine digital veins. *Vet. J.*, **192**, 368–373.
39. Bailey, S.R., Adair, H.S., Reinemeyer, C.R., *et al.* (2009) Plasma concentrations of endotoxin and platelet activation in the developmental stage of oligofructose-induced laminitis. *Vet. Immunol. Immunopathol.*, **129**, 167–173.
40. Weiss, D.J. and Evanson, O.A. (2002) Evaluation of lipopolysaccharide-induced activation of equine neutrophils. *Am. J. Vet. Res.*, **63**, 811–815.
41. Weiss, D.J., Evanson, O.A., McClenahan, D., *et al.* (1997) Evaluation of platelet activation and platelet-neutrophil aggregates in ponies with alimentary laminitis. *Am. J. Vet. Res.*, **58**, 1376–1380.
42. Weiss, D.J., Evanson, O.A., McClenahan, D., *et al.* (1998) Effect of a competitive inhibitor of platelet aggregation on experimentally induced laminitis in ponies. *Am. J. Vet. Res.*, **59**, 814–817.
43. Robertson, T.P., Bailey, S.R., and Peroni, J.F. (2009) Equine laminitis: a journal to the dark side of venous. *Vet. Immunol. Immunopathol.*, **129**, 164–166.
44. de la Rebière de Pouyade, G., Grulke, S., Detilleux, J., *et al.* (2009) Evaluation of low-molecular-weight heparin for the prevention of equine laminitis after colic surgery. *J. Vet. Emerg. Crit. Care (San Antonio)*, **19**, 113–119.
45. de la Rebière de Pouyade, G., Franek, T., Deby-Dupong, G., *et al.* (2008) Effects of unfractionated and fractionated heparins on myeloperoxidase activity and interactions with endothelial cells: possible effects on the pathophysiology of equine laminitis. *Vet. J.*, **178**, 62–69.
46. Cook, V.L., Neuder, L.E., Blikslager, A.T., *et al.* (2009) The effect of lidocaine on *in vitro* adhesion and migration of equine neutrophils. *Vet. Immunol. Immunopathol.*, **129**, 137–142.
47. Williams, J.M., Lin, Y.J., Loftus, J.P., *et al.* (2010) Effect of intravenous lidocaine administration on laminar inflammation in the black walnut extract model of laminitis. *Equine Vet. J.*, **42**, 261–269.
48. Faleiros, R.R. (2009) Laminitis research: Escika de Veterinària, Universidade Minas Gerais, Brazil. Proceedings of the Fifth International Equine Conference on Laminitis and Diseases of the Foot, November, pp. 40–41.
49. Loftus, J.P., Belknap, J.K., Stankiewicz, K.M., *et al.* (2007) Laminar xanthine oxidase, superoxide dismutase and catalase activities in the prodromal stage of black-walnut induced equine laminitis. *Equine Vet. J.*, **39**, 48–53.
50. Katz, L.M. and Bailey, S.R. (2011) A review of recent advances and current hypotheses on the pathogenesis of acute laminitis. *Equine Vet. J.*, **44**, 752–761.
51. Van Eps, A.W. and Pollitt, C.C. (2009) Equine laminitis model: cryotherapy reduces the severity of lesions evaluated seven days after induction with oligofructose. *Equine Vet. J.*, **41**, 741–747.
52. Van Eps, A.W., Leise, B.S., Watts, M., *et al.* (2012) Equine digital hypothermia inhibits early lamellar inflammatory signaling in the oligofructose laminitis model. *Vet. J.*, **44**, 230–237.
53. Kullmann, A., Holcombe, S.J., Hurcombe, S.D., *et al.* (2014) Prophylactic digital cryotherapy is associated with decreased incidence of laminitis in horses diagnosed with colitis. *Equine Vet. J.*, **46**, 554–559.
54. Reesink, H.L., Divers, T.J., Bookbinder, L.C., *et al.* (2012) Measurement of digital laminar and venous temperatures as a means of comparing three methods of topically applied cold treatment for digits of horses. *Am. J. Vet. Res.*, **73**, 860–866.
55. Van Eps, A.W., Pollitt, C.C., Underwood, C., *et al.* (2014) Continuous digital hypothermia initiated after the onset of lameness prevents lamellar failure in the oligofructose laminitis model. *Equine Vet. J.*, **46**, 625–630.

CHAPTER 32

Vasoactive Drug Therapy

Simon R. Bailey and Susan C. Eades

Introduction

Vascular changes have been observed both in the carbohydrate overload (CHO) and black walnut extract (BWE) models of acute sepsis-related laminitis (SRL) laminitis, and therefore it has been suggested that vasoconstriction or dysfunction may occur during the prodromal stage of laminitis, resulting in a decreased blood flow to the lamellar tissues. During the early stages of laminitis induced by starch overload, an increase in postcapillary resistance caused by digital venoconstriction reportedly occurs, resulting in a decreased blood flow to the lamellae [1]. In both the starch-overload and BWE model, an increase in capillary pressure was found which was proposed to cause transvascular fluid movement resulting in increased tissue pressure and edema formation [2,3]. Based on these findings, it was postulated that further increases in tissue pressure could collapse capillary beds and lead to tissue ischemia. However, it has been very difficult to establish whether these vascular changes play an important role in lamellar failure, or are merely associated with the inflammatory changes that are also observed. In more recent studies of sepsis-related laminitis (SRL), evidence of ischemia within the lamellar tissues has not been forthcoming, casting doubt on whether vascular disturbances are likely to be a primary initiating factor in the laminitis disease process [4]. Such disturbances could however play a contributing and synergistic pathophysiologic role in combination with inflammatory mechanisms [5].

Several vasoconstrictor agents have been identified that are released during laminitis, the most potent being serotonin (5-hydroxytryptamine; 5-HT), thromboxane and endothelin-1 (ET-1). 5-HT is a vasoactive amine released from activated platelets during acute laminitis [6], and is particularly potent in causing equine digital venoconstriction [7] (which would be consistent with the hemodynamic changes observed in a number of laminitis induction studies). Additional amine-type compounds with venoconstrictive actions similar to 5-HT have also been shown to be produced by bacteria in the equine hindgut in response to readily fermentable carbohydrate [8], with these compounds (including tyramine, tryptamine, and phenylethylamine) then being absorbed from the large intestine into the bloodstream [9].

Thromboxane, released from platelets, is also a very potent vasoconstrictor and may be released in sepsis/endotoxemia endotoxemia associated with SRL [6]. Many other prostanoid compounds are also released locally around the lamellar tissues and blood vessels. These include the vasoconstrictor prostaglandins PGF2α and PGE2, and the vasodilator prostacyclin (PGI2). In addition to prostanoids which have vasoconstrictor effects, isoprostanes may also be formed by the nonenzymatic free radical-catalyzed peroxidation of arachidonic acid. These agents, studied in the BWE model of SRL, cause vasoconstriction by stimulating thromboxane receptors and other prostanoid receptors [10].

Endothelial activation upregulates adhesion molecule expression on the luminal surface, which facilitates the adhesion of leukocytes to the endothelium followed by extravasation of neutrophils and other leukocytes into the lamellar tissues [4]. This may be further enhanced by chemotactic factors (chemokines) released locally [11]. The endothelium also releases vasoconstrictor mediators such as ET-1 which has been found to be a more potent vasoconstrictor of equine digital veins than arteries [7,12], and could therefore contribute to the selective venoconstriction proposed to occur during the developmental phases of laminitis [1].

A normal-functioning vascular endothelium is important for maintaining blood flow through the tissues, by releasing the endogenous vasodilator, nitric oxide (NO) [13]. Inflammation or activation of the endothelium can reduce NO production and induce the production of ET-1. There are also other vasodilatory defense mechanisms to promote the maintenance of blood flow through the equine digit. Substance P (SP) and calcitonin gene-related peptide (CGRP) are both important vasodilatory neuropeptides stored in endothelial cells as well as Sensory-motor nerves. Sensory-motor nerves are important mediators of peripheral vascular flow, and it has been suggested that dysregulation of this neuronal control might also be involved in the pathophysiology of equine acute laminitis [14,15].

Equine Laminitis, First Edition. Edited by James K. Belknap and Raymond Geor.

As well as some evidence of vasoconstriction being present during the early prodromal phases of acute laminitis, it is likely that vasodilation occurs in the acute phase, supported by increases in dorsal hoof wall temperature [16]. However, the increased blood flow may be primarily through the arteriovenous anastomoses, which are particularly numerous in this vascular bed [17], rather than through the nutrient capillaries. Vasodilation is consistent with the inflammatory changes observed during the acute phase of SRL, and one of the main inflammatory mediators causing vasodilation is prostacyclin (PGI2, released from the activated vascular endothelium) [18].

Vasoactive Drugs

A number of drugs with vasoactive properties have been used in the treatment of laminitis; these drugs have been used most in SRL, where lamellar ischemia was thought to be the central event resulting in lamellar failure during the early stages of laminitis. Most of these drugs are used with less frequency than in the past, both due to the fact that ischemia does not appear to be the major factor in SRL or endocrinopathic laminitis (although it still appears to be important in supporting limb laminitis), but also because the majority of these drugs have been proven to not increase lamellar blood flow. A major concern with the studies described below to assess the efficacy of the different drugs is the variability in scientific methodology, with none of the methods demonstrated unequivocally to assess lamellar microvascular blood flow.

Acepromazine

Acetylpromazine (acepromazine) is a phenothiazine derivative and is a frequently used tranquilizer in the horse. It is the most common vasodilator used for the treatment of laminitis [19]. Its sedative effects are explained by its actions as an alpha-adrenoceptor antagonist (with a short duration of action), and its vasodilator properties are also mainly associated with alpha$_1$-adrenoceptor blockade in vascular smooth muscle [20, 21]. Equine digital blood vessels are well-innervated and have many alpha$_1$- and alpha$_2$-adrenoceptors on their smooth muscle cells, with both mediating vasoconstriction [22, 23]. However, the class of drugs to which acetylpromazine belongs is relatively nonselective in its actions, and therefore there are also significant actions at several other receptor subtypes relevant to vasoconstriction and laminitis. For example, acepromazine also competitively inhibits the contractile effects of serotonin (5-HT) in both equine digital arteries and veins, by blocking 5-HT$_2$ receptors (S. Bailey, unpublished data). Serotonin may have significance in Equine Laminitis because it is released from activated platelets during the early prodromal stage [6] (see Chapter 12). Furthermore, as mentioned above, several compounds produced by bacteria in the equine hindgut in response to CHO can also cause vasoconstriction via these alpha-adrenoceptors and serotonin receptors [24,25]. After NSAIDs, acepromazine is likely to be the most common drug used by practitioners to treat laminitis; indeed, at one time, acepromazine was used in around one-third of laminitis cases in some areas [26]. In one study of laminitis cases observed in private practice in the United Kingdom, a somewhat weak association between acepromazine and survival was reported [27].

Research Regarding Acepromazine

Whether through local direct effects on blood vessel receptors, and/or via central effects on the sympathetic nervous system, the effects of acepromazine on blood flow in the distal limb may be quite profound, and have been demonstrated using ultrasonography [28]. Healthy horses instrumented with flow probes were also used to indicate that this drug had significant effects on improving digital vascular blood flow [29, 30]. In a recent study in which catheters were placed in the lamellar dermis to obtain interstitial fluid to assess metabolite concentration and urea clearance (as an indicator of blood flow in the lamellar microvasculature), acepromazine administration did not change lamellar blood flow [31]. Leise *et al.* [32] demonstrated very weak vasodilatory effects at low doses with minimal sedative effects. Therefore, it may be possible to slightly increase digital blood flow (of the large capacitance vessels) with acepromazine, without improving blood flow to the lamellae.

Phenoxybenzamine

Phenoxybenzamine is another phenothiazine derivative, which has also been used in the prevention and treatment of acute laminitis. Phenoxybenzamine is also principally an alpha$_1$-adrenoceptor antagonist, acting on the central nervous system (CNS) and also locally on smooth muscle of the peripheral vasculature, including that of the digit [21,33]. The main difference in the pharmacology of this compound, however, is that it binds irreversibly to and alkylates the receptors, producing much longer-lasting effects [34]. Like acetylpromazine, phenoxybenzamine has a wide range of pharmacological effects other than blocking alpha-adrenoceptors, including 5-HT$_2$ receptor antagonist properties in digital arteries and veins and also 5-HT$_1$ antagonist effects in digital arteries [35].

In one early study, phenoxybenzamine was reported to reduce the severity of CHO-induced laminitis and to prevent pedal bone rotation in a group of seven horses [36]; unfortunately, however, there was no control group (i.e., a group which received CHO but not phenoxybenzamine) with which to compare the results of the phenoxybenzamine-treated animals. Interestingly, in this study the beta-adrenoreceptor antagonist, propranolol (which also has 5-HT$_{1A}$ and 5-HT$_{1B}$ receptor blocking actions as well as blocking beta-adrenoceptors [35]), reportedly exacerbated the disease process [37].

Domperidone

Domperidone is a benzimidazole derivative which exhibits similar receptor antagonist profiles to acepromazine and phenoxybenzamine, and has been postulated to be of use in the treatment of laminitis, though clear evidence of efficacy in treating the disease has not yet been produced. The major difference between the clinical effects of domperidone, and the phenothiazines acepromazine and phenoxybenzamine, would be a lack of sedative effects with domperidone. It is thought that this compound does not cross the blood–brain barrier to a significant extent [38]. Domperidone is also known as a dopamine D_2 receptor antagonist, although it does not appear that D_2 receptors are present in equine digital blood vessels. *In-vitro* studies with equine digital arteries and veins have shown that it inhibits vascular contractions brought about by the stimulation of alpha$_1$-adrenoceptors and 5-HT_2 receptors (S. Bailey, unpublished data). *In vivo*, intravenous domperidone significantly increased digital lamellar microvascular blood flow in normal horses, as measured with laser Doppler flowmetry [39].

Pentoxifylline

Pentoxifylline is a nonspecific phosphodiesterase inhibitor belonging to the methylxanthine group of compounds. By boosting intracellular levels of the signaling secondary messengers, cyclic adenosine monophosphate (cAMP) and cyclic guanosine monophosphate (cGMP), it has numerous effects in different cell types throughout the body. cAMP causes vasodilation in vascular smooth muscle cells by inactivating the enzyme myosin light chain kinase [40]. In addition, pentoxifylline has documented hemorrheologic properties, improving the flexibility and deformability of erythrocytes to alter blood viscosity [41]. Pentoxifylline increased red blood cell (RBC) filtrability in horses, an effect that may be due to increased RBC deformability [42]. This drug may also be beneficial as an anti-inflammatory agent, because phosphodiesterase enzyme subtypes are important in leukocytes and platelets. It inhibits leukocyte activation in endotoxemia, reducing the production of proinflammatory cytokines such as tumor necrosis factor alpha (TNFα) [43], and also inhibits platelet aggregation [44].

Pentoxifylline administration (8.5 mg kg^{-1}, intravenous at 12-h intervals) also decreases lamellar matrix metalloprotease (MMP) concentrations; it had the most potent inhibitory effects on pro-MMP-9 and moderate inhibitory effects on pro-MMP-2 production, when compared with oxytetracycline, flunixin meglumine, and doxycycline in horses with experimentally induced endotoxemia [45]. Although the mechanism by which pentoxifylline reduced MMP production during endotoxemia is unknown, there are several actions of pentoxifylline that could play a role. A reduction in MMP production could be an indirect effect of leukocyte inhibition [46]. Pentoxifylline also decreases MMP mRNA synthesis [47]. Pentoxifylline (8.5 mg kg^{-1}, intravenous at 12-h intervals) also reduced the severity of lameness in horses with laminitis induced by corn starch overload [48]. There is also substantial evidence suggesting that pentoxifylline reduces blood glucose concentrations after diabetes induction in rats by improving insulin receptor sensitivity [49]; this would make it a potential therapeutic agent for laminitis associated with metabolic disease.

Isoxsuprine

Isoxsuprine hydrochloride was at one time widely used as a peripheral vasodilator, although its efficacy in the treatment of laminitis remains unproven [29,50]. It has been shown to act mainly as an alpha$_1$-adrenoceptor antagonist in equine digital blood vessels, but also had weak beta$_2$-adrenoceptor agonist and calcium channel antagonist properties [51, 52]. In one early study, isoxsuprine (0.6 mg kg^{-1}, intravenous) was shown to cause a decrease in systemic vascular resistance (indicative of peripheral vasodilation), but also caused CNS excitement [53]. However, when administered orally at the same dose twice daily, not only were there no cardiovascular effects but the drug could not be detected in the plasma (i.e., it was not absorbed) [53]. In another study, no pharmacological effect was observed in horses administered oral isoxsuprine at twice that dose (1.2 mg kg^{-1} b.i.d.) for eight days [54]. In one study using a laser Doppler flow probe to assess lamellar blood flow in healthy horses, although acetylpromazine increased blood flow to the digit, isoxuprine had no significant effect [29]. Therefore, the data overall suggest minimal absorption or vascular effects of isoxsuprine when administered orally, while the intravenous dose reported to cause a decrease in systemic vascular resistance is not acceptable due to CNS side effects.

Glyceryl Trinitrate

Glyceryl trinitrate (GTN; also known as nitroglycerine) was advocated as a treatment for laminitis during the late 1990s, based on earlier studies showing the contribution of NO to maintaining vasodilator tone in equine digital blood vessels. Nitric oxide is a labile endogenous vasodilator produced by the endothelium in vascular beds, including the equine digital circulation [55, 56]. GTN is a NO donor, which was administered as a gel on the skin above the hoof and reportedly absorbed transcutaneously [5]). Although initially it was suggested that this preparation would enhance perfusion within the hoof [58], it was later shown that transdermal application above the hoof, as an ointment or patches, was not effective in altering digital blood flow [59]. Furthermore, the finding that topical application of GTN over the pastern reduced the mean systemic blood pressure without increasing digital perfusion suggested that the compound was being absorbed into the subcutaneous and digital veins and cleared from the area in a proximal direction, without being delivered to the foot [60]. In an extracorporeal model of the distal limb using the starch overload laminitis model, nitroglycerine infusion into the arterial side of the (isolated) digital circulation caused a decrease in total vascular resistance but did not alter postcapillary resistance [61].

It should be noted that although boosting NO levels may not provide targeted vasodilation to the foot, it may nevertheless have some beneficial effects in systemic inflammation and inflammatory laminitis, including the inhibition of platelet aggregation and the scavenging of free radicals [62, 63].

Dimethyl Sulfoxide

Dimethyl sulfoxide (DMSO) has a number of pharmacologic actions which may be potentially beneficial in the treatment and prevention of acute laminitis [50]. It is reported to have properties as a free radical scavenger, an anti-inflammatory agent, and an inhibitor of platelet aggregation and endothelial cell protector [64, 65]. Although DMSO has been purported to cause vasodilation, evidence of vasodilation has not been substantiated. The cell membrane-stabilizing effects described for this compound may also be a factor. DMSO was of great interest as a therapeutic drug during the 1980s and 1990s in both human and veterinary medicine; in one study conducted during the early 1990s, DMSO was used in more than 25% of laminitis cases. However, interest in the drug has waned in human medicine, and there have been no conclusive studies to confirm any benefits in the treatment of horses for laminitis, including as a free radical scavenger (its major purported benefit during the 1980s) or as a vasodilator.

Experimental Drugs: Endothelin and 5-HT Receptor Antagonists, and Calcium Channel Blockers

Receptor antagonist drugs that block the vascular actions of the potent vasoconstrictors, endothelin and 5-HT, on the equine digit have been evaluated *in vitro* and *in vivo*. However, none of these drugs has been successfully trialed in laminitis models designed to evaluate lamellar pathology or lameness. In the CHO model of experimental laminitis, the nonselective endothelin receptor antagonist, PD145065, was infused into the digital arterial circulation and had significant vascular effects, decreasing postcapillary resistance [3]. The effect on lameness and lamellar damage could not be assessed in this terminal anesthesia model. In an equine low-dose endotoxin challenge model, the 5-HT_1 receptor antagonist, GR55562, was administered together with aspirin to counteract the digital hypoperfusion caused by 5-HT and thromboxane release from lipopolysaccharide (LPS)-activated platelets [66]. The combination of the two drugs inhibited LPS-induced digital hypoperfusion.

One of the very few reports which claimed efficacy for a drug in the reduction or prevention of clinical signs of acute laminitis was for the calcium channel blocker, BAYTG 1000 [67]. This dihydropyridine compound was reported to subjectively decrease the severity of lameness after CHO, although it did not reduce the incidence of lameness or laminitis. Although it was mainly thought to have a rheologic activity, the dihydropyridines are vasodilators with a relative selectivity towards vascular L-type calcium channels compared with the cardiac channels. No further investigations have been conducted with this drug.

Drugs with Indirect Vasoactive Properties: NSAIDs

Nonsteroidal anti-inflammatory drugs (NSAIDs) block two cyclo-oxygenase enzymes, COX-1 and COX-2, that are both involved in the generation of the same basic prostaglandin, PGH2. Different prostaglandin synthase enzymes present in different cell types produce specific prostanoids from PGH2. COX-1 is generally classed as a constitutive enzyme, because it is constantly expressed in many cell types, whereas COX-2 is generally more tightly controlled, being induced by many cell signaling events, including many inflammatory events. Prostaglandin release is an important feature of the inflammatory changes that occur in the CHO or BWE models of acute laminitis [68]. NSAIDs are commonly used in the treatment of this condition, indicated for their role as analgesics, but also have been purported to be protective of the digital vasculature by blocking the perceived cycle of pain and resulting hypertension [69]. However, as came to light with the cardiovascular crises with the human COX-2 inhibitor rofecoxib (Vioxx®), the effect of NSAIDs on the vasculature is more complex than that. Prostanoids produced in the vasculature include both potent vasodilators such as prostacyclin (and PGE2 depending on the PG receptors present), and potent vasoconstrictors such as thromboxane. Whereas, the vasoconstrictor thromboxane is mainly produced in platelets via COX-1 (platelets cannot produce COX-2 because of their lack of a nucleus), prostacyclin is primarily produced in the endothelial cells lining the vasculature which are more heavily regulated by COX-2 than COX-1. Therefore, nonselective NSAIDs such as phenylbutazone and flunixin will block the production of both vasodilators and vasoconstrictors by blocking COX-1 and COX-2, and it is therefore unknown what effect will occur regarding vasoconstriction or vasodilation. Some COX-2-selective NSAIDs may primarily block the production of vasodilators by the endothelium, thus more likely resulting in vasoconstriction by the continued production of thromboxane by the platelets (which are not affected by COX-2 inhibition); this was the result in an at-risk population of humans suffering heart attacks and treated with rofecoxib. This effect of COX-2 inhibitors again appears complex, as some appear to protect against a vasoactive environment within the vasculature [70]. It is not known whether firocoxib or meloxicam, the primary COX-2-selective NSAIDs used in horses (with firocoxib more COX-2-selective), result in: (i) a vasoactive environment prone to vasoconstriction (as seen with rofecoxib), or (ii) protection against such a vasoactive incident. It is possible that the nonselective NSAIDs are more protective due to inhibiting thromboxane production by platelets and therefore platelet aggregation (and possible vasoconstriction) in events such as endotoxemia documented to result in platelet activation [50,71].

In summary, there is no compelling evidence that any of the drugs discussed above and commonly used in the treatment of laminitis improve lamellar blood flow. As experimental techniques improve over the next few decades, hopefully it will become possible not only to definitively establish whether ischemia plays an important role in the disease process of the different types of laminitis, but also to accurately assess the effects of candidate drugs *in vivo* on lamellar microvascular flow dynamics.

References

1. Allen, D., Jr, Clark, E.S., Moore, J.N., and Prasse, K.W. (1990) Evaluation of equine digital Starling forces and hemodynamics during early laminitis. *Am. J. Vet. Res.*, **51** (12), 1930–1934.
2. Eaton, S.A., Allen, D., Eades, S.C., and Schneider, D.A. (1995) Digital Starling forces and hemodynamics during early laminitis induced by an aqueous extract of black walnut (*Juglans nigra*) in horses. *Am. J. Vet. Res.*, **56** (10), 1338–1344.
3. Eades, S.C., Stokes, A.M., and Moore, R.M. (2006) Effects of an endothelin receptor antagonist and nitroglycerin on digital vascular function in horses during the prodromal stages of carbohydrate overload-induced laminitis. *Am. J. Vet. Res.*, **67** (7), 1204–1211.
4. Loftus, J.P., Belknap, J.K., Stankiewicz, K.M., and Black, S.J. (2007) Laminar xanthine oxidase, superoxide dismutase and catalase activities in the prodromal stage of black-walnut induced equine laminitis. *Equine Vet. J.*, **39** (1), 48–53.
5. Brooks, A.C., Menzies-Gow, N., Bailey, S.R., Cunningham, F.M., and Elliott, J. (2010) Endotoxin-induced HIF-1alpha stabilisation in equine endothelial cells: synergistic action with hypoxia. *Inflamm. Res.*, **59** (9), 689–698.
6. Bailey, S.R., Adair, H.S., Reinemeyer, C.R., Morgan, S.J., Brooks, A.C., Longhofer, S.L., *et al.* (2009) Plasma concentrations of endotoxin and platelet activation in the developmental stage of oligofructose-induced laminitis. *Vet. Immunol. Immunopathol.*, **129** (3-4), 167–173.
7. Peroni, J.F., Moore, J.N., Noschka, E., Grafton, M.E., Aceves-Avila, M., Lewis, S.J., *et al.* (2006) Predisposition for venoconstriction in the equine laminar dermis: implications in equine laminitis. *J. Appl. Physiol.*, **100** (3), 759–763.
8. Bailey, S.R., Baillon, M.L., Rycroft, A.N., Harris, P.A., and Elliott, J. (2003) Identification of equine cecal bacteria producing amines in an in vitro model of carbohydrate overload. *Appl. Environ. Microbiol.*, **69** (4), 2087–2093.
9. Botteon, P.T.L., Ferraz, V.P., Glória, M.B.A., Melo, M.M., Paes Leme, F.O., Faleiros, R.R., *et al.* (2008) Plasma concentrations of tryptamine, tyramine and phenylethylamine in horses under the effect of carbohydrate overload and non-steroidal anti-inflammatory compounds. *Pesq. Vet. Bras.*, **28**, 299–302.
10. Noschka, E., Moore, J.N., Peroni, J.F., Lewis, S.J., Morrow, J.D., and Robertson, T.P. (2009) Thromboxane and isoprostanes as inflammatory and vasoactive mediators in black walnut heartwood extract induced equine laminitis. *Vet. Immunol. Immunopathol.*, **129** (3-4), 200–210.
11. Faleiros, R.R., Johnson, P.J., Nuovo, G.J., Messer, N.T., Black, S.J., and Belknap, J.K. (2011) Laminar leukocyte accumulation in horses with carbohydrate overload-induced laminitis. *J. Vet. Intern. Med./Am. Coll. Vet. Intern. Med.*, **25** (1), 107–115.
12. Katz, L.M., Marr, C.M., and Elliott, J. (2003) Characterization and comparison of the responses of equine digital arteries and veins to endothelin-1. *Am. J. Vet. Res.*, **64** (11), 1438–1443.
13. Berhane, Y., Bailey, S.R., Putignano, C., and Elliott, J. (2008) Characterization of agonist-induced endothelium-dependent vasodilatory responses in the vascular bed of the equine digit. *J. Vet. Pharmacol. Ther.*, **31** (1), 1–8.
14. Katz, L.M., Marr, C.M., and Elliott, J. (2003) Characterisation of the response of equine digital arteries and veins to substance P. *J. Vet. Pharmacol. Ther.*, **26** (5), 361–368.
15. Katz, L.M., Marr, C.M., and Elliott, J. (2011) Characterization of the responses of equine digital veins and arteries to calcitonin gene-related peptide. *Am. J. Vet. Res.*, **72** (7), 975–981.
16. Pollitt, C.C. and Davies, C.T. (1998) Equine laminitis: its development coincides with increased sublamellar blood flow. *Equine Vet. J. Suppl.*, **September**, 125–132.
17. Pollitt, C.C. and Molyneux, G.S. (1990) A scanning electron microscopical study of the dermal microcirculation of the equine foot. *Equine Vet. J.*, **22** (2), 79–87.
18. Bailey, S.R. and Elliott, J. (1999) The role of prostanoids and nitric oxide in endotoxin-induced hyporesponsiveness of equine digital blood vessels. *Equine Vet. J.*, **31** (3), 212–218.
19. Stashak, T.S. (1987) *Laminitis. Adams' Lameness in Horses*, 4th edition. Lea & Febiger Publications, Philadelphia, pp. 486–499.
20. Baxter, G.M., Tackett, R.L., and Moore, J.N. (1989) Reactivity of equine palmar digital arteries and veins to vasodilating agents. *Vet. Surg.*, **18** (3), 221–226.
21. Boosman, R. and Nemeth, F. (1988) Pathogenesis and drug-therapy of acute laminitis in horses – a review. *Tijdschr. Diergeneesk.*, **113** (22), 1237–1246.
22. Elliott, J. (1997) Alpha-adrenoceptors in equine digital veins: evidence for the presence of both alpha1 and alpha2-receptors mediating vasoconstriction. *J. Vet. Pharmacol. Ther.*, **20** (4), 308–317.
23. Zerpa, H., Bailey, S.R., Berhane, Y., and Elliott, J. (2006) Pharmacological characterization of alpha1-adrenoceptors in equine digital veins. *J. Vet. Pharmacol. Ther.*, **29** (1), 55–61.
24. Bailey, S.R., Menzies-Gow, N.J., Marr, C.M., and Elliott, J. (2004) The effects of vasoactive amines found in the equine hindgut on digital blood flow in the normal horse. *Equine Vet. J.*, **36** (3), 267–272.
25. Elliott, J., Berhane, Y., and Bailey, S.R. (2003) Effects of monoamines formed in the cecum of horses on equine digital blood vessels and platelets. *Am. J. Vet. Res.*, **64** (9), 1124–1131.
26. Slater, M.R., Hood, D.M., and Carter, G.K. (1995) Descriptive epidemiological study of equine laminitis. *Equine Vet. J.*, **27** (5), 364–367.
27. Menzies-Gow, N.J., Stevens, K., Barr, A., Camm, I., Elliot, S.B., and Longhofer, S.L. (2010) Severity and outcome of equine pasture-associated laminintis managed in first opinion practice in the UK. *Vet. Rec.*, **167** (10), 364–369.
28. Walker, M. and Geiser, D. (1986) Effects of acetylpromazine on the hemodynamics of the equine metatarsal artery, as determined by two-dimensional real-time and pulsed Doppler ultrasonography. *Am. J. Vet. Res.*, **47** (5), 1075–1078.
29. Ingle-Fehr, J.E. and Baxter, G.M. (1999) The effect of oral isoxsuprine and pentoxifylline on digital and laminar blood flow in healthy horses. *Vet. Surg.*, **28** (3), 154–160.
30. Adair, H.S., III, Goble, D.O., Shires, G.M., and Sanders, W.L. (1994) Evaluation of laser Doppler flowmetry for measuring coronary band and laminar microcirculatory blood flow in clinically normal horses. *Am. J. Vet. Res.*, **55** (4), 445–449.
31. Medina-Torres, C.E., Underwood, C., Pollitt, C.C., Castro-Olivera, E.M., Hodson, M.P., Richardson, D.W., *et al.* (2016) Microdialysis measurements of equine lamellar perfusion and energy metabolism in response to physical and pharmacological manipulations of blood flow. *Equine Vet. J.*, **48** (2), 246–252.
32. Leise, B.S., Fugler, L.A., Stokes, A.M., Eades, S.C., and Moore, R.M. (2007) Effects of intramuscular administration of acepromazine on

palmar digital blood flow, palmar digital arterial pressure, transverse facial arterial pressure, and packed cell volume in clinically healthy, conscious horses. *Vet. Surg.*, **36** (8), 717–723.

33. Baxter, G.M., Laskey, R.E., Tackett, R.L., Moore, J.N., and Allen, D. (1989) In vitro reactivity of digital arteries and veins to vasoconstrictive mediators in healthy horses and in horses with early laminitis. *Am. J. Vet. Res.*, **50** (4), 508–517.
34. Salles, J., Gascon, S., Ivorra, D., and Badia, A. (1994) In vivo recovery of alpha 1-adrenoceptors in rat myocardial tissue after alkylation with phenoxybenzamine. *Eur. J. Pharmacol.*, **266** (1), 35–42.
35. Bailey, S.R. (1998) A study of the vascular effects and factors regulating the concentration of 5-hydroxytryptamine in the equine digital circulation. Thesis, University of London.
36. Hood, D.M., Stephens, K.A., and Bowen, M.J. (1982) Phenoxybenzamine for the treatment of severe nonresponsive diarrhea in the horse. *J. Am. Vet. Med. Assoc.*, **180** (7), 758–762.
37. Hood, D.M., Stephens, K.A., and Amoss, M.S. (1982) The use of alpha- and beta-adrenergic blockade as a preventative in the carbohydrate model of laminitis: a preliminary report. *Am. Assoc. Equine Pract. Newsletter*, **2**, 142–146.
38. Tonini, M., Cipollina, L., Poluzzi, E., Crema, F., Corazza, G.R., and De Ponti, F. (2004) Review article: clinical implications of enteric and central D2 receptor blockade by antidopaminergic gastrointestinal prokinetics. *Aliment. Pharmacol. Ther.*, **19** (4), 379–390.
39. Castro, J.R., Adair, H.S., III, Radecki, S.V., Kiefer, V.R., Elliot, S.B., and Longhofer, S.L. (2010) Effects of domperidone on digital laminar microvascular blood flow in clinically normal adult horses. *Am. J. Vet. Res.*, **71** (3), 281–287.
40. Morgado, M., Cairrao, E., Santos-Silva, A.J., and Verde, I. (2012) Cyclic nucleotide-dependent relaxation pathways in vascular smooth muscle. *Cell. Mol. Life Sci.*, **69** (2), 247–266.
41. DePerri, T., Forconi, S., and Agnusdei, D. (1975) The effects of intravenous isoxsuprine on blood viscosity in patients with occlusive peripheral arterial disease. *Br. J. Clin. Pharmacol.*, **5**, 255–260.
42. Weiss, D.J., Evanson, O.A., and Geor, R.J. (1994) The effects of furosemide and pentoxifylline on the flow properties of equine erythrocytes: *in vitro* studies. *Vet. Res. Commun.*, **18** (5), 373–381.
43. Baskett, A., Barton, M.H., Norton, N., Anders, B., and Moore, J.N. (1997) Effect of pentoxifylline, flunixin meglumine, and their combination on a model of endotoxemia in horses. *Am. J. Vet. Res.*, **58** (11), 1291–1299.
44. Schroer, R.H. (1985) Antithrombotic potential of pentoxifylline. A hemorheologically active drug. *Angiology*, **36** (6), 387–398.
45. Fugler, L.A., Eades, S.C., Moore, R.M., Koch, C.E., and Keowen, M.L. (2013) Plasma matrix metalloproteinase activity in horses after intravenous infusion of lipopolysaccharide and treatment with matrix metalloproteinase inhibitors. *Am. J. Vet. Res.*, **74** (3), 473–480.
46. Loftus, J.P., Johnson, P.J., Belknap, J.K., Pettigrew, A., and Black, S.J. (2009) Leukocyte-derived and endogenous matrix metalloproteinases in the lamellae of horses with naturally acquired and experimentally induced laminitis. *Vet. Immunol. Immunopathol.*, **129** (3-4), 221–230.
47. Oger, S., Mehats, C., Dallot, E., Cabrol, D., and Leroy, M.J. (2005) Evidence for a role of phosphodiesterase 4 in lipopolysaccharide-stimulated prostaglandin E2 production and matrix metalloproteinase-9 activity in human amniochorionic membranes. *J. Immunol. (Baltimore, Md: 1950)*, **174** (12), 8082–8089.
48. Fugler, L.A., Eades, S.C., Koch, C.E., and Keowen, M.L. (2010) Clinical and matrix metalloproteinase inhibitory effects of pentoxifylline on carbohydrate overload laminitis: preliminary results. *J. Equine Vet. Sci.*, **30** (2), 106–107.
49. Garcia, F.A., Pinto, S.F., Cavalcante, A.F., Lucetti, L.T., Menezes, S.M., Felipe, C.F., *et al.* (2014) Pentoxifylline decreases glycemia levels and TNF-alpha, iNOS and COX-2 expressions in diabetic rat pancreas. *SpringerPlus*, **3**, 283.
50. Goetz, T.E. (1989) The treatment of laminitis in horses. *Vet. Clin. North Am. Equine Pract.*, **5** (1), 73–108.
51. Belloli, C., Carcano, R., Arioli, F., and Beretta, C. (2000) Affinity of isoxsuprine for adrenoreceptors in equine digital artery and implications for vasodilatory action. *Equine Vet. J.*, **32** (2), 119–124.
52. Elliott, J. and Soydan, J. (1995) Characterisation of beta-adrenoceptors in equine digital veins: implications of the modes of vasodilatory action of isoxsuprine. *Equine Vet. J. Suppl.*, **September**, 101–107.
53. Matthews, N.S., Gleed, R.D., Short, C.E., and Burrows, K. (1986) Cardiovascular and pharmacokinetic effects of isoxsuprine in the horse. *Am. J. Vet. Res.*, **47** (10), 2130–2133.
54. Harkins, J.D., Mundy, G.D., Stanley, S., Woods, W.E., Sams, R.A., Richardson, D.R., *et al.* (1998) Absence of detectable pharmacological effects after oral administration of isoxsuprine. *Equine Vet. J.*, **30** (4), 294–299.
55. Elliott, J., Bryant, C.E., and Soydan, J. (1994) The role of nitric oxide in the responses of equine digital veins to vasodilator and vasoconstrictor agents. *Equine Vet. J.*, **26** (5), 378–384.
56. Cogswell, A.M., Johnson, P.J., and Adams, H.R. (1995) Evidence for endothelium-derived relaxing factor nitric oxide in equine digital arteries. *Am. J. Vet. Res.*, **56** (12), 1637–1641.
57. Hinckley, K.A., Fearn, S., Howard, B.R., and Henderson, I.W. (1996) Nitric oxide donors as treatment for grass induced acute laminitis in ponies. *Equine Vet. J.*, **28** (1), 17–28.
58. Hinckley, K.A., Fearn, S., Howard, B.R., and Henderson, I.W. (1996) Glyceryl trinitrate enhances nitric oxide mediated perfusion within the equine hoof. *J. Endocrinol.*, **151** (2), R1–R8.
59. Gilhooly, M.H., Eades, S.C., Stokes, A.M., and Moore, R.M. (2005) Effects of topical nitroglycerine patches and ointment on digital venous plasma nitric oxide concentrations and digital blood flow in healthy conscious horses. *Vet. Surg.*, **34** (6), 604–609.
60. Hoff, T.K., Hood, D.M., and Wagner, I.P. (2002) Effectiveness of glyceryl trinitrate for enhancing digital submural perfusion in horses. *Am. J. Vet. Res.*, **63** (5), 648–652.
61. Eades, S.C., Stokes, A.M., and Moore, R.M. (2006) Effects of an endothelin receptor antagonist and nitroglycerin on digital vascular function in horses during the prodromal stages of carbohydrate overload-induced laminitis. *Am. J. Vet. Res.*, **67** (7), 1204–1211.
62. Furlong, B., Henderson, A.H., Lewis, M.J., and Smith, J.A. (1987) Endothelium-derived relaxing factor inhibits in vitro platelet aggregation. *Br. J. Pharmacol.*, **90** (4), 687–692.
63. Wang, Y., Mathews, W.R., Guido, D.M., Farhood, A., and Jaeschke, H. (1995) Inhibition of nitric oxide synthesis aggravates reperfusion injury after hepatic ischemia and endotoxemia. *Shock*, **4** (4), 282–288.

64. Alsup, E.M. and DeBowes, R.M. (1984) Dimethyl sulfoxide. *J. Am. Vet. Med. Assoc.*, **185** (9), 1011–1014.
65. Blythe, L.L, Craig, A.M., Appell, L.H., and Lassen, E.D. (eds) (1986) Intravenous use of dimethyl sulphoxide (DMSO) in horses: clinical and physiologic effects. Proceedings of the American Association of Equine Practitioners, pp. 441–446.
66. Menzies-Gow, N.J., Sepulveda, M.F., Bailey, S.R., Cunningham, F.M., and Elliott, J. (2008) Roles of thromboxane A2 and 5-hydroxytryptamine in endotoxin-induced digital vasoconstriction in horses. *Am. J. Vet. Res.*, **69** (2), 199–207.
67. Hood, D.M., Brumbaugh, G.W., and Wagner, I.P. (2002) Effectiveness of a unique dihydropyridine (BAYTG 1000) for prevention of laminitis in horses. *Am. J. Vet. Res.*, **63** (3), 443–447.
68. Blikslager, A.T., Yin, C., Cochran, A.M., Wooten, J.G., Pettigrew, A., and Belknap, J.K. (2006) Cyclooxygenase expression in the early stages of equine laminitis: a cytologic study. *J. Vet. Intern. Med.*, **20** (5), 1191–1196.
69. Baxter, G.M. (1994) Acute laminitis. *Vet. Clin. North Am. Equine Pract.*, **10** (3), 627–642.
70. Spektor, G. and Fuster, V. (2005) Drug insight: cyclo-oxygenase 2 inhibitors and cardiovascular risk – where are we now? Nat. Clin. Pract. Cardiovasc. *Med.*, **2** (6), 290–300.
71. Noschka, E., Moore, J.N., Peroni, J.F., Lewis, T.H., Lewis, S.J., and Robertson, T.P. (2010) Evaluation of the possible role of prostaglandin F(2 alpha) in laminitis induced in horses by nasogastric administration of black walnut heartwood extract. *Am. J. Vet. Res.*, **71** (2), 186–193.

CHAPTER 33

Analgesia

Bernd Driessen and Laura Zarucco

Introduction

Managing pain in horses afflicted by laminitis is often a great challenge because it is the dreadful suffering of the animals that frequently forces the veterinarian to end the battle with this disease. This chapter will highlight the rather complex mechanisms likely involved in generating and amplifying nociception in laminitis, thereby creating a state of maladaptive pain that is greatly resistant to conventional anti-inflammatory drug therapy. Based on this information, the concept of a multimodal approach to analgesia in the horse with laminitis is presented and targets for drug treatment are discussed.

Mechanisms of Pain in Laminitis

The majority of horses affected by laminitis eventually develop severe or chronic lameness and debilitation, and thus require pain treatment [1]. Understanding both the neuroanatomy of the equine foot and the pathophysiological processes involved in triggering and modifying nociception during the course of laminitis, even if still not known in their entirety, is crucial when prescribing pain therapy for the horse afflicted by this disease [2]. Inflammation emerges as the common pathological denominator in all cases of laminitis (especially after the severe tissue injury associated with displacement of the distal phalanx), and thus is likely the primary origin of disease-related pain [3]. Yet, nonsteroidal anti-inflammatory drug (NSAID) therapy often fails to sufficiently relieve pain once the digital lamellae which normally suspend the distal phalanx (DP) within the hoof capsule begins to collapse.

Sensory Innervation of the Foot

The distal forelimb and hindlimb of the horse are innervated by the medial and lateral digital nerves and their dorsal branches, all of which originate principally from spinal nerves C7–C8 and L6–S1–S2, respectively. Sensory innervation of the foot consists of thick myelinated A-fibers (largely $A_ß$ and maybe some $A_α$) transmitting low-threshold mechanical information, and small thin myelinated ($A_δ$-fibers) and unmyelinated afferents (C-fibers) which express a variety of peptides, and transmit high-threshold nociceptive (referring to pain usually due to tissue damage) information [4–8]. The $A_ß$ and potentially $A_α$ fibers innervate lamellated corpuscles (comparable with Pacinian corpuscles), mechanoreceptors clustered distal to the digital cushion in the heel segment of the hoof which normally function as proprioceptors, providing a secure gait [6, 8, 9]. Both, nociceptive $A_δ$- and C-fibers that stain immunohistochemically positive for the neuropeptides calcitonin gene-related peptide (CGRP) and substance P (SP) are widely distributed throughout the base of the dermal layer (especially dermal papillae in the solear and bulbar segments and dermal lamellae in the parietal segment) and run parallel to blood vessels without innervating them [6–8]. In addition, slow-conducting unmyelinated nerve fibers of the sympathetic nervous system accompany the dense network of blood vessels and arteriovenous anastomoses within the hoof capsule [8, 10]. These sympathetic nerves carry not only efferent fibers that regulate vasomotor tone but also afferent viscerosensory fibers that signal information about the vascular lumen, wall stress, and noxious stimulation or hypoxic/ischemic tissue conditions to the central nervous system (CNS) [10]. Hence, they may contribute to sympathetically maintained nociceptive stimulation that is generally unresponsive to conventional analgesics.

Collins *et al.* [9] described three distinct zones of innervation of the lamellar and sublamellar dermis of the dorsum of the foot. Zone 1 contains large multifascicular nerves that run in the sublamellar dermis adjacent and parallel to the parietal surface of the DP. Short branches of these nerves and longer ones from proximally located and lateral rami, run as neurovascular bundles within Zone 2 (the sublamellar dermis adjacent to the base of the dermal lamellae) and extend toward the primary lamellae, where single nerve fibers and small clusters emanate close to the dermoepidermal junction at the base of the primary epidermal lamellae. From there, they run along the axis of the primary dermal lamellae, associated with the small blood vessels, with small nerve endings penetrating into the secondary dermal lamellae (all lamellae in Zone 3).

Equine Laminitis, First Edition. Edited by James K. Belknap and Raymond Geor.

The sensory innervation of the DP is not well studied [9]. Deep branches of the medial and lateral digital nerves enter the solear foraminae of the DP, accompanying branches of the digital artery. Nerve fibers also enter the DP close to the insertion site of the deep digital flexor tendon, and the medullary spaces between the bone trabecula are richly populated with nerve fibers.

Transition from Inflammatory to Pathological (Neuropathic/Maladaptive) Pain

Signs of inflammation and vascular dysfunction are evident early in the developmental phase in experimental models of sepsis-related laminitis (SRL), when pain or other clinical symptoms are still absent [11–13]. During this prodromal phase, leukocyte extravasation and the development of platelet microthrombi are accompanied by upregulated gene expression for key inflammatory cytokines (e.g., interleukin [IL]-1β, IL-6), cyclooxygenase (COX)-2, and matrix metalloproteinases (MMPs) in the digital lamellae [13–17]. Although controversy still exists regarding the role of MMPs in lamellar failure, released and activated MMPs may mediate degradation of the collagen components of the basement membrane (BM) that is interposed between the secondary dermal lamellae (SDL) and secondary epidermal lamellae (SEL) and cause a separation of the SEL from the BM [12, 18–21]. Whilst reported to activate or sensitize peripheral nociceptors or to augment nociceptive signaling centrally [4, 22–24], the inflammatory mediators released in the lamellar tissues during the developmental phase of laminitis do not seem to evoke hoof pain. Histological data suggest that the disruption of the dermoepidermal lamellar bond is initially confined to the noninnervated BM and SEL (grade 1 histological laminitis) [12, 26]. Since the majority of sensory nerve terminals are clustered primarily at the base of the dermal lamellae, the distance between the terminals and the site of BM destruction and inflammatory reaction may be too great for nerve activation.

Unless the cause of laminitis is transient, histological changes at the dermal–epidermal interface progress further within 24–72 h, causing the BM to retract so much from the SEL that SDL connective tissue and SDL capillaries are injured by tension and shear forces (grade 2 histological laminitis) [12], as are the perivascular sensory nerve terminals near the base of the dermal lamellae. At this point, the developmental phase transits into the acute phase of laminitis that is hallmarked by the classical signs such as bounding digital pulses, increased hoof temperature, increased weight-shifting from one limb to another and sensitivity to hoof testers (indicating hyperalgesia), and lameness [11–13]. Although evidence for a marked increase in COX-2 enzyme activity could not be found in the acute phase in one study [16], concentrations of other vasoactive degradation products of arachidonic acid are elevated during the acute phase of experimentally induced laminitis [17]. In addition, extensive lamellar injury as evidenced by edema, separation of the dermal–epidermal junction, and, rarely, epidermal necrosis [26] has been reported during this phase. Thus, it is most likely that peripheral hyperalgesia develops secondary to the action of a variety of locally released inflammatory products [4, 5]. Furthermore, activated sensory nerve fibers in the dermal papillary layer are likely to release neuropeptides (e.g., CGRP) which target receptors on blood vessels and provoke neurogenic inflammation by causing vasodilation, plasma extravasation, and leukocyte emigration [7, 8]. As early as the acute phase of laminitis, persistent afferent nociceptive signaling from the peripheral nerves will initiate neural cellular events that eventually create a state of central (e.g., spinal cord) augmentation of the original nociceptive input being transmitted from the peripheral nerves to the brain (termed central hyperalgesia with increase in receptive fields) mediated in part by the spinal release of excitatory amino acids, tachykinins, prostanoids, and cytokines [5]. Some of these products reflect the activation not only of neurons but also of nearby non-neuronal cells (astrocytes, microglia) which contribute to the release of products (e.g., prostaglandins) that in turn increase the excitability of dorsal horn neurons in the spinal cord. Both, peripheral and early central hyperalgesia may explain the rapidly worsening pain that horses experience in the acute phase of laminitis.

Besides the local inflammatory processes promoting increased nociceptive signaling, a compartment injury/syndrome (tissue injury exacerbated by the inability of an injured tissue to expand/swell due to being encapsulated in noncompliant tissue) likely develops as a result of dermal edema and vasodilation; this occurs because the dermal tissues are constrained within the confines of the space between the hoof capsule and the distal phalanx. An increasing dermal pressure gradient associated with compartment injury affects the homeostasis of fascicular nerve fibers within the dermis [9]. Increasing interstitial pressures markedly reduce epineural venular blood flow and thus endoneural oxygen and nutrient supply, and eventually impair axoplasmic transport and the maintenance of myelin sheath integrity of the dermal nerve fibers. As a result, exposed nerve fibers in the lamellar tissue would become increasingly more mechanosensitive and convert pressure gradients arising within the hoof capsule into nociceptive signals. Hence, hyperexcitability due to increased lamellar pressure may generate pain via mechanoreceptors without nociceptor employment.

In transient/mild cases of laminitis, animals may pass through the acute phase of laminitis without having developed any gross structural changes to the dermal–epidermal lamellar apparatus, allowing for complete recovery from all symptoms including pain. If not, they enter – usually within two to three days – the chronic phase of laminitis that begins with the separation of the DP from the hoof wall and subsequent mechanical collapse of the foot [11–13]. It is during the early chronic or active chronic phase of the disease process that unrelenting pain may develop which often is very difficult to control with traditional NSAIDs and analgesic drug treatment [27, 28]. However, some animals may pass the early chronic phase rather rapidly and enter the stage of chronic stable laminitis without displaying any pronounced lameness [26].

The pain that animals with chronic laminitis suffer is multifactorial and greatly variable. The pathophysiological sequelae occurring after structural failure of the suspensory apparatus of the distal phalanx (SADP) in one animal may or may not occur to the same extent in another, and the type and scope of tissue repair and remodeling varies among individual horses [26]. A major component determining the degree of nociception is the extent of mechanical/structural failure of the foot's submural tissues, with distal displacement of the DP ('sinking') probably representing the worst scenario. Tearing of the dermal–epidermal lamellae with rotation or sinking of the DP results in widespread stretch injury to C- and A_δ-fibers in the dermal layers. Damaged sensory neurons respond with spontaneous impulse discharges that lead to sustained levels of excitability [4, 5]. These ectopic discharges begin to 'cross-talk' with adjacent uninjured nerve fibers, resulting in an amplification of the response to noxious stimulation as part of the *peripheral hyperalgesia* developing in the injured tissue. Distal phalanx displacement is likely to lead to increased submural pressure from further spreading edema accompanying inflammation and local hemorrhage [26]. The loss of digital stability with significant shifts in the distribution of strain and stress forces within the hoof capsule contribute to both mechano- (A_β) and nociceptor (A_δ, C) activities, as does elevated pressure on the coffin bone due to greater and longer-lasting contact between the internal surface of the sole and the distal phalanx during locomotion [26]. Furthermore, digital ischemia resulting from the tearing of SDL arterioles, vasoconstriction (primarily venoconstriction) in response to inflammatory mediators, arteriovenous blood shunting, thrombosis, and compression of the solear vascular bed after digital collapse are also likely to be important causative factors for pain [11–13,28,29]. Alternatively, dilation of hoof vessels in response to the release of neuropeptides (e.g., CGRP) from activated sensory nerve terminals may lead to a rapid increase in pressure within the hoof capsule (similar to the situation within the skull after vasodilation), thereby exacerbating foot pain [8, 10].

The factors mentioned above only partially explain why so many animals with chronic laminitis experience persistent and often worsening pain that is refractory to therapy, while others are spared or recover. While not studied in detail in horses, data obtained with laboratory animal models and clinical observations in human patients with severe tissue injury indicate that lesions to the peripheral somatosensory neurons can trigger a complex series of events that eventually alter peripheral nerve impulse signaling and central nervous sensory input processing. These processes result in a pain state commonly referred to as *neuropathic pain*; this is defined as pain that has its origin in a lesion in or a dysfunction of the sensory transmission pathways in the peripheral nervous system or CNS itself, and thus is considered a pathological condition in and of itself [4, 5, 30–33]. The changes may include: (i) large increases in spontaneous (ectopic) activity in injured afferent nerve fibers and dorsal root ganglia (DRG); (ii) ectopic activity in nociceptors after local increases in sodium channel expression and an enhanced sensitivity to excitatory inflammatory mediators; (iii) augmented synaptic neurotransmission in the dorsal horn resulting from an increased release of and response to excitatory neurotransmitters (glutamate); (iv) activation of astrocytes and microglia in the dorsal horn, facilitating neurotransmission; and (v) actions of MMPs capable of inducing neuropathic pain through microglial and astrocyte activation [4, 24, 30–33]. Ectopic neural firing activity occurs within 12–48 h after nerve injury, while sensitization and gene expression changes in spinal – and possibly supraspinal – neural networks begin later. Jones *et al.* [28] found in horses suffering from recurrent laminitis and laminitis refractory to treatment, neuromorphological changes and altered gene expression that are strikingly similar to those changes observed in animal models of peripheral nerve injury or in humans with neuropathic pain [5]. In addition, Collins *et al.* [9] found an increased expression of the calcium channel subunit $\alpha 2\delta$ (the target site for drugs such as gabapentin and pregabalin) in DRG neurons of laminitic horses. This ionophore protein is involved in signal transmission between first- and second-order sensory neurons in the dorsal horn of the spinal cord. In rodent pain models, $\alpha 2\delta$ expression is increased (independent of stimuli) in states of hyperalgesia and allodynia. Additionally, neuropeptide Y (NPY) expression was increased in DRG cells of large myelinated fibers innervating the laminitic hoof. Furthermore, an upregulated expression of activating transcription factor-3 (ATF3), a classical marker of peripheral nerve injury, was found in DRG cells of both large and small afferent fibers [28]. The abundant presence of MMPs from the developmental phase onwards may yet be another factor contributing to the development of neuropathic injury [12, 24]. Thus, it is likely that the mechanisms of peripheral and central sensitization and neuropathic remodeling described above play a central role in the development of the unrelenting pain experienced by many horses during chronic laminitis [5, 32, 33]. In this pain state, mildly noxious or subthreshold stimuli (transmitted by small A_δ- and C-afferent fibers) produce an exaggerated pain response due to amplified presynaptic and postsynaptic neuronal sensitivity and activity [28]. Thus, normally innocuous mechanical stimuli (such as those activating the lamellated corpuscles and low-threshold A_β fibers in the heel area when the foot touches the ground during locomotion) may be perceived as painful (tactile or mechanical *allodynia*) [30, 33]. This may explain the frequent limb shifting and high sensitivity to the hoof tester often observed in laminitic horses [28].

Concept of Multimodal Pain Therapy in Laminitis

For the past several decades, pain therapy in acute and chronic laminitis has largely been based on the proposed etiopathogenetic mechanisms underlying the disease (i.e., vascular or thromboembolic ischemia, inflammatory, metabolic, enzymatic, and biomechanical mechanisms), and consisted predominantly of NSAID administration [36–44]. In the acute phase, this therapy was often combined with other medications (e.g., acepromazine, pentoxifylline, isoxuprine, heparin, acetyl salicylic acid, nitroglycerine, dimethyl sulfoxide) addressing suspected ischemia and reperfusion injury (oxidative damage) in the dermal–epidermal lamellae, yet with conflicting results [37–41, 43–46]. This traditional approach often failed to control the multifactorial pain in horses with chronic laminitis, most likely because pain has been considered only a sign of laminitis rather than a pathological entity in itself. It is the abnormal neural signal processing due to damage to tissues (inflammatory pain) and nervous structures (neuropathic pain), and/or abnormal function of the nervous system as a whole (functional pain) that, over the course of the disease process, causes a state of nociception that is commonly referred to as pathological or *maladaptive pain* [5, 33, 46]. Conventional NSAIDs and other medications may not or may only partially target the neuropathophysiological mechanisms described above [4,5,32,34]. Therefore, a more holistic strategy aimed at preventing maladaptive pain or at least reducing the risk of its occurrence appears to be more reasonable [31,34,47]. This concept follows the notion that:

1. Events leading to acute pain, peripheral and central hyperalgesia, and neuropathic pain with or without allodynia occur simultaneously and are interrelated.
2. Drugs may exhibit a specific activity against only certain components of the pain syndrome.
3. Early integration of drugs with anti-hyperalgesic or anti-neuropathic pain activity into the treatment plan promises to reduce the risk of maladaptive pain development.
4. Loco-regional analgesia techniques may help to suppress the occurrence of hyperalgesia and neuropathic pain [34].

Accordingly, effective pain management in horses with laminitis favors a *multimodal* approach that involves, from the beginning, a combination of drugs with different pharmacological mechanisms of action and different target sites within the somatosensory neural conduit (Fig. 33.1). This concept entails also podiatric care and complementary treatment modalities including, but not limited to, electrotherapy, tenotomy, or

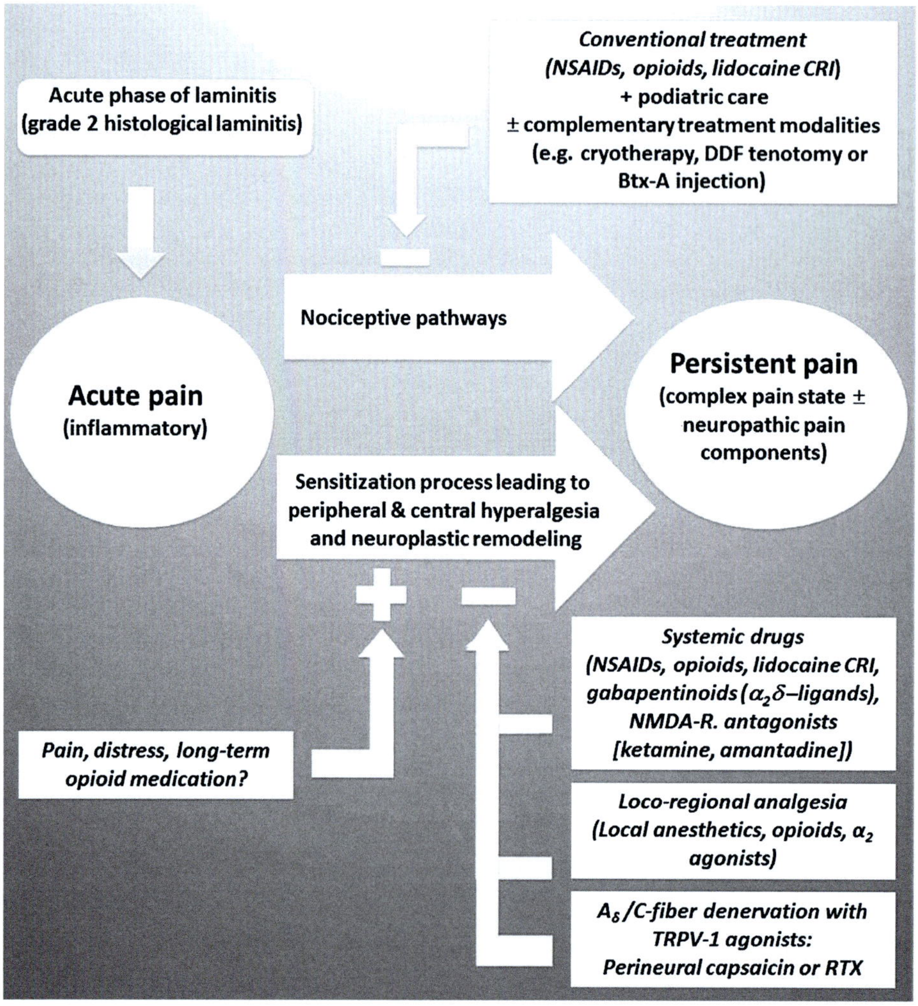

Figure 33.1 Amelioration of pain in acute and chronic laminitis employing a multimodal approach (see text for more details).

botulinum toxin (Btx-A)-induced relaxation of the deep digital flexor tendon, or physical therapy. Most of these treatments are aimed at altering biomechanical forces on the affected digit with the goal of decreased foot pain perception and improved recovery [34, 39, 40, 42, 43, 47–52].

For pain therapy in the horse with chronic laminitis to be successful, it has to accomplish multiple goals:

1 A reduction of nociceptive signal generation in sensory nerve terminals (NSAIDs, podiatric care).
2 Suppression of peripheral hyperalgesia (NSAIDs, local anesthesia and analgesia).
3 Inhibition/prevention of afferent nociceptive signal transmission to the CNS (loco-regional analgesia).
4 Inhibition of spinal nociceptive signal transmission and central hyperalgesia development (e.g., epidural/spinal anesthesia [using local anesthetics, opioids, α_2 agonists], systemic analgesia [using opioids, α_2 agonists, ketamine, NSAIDs, gabapentin, pregabalin]).
5 Prevention and/or inhibition of neuropathic pain (systemic lidocaine, opioids, NSAIDS, gabapentin, pregabalin).

Multi-modal pain therapy is mechanism-driven and should be evidence-based. It is a concept that supports the integration of new drugs and techniques whenever possible and meaningful.

Due to the current lack of data regarding the use of many of these treatment modalities in the horse, the equine veterinarian must rely primarily on findings in experimental animals and experiences in human medicine when developing an analgesic treatment plan for the horse with persistent foot pain. Experiences with neuropathic pain therapy in the human have demonstrated that:

1 Symptoms described by patients include but are not limited to allodynia (pain to a non-noxious stimulus such as light touch), hyperalgesia (exaggerated response to a mildly noxious stimulus), and hyperpathia (delayed and explosive response to a noxious stimulus), and therefore the diagnosis of neuropathic pain is often challenging and diagnostic criteria are still evolving.
2 Rarely, if ever, can a single pathophysiological mechanism be claimed responsible for generating and maintaining neuropathic pain.
3 Individual variation in the response to anti-neuropathic pain medications is substantial and unpredictable, thus favoring a stepwise process intended to identify the medication (or medication combination) that provides the greatest pain relief and fewest side effects while discontinuing drugs lacking analgesic efficacy.
4 Currently, first-line medications for neuropathic pain cannot be ranked by degree of efficacy.
5 No more than 40–60 % of patients with neuropathic pain will respond favorably to pharmacological treatments [53–57].

Whichever therapeutic approach (pharmacological and other approaches such as foot care) is chosen in an individual *multi-modal-* protocol, the ultimate objective is to achieve optimum pain control during each phase of laminitis, while at the same time minimizing the risk of negatively affecting the disease process itself or causing side effects of drug therapy [34].

Conventional Systemic Analgesics

Three different pharmacological classes of drugs are commonly administered systemically to treat pain in horses affected with laminitis: NSAIDs, opioids, and lidocaine. As described in more detail below, these drugs have also the potential to ameliorate nociceptive processes involved in the development of hyperalgesia and neuropathic pain.

Nonsteroidal Anti-Inflammatory Drugs (NSAIDs)

The basis of pharmacological therapy of laminitis and associated pain has been, and continues to be, treatment with NSAIDs (Table 33.1). The previously described evidence of increased

Table 33.1 Doses of commonly used nonsteroidal anti-inflammatory drugs (NSAIDs) in horses.

NSAID	Dose, route, and interval of drug administration*	Comments	References
Nonselective COX-1 and COX-2 inhibitors			
Phenylbutazone	2.2–4.4 (up to 6) mg kg^{-1} IV/PO, SID-BID	Highest toxicity among NSAIDs	[41, 42, 53, 60, 62, 66, 70]
Flunixine meglumine	1.1 mg kg^{-1} IV/PO, SID-BID	Cases of muscle necrosis reported with IM injection	[66, 70]
Ketoprofen	2.2–3.6 mg kg^{-1} IV/IM, SID-QID	Only parenteral administration	[53, 62, 66, 70]
Vedaprofen	1–2 mg kg^{-1} IV/PO, SID-BID	Limited experience	[70]
Eltenac	0.5–1 mg kg^{-1} IV, SID	Limited experience	[66, 70]
Naproxen	5 mg kg^{-1} IV 10 mg kg^{-1} PO, SID	Initially slow IV bolus, then PO	[70]
Preferential or selective COX-2 inhibitors			
Meloxicam	0.6 mg kg^{-1} IV/PO, SID-BID		[66, 70]
Etodolac	10–20 mg kg^{-1} IV/PO, SID-BID	Limited experience	[66, 70]
Firocoxib	0.1 mg kg^{-1} PO, SID	May require 0.3 mg kg^{-1} on 1st day of administration	[67, 68, 70]

*Routes and intervals of drug administration: IV, intravenous; IM, intramuscular; PO, per os (oral); SID, once daily; BID, twice daily.

cyclooxygenase (primarily COX-2) expression, concentrations of arachidonic acid degradation products, leukocyte emigration, and cytokine production in lamellar tissues during the developmental and acute phases of laminitis justifies the use of these agents (see Chapters 13 and 14).

It is well understood that prostaglandins reduce the activation threshold of peripheral nociceptors. Thus, NSAIDs, by reducing prostaglandin synthesis, decrease inflammatory hyperalgesia and allodynia. These drugs may also reduce the migration of leucocytes into the affected lamellar tissues, thereby limiting the production of numerous leukocyte-derived inflammatory mediators (e.g., cytokines) that contribute through their actions on the nervous system to pain sensation. While not appreciated by many clinicians, there is increasing evidence that common NSAIDs (e.g., phenylbutazone, flunixine meglumine, ketoprofen, naproxen) and the more recently marketed drugs (e.g., vedaprofen, meloxicam, firocoxib) mediate much of their potent antinociceptive effects centrally [38, 41, 44, 58]. By preventing the generation of prostaglandins that act as nociceptive signal-producing or -augmenting neuromodulators in the spinal cord dorsal horn, NSAIDs effectively suppress pain [59]. Unlike in peripheral tissues, where COX-1 is constitutively present for tissue homeostasis and COX-2 is inducible by inflammation [60], both COX isoforms are constitutively present in the CNS but with functionally different roles [61,62].

The concept that COX-2-preferential (meloxicam, Metacam®; etodolac, Etogesic®) or even COX-2-selective NSAIDS (firocoxib, Equioxx®) are therapeutically superior analgesics has been challenged recently [63–65]. Newly acquired laboratory data indicate that the suppression of inflammation-evoked central nociceptive activity and hyperalgesia by NSAIDs may be related to the selectivity for COX isoforms, since COX-2 seems to be only involved in the initiation but not necessarily in the maintenance of nociceptive spinal neuron activation, which may largely depend on COX-1 [62]. Under the premise of inflammation being the common pathological denominator [3], and hence the trigger for increased spinal sensory nerve excitability in all forms of laminitis (probably at least true after severe tissue injury associated with displacement of the DP), the use of nonselective NSAIDs promises to be more effective for analgesic therapy in laminitis. This idea is supported by two observations: (i) among clinicians the nonselective COX inhibitor phenylbutazone is considered the most potent and most consistent pain-relieving NSAID in laminitis [58, 65]; and (ii) only ketoprofen (3.63 mg kg^{-1}), a slightly COX-1-preferential NSAID [66], may reduce foot pain to a greater extent than phenylbutazone (2.2 mg kg^{-1}) [67]. Interestingly, the stereoisomers of ketoprofen are known to exert antinociceptive actions also through mechanisms other than COX inhibition. The R(−)-enantiomer of ketoprofen suppresses tactile allodynia via a yet to be defined mechanism of action, while the S(+)-enantiomer produces analgesia through mechanisms involving serotoninergic pathways both at the spinal and supraspinal level [68,69].

While high-dose NSAID administration may be desirable in the very early stages of laminitis, pain relief from NSAIDs in the acute phase must be balanced against the risks of exacerbated structural damage due to excessive movement and/or limb-loading of the horse [38]. In horses with chronic laminitis, effective analgesia frequently calls for high doses of NSAIDs, and an effect may still not be seen for up to three days after the initiation of treatment [38]. This must be considered when assessing the clinical response to NSAIDs, as must be the adverse effects associated with long-term NSAID administration (see Chapter 31 for further discussion of NSAIDs) [63,65,70].

Opiods

Opioids (Table 33.2) are generally indicated in moderate to severe pain [71, 72], but their analgesic efficacy in horses, if any, is much less well defined when administered systemically

Table 33.2 Doses of opioids and coadministered sedatives in horses.

Drug	Dose, route, and interval of drug administration*	References
Opioids		
Morphine	0.05–0.2 mg kg^{-1} IV/IM every 4–6 h or followed by IV CRI at 0.1–0.4 mg kg^{-1} h^{-1}	[70, 75]
Methadone	0.1–0.2 mg kg^{-1} IV/IM every 4–6 h	[70, 75]
Butorphanol	0.01–0.4 mg kg^{-1} IV, IM every 2–4 h	[74, 75, 83, 85]
	Bolus of 18 μg kg^{-1} followed by IV CRI at 13–24 μg kg^{-1} h^{-1}	[74, 75, 83, 84]
Buprenorphine	5–20 μg kg^{-1} IV/IM TID	[74, 75, 89–91]
	6 μg kg^{-1} sublingual BID	
Fentanyl	Two to three 10 mg (100 μg h^{-1}) patches to be changed every 3 days	[86–88]
Coadministered phenothiazine and/or α_2 agonist sedative/analgesic		
Acepromazine	0.01–0.08 mg kg^{-1} IV/IM BID/TID or CRI at 2–4 μg kg^{-1} h^{-1}	[74]
Detomidine	6 40 μg kg^{-1} IV/IM every 2–4 h	[74]
	Bolus of 5–40 μg kg^{-1} IV/IM followed by CRI at 7–36 μg kg^{-1} h^{-1}	
Medetomidine	5–7 μg kg^{-1} IM/IV every 2–4 h	[32, 73, 74]
	Bolus of 3–7 μg kg^{-1} IV/IM followed by CRI at 1.5–3.6 μg kg^{-1} h^{-1}	
Dexmedetomidine	Bolus of 1.5–3.0 μg kg^{-1} IV/IM followed by CRI at 0.75–1.8 μg kg^{-1} h^{-1}	

*Routes and intervals of drug administration: IV, intravenous; IM, intramuscular; SID, once daily; BID, twice daily; TID, three times daily; CRI, constant rate infusion.

in common clinical doses. At higher doses (i.e., ≥0.1 mg kg^{-1}) that have supporting experimental and clinical evidence for antinociceptive/analgesic efficacy, butorphanol, methadone, or morphine may provoke central excitatory responses and undesirable locomotor activity, requiring their combination with sedatives such as acepromazine or α_2 agonists (Table 33.2) [58, 73–76]. In addition, they decrease gastrointestinal motility and cause colon impaction [75, 77, 78], thus commonly limiting their long-term use. Combining lower doses of μ-opioids with low doses of α_2 agonists (preferably in the form of a constant rate infusion [CRI]) may achieve the desired level of analgesia by making use of the well-described synergism between the two drug classes, while avoiding profound CNS stimulatory effects of the opioids and hemodynamic effects of α_2 agonists (Table 33.2) [74]. However, impaired intestinal motility caused by opioids and α_2 agonists [79] remains a concern with long-term treatment. Whether opioids elicit fewer CNS stimulatory effects and are more effective in horses experiencing pain as a result of a naturally occurring disease compared to pain from experimental noxious stimulation, is controversial due to the fact that any scientific evidence for this claim is lacking [74, 75].

Controlled trials in human patients revealed efficacy of opioids against peripheral neuropathic pain and some components of central neuropathic pain [54, 55]. However, laboratory animal and human clinical evidence also exist that the long-term use of μ-opioid agonists such as morphine can trigger the development of a state of opioid-induced hyperalgesia (OIH), whereby a subject receiving opioids for the treatment of pain may actually become more sensitive to pain [80, 81]. Despite the facts that: (i) the mechanisms leading to OIH and its clinical relevance are still being debated, and (ii) the phenomenon is not described in horses [82], this potentially profound adverse effect should be considered when prescribing long-term opioid therapy in horses with chronic laminitis.

Butorphanol (Torbugesic®), a κ-opioid receptor agonist and μ-receptor antagonist, is probably the most widely used opioid in horses. However, due to the drug's low bioavailability after intramuscular administration (37%) and rapid decline in plasma levels after intravenous injection (to below the clinically effective threshold concentration of 10 ng ml^{-1}) [76, 83–85], its use in laminitis is limited. Even if administered intravenously at an analgesically effective dose of 0.1 mg kg^{-1}, the plasma concentration of butorphanol declines within 2 h to values below the 10 ng ml^{-1} mark [76], calling for a CRI to achieve persistent analgesia.

Transdermal administration of fentanyl (Duragesic®), a potent but very short-acting synthetic μ-opioid receptor agonist, has been found to not consistently alleviate musculoskeletal pain [86, 87]. If fentanyl patches were to be used as part of the multimodal pain management, at least as many patches as necessary should probably be applied to achieve plasma fentanyl levels generally considered to be analgesic in other species (i.e., ≥1 ng ml^{-1}) [88].

Buprenorphine (Buprenex®) is a μ-opioid agonist and κ-opioid antagonist. When applied as a sole analgesic agent in horses at doses of 10 μg kg^{-1} or greater, measurable antinociception has been reported to occur but with significant side effects including excitement, hemodynamic stimulation, and long-lasting reduction in gastrointestinal motility [89, 90]. The drug has been reported to provide clinically effective analgesia without provoking signs of excitement in a case of a filly with severe head and neck trauma that was administered buprenorphine (6 μg kg^{-1} twice daily) for five days via the sublingual/buccal mucosal route [91].

Systemic Lidocaine

The clinical use of systemic lidocaine for pain treatment in humans was first reported more than half a century ago, and, during the past decade, intravenous lidocaine has gained much popularity in equine practice [74, 91–94]. The current understanding of how the local anesthetic affects pain remains, however, unclear [74, 93–95].

The drug must be administered as a CRI due to its short half-life [96]. A loading dose of 1.3–1.5 mg kg^{-1} administered intravenously over 15 min followed by a CRI of 50–100 μg kg^{-1} min^{-1} is most commonly used [74, 94]. Data regarding the immediate analgesic effect of lidocaine on spontaneous (not evoked) pain in animals or patients are somewhat inconsistent when infused at clinically common doses [74, 92, 97, 98], and higher doses carry the risk of cardio- and neurotoxicity [99]. Since plasma concentrations achieved during long-term infusion vary widely among horses and may accumulate over time [74, 95, 96, 100, 101], monitoring of plasma levels (via a lidocaine ELISA kit; Neogen Corporation, Lansing, MI 48912, USA) is recommended, not only to avoid toxicity but also to ensure that analgesically effective concentrations (ca. ≥1 μg ml^{-1}) [92, 95] are being achieved.

Information from laboratory animal investigations indicates that any potential antinociceptive action of intravenous lidocaine is far more complex than previously thought. Besides its well-studied local anesthetic actions (i.e., Na^+ channel blockade) in the peripheral and central nervous systems, it also exerts multiple other mechanisms of action that target the spinal and supraspinal nociceptive systems [93, 102, 103]. Both, laboratory animal and controlled clinical trials in humans have found intravenous lidocaine to suppress the development of peripheral hyperalgesia as well as central nociceptive sensitization and allodynia [92, 93, 103–105], and therefore it can be also considered an antihyperalgesic agent (listed in Table 33.3).

Antihyperalgesic Pain Therapeutics

N-Methyl-D-Aspartate (NMDA) Receptor Antagonists

Persistent peripheral sensory nerve stimulation with ongoing nociceptive input to the spinal cord leads to activation of the *N*-methyl-D-aspartate (NMDA) receptor, a voltage- and

Table 33.3 Doses of antihyperalgesic and antineuropathic pain therapeutics in horses.

Drug	Dose, route, and interval of drug administration*	References
Local anesthetic		
Lidocaine	Bolus of 1.3–1.5 mg kg^{-1} IV over 15 min followed by a CRI of 50–100 µg kg^{-1} min^{-1}	[74, 94]
NMDA receptor antagonists		
Ketamine	0.1–0.2 mg kg^{-1} IV/IM every 1–4 h or CRI at 3–18 µg kg^{-1} h^{-1} or 60–120 µg kg^{-1} h^{-1}	[2, 110, 112]
Amantadine	5–10 mg kg^{-1} (split into two increments, 15 min apart), QID 20–120 mg kg^{-1} TID (dependent on individual bioavailability)	[118]
Calcium channel $\alpha_2\delta$-ligands		
Gabapentin	20 mg kg^{-1} IV (over 30 min), SID or BID, or ≥20 mg kg^{-1} PO, TID	[131]
Pregabalin	3–4 mg kg^{-1} PO, TID	[135, 136]

*Routes and intervals of drug administration: IV, intravenous; PO, per os (oral); SID, once daily; BID, twice daily; TID, three times daily; QID, four times daily; CRI, constant rate infusion.

ligand-gated ion channel complex on the postsynaptic membrane in spinal cord dorsal horn neurons [106]. The activation of spinal NMDA receptors is a key step in both the initiation and maintenance of activity-dependent central sensitization, and NMDA receptor antagonists have been shown experimentally to prevent and reverse the hyperexcitability of secondary afferent neurons that occurs soon after intense, repeated, or sustained nociceptive signal input to the dorsal horn [106–108]. Once activated, NMDA receptors allow a rapid inward current of Ca^{2+} ions, causing a cascade of intracellular events including the phosphorylation of NMDA receptors which results in a change in receptor activity and density; these changes contribute to postsynaptic hyperexcitability referred to as 'wind-up' [106, 108]. Changes in NMDA receptor activity are thought to contribute significantly to the severe pain that horses with chronic laminitis have to endure [109]. Therefore, the inclusion of NMDA receptor antagonists (examples discussed below) into a multimodal pain therapy is reasonable.

Ketamine

Ketamine is an NMDA receptor antagonist (see Table 33.3). At low doses, the drug seems to have specific selectivity for postsynaptic NMDA receptors in the dorsal horn of the spinal cord [110]. It is believed that the binding of ketamine to its receptor site is greatly facilitated when the NMDA receptor is in its open state because the high-affinity binding site is located within the channel pore. Due to the fact that prolonged afferent nociceptive signaling elicits a sustained activation of spinal NMDA receptors, it has been proposed that low-dose ketamine will preferentially bind to those activated receptors, thereby inhibiting or reversing the development of central hyperalgesia in states of persistent pain [107, 111, 112].

The pharmacokinetic characteristics of ketamine (rapid redistribution from the CNS to peripheral tissues and relatively short plasma half-life) [113] dictate that the drug is best administered as a CRI to obtain sustained effects. Infusion rates as low as 3–18 µg kg^{-1} h^{-1} are reported not as an analgesic treatment *per se* but as an antihyperalgesic/antiallodynic modality in multimodal analgesia for patients at risk of developing chronic maladaptive pain after major tissue damage [110–112]; these same rates may be suitable also as an adjunct in pain therapy for laminitic horses [2, 47]. Long-term administration of subanesthetic ketamine infusions as high as 400–1500 µg kg^{-1} h^{-1} in horses were not associated with signs of excitement or significant changes in measured physiological variables, and thus were considered safe [113, 114]. Even those higher infusion regimens are likely to only be effective as an antihyperalgesic/antiallodynic modality, as the measured plasma ketamine concentrations were approximately 10-fold below concentrations (2–4 µg ml^{-1}) associated with measurable acute antinociceptive effects [113].

Amantadine

Amantadine in doses known to exhibit antiviral (i.e., anti-influenza and anti-herpes virus) activity also acts as a non-competitive NMDA antagonist [115]. Unlike other NMDA antagonists, amantadine is clinically available for chronic use in both humans and horses [116–118]. It has no psychotropic side effects, is not a controlled substance, and is available in both injectable and oral (tablet) formulations. While there is evidence of a beneficial effect of amantadine in the treatment of painful peripheral neuropathies in human patients [116, 117], no such information exists yet in the horse. Since the pharmacology, pharmacokinetics, and neurological effects of amantadine in the horse are known [118], and antiviral doses appear to coincide with antihyperalgesic/antineuropathic activity (at least in the human), employing the drug as an adjunct to pain therapy in the laminitic horse might be considered. The intravenous administration of 5–10 mg kg^{-1} (split into two equal-volume increments injected 15 min apart, four times daily) seems to maintain safe and effective plasma concentrations [118]. Oral bioavailability in the horse is rather variable, and therefore individual animals may require oral doses as low as 20 mg kg^{-1} or as high as 120 mg kg^{-1} three times daily.

Anti-Neuropathic Pain Therapeutics

Neuropathic (neurogenic) pain has been defined as pain arising as a direct consequence of a lesion or disease affecting the somatosensory system [119]. Common types and causes of peripheral and central neuropathic pain syndromes have been reported in humans, but not in horses. To date, only postmortem findings in horses afflicted by chronic laminitis suggest that neuropathic pain exists in the equine species as well [28]. Unlike in human medicine, where guidelines for the diagnosis and grading of neuropathic (as opposed to non-neuropathic) pain are published and widely accepted [120, 121], no such guidelines have been developed in veterinary medicine. Thus, the prevalence of neuropathic pain in the horse are only speculative. Evidence-based consensus guidelines for the pharmacologic treatment of neuropathic pain in the human universally recommend tricyclic antidepressants (not tested in equine species) and calcium channel $\alpha_2\delta$-ligands (gabapentin, pregabalin) as first-line treatments for patients with neuropathic pain [55–57]. The guidelines suggest reserving opioid analgesics and NMDA receptor antagonists as second- or third-tier options in most cases, despite evidence of efficacy in certain forms of hyperalgesia and neuropathic pain [56]. In two of the guidelines, topical lidocaine has been recommended as a first-line treatment for patients with localized peripheral neuropathic pain [55–57].

Calcium Channel $\alpha_2\delta$-Ligands (Gabapentin, Pregabalin)

The anticonvulsant drugs gabapentin and pregabalin both bind with high affinity to the $\alpha_2\delta$-1 subunit of voltage-gated calcium channels in the spinal cord and brain [55, 122, 123], resulting in an inhibition of neuronal calcium currents. This inhibition ultimately causes a change in the release of neurotransmitters within the CNS such as glutamate, γ-aminobutyric acid (GABA), norepinephrine, and SP; these actions account for much of the analgesic activity of these compounds [124, 125]. Expression of the $\alpha_2\delta$-1 subunit has been shown in experimental neuropathic pain models to increase in chronic pain states in both afferent sensory neurons and in the spinal cord dorsal horn [126, 127]. Furthermore, recently reported preliminary findings in horses indicated significant expression of the $\alpha_2\delta$-1 subunit in DRG cells during chronic laminitis [9]. The observation of increased $\alpha_2\delta$-1 subunit expression in laboratory animals with nerve lesions promoting neuropathic pain development correlates well with the finding in those animal models that gabapentin exerts analgesic properties primarily in sensitized or hyperalgesic states [123, 127, 128]. More recently, gabapentin and pregabalin have been used clinically in humans to treat successfully a variety of neuropathic pain states [53–57]. Based on this evidence, it appears reasonable to include gabapentin in a multimodal pain treatment regimen for horses suffering from chronic laminitis.

Documented therapeutic use in horses refers only to oral administration of gabapentin (Neurontin®) in two animals which were thought to exhibit signs of neuropathic pain – one in conjunction with acute femoral nerve injury post surgery and one with a history of white line disease and chronic laminitis [47, 129]. Lacking information on pharmacokinetic properties of the drug in the equine species at that time, gabapentin doses were extrapolated from use in other species (2.5 mg kg^{-1} at intervals of 8, 12 or 24 h [129]; 2.0–3.3 mg kg^{-1} at intervals of 8 or 12 h [47]). In the meantime, two studies have been conducted in horses investigating the drug's pharmacokinetic properties as well as behavioral and cardiovascular parameters after intravenous oral administration [130, 131]. After intravenous (over 30 min) and oral administration of gabapentin (20 mg kg^{-1}), the median elimination half-lives were 8.5 and 7.7 h, respectively, which correspond well with data from other species [121]. After intravenous administration, plasma gabapentin concentrations remained above the 3–4 μg ml^{-1} range for approximately 15 h, similar to the dose associated with significant analgesic effects in adult human volunteers [131]. In the horse, the oral bioavailability of gabapentin is relatively poor (ca. 16%), and therefore plasma gabapentin concentrations decreased below the effective concentration threshold much more rapidly than after intravenous drug administration (i.e., within 2–3 h). Neither route of gabapentin administration was associated with effects on heart rate, rhythm or blood pressure, nor pronounced CNS effects, which concurs with data from other species [131]. In humans (where gabapentin is characterized by an oral bioavailability at least twice that in the horse), therapy for neuropathic pain usually entails three oral doses of 15–60 mg kg^{-1} of gabapentin per day [56, 133, 134]. It may therefore be predicted that oral gabapentin should be administered at a dose of at least 20 mg kg^{-1} three or more times daily to obtain a clinically relevant analgesic effect against neuropathic pain in the horse. Current clinical experiences of the present authors with oral gabapentin medication (20 mg kg^{-1}, t.i.d.) in laminitic horses have been rather disappointing, insofar as they added hardly any noticeable additional analgesia when administered in conjunction with NSAIDs such as phenylbutazone or ketoprofen. Clinical studies with intravenous administration of gabapentin and monitoring of plasma concentrations are warranted to explore whether this drug truly possesses significant analgesic efficacy in horses with chronic laminitis.

Pregabalin has not yet been used extensively in the horse under clinical conditions, and hence pharmacodynamic and dosing information is sparse [135]. The pharmacokinetic properties of pregabalin after intravenous and intragastric administration, respectively, of a single dose (4 mg kg^{-1}) have recently been reported [136]. After intravenous administration, initial plasma concentrations ranged from 20 to 28 μg ml^{-1}, and the elimination half-life was between 7 and 8 h. After intragastric administration, plasma concentrations reached a maximum of 4–7 μg ml^{-1} within 0.5–2.0 h and the median elimination half-life was 8 h. The median bioavailability of pregabalin (ca. 98%) was much higher than that reported for gabapentin (ca. 16%), and intragastric administration at 8-h dosing intervals produced steady-state plasma concentrations that were well within the therapeutic range reported for humans. However, therapeutic concentrations and safe dosing regimens of this drug have not yet been established in the horse.

Loco-Regional Anesthesia and Analgesia

The neuropathophysiological processes leading to the development of central hyperalgesia, neuropathic pain and allodynia are primarily triggered by increased spontaneous firing activity in ascending sensory nerve fibers during the first four to five days following peripheral nerve injuries [137,138]. Experimental evidence and clinical experiences in human medicine indicate that central hyperalgesia can be obliterated by no other treatment modality as effectively as it is by loco-regional anesthesia and analgesia aimed at interrupting or diminishing impulse trafficking from the site of tissue injury to the CNS and within the dorsal horn of the spinal cord [54,57,137–139]. These techniques may include topical local anesthetic application using 5% lidocaine patches (Lidoderm®); single, repetitive or continuous peripheral nerve blocks; and epidural or intrathecal anesthesia and analgesia.

Continuous Peripheral Nerve Blockade

Continuous peripheral nerve blockade (CPNB) is a treatment modality that has been long used in humans in orthopedic and trauma surgery [140]. The technique entails a continuous or intermittent low-dose administration of local anesthetics via catheters placed along peripheral nerves, thus providing persistent pain control while reducing the need for systemic medications. Techniques for the percutaneous placement of catheters close to the palmar nerves in the standing, sedated horse were recently developed, and provide a method for repeated or continuous perineural administration of low concentrations of local anesthetic solutions (e.g., bupivacaine or ropivacaine 0.125–0.5%) over a period of multiple days [140–143]. The therapy can continue for longer periods by exchanging catheters every four to eight days. With these techniques, significant analgesia can be obtained in horses with pain that is poorly responsive or even refractory to traditional systemic pain therapy [141,143]. These techniques further offer the advantage of determining the intensity of the analgesic effect by adjusting the concentration of the local anesthetic solution and/or the rate of drug administration to a desired level of comfort, without causing complete sensory blockade. The CPNB catheters can also be placed more proximal on the thoracic limb in close proximity to the ulnar and median nerves [144]. This technique may then provide a significant reduction of pain perception in the entire distal forelimb [145]. However, the use of either CPNB technique in the acute and early chronic phase of laminitis is controversial and warrants further clinical study due to the fact that a pronounced nociceptive blockade of the affected limb will allow the horse to increase the load on the foot and potentially exacerbate lamellar injury.

Caudal Epidural Analgesia

In horses experiencing severe pain due to chronic laminitis primarily in their hind limb(s), caudal epidural (sacrococcygeal or first intercoccygeal space) administration of analgesics such as opioids (e.g., morphine 0.05–0.2 mg kg^{-1}; methadone 0.1 mg kg^{-1}), α_2-agonists (e.g., xylazine 0.17 mg kg^{-1}; detomidine 20–40 μg kg^{-1}; medetomidine 2–5 μg kg^{-1}) or a combination thereof with or without low doses of local anesthetic (e.g., bupivacaine or ropivacaine 0.125–0.25%) provides long-term pain control [146, 147]. Unlike local anesthetics and α_2-agonists, morphine is characterized by slow onset of action (1–2 h) but a long duration of effect (3–8 h and longer). To allow repeated drug administration, it is recommended to place an epidural catheter that is advanced from the sacrococcygeal or first intercoccygeal space up to 30 cm cranially [146, 147]. Medications may be administered as intermittent boluses (15–30 ml per average adult horse) or as an infusion (0.5–3.0 ml h^{-1}). When administered in volumes of 50–90 ml epidurally, opioids (e.g., morphine 0.05–0.2 mg kg^{-1}; methadone 0.1 mg kg^{-1}) spread far enough cranially to reach the thoracic and cervical segments of the spinal cord [148, 149]. Therefore, these opioids can also inhibit nociception originating from the forelimbs affected by laminitis, and hence can complement or even replace other loco-regional techniques such as CPNB. Based on their clinical experience, the present authors consider repetitive or continuous epidural administration of morphine to be the most effective analgesic adjunct to systemic NSAID administration and the most valuable alternative to the CPNB technique, also in horses afflicted by forelimb laminitis. In most laminitic horses with moderate to severe pain, constant-rate infusions of lidocaine, ketamine, butorphanol (or morphine), or a combination thereof, are therapeutically less effective than high-volume caudal-epidural morphine. However, the risks of side effects associated with epidural morphine must be weighed against the potential benefit of better analgesia.

TRPV-1 Receptor Agonists (Capsaicin, Resiniferatoxin)

The transient receptor potential cation channel, subfamily V, member 1 (TRPV-1) is a membrane ion channel that, in most species, is highly expressed in sensory neurons of the dorsal root and trigeminal ganglia giving rise to the A_δ and C fibers of the primary nociceptive afferents [150, 151]. Also referred to as the vanilloid receptor, this polymodal cation channel is involved in various modes of sensory signaling, ranging from thermal and mechanical nociception to vision, taste, olfaction, touch, and osmosensation. The TRPV-1channel has been identified in horses and is likely more expressed in horses with laminitis [9, 109, 152].

Current thoughts are that peripheral perineural (i.e., remote from the neuronal perikarya in the DRG) administration of TRPV-1 agonists, such as capsaicin or resiniferatoxin (RTX), will initially produce nociceptor depolarization and hence pain as a result of TRPV-1 channel activation. However, receptor desensitization, accompanied by long-term but reversible blockade of a portion of nociceptive afferent fibers within peripheral nerves, will likely subsequently ensue [153, 154]. Therefore, treatment with TRPV-1 agonists may serve as a method for regional pain control in horses with laminitis [9, 109]. Studies in laboratory animals indicate that perineural capsaicin and RTX application produces a significant inhibition of inflammatory nociception (including hyperalgesia) that is both dose- and time-dependent, without changing proprioceptive sensations and motor control [153]. Recovery studies showed that the physiological sensory function can return as early as two weeks post-RTX or capsaicin treatment; however, immunohistochemical examination of the DRG revealed a partial, but significant, reduction in the number of the TRPV-1-positive neurons post treatment.

While the use of RTX in horses has not yet been described, the effects of local administration of capsaicin in equines have been reported [155]. Compared to no treatment, a single topical application of capsaicin ointment (Equi-Block® containing capsaicin 0.25%) over the medial and lateral palmar digital nerves, significantly attenuated signs of pain in a reversible model of severe (non-weight-bearing) foot lameness. This effect lasted for up to 4 h. Some horses initially displayed an episode of increased pain sensation, likely due to the initial agonistic action of capsaicin on TPRV-1 receptors described above. This response can likely be obliterated by prior perineural local anesthetic drug infiltration proximal to the site of capsaicin application. Berardinelli *et al.* [156] injected an 8% capsaicin solution along the medial and lateral palmar nerves in horses to study whether selective deafferentiation of sensory fibers (A_δ- and C-fibers) in the distal part of the forelimb would alter the muscle fiber composition in the muscles of the same limb. Indeed, a shift in the muscle fiber composition from fast (type II) to slow contracting (type I) fibers in the flexor carpi radialis muscle was observed within 120 days post-treatment. This indicates that the long-term deafferentiation of sensory nerve fibers produces a plastic remodeling of the spinal cord and indirectly influences motor neuron activity, enhancing their tonic discharge. Further equine studies with capsaicin and RTX are warranted before the risks and long-term success of local treatment with these TRPV-1 ligands in animals suffering from persistent pain can be assessed.

References

1. Moore, R.M. (2009) Laminitis vision: 20/20 by 2020. Proceedings of the Fifth International Equine Conference on Laminitis and Diseases of the Foot. Palm Beach, FL, USA, pp. 15–20.
2. Driessen, B., Bauquier, S.H., and Zarucco, L. (2010) Neuropathic pain management of chronic laminitis. *Vet. Clin. Equine*, **26**, 315–337.
3. Orsini, J., Galantino-Homer, H., and Pollitt, C.C. (2009) Laminitis in horses: through the lens of systems theory. *J. Equine Vet. Sci.*, **29**, 105–114.
4. Yaksh, T.L. (2009) Pain Management I: Basic mechanisms in pain processing. Proceedings of the Fifth International Equine Conference on Laminitis and Diseases of the Foot. Palm Beach, FL, USA. pp. 84–85.
5. Yaksh, T.L. (2009) Pain Management II: Current thinking on the mechanisms underlying laminitic pain. Proceedings of the Fifth International Equine Conference on Laminitis and Diseases of the Foot. Palm Beach, FL, USA, pp. 86–88.
6. Bowker, R.M., Brewer, A.M., Vex, K.B.A„ *et al.* (1993) Sensory receptors in the equine foot. *Am. J. Vet. Res.*, **54**, 1840–1844.
7. Van Wulfen, K.K. and Bowker, R.M. (2002) Evaluation of tachykinins and their receptors to determine sensory innervation in the dorsal hoof wall and insertion of the distal sesamoidean impar ligament and deep digital flexor tendon on the distal phalanx in healthy feet of horses. *Am. J. Vet. Res.*, **63**, 222–228.
8. Buda, S. and Budras, K.D. (2005) Segment specific nerve supply of the equine hoof. *Pferdeheilkunde*, **21**, 280–284.
9. Collins, S.N., Pollitt, C., Wylie, C.E., *et al.* (2010) Laminitic pain: Parallels with pain states in humans and other species. *Vet. Clin. Equine*, **26**, 643–671.
10. Molyneux, G.S., Haller, C.J., Mogg, K., *et al.* (1994) The structure, innervation and location of arteriovenous anastomoses in the equine foot. *Equine Vet. J.*, **26**, 305–312.
11. Hood, D.M. (1999) Laminitis in the horse. *Vet. Clin. North Am. Equine Pract.*, **15**, 287–294.
12. Pollitt, C.C. (2004) Equine laminitis. *Clin. Tech. Equine Pract.*, **3**, 34–44.
13. Rendle, D. (2006) Equine laminitis. 1. Management in the acute stage. *In Practice*, **28**, 434–443.
14. Fontaine, G.L., Belknap, J.K., Allen, D., *et al.* (2001) Expression of interleukin-1β in the digital laminae of horses in the prodromal stage of experimentally induced laminitis. *Am. J. Vet. Res.*, **62**, 714–720.
15. Waguespack, R.W., Cochran, A., and Belknap, J.K. (2004) Expression of the cyclooxygenase isoforms in the prodromal stage of black walnut-induced laminitis in horses *Am. J. Vet. Res.*, **65**, 1724–1729.
16. Blikslager, A.T., Yin, C.L., Cochran, A.M., *et al.* (2006) Cyclooxygenase expression in the early stages of equine laminitis: a cytologic study. *J. Vet. Intern. Med.*, **20**, 1191–1196.
17. Noschka, E., Moore, J.N., Peroni, J.F., *et al.* (2009) Thromboxane and isoprostanes as inflammatory and vasoactive mediators in black walnut heartwood extract induced equine laminitis. *Vet. Immunol. Immunopathol.*, **129**, 200–210.
18. Pollitt, C.C. (1996) Basement membrane pathology: a feature of acute equine laminitis. *Equine Vet. J.*, **28**, 38–46.
19. Pollitt, C.C. and Daradka, M. (1998) Equine laminitis basement membrane pathology: loss of type IV collagen, type VII collagen and laminin immunostaining. *Equine Vet. J. Suppl.*, **26**, 139–144.
20. Johnson, P.J., Tyagi, S.C., Katwa, L.C., *et al.* (1998) Activation of extracellular matrix metalloproteinases in equine laminitis. *Vet. Rec.*, **14**, 392–396.
21. Johnson, P.J., Kreeger, J.M., Keeler, M., *et al.* (2000) Serum markers of lamellar basement membrane degradation and lamellar histopathological changes in horses affected with laminitis. *Equine Vet. J.*, **32**, 462–468.
22. Binshtok, A.M., Wang, H., Zimmermann, K., *et al.* (2008) Nociceptors are interleukin-1beta sensors. *J. Neurosci.*, **28**, 14062–14073.
23. De Jongh, R.F., Vissers, K.C., Meert, T.F., *et al.* (2003) The role of interleukin-6 in nociception and pain. *Anesth. Analg.*, **96**, 1096–1103.
24. Kawasaki, Y., Xu, Z.Z., Wang, X., *et al.* (2008) Distinct roles of matrix metalloproteases in the early- and late-phase development of neuropathic pain. *Nat. Med.*, **14**, 331–336.
25. Kyaw-Tanner, M. and Pollitt, C.C. (2004) Equine laminitis: increased transcription of matrix metalloproteinase-2 (MMP-2) occurs during the developmental phase. *Equine Vet. J.*, **36** (3), 221–225.
26. Morgan, S.J., Grosenbaugh, D.A., and Hood, D.M. (1999) The pathophysiology of chronic laminitis. *Vet. Clin. North Am. Equine Pract.*, **15**, 395–417.

27. Orsini, J.A., Galantino-Homer, H., and Pollitt, C.C. (2009) Hot topics at the Fourth International Equine Conference on laminitis and diseases of the foot. Large animal Proceedings of the North American Veterinary Conference, Orlando, Florida, USA, pp. 216–217.
28. Jones, E., Viñuela-Fernandez, I., Eager, R.A., *et al.* (2007) Neuropathic changes in equine laminitis pain. *Pain*, **132**, 321–331.
29. Moorc, J.N. and Allen, D. (1996) The pathophysiology of acute laminitis. *Vet. Med.*, **10**, 936–939.
30. Doubell, T.P., Mannion, R.J., and Wolf, C.J. (1999) The dorsal horn: state dependent sensory processing, plasticity, and the generation of pain, in *Textbook of Pain*, 4th edition (eds P.D. Wall and R. Melzak), Churchill-Livingstone, New York, NY, USA, pp. 165–182.
31. Klusakova, I. and Dubovy, P. (2009) Experimental models of peripheral neuropathic pain based on traumatic nerve injuries – an anatomical perspective. *Ann. Anat.*, **191**, 248–259.
32. Costigan, M., Scholz, J., and Woolf, C.J. (2009) Neuropathic pain: a maladaptive response of the nervous system to damage. *Annu. Rev. Neurosci.*, **32**, 1–32.
33. Driessen, B. (2007) Pain: From sign to disease. *Clin. Tech. Equine Pract.*, **6**, 120–125.
34. Driessen, B. and Zarucco, L. (2007) Pain: From diagnosis to effective treatment. *Clin. Tech. Equine Pract.*, **6**, 126–134.
35. Hood, D.M., Wagner, I.P., Taylor, D.D., *et al.* (2001) Voluntary limb-load distribution in horses with acute and chronic laminitis. *Am. J. Vet. Res.*, **66**, 1393–1398.
36. Hunt, R.J. (1996) Diagnosing and treating chronic laminitis in horses. *Vet. Med.*, **91**, 1025–1032.
37. Brumbaugh, G.W., Sumano Lopez, H., and Hoyos Sepulveda, M.L.H. (1999) The pharmacologic basis for the treatment of developmental and acute laminitis. *Vet. Clin. North Am. Equine Pract.*, **15**, 345–362.
38. Sumano Lopez, H., Hoyos Sepulveda, M.L., and Brumbaugh, G.W. (1999) Pharmacologic and alternative therapies for the horse with chronic laminitis. *Vet. Clin. North Am. Equine Pract.*, **15**, 495–516.
39. Parks, A.H. (2003) Treatment of acute laminitis. *Equine Vet. Educ.*, **15**, 273–280.
40. Parks, A. and O'Grady, S.E. (2003) Chronic laminitis: current treatment strategies. *Vet. Clin. North Am. Equine Pract.*, **19**, 393–416.
41. Belknap, J.K. (2006) Treatment of the acute laminitis case. Large animal Proceedings of the North American Veterinary Conference, Orlando, Florida, USA, pp. 76–78.
42. Belknap, J.K. (2006) Treatment of the chronic laminitis case. Large animal Proceedings of the North American Veterinary Conference, Orlando, Florida, USA, pp. 79–80.
43. Piccot-Crezollet, C., Olive, J., and Cadore, J.L. (2008) Diagnostic and therapeutic approaches in the face of acute laminitis in horses. *Le Nouveau Praticien Veterinaire – Equine*, **5**, 17–23.
44. Moore, R.M. (2008) Evidence-based treatment for laminitis - what works? *J. Equine Vet. Sci.*, **28**, 176–179.
45. Divers, T.J. (2006) Medical treatment of acute laminitis. Large Animal Proceedings of the North American Veterinary Conference, Orlando, Florida, USA, pp. 174.
46. Siddall, P.J. and Cousins, M.J. (2004) Persistent pain as a disease entity: implications for clinical management. *Anesth. Analg.*, **99**, 510–520.
47. Dutton, D.W., Lashnits, K.J., and Wegner, K. (2009) Managing severe hoof pain in a horse using multimodal analgesia and a modified composite pain score. *Equine Vet. Educ.*, **21**, 37–43.
48. Hansen, N., Buchner, F., Haller, J., *et al.* (2005) Evaluation using hoof wall strain gauges of a therapeutic shoe and a hoof cast with a heel wedge as potential supportive therapy for horses with laminitis. *Vet. Surg.*, **34**, 630–636.
49. Morrison, S. (2006) Rehabilitating the laminitic foot. Large Animal Proceedings of the North American Veterinary Conference, Orlando, Florida, USA, pp. 186–189.
50. Hunt, R.J., Allen, D., Baxter, G.M., *et al.* (1991) Mid-metacarpal deep digital flexor tenotomy in the management of refractory laminitis in horses. *Vet. Surg.*, **20**, 15–20.
51. Vasko, K.A., Spauchus, A., and Lowry, M. (1986) Laminitis treatment with electrotherapy. *Equine Pract.*, **8**, 28–31.
52. Carter, D.W. and Renfroe, J.B. (2009) A novel approach to the treatment and prevention of laminitis: botulinum toxin type A for the treatment of laminitis. *J. Equine Vet. Sci.*, **29**, 595–600.
53. Galluzzi, K.E. (2005) Management of neuropathic pain. *J. Am. Osteopath. Assoc.*, **105**, S12–S19.
54. Finnerup, N.B., Otto, M., McQuay, H.J., *et al.* (2005) Algorithm for neuropathic pain treatment: An evidence-based proposal. *Pain*, **118**, 289–305.
55. Dworkin, R.H., O'Connor, A.B., Backonja, M., *et al.* (2007) Pharmacologic management of neuropathic pain: evidence-based recommendations. *Pain*, **132**, 237–251.
56. O'Connor, A.B. and Dworkin, R.H. (2009) Treatment of neuropathic pain: an overview of recent guidelines. *Am. J. Med.*, **122** (10 Suppl.), S22–S32.
57. McGeeney, B.E. (2009) Pharmacological management of neuropathic pain in older adults: an update on peripherally and centrally acting agents. *J. Pain Symptom Manag.*, **38** (2 Suppl.), S15–S27.
58. Clark, J.O. and Clark, T.P. (1999) Analgesia. *Vet. Clin. North Am. Equine Pract.*, **15**, 705–723.
59. Griffin, R.S. and Woolf, C.J. (2008) Pharmacology of Analgesia, in *Principles of Pharmacology: The Pathophysiologic Basis of Drug Therapy*, 2nd edition (eds D.E. Golan, A.H. Tashjian, E.J. Armstrong, and A.W. Armstrong), Wolters Kluwer, Lippincott Williams & Wilkins, Philadelphia, pp. 263–281.
60. Rouzer, C.A. and Marnett, L.J. (2005) Structural and functional differences between cyclooxygenases: fatty acid oxygenases with a critical role in cell signaling. *Biochem. Biophys. Res. Commun.*, **338**, 34–44.
61. Yaksh, T.L., Dirig, D.M., Conway, C.M., *et al.* (2001) The acute antihyperalgesic action of nonsteroidal, anti-inflammatory drugs and release of spinal prostaglandin E_2 is mediated by the inhibition of constitutive spinal cyclooxygenase-2 (COX-2) but not COX-1. *J. Neurosci.*, **21**, 5847–5853.
62. Urdaneta, A., Siso, A., Urdaneta, B., *et al.* (2009) Lack of correlation between the central anti-nociceptive and peripheral anti-inflammatory effects of selective COX-2 inhibitor parecoxib. *Brain Res. Bull.*, **80**, 56–61.
63. Simon, L.S. (1998) Biology and toxic effects of nonsteroidal anti-inflammatory drugs. *Curr. Opin. Rheumatol.*, **10**, 153–158.
64. Blikslager, A. (2009) Role of NSAIDs in the management of pain in horses. Proceedings of the American Association of Equine Practitioners - Focus Meeting, Raleigh, North Carolina, USA, pp. 218–223.

65. Divers, T.J. (2008) COX inhibitors: Making the best choice for the laminitic case. *J. Equine Vet. Sci.*, **28**, 367–369.
66. Cryer, B. and Feldman, M. (1998) Cyclooxygenase-1 and cyclooxygenase-2 selectivity of widely used nonsteroidal anti-inflammatory drugs. *Am. J. Med.*, **104**, 413–421.
67. Owens, J.G., Kamerling, S.G., Stanton, S.R., *et al.* (1995) Effects of ketoprofen and phenylbutazone on chronic hoof pain and lameness in the horse. *Equine Vet. J.*, **27**, 296–300.
68. Ossipov, M.H., Jerussi, T.P., Ren, K., *et al.* (2000) Differential effects of spinal (R)-ketoprofen and (S)-ketoprofen against signs of neuropathic pain and tonic nociception: evidence for a novel mechanism of action of (R)-ketoprofen against tactile allodynia. *Pain*, **87**, 193–199.
69. Diaz-Reval, M.I., Ventura-Martinez, R., Deciga-Campos, M., *et al.* (2004) Evidence for a central mechanism of action of S-(+)-ketoprofen. *Eur. J. Pharmacol.*, **483**, 241–248.
70. Moses, V.S. and Bertone, A.L. (2002) Nonsteroidal anti-inflammatory drugs. *Vet. Clin. North Am. Equine Pract.*, **18**, 21–37.
71. Martin, W.R. (1983) Pharmacology of opioids. *Pharmacol. Rev.*, **35**, 283–323.
72. Inturrisi, C.E. (2002) Clinical pharmacology of opioids for pain. *Clin. J. Pain*, **18** (Suppl.), S3–S13.
73. Bennett, R.C. and Steffey, E.P. (2002) Use of opioids for pain and anesthetic management in horses. *Vet. Clin. North Am. Equine Pract.*, **18**, 46–60.
74. Driessen, B. (2007) Pain: systemic and local/regional drug therapy. *Clin. Tech. Equine Pract.*, **6**, 135–144.
75. Clutton, R.E. (2010) Opioid analgesia in horses. *Vet. Clin. Equine*, **26**, 493–514.
76. Knych, H.K., Casbeer, H.C., McKemie, D.S., *et al.* (2013) Pharmacokinetics and pharmacodynamics of butorphanol following intravenous administration to the horse. *J. Vet. Pharmacol. Ther.*, **36** (1), 21–30.
77. Roger, T., Bardon, T., and Ruckebusch, Y. (1985) Colonic motor responses in the pony: relevance of colonic stimulation by opiate antagonists. *Am. J. Vet. Res.*, **46**, 31–36.
78. Boscan, P., Van Hoogmoed, L.M., Farver, T.B., *et al.* (2006) Evaluation of the effects of the opioid agonist morphine on gastrointestinal tract function in horses. *Am. J. Vet. Res.*, **67**, 992–997.
79. Sasaki, N., Yoshihara, T., and Hara, S. (2000) Difference in the motile reactivity of jejunum, cecum, and right ventral colon to xylazine and medetomidine in conscious horses. *J. Equine Sci.*, **11**, 63–68.
80. Angst, M.S. (2006) Opioid-induced hyperalgesia: a qualitative systematic review. *Anesthesiology*, **104**, 570–587.
81. Silverman, S.M. (2009) Opioid induced hyperalgesia: clinical implications for the pain practitioner. *Pain Physician*, **12**, 679–684.
82. Fishbain, D.A.A. (2009) Do opioids induce hyperalgesia in humans? An evidence-based structured review. *Pain Med.*, **10**, 829–839.
83. Sellon, D.C., Monroe, V.L., Roberts, M.C., *et al.* (2001) Pharmacokinetics and adverse effects of butorphanol administered by single intravenous injection or continuous intravenous infusion in horses. *Am. J. Vet. Res.*, **62**, 183–189.
84. Sellon, D.C., Roberts, M.C., Blikslager, A.T., *et al.* (2004) Effects of continuous rate intravenous infusion of butorphanol on physiologic and outcome variables in horses after celiotomy. *J. Vet. Intern. Med.*, **18**, 555–563.
85. Sellon, D.C., Papich, M.G., Palmer, L., *et al.* (2008) Pharmacokinetics of butorphanol in horses after intramuscular injection. *J. Vet. Pharmacol. Ther.*, **32**, 62–65.
86. Wegner, K., Franklin, R.P., Long, M.T., *et al.* (2002) How to use fentanyl transdermal patches for analgesia in horses. Proceedings of the 48th Annual Convention of the American Association of Equine Practitioners, Orlando, Florida, USA, pp. 291–294.
87. Thomasy, S.M., Slovis, N., Maxwell, L.K., *et al.* (2004) Transdermal fentanyl combined with non-steroidal anti-inflammatory drugs for analgesia in horses. *J. Vet. Intern. Med.*, **18**, 550–554.
88. Orsini, J.A., Moate, P.J., Kuersten, K., *et al.* (2006) Pharmacokinetics of fentanyl delivered transdermally in healthy adult horses – variability among horses and its clinical implications. *J. Vet. Pharmacol. Ther.*, **29**, 539–546.
89. Carregaro, A.B., Luna, S.P., Mataqueiro, M.I., *et al.* (2007) Effects of buprenorphine on nociception and spontaneous locomotor activity in horses. *Am. J. Vet. Res.*, **68**, 246–250.
90. Davis, J.L., Messenger, K.M., LaFevers, D.H., *et al.* (2011) Pharmacokinetics of intravenous and intramuscular buprenorphine in the horse. *J. Vet. Pharmacol. Ther.*, **35**, 52–58.
91. Walker, A.F. (2007) Sublingual administration of buprenorphine for long-term analgesia in the horse. *Vet. Rec.*, **160**, 808–809.
92. Mao, J. and Chen, L.L. (2000) Systemic lidocaine for neuropathic pain relief. *Pain*, **87**, 7–17.
93. Lauretti, G.R. (2008) Mechanisms of analgesia of intravenous lidocaine. *Rev. Bras. Anestesiologia*, **58**, 280–286.
94. Doherty, T.J. and Seddighi, M.R. (2010) Local anesthetics as pain therapy in horses. *Vet. Clin. Equine*, **26**, 533–549.
95. Robertson, S.A., Sanchez, L.C., Merritt, A.M., *et al.* (2005) Effect of systemic lidocaine on visceral and somatic nociception in conscious horses. *Equine Vet. J.*, **37**, 122–127.
96. Feary, D.J., Mama, K.R., Wagner, A.E., *et al.* (2005) Influence of general anaesthesia on pharmacokinetics of intravenous lidocaine infusion in horses. *Am. J. Vet. Res.*, **66**, 574–580.
97. Gottrup, H., Bach, F.W., Juhl, G., *et al.* (2006) Differential effect of ketamine and lidocaine on spontaneous and mechanical evoked pain in patients with nerve injury pain. *Anesthesiology*, **104**, 527–536.
98. Gormsen, L., Finnerup, N.B., Almqvist, P.M., *et al.* (2009) The efficacy of the AMPA receptor antagonist NS1209 and lidocaine in nerve injury pain: a randomized, double-blind, placebo-controlled, three-way crossover study. *Anesth. Analg.*, **108**, 1311–1319.
99. Meyer, G.A., Lin, H.C., Hanson, R.R., *et al.* (2001) Effects of intravenous lidocaine overdose on cardiac electrical activity and blood pressure in the horse. *Equine Vet. J.*, **33**, 434–437.
100. De Solis, C.N. and McKenzie, H.C., III. (2007) Serum concentrations of lidocaine and its metabolites MEGX and GX during and after prolonged intravenous infusion of lidocaine in horses after colic surgery. *J. Equine Vet. Sci.*, **27**, 398–404.
101. Dickey, E.J., McKenzie, H.C., III, Brown, K.A., *et al.* (2008) Serum concentrations of lidocaine and its metabolites after prolonged infusion in healthy horses. *Equine Vet. J.*, **40**, 348–352.
102. Woolf, C.J. and Wiesenfeld-Hallin, Z. (1985) The systemic administration of local anaesthetics produces a selective depression of

C-afferent fibre evoked activity in the spinal cord. *Pain*, **23**, 361–374.
103. Ness, T. (2000) Intravenous lidocaine inhibits visceral nociceptive reflexes and spinal neurons in the rat. *Anesthesiology*, **92**, 1685–1691.
104. Abram, S.E. and Yaksh, T.L. (1994) Systemic lidocaine blocks nerve injury-induced hyperalgesia and nociceptor-driven spinal sensitization in the rat. *Anesthesiology*, **80**, 383–391.
105. Attal, N., Rouaud, J., Brasseur, L., *et al.* (2004) Systemic lidocaine in pain due to peripheral nerve injury and predictors of response. *Neurology*, **62**, 218–225.
106. Giordano, J. (2001) The neurobiology of pain, in *Pain Management: A Practical Guide for Clinicians*, 6th edition (ed. R.S. Weiner), CRC Press, Boca Raton, FL, pp. 1089–1100.
107. Latremoliere, A. and Woolf, C.J. (2009) Central sensitization: a generator of pain hypersensitivity by central neural plasticity. *J. Pain*, **10**, 895–926.
108. Woolf, C.J. (2011) Central sensitization: Implications for the diagnosis and treatment of pain. *Pain*, **152**, S2–S15.
109. Yaksh, T.L. (2010) The pain state arising from the laminitic horse: insights into future analgesic therapies. *J. Equine Vet. Sci.*, **30**, 79–82.
110. Berti, M., Baciarello, M., Troglio, R., *et al.* (2009) Clinical uses of low-dose ketamine in patients undergoing surgery. *Curr. Drug Targets*, **10**, 707–715.
111. Visser, E. and Schug, S.A. (2006) The role of ketamine in pain management. *Biomed. Pharmacother.*, **60**, 341–348.
112. Richebe, P., Rivat, C., and Rivalan, B. (2005) Low-dose ketamine: antihyperalgesic drug, non-analgesic. *Annu. Fr. Anesth. Reanim.*, **24**, 1349–1359.
113. Lankveld, D.P.K., Driessen, B., Soma, L.R., *et al.* (2006) Pharmacodynamic effects and pharmacokinetic profile of a long-term continuous rate infusion of racemic ketamine in healthy conscious horses. *J. Vet. Pharmacol. Ther.*, **29**, 477–488.
114. Fielding, C.L., Brumbaugh, G.W., Matthews, N.S., *et al.* (2006) Pharmacokinetics and clinical effects of a subanesthetic continuous rate infusion of ketamine in awake horses. *Am. J. Vet. Res.*, **67**, 1484–1490.
115. Korenhuber, J., Quack, G., Danysz, W., *et al.* (1995) Therapeutic brain concentration of the NMDA receptor antagonist amantadine. *Neuropharmacology*, **34**, 713–721.
116. Pud, D., Eisenberg, E., Spitzer, A., *et al.* (1998) The NMDA receptor antagonist amantadine reduces surgical neuropathic pain in cancer patients: a double blind, randomized, placebo controlled trial. *Pain*, **75**, 349–354.
117. Amin, P. and Sturrock, N.D. (2003) A pilot study of the beneficial effects of amantadine in the treatment of painful diabetic peripheral neuropathy. *Diabet. Med.*, **20**, 114–118.
118. Rees, W.A., Harkins, J.D., Woods, W.E., *et al.* Amantadine and equine influenza: pharmacology, pharmacokinetics and neurological effects in the horse. *Equine Vet. J.*, **29**, 104–110.
119. Treede, R.D., Jensen, T.S., Campbell, J.N., *et al.* (2008) Neuropathic pain: Redefinition and a grading system for clinical and research purposes. *Neurology*, **70**, 1630–1635.
120. Cruccu, G. and Truini, A. (2009) Tools for assessing neuropathic pain. *PLoS Medicine/Public Library of Science*, **6**, e1000045.
121. Haanpaa, M., Attal, N., Backonja, M., *et al.* (2011) NeuPSIG guidelines on neuropathic pain assessment. *Pain*, **152**, 14–27.
122. Taylor, C.P. (2004) The biology and pharmacology of calcium channel α_2-δ proteins. *CNS Drug Rev.*, **10**, 183–188.
123. Maneuf, Y.P., Luo, Z.D., and Lee, K. (2006) α2δ and the mechanism of action of gabapentin in the treatment of pain. *Semin. Cell Dev. Biol.*, **17**, 565–570.
124. Dixit, R.K. and Bhargava, V.K. (2002) Neurotransmitter mechanisms in gabapentin antinociception. *Pharmacology*, **65**, 198–203.
125. Sills, G.J. (2006) The mechanisms of action of gabapentin and pregabalin. *Curr. Opin. Pharmacol.*, **6**, 108–113.
126. Luo, Z.D., Chaplan, S.R., Higuera, E.S., Sorkin, L.S., *et al.* (2001) Upregulation of dorsal root ganglion α2δ calcium channel subunit and its correlation with allodynia in spinal nerve-injured rats. *J. Neurosci.*, **21**, 1868–1875.
127. Newton, R.A., Bingham, S., Case, P.C., *et al.* (2001) Dorsal root ganglion neurons show increased expression of the calcium channel α2δ-1 subunit following partial sciatic nerve injury. *Mol. Brain Res.*, **95**, 1–8.
128. Harding, L.M., Kristensen, J.D., and Baranowski, A.P. (2005) Differential effects of neuropathic analgesics on wind-up-like pain and somatosensory function in healthy volunteers. *Clin. J. Pain*, **21**, 127–132.
129. Davis, J.L., Posner, L.P., and Elce, Y. (2007) Gabapentin for the treatment of neuropathic pain in a pregnant horse. *J. Am. Vet. Med. Assoc.*, **231**, 755–758.
130. Dirikolu, L., Dafalla, A., Ely, K.J., *et al.* (2008) Pharmacokinetics of gabapentin in horses. *J. Vet. Pharmacol. Ther.*, **31**, 175–177.
131. Terry, R., McDonnell, S.M., van Eps, A.W., *et al.* (2010) Pharmacokinetic profile and behavioral effects of gabapentin in the horse. *J. Vet. Pharmacol. Ther.*, **33**, 485–494.
132. Eckhardt, K., Ammon, S., Hofmann, U., *et al.* (2000) Gabapentin enhances the analgesic effect of morphine in healthy volunteers. *Anesth. Analg.*, **91**, 185–191.
133. Moulin, D.E., Clark, A.J., Gilron, I., *et al.* (2007) Pharmacological management of chronic neuropathic pain – Consensus statement and guidelines from the Canadian Pain Society. *Pain Res. Manag.*, **12**, 13–21.
134. Bohlega, S., Alsaadi, T., Amir, A., *et al.* (2010) Guidelines for the pharmacological treatment of peripheral neuropathic pain: expert panel recommendations for the Middle East region. *J. Int. Med. Res.*, **38**, 295–317.
135. Divers, T.J. and DeLahunta, A. (2008) Neurologic emergencies, in *Equine Emergencies*, 3rd edition (eds J.A. Orsini and T.J. Divers), Saunders Elsevier, St Louis, MO, pp. 331–374.
136. Mullen, K.R., Schwark, W., and Divers, T.J. (2013) Pharmacokinetics of single-dose intragastric and intravenous pregabalin administration in clinically normal horses. *Am. J. Vet. Res.*, **74**, 1043–1048.
137. Xie, W., Strong, J.A., Meij, J.T., *et al.* (2005) Neuropathic pain: early spontaneous afferent activity is the trigger. *Pain*, **116**, 243–256.
138. Reuben, S.S. and Buvanendran, A. (2007) Preventing the development of chronic pain after orthopaedic surgery with preventive multimodal analgesic techniques. *J. Bone Joint Surg.*, **89**, 1343–1358.
139. Boezaart, A.P. (2006) Perineural infusion of local anesthetics. *Anesthesiology*, **104**, 872–880.
140. Driessen, B., Scandella, M., and Zarucco, L. (2008) Development of a technique for continuous perineural blockade of the palmar nerves in the distal equine thoracic limb. *Vet. Anaesth. Analg.*, **35**, 432–448.

141. Zarucco, L., Driessen, B., Scandella, M., *et al.* (2007) Continuous perineural block of the palmar nerves: A new technique for pain relief in the distal equine forelimb. *Clin. Tech. Equine Pract.*, **6**, 154–164.
142. Zarucco, L., Driessen, B., Scandella, M., *et al.* (2010) Sensory nerve conduction and nociception in the equine lower forelimb during perineural bupivacaine infusion along the palmar nerves. *Can. J. Vet. Res.*, **74**, 305–313.
143. Watts, A.E., Nixon, A.J., and Reesink, H.L. (2011) Continuous peripheral neural blockade to alleviate signs of experimentally induced severe forelimb pain in horses. *J. Am. Vet. Med. Assoc.*, **238**, 1032–1039.
144. Driessen, B. and Zarucco, L. (2013) Treatment of acute and chronic pain in horses, in *Pain Management in Veterinary Practice* (eds C. Egger, L.C. Love, and T.J. Doherty), Wiley-Blackwell, Ames, Iowa, pp. 323–348.
145. Driessen, B., Zarucco, L., Scandella, M., *et al.* (2008) Antinociceptive efficacy of continuous perineural blockade of median and ulnar nerves in the equine forelimb. Proceedings of the Association of Veterinary Anaesthetists' Autumn 2008 Meeting, Barcelona, Spain.
146. Natalini, C.C. and Driessen, B. (2007) Epidural and spinal anesthesia and analgesia in the equine. *Clin. Tech. Equine Pract.*, **6**, 144–153.
147. Natalini, C.C. (2010) Spinal anesthetics and analgesics in the horse. *Vet. Clin. Equine*, **26**, 551–564.
148. Hendrickson, D.A., Southwood, L.L., Lopez, M.J., *et al.* (1998) Cranial migration of different volumes of new-methylene blue after caudal epidural injection in the horse. *Equine Pract.*, **20**, 12–14.
149. Bellei, M.H., Kerr, C., Johnson, R., *et al.* (2009) Pharmacokinetics of epidural morphine in awake and isoflurane-anesthetized horses. *Vet. Anaesth. Analg.*, **36**, 14.
150. Grimm, C., Aneiros, E., and de Groot, M. (2011) Dissecting TRPV1: lessons to be learned. *Channels*, **5**, 201–204.
151. Xia, R., Dekermendjian, K., Lullau, E., *et al.* (2011) TRPV1: a therapy target that attracts the pharmaceutical interests. *Adv. Exp. Med. Biol.*, **704**, 637–665.
152. DaCunha, A.F., Chirgwin, S.R., Stokes, A.M., *et al.* (2008) Quantitative expression of the TRPV-1 Gene in central and peripheral nervous tissue in horses. *Int. J. Appl. Res. Vet. Med.*, **6**, 15–23.
153. Neubert, J.K., Mannes, A.J., Karai, L.J., *et al.* (2008) Perineural resiniferatoxin selectively inhibits inflammatory hyperalgesia. *Mol. Pain*, **4**, 3 open access journal ; doi:10.1186/1744-8069-4-3.
154. Wong, G.Y. and Gavva, N.R. (2009) Therapeutic potential of vanilloid receptor TRPV1 agonists and antagonists as analgesics: Recent advances and setbacks. *Brain Res. Rev.*, **60**, 267–277.
155. Seino, K.K., Foreman, J.H., Greene, S.A., *et al.* (2003) Effects of topical perineural capsaicin in a reversible model of equine foot lameness. *J. Vet. Intern. Med.*, **17**, 563–566.
156. Berardinelli, P., Barazzoni, A.M., Russo, V., *et al.* (2003) Selective deafferentation of hand cutaneous territory is followed by changes in fibre type distribution of a forearm muscle in the horse. *Arch. Italiennes de Biologie*, **141**, 19–25.

CHAPTER 34
Digital Hypothermia

Andrew W. van Eps and Christopher C. Pollitt

Introduction

A multitude of treatments have been suggested and used for laminitis in horses, dating back to the beginning of recorded history. Amongst those, a traditional treatment for acute laminitis was to stand the affected horse in a cool stream. The effect of cooling the feet (cryotherapy/therapeutic hypothermia) has only recently been tested in experimental models of laminitis, and it is the only therapeutic modality for laminitis that has stood up to repeated scientific scrutiny. The effects of hypothermia on tissue are complex, powerful, and difficult to replicate pharmaceutically. The value of therapeutic hypothermia in the modern clinical setting was first recognized and utilized in humans undergoing cardiac bypass surgery, the objective being protection and preservation of organs (particularly the heart and brain) during planned operative ischemia [1]. Therapeutic hypothermia has since been studied extensively and has achieved variable clinical adoption as a preventive as well as a therapeutic agent in human patients with traumatic brain injury, stroke, cardiac arrest, and neonatal encephalopathy [2–4]. There is some evidence from rodent sepsis models that therapeutic hypothermia may help to prevent and treat acute lung injury [5–7], an important manifestation of end-organ damage in human sepsis. Protocols for whole-body and regional hypothermia are currently evolving, though ideal methods, temperature and duration are still not clear. Hypothermia can have detrimental effects, which are perhaps most important where cooling of the target organ requires cooling of the whole body, and particularly when cooling is more profound. The equine distal limb offers a unique opportunity for the use of therapeutic hypothermia: the target organ (lamellar tissue) can be cooled selectively, in isolation from other tissues. The equine distal limb is also adapted to extreme environmental cold, allowing more profound local hypothermia without apparent side effects and with excellent tolerance from the horse.

Therapeutic Mechanisms of Hypothermia

Analgesic and Hypometabolic Effects

The major effects of hypothermia on tissue reported in the human literature include analgesia, reduced metabolism, and a vascular response [8]. Cold has a direct effect on peripheral nerves, reducing conduction velocity, raising the threshold for stimulation, and increasing the refractory period after stimulation [9]. Tissue metabolic rate and oxygen consumption are directly related to temperature [10], and this hypometabolic effect was traditionally credited as the major basis for the therapeutic effects of hypothermia. Hypothermia has been intensively studied in brain tissue for its neuroprotective effects following traumatic and ischemic brain injury [11]. Cerebral metabolism decreases by 6–10% for each 1 °C decrease in body temperature [12–14]. A reduced requirement of cooled tissue for oxygen, glucose, and other metabolites enhances the survival of cells during periods of ischemia, protecting tissues from secondary hypoxic damage [8] and maintaining tissue viability during organ transplant surgery [15]. Hypothermia reduces apoptosis, mitochondrial failure and inflammation after cerebral ischemia–reperfusion [11]. Likewise, reductions in enzymatic activity, including that of collagenases, are observed at lower temperatures [16, 17].

Anti-Inflammatory Effects

Regional hypothermia (cryotherapy) is well established as a treatment for reducing inflammation and providing analgesia in acute musculoskeletal injury and following orthopedic surgery in humans [8, 18, 19]. The array of potent anti-inflammatory effects exerted by hypothermia is also proving useful in other disease scenarios where inflammation plays a major role, including both in the treatment of primary inflammatory conditions and also in protecting tissue from inflammatory damage post-ischemia. The primary anti-inflammatory effects of

Equine Laminitis, First Edition. Edited by James K. Belknap and Raymond Geor.

hypothermia demonstrated in rodent models of human disease include the reduced production and activity of proinflammatory cytokines [7, 20, 21], increased production of anti-inflammatory cytokines (particularly interleukin [IL]-10) [7, 22], reduced adhesion and extravasation of leukocytes from the microvasculature into affected tissues [23, 24], and a reduced production of free radicals of oxygen or reactive oxygen species (ROS) by polymorphonuclear leukocytes [25]. In addition, hypothermia had an inhibitory effect on matrix metalloproteinase (MMP) expression (leukocyte-derived MMP-9) in studies of brain trauma [26] and cardiac arrest [27]. The anti-inflammatory effects of hypothermia are thought to play an important role in reducing the prolonged phase of inflammatory tissue damage in the brain associated with reperfusion after ischemia [28].

Preventing End-Organ Damage in Sepsis

Of particular interest, and a topic of much recent research, is the potential for hypothermia to protect against end-organ damage during systemic inflammatory conditions, including sepsis. Mild, whole-body hypothermia (5–6 °C below normal) has been shown to increase survival in rodent models of sepsis [5, 29], and the experimental evidence is prompting discussions of clinical applications of therapeutic hypothermia in septic human patients [30, 31]. The preservation of cellular energy metabolism and mitochondrial function [32], reduced inflammation [6, 7, 22, 33], and inhibition of apoptotic pathways [34] are effects of hypothermia that are proposed to protect against end-organ damage in the liver, lung, and heart. Pre-emptive hypothermia (10 °C below normal) markedly reduced the severity of acute lung injury in a rat model of sepsis by reducing neutrophil emigration, inhibiting proinflammatory cytokine activity, and increasing anti-inflammatory cytokine activity [7]. In a subsequent study, less-profound hypothermia (5 °C below normal) applied after the induction of neutrophilic inflammation in the lung decreased the severity of acute lung injury, suggesting a potential therapeutic role for hypothermia beyond its preventive effect [6].

Vascular Effects

Hypothermia in most tissues generally results in local vasoconstriction [35]. This is largely mediated by sympathetic nervous control; however, a direct constrictive effect on blood vessel walls may occur, particularly when the tissue temperature approaches 0 °C [36]. A scintigraphic study demonstrated a significant reduction in soft tissue perfusion when the equine digit was immersed in 4 °C iced water for a short period of 30 min [37]. Based on hoof temperature measurements, digital vasoconstriction appears to predominate when distal limb cryotherapy is applied continuously for longer periods [38–41] and when horses are maintained in a controlled, low-ambient temperature (10 °C) environment [42]; however intermittent, spontaneous increases in hoof temperature (up to 12 °C during cold water immersion at 5 °C and up to 25 °C in a 10 °C climate-controlled room) were noted in four of six and four of eight horses in respective studies [41, 42]. These 1- to 12-h periods of increased hoof temperature can occur synchronously or asynchronously in the forelimbs (Fig. 34.1). The phenomenon is similar to that noted in horses living in natural environments below freezing (C. Pollitt, unpublished data). The function or reason for this periodic hoof temperature increase in the face of environmental or local hypothermia is unclear. The increases in hoof temperature most likely represent transient increases in perfusion, metabolism, or both [43], and may be associated with opening of arteriovenous anastomoses (AVAs). The fact that these periods are not reliably synchronous suggests that the trigger is a local phenomenon, possibly local tissue temperature or accumulation of metabolic intermediates normally removed during adequate blood flow. In other tissues, periods of transient vasodilation (cold-induced vasodilation; CIVD) are observed when temperatures are reduced below approximately 18 °C [44]. A cyclic pattern of increasing and decreasing blood flow (the 'hunting' reaction) may be noted [45]. The phenomenon of CIVD has been studied mostly in the human hand, but it has also been noted in the face, forearms, and feet [46]. In the human finger, CIVD appears to occur as a result of dilation of the AVAs, whereas cold-induced vasoconstriction seems to result from the constriction of AVAs as well as the arteries supplying the finger [47].

Rationale and Evidence for Use of Digital Hypothermia in Laminitis

The present understanding of the pathophysiology of laminitis has evolved dramatically during recent years, as has the understanding of the mechanisms by which hypothermia can alter disease progression. Eighteenth century references to the use of digital hypothermia for the treatment of laminitis have been cited by Wagner [48], but it was the study of Pollitt and Davies [42] that prompted scientific evaluation of its effects. In this study, the investigators used a carbohydrate overload (CHO) model of laminitis in a climate-controlled room (10 °C) to demonstrate increased hoof temperature (indicative of vasodilation) during the developmental phase in horses that went on to develop laminitis (compared with those that did not), prompting the hypothesis that digital vasoconstriction might be protective. At the time of that study, vascular changes (vasoconstriction and ischemia) were thought to be major initiating events in laminitis, regardless of the inciting cause. During recent years, investigators have come to realize that there are important differences in the pathophysiology of laminitis, depending on the inciting cause. This has resulted in laminitis being divided into essentially three forms, based up the purported basic mechanisms of disease, namely sepsis, hyperinsulinemia/endocrinopathy, and supporting limb laminitis. The mechanisms that lead to the different forms of laminitis are now better defined (see relevant chapters), allowing a more informed exploration of the opportunities for therapeutic intervention with hypothermia in the clinical setting.

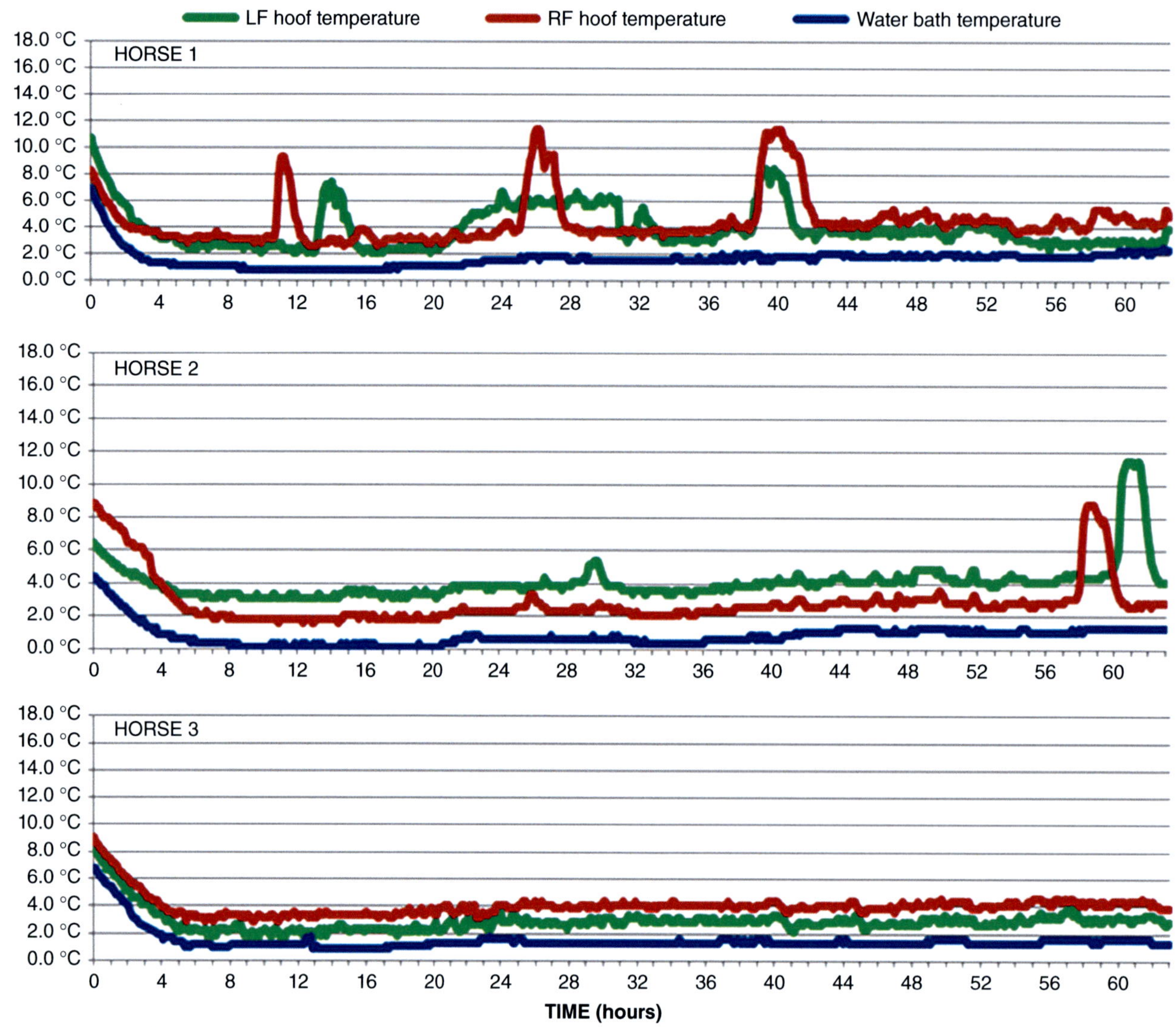

Figure 34.1 Hoof temperature traces from both front limbs of three horses during cold water immersion of all four feet over a three-day period. Intermittent, spontaneous increases in hoof temperature are noted regularly in some horses (Horse 1), rarely in others (Horse 2), and not at all in some horses (Horse 3). These 1- to 12-h periods of increased hoof temperature occur sometimes synchronously in the forelimbs, and sometimes asynchronously, and are also seen in horses living in natural environments below freezing (C. Pollitt, unpublished data). The increases in hoof temperature may be associated with the opening of arteriovenous anastomoses (AVAs). The fact that these periods are not reliably synchronous suggests that the trigger is a local phenomenon, possibly local tissue temperature or accumulation of metabolic intermediates (e.g., lactate).

Studies evaluating the effects of digital hypothermia on the development of laminitis have been performed exclusively in the oligofructose (OF) experimental model of sepsis-related laminitis (SRL). These studies have utilized ice and water or refrigerated water immersion of the distal limb, leading to internal hoof temperatures of 3–8 °C (at least a 20 °C decrease below normal foot temperature). This is dramatically more profound than the 3–5 °C reduction in body temperature that is commonly targeted for whole-body hypothermia used in human medicine for a variety of disease processes [1, 11]. In an initial study in which hypothermia was initiated at the time of OF administration, continuous cooling of a single limb during the developmental phase dramatically reduced both the severity of clinical signs of lameness and the severity of lamellar injury (on histopathology) when evaluated 48 h after the OF dose [39]. That study proved the principle of prophylactic hypothermia as a viable preventive treatment for animals at risk of SRL. A follow-up study showed that digital hypothermia of all four limbs maintained for 72 h after OF dosing resulted in a reduced severity of lameness and lamellar injury evaluated four days after cooling ceased [41]. The study also showed that the prophylactic effect of digital hypothermia does not merely delay the appearance of laminitis pathology, but rather has a lasting protective effect. In both studies, pathologic changes to the lamellae were not completely absent in the hypothermic limbs, but were ameliorated to an extent that would translate into a meaningful clinical effect. The current evidence for the use of therapeutic digital hypothermia in laminitis is based solely on these controlled experimental studies with small treatment and control groups (six to eight horses): what remained lacking until recently was a clinical trial evaluating the effects of digital hypothermia in the clinical setting. Kullman *et al.* described a multicenter retrospective series of 130 colitis cases, with an overall acute laminitis incidence of 21% [49]. Horses treated with digital hypothermia in that study had 10-fold lower odds of developing laminitis compared to horses that did not have their feet cooled, demonstrating that prophylactic cooling is an effective laminitis preventative in clinical colitis cases.

There are several possible mechanisms by which hypothermia protects lamellar tissue from damage and reduces the progression of laminitis in the OF model (and likely the clinical case) of SRL [50–52]. Inflammation and protease activity are implicated in the developmental as well as acute phases of SRL [53–59]. When applied before the onset of clinical lameness in the OF model, continuous digital hypothermia dramatically inhibited gene expression of a wide range of inflammatory mediators that included cytokines, chemokines, and cyclooxygenase-2 in lamellar tissue [60]. In addition, hypothermia had an inhibitory effect on lamellar matrix metalloproteinase (MMP) expression in the OF model [39], a finding consistent with experimental studies of hypothermia in brain trauma [26] and cardiac arrest [27]. In other animal models of sepsis, the preservation of cellular energy metabolism and mitochondrial function [32], reduced inflammation [6, 7, 22, 33], and inhibition of apoptotic pathways [34] are effects of hypothermia that protect against end-organ damage in the liver, lung, and heart. The contribution of cellular energy failure (non-ischemic) to the different forms of laminitis is unclear, but hypothermia of the equine digit may also exert protective effects on lamellar tissue by modulating mitochondrial function and reducing metabolic demands.

It is unclear whether digital hypothermia would have a preventive effect on the development of supporting limb or endocrinopathic laminitis, as in the clinical setting both of these forms have a developmental phase that is much less predictable than that associated with the septic form, with little evidence of the marked lamellar inflammatory signaling documented in SRL. However, inflammation, protease activation, and pain are likely to be features of the early laminitis case beginning to undergo lamellar failure/injury and digital displacement, regardless of the inciting cause. It is therefore rational to expect that digital hypothermia might have beneficial effects in acute laminitis, once lameness is already evident. Due to the concern that veterinarians in clinical practice often do not attend cases of any type of laminitis until the animal is already demonstrating clinical signs of lameness, a recent study was performed in which digital hypothermia was not initiated until after the onset of lameness in the OF model. In this study, a profound therapeutic effect was still observed with digital hypothermia [61], with only mild to undetectable lesions present in the hypothermic limb (Fig. 34.2) in the face of total lamellar failure (complete separation of lamellar epidermis from dermis; 'sinking') in untreated control limbs. As the goal in the treatment of acute laminitis should be to reduce progression of the lesion (lamellar separation and ultimately mechanical failure of the suspensory apparatus of the distal phalanx), this study documented that digital hypothermia instituted at the onset of clinically apparent lameness is an effective therapy. Digital hypothermia also exhibited analgesic effects in that study, which would clearly be beneficial in the acute laminitis patient.

Digital Hypothermia in Clinical Cases

Case Selection

Once established, laminitis causes derangements of lamellar structure that are largely irreversible; therefore efforts should be aimed at prevention. It follows that digital hypothermia is likely to be most effective prior to the onset of clinical signs, but this is often not possible or practical in the clinical setting. Any horse that is at immediate risk of developing acute laminitis is an appropriate candidate for continuous distal limb hypothermia. Conditions associated with a high risk of laminitis development include colitis, enteritis, complicated gastrointestinal obstructions, metritis, pneumonia, and alimentary carbohydrate (grain) overload [62–66]. Horses exhibiting clinical signs consistent with endotoxemia/sepsis should be considered at particularly high risk [62]. The most recent study described above suggests that digital hypothermia is also indicated in acute laminitis [61]. Regardless of the inciting cause, digital hypothermia will provide analgesia and may help to reduce lesion progression in horses with acute laminitis (or chronic laminitis with a recrudescent, acute episode).

Timing and Duration of Treatment

The ideal target period to initiate treatment is the developmental phase (defined as the period between the initial causative event and the appearance of acute lameness). The duration of the developmental phase is highly variable, lasting between 18 and 72 h in CHO models, up to five days in clinical colitis, enteritis, and metritis cases, or longer with other diseases such as pleuropneumonia. The difficulty in identifying the developmental phase (there is a current lack of any suitable biomarker) means that the perceived risk of laminitis and the logistics of application (constant digital hypothermia is a very labor-intensive therapy for owners/technicians) will govern the decision to treat prophylactically in most cases. Resolution of the primary disease may be used as an indicator for ceasing digital hypothermia in individual cases. It is prudent to continue therapy for 24–48 h after resolution of the clinical signs of sepsis (fever, mucous membrane hyperemia) and normalization of laboratory indicators (leukopenia and perhaps serum amyloid A concentration) of systemic inflammation.

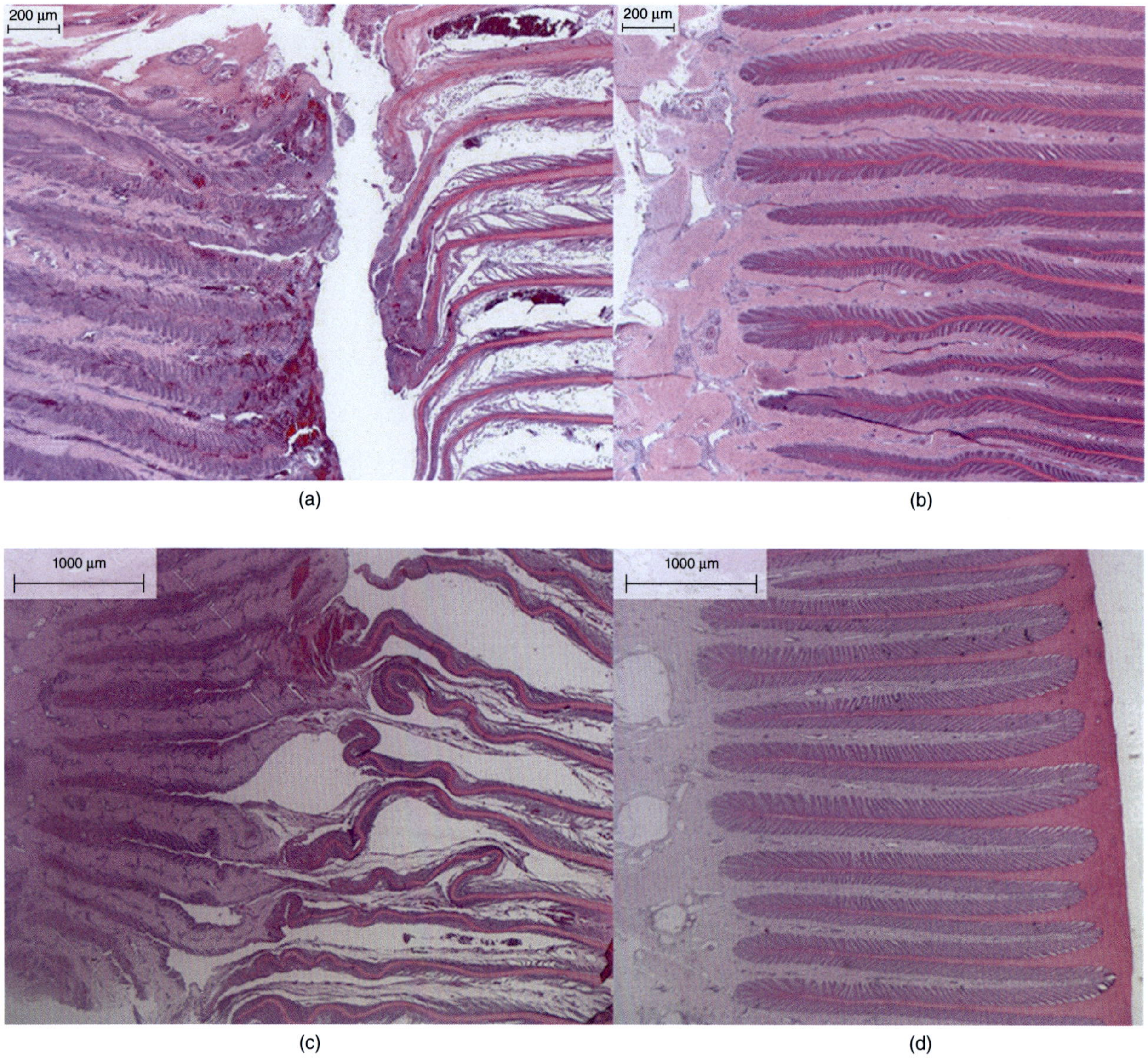

Figure 34.2 Digital hypothermia can protect lamellar tissue from complete separation/mechanical failure. The upper images represent the histological appearance of an uncooled hind limb (a) and a cooled forelimb (b) from the same horse: this was a clinical case of colitis that was euthanized due to the development of laminitis in the uncooled hind limbs. A similar effect has been shown in experimental models, even when cooling is delayed until after the onset of laminitis: complete separation of lamellar epidermis is noted in the uncooled forelimb (c) compared with almost no appreciable structural change in the cooled limb (d) [61].

When treating acute cases of laminitis, it is rational to use digital hypothermia as part of a first aid strategy. Cooling for two to three days or more may be warranted in the acute laminitis case, although there is currently no evidence to guide cessation of therapy in these cases. Anecdotal evidence from clinical cases suggests that digital hypothermia can be maintained for days to weeks, without ill effect. There is no evidence to support the use of intermittent cooling, and all experimental studies have thus far have used continuous digital hypothermia. Studies conducted in other species suggests that (ideally) rewarming should be gradual (over 12–24 h), as rapid rewarming after therapeutic hypothermia may negate the protective effect [11]. However, in most clinical cases, cryotherapy is ceased without gradual rewarming, without apparent negative effects.

Cooling Methods

To maximize the clinical effect and minimize any side effects, therapeutic hypothermia should be targeted as much as possible to the tissue of interest. The equine distal limb presents a unique opportunity, as, distal to the carpus and tarsus, there is no muscle and the major blood vessels are superficial, seemingly ideal for inducing deep hypothermia of the foot. However, the hair coat and hoof provide a barrier to the effective conduction of thermal energy in and out of the limb, and blood flowing through the major arteries constantly replenishes the rich vascular network within the corium with warmed (or cooled) blood. The numerous lamellar AVAs [67], typical of a thermoregulatory organ, mean that rapid increases in net perfusion of the foot with warm blood can occur.

Numerous modalities are used for distal limb cryotherapy in horses, and there are several commercially available devices for this purpose, although most are suited to short-term (30–60 min) applications for therapies unrelated to laminitis. Reported studies focused on limb structures other than the foot have used commercial cold gel wraps and cold cuffs as well as ice water immersion [68, 69]. In order to achieve consistently low temperatures within the target (lamellar) tissue, the requirements for cooling methods appear to differ significantly from those most commonly used for distal limb tendon/skeletal cooling.

Studies with experimental models of laminitis have shown a preventive effect when hoof temperatures (measured by a probe embedded in the hoof wall or on the hoof surface) were maintained consistently at 3–5 °C using cold water alone or ice and water slurries, immersing the limb up to the proximal metacarpus (just below the carpus). As discussed earlier, this technique usually results in a 20 °C or more decrease below normal foot temperature. When applied after the onset of lameness in the OF laminitis model, the same method resulted in hoof wall surface temperatures of 6–8 °C, and still achieved a significant therapeutic effect. Recent human medical-related studies suggested a superior effect when mild to moderate (3–5 °C reduction below normal temperature) therapeutic hypothermia is used compared with traditional, more profound (>5 °C reduction) hypothermia in a variety of disease processes [1,11]. However, this may be due mostly to reduced human side effects at warmer temperatures, particularly with whole-body hypothermia. A critical temperature for laminitis prevention and treatment has not been established, although it is possible that even mild decreases in lamellar temperature may have some beneficial effect.

Based on currently available data, clinical distal limb cryotherapy should be aimed at achieving hoof wall surface temperatures that are (at least) consistently below 10 °C. In order to effectively cool the lamellae, it appears that the hoof and its solear surface, as well as the pastern, fetlock and metacarpal/metatarsal region, must be included to cool incoming arterial blood. A water interface against the limb overcomes the conduction barrier of the hair coat and negates the difficulty in achieving a consistent contact between the heat exchanger and the uneven surface of the equine distal limb. Immersion of the limb from the upper metacarpus/metatarsus distally in an ice and water mixture effectively achieves this, although constant ice replenishment is labor-intensive. In a recent study, temperature was measured directly in the lamellar tissue and the digital vein during cryotherapy application to compare three different cooling methods [40]. The results obtained indicated that immersion in an ice and water slurry to the level of the upper pastern (using a 5-liter fluid bag) or the mid to upper cannon (using a wader-style vinyl boot) achieved rapid cooling to around 11 °C (approximately a 24 °C decrease), and the two methods were not significantly different over the 2-h treatment period. Application methods that use gel or ice packs wrapped around the distal limb/digit tend to perform poorly, even when replaced as frequently as every 30 min [70]. A summary of the efficacy of different methods currently available for digital hypothermia is shown in Figure 34.3. A commercial equine ice boot (designed for laminitis cases) which incorporates a digital cushion and allows cooling to the proximal metacarpus/metatarsus has recently become available (Soft-Ride Company). Immersion of the distal limb in this boot has been documented to reach the target temperature of 5–8 degrees Celsius.

Although laminitis is more common and more severe in the forelimbs, it is important to cool hindlimbs as well as forelimbs in cases at risk. The present authors have received specimens and reports from clinical cases where laminitis has developed exclusively in the uncooled hindlimbs when cryotherapy was applied only to the forelimbs. A tub, 200 cm long, 80 cm wide and 50 cm high, as used in a previous study [41], offers a practical method for the prolonged, continuous application of cryotherapy to all four limbs that can be used clinically. A water-tight door at one end for ease of access, and a rubber floor are suggested. Temporary or permanent stocks, together with cross-tying the head may assist in keeping the horse stationary. A refrigerated pump, recirculating water at around 1–2 °C, can reduce or replace the requirement for ice (Fig. 34.3). The disadvantages of this system are the inability of the horse to lie down, the need for constant supervision, a lack of portability, and potential biosecurity issues (particularly in colitis cases). A system capable of cooling all four limbs effectively, that allows ambulation and is linked to a refrigeration system, would be ideal for hospitals and requires development. Most of the currently available cooling cuff devices made for the equine distal limb are either untested or unable to reduce temperatures within the digit to the desired levels for laminitis prevention, without major modification.

Side Effects and Contraindications

The equine distal limb appears resilient in the face of extreme, continuous hypothermia: there are no reports in the literature of complications directly related to therapeutic hypothermia of the equine distal limb, and no adverse effects are reported in polar climates where the distal limbs of horses and ponies are continuously immersed in snow and sub-zero ambient temperatures. Cold-induced pain, observed in human patients when cryotherapy is applied at 5 °C or less [19], is not observed in horse studies. Adverse effects of local therapeutic hypothermia in people are rare but may include frostbite and nerve palsy [8]. The temperatures and duration of exposure required to induce frostbite are unclear. Nerve palsy in humans usually involves large superficial nerves, and it may be that compression (often

	Method	Mean hoof temperature (°C)	Mean reduction from control group (°C)
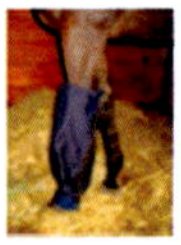	Ice boot distal limb (not including foot)	**25.7**	**6.6**
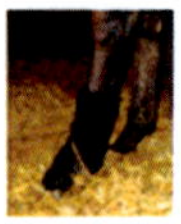	Frozen gel pack wrap distal limb (including foot)	**19.8**	**12.5**
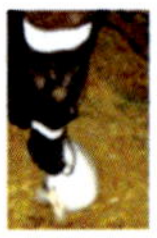	Rectal sleeve tied around coronet filled with crushed ice	**17.9**	**14.4**
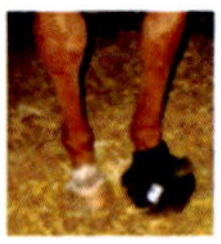	Frozen gel pack boot (foot only)	**16.2**	**16.1**
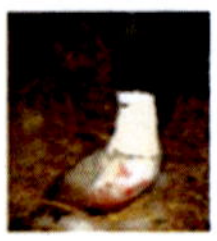	5 L Fluid bag filled with ice	**5.5**	**26.8**
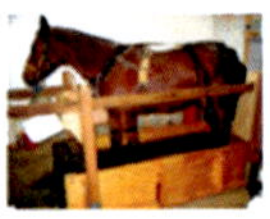	Water bath to upper metacarpus (1 °C refrigerated water, all 4 limbs)	**3.9**	**28.6**
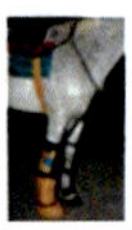	Ice boot filled with ice and water to upper metacarpus	**2.7**	**29.6**

Figure 34.3 Comparison of several different methods used for digital hypothermia over an 8- h study period. Where ice packs and crushed or cubed ice was used, this was replenished every 30 min. Hoof temperature was measured using probes embedded in the dorsal hoof wall. Methods with a water interface that include the distal limb and foot achieved a lower hoof temperature (A. van Eps, unpublished data).

used in conjunction with cryotherapy in human patients) contributes to nerve palsy. Prolonged exposure to cold and moisture (days to weeks) is associated with the development of 'immersion foot' and 'trench foot' in human patients [71]. Local swelling and pain are features of these conditions, which may progress to blistering of the skin, nerve damage, and gangrene [72]. There are anecdotal reports of a similar phenomenon in horses being treated with digital hypothermia: dermatitis of the pastern and maceration of the coronary band can occur particularly when cooling for more than five days, but in most cases this resolves with no or minimal treatment once the cooling is ceased. On rare occasions the dermatitis progresses to more severe necrosis of the skin (Fig. 34.4). Profound whole-body hypothermia (more than 10 °C below normal) can result in severe side effects associated with cardiac, endocrine, and metabolic function [11]. Hypothermia has also been associated with coagulopathy and an increased risk of infection [11]. The association between whole-body hypothermia and a reduced ability to clear infection is based on the results of one rodent study conducted during the 1960s [73]. More recent studies have not demonstrated adverse effects of hypothermia on bacterial growth in rodent models of sepsis [32], and the benefits of hypothermia are now thought to outweigh the risks in sepsis [31]. Unfortunately, it is difficult to extrapolate the results of these studies to the profound local hypothermia achieved in the digits of horses, and it may be prudent to avoid this for prolonged periods in cases where laminitis is associated with infection within the foot (e.g., laminitis accompanied by subsolear or submural abscessation, septic osteitis, or seedy toe).

Overall, distal limb cryotherapy for equine SRL is the only therapy or prevantative strategy in either humans or animals to withstand the rigors of both experimental and clinical studies for the prevention (or amelioration) of end organ damage in the septic patient. Distal limb cryotherapy has not only greatly reduced the incidence of laminitis in septic equine patients, but has also improved survival rates in these patients due to the fact that laminitis is the primary reason for treatment failure and euthanasia in septic conditions such as enterocolitis.

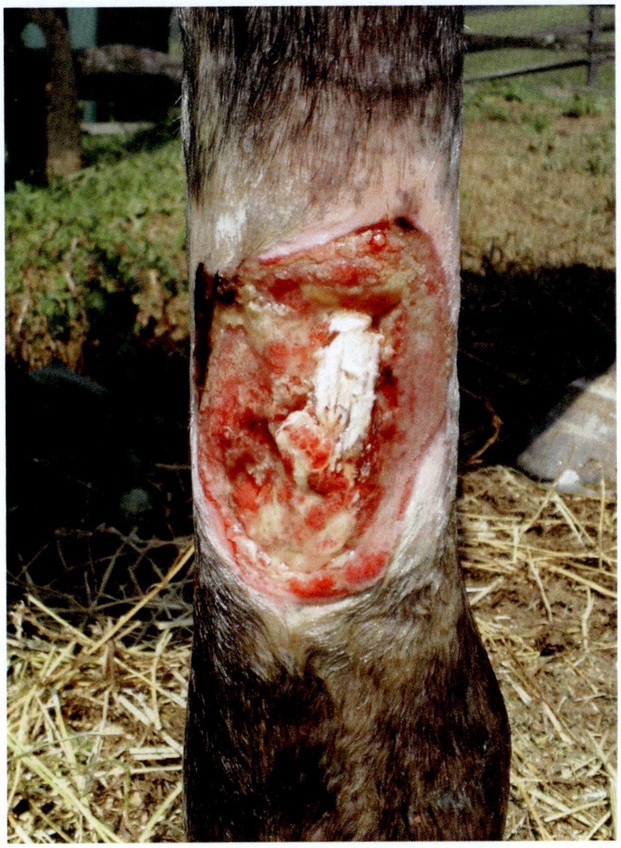

Figure 34.4 Complications from digital hypothermia in horses are extremely rare, although with longer application (>5 days) there are anecdotal reports of dermatitis and coronary band maceration. Occasionally, severe dermatitis can progress to necrosis of skin and deeper structures. This photograph depicts a lesion on the dorsal metacarpal region of a gelding that had been treated for colitis and had digital hypothermia applied for nine days to all four limbs, using cubed ice and wader-style boots. The ice boots were removed on day 9 due to developing cellulitis/dermatitis. This progressed to necrosis and required debridement of skin and part of an extensor tendon. The lesion healed eventually and the horse returned to athletic activity. The probability of this type of complication may be increased with longer application times (>5 days) and when ice is applied directly to the skin (without a water interface). Photograph courtesy of Dr Joy Tomlinson, University of Pennsylvania.

References

1. Varon, J. and Acosta, P. (2008) Therapeutic hypothermia: past, present, and future. *Chest*, **133** (5), 1267–1274.
2. Crossley, S., Reid, J., McLatchie, R., Hayton, J., Clark, C., MacDougall, M., and Andrews, P.J. (2014) A systematic review of therapeutic hypothermia for adult patients following traumatic brain injury. *Crit. Care*, **18** (2), R75.
3. Rossouw, G., Irlam, J., and Horn, A.R. (2014) Therapeutic hypothermia for hypoxic ischaemic encephalopathy using low-technology methods: a systematic review and meta-analysis. *Acta Paediatr.*, **104** (12), 1217–1228.
4. Xiao, G., Guo, Q., Shu, M., Xie, X., Deng, J., Zhu, Y., and Wan, C. (2013) Safety profile and outcome of mild therapeutic hypothermia in patients following cardiac arrest: systematic review and meta-analysis. *Emerg. Med. J.*, **30** (2), 91–100.
5. Rim, K.P., Kim, K., Jo, Y.H., Lee, J.H., Rhee, J.E., Kang, K.W., Suh, G.J., Kwon, W.Y., Lee, M.J., and Lee, H.S. (2012) Effect of therapeutic hypothermia according to severity of sepsis in a septic rat model. *Cytokine*, **60** (3), 755–761.
6. Chin, J.Y., Koh, Y., Kim, M.J., Kim, H.S., Kim, W.S., Kim, D.S., Kim, W.D., and Lim, C.M. (2007) The effects of hypothermia on endotoxin-primed lung. *Anesth. Analg.*, **104** (5), 1171–1178.
7. Lim, C.M., Kim, M.S., Ahn, J.J., Kim, M.J., Kwon, Y., Lee, I., Koh, Y., Kim, D.S., and Kim, W.D. (2003) Hypothermia protects against endotoxin-induced acute lung injury in rats. *Intensive Care Med.*, **29** (3), 453–459.
8. Swenson, C., Sward, L., and Karlsson, J. (1996) Cryotherapy in sports medicine. *Scand. J. Med. Sci. Sports*, **6** (4), 193–200.
9. Douglas, W.W. and Malcom, J.L. (1955) The effect of localized cooling on mammalian muscle spindles. *J. Physiol.*, **130**, 53–71.
10. Fuhrman, G.J. and Fuhrman, F.A. (1959) Oxygen consumption of animals and tissues as a function of temperature. *J. Gen. Physiol.*, **42**, 715–722.
11. Polderman, K.H. (2009) Mechanisms of action, physiological effects, and complications of hypothermia. *Crit. Care Med.*, **37** (7 Suppl.), S186–S202.
12. Erecinska, M., Thoresen, M., and Silver, I.A. (2003) Effects of hypothermia on energy metabolism in mammalian central nervous system. *J. Cereb. Blood Flow Metab.*, **23** (5), 513–530.
13. Hagerdal, M., Harp, J., Nilsson, L., and Siesjo, B.K. (1975) The effect of induced hypothermia upon oxygen consumption in the rat brain. *J. Neurochem.*, **24** (2), 311–316.
14. Palmer, C., Vannucci, R.C., Christensen, M.A., and Brucklacher, R.M. (1989) Regional cerebral blood flow and glucose utilization during hypothermia in newborn dogs. *Anesthesiology*, **71** (5), 730–737.
15. Griepp, R.B., Stinson, E.B., and Shumway, N.E. (1973) Profound local hypothermia for myocardial protection during open-heart surgery. *J. Thorac. Cardiovasc. Surg.*, **66** (5), 731–741.
16. Harris, E.D., Jr and McCroskery, P.A. (1974) The influence of temperature and fibril stability on degradation of cartilage collagen by rheumatoid synovial collagenase. *N. Engl. J. Med.*, **290** (1), 1–6.
17. Zachariassen, K.E. (1991) Hypothermia and cellular physiology. *Arctic Med. Res.*, **50** (Suppl. 6), 13–17.
18. Knight, K.L. (1995) Metabolism and inflammation, in *Cryotherapy in Sports Injury Management* (ed. K.L. Knight), Human Kinetics, Champaign, IL, pp. 77–84.
19. Ohkoshi, Y., Ohkoshi, M., Nagasaki, S., Ono, A., Hashimoto, T., and Yamane, S. (1999) The effect of cryotherapy on intraarticular temperature and postoperative care after anterior cruciate ligament reconstruction. *Am. J. Sports Med.*, **27** (3), 357–362.
20. Westermann, S., Vollmar, B., Thorlacius, H., and Menger, M.D. (1999) Surface cooling inhibits tumor necrosis factor-alpha-induced microvascular perfusion failure, leukocyte adhesion, and apoptosis in the striated muscle. *Surgery*, **126** (5), 881–889.
21. Webster, C.M., Kelly, S., Koike, M.A., Chock, V.Y., Giffard, R.G., and Yenari, M.A. (2009) Inflammation and NFkappaB activation is decreased by hypothermia following global cerebral ischemia. *Neurobiol. Dis.*, **33** (2), 301–312.
22. Scumpia, P.O., Sarcia, P.J., Kelly, K.M., DeMarco, V.G., and Skimming, J.W. (2004) Hypothermia induces anti-inflammatory cytokines and inhibits nitric oxide and myeloperoxidase-mediated

damage in the hearts of endotoxemic rats. *Chest*, **125** (4), 1483–1491.
23. Prandini, M.N., Neves Filho, A., Lapa, A.J., and Stavale, J.N. (2005) Mild hypothermia reduces polymorphonuclear leukocytes infiltration in induced brain inflammation. *Arq. Neuropsiquiatr.*, **63** (3B), 779–784.
24. Kamler, M., Goedeke, J., Pizanis, N., Milekhin, V., Schade, F.U., and Jakob, H. (2005) In vivo effects of hypothermia on the microcirculation during extracorporeal circulation. *Eur. J. Cardiothorac. Surg.*, **28** (2), 259–265.
25. Novack, T.A., Dillon, M.C., and Jackson, W.T. (1996) Neurochemical mechanisms in brain injury and treatment: a review. *J. Clin. Exp. Neuropsychol.*, **18** (5), 685–706.
26. Jia, F., Pan, Y.H., Mao, Q., Liang, Y.M., and Jiang, J.Y. (2010) Matrix metalloproteinase-9 expression and protein levels after fluid percussion injury in rats: the effect of injury severity and brain temperature. *J. Neurotrauma*, **27** (6), 1059–1068.
27. Hastbacka, J., Tiainen, M., Hynninen, M., Kolho, E., Tervahartiala, T., Sorsa, T., Lauhio, A., and Pettila, V. (2012) Serum matrix metalloproteinases in patients resuscitated from cardiac arrest. The association with therapeutic hypothermia. *Resuscitation*, **83** (2), 197–201.
28. Gonzalez-Ibarra, F.P., Varon, J., and Lopez-Meza, E.G. (2011) Therapeutic hypothermia: critical review of the molecular mechanisms of action. *Front. Neurol.*, **2**, 4.
29. Chang, Y.T., Wann, S.R., Tsai, J.S., Kao, C.H., Lee, P.T., Huang, N.C., Yen, C.C., Huang, M.S., and Chang, H.T. (2013) The role of autonomic nervous system function in hypothermia-mediated sepsis protection. *Am. J. Emerg. Med.*, **31** (2), 375–380.
30. Crouser, E.D. (2012) Warming up to hypothermia for treatment of severe sepsis. *Crit. Care Med.*, **40** (3), 1020–1022.
31. Acosta-Lara, P. and Varon, J. (2013) Therapeutic hypothermia in sepsis: to use or not to use? *Am. J. Emerg. Med.*, **31** (2), 381–382.
32. Beurskens, C.J., Aslami, H., Kuipers, M.T., Horn, J., Vroom, M.B., van Kuilenburg, A.B., Roelofs, J.J., Schultz, M.J., and Juffermans, N.P. (2012) Induced hypothermia is protective in a rat model of pneumococcal pneumonia associated with increased adenosine triphosphate availability and turnover. *Crit. Care Med.*, **40** (3), 919–926.
33. Fujimoto, K., Fujita, M., Tsuruta, R., Tanaka, R., Shinagawa, H., Izumi, T., Kasaoka, S., and Maekawa, T. (2008) Early induction of moderate hypothermia suppresses systemic inflammatory cytokines and intracellular adhesion molecule-1 in rats with caerulein-induced pancreatitis and endotoxemia. *Pancreas*, **37** (2), 176–181.
34. Lee, J.H., Kim, K., Jo, Y.H., Kim, M.A., Rim, K.P., Kang, K.W., Rhee, J.E., Lee, M.J., Lee, H.S., Kwon, W.Y., and Suh, G.J. (2013) Therapeutic hypothermia attenuates liver injury in polymicrobial sepsis model of rats via Akt survival pathway. *J. Surg. Res.*, **181** (1), 114–120.
35. Lehmann, J.F. and de Lateur, B.J. (1990) Cryotherapy, in *Therapeutic Heat and Cold* (ed. J.F. Lehmann), Williams & Wilkins, Baltimore, pp. 590–631.
36. Perkins, J.F., Li, M.C., and Hoffman, F. (1948) Sudden vasoconstriction in denervated or sympathectomized paws exposed to cold. *Am. J. Physiol.*, **155**, 165–178.
37. Worster, A.A., Gaughan, E.M., Hoskinson, J.J., Sargeant, J., and Erb, J.H. (2000) Effects of external thermal manipulation on laminar temperature and perfusion scintigraphy of the equine digit. *N. Z. Vet. J.*, **48** (4), 111–116.
38. Pollitt, C.C. and Van Eps, A.W. (2004) Prolonged, continuous distal limb cryotherapy in the horse. *Equine Vet. J.*, **36** (3), 216–220.
39. Van Eps, A.W. and Pollitt, C.C. (2004) Equine laminitis: cryotherapy reduces the severity of the acute lesion. *Equine Vet. J.*, **36** (3), 255–260.
40. Reesink, H.L., Divers, T.J., Bookbinder, L.C., van Eps, A.W., Soderholm, L.V., Mohammed, H.O., and Cheetham, J. (2012) Measurement of digital laminar and venous temperatures as a means of comparing three methods of topically applied cold treatment for digits of horses. *Am. J. Vet. Res.*, **73** (6), 860–866.
41. Van Eps, A.W. and Pollitt, C.C. (2009) Equine laminitis model: cryotherapy reduces the severity of lesions evaluated seven days after induction with oligofructose. *Equine Vet. J.*, **41** (8), 741–746.
42. Pollitt, C.C. and Davies, C.T. (1998) Equine laminitis: its development coincides with increased sublamellar blood flow. *Equine Vet. J. Suppl.*, **26** (26), 125–132.
43. Hood, D.M., Wagner, I.P., and Brumbaugh, G.W. (2001) Evaluation of hoof wall surface temperature as an index of digital vascular perfusion during the prodromal and acute phases of carbohydrate-induced laminitis in horses. *Am. J. Vet. Res.*, **62** (7), 1167–1172.
44. Clarke, R.S.J., Hellon, R.F., and Lind, A.R. (1958) Vascular reactions of the human forearm to cold. *Clin. Sci.*, **17**, 165–179.
45. Lewis, T. (1930) Observations upon the reactions of the vessels of the human skin to cold. *Heart*, **15**, 177–208.
46. Daanen, H.A. (2003) Finger cold-induced vasodilation: a review. *Eur. J. Appl. Physiol.*, **89** (5), 411–426.
47. Bergersen, T.K., Hisdal, J., and Walloe, L. (1999) Perfusion of the human finger during cold-induced vasodilatation. *Am. J. Physiol.*, **276** (3 Pt 2), R731–R737.
48. Wagner, I.P. and Heymering, H. (1999) Historical perspectives on laminitis. *Vet. Clin. North Am. Equine Pract.*, **15** (2), 295–309.
49. Kullmann, A., Holcombe, S.J., Hurcombe, S.D., Roessner, H.A., Hauptman, J.G., Geor, R.J., and Belknap, J. (2014) Prophylactic digital cryotherapy is associated with decreased incidence of laminitis in horses diagnosed with colitis. *Equine Vet. J.*, **46** (5), 554–559.
50. Pollitt, C.C. and Visser, M.B. (2010) Carbohydrate alimentary overload laminitis. *Vet. Clin. North Am. Equine Pract.*, **26** (1), 65–78.
51. Van Eps, A.W. and Pollitt, C.C. (2006) Equine laminitis induced with oligofructose. *Equine Vet. J.*, **38** (3), 203–208.
52. Bailey, S.R., Adair, H.S., Reinemeyer, C.R., Morgan, S.J., Brooks, A.C., Longhofer, S.L., and Elliott, J. (2009) Plasma concentrations of endotoxin and platelet activation in the developmental stage of oligofructose-induced laminitis. *Vet. Immunol. Immunopathol.*, **129** (3-4), 167–173.
53. Belknap, J.K., Giguere, S., Pettigrew, A., Cochran, A.M., Van Eps, A.W., and Pollitt, C.C. (2007) Lamellar pro-inflammatory cytokine expression patterns in laminitis at the developmental stage and at the onset of lameness: innate vs. adaptive immune response. *Equine Vet. J.*, **39** (1), 42–47.
54. Blikslager, A.T., Yin, C., Cochran, A.M., Wooten, J.G., Pettigrew, A., and Belknap, J.K. (2006) Cyclooxygenase expression in the early stages of equine laminitis: a cytologic study. *J. Vet. Intern. Med./Am. Coll. Vet. Intern. Med.*, **20** (5), 1191–1196.
55. Johnson, P.J., Tyagi, S.C., Katwa, L.C., Ganjam, V.K., Moore, L.A., Kreeger, J.M., and Messer, N.T. (1998) Activation of extracellular

matrix metalloproteinases in equine laminitis. *Vet. Rec.*, **142** (15), 392–396.

56. Leise, B.S., Faleiros, R.R., Watts, M., Johnson, P.J., Black, S.J., and Belknap, J.K. (2011) Laminar inflammatory gene expression in the carbohydrate overload model of equine laminitis. *Equine Vet. J.*, **43** (1), 54-61.
57. Coyne, M.J., Cousin, H., Loftus, J.P., Johnson, P.J., Belknap, J.K., Gradil, C.M., Black, S.J., and Alfandari, D. (2009) Cloning and expression of ADAM-related metalloproteases in equine laminitis. *Vet. Immunol. Immunopathol.*, **129** (3-4), 231–241.
58. Visser, M.B. and Pollitt, C.C. (2012) The timeline of metalloprotease events during oligofructose induced equine laminitis development. *Equine Vet. J.*, **44** (1), 88–93.
59. Visser, M.B. and Pollitt, C.C. (2011) Lamellar leukocyte infiltration and involvement of IL-6 during oligofructose-induced equine laminitis development. *Vet. Immunol. Immunopathol.*, **144** (1-2), 120–128.
60. Van Eps, A.W., Leise, B.S., Watts, M., Pollitt, C.C., and Belknap, J.K. (2012) Digital hypothermia inhibits early lamellar inflammatory signalling in the oligofructose laminitis model. *Equine Vet. J.*, **44** (2), 230–237.
61. Van Eps, A.W., Pollitt, C.C., Underwood, C., Medina-Torres, C.E., Goodwin, W.A., and Belknap, J.K. (2014) Continuous digital hypothermia initiated after the onset of lameness prevents lamellar failure in the oligofructose laminitis model. *Equine Vet. J.*, **46** (5), 625–630.
62. Parsons, C.S., Orsini, J.A., Krafty, R., Capewell, L., and Boston, R. (2007) Risk factors for development of acute laminitis in horses during hospitalization: 73 cases (1997–2004). *J. Am. Vet. Med. Assoc.*, **230** (6), 885–889.
63. Cohen, N.D., Parson, E.M., Seahorn, T.L., and Carter, G.K. (1994) Prevalence and factors associated with development of laminitis in horses with duodenitis/proximal jejunitis: 33 cases (1985–1991). *J. Am. Vet. Med. Assoc.*, **204** (2), 250–254.
64. Cohen, N.D. and Woods, A.M. (1999) Characteristics and risk factors for failure of horses with acute diarrhea to survive: 122 cases (1990–1996). *J. Am. Vet. Med. Assoc.*, **214** (3), 382–390.
65. Slater, M.R., Hood, D.M., and Carter, G.K. (1995) Descriptive epidemiological study of equine laminitis. *Equine Vet. J.*, **27** (5), 364–367.
66. Alford, P., Geller, S., Richrdson, B., Slater, M., Honnas, C., Foreman, J., Robinson, J., Messer, M., Roberts, M., Goble, D., Hood, D., and Chaffin, M. (2001) A multicenter, matched case-control study of risk factors for equine laminitis. *Prevent. Vet. Med.*, **49** (3-4), 209–222.
67. Pollitt, C.C. and Molyneux, G.S. (1990) A scanning electron microscopical study of the dermal microcirculation of the equine foot. *Equine Vet. J.*, **22** (2), 79–87.
68. Kaneps, A.J. (2000) Tissue temperature response to hot and cold therapy in the metacarpal region of a horse. Proceedings of the Forty-Sixth Annual Convention of the American Association of Equine Practitioners, San Antonio, Texas.
69. Turner, T.A., Wolfsdorf, K., Jourdenais, J., and Blake, C.L. (1992) Effects of heat, cold, biomagnets and ultrasound on skin circulation in the horse. Proceedings of the Thirty-Seventh Annual Convention of the American Association of Equine Practitioners, San Francisco, California.
70. Van Eps, A.W. and Orsini, J.A. (2016) A comparison of seven methods for continuous therapeutic cooling of the equine digit. *Equine Vet. J.*, **48** (1), 120–124.
71. DeGroot, D.W., Castellani, J.W., Williams, J.O., and Amoroso, P.J. (2003) Epidemiology of U.S. Army cold weather injuries, 1980–1999. *Aviat. Space Env. Med.*, **74**, 564–570.
72. Ungley, C.C., Channell, G.D., and Richards, R.L. (2003) The immersion foot syndrome. 1946. *Wilderness Environ. Med.*, **14**, 135–141; discussion 134.
73. Webb, W.R., Deguzman, V.C., Grogan, J.B., and Artz, C.P. (1962) Hypothermia: its effects upon hematologic clearance in experimentally induced staphylococcal bacteremia. *Surgery*, **52**, 643–647.

CHAPTER 35
Equine Sepsis

Samuel D. Hurcombe and Susan J. Holcombe

Introduction

Horses with inflammatory diseases such as an acute abdominal crisis, enterocolitis, septic endometritis and pleuritis risk developing laminitis [1]. These horses frequently exhibit clinical signs of endotoxemia/sepsis and associated systemic inflammation which are considered hazards for the development of acute laminitis [1]. The presumption of endotoxemia and/or sepsis in these patients is frequently made without confirmation of free endotoxin or bacteria in the blood. The diagnosis of endotoxemia and/or sepsis is most commonly based on clinical evidence and indices of a systemic inflammatory response with confirmed gastrointestinal injury or bacterial infection. The pathophysiology of sepsis-related laminitis (SRL) is unclear, but it may share characteristics of each of the three experimental models of laminitis including oral administration of excessive carbohydrate in the form of corn starch or oligofructose (see Chapters 7 and 8), the administration of black walnut extract (BWE; see Chapter 9), or intravenous hyperinsulinemia (see Chapter 10) [2–4]. Sepsis-related laminitis is most closely related to the carbohydrate overload (CHO) models of laminitis due to the associated injury to the hindgut and documented absorption of endotoxin (and possibly other toxins) into the systemic circulation [2]. However, septic/endotoxic horses are frequently hyperglycemic and potentially insulin-resistant [5]. Data from the hyperinsulinemic laminitis model may be useful when treating horses with sepsis-associated disease, even if recommendations are limited to minimizing the duration of insulin dysregulation by treating the acute inflammation and hemodynamic crisis. Finally, BWE, although known to contain small amounts of endotoxin (thought to be the result of contamination during soaking of the black walnut shavings in a nonsterile environment), most likely functions through other biologically active toxins present in black walnut heartwood, and possibly also through the production of reactive oxygen species (ROS) (see Chapter 9) [6]. Factors involved in acute laminitis occur to varying degrees in these models of laminitis, and include inflammation, degradation of the elements of the lamellar extracellular matrix, endothelial/ vascular dysfunction, and systemic and metabolic disruption of homeostasis [2]. Many of these events occur in septic horses, and form the basis for therapeutic interventions.

The aim of this chapter is to present medical therapeutic options for septic/endotoxic horses with presumptive acute developmental laminitis. Treatment recommendations will be verified based on evidence provided by elegant research from several renowned laboratories. Occasionally, strategies based on standard of care (and widespread anecdotes) may be described as such. First, the patient population will be clarified, after which factors associated with sepsis, endotoxemia, and systemic inflammatory response implicated in the pathogenesis of laminitis will be discussed. The epidemiology of 'at-risk' septic horses will also be described.

Sepsis versus Endotoxemia and its Role in Laminitis

Sepsis in human medicine is defined as an infection causing a systemic inflammatory response, based on the presence of at least two systemic inflammatory response criteria. These criteria, translated loosely from human to horse include: (i) tachycardia with heart rate ≥60 beats per min; (ii) fever (≥39 °C or 101 °F) or hypothermia (≤37 °C or 98 °F); (iii) leukocytosis ≥12 000 cells μl^{-1} or leucopenia ≤4000 cells μl^{-1} or >10% band neutrophils; and (iv) $PaCO_2$ <32 mmHg (hypocapnia/hypocarbia) or respiratory rate ≥20 breaths per min [7]. The systemic inflammatory response in sepsis is most commonly due to the presence of one or more bacterial products termed pathogen-associated molecular pattern proteins (PAMPs) such as endotoxin/lipopolysaccharide, flagellin, and lipoproteins in the bloodstream [1]. Although the terms sepsis and endotoxemia are used somewhat interchangeably in human and veterinary medicine, endotoxemia is truly just one type of sepsis and is, by definition, the presence of free endotoxin in the blood. The gastrointestinal contents are the largest source of endotoxin. Endotoxin is liberated from the cell wall of Gram-negative bacteria when the organisms (most enteric bacteria) replicate or divide, and also when there is a die-off of Gram-negative bacteria, as occurs with CHO (see Chapter 7). Endotoxin and

Equine Laminitis, First Edition. Edited by James K. Belknap and Raymond Geor.

other bacterial products/PAMPs enter the systemic circulation and bind to effector cells of the innate immune system, including mononuclear cells. Proinflammatory cytokines and chemokines are produced following the activation of pathways, and include nuclear factor kappa B (NF-κB) and the three mitogen-activated protein kinase (MAPK) pathways [8]. Activation of these pathways results in the production of proinflammatory mediators that are responsible for the clinical signs of endotoxemia and sepsis. These same factors are also increased in lamellar tissue during acute developmental laminitis. Specifically, the expression of proinflammatory cytokines such as interleukin (IL)-1β and IL-6, and the chemokine IL-8 correlate with the clinical severity of sepsis in people and laminitis in horses [2, 8]. Arachidonic acid products of the cyclooxygenase and lipoxygenase pathways, including prostaglandins and leukotrienes, are associated with enhanced inflammatory response, clinical signs of sepsis and endotoxemia, and laminitis. Lesions associated with lamellar dysfunction and failure may result from the same events documented to be involved in organ injury in human sepsis, including dysoxia (defined as a condition in which tissues cannot make full use of the available oxygen), inflammation, and/or hypercoagulation. Other lamellar changes resembling those present in sepsis-associated organ injury include leukocyte and endothelial activation, leukocyte adhesion and emigration through the capillaries, and inflammation evidenced by proinflammatory cytokine expression and possibly oxidant injury [2]. Identifying common factors in systemic and lamellar pathology aids in therapeutic planning.

Gastrointestinal injury is closely associated with the development of endotoxemia and sepsis in people and horses [1, 7, 9, 10]. Sepsis and endotoxemia can occur together, especially if the hemodynamic instability of septic shock leads to diminished gastrointestinal perfusion and gut ischemia. Damage to the gastrointestinal mucosa weakens normal defenses against the absorption/translocation of bacteria and bacterial products including endotoxin, flagellin, and other toxins. Exaggerated systemic host response to these products causes the clinical signs of sepsis (can be termed endotoxemia when the specific toxin is endotoxin). Lipopolysaccharide (LPS) was detected in the blood of 25–41% of horses admitted to referral centers for colic. Bacteremia was confirmed in 29% of horses with colitis/typhlocolitis [9]. Bacterial translocation from the ischemic small intestine occurred in 13.8% of horses with small intestinal incarceration [10]. Determining whether sick horses with gastrointestinal disease – be it colic or entero(typhlo)colitis – are septic, endotoxemic, or both, may not be important. Indeed, many investigators have administered LPS infusions to horses, but none of these have ever developed laminitis. However, LPS had a concentration-dependent effect on the hoof lamellar integrity when equine lamellar explants were cultured with 10 and 100 $\mu g\ ml^{-1}$ LPS [11]. In the study conducted by Reisinger and colleagues, lamellar explants treated with 10 and 100 $\mu g\ ml^{-1}$ LPS required less force to separate compared to control explants. However, LPS did not exhibit any cytotoxic effects on epidermal or dermal cells at any of the concentrations tested [11]. Factors other than, or in addition to, endotoxin likely provide key triggers for laminitis. Recognizing that these horses have clinical signs of sepsis/endotoxemia and are at risk for laminitis is important.

Horses with early sepsis/endotoxemia may show vague clinical signs that include inappetance, reduced activity, and reduced water intake. Mild-moderate tachycardia, tachypnea and bright red mucous membranes with a brisk capillary refill time (e.g., ≤1 s) may be observed. These signs are consistent with a *hyperdynamic phase* of toxemia, wherein systemic vasodilation, a reduced cardiac afterload and an increase in rate-dependent cardiac output develop. At this time point, changes in the effective circulating volume are minimal and result in an almost hyperperfused state (i.e., increased tissue perfusion). Some of the milder types of equine sepsis, such as acute metritis due to retained fetal membranes, may only exhibit the hyperdynamic state and not progress to the more severe hypodynamic phase. It is important to realize that animals with even this milder phase of sepsis still commonly develop laminitis.

With time and progression of sepsis in the absence of therapy, the hyperdynamic phase is followed by a *hypodynamic phase*. The vascular volume to the periphery contracts and blood is pooled to a central reservoir in order to preserve essential organ perfusion (heart and brain, but not the gastrointestinal system). These horses are severely depressed, with cool appendages, anorexia, alterations in core body temperature (either fever or hypothermia may be observed), tachycardia, tachypnea, and reduced to absent borborygmi. The mucous membranes are often dark pink to purple, tacky and cool with a prolonged capillary refill time (>2 s). Small vessel injection is caused by elevated levels of prostacyclin (PGI), histamine, and complement (C3 and C5a). A blue discoloration to the gingival margin, frequently referred to as a toxic line, is caused by desaturated hemoglobin in erythrocytes sluggishly flowing through mucous membrane capillaries. Cardiac output decreases, pulse pressure (systolic–diastolic pressure) is poor and jugular vein fill is prolonged in affected horses. Urine production ceases and manure may be very dry as reserve fluid is absorbed from the gastrointestinal tract. Conversely, these horses may have diarrhea or impaired gastric emptying with nasogastric reflux. Sodium- and chloride-rich gastrointestinal secretions directly deplete the plasma volume, which exacerbates the hypovolemic state. Systemic hypotension and decreased cardiac output lead to hypoperfusion of the organs and tissue beds. If poor tissue perfusion persists, organ dysfunction and failure may result, including lamellar failure. Clinical pathology testing may reveal evidence of hemoconcentration, including elevated packed cell volume (PCV >40%) with diminished total protein (TP <5.5 $g\ dl^{-1}$). Leukopenia largely due to neutropenia results from margination and diapedesis of polymorphonuclear cells and mononuclear cells toward chemotactins. Occasionally, horses may develop leukocytosis and neutrophilia prior to white blood cell numbers plummeting. Blood L-lactate may be increased due to poor systemic perfusion and regional anaerobic metabolism, gut ischemia, or increased circulating catecholamines caused by the systemic stress response [12]. In a retrospective study of horses with enterocolitis and systemic inflammatory response syndrome (SIRS), those that developed laminitis had higher blood L-lactate concentrations at the time of hospital admission compared to values measured in those that did not develop laminitis [13]. Specific measures of organ function available from the serum chemistry aid in assessing kidney and liver injury and help direct therapy. Occasionally, septic/endotoxemic horses will demonstrate strange behaviors, including head pressing or other signs of dementia. These central cerebral responses may be due to severe metabolic acidosis or hyperammonemia associated with gastrointestinal disturbance [14].

Therapy goals include minimizing or reversing organ dysfunction by reducing the detrimental effects of dysoxia, hypoperfusion, and dysregulated inflammation. The digital lamellae of the horse may be considered a 'shock' organ [2]. In septic/endotoxemic horses, medical therapy is largely aimed at controlling infection, minimizing the effects of endotoxin/exotoxin liberation, improving global and microvascular perfusion, and reducing inflammation. If these targets are achieved, many secondary sequelae such as coagulopathy, multiple organ dysfunction, and immunocompromise, are prevented or minimized.

Epidemiology of the Septic Horse At-Risk for Laminitis

In one study, the odds of a horse with clinical evidence of endotoxemia/sepsis developing laminitis during hospitalization were fivefold those of a horse with no clinical signs or clinicopathologic evidence of endotoxemia/sepsis [1]. Clinical diagnoses of underlying/predisposing diseases in laminitic patients included pneumonia, diarrhea, medical and surgical colic, acute renal failure, vascular abnormalities, retained placenta and pituitary pars intermedia dysfunction (PPID) [1]. The prevalence of laminitis in horses with conditions causing endotoxemia varies depending on the primary lesion, and is reported to be between 3% and 30% [14–18]. Obesity, increased age, and evidence of metabolic syndrome are likely to enhance the proinflammatory response and likely the risk of acute laminitis in horses with clinical illness and evidence of systemic inflammation [19]. Between 2.4% and 4.4% of horses were reported to develop laminitis following surgical evaluation and/or the correction of acute abdominal disease [20, 21]; horses were significantly less likely to return to intended use or performance following exploratory celiotomy for colic if they developed laminitis [20]. Ten of 195 horses (5.1%) developed laminitis between the time of surgery and six-month follow-up [20]. Whereas five of those 10 horses developed laminitis in hospital, the other five developed laminitis at home following hospital discharge [20]. A post-mortem study conducted by Laskoski *et al.* confirmed the association between colic and lamellar injury [22]. Eighteen horses with lethal gastrointestinal disease were divided into two groups based on evidence of leukopenia or normal total systemic white blood cell counts. Lamellar lesions were observed in both leukopenic and non-leukopenic horses, with no difference in lamellar lesion severity between the groups. Interestingly, of five horses with the most severe lamellar lesions, only one horse had clinical signs of laminitis prior to death; this suggested that horses may develop lamellar injury in hospital but will not show clinical signs of laminitis until being discharged from the hospital [22]. In the case of surgical colic, the high-risk period is often the postoperative period where reperfusion of compromised tissue in addition to an impaired mucosal barrier allows for translocation (defined as the passage of from the gastrointestinal tract to extraintestinal sites, such as the mesenteric lymph nodes and bloodstream) of bacteria, bacterial components, and toxins. The administration of analgesics in the postoperative period may mask early clinical signs of laminitis. Therefore, if horses are released from hospital within 24–72 h of surgery, clinical evidence of lamellar insults may be noticed for the first time by the owners at home.

Laminitis is more prevalent in horses with entero(typhlo) colitis and diarrhea than horses with surgical acute abdomen. In one study, 11.5% (14/122) of horses admitted for acute onset of diarrhea had or developed laminitis [17]. By comparison, 21% (27/130) of horses admitted for evaluation and treatment of colitis with evidence of systemic inflammatory response and diagnosed with either Potomac Horse Fever (*Neorickettsia risticii*), enteric clostridiosis or salmonellosis had or developed signs of acute laminitis based on increased digital pulses and lameness [13]. The severity of clinical signs or cause of sepsis has not been correlated with odds of developing laminitis. Again, whereas many investigators have administered various doses of endotoxin to numerous horses resulting in mild to severe endoxemia [23, 24], none of these horses have ever developed laminitis [23, 24].

Treatment

Therapeutic targets in horses with evidence of sepsis and risk of acute laminitis include: (i) resolving infection, (ii) restoration of circulation and oxygen delivery, (iii) minimizing inflammation, (iv) suppressing toxin absorption and action, and (v) providing sufficient and appropriate analgesia. Specific treatment of the lamellae includes cryotherapy and digital support.

Infection Control

Antimicrobials

Antimicrobial therapy makes intuitive sense in the face of bacterial sepsis. The administration of antimicrobials within 60–180 min of sepsis diagnosis in the emergency department is significantly associated with improved survival [25]. *This point cannot be overstated.* The choice, route of administration, duration of administration, source of infection and microbial isolate(s) involved should be considered when establishing a treatment regimen. Frequently, broad-spectrum antibiosis is initiated pending the results of culture and sensitivity. The negative effects of antibiotic administration should also be considered. Worsening bacterial floral disruption is a concern when administering antibiotics (see Table 35.1) to horses with gastrointestinal insults [26, 27], with negative effects including antibiotic-associated colitis. A recent study showed that antibiotic-associated colitis occurs infrequently (incidence 0.6%), but the mortality rate among these horses was significant at 18.8% [27]. In certain diseases such as Potomac Horse Fever (*Neorickettsia risticii*), in which acute lamellar inflammation is common, oxytetracycline (6.6 mg kg^{-1}, intravenous once daily, generally as an infusion) is indicated in order to treat the infection and hasten resolution of the inflammatory insult. Metronidazole (25 mg kg^{-1}, oral q. 6 h) is warranted in horses with hemorrhagic diarrhea, at risk for or with a confirmed diagnosis of clostridial enterocolitis.

Surgical Management

Surgery is performed to remove devitalized tissue, including sections of the gastrointestinal tract in horses with colic. The evacuation of luminal contents (feed impactions, sand, enteroliths or fecaliths) damages the intestinal mucosa and may exacerbate signs of sepsis/endotoxemia. Perioperative therapy to diminish these effects is warranted, though evidenced-based medical data are lacking to support the use of many of these treatments.

The debridement of infected wounds is critical to healing and limiting the systemic response to the infection. Debridement, to facilitate the drainage of exudates, and lavage of contaminated wounds/surgical sites are recommended following sampling for bacterial culture. The rate of wound repair and resolution of infection is enhanced by surgical debridement and drainage. Debridement and effective drainage also facilitate antibiosis and may limit the duration of administration. For example, a celiotomy incision infection may produce signs of systemic sepsis including fever, tachycardia, and decreased appetite. Appropriate management includes drainage, culture and sensitivity, and subsequent antimicrobial therapy based on culture and sensitivity results. Treatment is continued until the signs of infection (e.g., drainage, local hyperemia, and fever) resolve.

Table 35.1 Typical antibiotic choices used in adult horses.

Systemic antibiotics for adult horses	Dose rate; Route of administration; Frequency of administration*	Comments
β-Lactams		Broad-spectrum, time-dependent, bactericidal, synergistic with aminoglycosides.
Sodium ampicillin	15–40 mg kg^{-1}, IV/IM, q. 6–8 h	Cephalosporins show enhanced efficacy against Gram-negative bacteria with higher-generation drugs.
Potassium/sodium penicillin	22 000–44 000 IU kg^{-1}, IV, q. 4–6 h	
Procaine penicillin	22–44 mg kg^{-1}, IM, q. 12 h	
Sodium ceftiofur	2.2–4.4 mg kg^{-1}, IV/IM, q. 12 h	
Sodium cefazolin	11–22 mg kg^{-1}, IV, q. 6–8 h	
Aminoglycosides		Gram-negative aerobes primarily, concentration dependent, bactericidal, synergistic with β-lactams. Nephrotoxic; use in well- hydrated animals.
Gentamicin sulfate	6.6 mg kg^{-1}, IV, q. 24 h	
Amikacin sulfate	15–20 mg kg^{-1}, IV, q. 24 h	
Folate synthesis inhibitors		Broad-spectrum with good absorption. Do not administer parenteral formulations if the patient has ileus or has recently received α_2 agonist (e.g., detomidine) medications.
Trimethoprim–sulfamethoxazole	15–25 mg kg^{-1}, IV/PO, q. 12 h	
Trimethoprim–sulfadiazine		
Fluoroquinolones		Effective against Gram-negative aerobes and some Gram-positive aerobes (*Staphylococcus* sp., including many methicillin-resistant strains in horses). No efficacy against anaerobes.
Enrofloxacin	7.5 mg kg^{-1}, IV, q. 24 h 5–7.5 mg kg^{-1}, PO, q. 24 h	Care when using parenteral preparations orally. Dilute or mix with diluents to reduce gingival ulcerations. Rapid administration intravenously may cause transient ataxia and further neurologic signs.
Marbofloxacin	2 mg kg^{-1}, PO/IV, q. 24 h (Europe)	
Tetracyclines		Broad-spectrum including *Rickettsia*, *Chlamydophila*, and Spirochaetes. Variable absorption when given enterally. Do not administer doxycycline IV. Nephrotoxic; use in well-hydrated animals.
Oxytetracycline	6.6 mg kg^{-1}, IV, q. 12 h	Doxycycline may also have anti-MMP properties.
Doxycycline	5–10 mg kg^{-1}, PO, q. 12 h	
Minocycline	4 mg kg^{-1}, PO, q. 12 h	
Other		
Metronidazole	15–25 mg kg^{-1}, PO, q. 8 h 45–60 mg kg^{-1}, per rectum, q. 8 h	Efficacious against most anaerobes and flagellated protozoa. Rectal bioavailability is 33–50%.
Chloramphenicol palmitate	15–20 mg kg^{-1}, IV, q. 8–12 h 50 mg kg^{-1}, PO, q. 6–8 h	Broad-spectrum, high volume of distribution. Bacteriostatic. Human health issue. Compounded paste may decrease human contact and minimize idiosyncratic aplastic anemia risk.
Chloramphenicol succinate	25–50 mg kg^{-1}, IV, q. 6–8 h	

Dose rates provided are a guide. Specific indications and contraindications may exist in certain patients. All antibiotics have the potential to disrupt the gastrointestinal flora and cause antibiotic-associated colitis. All patients should be monitored for signs of gastrointestinal upset including depression, decreased appetite, and altered fecal consistency and adjustments to the treatment plan made accordingly.

*Routes and intervals of drug administration: IV, intravenous; IM, intramuscular; PO, per os (oral).

MMP = matrix metalloproteinase.

Retained fetal membranes and subsequent metritis put mares at risk for the development of laminitis [1]. The administration of broad-spectrum antimicrobial drugs, the judicious use of flunixin meglumine, and local foot therapy are fundamental strategies to treat infection, inflammation, and limit laminitis risk. Direct uterine therapy is controversial among theriogenologists. Some advocate intrauterine lavage with warm, sterile, polyionic solution, while others recommend minimum intrauterine therapy. Most suggest systemic oxytocin (intravenous, subcutaneous, intramuscular, or constant rate infusion [CRI]) to stimulate uterine evacuation.

Fluid Therapy

Horses are exquisitely sensitive to the effects of endotoxin in the systemic circulation, making maldistributive shock a commonly encountered problem in the septic/endotoxemic equine patient. The term 'maldistributive' refers to an abnormal shunting, pooling and sequestration of vascular volume such that the uniform delivery of nutrients is decreased [28, 29]. The venous system, which is well-known for having a high capacitance, pools blood under venodilatory states, thereby reducing venous return to the heart and therefore cardiac output. Specific tissue beds are affected differently.

Perfusion of the lamellae is essential to tissue health. The lamellae are contained within the rigid hoof capsule such that: {lamellar perfusion pressure = digital artery pressure (mean arterial pressure) – intracapsular pressure of the hoof}. However, the urgency to restore general organ perfusion may not apply to the lamellae. Minimizing the invasion of activated leukocytes to the lamellae in septic/endotoxic horses may be a critical step in preventing laminitis. Therefore, digital cryotherapy (the application of ice to the feet) is recommended prior to or during volume resuscitation. Appropriately performed digital cooling will reduce hoof and digital vein temperature, reduce lamellar metabolism, and decrease the activation of leukocytes and subsequent proinflammatory cytokine production [30]. More simply stated, the feet should be placed in ice water prior to or during rapid, aggressive administration of fluids in horses at risk for SRL.

The acute hemodynamic consequences of endotoxemia in horses include an increased cardiac index due to an increased heart rate, a decreased systemic vascular resistance, and thus a reduced afterload to ventricular ejection. Clinically, the early stages of maldistributive shock may be recognized by tachycardia, poor peripheral pulse quality (except in the digital vessels), warm extremities, and bright pink/red mucous membranes. The capillary refill time is brisk (<1 s), indicating marked vasodilation and an increased flow through the gingival vascular beds.

As blood begins to shunt to essential organs, the peripheral vascular beds are bereaved of flow. Cool extremities, dark pink, muddy, purple-tinged mucous membranes, gingival congestion (toxic gingival margin), vascular injection and prolonged capillary refill time (>2 s) are recognized. The cardiac index and arterial blood pressure are decreased despite the presence of tachycardia, and organ perfusion diminishes. These findings herald a decompensated hemodynamic state and represent a failing heart, vasoplegia, and a failure to maintain blood pressure and perfusion. If oxygen delivery to the organs cannot meet oxygen utilization to maintain aerobic metabolism, glycolysis begins and L-lactate production rises. Aggressive therapy is required to improve oxygen delivery, vascular volume, tissue perfusion, and removal of accumulating acids, metabolites and toxins. Otherwise, organ dysfunction will soon be followed by organ failure and subsequent death.

Volume Repletion

Optimization of the effective circulating volume is the first goal in treating shock and hypoperfusion. Perfusion is inextricably linked to volume status, and the clinician does not necessarily need sophisticated methodologies to document hypoperfusion, shock, and the need for volume replacement. Suggested volumes and flow rates for various fluid solutions that may be used in management of the hypoperfusing septic/endotoxemic horse are shown in Table 35.2.

Isotonic Crystalloid Fluids

Isotonic, polyionic crystalloid solutions form the foundation in a fluid therapy regimen, and are an excellent choice for simple dehydration as they diffuse freely between fluid compartments (extracellular and intracellular). Lactated Ringer's solution, Plasmalyte-148, Normosol-R are such proprietary fluids. Normal saline (0.9% sodium chloride) should be reserved for situations where balanced polyionic crystalloids are not available, or in cases of hyponatremia and hypochloremia.

Determining the volume required and rate of administration is probably the single most important aspect of formulating a fluid therapy plan. Adequate volume replenishment to account for dehydration, third spacing of fluids within the gut/peritoneal space, maintenance requirements and ongoing losses is essential. The maintenance fluid rate is approximately 2 ml kg^{-1} h^{-1}, while a shock bolus of fluid is administered at 90 ml kg^{-1} h^{-1}. Almost all of the available isotonic crystalloid solutions are considered replacement solutions rather than maintenance solutions, as their electrolyte composition is designed to be similar to the composition of the extracellular fluid and not the daily replacement needs. Suggested flow rates for isotonic crystalloid solutions in horses are shown in Table 35.2.

Hypertonic Crystalloid Fluids

Hypertonic saline solution (HSS) is available in a variety of concentrations. Typically, 7.2% solutions are used for fast, effective intravascular volume recruitment. The ability for hyperosmolar solutions to recruit volume relates to the number of effective osmoles in solution, which translates to its 'water-holding' ability. Water is recruited from the intracellular space to expand the vascular volume. The increase in intravascular volume following the administration of hypertonic saline is short-lived (e.g.,

Table 35.2 Fluid choices and rates of administration for horses.

Fluid type	Dose rates	Example of product	Comments
Isotonic crystalloid solutions	Calculate the fluid deficit and administer 10–20 ml kg^{-1} aliquots and re-assess after each administration	Lactated Ringer's solution Hartmann's solution Plasmalyte-148 Normosol-R	High flow rates will cause dilution of blood constituents including clotting factors, platelets, and proteins, and may lead to coagulopathy and decreases in colloid osmotic pressure.
Bicarbonate replacement therapy	Calculate the deficit: Desired – Current × 0.3 (coefficient for the ECF). Divide deficit by the concentration of product chosen. For example, 8.4% sodium bicarbonate has 1 Eq ml^{-1}. Administer 50% of the deficit immediately (1–2 h), and the remainder over the following 24 h	8.4% sodium bicarbonate solution (1 mEq ml^{-1})	Recheck blood gas and serum chemistry every 6–12 h (or more frequently) to adjust dose and/or rate of administration.
Colloid Natural plasma Synthetic Hydroxyethyl starch	Variable dose rates. 4–12 ml kg^{-1} (2–6 l in 500 kg horse) IV every 24–48 h Up to 20 ml kg^{-1} IV every 24 h as a bolus. Can be combined with hypertonic saline solution for resuscitation	Commercial products include: 1. Higamm (hyperimmune plasma) Hetastarch® 6% solution	Clinical identification of edema formation and clinicopathological evidence of hypoproteinemia and decreased COP may help guide the need for colloid solutions as well as repeat dosing. Monitor for hypersensitivity reactions with plasma administration. Start slowly. Note: when using synthetic colloids, refractometric measurements of total solids protein will decrease despite an increase in COP due to relative dilution of remaining plasma proteins.
Hypertonic crystalloid solutions	2–4 ml kg^{-1} IV as a bolus for fast volume recruitment into the vascular space.	7.2% sodium chloride solution	Rapid but short-lived volume recruitment. Can be combined with colloid solutions for resuscitation. Check serum sodium concentrations prior to repeat dosing to prevent hypernatremia.

COP, colloid osmotic pressure.

20–30 min) because there are no high-molecular-weight components in these hypertonic solutions. Sodium and chloride ions redistribute between all compartments within the extracellular fluid space (intravascular and interstitial), and the osmotic pressure within the vascular space decreases. These solutions essentially recruit volume rapidly for a short period of time, but should be followed by isotonic fluids (see Isotonic Crystalloid Fluids) and/or colloid solutions.

In addition to restoring microvascular perfusion, small volumes of hypertonic saline may help balance immune cell responses. The administration of hypertonic saline to preclinical models of sepsis (generally cecal ligation and puncture models in rodents) demonstrated improved regional organ blood flow by reducing endothelial cell edema and vascular resistance by modifying nitric oxide expression [31]. Hypertonic saline resuscitation reportedly diminishes neutrophil activation, decreased selectin expression, leukocyte adhesion and emigration, and the production of proinflammatory cytokines, but augments the production of IL-10 (an 'anti-inflammatory' cytokine) [31]. Studies using the black walnut and oligofructose models of laminitis demonstrated that endothelial cell activation and lamellar inflammation occur early in developing laminitis [2,3]. The efficacy of hypertonic solutions in naturally occurring (or experimentally induced) laminitis has not been tested, but the combined data from research models is compelling. Dosing, administration frequency, and effective tonicity remain speculative.

Other hypertonic fluids (e.g., sodium bicarbonate) *should not be used to expand the effective circulating volume.* Hypertonic sodium bicarbonate should be reserved for correcting acidemia, wherein the primary cause is a loss of buffer base. Lactic acidosis secondary to hypoperfusion often results in hypobicarbonatemia; however, by simply improving perfusion through volume replenishment, serum bicarbonate concentration often normalizes without bicarbonate therapy.

Some diseases (e.g., typhlocolitis, renal tubular acidosis) result in absolute loss of base, and affected animals may benefit from bicarbonate administration. Methods to calculate the base deficit and amount of bicarbonate needed to restore bicarbonate to normal are shown in Table 35.2. However, this calculation assumes no ongoing losses or utilization of buffer base. In clinical practice, many patients continue to lose or utilize large amounts of base. Some clinicians have advocated a multiplication factor to take into account ongoing losses that cannot be accounted for by a simple replacement formula, for example doubling the calculated deficit. Whichever method is chosen, repeated assessments of pH and bicarbonate concentrations should be made every 6–12 h to gauge the response to therapy and to make any dosage/rate adjustments when administering buffer base.

Colloid Fluids

Colloids are solutions that contain high-molecular-weight molecules (sugars or proteins) suspended in a crystalloid solution containing electrolytes. These solutions are designed to stay principally within the intravascular space and augment volume retention by their charge and size. The normal colloid osmotic pressure (COP) of equine plasma is approximately 20 mmHg. In many disease states in horses – notably inflammatory or ischemic lesions of the gastrointestinal tract – decreases in the COP are often observed. Tissue edema may result from the increased intravascular hydrostatic pressure, leading to fluid egress into the interstitium. Vascular volume retention is favored, theoretically, and the flow of fluid out of the vessel is minimized by increasing the intravascular colloidal pressure by administering colloids. For instance, when aggressive crystalloid therapy is performed (such as during anesthesia for colic surgery), the COP is reduced and intravascular hydrostatic pressure is increased, favoring interstitial fluid accumulation [32,33]. In theory, colloid administration helps to offset this loss of circulating volume and promote a better blood flow, pressure, and thus organ perfusion. However, a recent report showed that these effects may be limited in horses [34,35]. The administration of synthetic colloids and balanced polyionic crystalloid solutions, randomly, to horses with gastrointestinal disease resulted in an increased COP, but there was no significant difference in survival rates between the groups [35]. Additionally, hydroxyethyl starch solutions are associated with increased mortality and severe kidney injury and dysfunction when used in humans with sepsis and severe sepsis [36]. The use of synthetic colloids in human and veterinary medicine has diminished as complications associated with kidney function, coagulation, liver function, dermatologic issues, and survival have been reported.

Natural colloids used in horses include fresh plasma, fresh-frozen plasma, and whole-blood. The use of these products is not without some risk, as hypersensitivity reactions are reported in 10% of horses receiving plasma and in 16% of horses receiving whole-blood [37, 38]. However, several benefits of natural colloids exist, including the replenishment of clotting factors, plasma proteins, soluble anti-inflammatory mediators, and complement. Given that endotoxemia is a consumptive disorder (consuming both clotting factors and natural anticoagulants), a combined approach to colloid therapy may confer the most benefit for horses with endotoxemia where a combination of both plasma and synthetic colloid administration can provide both COP support and replace much-needed biological substances.

Monitoring the Response to Fluid Therapy

Clinical markers of improvement of global perfusion include a gradual normalization of the heart rate, mucous membrane color and capillary refill time, warming of the ears and limb extremities (if they were previously cool), as well as improved attitude and demeanor. With improved splanchnic perfusion, borborygmi may be ausculted. Urine production signals improved renal perfusion and is an excellent marker of glomerular filtration and tubular flow.

Clinicopathologic variables may begin to normalize in response to perfusion improvement fairly quickly. A decrease in peripheral blood L-lactate concentration would be expected as lactate clearance increases alongside improvements in global perfusion and oxygenation.

Anti-Endotoxin Therapy

Limiting the absorption, liberation, and dissemination of LPS systemically is an important target in the management of horses with sepsis/endotoxemia. Therapies can be classified into several groups based on their mechanism of action.

Reducing Intestinal LPS Absorption

Data from CHO models of laminitis suggest that signs of sepsis and endotoxemia precede the development of laminitis [2]. CHO causes a deterioration of the cecal and colonic mucosa [39], and mucosal damage and increased permeability to toxins and bacteria are associated with bacterial population changes within the gut, altered bacterial fermentation, increased lactate production, and acidosis [39, 40]. These luminal changes disrupt the colonic mucosal defenses against bacteria and bacteria toxins entering the systemic circulation. Substances meant to neutralize toxins within the gastrointestinal lumen and limit mucosal injury are administered orally to horses at risk of entero(typhlo)colitis. Mineral oil, activated charcoal, and di-tri-octahedral (DTO) smectite (Biosponge®) are given via a nasogastric tube to horses following the ingestion of excessive carbohydrate (grain overload) or presumed hindgut mucosal damage to bind toxins, thus preventing their hematogenous absorption. Some available data support these treatments. In a study in which DTO smectite was randomly administered to horses following surgical treatment of ascending colon disease, horses that received the DTO smectite had significantly less diarrhea (10.8%) compared to horses that did not receive smectite (41.4%) [37]. The development of laminitis in the study population was not described. No direct evidence exists to support the use of intestinal protectants in septic horses for laminitis prevention; however, horses receiving DTO smectite had an improved mucous membrane color, suggesting recovery from sepsis/toxemia [41]. The decreased incidence of diarrhea in treated horses may diminish laminitis risk. Recommendations for DTO smectite administration are 0.5 kg DTO smectite in 4 liters of water per nasogastric tube once or twice daily for three days [41].

Alimentary CHO causes changes in the gastrointestinal microbiome [42, 43]. Similar disruptions likely occur in horses with sepsis/endotoxemia, especially when clinical signs are the result of gastrointestinal injury. However, there are no data to support this assumption. The administration of *Saccharomyces boulardii* to horses with acute enterocolitis was associated with a decreased severity of clinical signs and duration of diarrhea in one study [44]. The anecdotal use of pre- and probiotic therapy in horses (and humans) is widespread, with many products being available though their clinical usefulness remains untested. It is also unknown whether or not the administration of probiotics is superior to resuming adequate nutrition and fiber.

Binding Circulating LPS in Plasma

Treatments are administered to horses in an attempt to bind endotoxin, blocking its systemic effects. At present, no data exist supporting the use of these therapies to prevent or diminish laminitis. Data refuting the use of endotoxin-binding drugs include the absence of horses developing laminitis following the systemic administration of endotoxin [23, 24]. Additionally, horses develop tolerance to the clinical and cellular effects of endotoxin after approximately 24 h [24]. If used, products that bind endotoxin should be administered acutely and probably discontinued after 24 h.

Products that bind circulating endotoxins include polymixin B, lipid emulsions, and anti-endotoxin serum and plasma. Polymixin B (PMB) is a cationic antimicrobial capable of binding and neutralizing endotoxin. In one study, horses received 20 ng kg^{-1} LPS followed by 5000 units of PMB [45]; treatment with PMB after the administration of endotoxin significantly reduced fever, tachycardia, and serum TNF levels compared to saline controls [45]. No signs of neurotoxicity or kidney toxicity were noted, and the urinary GGT:creatinine ratio (a sensitive indicator of kidney injury) did not change [45]. However, as renal compromise is not uncommon in the septic equine patient, these patients may be more at risk of nephrotoxicity than the normal horses used in these studies. The administration of PMB may be indicated, acutely, in horses with evidence of endotoxemia. PMB dosing is 1000–6000 units kg^{-1} in 1 liter of 0.9% saline, infused as a bolus every 8–12 h [46]. Anecdotally, surgeons and anesthetists administer PMB intraoperatively to combat the systemic effects of endotoxin on cardiopulmonary parameters as gastrointestinal lesions are corrected. This earlier use of the medication is sensible given the potential absorption of endotoxin during abdominal surgery and the quick development of tolerance. However, preclinical studies in human medicine have shown that PMB does not bind all endotoxin equally [47]. Rabbits treated with PMB were protected against *Escherichia coli* LPS but not against other Gram-negative bacterial LPS sources; these data likely indicate that PMB will only function with *E. coli* endotoxin in the horse and will not be effective with other common sources of endotoxin in equine sepsis (e.g., *Salmonella* endotoxin in salmonella enterocolitis) [48]. Lipid emulsions have been used *in vivo* in pretreatment endotoxin research models to attenuate the effects of equine endotoxemia [49]; the administration of 100 mg kg^{-1} phospholipid emulsion followed by 30 ng kg^{-1} LPS improved the clinical signs of endotoxemia including reductions in heart rate, rectal temperature, serum TNFα level, and the degree of leucopenia [49]. Potential complications associated with administration of lipid emulsions include hemolysis and anaphylaxis. No commercial products are currently available for horses. Anti-endotoxin plasma and sera (Endoserum®, *Salmonella typhimurium* antiserum, Imvacc; Equiplas *J Escherichia coli* plasma, Plasvacc) containing antibodies against LPS have been used in an attempt to bind endotoxin and diminish associated clinical signs. Evidence is lacking to support the use of these products.

Anti-Inflammatory Therapy

Anti-inflammatory drugs mitigate signs of the systemic inflammatory response associated with sepsis/endotoxemia, provide analgesia, and possibly limit lamellar inflammation. Cyclooxygenase (COX) enzyme expression is increased in the blood and tissues of patients with sepsis/endotoxemia and in the lamellae of horses with laminitis. Cyclooxygenase 2 gene expression was increased in lamellar samples following both oligofructose and BWE-induced laminitis [3, 30, 50]. The administration of flunixin meglumine, a non-selective COX-1 and COX-2 inhibitor, diminishes clinical signs and pain associated with colic and endotoxemia in horses [51, 52]. Flunixin meglumine (1.1 mg kg^{-1}, intravenous) administered 30 min after LPS infusion diminished TNFα gene expression in whole blood [52]. However, the administration of flunixin meglumine was associated with significantly increased IL-6 gene expression [52]. Expression of IL-6 was also increased in lamellar tissue in three different experimental models of SRL, and was associated with increased pro-matrix metalloproteinase 9 levels in lamellar explants [53]. The effects of IL-6 on tissues is unclear because this cytokine has both inflammatory and anti-inflammatory actions [54]. Other nonsteroidal anti-inflammatory drugs (NSAIDs) used in horses with sepsis/endotoxemia include phenylbutazone, ketoprophen, and the COX-2-selective medication, firocoxib. Experimental studies [2, 3] and anecdotal clinical evidence suggests that flunixin meglumine is superior to the other NSAIDs at diminishing signs of endotoxemia. *In-vivo* studies suggest that firocoxib is associated with improved gastrointestinal mucosal healing and restitution following ischemic insult to the gastrointestinal tract compared to flunixin meglumine [55]. The "anti-endotoxic" effects of firocoxib, as well as its effectiveness in acute and developmental laminitis, are unclear. Anecdotal reports suggest that flunixin meglumine is a superior analgesic in cases of equine sepsis/endotoxemia and laminitis compared to firocoxib.

Lidocaine, a local anesthetic and sodium channel blocker, is used to treat horses with sepsis/endotoxemia caused by gastrointestinal insult [56]. Lidocaine (1.3 mg kg^{-1} intravenous infusion over 15 min followed by 0.3 mg kg^{-1} h^{-1}, continuous rate infusion) improved the healing of ischemically injured intestine by reducing inflammation and blocking sodium channels, thereby limiting intracellular calcium and cellular injury [56–58]. Lidocaine diminished neutrophil emigration to the mucosa and reduced prostanoid production. The coadministration of lidocaine and flunixin meglumine blocked the deleterious effects of flunixin meglumine on mucosal healing [57, 58]. However, lidocaine was ineffective *in vivo* at preventing neutrophil activation or preventing inflammatory events associated with the BWE model of SRL [3,59]. No clinical studies have evaluated the efficacy of lidocaine as a preventive therapy for laminitis in clinical cases of equine sepsis/endotoxemia.

Pentoxyfylline is a trisubstituted xanthine derivative and nonspecific phosphodiesterase inhibitor. Horses with sepsis/endotoxemia are treated with pentoxifylline (8.5 mg kg^{-1} oral, q. 12 h) to diminish inflammatory effects associated with TNFα expression [60]. Additionally, pentoxifylline improved microvascular flow and tissue oxygen delivery by increasing erythrocyte deformability [61]. Pentoxifylline may have direct effects on the digital vasculature in septic horses. *In-vitro* studies showed that pentoxifylline induced digital vein relaxation through the nitric oxide synthase and COX pathways [62]. Vasodilation was partially blocked by the application of indomethacin, a COX-nonspecific inhibitor. The therapeutic effects of pentoxifylline and flunixin meglumine were assessed in a pretreatment *in vivo* endotoxemia model [63]. Treatment with flunixin meglumine versus a combination of flunixin meglumine and pentoxifylline prior to LPS administration diminished the proinflammatory cytokine and prostanoid response and improved the hemodynamics [63]. The efficacy of pentoxifylline *in vivo* as a treatment in clinical sepsis/endotoxemia or its actions in SRL are unknown.

Anecdotal reports suggest that doxycycline (5 mg kg^{-1} oral, q. 12 h for five doses) [64] may reduce the signs of acute laminitis by suppressing matrix metalloproteinase (MMP) activity. However, MMPs may not play an active role in developmental laminitis [65].

Local Treatment of the Digit

Hypothermia

Prophylactic digital hypothermia has become the centerpiece of treatment for SRL due to the fact that it is the only treatment consistently demonstrated to be efficacious in both experimental models and a retrospective clinical study of SRL (see Chapter 34) [13]. Importantly, it is the only therapy which has withstood scientific rigor in either human or veterinary research as being an effective treatment to decrease organ/tissue injury in sepsis. In distinction to human hypothermia protocols in which the target temperature for tissues is usually greater than 25 °C, digital hypothermia used in Equine Laminitis is a profound hypothermia in which immersion of the distal limb in ice water maintains the hoof wall/lamellar temperature at approximately 5 °C. As discussed in detail in Chapter 34, hypothermia has been demonstrated experimentally to protect the structural integrity of the lamellae when used prophylactically (i.e., initiated at the time a carbohydrate bolus is given to the horse to induce laminitis) or when initiated at the onset of clinical signs of laminitis [30, 66]. Using the oligofructose model, digital hypothermia exhibited a dramatic inhibition of multiple lamellar inflammatory signaling events including expression of chemokines, proinflammatory cytokines, COX-2, MMP-2 and endothelial adhesion molecules [30, 66]. Other factors proposed to play a protective role with digital hypothermia include the induction of analgesia, decreased tissue metabolism, and decreased lamellar perfusion (this is purported to result in less toxin delivery to the lamellae in the septic horse) [66, 67]. In addition to efficacy exhibited in experimental models of SRL, a retrospective study of enterocolitis cases in two referral hospitals demonstrated a dramatic decrease in the incidence of laminitis in cases treated prophylactically with digital hypothermia [13]. Effective digital hypothermia in the clinical situation has been achieved using ice bags (5-liter fluid bag filled with ice water) and boots filled with ice/ice water slurry and continuously applied [67]. Ice should be replenished every 1–2 h to maintain the ice/ice slurry within the boot. Anecdotally, forelimbs are iced more frequently than the fore and hind limbs; convenience and lack of patient compliance detract from hind foot icing. However, as similar inflammatory responses in both front and hind limb lamellae occur in the CHO laminitis model [68], hindlimbs should also be included when possible. Therefore, recommendations for limb hypothermia include: (i) the application of ice boots to horses at risk for SRL very early (within 5–60 min of hospital admission or recovery from general anesthesia when application is safe); (ii) application of continuous ice/ice slurry to maintain consistent hypothermia for 24–48 h beyond the resolution of clinical signs of sepsis/endotoxemia; and (iii) application of cryotherapy to all four limbs when possible [30, 65].

Hoof Support

As discussed in more detail in other chapters, hoof support to redistribute the load placed on the lamellae is indicated in horses with or at risk for SRL. The application of padding to the feet and/or enhanced footing and bedding can help to support the foot. Choices of bedding material include shavings, sawdust, paper, straw, tan bark, peat moss, and sand. Whatever is chosen, it should be adequately deep to not only protect the digit but also to supply a comfortable and protective surface to encourage recumbency while protecting pressure points from decubital ulceration. The removal of shoes is recommended and helpful in at-risk horses, and certainly in horses with increased digital pulses and pain (as discussed in Chapter 7). Many types of pad exist to help distribute weight across the foot. However, it is difficult with some modes of digital hypothermia to have room both for ice water and a pad (especially if 5-liter fluid bags are used). In this circumstance, it may be preferable to provide a deep soft bedding (e.g., peat moss) to support the foot in lieu of a pad, so as to allow adequate room in the bag for ice and water. Slings can be used to decrease the load on the horse's feet. However, the use of slings in SRL is uncommon due to the cost, horse compliance, and numerous biosafety issues. Effective use of slings in the acute treatment of laminitis requires the horse to use the sling, thus unweighting the limbs. Some horses develop anxiety and agitation in slings, which defeats the proposed benefit.

Pain Control

Analgesia to relieve the pain associated with lamellar injury and/or failure is a critical adjunct to therapy in the endotoxic/septic horse for both physiologic and humane reasons. Affected horses are reluctant to move around their stalls and may refuse to eat or drink. Tachycardia, tachypnea, changes in posture, sweating and altered mentation may occur in affected horses. NSAIDs are frequently administered to horses with laminitis as part of a multi-model analgesic plan. Continuous rate infusions of lidocaine, ketamine, detomidine, and morphine in various combinations may be administered [69]. The reader is referred to Chapter 33, in which analgesic therapy is described in detail. Cryotherapy of affected digits is recommended for its analgesic properties.

Thromboprophylaxis

There is an intrinsic link between coagulation and inflammation in SIRS patients. Hypercoagulability may result in dysregulated thrombin formation and lead to the generation of microthrombi [7]. Microthrombi have been found in lamellar tissue during the early stages of laminitis and represent a potential link between lamellar microvascular flow disturbances and lamellar failure in horses with overwhelming inflammation and coagulation due to sepsis [39, 70]. Tissue fibrin deposition, notably capillary microthrombus formation, has also been documented in septic foals and reflects a hypercoagulable state [71].

Inflammatory changes in vascular tone in the foot may be permissive for thrombotic events. Levels of endothelin-1, a potent vasoconstrictor, were increased in lamellar tissue samples during the inflammatory response as a result of endothelial cell activation [72]. The mechanism linking sepsis/endotoxemia, vascular changes and laminitis is unclear.

Platelet activation promotes endothelial activation and leukocyte margination into tissues (thus exacerbating inflammatory injury) in human sepsis; this response likely occurs in the lamellae of horses [73]. Laminitis may thus be linked to platelet activation leading to local lamellar microthrombus formation, hemodynamic alterations, and an exacerbation of inflammatory signaling in lamellar tissues [39, 74]. Anticoagulant drugs (see Table 35.3) such as heparins and platelet inhibitors are used to treat/prevent Equine Laminitis. Heparins potentiate anti-thrombin activity and inhibit tissue factor liberation and thrombin generation [75]. Several clinical studies have advocated the use of heparins to prevent or limit the development of laminitis in horses with inflammatory lesions [15, 17, 73, 75, 76]. Horses diagnosed with duodenitis/proximal jejunitis treated with heparin had a lower incidence of laminitis compared to horses diagnosed with enteritis that did not receive heparin [17]. Pouyade *et al.* reported that the administration of low-molecular-weight heparin (LMWH; enoxaparin) was effective in preventing laminitis following colic surgery [15]. The investigators speculate that LMWH may prevent laminitis by acting as both an anticoagulant and MMP inhibitor [15]. Perhaps the efficacy of thromboprophylactic therapy in preventing Equine Laminitis depends on the cause of the sepsis/endotoxemia and the specific colic lesion.

Table 35.3 Anticoagulant medications used in horses to prevent microthrombi generation.

Drug	Suggested dosage*	Comments
Heparin (unfractionated; UFH)	40–100 IU kg^{-1}, IV/SQ q. 6–8 h	Severe anemia can develop due to RBC agglutination, monitor PCV/HCt when using UFH. Protamine sulfate can be used as an effective reversal agent.
Heparin (low- molecular-weight)	Dalteparin 50–100 IU kg^{-1}, SC, q. 24 h Enoxaparin 40–80 IU kg^{-1}, SC, q. 24 h	Monitor efficacy by anti-factor Xa activity [76]
Aspirin	10–20 mg kg^{-1}, PO, q. 36–48 h	Less efficacious in inhibiting platelet aggregation as thromboxane A_2 is of lesser importance in equine platelet aggregation [77]
Clopidogrel	2 mg kg^{-1}, PO, q. 24 h	Inhibits platelet aggregation by inhibiting the P2Y12 ADP receptor of equine platelets [78]

Dose rates provided are a guide. Specific indications and contraindications may exist in certain patients.
*Routes of drug administration: IV, intravenous; IM, intramuscular; PO, per os (oral); SQ, subcutaneous.
HCt, hematocrit; PCV, packed cell volume; RBC, red blood cell.

The decision to use thromboprophylactic medications should be based on whether the patient has clinical evidence of thromboses (i.e., venepuncture or catheter-associated thrombosis) and clinicopathologic evidence of hypercoagulability (i.e., decreased prothrombin time [PT], activated partial thromboplastin time [APTT], hypercoagulable thromboelastograph trace, etc.). Careful monitoring of the response to therapy should also be instituted to ensure that the patient does not become hypocoagulable, particularly when using unfractionated heparin [75,76].

Outcomes and Expectations

Treating horses with sepsis/endotoxemia, whatever the cause, is expensive and has an uncertain outcome. Client education regarding the risk of SRL, prevention and treatment strategies, and prognosis – including a discussion about managing the chronically founder horse – is warranted.

Athleticism

Limited studies exist specifically assessing the prognosis for athleticism in SRL. A recent clinical study evaluating horses presenting for acute surgical colic showed the incidence of laminitis to be approximately 3%. Horses that developed laminitis while in the hospital were 10.1-fold more likely to not return to use and performance than those that did not develop laminitis. Moreover, if the horse developed laminitis following discharge from the hospital, it was 5.4-fold less likely to return to the intended athletic use [19].

Quality of Life

Unfortunately, many horses recover from the primary cause of sepsis but succumb to lamellar failure. Acute lamellar inflammation without resultant mechanical failure may carry a better prognosis. The goal of therapy is to resolve the primary insult (i.e., surgical or medical treatment of acute abdomen or enterocolitis, respectively) as well as reduce lamellar inflammation/injury before failure occurs. If the inflammatory process can be quickly subdued with limited mechanical damage to the foot, the horse has the potential for recovery. However, when lamellar failure occurs (rotation, sinking) the prognosis worsens dramatically. Large body size [1], multiple limb involvement, as well as mechanical sinking of the third phalanx within the hoof are grave prognostic signs. Anecdotally, hindlimb laminitis may be associated with a worse prognosis than forelimb laminitis, particularly when mechanical failure occurs.

References

1. Parsons, C.S., Orsini, J.A., Krafty, R., *et al.* (2007) Risk factors for development of acute laminitis in horses during hospitalization: 73 cases (1997–2004). *J. Am. Vet. Med. Assoc.*, **230**, 885–889.
2. Belknap, J.K., Moore, J.N., and Crouser, E.C. (2009) Sepsis: from human organ failure to lamellar failure. *Vet. Immunol. Immunopathol.*, **129**, 155–157.
3. Loftus, J.P., Black, S.J., Pettigrew, A., *et al.* (2007) Early lamellar events involving endothelial activation in horses with black walnut-induced laminitis. *Am. J. Vet. Res.*, **68** (11), 1205–1211.
4. De Laat, M.A., McGowan, C.M., Sillence, M.N., and Pollitt, C.C. (2010) Hyperinsulinemic laminitis. *Vet. Clin. North Am. Equine Pract.*, **26** (2), 257–264.
5. Toth, F., Frank, N., Elliott, S.B., *et al.* (2008) Effects of an intravenous endotoxin challenge on glucose and insulin dynamics in horses. *Am. J. Vet. Res.*, **62**, 82–88.
6. Hurley, D.J., Berghaus, L.J., Hurley, K.A., *et al.* (2011) Evaluation of the in vitro effects of aqueous black walnut extract on equine mononuclear cells. *Am. J. Vet. Res.*, **72** (3), 318–325.
7. American College of Chest Physicians/Society of Critical Care Medicine Consensus Conference: Definitions for sepsis and organ failure and guidelines for the use of innovative therapies in sepsis. *Crit. Care Med.*, **20** (6), 864–874.
8. Gille-Johnson, P., Smedman, C., Gudmundsdotter, L., *et al.* (2012) Circulating monocytes are not the major source of plasma cytokines in patients with sepsis. *Shock*, **38** (6), 577–583.
9. Johns, I., Tennent-Browns, B., Shaer, B.D., *et al.* (2009) Blood culture status in mature horses with diarrhea: a possible association with survival. *Equine Vet. J.*, **41**, 160–164.
10. Hurcombe, S.D., Mudge, M.C., and Daniels, J.B. (2012) Presumptive bacterial translocation in horses with strangulating small intestinal lesions requiring resection and anastomosis. *J. Vet. Emerg. Crit. Care (San Antonio)*, **22** (6), 653–660.
11. Reisinger, N., Schaumberger, S., Nagl, V., *et al.* (2015) Concentration-dependent influence of lipopolysaccharides on separation of hoof explants and supernatant lactic acid concentration in an ex-vivo/in-vitro laminitis model. *PLoS ONE*, **10** (11), e0143754.
12. Tennent-Brown, B.S. (2012) Interpreting lactate measurement in critically ill horses: diagnosis, treatment, and prognosis. *Compend. Contin. Educ. Vet.*, **34** (1), E1–E6.
13. Kullmann, A., Holcombe, S.J., Hurcombe, S.D., *et al.* (2014) Prophylactic digital cryotherapy is associated with decreased incidence of laminitis in horses diagnosed with colitis. *Equine Vet. J.*, **46** (5), 554–559.
14. Dunkel, B., Chaney, K.P., Dallap-Schaer, B.L, *et al.* (2011) Putative intestinal hyperammonaemia in horses: 36 cases. *Equine Vet. J.*, **43** (2), 133–140.
15. Pouyade, G., Grulke, S., Detilleux, J., *et al.* (2009) Evaluation of low-molecular-weight heparin for the prevention of equine laminitis after colic surgery. *J. Vet. Emerg. Crit. Care*, **19**, 113–119.
16. Cohen, N.D., Parson, E.M., Seahorn, T.L., *et al.* (1994) Prevalence and factors associated with development of laminitis in horses with duodenitis/proximal jejunitis: 33 cases (1985–1991). *J. Am. Vet. Med. Assoc.*, **204**, 250–254.
17. Cohen, N.D. and Woods, A.M. (1999) Characteristics and risk factors for failure of horses with acute diarrhea to survive: 122 cases (1990–1996). *J. Am. Vet. Med. Assoc.*, **214**, 382–390.
18. Stewart, M.C., Hodgson, J.L., Kim, H., *et al.* (1995) Acute febrile diarrhea in horses: 86 cases (1986–1991). *Aust. Vet. J.*, **72**, 41–44.
19. Vick, M.M., Adams, A.A., Murphy, B.A., *et al.* (2007) Relationships among inflammatory cytokines, obesity, and insulin sensitivity in the horse. *J. Anim. Sci.*, **85**, 1144–1155.

20. Davis, W., Fogle, C.A., Gerard, M.P., *et al.* (2013) Return to use and performance following exploratory celiotomy for colic in horses: 195 cases (2003–2010). *Equine Vet. J.*, **45** (2), 224–228.
21. Tomlinson, J.E., Boston, R.C., and Brauer, T. (2013) Evaluation of racing performance after colic surgery in Thoroughbreds: 85 cases (1996–2010). *J. Am. Vet. Med. Assoc.*, **243** (4), 532–537.
22. Laskoski, L.M., Locatelli-Dittrich, R., Valadao, C.A.A., *et al.* (2015) Systemic leukopenia, evaluation of lamellar leukocyte infiltration and lamellar lesions in horses with naturally occurring colic syndrome. *Res. Vet. Sci.*, **101**, 15–21.
23. Wylie, C.E., Collins, S.N., Verheyen, K.L.P., *et al.* (2011) Frequency of equine laminitis: A systematic review with quality appraisal of published evidence. *Vet. J.*, **189**, 248–256.
24. Tadros, E.M., Frank, N., Newkirk, K.M., *et al.* (2012) Effects of a 'two-hit' model or organ damage on the systemic inflammatory response and development of laminitis in horses. *Vet. Immunol. Immunopathol.*, **150**, 90–100.
25. Dellinger, R.P., Levy, M.M., Carlet, J.M., *et al.* (2008) Surviving sepsis campaign: international guidelines for management of severe sepsis and septic shock. *Crit. Care Med.*, **36**, 296–327.
26. McGorum, B.C. and Pirie, R.S. (2009) Antimicrobial associated diarrhea in the horse. Part 1: Overview, pathogenesis and risk factors. *Equine Vet. Educ.*, **21**, 610–616.
27. Barr, B.S., Waldridge, B.M., Morresey, P.R., *et al.* (2013) Antimicrobial-associated diarrhoea in three equine referral practices. *Equine Vet. J.*, **45** (2), 145–148.
28. Mark, P.E. (2014) Early management of severe sepsis: concepts and controversies. *Chest*, **145** (6), 1407–1418.
29. Ince, C. (2014) The rationale for microcirculatory guided fluid therapy. *Curr. Opin. Crit. Care*, **20** (3), 301–308.
30. Van Eps, A.W., Leise, B.S., Watts, M., *et al.* (2012) Digital hypothermia inhibits early lamellar inflammatory signaling in the oligofructose laminitis model. *Equine Vet. J.*, **44** (2), 230–237.
31. Shih, C.C., Tsai, M.F., Chen, S.J., *et al.* (2012) Effects of small-volume hypertonic saline on acid-base and electrolyte balance in rats with peritonitis-induced sepsis. *Shock*, **38** (6), 649–655.
32. Boscan, P., Watson, Z., and Steffey, E.P. (2007) Plasma colloid osmotic pressure and total protein trends in horses during anesthesia. *Vet. Anaesth. Analg.*, **34**, 275–283.
33. Boscan, P. and Steffey, E.P. (2007) Plasma colloid osmotic pressure and total protein in horses during colic surgery. *Vet. Anaesth. Analg.*, **34**, 408–415.
34. Wendt-Hornickle, E.L., Snyder, L.B., Tang, R., *et al.* (2011) The effects of lactated Ringer's solution (LRS) or LRS and 6% hetastarch of the colloid osmotic pressure, total protein and osmolality in healthy horses undergoing general anesthesia. *Vet. Anaesth. Analg.*, **38**, 336–343.
35. Bellezzo, F., Kuhnmuench, T., and Hackett, E.S. (2014) The effect of colloid formulation on colloid osmotic pressure in horses with naturally occurring gastrointestinal disease. *BMC Vet. Res.*, **10** (Suppl.1), 1–5.
36. Seymour, C.W. and Rosengart, M.R. (2015) Septic shock: advances in diagnosis and treatment. *J. Am. Med. Assoc.*, **314** (7), 708–717.
37. Wilson, E.M., Holcombe, S.J., Lamar, A., *et al.* (2010) Incidence of transfusion reactions and retention of procoagulant and anticoagulant factor activities in equine plasma. *J. Vet. Intern. Med.*, **23**, 323–328.
38. Hurcombe, S.D., Mudge, M.C., and Hinchcliff, K.W. (2007) Clinical and clinicopathologic variables in adult horses receiving blood transfusions: 31 cases (1999–2005). *J. Am. Vet. Med. Assoc.*, **231**, 267–274.
39. Krueger, A.S., Kindern, D.A., Garner, H.E., and Sprouse, R.F. (1986) Ultrastructural study of the equine cecum during onset of laminitis. *Am. J. Vet. Res.*, **47** (8), 1804–1812.
40. Weiss, D.J., Geor, R.J., Johnston, G., *et al.* (1994) Microvascular thrombosis associated with onset of acute laminitis in ponies. *Am. J. Vet. Res.*, **55**, 606–612.
41. Hassel, D.M., Smith, P.A., Nieto, J.E., *et al.* (2009) Di-tri-octahedral smectite for the prevention of post-operative diarrhea in equids with surgical disease of the large intestine: Results of a randomized clinical trial. *Vet. J.*, **182**, 210–214.
42. Onishi, J.C., Park, J.W., Prado, J., *et al.* (2012) Intestinal bacterial overgrowth includes potential pathogens in the carbohydrate overload models of equine acute laminitis. *Vet. Microbiol.*, **159**, 354–363.
43. Milinovich, G.J., Burrell, P.C., Pollitt, C.C., *et al.* (2008) Microbial ecology of the equine hindgut during oligofructose-induced laminitis. *ISME J.*, **2**, 1089–1100.
44. Desrochers, A.M., Dolente, B.A., Roy, M.F., *et al.* (2005) Efficacy of *Saccharomyces boulardii* for treatment of horses with acute enterocolitis. *J. Am. Vet. Med. Assoc.*, **227**, 954–959.
45. Barton, M.H., Parviainen, A., and Norton, N. (2004) Polymixin B protects horses against induced endotoxaemia in vivo. *Equine Vet. J.*, **36** (5), 397–401.
46. Morresey, P.R. and MacKay, R.J. (2006) Endotoxin-neutralizing activity of polymyxin B in blood after IV administration in horses. *Am. J. Vet. Res.*, **67**, 642–647.
47. Cavaillon, J.M. (2011) Polymyxin B for endotoxin removal in sepsis. *Lancet*, **11**, 426–427.
48. Baldwin, G., Alperta, G., Caputa, G.I., *et al.* (1991) Effect of polymyxin B on experimental shock from meningococcal and *Escherichia coli* endotoxins. *J. Infect. Dis.*, **164**, 542–549.
49. Moore, J.N., Barton, M.H., Hurley, D.J., *et al.* (2007) Rapid infusion of a phospholipid emulsion attenuates the effects of endotoxaemia in horses. *Equine Vet. J.*, **39** (3), 243–248.
50. Blikslager, A.T., Yin, C., Cochran, A.M., *et al.* (2006) Cyclooxygenase expression in the early stages of equine laminitis: a cytologic study. *J. Vet. Intern. Med.*, **20**, 1191–1196.
51. Jochle, W., Moore, J.N., Brown, J., *et al.* (1989) Comparison of detomidine, butorphanol, flunixin meglumine, and xylazine in clinical cases of equine colic. *Equine Vet. J. Suppl.*, **7**, 111–116.
52. Jacobs, C.C., Holcombe, S.J., Cook, V.L., *et al.* (2013) Ethyl pyruvate diminishes the inflammatory response to lipopolysaccharide infusion in horses. *Equine Vet. J.*, **45** (3), 333–339.
53. Visser, M.B. and Pollitt, C.C. (2011) Lamellar leukocyte infiltration and involvement of IL-6 during oligofructose-induced equine laminitis development. *Vet. Immunol. Immunopathol.*, **144**, 120–128.
54. Remick, D.G., Bolgos, G.R., Siddiqui, J., *et al.* (2002) Six at six: interleukin-6 measured 6 hours after the initiation of sepsis predicts mortality over 3 days. *Shock*, **17**, 463–467.
55. Cook, V.L. and Blikslager, A.T. (2008) Use of systemically administered lidocaine in horses with gastrointestinal tract disease. *J. Am. Vet. Med. Assoc.*, **232** (8), 1144–1148.
56. Cook, V.L., Jones, S.J., McDowell, M.R., *et al.* (2009) Anti-inflammatory effects of systemically administered lidocaine in ischemic-injured equine jejunum. *Am. J. Vet. Res.*, **10**, 1259–1268.

57. Cook, V.L., Neuder, L.E., and Blikslager, A.T. (2009) The effect of lidocaine on in vitro adhesion and migration of equine neutrophils. *Vet. Immunol. Immunopathol.*, **129**, 137–142.
58. Williams, J.M., Lin, Y.J., Loftus, J.P., *et al.* (2010) Effect of intravenous lidocaine administration on lamellar inflammation in the black walnut extract model of laminitis. *Equine Vet. J.*, **42** (3), 261–269.
59. Barton, M.H., Moore, J.N., and Norton, N. (1997) Effects of pentoxifylline infusion on responses of horses to in vivo challenge exposure with endotoxin. *Am. J. Vet. Res.*, **58** (11), 1300–1307.
60. Geor, R.J., Weiss, D.J., Burris, S.M., *et al.* (1992) Effects of furosemide and pentoxifylline on blood flow properties in horses. *Am. J. Vet. Res.*, **53** (11), 2043–2049.
61. Kabbesh, N., Gogny, M., and Chatagnon G. (2012) Vasodilatory effect of pentoxifylline in isolated equine digital veins. *Vet. J.*, **192** (3), 368–373.
62. Baskett, A., Barton, M.H., Norton, N., *et al.* (1997) Effect of pentoxifylline, flunixin meglumine, and their combination on a model of endotoxemia in horses. *Am. J. Vet. Res.*, **58** (11), 1291–1299.
63. Schnabel, L.V., Papich, M.G., Watts, A.E., *et al.* (2010) Orally administered doxycycline accumulates in synovial fluid compared to plasma. *Equine Vet. J.*, **42** (3), 208–212.
64. Visser, M.B. and Pollitt, C.C. (2012) The timeline of metalloprotease events during oligofructose induced equine laminitis development. *Equine Vet. J.*, **44**, 88–93.
65. Van Eps, A.W. and Pollitt, C.C. (2004) Equine laminitis: cryotherapy reduces the severity of the acute lesion. *Equine Vet. J.*, **36**, 255–260.
66. Worster, A.A., Gaughan, E.M., Hoskinson, J.J., *et al.* (2000) Effects of external thermal manipulation on lamellar and perfusion scintigraphy of the equine digit. *N. Z. Vet. J.*, **48**, 111–116.
67. Reesink, H.L., Divers, T.J., Bookbinder, L.C., *et al.* (2012) Measurement of digital lamellar and venous temperatures as a means of comparing three methods of topically applied cold treatment for digits of horses. *Am. J. Vet. Res.*, **73**, 860–866.
68. Leise, B.S., Faleiros, R.R., Watts, M. *et al.* (2012) Hind limb lamellar inflammatory response is similar to that present in forelimbs after carbohydrate overload in horses. *Equine Vet. J.*, **44**, 633–639.
69. Sanchez, L.C. and Robertson, S.A. (2014) Pain control in horses: what do we really know? *Equine Vet. J.*, **46** (4), 517–523.
70. Weiss, D.J., Trent, A.M., and Johnston, G. (1995) Prothrombotic events in the prodromal stages of acute laminitis in ponies. *Am. J. Vet. Res.*, **56**, 986–991.
71. Cotovio, M., Monreal, L., Armengou, L., *et al.* (2008) Fibrin deposits and organ failure in newborn foals with severe septicemia. *J. Vet. Intern. Med.*, **22**, 1403–1410.
72. Eades, S.C., Holm, A.S., Moore, R.M., *et al.* (2002) A review of the pathophysiology and treatment of acute laminitis: pathophysiology and therapeutic implications of endothelin-1. Proceedings American Association of Equine Practitioners Annual Convention, Orlando, Florida, pp. 353–361.
73. Belknap, J.K. and Moore, J.N. (1989) Evaluation of heparin for prophylaxis of equine laminitis: 71 cases (1980–1986). *J. Am. Vet. Med. Assoc.*, **195**, 505–507.
74. Hood, D.M., Grosenbaugh, D.A., Mostafa, M.B., *et al.* (1993) The role of vascular mechanisms in the development of acute equine laminitis. *J. Vet. Intern. Med.*, **7**, 228–234.
75. Moore, B.R. and Hinchcliff, K.W. (1994) Heparin: a review of its pharmacology and therapeutic use in horses. *J. Vet. Intern. Med.*, **8**, 26–35.
76. Feige, K., Schwartzwald, C.C., and Bombeli, T. (2003) Comparison of unfractioned and low molecular weight heparin for prophylaxis of coagulopathies in 52 horses with colic: a randomized double-blind clinical trial. *Equine Vet. J.*, **35**, 506–513.
77. Heath, M.F., Evans, R.J., Poole, A.W., *et al.* (1994) The effects of aspirin and paracetamol on the aggregation of equine blood platelets. *J. Vet. Pharmacol. Ther.*, **17**, 374–378.
78. Brainard, B.M., Epstein, K.L., LoBato, D., *et al.* (2011) Effects of clopidogrel and aspirin on platelet aggregation, thromboxane production, and serotonin secretion in horses. *J. Vet. Intern. Med.*, **25**, 116–122.

CHAPTER 36

Equine Metabolic Syndrome

Andy E. Durham

Pharmacologic Treatment of the Equine Metabolic Syndrome

Equine metabolic syndrome (EMS) describes the clustering of several risk factors for laminitis [1] which, if not subsequently controlled, predicts a recurrence of the condition. When laminitis cases are encountered, it is essential that they are examined for the presence of such risk factors so that further control measures can be implemented. Potential recognized targets for management-related and therapeutic interventions include diet (quality and quantity), obesity, aerobic fitness, and insulin dysregulation. Although anecdotal observations and experiences indicate that laminitis risk is frequently reduced following effective control of these factors, there is currently no scientific proof of such. Obesity and consequent insulin dysregulation are highly prevalent and fundamental risk factors in EMS cases; therefore, weight reduction is an essential goal of management. In the author's view, one of the major advances in EMS management in practice is the growing confidence and ability of practitioners to offer specific dietary advice to owners of obese horses following evidence-based recommendations (see Chapter 50) [2–5]. Although options for pharmacologic treatment of EMS are discussed in this chapter, these treatments should never be regarded as a substitute for management-related countermeasures. There is a danger that, given the practical difficulties of achieving weight loss in extremely metabolically efficient individuals ('easy keepers' [3]), some owners might regard pharmacologic assistance as an easier alternative to dietary and exercise control. This suggestion should be firmly repudiated in preliminary discussions with the owner or trainer of the proposed EMS-management plan as sole reliance on pharmaceutical interventions is highly likely to fail.

Pharmacologic management of the metabolic syndrome in humans is common and dependent on many different drug classes and actions. Although of interest to the equine practitioner, products found to be useful in human patients may frequently be inappropriate for EMS cases due to inherent species differences in pharmacodynamics and pharmacokinetics, in addition to further important physiologic and pathophysiologic differences relating to nutrition, nutrient metabolism, EMS, and the metabolic syndrome. To date, the only pharmacologic agents that have received significant attention in EMS cases are L-thyroxine, metformin hydrochloride and pioglitazone.

L-Thyroxine (Levothyroxine)

Early mistaken suspicions that obese, lethargic, laminitis-prone individuals were clinically hypothyroid first led to the use of L-thyroxine (e.g., Thyro L; Lloyd Inc., Shenandoah, Iowa, USA; Soloxine; Virbac Ltd, Bury St Edmunds, Suffolk, UK) for the intention of replacement therapy in such cases. Although it is now accepted that hypothyroidism does not play a role in laminitis susceptibility, evidence suggests that exogenous thyroid hormone may nevertheless have beneficial effects in obese laminitis-prone animals. One study found that mares typically lost approximately 0.5% bodyweight weekly when treated with L-thyroxine on an increasing dosage regime from 0.05 to 0.20 mg kg^{-1} daily over eight weeks [6]. In a further, more prolonged study by the same group, the daily administration of 0.1 mg kg^{-1} L-thyroxine was associated with an approximate 0.6% bodyweight loss per week over the course of 16 weeks; however, weight loss did not continue with longer-term treatment for up to 48 weeks [7]. It was suggested that L-thyroxine leads to lipolysis and the mobilization of adipose stores due to an increased basal metabolic rate [7]. In association with the weight loss, serum insulin concentrations decreased slightly and insulin sensitivity approximately doubled during treatment in the same study [7]. Significant adverse health effects of exogenous L-thyroxine were not seen in a related report [8]. The use of L-thyroxine in EMS cases is recommended alongside dietary restriction, not only to augment the effect on weight loss but also to guard against the possible adverse effects of increased appetite during treatment [9]. Typically, a dose of approximately 0.1 mg kg^{-1} L-thyroxine orally q. 24 h is recommended for between three and six months, depending on response in terms of body condition. At the end of the treatment period, the drug should be gradually withdrawn over two to four weeks to allow the re-establishment

Equine Laminitis, First Edition. Edited by James K. Belknap and Raymond Geor.

of normal responsiveness of the pituitary–thyroid axis. Outside of the USA, the use of L-thyroxine is greatly limited by cost.

Metformin Hydrochloride

Use and Effects in Other Species

Metformin, an inexpensive biguanide drug, has become the mainstay of medical therapy for human patients with the metabolic syndrome over the past 50 years [10]. For such a widely prescribed product, its mode of action is poorly understood (although it is one of few pharmaceutical agents shown to decrease cardiovascular disease, the major morbidity and cause of mortality in humans with the metabolic syndrome [11]). Metformin promotes the phosphorylation of adenosine monophosphate (AMP)-activated protein kinase (AMPK), an important regulator of energy metabolism. Biguanide drugs have antihyperglycemic effects, with the most widely quoted action of metformin being as an insulin-sensitizer leading to the inhibition of hepatic gluconeogenesis and stimulation of glucose uptake in muscle and adipose tissue [12–14]. However, several other pharmacologic effects of metformin are recognized, and the relative importance of the insulin-sensitizing effect of biguanides was initially brought into question many years ago [15]. Furthermore, it is evident that metformin exhibits unusual pharmacokinetic and pharmacodynamic properties worthy of consideration.

There is a lack of correlation between systemic plasma drug concentrations and glycemic control in humans treated with metformin [16]; this is probably explained by the particular affinity that metformin and other biguanides have for enterocytes. In both mice and humans, biguanides have been shown to accumulate in the gastrointestinal mucosa (especially the jejunum and ileum) at approximately 100-fold the concentrations found in plasma and other tissues following oral administration [17–20]. Plasma membrane monoamine transporter (PMAT), identified on the apical membrane of human enterocytes, has been shown to have a high affinity for metformin and is responsible for intestinal uptake of the drug [21]. Minor intestinal metformin accumulation also occurs following intravenous administration, albeit with lower tissue concentrations compared to oral dosing [19]. This deep enterocytic compartment of drug accumulation is also clearly functionally important, as demonstrated in rodent studies in which a more profound and prolonged antihyperglycemic effect of metformin occurred when administered intraduodenally compared to the intravenous route [22]. This finding led to the description of an important 'first-pass pharmacodynamic effect' of metformin prior to any systemic pool of drug being established.

Consistent with enteric accumulation, several studies have shown that metformin and other biguanides have marked effects on intestinal glucose uptake, utilization, and systemic absorption. Numerous *in-vivo* studies have demonstrated a decreased glycemic response to oral glucose dosing when humans, dogs, guinea pigs, hamsters, or rats are pretreated with metformin and other biguanides [15, 23–28]. However, this is not a result of glucose malabsorption but rather an increased glucose uptake and utilization by enterocytes in the presence of metformin [20,28,29]. Enterocytes normally show high levels of glucose utilization via glycolytic pathways [30], which is further augmented in the presence of metformin in both fed and fasted states [31]. Thus, absorbed glucose is primarily metabolized by enterocytes into lactate rather than being assimilated into the systemic circulation [15,27,31–33].

Consistent with the effects of metformin described above, there is a detectable postprandial hyperlactemia noted during metformin therapy, but this is generally mild and not clinically concerning [20, 27, 31]. Lactic acidosis was recognized as an important adverse effect of phenformin, a predecessor of metformin [34]. This does not appear to be a significant concern with metformin use in humans with normal renal and hepatic function [35], although it does perhaps merit further investigation in horses. In humans, metformin is not protein-bound and is excreted entirely via the kidneys unchanged via the urine [36]; therefore, its use in patients with renal insufficiency is not recommended.

Studies of intestinal glucose absorption have indicated the presence of both an active sodium glucose transporter-1 (SGLT-1) and a passive glucose (GLUT-2) transporter that enable the uptake of glucose from the intestinal lumen; both are expressed in response to the presence of sugars in the intestinal lumen [37, 38]. Metformin treatment in rats was associated with increased SGLT-1 gene expression in the small intestine, but had no effect on the expression of GLUT-2 genes in one study [39]. In contrast, another study [28] found that metformin decreased SGLT-1 and increased GLUT-2 abundance in the rat jejunum, an effect that was dependent on metformin causing AMPK phosphorylation (resulting in the activation of AMPK). Thus, the precise interaction between metformin and glucose transporters has yet to be clarified.

Use and Effects in Equids

A study of laminitis-prone horses and ponies reported a significant decrease in plasma glucose and insulin within two weeks of beginning metformin therapy at 15 mg kg^{-1} q. 12 h [40]. However, subsequent studies indicated very poor oral bioavailability of metformin in horses of only 7% following fasting [41], compared with 50–60% in humans and rats [19, 22, 36]. Further studies found no detectable effect of 15 mg kg^{-1} metformin on peripheral insulin sensitivity in both normal horses [42] and insulin-resistant ponies [43], casting doubt on the existence of any real clinical benefits of the drug in EMS cases.

However, all of the findings in the above studies may be reconciled by hypothesizing that metformin in horses may have negligible systemic effects due to poor bioavailability, but may well have significant direct enteric effects as described in other species above. In the original study of the use of metformin in laminitis-prone horses and ponies, an acute mild hypoglycemic effect was noted following metformin with an approximate 10% decrease in plasma glucose 3 h following drug administration [40]. A further study has recently confirmed a significant moderation of hyperglycemia and hyperinsulinemia in horses when metformin was administered at a dose of 30 mg kg^{-1} prior to oral glucose dosing [44] which was also consistent with the findings in other species. This effect was found in normal horses, horses with dexamethasone-induced insulin resistance, and in horses with naturally occurring insulin resistance. Thus, there is accumulating evidence that metformin decreases enteric glucose absorption and subsequent insulinemia in horses as well as other species.

It is relevant that current suspicions of the apparent pathogenetic links between insulin dysregulation and laminitis focus on diet-induced hyperinsulinemia rather than tissue insulin insensitivity *per se* [45–47]. In this respect, the lack of any detectable insulin-sensitizing effect of metformin in horses [42, 43], yet the demonstration of moderation of hyperglycemia and hyperinsulinemia [40,44] maintains clinical interest in the drug. However, this would imply that the use of metformin may not be as effective in horses or ponies where diet is controlled as per recommendations (i.e., low nonstructural carbohydrate [NSC] content with low-to-moderate glycemic/insulinemic effects). The drug might be best applied in subjects that are still ingesting significant NSC from grazing, for example pituitary pars intermedia dysfunction (PPID) cases or EMS cases that are being allowed some limited grazing following on from an effective weight loss and exercise program. The moderation of glucose absorption might also be expected to assist weight control in such individuals. Rather than regular interval dosing, it might be wise to target drug administration pre-turnout to limit the subsequent glycemic and insulinemic effect of grazing. However, it should also be stated that any putative clinical benefits of metformin in horses are still based largely on anecdote (although one study commented that laminitis was improved in 14/18 [78%] treated subjects [40]). Further studies are clearly required.

Despite frequent gastrointestinal symptoms in human patients treated with metformin, no adverse effects of oral therapy have been reported in horses using doses up to 30 mg kg^{-1} [40–44]. Given the relative unimportance of achieving high plasma drug concentrations (due to effects occurring at the level of the luminal surface of the enterocyte), along with the commonly encountered practical problem of poor palatability in horses, further investigations of lower doses of metformin in horses might be warranted.

Thiazolodinediones

Thiazolidinediones (TZDs) are commonly prescribed insulin-sensitizing drugs used in human metabolic syndrome patients [13]. Recent investigations of pioglitazone in horses have revealed a reasonable pharmacokinetic profile [48] and some potential clinical benefits. In one study in which pioglitazone was administered at a dose of 1 mg kg^{-1} daily to lean, healthy horses [49], it was found that, although insulin sensitivity was not changed significantly by the treatment either before or after lipopolysaccharide (LPS)-induced insulin resistance, pioglitazone was associated with an increased abundance of GLUT-1 (a glucose transporter) and CD36 (a fatty acid transporter important in insulin-sensitizing actions of pioglitazone in humans) proteins and insulin receptor transcripts in skeletal muscle. Additionally, apparent protection against the endotoxin-induced suppression of GLUT-4 was seen in adipose tissue. No effects of pioglitazone on LPS-induced inflammatory markers was detected in a further study [50]. Further studies are required in different equine models relevant to EMS and insulin dysregulation prior to promotion of use of this drug (or class of drugs) to treat EMS-associated laminitis.

References

1. Frank, N., Geor, R.J., Bailey, S.R., Durham, A.E., and Johnson, P.J. (2010) Equine metabolic syndrome. *J. Vet. Intern. Med.*, **24**, 467–475.
2. Dugdale, A.H., Curtis, G.C., Cripps, P., Harris, P.A., and Argo, C.M. (2010) Effect of dietary restriction on body condition, composition and welfare of overweight and obese pony mares. *Equine Vet. J.*, **42**, 600–610.
3. Argo, C.M., Curtis, G.C., Grove-White, D., Dugdale, A.H., Barfoot, C.F., and Harris, P.A. (2012) Weight loss resistance: a further consideration for the nutritional management of obese Equidae. *Vet. J.*, **194**, 179–188.
4. Geor, R.J. and Harris, P. (2013) Laminitis, in *Equine Applied and Clinical Nutrition* (eds R.J. Geor, P.A. Harris, and M. Coenen), Saunders Elsevier, pp. 469–486.
5. Geor, R.J. and Harris, P. (2013) Obesity, in *Equine Applied and Clinical Nutrition* (eds R.J. Geor, P.A. Harris, and M. Coenen), Saunders Elsevier, pp. 487–502.
6. Sommardahl, C.S., Frank, N., Elliott, S.B., Webb, L.L., Refsal, K.R., Denhart, J.W., and Thompson, D.L., Jr. (2005) Effects of oral administration of levothyroxine sodium on serum concentrations of thyroid gland hormones and responses to injections of thyrotropin-releasing hormone in healthy adult mares. *Am. J. Vet. Res.*, **66**, 1025–1031.
7. Frank, N., Elliott, S.B., and Boston, R.C. (2008) Effects of long-term oral administration of levothyroxine sodium on glucose dynamics in healthy adult horses. *Am. J. Vet. Res.*, **69**, 76–81.
8. Frank, N., Buchanan, B.R., and Elliott, S.B. (2008) Effects of long-term oral administration of levothyroxine sodium on serum thyroid hormone concentrations, clinicopathologic variables, and echocardiographic measurements in healthy adult horses. *Am. J. Vet. Res.*, **69**, 68–75.
9. Frank, N. (2011) Equine metabolic syndrome. *Vet. Clin. North Am. Equine Pract.*, **27**, 73–92.
10. Nathan, D.M., Buse, J.B., Davidson, M.B., Ferrannini, E., Holman, R.R., Sherwin, R., and Zinman, B. (2009) Medical management of hyperglycemia in type 2 diabetes: a consensus algorithm for the initiation and adjustment of therapy. *Diabetes Care*, **32**, 193–203.

11. UK Prospective Diabetes Study (UKPDS) Group. (1998) Effect of intensive blood-glucose control with metformin on complications in overweight patients with type 2 diabetes (UKPDS 34). *Lancet*, **352**, 854–865.
12. Stumvoll, M., Nurjhan, N., Perriello, G., Dailey, G., and Gerich, J.E. (1995) Metabolic effects of metformin in non-insulin dependent diabetes mellitus. *N. Engl. J. Med.*, **333**, 550–554.
13. Bailey, C.J. (2005) Treating insulin resistance in type 2 diabetes with metformin and thiazolidinediones. *Diabetes Obesity Metab.*, **7**, 675–691.
14. Hays, N.P., Galassetti, P.R., and Coker, R.H. (2008) Prevention and treatment of type 2 diabetes: current role of lifestyle, natural product, and pharmacological interventions. *Pharmacol. Ther.*, **118**, 181–191.
15. Caspary, W.F. and Creutzfeldt, W. (1973) Inhibition of intestinal amino acid transport by blood sugar lowering biguanides. *Diabetologia*, **9**, 6–12.
16. Marchetti, P., Benzi, L., Cecchetti, P., Giannarelli, R., Boni, C., Ciociaro, D., Ciccarone, A.M., Di Cianni, G., Zappella, A., and Navalesi, R. (1987) Plasma biguanide levels are correlated with metabolic effects in diabetic patients. *Clin. Pharmacol. Ther.*, **41**, 450–454.
17. Wick, A.N., Stewart, CJ., and Serif, G.S. (1960) Tissue distribution of C^{14}-1abeled beta-phenethylbiguanide. *Diabetes*, **9**, 163–169.
18. Yoh, Y.J. (1967) Distribution of n-butylbiguanide-^{14}C-hydrochloride in mouse tissues. *Jap. J. Pharmacol.*, **17**, 439–449.
19. Wilcock, C. and Bailey, C.J. (1994) Accumulation of metformin by tissues of the normal and diabetic mouse. *Xenobiotica*, **24**, 49–57.
20. Bailey, C.J., Wilcock, C., and Scarpello, J.H. (2008) Metformin and the intestine. *Diabetologia*, **51**, 1552–1553.
21. Zhou, M., Xia, L., and Wang, J. (2007) Metformin transport by a newly cloned proton-stimulated organic cation transporter (plasma membrane monoamine transporter) expressed in human intestine. *Drug Metab. Dispos.*, **35**, 1956–1962.
22. Stepensky, D., Friedman, M., Raz, I., and Hoffman, A. (2002) Pharmacokinetic-pharmacodynamic analysis of the glucose-lowering effect of metformin in diabetic rats reveals first-pass pharmacodynamic effect. *Drug Metab. Dispos.*, **30**, 861–868.
23. Czyzyk, A., Lawecki, J., Sadowski, J., Ponikowska, I., and Szczepanik, Z. (1968) Effect of biguanides on intestinal absorption of glucose. *Diabetes*, **17**, 492–498.
24. Love, A.H.G. (1969) The effect of biguanides on intestinal absorption. *Diabetologia*, **5**, 422.
25. Hollobaugh, S.L., Rue, M.B., and Kriger, F.A. (1970) Studies on the site and mechanism of action of phenformin. I. Evidence for significant 'non-peripheral' effects of phenformin on glucose metabolism in normal subjects. *Diabetes*, **19**, 45–49.
26. Lorch, E. (1971) Inhibition of intestinal absorption and improvement of oral glucose tolerance by biguanides in the normal and in the streptozotocin-diabetic rat. *Diabetologia*, **7**, 195–203.
27. Bailey, C.J., Wilcock, C., and Day, C. (1992) Effect of metformin on glucose metabolism in the splanchnic bed. *Br. J. Pharmacol.*, **105**, 1009–1013.
28. Sakar, Y., Meddah, B., Faouz, M.A., Cherrah, Y., Bado, A., and Ducroc, R. (2010) Metformin-induced regulation of the intestinal D-glucose transporters. *J. Physiol. Pharmacol.*, **61**, 301–307.
29. Mithieux, G., Rajas, F., and Zitoun, C. (2006) Glucose utilization is suppressed in the gut of insulin-resistant high fat-fed rats and is restored by metformin. *Biochem. Pharmacol.*, **72**, 1757–1762.
30. Krebs, H.A. (1972) Some aspects of the regulation of fuel supply in omnivorous animals. *Adv. Enzyme Regul.*, **10**, 397–420.
31. Wilcock, C. and Bailey, C.J. (1990) Sites of metformin-stimulated glucose metabolism. *Biochem. Pharmacol.*, **39**, 1831–1834.
32. Berger, W. and Kunzli, H. (1970) Effect of dimethylbiguanide on insulin, glucose and lactic acid contents in portal vein blood and peripheral venous blood in the course of intraduodenal glucose tolerance test. *Diabetologia*, **6**, 37.
33. Pénicaud, L., Hitier, Y., Ferré, P., and Girard, J. (1989) Hypoglycaemic effect of metformin in genetically obese (fa/fa) rats results from an increased utilization of blood glucose by intestine. *Biochem. J.*, **262**, 881–885.
34. Bergman, U., Boman, G., and Wiholm, B.E. (1978) Epidemiology of adverse drug reactions to phenformin and metformin. *Br. Med. J.*, **11**, 464–466.
35. Bailey, C.J. and Turner, R.C. (1996) Metformin. *N. Engl. J. Med.*, **334**, 574–579.
36. Pentikäinen, P.J., Neuvonen, P.J., and Penttilä, A. (1979) Pharmacokinetics of metformin after intravenous and oral administration to man. *Eur. J. Clin. Pharmacol.*, **16**, 195–202.
37. Merediz, E.F., Dyer, J., Salmon, K.S., and Shirazi-Beechey, S.P. (2004) Molecular characterisation of fructose transport in equine small intestine. *Equine Vet. J.*, **36**, 532–538.
38. Kellett, G.L., Brot-Laroche, E., Mace, O.J., and Leturque, A. (2008) Sugar absorption in the intestine: the role of GLUT2. *Annu. Rev. Nutr.*, **28**, 35–54.
39. Lenzen, S., Lortz, S., and Tiedge, M. (1996) Effect of metformin on SGLT1, GLUT2, and GLUT5 hexose transporter gene expression in small intestine from rats. *Biochem. Pharmacol.*, **51**, 893–896.
40. Durham, A.E., Rendle, D.I., and Newton, J.E. (2008) The effect of metformin on measurements of insulin sensitivity and beta cell response in 18 horses and ponies with insulin resistance. *Equine Vet. J.*, **40**, 493–500.
41. Hustace, J.L., Firshman, A.M., and Mata, J.E. (2009) Pharmacokinetics and bioavailability of metformin in horses. *Am. J. Vet. Res.*, **70**, 665–668.
42. Firshman, A.M., Hustace, J.L., Peterson, K., and Mata, J. (2009) The effect of metformin on insulin sensitivity in horses. (abstract #340). *J. Vet. Intern. Med.*, **23**, 782.
43. Tinworth, K.D., Boston, R.C., Harris, P.A., Sillence, M.N., Raidal, S.L., and Noble, G.K. (2012) The effect of oral metformin on insulin sensitivity in insulin-resistant ponies. *Vet. J.*, **191**, 79–84.
44. Rendle, D.I., Rutledge, F., Hughes, K.J., and Durham, A.E. (2013) Effects of metformin hydrochloride on glucose and insulin responses in horses. *Equine Vet. J.*, **45**, 751–754.
45. Asplin, K.E., Sillence, M.N., Pollitt, C.C., and McGowan, C.M. (2007) Induction of laminitis by prolonged hyperinsulinaemia in clinically normal ponies. *Vet. J.*, **174**, 530–535.
46. de Laat, M.A., McGowan, C.M., Sillence, M.N., and Pollitt, C.C. (2010) Equine laminitis: induced by 48 h hyperinsulinaemia in Standardbred horses. *Equine Vet. J.*, **42**, 129–135.
47. de Laat, M.A., Sillence, M.N., McGowan, C.M., and Pollitt, C.C. (2012) Continuous intravenous infusion of glucose induces endogenous hyperinsulinaemia and lamellar histopathology in Standardbred horses. *Vet. J.*, **191**, 317–322.
48. Wearn, J.M., Crisman, M.V., Davis, J.L., Geor, R.J., Hodgson, D.R., Suagee, J.K., Ashraf-Khorassani, M., and McCutcheon, L.J. (2011)

Pharmacokinetics of pioglitazone after multiple oral dose administration in horses. *J. Vet. Pharmacol. Ther.*, **34**, 252–258.

49. Suagee, J.K., Corl, B.A., Wearn, J.G., Crisman, M.V., Hulver, M.W., Geor, R.J., and McCutcheon, L.J. (2011) Effects of the insulin-sensitizing drug pioglitazone and lipopolysaccharide administration on insulin sensitivity in horses. *J. Vet. Intern. Med.*, **25**, 356–364.
50. Wearn, J.G., Suagee, J.K., Crisman, M.V., Corl, B.A., Hulver, M.W., Hodgson, D.R., Geor, R.J., and McCutcheon, L.J. (2012) Effects of the insulin-sensitizing drug, pioglitazone, and lipopolysaccharide administration on markers of systemic inflammation and clinical parameters in horses. *Vet. Immunol. Immunopathol.*, **145**, 42–49.

CHAPTER 37

Pituitary Pars Intermedia Dysfunction

Dianne McFarlane, Philip J. Johnson and Harold C. Schott, II

Introduction

Endocrinopathic laminitis is the most common type of laminitis encountered in equine practice, accounting for approximately 70–90% of all cases [1,2]. Endocrinopathic laminitis may arise in the context of either equine metabolic syndrome (EMS) or pituitary pars intermedia dysfunction (PPID). An increased awareness of risk factors and an ability to both recognize and diagnose these endocrinopathic conditions should lead to a lessening of the incidence and severity of this common form of laminitis. It is becoming clear that abnormal glucose and insulin homeostasis ('insulin dysregulation') appears to represent the critical mediator of laminitis in both conditions [3–5]. Both insulin resistance (IR) and hyperinsulinemia have been suggested as plausible independent mediators of laminitis in EMS and PPID [3–5].

Pituitary pars intermedia dysfunction is a neurodegenerative condition resulting from a loss of dopaminergic neurons that originate in the hypothalamus [5]. In the healthy state, dopamine released by these neurons is inhibitory to cells in the pars intermedia termed *melanotropes* (see Fig. 16.1). In PPID, diminished dopamine release results in: (i) the proliferation (by clonal expansion) of melanotropes; (ii) an increased secretion by melanotropes of proopiomelanocortin peptides (melanocortins, including corticotropin [ACTH], beta-endorphin, alpha-melanocyte stimulating hormone, and corticotropin-like intermediate peptide); see Fig. 16.1 in Chapter 16; and (iii) the development of a pituitary adenoma.

Pituitary-derived melanocortin hypersecretion represents the principal endocrinopathic perturbation in horses affected with PPID. Unlike dogs and humans in which pituitary-dependent Cushing's disease results principally from the actions of ACTH derived from the corticotropes of the pars distalis, adrenal cortical hypertrophy is reported in only approximately 20% of PPID-affected horses [7–11]. Moreover, the biological activity of PPID-derived ACTH produced by melanotropes appears to be significantly reduced compared to ACTH derived from corticotropes [12–15].

Aside from an increased risk of laminitis, the other clinical manifestations of PPID, which include abnormalities of the haircoat, abnormal body fat distribution, fluctuations in body composition, immune compromise, and polyuria/polydipsia, have been extensively reviewed elsewhere [16–18]. Donaldson *et al.* reported that laminitis may represent one of the earliest signs of PPID, and that younger horses with laminitis may have PPID without other clinical signs commonly associated with the disease [1]. However, it should be noted that laminitis is not present in all PPID-affected horses, and may occur only in those horses with concurrent insulin dysregulation (see Chapter 16). Epidemiological estimates suggest about 30% of horses with PPID also have hyperinsulinemia, and 25% suffer laminitis [2,19].

Therefore, it appears that insulin dysregulation represents the critical risk factor for endocrinopathic laminitis in both PPID and in EMS. Current research is focused on obtaining an improved understanding of the pathophysiological link between insulin dysregulation and endocrinopathic laminitis. The observation that prolonged hyperinsulinemia can induce laminitis in healthy horses has suggested that hyperinsulinemia is an independent risk factor for endocrinopathic laminitis [3,4,20]. Heightened levels of circulating insulin (hyperinsulinemia) are thought to adversely affect the integrity of the digital lamellae by insulin-mediated activation of insulin-like growth factor-1 (IGF-1) receptors on basal epidermal cells in the hoof [21]. Furthermore, hyperinsulinemia may also cause increased vascular resistance and endothelin-1 expression in the equine digit, suggesting that the risk of endocrinopathic laminitis might also result from abnormalities of perfusion [22].

Insulin dysregulation may be present in the absence of PPID (when it is referred to as EMS), or as a component of the multiple clinical abnormalities in horses affected with PPID. Therefore, in order to prevent or reduce the risk of endocrinopathic laminitis in horses and ponies affected with PPID, veterinarians must address *both* insulin dysregulation *and* melanocortin hypersecretion.

The action of insulin may be more important in terms of laminitis risk than other endocrinopathic aspects of PPID. Although the likely role of cortisol as a 'cause' of laminitis has diminished during recent years, further investigations are required to assess the role of melanocortins on both laminitis

Equine Laminitis, First Edition. Edited by James K. Belknap and Raymond Geor.

risk and insulin sensitivity. A satisfactory explanation for the relationship between EMS and PPID is still lacking, but EMS may represent a risk factor for the development of PPID (endocrinopathic convergence). It is interesting to note that insulin dysregulation associated with EMS has been proposed to be a 'proinflammatory state' that might promote clinical expression of lamellar injury, whereas PPID is an inherently 'anti-inflammatory state' in which the clinical expression (pain, lameness) of laminitis is often subdued [23,24].

Early Recognition of Patients At-Risk for PPID and Endocrinopathic Laminitis

Veterinarians should be alert to the fact that laminitis in mature to older ponies and horses is commonly associated with either or both EMS and PPID [1,2]. Results of endocrinological evaluations of almost 90% of 36 horses presented for laminitis to the Helsinki University Equine Teaching Hospital over a 16-month period were consistent with a diagnosis of endocrinopathic laminitis [2]. Of those horses, approximately two-thirds showed basal hyperinsulinemia and an absence of hypertrichosis (consistent with EMS), and one-third had a diagnosis of PPID. Hyperinsulinemia was evident in almost all (10/11) of the PPID-affected horses with laminitis. Pony breeds are at greater risk than horses for development of endocrinopathic laminitis [2,25].

Age represents an independent risk factor for laminitis [2,25, 26]. Other age-related risk factors for the development of laminitis include diminishing insulin sensitivity and the onset of PPID [27,28]. Older horses may be at greater risk for 'other' causes of laminitis (risk factors such as sepsis), especially during hospitalization [29].

In addition to changes in the growth pattern of the hooves resulting from chronic endocrinopathic laminitis, abnormalities identified on physical examination that are potentially implicative for PPID include an abnormal body condition (including generalized or regional adiposity), or a poor body condition due to loss of skeletal (especially epaxial) musculature, abnormalities of the haircoat (including regional hypertrichosis, complete or incomplete failure of [or delayed] shedding in the spring, and a lightening of the coat color), chronic infections resulting from immune compromise, and altered behavior (lethargy). Other clinical abnormalities include poorly healing skin or corneal injuries, abnormalities regarding sweating (hyperhidrosis, hypohidrosis, and anhidrosis), infertility, and polyuria/polydipsia [16–19,27].

The development of PPID should be considered in horses that are already being managed for EMS that begin to lose body condition to an unexpected degree. If baseline insulin or results of dynamic glucose/insulin studies are being undertaken on a regular basis as a part of routine wellness examinations, the development of PPID should be suspected if evidence of worsening insulin sensitivity is detected in otherwise well-managed patients (where PPID may be a contributing factor in the worsening of insulin dysregulation) [30].

The diagnosis of PPID, including endocrinological testing, is detailed in Chapter 24 and in other relevant publications [16,17, 27,30–34].

Prevention of Laminitis in PPID-Affected Equids

Logical strategies aimed at reducing the risk of laminitis in horses and ponies that are either affected with or at risk of developing PPID can be summarized thus:

- Proactively increased vigilance by veterinarian and client for early signs of PPID and insulin dysregulation in horses and ponies, especially after 12–15 years of age:
  - Recognition that endocrinopathic laminitis might be the first and only sign of underlying PPID in mature horses and ponies;
  - Recognition of the fact that morphological/radiographic changes in the appearance of the hoof commonly result from underlying endocrinopathic laminitis in the absence of pain and lameness, and that these animals are at increased risk for all types of laminitic pain;
  - Vigilance and awareness that the risk of endocrinopathic laminitis in certain animals is greater in some than others (see below).
- Institution of regular hoof care:
  - Vigilant and knowledgeable farrier–veterinarian teams can detect early-onset endocrinopathic laminitis;
  - Routine and appropriate farriery/hoof trimming should be used to optimize hoof structure and reduce the risk of laminitis.
- Routine employment of appropriate diagnostic tests for PPID and insulin dysregulation on a regular basis for horses and ponies after 12–15 years of age:
  - Annual monitoring of the plasma ACTH concentration
    - Best performed during the month of September
  - Annual monitoring of the plasma insulin concentration or use of dynamic glucose/insulin testing (e.g. the oral sugar test).
- Institution of treatment using pergolide mesylate for mature horses and ponies in which increased plasma ACTH concentration has been demonstrated, or in which PPID has been diagnosed based on other diagnostic test strategies or the development of the clinical phenotype.
- Critical assessment of body condition on a regular basis:
  - Changes in body condition may be implicative for underlying early endocrinopathy (EMS and PPID);
  - Dietary strategies intended to optimize body condition should be instituted when appropriate.
- Institution of dietary strategies intended to prevent obesity and to improve insulin sensitivity.

- Exercise for those mature horses and ponies that are at risk for endocrinopathic laminitis (both EMS and PPID):
  - Unless precluded by the presence of lameness due to pre-existing laminitis.
- Annual photographic and radiographic recording of the external and internal appearance of the hoof:
  - Early laminitis may be detected sooner during the course of PPID if better records are maintained and proactive evaluation of the relationship between P3 and the dorsal aspect of the hoof wall is undertaken (see Chapter 27).
- Diligent preventive strategies for laminitis associated with sepsis/systemic inflammation or severe lameness in one limb should be instituted in horse with PPID or EMS:
  - Reduced mobility, working with farrier to promote healthy P3/hoof angles, appropriate treatment of the primary disease, etc.;
  - Horses and ponies with PPID (and/or insulin dysregulation) are likely at increased risk for laminitis resulting from all possible causes.
- Consider dietary supplementation with antioxidants:
  - Vitamin E (5000 units, daily, given orally) and/or resveratrol (400 mg, daily, given orally) may be considered in order to mitigate laminitis risk in PPID-affected equids;
  - Evidence for efficacy is presently lacking.

Nutritional Management

Insulin dysregulation represents a very important risk factor for endocrinopathic laminitis when it is identified in PPID-affected patients. Therefore, dietary recommendations intended to improve insulin sensitivity should be considered when making treatment recommendations for horses and ponies affected with PPID [35–37]. As detailed in Chapter 36 and in recent reviews [30, 38, 39], targeted weight loss (reversal of obesity, when present) and provision of a ration with a low nonstructural carbohydrate (NSC) content (intended to minimize elevations in the plasma insulin concentration) represent the two major principles of dietary adjustment for insulin-dysregulated horses.

In brief, PPID-affected horses that are at risk for endocrinopathic laminitis should not be fed starch-rich cereal grain rations or high-NSC content forage. The NSC content of pasture grasses can provoke or aggravate endocrinopathic laminitis in insulin-dysregulated, PPID-affected equids (the resulting laminitis is referred to as pasture-associated laminitis). Therefore, unrestricted pasture grazing should be avoided, especially at certain times of the year (spring, fall, and summer following rainfall). The risk of pasture-associated laminitis is sufficiently high for some insulin-insensitive PPID-affected horses that pasture grazing should probably not be allowed whatsoever.

The ration of horses at risk of endocrinopathic laminitis (insulin-dysregulated and/or PPID) should be constituted based on a grass hay source with low (<10–12%) NSC content. Ideally, the NSC content of provided forage should be determined by forage analysis (the analysis of a hay sample can be performed by many commercial laboratories). Alternatively, proprietary rations (with guaranteed low NSC content) that have been developed specifically for insulin-dysregulated-affected equids may be fed. When practical, soaking of forage under water for 30–60 min may reduce the NSC content of some (but not all) batches of hay to some extent [40]. Soaking of forage under water for longer periods of time (12–15 h) has been shown to significantly reduce the NSC content more reliably [41].

The body condition score of PPID-affected horses and ponies may be high (obese) or low (thin). Therefore, dietary adjustment should be provided to either address the reversal of obesity or to promote weight gain. If there is a need for weight gain, a forage-based ration (intended to promote insulin sensitivity) may not completely meet the patient's energy requirements and dietary supplementation with either vegetable oil or a commercial low NSC (complete pelleted) ration may be used.

Value of Exercise

Many studies have demonstrated that exercise leads to improvements in insulin sensitivity in both human and equine patients [42–47]. Therefore, the fact that insulin dysregulation appears to be very important regarding the development of laminitis suggests that exercise may be useful in terms of reducing the risk of laminitis in PPID-affected equids. Although specific studies regarding the effect of exercise on the risk and clinical expression of laminitis in PPID-affected equids have not been reported, multiple studies have demonstrated the beneficial effects of exercise on insulin sensitivity in horses [42–47]. Of note, improved insulin sensitivity was observed in both obese and lean aged mares following only seven days of light trotting exercise (on a lunge line) in one study [43]. Therefore, the development of pain associated with laminitis may be reduced for those PPID-affected equids that can be lightly exercised on a regular basis if exercise is not medically precluded by other conditions associated with advancing age (such as pre-existing laminitis and arthritis).

Pharmacological Management of PPID

Pergolide

The drug of choice for the specific treatment of PPID is pergolide mesylate. Pergolide is a dopaminergic agonist with considerably greater affinity for D_2 rather than D_1 receptors [48]. It was manufactured for the purpose of treating Parkinson's disease in people, a disease characterized by the progressive loss of dopaminergic neurons. Because a loss of hypothalamic dopaminergic innervation appears to be the underlying mechanism for the development of PPID in equids, treatment with dopaminergic agonists was a logical approach to therapy. Experimentally, Orth and coworkers showed in 1982 that pergolide administration caused a decrease in plasma immunoreactive pro-opiomelanocortin (POMC)-derived peptides in a pony with PPID [48]. The clinical use of pergolide to treat PPID has been reported since the 1990s [49, 50].

The efficacy of manufactured (as opposed to compounded) pergolide in horses with PPID was demonstrated in an open-field clinical efficacy study of 122 equids with physical examination findings (hypertrichosis, hyperhidrosis, polyuria–polydipsia, abnormal fat distribution, and muscle wasting) and endocrine testing results (either plasma adrenocorticotrophic hormone [ACTH] concentration >50 pg ml^{-1} or failure of an overnight dexamethasone suppression test) supportive of PPID [51]. Treatment with pergolide mesylate was started at 2 μg kg^{-1} (oral, q. 24 h) and equids were re-evaluated after 90 and 180 days of treatment. When endocrine test results remained abnormal at 90 days ($n = 47$), the dose was increased to 4 μg kg^{-1} (oral, q. 24 h). Treatment success after 180 days was defined as either a normalization of dexamethasone suppression test results (<1.0 μg dl^{-1}) or a decrease in plasma ACTH concentration by 50% (or to <50 pg ml^{-1} when the initial value was <100 pg ml^{-1}) and improvement in clinical signs. In all, 76% equids were treatment successes. Both the median score of clinical signs and mean concentrations of ACTH and cortisol following dexamethasone administration were decreased during the study period.

The most common adverse event reported was transient inappetance which was observed in one-third of the cases, mostly during the initial 30 days of treatment [51]. Other adverse events were reported in less than 10% of the cases and included lethargy, colic, diarrhea, lameness, and weight loss. It was unclear whether or not these events were related to use of the drug. There were ten reports of laminitis during the study: seven were considered flare-ups of chronic laminitis, and three were apparently new cases of laminitis. The results of the open-field efficacy study showed clearly that pergolide is effective in improving clinical signs of PPID; however, not all clinical problems may be fully corrected (e.g. laminitis).

Limited information exists regarding the pharmacokinetics of pergolide in horses. In one study it was shown that, following the administration of a single oral dose (10 μg kg^{-1}) to fasted adult, healthy horses, the plasma concentrations of the drug were four- to 10-fold greater than in humans after a similar dose, suggesting a greater bioavailability in equids [52]. The study authors concluded that a daily dose of 1–2 μg kg^{-1} (0.5–1 mg to a 500-kg horse) would be expected to produce drug levels in equids similar to therapeutic plasma concentrations in humans with Parkinson's disease. In a second study investigating drug disposition in fed, aged PPID horses, a similar plasma concentration was achieved when adjusted for the lower dose (2 μg kg^{-1}) administered [53]. In this study, concurrent plasma hormone concentrations (ACTH) were observed to decrease in the pergolide-treated horses, which suggested that the achieved plasma drug concentrations were adequate to evoke a therapeutic response. Regardless of the reported bioavailability in these two studies, it is important to note that the target dopaminergic nerve terminals in PPID, the periventricular neurons, are outside the blood–brain barrier, while the target nerve terminals in Parkinson's disease are in the midbrain. Therefore, the extrapolation of drug target concentrations between the two diseases may not be justified.

Three studies have reported a mean plasma half-life of pergolide in horses; two of these suggested a 24-h half-life [52, 53], while one found a shorter half-life of only 5 h [54]. The discordant results are likely due to differences in study design, population characteristics, and drug analysis methodology. The shorter half-life reported by Rendle and colleagues led to the suggestion that more frequent dosing may be clinically advantageous. However, a recent pharmacodynamic study found that plasma ACTH concentrations remained unchanged for a minimum of two days after discontinuation of chronic oral pergolide treatment (this study was limited by a small sample size [$n = 6$] and marked inter-animal variation) [53]. Anecdotal reports suggest that some horses have an improved clinical response when pergolide is administered twice daily. Therefore, in individual clinical cases of horses with PPID that do not respond adequately to pergolide therapy, splitting the daily dose into two portions administered every 12 h may prove beneficial. In general, it is considered advisable to adjust pergolide dose and dose frequency based on response to therapy in the individual animal using clinical response and diagnostic test results (e.g., ACTH concentration) rather than adjusting dose based on predicted pharmacokinetic properties.

Adverse effects of pergolide, identified in the efficacy study and in clinical field cases, include anorexia and less commonly diarrhea and colic, with the latter problems more often associated with higher doses of the drug [16, 49, 51]. Transient anorexia is usually recognized during the initial few weeks of pergolide treatment, and can be overcome by stopping treatment for a few days and starting back at half the dose or splitting the daily dose into two treatments, then slowly increasing to the desired dose. Many clinicians elect to start all horses on low doses and increase incrementally over the first one to two weeks, rather than risk anorexia. Although pregnant mares have been treated with the drug, the safety of pergolide use during pregnancy has not been studied in equids. In people, chronic use of pergolide was associated with a cardiac valvulopathy, though this has not been reported in horses.

Currently, it is the present authors' recommendation that the initial medical treatment for equids with PPID should be pergolide at a dose of 2 μg kg^{-1}, oral, q. 24 h (1 mg per day for a 500-kg horse). If no improvement is noted within 30 days, the daily dose can be increased by 1–2 μg kg^{-1} (to 1.5–2 mg per day for a 500-kg horse) with reassessment after 30 days. The timing of clinical improvement may depend on season, as hair coat changes will vary with the time of year that treatment is initiated. If no improvement or limited improvement is observed at a total pergolide dose of 6 μg kg^{-1} (3 mg per day for a 500-kg horse), the addition of cyproheptadine (0.5 mg kg^{-1}, oral, q. 24 h) along with the pergolide may provide additional benefit beyond pergolide alone. A maximum pergolide dose has not been established, and while some clinicians report administering total doses in excess of 5 mg per day per horse [49], the present authors have limited to no direct experience with doses this high.

It is also important to recognize that the rate of clinical improvement is higher than that for the normalization of endocrine test results. For example, 13 of 20 pergolide-treated horses in one study were reported to have improved clinically, while only seven of 20 had normalization of endocrine test results [55]. It is prudent to regularly perform follow-up endocrine testing when managing equids with PPID. The present authors currently recommend measuring plasma ACTH concentrations (endogenous or TRH-stimulated) once or twice yearly in horses that appear to be stable, and 30 days after a change in medication dose or addition of cyproheptadine. Measurements of endogenous ACTH concentrations in the fall when horses are experiencing a seasonal spike in hormone release may facilitate the seasonal management of pergolide doses to avoid undue risk of laminitis or other PPID complications. Although the therapeutic goal is to return plasma ACTH concentrations to within the normal reference interval (or to normalize cortisol suppression in response to dexamethasone administration), this goal may not be achievable in all cases, particularly late-stage cases. In such animals, improvements in clinical signs and quality of life should be the therapeutic goal.

Cyproheptadine

Cyproheptadine has been suggested as a second-line drug, used in combination with pergolide when maximal tolerated doses of pergolide alone are insufficient to resolve clinical signs. When only a minimal response has been observed at a pergolide dose of 3–5 mg per day, the addition of cyproheptadine (0.3–0.5 mg kg^{-1}, oral, q. 24 h) to pergolide therapy may produce additional clinical improvements. Cyproheptadine is a serotonin antagonist with additional antihistamine, antimuscarinic, and calcium channel-blocking actions. Several small studies have shown a limited efficacy of cyproheptadine for improving clinical signs of PPID when used as a monotherapy at 0.25–0.5 mg kg^{-1}, oral, q. 24 h [56,57]; to date, no non-empirical data are available evaluating the efficacy of pergolide and cyproheptadine combination therapy. Cyproheptadine lowers the seizure threshold in mice [58]. Therefore, although direct information is not available regarding the potentiation of seizures in horses, the use of cyproheptadine in horses with a history of seizures or central neurologic disease is not advised and the drug should be discontinued in horses that develop neurologic signs while on treatment.

Nutraceuticals

Many nutraceuticals, botanicals, and natural remedies have been marketed for the treatment of PPID. A lack of efficacy and safety evidence, in conjunction with the absence of product regulation and standardization, make these remedies contraindicated for the treatment of horses with PPID. One of the more popular natural remedies is *Vitex agnus castus* extract, also known as 'chasteberry extract.' 'The latter has been shown to bind dopamine D_2 receptors and to decrease prolactin release in rodents, similar to the synthetic dopamine agonist lusuride [59]. However, in a study of 14 horses with PPID, a commercial 'chasteberry extract' failed to resolve clinical signs or to improve diagnostic test results [60]. Furthermore, the overall condition of several animals deteriorated while on the Vitex treatment, and use of the extract needed to be discontinued prior to completion of the study. In contrast, eight of nine of the same horses improved when subsequently treated with pergolide (Permax®; Eli Lilly). The results of this single small study support the use of pergolide rather than chasteberry extract in the treatment of horses with PPID.

Pharmacological Management of Insulin Dysregulation

The importance of the fact that elevated insulin represents a major risk factor for endocrinopathic laminitis cannot be overstated. In some cases, recommended management changes (adjusting the ration, enhanced exercise, and limiting or reducing access to pasture) intended to reduce potentially dangerous postprandial insulin spiking or hyperinsulinemia resulting from peripheral tissue insensitivity to insulin may be impractical or impossible to achieve to an optimal extent. Moreover, the employment of drug therapy may be critical to reduce the damaging effects of laminitis before changes to the patient's management have had sufficient time to work (typically three to six months).

Two pharmacological strategies have been introduced and may be helpful in the management of insulin dysregulation associated with either or both EMS and PPID. Mild to moderate weight loss and improvements in insulin sensitivity can be achieved using levothyroxine sodium (Thyro-L™; Lloyd, Inc., Shenandoah, Iowa, USA) at a dosage of 48 mg per day for three to six months [61]. Alternatively, metformin (1,1-dimethylbiguanide hydrochloride), one of the most widely prescribed type-2 diabetes therapeutic agents in human medicine, may be administered. Although metformin acts to improve tissue sensitivity to insulin in human diabetic patients, it has low oral bioavailability in horses and has not been demonstrated to improve insulin sensitivity in this species [62]. However, by virtue of local action in the intestinal epithelium, metformin is useful for the purpose of blunting postprandial glucose and insulin spiking in horses (see Chapter 36 for further discussion) [63]. It is currently recommended that metformin (30 mg kg^{-1}, oral, q. 8–12 h) should be administered to at-risk horses at approximately 1 h prior to feeding or turnout at pasture [64].

References

1. Donaldson, M.T., Jorgensen, A.J., and Beech, J. (2004) Evaluation of suspected pituitary pars intermedia dysfunction in horses with laminitis. *J. Am. Vet. Med. Assoc.*, **224** (7), 1123–1127.

2. Karikoski, N.P., Horn, I., McGowan, T.W., and McGowan, C.M. (2011) The prevalence of endocrinopathic laminitis among horses presented for laminitis at a first-opinion/referral equine hospital. *Domest. Anim. Endocrinol.*, **41** (3), 111–117.
3. de Laat, M.A., McGowan, C.M., Sillence, M.N., and Pollitt, C.C. (2010) Equine laminitis: induced by 48 h hyperinsulinaemia in Standardbred horses. *Equine Vet. J.*, **42** (2), 129–135.
4. Asplin, K.E., Sillence, M.N., Pollitt, C.C., and McGowan, C.M. (2007) Induction of laminitis by prolonged hyperinsulinaemia in clinically normal ponies. *Vet. J.*, **174** (3), 530–535.
5. Carter, R.A., Treiber, K.H., Geor, R.J., Douglass, L., and Harris, P.A. (2009) Prediction of incipient pasture-associated laminitis from hyperinsulinaemia, hyperleptinaemia, and generalized and localized obesity in a cohort of ponies. *Equine Vet. J.*, **41**, 171–178.
6. McFarlane, D., Dybdal, N., Donaldson, M.T., Miller, L., and Cribb, A.E. (2005) Nitration and increased alpha-synuclein expression associated with dopaminergic neurodegeneration in equine pituitary pars intermedia dysfunction. *J. Neuroendocrinol.*, **17** (2), 73–80.
7. de Bruin, C., Meij, B.P., Kooistra, H.S., Hanson, J.M., Lamberts, S.W., and Hofland, L.J. (2009) Cushing's disease in dogs and humans. *Horm. Res.*, **71** (Suppl.1), 140–143.
8. Heinrichs, M., Baumgartner, W., and Capen, C. (1990) Immunocytochemical demonstration of proopiomelanocortin-derived peptides in pituitary adenomas of the pars intermedia in horses. *Vet. Pathol.*, **27**, 419–425.
9. Boujon, C.E., Bestetti, G.E., Meier, H.P., Straub, R., Junker, U., and Rossi, G.L. (1993) Equine pituitary adenoma: a functional and morphological study. *J. Comp. Pathol.*, **109** (2), 163–178.
10. Okada, T., Shimomuro, T., Oikawa, M., Nambo, Y., Kiso, Y., Morikawa, Y., *et al.* (1997) Immunocytochemical localization of adrenocorticotropic hormone-immunoreactive cells of the pars intermedia in Thoroughbreds. *Am. J. Vet. Res.*, **58** (8), 920–924.
11. Glover, C.M., Miller, L.M., Dybdal, N.O., Lopez, A., Duckett, W.M., and McFarlane, D. (2009) Extrapituitary and pituitary pathological findings in horses with pituitary pars intermedia dysfunction: a retrospective study. *J. Equine Vet. Sci.*, **29**, 146–153.
12. Orth, D.N. and Nicholson, W.E. (1982) Bioactive and immunoreactive adrenocorticotropin in normal equine pituitary and in pituitary tumors of horses with Cushing's disease. *Endocrinology*, **111** (2), 559–563.
13. Sommer, K. (2003) Das Equine Cushing-Sydrom: Entwicklung eines ACTH-bioassays für die Ermittlung des biologisch-immunreaktiven Verkaltnisses von endogenem ACTH in equinen Blutproben (The equine Cushing syndrome: development of an ACTH- bioassay for determination of the biological-immunoreactive-ratio of endogenous ACTH in equine blood samples). Dissertation, Stiftung Tierarztliche Hochschule Hannover, School of Veterinary Medicine, Hannover, Germany.
14. Cordero, M., Shrauner, B., and McFarlane, D. (2011) Bioactivity of plasma ACTH from horses with PPID compared to normal horses (abstract). *J. Vet. Intern. Med.*, **25**, 664.
15. Beech, J., Boston, R., and Lindborg, S. (2011) Comparison of cortisol and ACTH responses after administration of thyrotropin-releasing hormone in normal horses and those with pituitary pars intermedia dysfunction. *J. Vet. Intern. Med.*, **25** (6), 1431–1438.
16. Schott, H.C., II. (2002) Pituitary pars intermedia dysfunction: equine Cushing's disease. *Vet. Clin. North Am. Equine Pract.*, **18** (2), 237–270.
17. McFarlane, D. (2011) Equine pituitary pars intermedia dysfunction. *Vet. Clin. North Am. Equine Pract.*, **27** (1), 93–113.
18. McFarlane, D. (2014) Pathophysiology and clinical features of pituitary pars intermedia dysfunction. *Equine Vet. Educ.*, **26**, 592–598.
19. McGowan, T.W., Pinchbeck, G.P., and McGowan, C.M. (2013) Prevalence, risk factors and clinical signs predictive for equine pituitary pars intermedia dysfunction in aged horses. *Equine Vet. J.*, **45** (1), 74–79.
20. de Laat, M.A., Sillence, M.N., McGowan, C.M., and Pollitt, C.C. (2012) Continuous intravenous infusion of glucose induces endogenous hyperinsulinaemia and lamellar histopathology in Standardbred horses. *Vet. J.*, **191** (3), 317–322.
21. de Laat, M.A., Pollitt, C.C., Kyaw-Tanner, M.T., McGowan, C.M., and Sillence, M.N. (2013) A potential role for lamellar insulin-like growth factor-1 receptor in the pathogenesis of hyperinsulinaemic laminitis. *Vet. J.*, **197** (2), 302–306.
22. Gauff, F., Patan-Zugaj, B., and Licka, T.F. (2013) Hyperinsulinaemia increases vascular resistance and endothelin-1 expression in the equine digit. *Equine Vet. J.*, **45** (5), 613–618.
23. Vick, M.M., Adams, A.A., Murphy, B.A., Sessions, D.R., Horohov, D.W., Cook, R.F., *et al.* (2007) Relationships among inflammatory cytokines, obesity, and insulin sensitivity in the horse. *J. Anim. Sci.*, **85** (5), 1144–1155.
24. McFarlane, D. and Holbrook, T.C. (2008) Cytokine dysregulation in aged horses and horses with pituitary pars intermedia dysfunction. *J. Vet. Intern. Med.*, **22** (2), 436–442.
25. Alford, P., Gellar, S., Richardson, B., Slater, M., Honnas, C., Foreman, J., *et al.* (2001) A multicenter, matched case-control study of risk factors for equine laminitis. *Prev. Vet. Med.*, **49**, 209–222.
26. Polzer, J. and Slater, M.R. (1996) Age, breed, gender and seasonality as risk factors for equine laminitis. *Prev. Vet. Med.*, **29**, 179–184.
27. Messer, N.T., IV and Johnson, P.J. (2007) Evidence-based literature pertaining to thyroid dysfunction and Cushing's syndrome in the horse. *Vet. Clin. North Am. Equine Pract.*, **23** (2), 329–364.
28. McGowan, C.M., Geor, R.J., and McGowan, T.W. (2008) Prevalence and risk factors for hyperinsulinemia in ponies (abstract). *J. Vet. Intern. Med.*, **22**, 734.
29. Parsons, C.S., Orsini, J.A., Krafty, R., Capewell, L., and Boston, R. (2007) Risk factors for development of acute laminitis in horses during hospitalization. *J. Am. Vet. Med. Assoc.*, **230**, 885–889.
30. Frank, N. (2011) Equine metabolic syndrome. *Vet. Clin. North Am. Equine Pract.*, **27** (1), 73–92.
31. Frank, N., Geor, R.J., Bailey, S.R., Durham, A.E., and Johnson, P.J. (2010) Equine metabolic syndrome. *J. Vet. Intern. Med.*, **24** (3), 467–475.
32. Beech, J., Boston, R., Lindborg, S., and Russell, G.E. (2007) Adrenocorticotropin concentration following administration of thyrotropin-releasing hormone in healthy horses and those with pituitary pars intermedia dysfunction and pituitary gland hyperplasia. *J. Am. Vet. Med. Assoc.*, **231** (3), 417–426.
33. Copas, V.E. and Durham, A.E. (2012) Circannual variation in plasma adrenocorticotropic hormone concentrations in the UK in normal horses and ponies, and those with pituitary pars intermedia dysfunction. *Equine Vet. J.*, **44** (4), 440–443.
34. Durham, A.E., McGowan, C.M., Fey, K., Tamzali, Y., and van der Kolk, J.H.I. (2014) Pituitary pars intermedia dysfunction: Diagnosis and treatment. *Equine Vet. Educ.*, **26**, 216–223.

35. Treiber, K., Carter, R., Gay, L., Williams, C., and Geor, R. (2009) Inflammatory and redox status of ponies with a history of pasture-associated laminitis. *Vet. Immunol. Immunopathol.*, **129**, 216–220.
36. Pratt, S.E., Geor, R.J., and McCutcheon, L.J. (2006) Effects of dietary energy source and physical conditioning on insulin sensitivity and glucose tolerance in standardbred horses. *Equine Vet. J. Suppl.*, **36**, 579–584.
37. Vervuert, I., Voigt, K., Hollands, T., Cuddeford, D., and Coenen, M. (2009) Effect of feeding increasing quantities of starch on glycaemic and insulinaemic responses in healthy horses. *Vet. J.*, **182** (1), 67–72.
38. Geor, R.J. (2010) Current concepts on the pathophysiology of pasture-associated laminitis. *Vet. Clin. North Am. Equine Pract.*, **26** (2), 265–276.
39. McGowan, C.M., Dugdale, A.H., Pinchbeck, G.L., and Argo, C.M. (2013) Dietary restriction in combination with a nutraceutical supplement for the management of equine metabolic syndrome in horses. *Vet. J.*, **196**, 153–159.
40. Longland, A.C., Barfoot, C., and Harris, P.A. (2009) The loss of water-soluble carbohydrate and soluble protein from nine different hays soaked in water for up to 16 hours. *J. Equine Vet. Sci.*, **29** (5), 383–384.
41. Mack, S.J., Dugdale, A.H., Argo, C.M., Morgan, R.A., and McGowan, C.M. (2014) Impact of water-soaking on the nutrient composition of UK hays. *Vet. Rec.*, **174** (18), 452–454.
42. Gordon, M.E., McKeever, K.H., Betros, C.L., and Manso Filho, H.C. (2007) Exercise-induced alterations in plasma concentrations of ghrelin, adiponectin, leptin, glucose, insulin, and cortisol in horses. *Vet. J.*, **173** (3), 532–540.
43. Powell, D.M., Reedy, S.E., Sessions, D.R., and Fitzgerald, B.P. (2002) Effect of short-term exercise training on insulin sensitivity in obese and lean mares. *Equine Vet. J. Suppl.*, **34**, 81–84.
44. Stewart-Hunt, L., Geor, R.J., and McCutcheon, L.J. (2006) Effects of short-term training on insulin sensitivity and skeletal muscle glucose metabolism in standardbred horses. *Equine Vet. J. Suppl.*, **36**, 226–232.
45. Treiber, K.H., Hess, T.M., Kronfeld, D.S., Boston, R.C., Geor, R.J., Friere, M., *et al.* (2006) Glucose dynamics during exercise: dietary energy sources affect minimal model parameters in trained Arabian geldings during endurance exercise. *Equine Vet. J. Suppl.*, **36**, 631–636.
46. Freestone, J.F., Beadle, R., Shoemaker, K., Bessin, R.T., Wolfsheimer, K.J., and Church, C. (1992) Improved insulin sensitivity in hyperinsulinaemic ponies through physical conditioning and controlled feed intake. *Equine Vet. J.*, **24** (3), 187–190.
47. de Graaf-Roelfsema, E., van Ginneken, M.E., van Breda, E., Wijnberg, I.D., Keizer, H.A., and van der Kolk, J.H. (2006) The effect of long-term exercise on glucose metabolism and peripheral insulin sensitivity in standardbred horses. *Equine Vet. J. Suppl.*, **36**, 221–225.
48. Orth, D.N., Holscher, M.A., Wilson, M.G., Nicholson, W.E., Plue, R.E., Mount, C.D. (1982) Equine Cushing's disease: plasma immunoreactive proopiolipomelanocortin peptide and cortisol levels basally and in response to diagnostic tests. *Endocrinology*, **110** (4), 1430–1441.
49. Beech, J. (1994) Treatment of hypophysial adenomas. *Compend. Contin. Educ. Pract. Vet.*, **16**, 921–923.
50. Peters, D.F., Erfle, J.B., and Slobojan, G.T. (2011) Low-dose pergolide mesylate treatment for equine hypophyseal adenomas (Cushing's syndrome). Proceedings of the 41st Annual Convention of the American Association of Equine Practitioners, pp. 154–155.
51. FDA Freedom of Information Summary Prascend (2011) Available at: http://www.fda.gov/downloads/Animal Veterinary/Products/ApprovedAnimal DrugProducts/FOIADrugSummaries/UCM280354.pdf.
52. Gehring, R., Beard, L., Wright, A., Coetzee, J., Havel, J., and Apley, M.I. (2010) Single-dose oral pharmacokinetics of pergolide mesylate in healthy adult mares. *Vet. Ther.*, **11** (1), E1–E8.
53. McFarlane, D., Banse, H.E., Yang, F., and Maxwell, L.K. (2014) Pharmacokinetics and pharmacodynamics of pergolide mesylate after chronic oral administration in horses with PPID (abstract). *J. Vet. Intern. Med.*, **28**, 1104.
54. Rendle, D., Hughes, K.J., Doran, G.S., and Edwards, S.H. (2015) Pharmacokinetics of pergolide after intravenous administration. *Am. J. Vet. Res.*, **76**, 155–160.
55. Schott, H.C., Coursen, C.L., Eberhart, S.W., Nachreiner, R.J., Refsal, K.R., Ewart, S.L., *et al.* (2001) The Michigan Cushing's Project. Proceedings of the 47th Annual Convention of the American Association of Equine Practitioners, pp. 22–24.
56. Perkins, G.A., Lamb, S., Erb, H.N., Schanbacher, B., Nydam, D.V., and Divers, T.J. (2002) Plasma adrenocorticotropin (ACTH) concentrations and clinical response in horses treated for equine Cushing's disease with cyproheptadine or pergolide. *Equine Vet. J.*, **34**, 679.
57. Donaldson, M.T., LaMonte, B.H., Morresey, P., Smith, G., and Beech, J. (2002) Treatment with pergolide or cyproheptadine of pituitary pars intermedia dysfunction (Equine Cushing's Disease). *J. Vet. Intern. Med.*, **16**, 742–746.
58. Singh, D. and Goel, R.K. (2010) Proconvulsant potential of cyproheptadine in experimental animal models. *Fundam. Clin. Pharmacol.*, **24**, 451–455.
59. Sliutz, G., Speiser, P., Schultz, A.M., Spona, J., and Zeillinger, R. (1993) Agnus castus extracts inhibit prolactin secretion of rat pituitary cells. *Horm. Metab. Res.*, **25** (5), 253–255.
60. Beech, J. (2002) Comparison of *Vitex agnus castus* extract and pergolide in treatment of equine Cushing's syndrome. Proceedings of the 48th Annual Convention of American Association of Equine Practitioners, pp. 175–177.
61. Frank, N., Sommardahl, C.S., Eiler, H., Webb, L.L., Denhart, J.W., and Boston, R.C. (2005) Effects of oral administration of levothyroxine sodium on concentrations of plasma lipids, concentration and composition of very-low-density lipoproteins, and glucose dynamics in healthy adult mares. *Am. J. Vet. Res.*, **66** (6), 1032–1038.
62. Hustace, J.L., Firshman, A.M., and Mata, J.E. (2009) Pharmacokinetics and bioavailability of metformin in horses. *Am. J. Vet. Res.*, **70**, 665–668.
63. Rendle, D.I., Rutledge, F., Hughes, K.J., Heller, J., and Durham, A.E. (2013) Effects of metformin hydrochloride on blood glucose and insulin responses to oral dextrose in horses. Equine Vet. *J.*, **45** (6), 751–754.
64. Frank, N. and Tadros, E.M. (2014) Insulin dysregulation. Equine Vet. *J.*, **46** (1), 103–112.

PART 6

Treatment of Laminitis: Digital Support and Stabilization of the Distal Phalanx

Equine Laminitis, First Edition. Edited by James K. Belknap and Raymond Geor.

CHAPTER 38

Therapeutic Shoes: Application of Principles

Stephen E. O'Grady

Introduction

Many of the therapeutic shoes used to treat laminitis are steeped in tradition and empirically based on the past experience of the attending clinician/farrier. Unfortunately, there are no controlled studies to verify the effectiveness of these shoeing techniques from either profession. The application of therapeutic farriery requires each case of laminitis to be approached on an individual basis, noting the clinical signs, the amount of pain, movement, foot conformation, and the structures of the foot that can be used to change the forces placed on or within the hoof capsule. These observations, coupled with high-quality radiographs and a thorough examination of the foot, will then suggest overall goals of treatment and address the anatomical and functional abnormalities identified [1, 2]. The approach to farriery should be based on biomechanical principles aimed at restoring the form and function in a given laminitic foot rather than using any one method of farriery, product, or shoe [1]. As the present author does not recommend shoes in the acute stage of laminitis, this chapter will focus on chronic laminitis defined by the presence of mechanical collapse of the lamellae and displacement of the distal phalanx (DP) within the hoof capsule [1, 3, 4].

Therapeutic Shoes

In order to discuss therapeutic shoes, it becomes necessary to present an overview assessment of the term *therapeutic farriery*. The latter could be described as 'the art and science of affecting/influencing the structures of the foot.' This certainly bears relevance when considering farriery for the laminitic horse, but it must be remembered that trimming is the mainstay of therapeutic farriery [1–5]. Furthermore, trimming will be dependent on the structures present, the integrity of those structures, and the mass or density of the foot present. Various shoes are then applied to protect what has been trimmed, to compliment what has been trimmed, and to change the basic biomechanical forces on the foot. Therapeutic shoeing techniques can be used to increase the ground surface of the foot, unload areas of the foot, effect or reposition breakover, provide heel elevation, and perhaps decrease concussion to some degree [4–8]. Biomechanically, these techniques can: (i) change the dorsopalmar or mediolateral orientation of the foot thus changing forces by moving the center of pressure (COP; see Chapter 5); (ii) change the forces (e.g., associated with breakover); and (iii) decrease the stresses associated with the deep digital flexor tendon by adding heel elevation when necessary (see Fig. 41.1). Lastly, there are materials such as the various deformable impression materials and urethane products that not only increase the surface area on the solear surface of the foot but also decrease the concussive forces placed on the foot during motion (as discussed in Chapter 39). There are a myriad of shoes used to treat laminitis, such as the rail shoe, the egg bar shoe, the heart bar shoe, the reverse shoe and, more recently, the wooden shoe. However, none of these shoes will be consistently successful in treating the laminitic case unless the conformation of the foot, the trim, and the biomechanical forces placed on the foot are understood and considered. As can be noted from above, the principles for the appropriate trim and the application of a shoe are interdependent, cannot be separated, and therefore must be considered together. The principles that will be used in this text are: (i) to reduce the load on the most severely affected wall/lamellae and transfer load to a less compromised section of the foot; (ii) to recruit all available ground surface of the foot to bear weight; and (iii) to decrease the moment about the distal interphalangeal joint as necessary (see Chapter 5). Simplistically stated in farrier terms, the aim is to reposition the load on the ground surface of the foot, position breakover appropriately, and provide heel elevation if necessary.

Radiology

Farriery for the laminitic horse will always be contingent on good-quality radiographs consisting of both a lateral and dorsopalmar (0 degree horizontal) view (described in detail in Chapter 27) [1–5]. As important as the quality of the radiographs is the correct positioning of the horse's foot when taking the radiographs. The feet should be placed on two wooden blocks of equal height that are compatible with the orientation of the

Equine Laminitis, First Edition. Edited by James K. Belknap and Raymond Geor.

primary beam of the radiograph generator directed on the foot. The position of the limb (MC3) should be perpendicular with the ground when taking both the lateral and dorsopalmar views. The lateral radiograph has always been considered the 'gold standard' for evaluating laminitis, but it limits the evaluation of the distal phalanx (DP) to one plane. It does not allow identification of asymmetrical medial or lateral distal displacement of the DP. Therefore, the present author considers it crucial that a dorsopalmar (zero-degree-horizontal) radiographic projection be included as part of the radiographic study for chronic laminitis. If necessary, a dorsopalmar oblique view may also be included to evaluate the solear margin and integrity of the DP.

The radiographic features of chronic laminitis are well documented elsewhere in this book (see Chapter 27), but the following observations from the lateral radiograph are important in guiding therapeutic farriery:

- The degree of dorsal capsular rotation.
- The angle of the solear surface of the DP relative to the ground.
- The distance between the dorsal, distal margin of the DP and the ground (sole thickness).
- The position of the distal interphalangeal joint.

Furthermore, the center of rotation can be ascertained from the radiograph along with the areas of the hoof such as the heel that can be trimmed in an attempt toward biomechanical congruency. As the center of rotation is located a few millimeters palmar to the widest part of the foot, the widest part of the foot can be used as a consistent guideline when using the center of rotation to guide therapeutic trimming and shoeing.

The dorsopalmar radiograph (as discussed in Chapter 27) is examined to determine the horizontal position of the DP in the frontal plane. Asymmetrical distal displacement of the DP on either the lateral or medial side is present if: (i) an imaginary line is drawn across the articular surface of the distal interphalangeal joint or between the foramens of the semilunar canal of the DP is not parallel to the ground; (ii) the joint space is widened on the affected side and narrowed on the opposite side; and (iii) the width of the hoof wall always appears thicker than normal on the affected side (see Chapter 27). If the position of the coronary band is visible on the radiograph, then the distance between the coronary band and the palmar processes of the DP will be greater on the affected than the unaffected side. The location of lucent areas or gas pockets is determined by correlating the findings of the lateral and dorsopalmar radiographs.

Therapeutic Farriery

The Trim: Rotation

The trim is the underlying basis for treatment of all horses with chronic rotation of the DP. Rotation of the DP can be divided into dorsal capsular rotation and phalangeal rotation [1, 6]. In dorsal capsular rotation, the DP diverges distally away from the hoof capsule, while the alignment of the DP remains in a straight line with the second phalanx (i.e., there is no flexion of the distal interphalangeal joint). In contrast, with phalangeal rotation, the DP diverges away from the hoof capsule but, in this displacement, there is flexion present in the distal interphalangeal joint signifying a shortening of the deep digital flexor muscle tendon unit. Phalangeal rotation will generally require heel elevation as part of the recommended farriery. The immediate objective of the trim is to re-align the ground surface of the hoof capsule with the solear surface of the DP. To do this accurately and consistently requires radiographic guidance and the ability to apply the information gained from the images to the foot. The long-term objective of trimming is to restore the best anatomical relationship between the DP and the hoof capsule. Before initiating the trim, the horse should be observed walking in a straight line and on turns. The degree of lameness, especially on turns, and the landing pattern of each foot should be assessed and noted.

To place the trim in a practical perspective, the frog is trimmed to the point where it is solid and pliable. A line is now drawn across the widest part of the foot with a felt-tipped marker (Fig. 38.1a). This line gives a referable guideline as it remains fairly constant and is consistent with the center of rotation (COR); the COR will be a few millimeters palmar or plantar to this line. As discussed above, this line is the point where information from the radiograph can be transferred to the foot. From this line, the heels are trimmed lower or moved

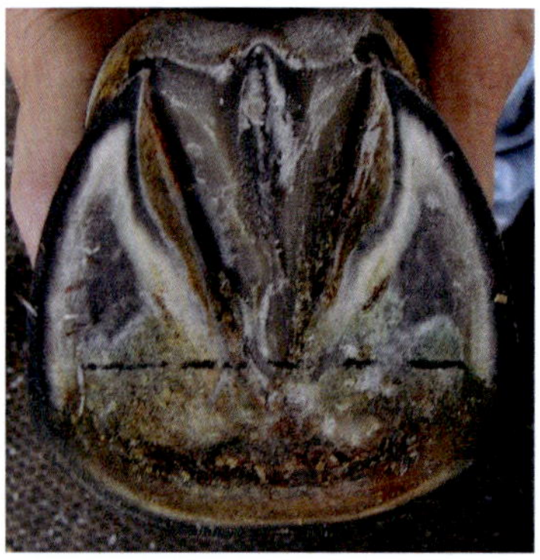

(a)

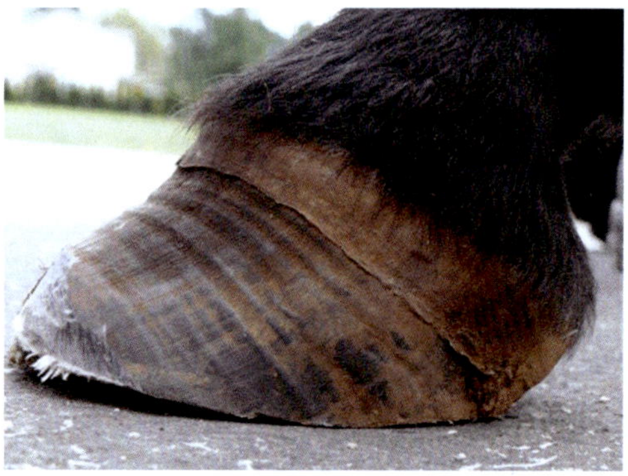

(b)

Figure 38.1 (a) Note the use of a line drawn across the widest part of the foot, indicative of the center of rotation COR) of the foot. This line is used as a reference guideline for shoeing and trimming. (b) Note the two planes created on the solear surface by trimming the solear surface caudal to the COR line.

palmarly/plantarly according to the depth of the sole noted on the radiograph. It is desirable to complete the trim with the heels of the hoof capsule and the frog on the same plane if possible. This method of trimming will produce two planes on the solear surface of the foot (Fig. 38.1b), thus shifting the load palmarly and unloading the toe. There should be no trimming performed dorsal to the line drawn across the widest part of the foot. The toe length (the distance the toe of the hoof capsule has diverged from the parietal surface of the distal phalanx) is reduced by trimming the outer surface of the dorsal hoof wall according to the radiograph. The amount of toe length to be removed can further be determined by assessing the distance dorsal to the line across the widest part of the foot to the perimeter of the hoof capsule at the toe. This distance dorsal to the widest part of the foot should approximate the distance from the line (at the widest part of the foot) palmarly/plantarly to the widest part of the frog. Breakover will be created in the shoe and the position of breakover will be determined with the placement of the shoe.

The Trim: Symmetrical and Asymmetrical Distal Displacement

The trim for symmetrical distal displacement, referred to as 'sinking,' will depend on the individual hoof conformation [2]. Here, the circumferential damage to the lamellae combined with the weight of the horse causes the DP to descend symmetrically within the hoof capsule rather than rotate. The deep digital flexor tendon (DDFT) appears to have minimal influence on this process. The heels are trimmed if necessary to create as much ground surface as possible in the palmar/plantar section of the foot, and the toe is shortened from the outer dorsal hoof wall to decrease the moment (Moment or vector = force × length; see Chapter 5) on the distal interphalangeal joint created at breakover. Following the trim, the farriery will focus on recruiting all available structures of the foot to share load in an attempt to decrease the load on the lamellae.

When trimming a foot with asymmetrical distal displacement, there is always a tendency to excessively trim the unaffected side of the foot opposite the displacement in an attempt to counter the displacement and 'balance the foot,' but this practice should be discouraged. Here, the frog is trimmed to remove any exfoliating horn, and the heels of the hoof capsule are trimmed such that the frog and the entire hoof wall are on the same plane. The toe is reduced as previously described. A shoe or device will be used to move the center of pressure (COP) towards the contralateral (unaffected) side of the foot, thus unloading the lamellae on the affected side of the foot [1, 10].

Shoes

It is readily apparent that no single method, prescription, shoe type or device is effective in treating all horses with all types of displacement due to a number of variables such as: the severity of the initial insult; the severity and type of displacement of the DP; the difference in individual foot conformation; the stage in the disease process; the variability in progression of different animals following treatment; and the types of previous treatments used in animals [2, 4]. However, there are guidelines that have proved useful and can be adapted to the needs of the individual horse.

General Principles for Farriery

There are many considerations involved in shoe selection and the shoeing technique: (i) where and how to position the shoe on the trimmed foot; (ii) where to position the point of breakover; (iii) whether to provide support for the ground surface of the frog and sole, and, if so, which type of material and how; and (iv) whether to elevate the heels. A brief discussion of these considerations, as they apply to the practical treatment of chronic laminitis, may be helpful.

The initial placement or position of the shoe on the foot allows the remainder of the biomechanical principles to be applied accurately. The present author considers the COR (discussed above), not only when trimming the foot but when fitting and placing the shoe. The shoe is fitted and placed on the foot with the line or widest part of the foot located in the middle of the shoe. The distance from this line to the perimeter of the toe and to the end of the heel of the shoe will generally be in approximate proportions [1, 2]. The objective of moving the point of breakover palmarly/plantarly, compared to normal shoeing practices, is to improve the ease of movement (i.e., rollover) at the toe by decreasing the stresses within the dorsal lamellae. Thinking biomechanically, it will effectively decrease the moment exerted on the distal interphalangeal joint (DIPJ) (described in Chapter 5). There is some debate as to what the optimal position for the point of breakover should really be in horses with displacement of the DP. Generally, a good guideline, as described in Chapter 41 in more detail (see Fig. 41.6), is to draw a line on the radiograph from the distal, dorsal margin of the DP perpendicular to the line drawn approximately 15 mm distal and parallel to the DP which indicates the desired plane of the trim (Fig. 38.2a). The point of breakover is then positioned approximately 6–9 mm dorsal to the junction of the two lines. Another practical method to establish the point of breakover is to place the trimmed foot on the ground and place a rasp or some type of straight edge vertically against the foot from just dorsal to the dorsal aspect of the coronet to the ground (Fig. 38.2b). Mark the spot on the outside of the hoof capsule where the rasp bisects the foot at the ground surface. This mark can be transferred to the shoe and will consistently place the point of breakover just dorsal to the margin of the dorsodistal aspect of the DP (Fig. 38.2b). Some clinicians will attempt to position the point of breakover palmar to the dorsal margin of the DP, but this can significantly decrease the surface area of the ground surface of the foot available to accept weight and render the foot unstable for weight-bearing. Additionally, positioning of the dorsal margin of the shoe warrants attention. The position of the dorsal margin of the shoe should be placed at the toe in relationship to

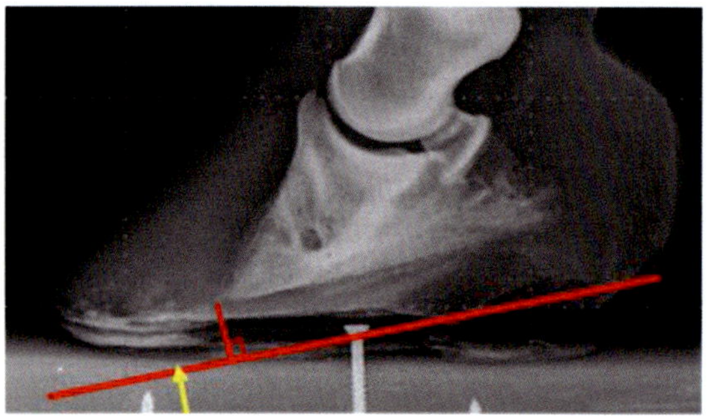
(a)

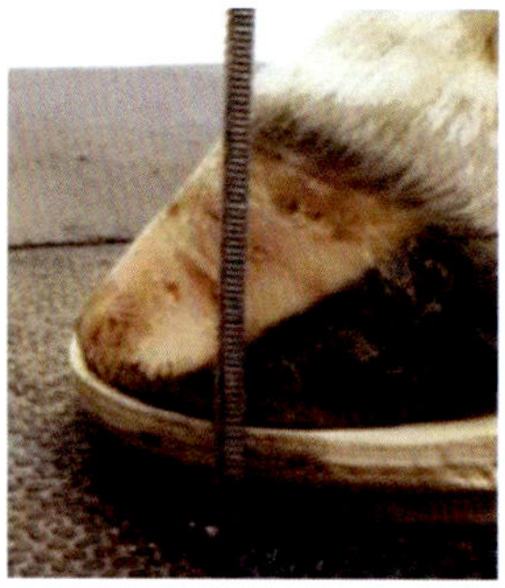
(b)

Figure 38.2 Determination of the point of breakover. Note the use of two lines drawn on the radiograph (a) (line placement discussed in text and in Chapter 41), with the point of breakover being 6–9 mm dorsal (a, arrow) to the junction of these two lines. (b) Alternatively, a rasp is placed even with the dorsal aspect of the coronet to indicate placement of breakover on the solear surface.

the widest part of the foot which will generally be the same distance as that from the widest part of the foot to the heels of the shoe (Fig. 38.1a), the position of the point of breakover can be created in the shoe and moved palmarly as necessary by rolling the toe of the shoe either by forging or with a grinder. Appropriate breakover created in the shoe should be characterized by a marked taper from the point of breakover to the outer margin of the shoe (Fig. 38.3).

The goal of supporting the sole, bars, and frog is to reduce weight-bearing by the dorsal hoof wall and thereby reduce the stress on the lamellae [1, 2, 5]. Adding support to this area increases the weight-bearing surface area of the solear surface of the foot, effectively utilizing a greater percentage of structures such as the sole, bars, and frog for 'load-sharing.' Moreover, this concept is utilized to redistribute the weight-bearing function on the bottom of the foot, placing less load on those structures that are compromised. The ground surface of the sole, bars, and frog can be supported – either fully or partially – by various bar shoes,

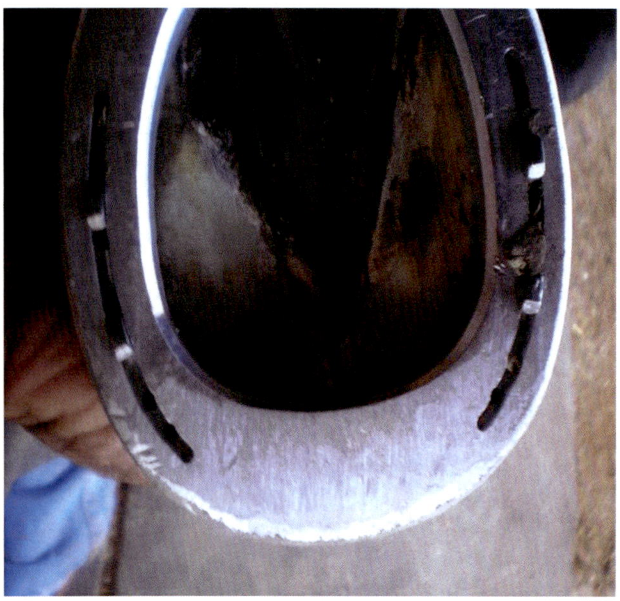

Figure 38.3 Note the breakover in the shoe created by tapering the shoe from the ground surface to the outer margin of the shoe.

pads, or some type of deformable synthetic silastic material (see Chapter 39). The bar segment of the various bar shoes only support small sections/structures on the ground surface of the foot, and pads – if placed between the shoe and ground surface of the foot – provide protection but do not usually extend into any concave space between the branches of the shoe (nor do they conform to the structures on the solear surface of the foot). Synthetic polymers, such as impression material or polyurethane products (see Chapter 39), conform to the ground surface of the foot and fill the space between the branches of the shoe, and therefore provide the greatest amount of support to the ground surface of the foot under the sole, bars, and frog. However, if the integrity of the structures being loaded (for example thin soles or collapsed heels) is inadequate, or if discomfort is noted when hoof testers are applied to these structures, the use of polymers will not be effective and may be detrimental. A compromise here is to use a leather or plastic pad and selectively place impression material under the pad over an area which will employ those structures capable of accepting load.

In addition to sole support, another technique used to decrease lamellar stress is *heel elevation*. The objective of elevating the heels is to decrease the tension in the deep digital flexor tendon, which decreases the moment about the distal interphalangeal joint with the intention of decreasing the stresses within the dorsal lamellae. There are various ways to determine the necessity for heel elevation, including: (i) increased lameness following the trim that was not present prior to the trim; (ii) a 'toe-first' landing following the trim; and (iii) by placing the trimmed foot 6–10 inches (15–25 cm) palmar to the other foot. If the horse cannot place the heel on the ground and a space is created between the ground and the caudal hoof capsule with the foot in this position, increased tension in (or a shortening of) the musculotendinous unit of the DDFT is likely present and heel elevation will be necessary. Heel elevation is usually appropriate phalangeal rotation (i.e., flexural deformity of the DIPJ) that are landing toe-first when walking in a straight line. In the present author's opinion, the amount of heel elevation required generally varies between 2° and 4°. Heel elevation may be obtained with wedged shoes, wedge pads, wedge inserts, or by attaching rails to the shoe (described below). The efficacy of heel elevation is best judged by the comfort of the horse – whether at rest, walking, or making turns – after heel elevation is applied. Ideally, the heel elevation applied is such that the horse lightly lands heel first. If a horse lands markedly heel first, there is too much heel elevation, while if it lands toe first there is not enough heel elevation. This assumes that other causes of pain have been precluded, particularly dorsal sole pressure. Unfortunately, prolonged heel elevation can cause heel contracture, which potentially causes the heels themselves to become painful. *Therefore, use the least heel elevation necessary and remove it as rapidly as possible compatible with the improvement in lameness.*

A clinician may have a good idea of what measures will be effective based on history, physical examination, foot conformation, and the severity of displacement noted on radiographs. For horses with dorsal capsular or phalangeal rotation: (i) moving the point of breakover palmarly will benefit all horses; (ii) increasing the ground surface with sole, bars, and frog support (e.g., with a silastic putty) will be based on the severity of the gait, the thickness of the sole, and the response of the horse to hoof tester application over the sole; and (iii) elevating the heels may benefit the horse, with the degree of elevation based on the severity of the lameness, and whether the foot lands heel first, flat, or toe first.

Types of Shoes

Similar results may be obtained with several, if not many, different types of shoes. Success with any given technique increases with the experience of both the veterinarian and the farrier continually applying that particular method. Shoes such as egg-bar shoes, heart-bar shoes, reverse shoes, aluminum shoes (with or without rails), and the wooden shoe all have merit, and all have had their successes and failures. However, any of these shoes has to be coupled with the appropriate trim and the fundamental guidelines for application with special attention paid to size, fitting and placement. The present author has been most successful using a wide web aluminum shoe or a wooden shoe.

Wide Web Aluminum Shoe

The guidelines described here for fitting and placing the wide web aluminum shoe (Fig. 38.4) can be used to apply any of the shoes described below for shoeing a horse with chronic laminitis. A wide web aluminum shoe forms an inexpensive, simple, and basic therapeutic shoe which can be modified to obtain the desired biomechanical effects. Any one of the various brands of aluminum shoes that are manufactured can be used. The aluminum shoe is lightweight but the web is wide and sturdy, the shape can be easily altered, and it can be glued onto the foot with a composite (an acrylic or urethane substance with adhesive properties) if desired. The toe of the shoe is changed into a blunt shape and it is fitted to the appropriately trimmed foot, again using the radiograph as a template. As described above, the line drawn across the widest part of the foot can act as a guideline for placing the shoe. The thickness of the web of the shoe is tapered using a grinder to move the point of breakover in a palmar/plantar direction. The ground surface of the branches of the shoe at the quarters can also be beveled with a grinder to provide enhanced mediolateral breakover. The heels of the shoe should not extend excessively beyond the heels of the hoof capsule, as excessive length will result in unnecessary leverage. Heel elevation can be added by the use of rails (Fig. 38.5a) or by inserting a bar wedge (Fig. 38.5b and c) or a full wedge pad, using varying degrees of wedging between the shoe and the foot. Rails are narrow, wedge-shaped distal extensions that are applied to the axial side of the ground surface of the shoe. As such, they elevate the heels and ease medial and lateral breakover. The rails can be made in different heights and can be attached to the ground surface of the shoe with screws, by welding, or by gluing the rails to the shoe with a composite. Sole, bar, and frog support is achieved by applying impression material between the branches of the shoe. It has been the present author's observation that the rails sink into a deformable surface and do not exert the same biomechanical effect as when other methods of heel elevation are incorporated with or within the shoe itself. Hence, the flat, wide web aluminum shoe can be used to provide improved breakover, heel elevation, and increased ground surface area.

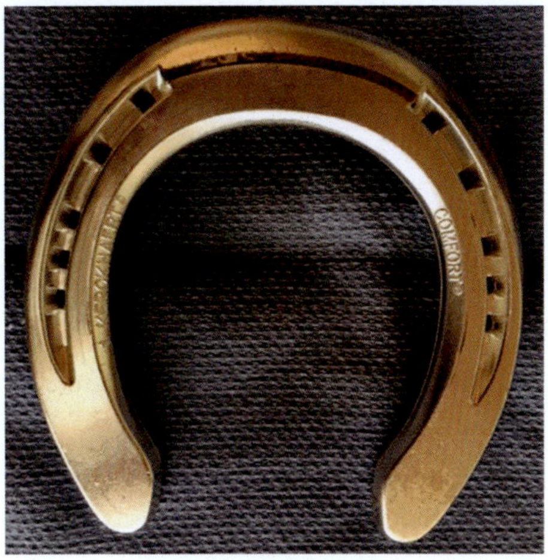

Figure 38.4 Example of a wide-webbed aluminum shoe used by the present author as a basic shoe which can be adjusted to apply wanted biomechanical principles for therapeutic shoeing of the laminitis case.

Bar Shoes

The *egg-bar shoe* (Fig. 38.6) is a closed-heel shoe shaped in the form of an egg, as the name implies, with the bar extending in a palmar direction. This palmar extension may increase the ground surface of the foot, mildly decreasing tension in the DDFT, but may also function as an unwanted lever placing excess pressure on the heel structures of the hoof capsule. However, if the horse is kept on deep soft bedding, the egg bar section of the shoe creates a flotation of the heel (rather like a snowshoe on snow) which causes the heels to remain higher on the substrate than the toe, and thus functions as a heel wedge in soft substrate. The toe of the shoe may be squared or rolled to position the point of breakover appropriately. In horses with

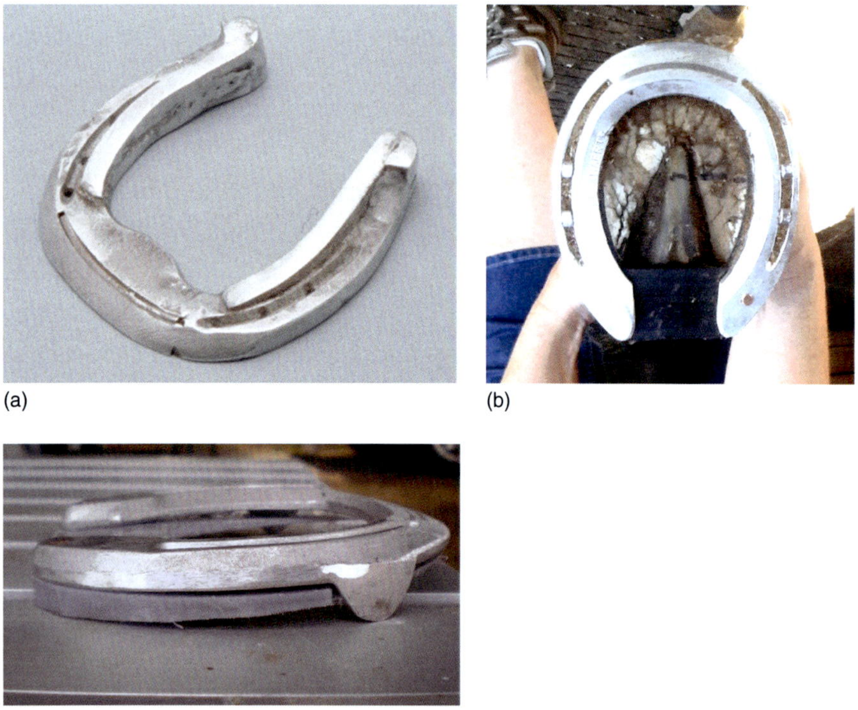

(a) (b) (c)

Figure 38.5 Note the attachment of rails (a) or a bar wedge (b,c) to the aluminum shoe to provide heel elevation.

chronic laminitis, egg-bar shoes can be used in conjunction with a synthetic polymer to increase the ground surface area of the foot, depending on the degree of stability of the DP and the amount of sole thickness present (Fig. 38.6). Additional heel elevation may be obtained by using a wedge pad/insert or a manufactured egg-bar shoe incorporating a heel wedge (e.g., a 3° egg-bar shoe). Caution must be applied in the horse with ongoing lamellar instability; if the manufactured egg-bar shoe is used without some form of silastic material placed between the branches of the shoe, the weight of the horse may cause the unsupported structures on the solear surface of the foot to descend distally between the heightened branches of the shoe and place excessive load on the hoof wall.

The *heart-bar shoe* (Fig. 38.7a) should be fitted and positioned on the foot in relation to the solear margin of the DP, as previously described. Its toe can be squared or rolled to position the point of breakover appropriately. It is often cited that the point of the frog plate should extend to a point 9 mm palmar to the trimmed apex of the frog; however, it may be more realistic to create the frog plate as a mirror image of the trimmed

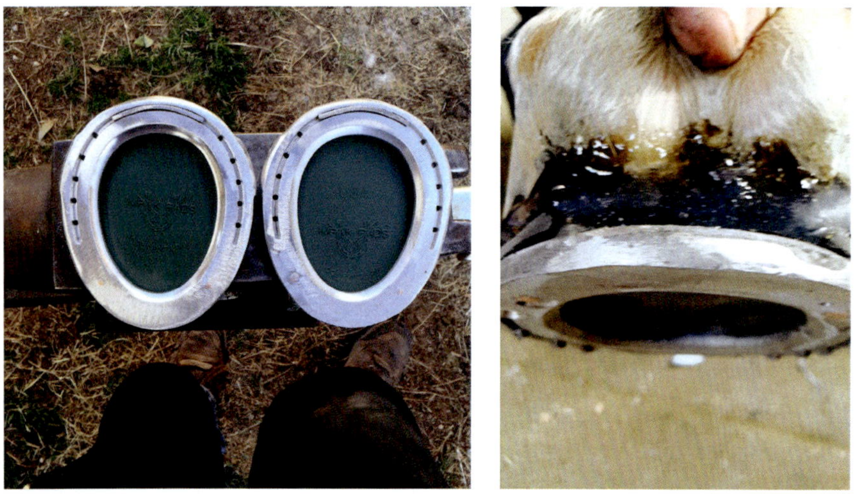

(a) (b)

Figure 38.6 (a) An egg-bar shoe. (b) Application of the egg-bar shoe by combined use of synthetic polymer on the sole. Illustrations courtesy of Dave Gilliam.

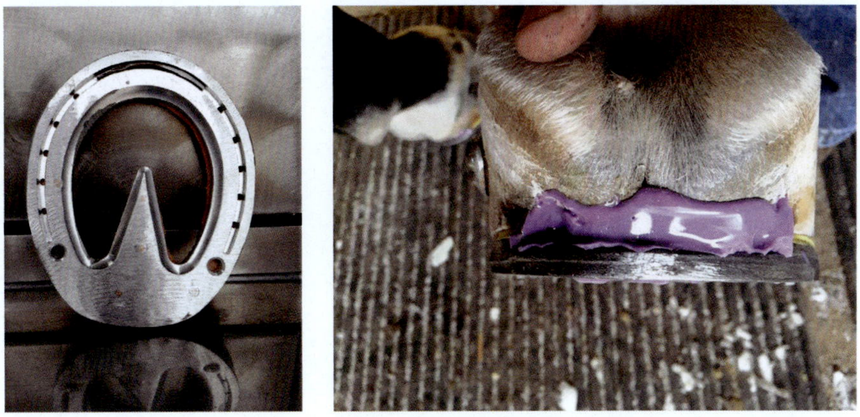

(a) (b)

Figure 38.7 (a) Example of a heart-bar shoe. (b) Combination of sole support with the heart-bar shoe.

frog. The heart-bar shoe is thought to enable the frog to load and share some of the weight-bearing function which would redistribute some of the weight borne by the foot away from the wall. It must be remembered that, in order to perform this function, the frog must be healthy, of sufficient density, and located on the same plane as the hoof wall at the heels. If the frog is of insufficient size and is receded below the level of the hoof wall, another type of shoe should be considered. It is unknown if the heart-bar shoe provides any other benefit. Heart-bars shoes are frequently welded into an egg-bar shoe (commonly referred to as a 'full support' shoe). This provides the added benefit of functioning like a wedge in soft substrate, as previously described. Heart-bar shoes can also be used in combination with other forms of foot support to increase the surface area that is either poured (e.g., polyurethane pour-in pad) or pressed (e.g., silicone putty) into the cavity formed between the branches of the shoe and the frog plate to provide additional support to the ground surface of the foot (Fig. 38.7b).

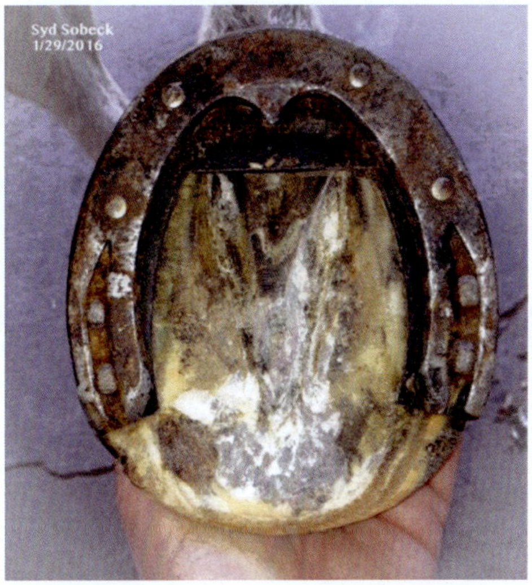

Figure 38.8 An example of a reverse shoe.

Reverse Shoe

The reverse shoe (Fig. 38.8) is based on the principle that it moves the breakover in a palmar direction because the toe of the shoe is open, it puts no pressure on the dorsal sole, and it functions as an egg-bar shoe at the heels. Although commonly used during the last two decades of the last century, its use has decreased in popularity due to the following concerns. The first function of any shoe is to offer protection, and the open toe of the reverse shoe leaves the compromised section of the toe just dorsal to the DP vulnerable. Second, the sole with the compromised lamellae, commonly present in the dorsal aspect of the foot, is relatively unsupported with a reverse shoe, and can descend down between the two branches of the shoe; this results in further digital displacement and soft tissue trauma to the foot. Depending on the degree of stability within the foot, the reverse shoe must be used with appropriate ground or solear support; however, inserting some form of solear support often results in excessive pressure on the sole. Another disadvantage of this style of shoeing is that it concentrates stress where the dorsal margins of the branches of the shoe contact the wall, commonly at a point where the lamellae/white line are severely compromised in the horse with rotation of the DP.

Wooden Shoe

The present author uses the wooden shoe (Fig. 38.9a) as a transitional device to promote hoof wall and sole growth in order to realign the DP within the hoof capsule [1, 2, 4, 8–11]. Once the shape and conformation of the hoof capsule is acceptable, the wooden shoe will be replaced by one of the traditional shoes described above, or the horse will be allowed to go barefoot. The wooden shoe may provide additional advantages to the traditional shoes commonly used to treat chronic laminitis. One major advantage of the wooden shoe, which is due to its flat solid construction, is its ability to distribute weight-bearing evenly over a specified section of the foot. This is helpful when trying to recruit ground surface in the palmar/plantar foot in order to shift the load from the dorsal lamellae when the structures in

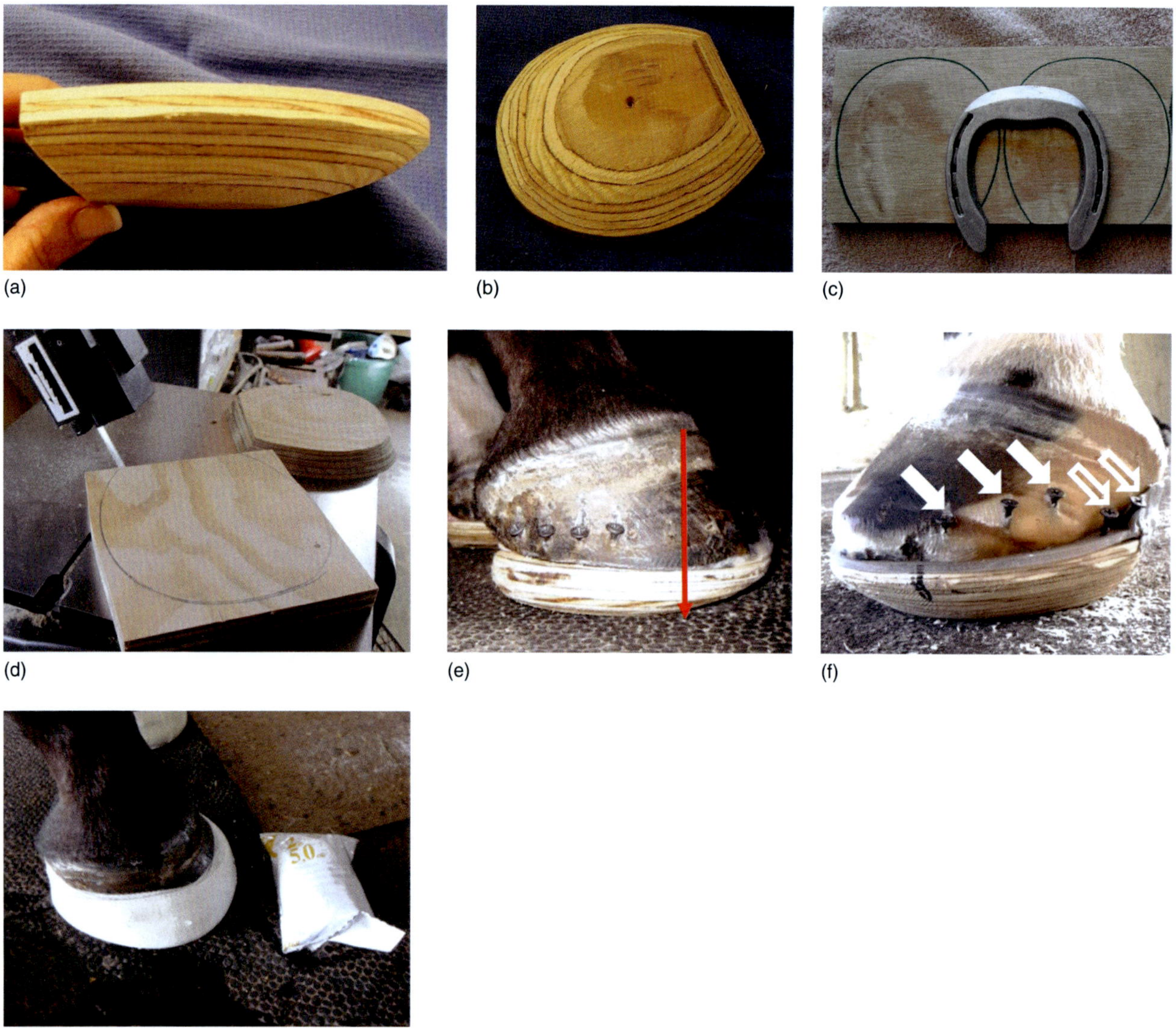

(a) (b) (c) (d) (e) (f) (g)

Figure 38.9 (a,b) The wooden shoe can be made using the Natural Balance Shoe as a template to draw the border of the wooden shoe on 1.125-inch (30-mm) plywood (c), followed by cutting the plywood at a 45° angle with an angle saw (d). The bevel on the dorsal aspect of the shoe is placed directly distal to the dorsal limit of the coronary band (see line in panel e). The wooden shoe can be applied with screws through the distal hoof wall (f, solid arrows) and adjacent to the margin of the hoof wall (f, open arrows), or with a combination of a smaller number of screws and 2-inch (50-mm) casting tape (g).

this section of the foot are less than optimal. Additionally, in the horse with focal sources of solear pain or an unhealthy thin or prolapsed sole, that area of the foot surface of the wooden shoe can be removed to increase the comfort of the horse (discussed further below regarding prolapsed sole).

Other advantages are:

- Simplicity of construction – simple plywood.
- Mechanics such as breakover and heel elevation can be fabricated into the shoe.
- Beveled perimeter of the shoe concentrating the load under the DP.
- Solid base of shoe allowing maximum recruitment of surface area in the palmar/plantar section of the foot to accept load.
- Solid base combined with an appropriate amount of impression material places even pressure and load across the palmar/plantar section of the foot.

The present author derives the shape of the wooden shoe (Fig. 38.9a) by using the Natural Balance (EDSS, Inc., Penrose, CO, USA) shoe as a template (Fig. 38.9b). In this case, 1.125-inch (30-mm) plywood is cut out using an angle saw, with the perimeter being beveled at an angle of 45° (Fig. 38.9c). This bevel not only moves the breakover palmarly, but also moves the medial and lateral weight-bearing surfaces axially, enhancing medial and lateral breakover. After the foot has been trimmed as described above, the appropriate size of wooden shoe is fitted to the trimmed foot and placement of the shoe is determined by superimposing corresponding lines drawn across the widest part of the foot and a line drawn across the middle of the block. The bevel on the front of the shoe is then increased with a rasp until the point of breakover is positioned to correspond to an imaginary vertical line drawn through the dorsal limit of the coronary band to the ground (see Fig. 38.9d). The present author applies a thin layer of impression material between the ground surface of the foot palmar to the apex of the frog, and just enough impression material to fill the frog sulci and create a level plane in the palmar section of the foot. The impression material is allowed to set with the horse in a weight-bearing position. The shoe is attached with screws inserted through pilot holes previously drilled in the distal hoof wall (Fig. 38.9e, f). Screws are placed just palmar to the widest part of the foot in order to maintain the two planes created during the trim. Alternatively, screws can be screwed into the plywood adjacent to the margin of the distal hoof wall, and the shoe secured by incorporating the screw heads into 2-inch (5-cm) casting tape that is placed around the perimeter of the foot (this allows for a smaller number of screws to be used; Fig. 38.9g). A wedge pad may be applied to the foot surface of the shoe to provide heel elevation if needed. If the sole has prolapsed below the level of the dorsal hoof wall, or if the DP has penetrated the sole, the foot surface of the shoe is recessed using a motorized burr or grinder to remove any direct pressure from the sole. The present author uses the wooden shoe as a transient device to help produce hoof wall at the coronet and create the sole depth necessary to realign the DP.

Glue-On Shoes

Glue-on technology provides another option for shoeing chronically laminitic horses [6]. The technique is relatively simple, atraumatic, and inexpensive. The same farriery principles apply; using radiographic guidance and the appropriate trim, the shoe is bonded to the foot in a manner that realigns the DP relative to the ground surface. The present author uses the direct method where a wide web aluminum shoe is glued directly to the foot using an acrylic adhesive (Equilox®, Pine Island, MN, USA)[a]. The foot is trimmed as described and the shoe is fitted to the foot with breakover ground into the toe of the shoe. Shredded fiberglass is mixed with the composite and molded into two tubular shapes. The composite rolls are placed on foot over the area that was trimmed (where the shoe will contact it), starting at the widest part of the foot. The shoe is pressed into the composite and the amount of heel elevation is attained by the amount of pressure applied. The ground surface of the foot between the branches of the shoe is filled with silastic material to provide sole support. The silastic material is extended dorsally between the hoof and the shoe if a space is present from the trim. Glue-on technology can be very effective in the initial stages of chronic laminitis, and may allow more flexibility and precision in realigning the DP than other techniques. It can be tailored to the specific requirements of each foot simply by using more or less of the composite as needed.

[a] Equilox®, Pine Island, MN, USA.

Follow-Up Farriery

Horses with chronic laminitis will have had shoes applied with adjusted breakover, solear support, and heel elevation. As the tissues heal, the horse becomes more comfortable and the foot conformation improves, and the farriery principles can be slowly modified and eliminated in reverse order. In the present author's experience, there appears to be some intrinsic shortening of the musculotendinous deep digital flexor unit over time when heel elevation is maintained continuously. Therefore, when increased stability and comfort is achieved, heel elevation should be gradually removed. However, if the shortening of the musculotendinous unit is significant, some degree of heel elevation may have to be continued indefinitely. With additional stability and the increased sole depth/thickness, the solear support can gradually be removed in most cases. Eventually, the horse may be shod in a routine fashion or left barefoot. However, in some horses with permanent dorsal capsular rotation and compromised lamellae, the shoes may need to be repeatedly reset with the aid of radiographs, although heel elevation, and solear support may no longer be needed.

Asymmetrical Distal Displacement/ Mediolateral Rotation of the Distal Phalanx

Assymetrical distal displacement (the present author also uses the term mediolateral [unilateral] rotation) of the DP is a less common condition than dorsal capsular rotation, and less is known about treating horses with this type of displacement. Assymetrical distal displacement often occurs concurrently with dorsal capsular rotation and, if recognized, should be addressed immediately as it appears to respond best in the early stages. The increased use of the dorsopalmar radiograph view reveals a higher incidence in this condition than was previously recognized. In the present author's opinion, asymmetrical distal displacement/medial lateral rotation is driven by foot conformation as it has only been observed when the foot is offset to the lateral side, placing a disproportionate load on the medial side of the foot. One of the early signs of mediolateral displacement is a noticeable lack of hoof wall growth at the coronet on the affected side the dorsal part of the hoof capsule, which can be readily palpated at the coronet (the hair at the coronet will be observed to be protruding straight out rather than lying flat against the hoof wall; Fig. 38.10c). The incidence of mediolateral/asymmetrical displacement appears to increase when horses with the offset foot conformation have had excessive heel elevation applied in the earlier stage of laminitis. Theoretically, the hoof capsule can be stabilized in relation to the DP by reducing the weight-bearing on the affected side (e.g., the medial

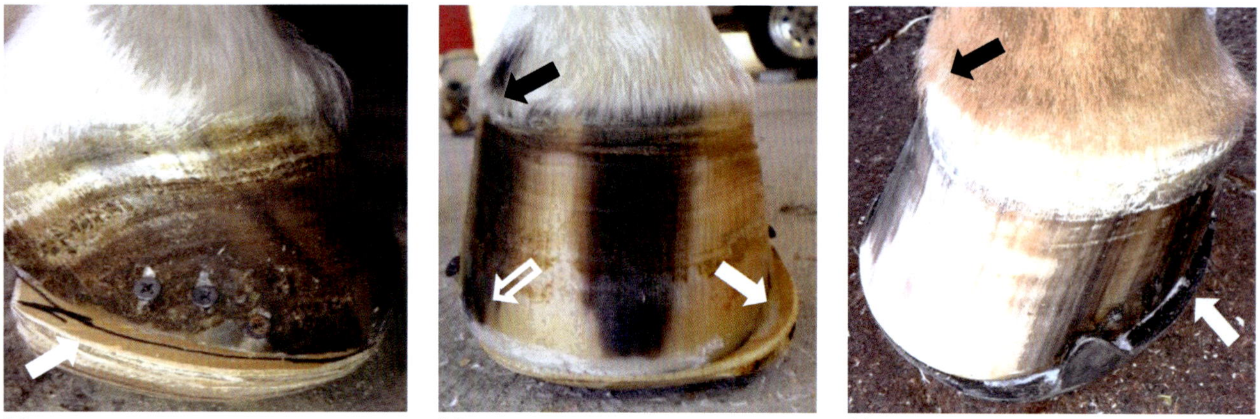

(a) (b) (c)

Figure 38.10 (a) Extension on unaffected side of foot for asymmetrical distal displacement. Note the characteristic appearance of the coronary band on the affected side with decreased hoof growth distal to the coronary band on that side [and hair immediately above coronary band protruding outward] (black arrows in panels b and c) in the case of asymmetric distal displacement and the placement of the shoes tight on the affected side of the foot (medial side on panel, open white arrow in panel b) and wide on the unaffected side of the foot (solid white arrows, wooden shoe in panels a and b, and aluminum shoe in panel c) to take the pressure off the medial aspect of the hoof wall.

side) by increasing weight-bearing on the opposite side (e.g., the lateral side). In other words, the COP can be shifted toward the non-affected or less-affected side of the foot (Fig. 38.10) [10]. This is best accomplished by extending the shoe on the opposite side of the foot to act as a lever, and hence act as a mild wedge. The present author has had success in controlling mediolateral rotation in a limited number of horses by applying either the wide web aluminum shoe or the wooden shoe in this manner, setting the shoe tight on the affected side and wide on the unaffected side (Fig. 38.10b and c); this method is usually combined with the use of impression material. When the wooden shoe is used, increasing the bevel on the lateral side of the shoe (in the horse with medial displacement) appears to increase the benefit. Before applying the shoe, any flare should be reduced on the affected side by using a rasp on the adjacent outer hoof wall.

This trimming and shoeing technique has visibly improved comfort, promoted hoof wall growth at the coronet on the affected side, and/or abolished the evidence of mediolateral rotation over time. This technique appears promising, but because the complication rate with this condition appears to be high, the prognosis for treating asymmetrical distal displacement is still less favorable than it is with dorsal capsular/phalangeal rotation. Unless the hoof wall on the medial side is completely detached, the present author has been reluctant to resect the hoof wall as it may provide some stability and prevent collapse. If the margin of the hoof capsule is detached and impinging into the coronet, a thin strip of hoof wall can be removed which will immediately increase comfort (see Chapter 44 for further discussion on hoof wall resections). Identifying and aggressively treating this type of displacement of the DP in the early stage may change the outcome in many cases.

Symmetrical Distal Displacement/'Sinking' of the Distal Phalanx

Cases with symmetrical distal displacement (sinking) of the DP are often very unrewarding cases to treat. The essential difference between the farriery of a horse with distal displacement of the DP and a horse with capsular or phalangeal rotation is that neutralizing the moment about the distal interphalangeal joint is less important with symmetrical distal displacement. The present author approaches these cases with either the wooden shoe or a distal limb fiberglass cast. Either mode of therapy must be employed as soon as possible for any chance of success. If appropriate, the length of the dorsal hoof wall is reduced and the wooden shoe is applied (as described above) with the screws being placed around the perimeter of the hoof wall rather than through it. There have also been reports describing the successful use of a fiberglass cast with a composite being formed in the shape of a dome and applied to the ground surface of the cast (see Chapter 42). If the horse survives the acute stage, or if any improvement is noted in horses with distal displacement, the present author may continue this therapy for a considerably longer period of time (two to four months if necessary) before shoeing the horse with a metal shoe. When shoes are applied, the toe of the shoes are similarly blunted, rolled, and fitted as previously described for horses with capsular rotation. The heels are seldom elevated as there is minimal involvement of the DDFT. The solear cavity, sulci of the frog, and space between the branches of the shoe are similarly filled with a silastic material if the integrity of the structures can accommodate an additional load. After four to eight months, the sole support can be removed; after eight to twelve months, it should be possible to revert to routine shoeing or allow the horse to go barefoot.

Treatment Failure

There are many reasons why the treatment of chronic laminitic horses is not successful. The overwhelming severity of the initial disease is the most important, particularly when followed by persistent infection [1–4, 8, 12]. Financial constraints are also important because the treatment can be very expensive, long, and exhausting. Therefore, many owners stop treatment as the full implications of the cost, or the psychological or physical toll of the rehabilitation process become apparent [12]. The failure of owners to comply with recommendations from veterinarians and farriers is not uncommon. On the other hand, a successful outcome is invariably enhanced by merging the veterinary and farrier expertise along with owner compliance.

References

1. O'Grady, S.E. (2010) Farriery for Chronic Laminitis, in *The Veterinary Clinics of North America* (ed. C.C. Pollitt), vol. 26 (2), W.B. Saunders, Philadelphia, pp. 407–423.
2. Parks, A.H. and O'Grady, S.E. (2015) Chronic Laminitis, in *Current Therapy in Equine Medicine* (eds N.E. Robinson and K. Sprayberry), vol. 7, W.B. Saunders, St Louis, MO, pp. 869–878.
3. Hunt, R.J. (1998) Chronic Laminitis, in *Current Techniques in Equine Surgery and Lameness*, 2nd edition (eds N.A. White and J.N. Moore), W.B. Saunders, Philadelphia, pp. 548–552.
4. O'Grady, S.E. and Parks, A.H. (2008) Farriery options for acute and chronic laminitis. *Proceedings of the American Association of Equine Practice*, Vol. **54**, pp. 355–363.
5. Parks, A.H. and O'Grady, S.E. (2008) Chronic Laminitis, in *Current Therapy in Equine Medicine* (eds N.E. Robinson and K. Sprayberry), vol. 6, W.B. Saunders, St Louis, MO, pp. 550–560.
6. O'Grady, S.E. (2006) Realignment of P3 – the basis for treating chronic laminitis. *Equine Vet. Educ.*, **8**, 272–276.
7. Hunt, R.J. (2008) Equine Laminitis: Practical Clinical Considerations. *Proceedings of the American Association of Equine Practice*, Vol. **54**, pp. 347–353.
8. Parks, A.H. and O'Grady, S.E. (2003) Chronic laminitis: current treatment strategies, in *The Veterinary Clinics of North America* (ed. S.E. O'Grady), vol. 19 (2), W.B. Saunders, Philadelphia, pp. 393–416.
9. O'Grady, S.E. and Steward, M.L. (2009) The Wooden shoe as an option for treating chronic laminitis. *Equine Vet. Educ.*, **21**, 393–416.
10. O'Grady, S.E., Steward, M., and Parks, A.H. (2007) How to construct and apply the wooden shoe for treating three manifestations of chronic laminitis. Proceedings of the American Association of Equine Practice, vol. 53, pp. 423–429.
11. Nickels, F.A. (2011) Hoofcare of the laminitic horse, in *Diagnosis and Management of Equine Lameness*, 2nd edition (eds M.W. Ross and S.J. Dyson), Elsevier (Saunders), St Louis, MO, pp. 379–382.
12. Moyer, W., Schumacher, J., and Schumacher, J. (2000) Chronic Laminitis: Considerations for the Owner and Prevention of Misunderstandings. Proceedings of the American Association of Equine Practice, vol. 46, pp. 59–61.

CHAPTER 39

Solear Support Techniques

Raul J. Bras

History

Therapeutic farriery techniques on the feet of laminitic horses, which have included supporting the coffin bone and sole, have been discussed since before the eighteenth century [1]. Proper trimming techniques recommended rounding the toe to conserve the sole, and rasping the heels and quarters, thus enabling the frog to bear weight [2]. In 1898, reference was made to a shoe that would provide frog pressure; this appears to be first mention of a heart-bar shoe in the literature [3] (Fig. 39.1). During the late 1800s into the early 1900s, most treatments incorporated the use of a wide-webbed heart-bar shoe which was beveled to relieve sole pressure, and introduced the concept of packing the bottom of the foot with tar or oakum under a leather pad in order to provide further support for the coffin bone and sole [4, 5]. Until the late 1980s, the majority of therapies regarding support of the ground surface of the foot revolved around frog support, either with shoes such as the heart-bar or temporary padding over the frog in acute cases. A driving reason for commonly not incorporating the sole previous to this time appears to have been the concern of compressing the digital vasculature on the solear surface of the distal phalanx (DP). Over the past 25 years, the concept of supporting not only the frog but also the bars and sole of the foot with a pliable substance in acute laminitis cases has become somewhat routine. Whereas, Styrofoam was the first substance to enjoy widespread use to provide solear support, other longer-lasting substances (e.g., silastic putties and 'pour-in' polyurethane pads) are more commonly used today to provide similar solear support.

Current Understandings

The current scientific understanding of the foot is inadequate to properly explain many of the practices that are commonly performed when dealing with laminitis. Many practical modifications to the foot are performed to alter the distribution of forces acting on the foot. The sum of all the forces acting on the ground surface of the foot are represented by the ground reaction force (GRF), a vector with both a magnitude and direction. The vector acts through a point, frequently referred to as the center of pressure (COP; see Fig. 5.2 in Chapter 5). However, the clinician needs to realize that the term COP denotes that there is pressure on a large area of the sole – in all directions from the center of pressure – which is 'centered' at this point. Therefore, in an attempt to adequately address the GRF and COP by increasing the solear surface in contact with the ground, the sole support applied would best address the forces on the solear surface if placed in all directions from the center or pressure on the solear surface. The role of the sole, frog, and bars in normal weight-bearing and transmission of the GRFs to the internal structures of the foot is only partially understood. Altering the distribution of forces across the ground surface of the foot cannot be achieved without regard to the COP. The distribution of forces may be changed to increase or decrease weight-bearing by one area of the foot to reduce or increase weight-bearing by another part of the foot. One main goal to be implemented during laminitis is to move the COP away from the most compromised area of the foot.

An understanding of load distribution across the solear surface of the foot is important in laminitis. The DP is considered to be suspended within the hoof by the digital lamellae, even though it is known that the entire ground surface of the foot, and not just the wall, is normally capable of some degree of bearing weight [6]. The loading patterns observed in the horse with laminitis can be significantly different from those in the normal horse. One prevalent change is an increase in the load distributed across the sole that is caused by the mechanical failure of the digital lamellae. During displacement of the DP in laminitis, the horse's weight forces the DP distally within the foot, without adequate support from the lamellae. As this occurs, there is a loss of structural integrity that limits the ability of the DP and hoof capsule to act as an integrated structure. This loss of structural integrity decreases the percentage by which the DP is suspended by the lamellae, and purportedly increases the percentage by which it must be supported on its solear surface; however, it is not known if the sole can truly support the DP in these circumstances. As the loss of lamellar integrity reaches the point in which there is a decreased ability to transfer loading

Equine Laminitis, First Edition. Edited by James K. Belknap and Raymond Geor.

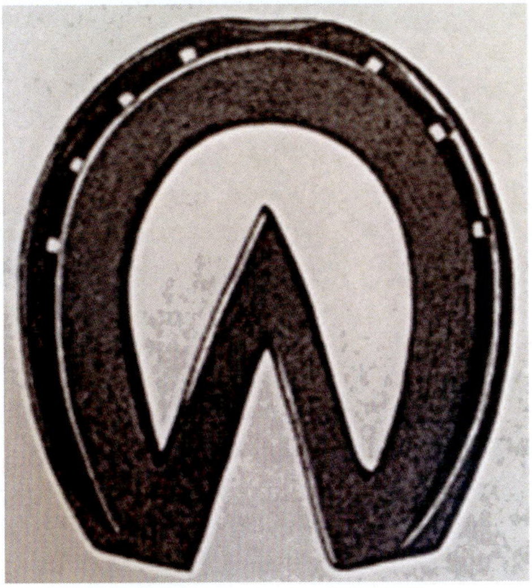

Figure 39.1 In 1898, a reference was made to a heart-bar shoe designed to provide pressure in the frog region. Illustration reproduced from Dollar, J.A.W. (1898) Shoeing after laminitis, in *A Handbook of Horseshoeing*, William R. Jenkins, New York, p. 352.

forces among components, further failure occurs as individual structures (e.g., remaining intact lamellae) are subjected to loads exceeding their limits [7].

Foot pain in laminitis is thought to be the product of the altered forces incurred as the foot fails mechanically. The foot's structural collapse produces compressive and shear forces in the subsolear region, with the primary result of these forces being the compression of the sole by the DP. These compressive and shear forces can result in several lesions affecting the vasculature supplying the solear tissue (see Figs 27.1 and 27.2), which is located in the thin dermis between the DP and the keratinized sole. Once structural integrity of the lamellar support of the DP is lost, there is no longer protection of the inner structures under the sole from the load imposed by the descending DP [7]. The primary goal of rehabilitation is to reduce or redistribute the abnormal forces, with the intention of regaining the foot's structural integrity. As many horses suffering from lamellar instability initially appear relatively comfortable with shoes on because the sole is unloaded, it is tempting to leave the shoes on or to apply shoes for temporary relief. Unfortunately, this permits the unsupported sole to prolapse further. A general approach is to provide a greater surface area for weight-bearing in less painful/less compromised areas of the foot. Frog and solear support may be provided either to stabilize the DP within the hoof capsule or in effort to address regional pain by unloading a specific area of the solear surface of the foot [8].

Sole Support Material

The application of a material to all or part of the ground surface of the foot is performed in an attempt to provide relief to the digital lamellae by recruiting other parts of the foot to bear weight (Fig. 39.2). The use of sole support material to increase the weight-bearing surface area of the palmar/plantar hoof can purportedly provide for weight-sharing and support of the DP. A foot loaded within a small surface area will produce higher compressive forces in the underlying tissue structures than an identical load applied to a greater surface area [9]. Sole support material can be applied to the entire solear surface of the foot (Figs 39.2a and 39.3) or only to the caudal solear surface (most

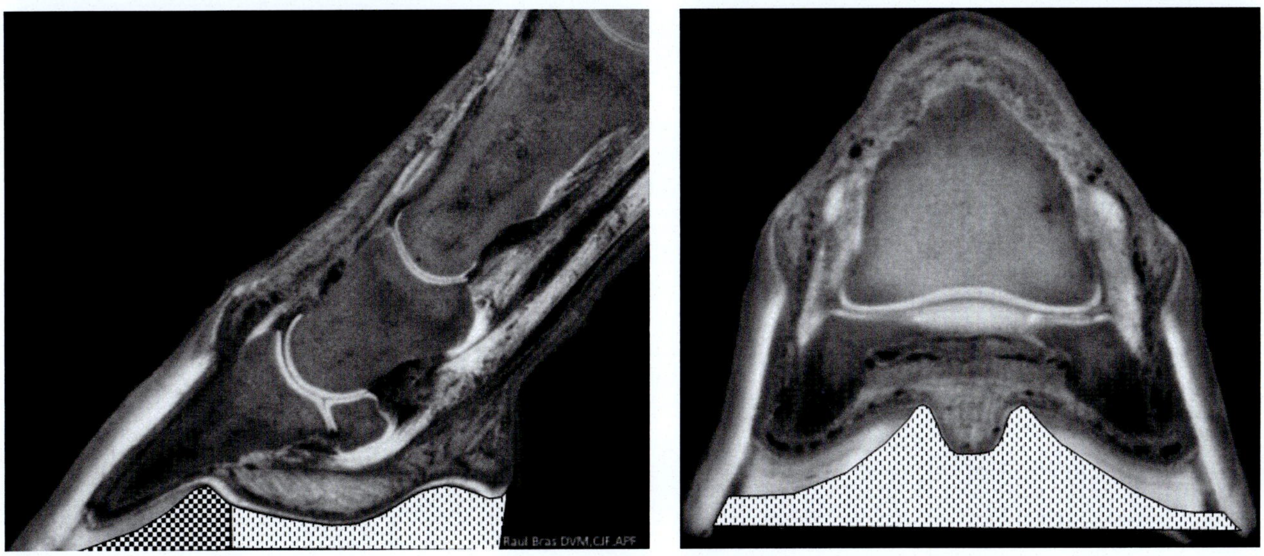

(a) (b)

Figure 39.2 A schematic representation of the recruitment of the solear surface to bear weight and thus support the distal phalanx. (a) Sagittal view of the solear area under the distal phalanx when cushion support material is placed in the caudal aspect of the foot (caudal to the apex of the frog). (b) The increased area of the distal phalanx (checkered area) when the entire sole is incorporated in some type of cushion support.

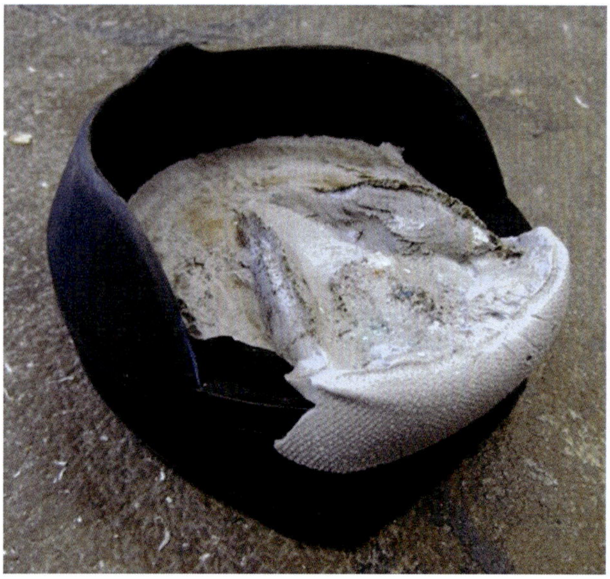

Figure 39.3 An example of incorporating the majority of the solear surface as a weight-bearing surface using cushion support material.

commonly from approximately the apex of the frog caudally (Figs 39.4 and 39.2a and b) in cases in which there is concern that displacement of the DP (usually rotation) will result in excess pressure on the dorsal sole. The sole support material is usually applied even with the ground surface of the shoe in order for there only to be 'passive loading' (loading that only occurs when the horse is weight-bearing on that foot) of the sole, digital cushion, and frog in the caudal aspect of the foot

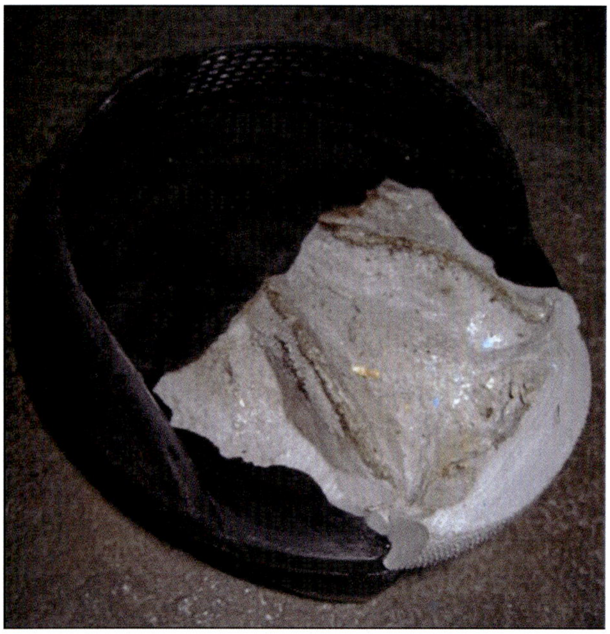

Figure 39.4 An example of incorporating the caudal aspect of the solear surface as a weight-bearing surface using cushion support material.

(Fig. 39.4). Passive loading is accomplished by loading the sole impression material before it sets (allowing the excess material to exit caudally), the result being that sole support material is approximately even with the ground surface of the shoe. The load is distributed as evenly and atraumatically as possible over the sole, bars, frog, digital cushion, and wall in attempt to support (indirectly) the DP [10]. Whereas it is likely that the application of sole support material to the entire solear surface of the foot will provide support to the DP, it has not been proven that placing support in only the caudal aspect of the foot greatly improves support of the DP. As can be seen in Figure 39.2a, supporting the solear surface behind the apex of the frog at best only provides support to the caudal half of the DP, with a great deal of the support material only having the navicular bone, deep digital flexor tendon, and digital cushion above it. Additionally, if the most cranial aspect of the putty/padding is near the apex of the frog, support will barely reach the COP of the GRF (see Fig. 5.2). Thus, when possible, it may be more effective to provide support to the entire sole and therefore the entire solear surface of the DP (approximately, even with the dorsal aspect of the coronary band from the side). This provides for the breakover to still be brought to the appropriate spot caudal to the toe (see Chapter 38), while incorporating the entire solear surface area directly distal to the DP. As mentioned above, the concern with extending solear support through the toe of the solear surface is that the material may exacerbate compression of the solear tissue under the dorsal tip of the DP in the digit; this is especially a concern in the foot undergoing palmar rotation of the DP. Therefore, the decision to use cushion support material cranial to the frog apex should be based on results from radiography, and physical/lameness examinations (especially hoof testers and assessing the comfort of the horse when walking with the pads in place) to ensure that excessive pressure is not placed on the ground surface of the sole in a region which is already compromised due to pressure from a displacing DP above the sole.

An important point with sole support is that caution must be exercised not only regarding the toe in palmar rotation of the DP but also regarding the palmar aspects of the foot in symmetrical or asymmetrical distal displacement. The increased pressure on the solear surface of the foot obtained by adding a material to the solear surface may cause excessive pressure on the dermal and epidermal tissue between the margin of the DP and the ground surface of the sole. This is likely to be more of a concern in the animal which is actively undergoing distal displacement of the DP. Excessive pressure from sole support material pushing up from the ground surface could cause further damage to the internal soft tissue structures (i.e., by compromising both the blood supply to the sole distal to the margin of the DP phalanx and the viability of the solear epithelium) [11]. Additionally, some horses have regions of the foot that are too painful to be used for weight-bearing (or focal areas of sepsis), which requires either (i) a combination of products of different hardness or (ii) trimming material away from the painful areas. A thorough examination of the foot is essential to determine which support method is the most appropriate [12].

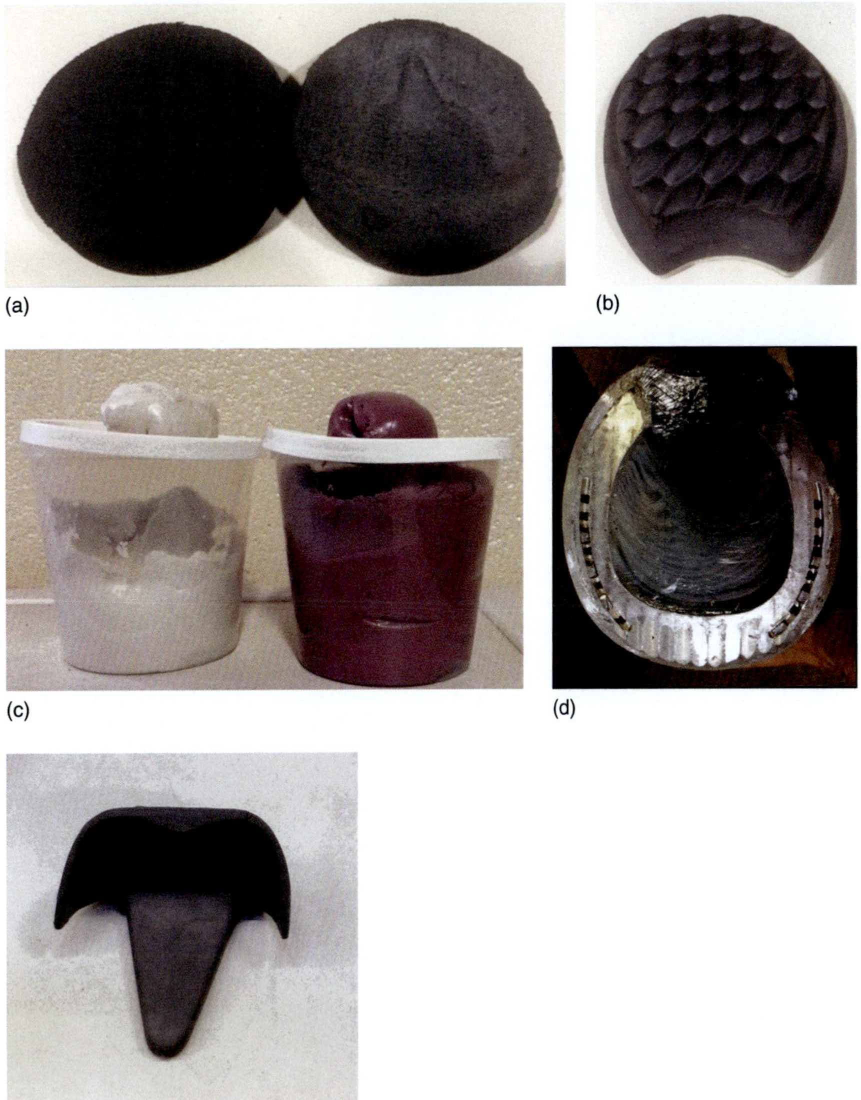

(a) (b) (c) (d) (e)

Figure 39.5 Different options for material to provide sole support include: (a) closed-cell foam; (b) EVA pads; (c) commercial impression material; (d) commercial polyurethane pour-in pads; and (e) lily pads.

A wide range of materials have been used in attempt to effectively level the ground surface of the foot with the hoof wall, and therefore support the foot's solear surface. There is a large variation in the hardness of the different materials available. The firmer materials offer more support but are less forgiving to thin, weak, painful areas, whereas the softer materials are more forgiving but offer less support. In the author's opinion, most horses respond well to materials that are close to the hardness of a freshly trimmed frog. The materials commonly used include high-density Styrofoam, closed cell foam, ethyl vinyl acetate (EVA) foam, silicone putties (many two-part systems are available commercially of different stiffness characteristics), and polyurethane pour-in pads. High-density Styrofoam (housing insulation) conforms to the foot reasonably well but is difficult to maintain evenly on the foot and requires frequent replacement due to crushing (or the addition of multiple pieces). Using this material can result in a reasonable sole support and comfort for a light horse, but newer materials and supportive appliances have decreased the use of this product. Closed-cell foam (Fig. 39.5a) is used more frequently to make digital pads; it is available from distributors in multiple densities (the 4 lb in^{-2} density is commonly used for horses). The advantages of closed-cell foam are: (i) it is deformable to mold to the solear surface to provide solear support; (ii) it does not crush (see Fig. 39.5a); and (iii) it can be cut/shaped to the veterinarian's/farrier's preference (e.g., beveled dorsally for breakover, trimmed to unweight specific areas). EVA pads (Fig. 39.5b) are more stiff than closed-cell pads, and can be more easily formed into desired shapes (e.g., beveled on all sides like a wooden shoe/clog). Due to the increased stiffness, the material may not mold as well to the sole as other materials, such as closed-cell foam. Putty-like impression material (Figs 39.3, 39.4, and 39.5c; also termed cushion support material) is commonly used and allows incorporation of the entire frog and the majority of the sole; it is a much more stable appliance and easier to maintain. The impression material is a two-part material that is kneaded together in equal parts

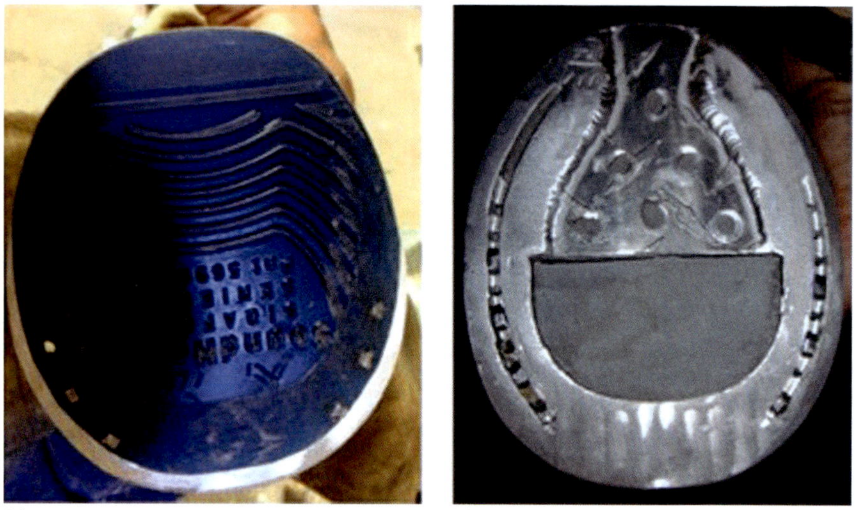

(a) (b)

Figure 39.6 Examples of combinations of solid plates with sole support material: a) an example of a solid aluminum plate shoe coated with urethane to provide support and protection to the entire sole; b) an example of an aluminum shoe with a solid heel aluminum plate to provide protection to the caudal part of the foot. It must be noted that impression material was used for support to the entire sole.

(Fig. 39.5c) and is most commonly conformed to the palmar two-thirds of the foot extending from the apex of the frog to the palmar heels. As the material is formed to the periphery of the sole, care is taken to extend the material only to the white line and leave the hoof wall unloaded. Another advantage of the impression material is that its depth can be adjusted to the desired thickness. Once the material sets, it tends to be very durable and can be removed periodically to evaluate and clean the foot and reapplied, maintaining a snug fit. If used with a shoe, some type of mesh is commonly incorporated between the sole and shoe; the mesh is then incorporated into the silicone putty when it is applied to the bottom of the foot so that the putty will not fall out. The primary disadvantage of the putty is that the sole can collect moisture between the putty and the sole, which may result in thrush or maceration of the solear epithelium. Some clinicians treat the sole with a stringent substance (e.g., copper sulfate) prior to application of the putty. Polyurethane pour-in pads (Fig. 39.5d), which bind to the solear surface, do not have the disadvantage of moisture build-up between the pad and sole. Due to the liquid nature of the substance prior to it setting up, it is more difficult to mold into the desired shape. However, it is still a valuable addition to provide sole support with shoeing.

When used with shoes, most sole support materials are placed in the sole even with the ground surface of the shoe (see Fig. 39.5d). However, sole support material can also be used under a solid-plate customized shoe (Fig. 39.6); this method provides even, constant loading in a controlled and protected manner. Additionally, a firmer product with more support can be used when it does not have direct contact with the uneven ground surface [12]. Although it is questionable how much support frog pressure provides to the DP, specific frog pressure can be applied using either silicone putties to form a resilient frog pads or commercial pads that fit directly over the frog (e.g., Lily pads; Fig. 39.5e). Similar frog support has been achieved by applying roll gauze or multiple layers of plaster casting material conformed to the frog. These materials are held in place with an elastic tape, and caution should be taken to avoid excessive pressure around the coronary band when applying the tape. These methods can be frustrating to maintain due to the shifting of the material as the horse moves around. Importantly, no studies have confirmed that frog support provides support to the DP.

In conclusion, although sole support is currently incorporated in the digital management of most laminitis cases, adequate studies have not been performed to confirm the degree of physical support to the DP provided by the different methods of sole/frog support. Due to the anatomic relationship of the DP to the sole, it is likely that the greater surface area of the sole addressed by the sole support (especially the dorsal aspect of the sole), the more support will be provided to the DP. However, it is critical for the caregiver to contemplate the possible adverse effects of providing sole pressure to a solear corium already undergoing compression by a distally displacing DP, and to adjust both the type of support (e.g., choosing between materials of different 'stiffnesses') and the areas of the sole to which pressure is applied in each individual case.

References

1. Wagner, I.P. (1999) Historical Perspective on Laminitis, in *The Veterinary Clinics of North America, Laminitis*, vol. 15 (2). W.B. Saunders Co., pp. 295–309.
2. Freeman, S. (1796) Description of different sorts of feet and of the proper management of those which are most liable to be foundered, in *Observations on the Mechanics of the Horse's Foot*. W. Bulmer and Co., London, p. 46.
3. Dollar, J.A.W. (1898) Shoeing after Laminitis, in *Handbook of Horseshoeing*. William R. Jenkins, New York, p. 352.
4. Percivall, W. (1871) Laminitis, in *Hippopathology – Lameness in the Horse*. Longmans, Green, Reader and Dyer, London.
5. Churchill, P.G. (1926) Laminitis, in *American Methods of Horseshoeing*. Republic Press, Junction City, p. 94.
6. Goetz, T. (1987) Anatomic, hoof, and shoeing considerations for the treatment of laminitis in horses. *J. Am. Vet. Med. Assoc.*, **190**, 1323–1332.

7. Hood, D.M. (1999) The Mechanism and Consequences of Structural Failure of the Foot, in *The Veterinary Clinics of North America, Laminitis*, vol. 15 (2). W.B. Saunders Co., pp. 437–461.
8. Curtis, S. (1999) Trimming and Shoeing the Chronically Affected Horse, in *The Veterinary Clinics of North America, Laminitis*, vol. 15 (2). W.B. Saunders Co., pp. 463–480.
9. Bowker, R.M. (2003) Contrasting structural morphologies of 'good and bad' footed horses. Proceedings 49th American Association of Equine Practitioners, New Orleans, LA.
10. Steward, M.L. (1999) The Use of the Wooden Shoe (Steward Clog) in Treating Laminitis, in *The Veterinary Clinics of North America, Laminitis*, vol. 15 (2). W.B. Saunders Co., pp. 207–214.
11. Parks, A.H. (1999) Treatment of Acute Laminitis – Supportive Therapy, in *The Veterinary Clinics of North America, Laminitis*, vol. 15 (2). W.B. Saunders Co., pp. 363–374.
12. Morrison, S.E. (2010) Chronic Laminitis – Foot Management, in *The Veterinary Clinics of North America, Advances in Laminitis, Part II*, vol. 26 (2). W.B. Saunders Co., pp. 425–446.

CHAPTER 40

Approaching Digital Management Prior to Displacement of the Distal Phalanx

Randy B. Eggleston

Introduction

The cliché "...an ounce of prevention is worth a pound of cure" is an appropriate description of the vital importance of avoiding or minimizing digital displacement due to laminitis. Although there is some variability in the literature regarding the value of using different degrees/types of displacement of the distal phalanx (DP) for determination of the prognosis of the laminitis patient, there is little question that minimizing displacement of the phalanx is critical to the athletic future, if not the survival, of the horse. The two instances in which the veterinarian is confronted with digital management prior to distal phalangeal displacement are: (i) the horse known to be at risk of laminitis; and (ii) the horse exhibiting early clinical signs of laminitis but not yet exhibiting radiographic evidence of displacement of the DP. Early recognition and identification of horses at risk of developing laminitis are imperative to the success of treatment and reducing the chronic changes that occur and have a significant impact on the horse's long-term prognosis. Due to extensive clinical and basic research investigations conducted over several decades, the ability to identify animals at risk of the different types of laminitis is much greater, and includes those animals with: (i) systemic inflammatory disease/sepsis, (ii) endocrinopathic disease and (iii) orthopedic disease (or other causes of severe unilateral lameness [e.g., septic joint or tendon sheath]) resulting in excessive support borne by the opposite limb. It is often difficult to predict which one of these horses will develop laminitis; most clinicians have witnessed 'at-risk' clinical cases which appeared to be exposed to a similar inciting cause of laminitis, yet one animal succumbs to the disease while the other exhibits no signs of the disease. This also occurs in experimental models of laminitis, with only approximately 75–80% of animals responding to the identical inciting stimulus given to induce laminitis. Because it is not possible to clinically delineate the at-risk animals which will not develop laminitis, the prophylactic treatment of all suspected high-risk cases is necessary with the hope of preventing the disease itself or at least limiting displacement of the DP.

The second clinical presentation – the equid demonstrating clinical signs of laminitis but no radiographic evidence of displacement of the DP – is an even more compelling case for aggressive digital management. This was realized from recent research which showed that, by the time the horse shows clinical signs and the veterinarian is notified, the injury and destructive changes are occurring within the lamellae and may have been triggered 8–12 h earlier. Although radiographic imaging during the developmental and acute phase of the disease is still the 'gold standard' for assessing the displacement of the DP, it is now realized that it is unreliable for predicting and consistently diagnosing active disease. Research comparing radiographic evaluation with that of high-field magnetic resonance imaging (MRI) during the developmental and acute phases of laminitis showed a low sensitivity for positively identifying and diagnosing laminitis. MRI was used to identify five different changes that correlated strongly with the histologic diagnosis of laminitis, and therefore are likely consistent with early active stage laminitis: (i) a loss of normal sublamellar corium architecture; (ii) a loss of lamellar architecture; (iii) increased signal intensity in the corium; (iv) increased signal intensity in the lamellae; and (v) separation within the lamellae [1]. In some animals, total separation of the dorsal lamellae was apparent on MRI, although radiographic measurements (used to assess for displacement of the DP) were still normal. Therefore, even with no radiographic evidence of displacement of the DP, it is likely that the horse exhibiting clinical signs of laminitis may have lamellar instability making digital management an emergent issue.

Currently, there is no effective systemic medical treatment regimen that will consistently prevent triggering of the different types of laminitis. Those horses at risk of developing laminitis should be confined to a well-bedded stall, taken out of work (strict stall rest), and their nutritional status thoroughly evaluated. The initial goals of preventing laminitis include:

Equine Laminitis, First Edition. Edited by James K. Belknap and Raymond Geor.

(i) appropriate treatment of any primary systemic disease putting the horse at risk (e.g., antibiotics for pneumonia, acute metritis); (ii) controlling systemic inflammation/sepsis; (iii) stabilizing any underlying metabolic disease; (iv) maintaining relatively equal weight-bearing in the orthopedic patient; and (v) performing digital support for the patient (discussed below).

A mainstay of therapy, whether for prevention or treatment of the active disease, is local supportive therapy of the foot. The normal function of the horse's foot is a well-orchestrated balance between the exceedingly functional capacity of the lamellar suspensory apparatus (suspension of the DP within the hoof capsule by adhesion of the dermal and epidermal lamellae) and the external and internal forces placed on the foot. The normal foot sustains the forces of weight-bearing, ground reaction forces, and the tension of the deep digital flexor tendon. A detailed description of these forces and the effects they have on the lamellar suspensory apparatus of the foot are explained in detail in Chapters 3, 4, and 5). Horses suffering from the destructive effects of laminitis and breakdown of the lamellar suspensory apparatus experience a significant shifting of the normal balance, where the forces normally placed on the foot now become greater than that which the deficient functional capacity of the injured lamellae can withstand. Depending on multiple factors that include the horse's weight, the conformation of the distal limb, and the location and degree of lamellar injury, the digit may undergo symmetrical distal displacement, asymmetrical distal displacement (e.g., 'medial sinking'), or dorsal rotation of the DP (see Chapter 20 for further discussion). The challenge in treating the laminitis patient prior to displacement is that it is usually impossible for the clinician (veterinarian or farrier) to forecast the type of displacement that may occur in that horse. The general goals of supportive therapy of the foot are interrelated and include: (i) to reduce the normal stresses on the foot (and especially the affected lamellae); and (ii) to alter the load on the foot, reducing the load in the more severely affected portion of the foot and transferring that load to the portions less affected. Two techniques used to accomplish these goals are: (i) incorporating more sole surface to bear weight; and (ii) decreasing the moment about the distal interphalangeal joint (see Chapters 5 and 41 for descriptions of moments). Appropriate supportive therapy of the digit may also have a significant impact on pain control.

A complete examination of the foot should be performed and evaluated for potential signs of impending laminitis or characteristics that can potentially add to the risk of developing the different types of displacement of the DP. The foot should be evaluated for size and shape with respect to the size of the horse. If the foot is small in relationship to the size and weight of the horse, then consideration of earlier or more aggressive changes to the support of the foot may be made. The external wall should be evaluated for any flaring, distortion, or excessive toe length. Any of these abnormalities to the wall can increase the stress to that portion of the wall and potentially to the underlying lamellae, and should be trimmed or dressed down to be in line with the true angle of the wall.

Reducing the Overall Stress on the Entire Foot

The first step in removing the overall stress is purely a management issue, stall-resting the horse to avoid lamellar injury likely to occur with the greater impact sustained by the foot when the animal is constantly ambulating at different speeds. The second step (described in depth in Chapter 30) is to establish some type of deformable bedding material such as wood shavings/mulch, sawdust, or sand. These materials will conform to the concavity of the foot, thereby incorporating the sole as a weight-bearing structure and thus reducing the concentrated stress on one particular portion of the foot, more commonly the wall. Allowing the foot to sink into the bedding redistributes the weight evenly throughout the entire foot. Interestingly, horses that are in active laminitis and housed on deep bedding material can sometimes be observed rearranging the material and positioning themselves in peaks and valleys, placing their feet in a way that alters weight-bearing away from more painful areas of the foot. Soft, deep, comfortable bedding will also entice some horses to lie down, which is the best way to decrease the stress on lamellae. Sand stalls are the most effective way to gain sole support, but these can be difficult to clean and manage, and may dissuade the animal used to other types of bedding from laying down. A third important step is to remove the shoes if the horse is shod, due to the fact that shoes concentrate the stresses along the perimeter of the hoof wall, potentially adding risk of lamellar failure by concentrating more stress on the digital lamellae. It is important that the shoes be pulled properly to avoid any damage to the wall and further damage to the underlying lamella. Optimally, the shoes should be pulled early in the disease process not only to decrease forces on the digital lamella but also because, if delayed until the horse starts to show clinical signs of lameness, the removal of shoes becomes more difficult and causes more discomfort and possibly further lamellar injury (due to having to place all the weight on one limb). Although slinging horses in active laminitis is also an effective way to reduce the overall stress within the foot, it is usually not necessary in the early stages of the disease. Additionally, it is difficult to predict how an individual animal will respond to the sling, making it potentially dangerous to the patient and personnel in many cases.

Changing the Load Dynamics

Changing the load dynamics away from the most severely affected portion of the foot will further redistribute weight onto healthier and more comfortable portions of the foot. The dorsal portion of the sole and the dorsal hoof wall are the areas usually most affected by the destruction and instability of laminitis. Common methods used to attempt to reduce the load on the hoof wall include: (i) incorporating weight-bearing through the sole and frog; (ii) decreasing the moment arm by bringing the breakover to a more caudal point; (iii) decreasing the pull of the deep digital flexor tendon on the distal phalanx (a cause of increased distracting forces to the dorsal lamellae); and (iv) moving the shoe away from the injured lamellae, placing more weight on a less-affected part of the hoof wall.

Incorporating Weight-Bearing Through the Sole and Frog

Different techniques to accomplish this include (as described in Chapter 39): (i) packing the sole and frog of the foot with an assortment of impression materials (silicone putties) which mold to the ground surface of the foot, or (ii) applying padding to the sole and frog through either foam pads or commercial shoes containing pads (e.g., Soft-Ride™). The goal of all of these products is to apply a product that will mold into the concavities in the solear surface of the hoof capsule, and span the distance to the ground, thus allowing the solear surface to support some of the weight normally born by the hoof wall. A high-density foam made from ethylene vinyl acetate (EVA) is a product which is more rigid and durable than other foam materials. It tends to hold shape and resist breakage under the weight stress of the horse; it can also be shaped to a greater extent than the other foams, allowing it to be beveled dorsally (to decrease the extensor moment arm) or around the majority of the circumference in the shape of a Steward clog/wooden shoe to decrease the forces on the quarters and heels also. A number of therapeutic boots are commercially available for use with various foot conditions. The one that seems to be most widely used is the Soft-Ride boot. This boot, which primarily provides a gel orthotic insert (as with the other padding described above) to mold to the sole and frog provide both cushioning and support to the foot by incorporating the entire sole surface into a weight-bearing surface. Soft-Rides are popular due to a design which keeps them fairly firmly in place, and the shoes' availability in multiple sizes and orthotic inserts of different stiffnesses, depending on the desired effect. An *in-vitro* study looking at microstrain across the lamellae suggested that application of a Soft-Ride boot decreased the mean microstrain on the dorsal surface of the hoof capsule, while increasing the mean microstrain on the DP [2]. Therefore, the difference in strain across the lamellae is less following application of the Soft Ride boot.

Decreasing the Moment Arm of the Distal Interphalangeal Joint

The second method involves decreasing the extensor moment arm of the distal interphalangeal joint by bringing the breakover to a more caudal point. Because the dorsal hoof is the most common region of the foot to experience the destructive mechanisms of laminitis and lamellar detachment, unloading this region of the foot by either trimming the foot or applying a temporary shoe to accomplish this will reduce the forces on the dorsal lamellae and likely help to reduce pain and lamellar injury. Rasping or nipping a 45° bevel in the dorsal aspect of the toe from the white line dorsally will not only move the breakover caudally, but will effectively decrease the load at the dorsal aspect of the hoof wall by unweighting the toe. Additionally, applying a dramatically beveled temporary shoe (e.g., the Nanric Ultimate or EVA clog) will accomplish the same goal. In horses confined to a stall and with reduced mobility, the effects of shortening the point of breakover are unknown (a greater effect is likely in the horse at pasture or at work).

Decreasing the Pull of the Deep Digital Flexor Tendon on the DP

Heel elevation is the most common method of reducing lamellar stress by neutralizing the tension of the deep digital flexor tendon (which also decreases the moment caused by tension of the tendon). In a bare-footed horse, there are a number of ways to achieve heel elevation. Using standard wedge pads cut to the desired size and bonded or taped the foot can work well. The disadvantage in using this method is that there tends to be some shifting and instability to the pads. The Nanric Ultimate is a commercial option that, in addition to decreasing lamellar stress by decreasing breakover, incorporates both an 18° heel wedge and a short cuff around the toe which greatly increases the stability and reliability of wedging (versus only applying wedge pads).

Moving the Shoe Away from the Injured Lamellae

Moving the shoe away from the injured lamellae and placing more weight on a less-affected part of the hoof wall is most commonly used in the horse with asymmetrical distal displacement (the medial aspect of the foot is usually affected). In this case, one technique used in attempting to decrease the pressure on the affected side is to pull whatever apparatus that is applied to the foot towards the opposite side, so that it actually overlaps the hoof wall on the opposite side (see Chapters 38 and 41).

Other methods of supportive therapy that can be considered in these cases (although beyond the scope of this chapter) include using foot casts (see Chapter 42), EVA or wooden shoes/clogs (see Chapter 38), and possibly other types of therapeutic shoeing (although the trauma of applying a shoe in horses with ongoing lamellar injury makes this choice questionable). Foot casts work well in some horses that are experiencing severe pain. The casts tend to add stability to the foot and alleviate some degree of discomfort (discussed in Chapter 42). Wooden shoes/clogs, although used more frequently several weeks after the onset of laminitis, can be applied relatively atraumatically (see Chapter 38) and provide biomechanical advantages difficult to obtain with more temporary types of treatment. The combination of EVA and wood in a clog may be of more benefit to the early cases being described in this chapter, as the EVA will provide somewhat of a cushion for the animal.

Secondary to the vascular damage that occurs within the foot in the laminitic horse, there is a propensity for limb edema that may exacerbate the already abnormal hemodynamics within the foot. Maintaining the horse in well-padded support wraps will help control limb edema.

In the high-risk horse that has not yet exhibited clinical signs of laminitis, the present author commonly uses distal limb cryotherapy/digital hypothermia (see Chapter 34) in conjunction with the Soft-Ride boots. Distal limb cryotherapy, the only treatment that has been shown to protect against lamellar destruction in horses at risk and in early clinical stages of laminitis.

The success of preventing or treating acute laminitis depends on the recognition of the at-risk patient and an early initiation of therapy for those cases that are showing clinical signs; laminitis should always be considered a medical emergency. The goals of treatment should always encompass the whole horse, treating any underlying systemic disease (inflammatory or endocrinopathic) and focusing on aggressive medical therapy and supportive care of the foot.

References

1. Arble, J.B., Mattoon, J.S., Drost, W.T., Weisbrode, S.E., Wassenaar, P.A., Pan, X., *et al.* (2009) Magnetic resonance imaging of the initial active stage of equine laminitis at 4.7 T. *Vet. Radiol. Ultrasound*, **50** (1), 3–12.
2. Williams, J.M. (2013) A biomechanical assessment of clinical conditions in the horse. Thesis, Ohio State University.

CHAPTER 41

Hoof Care Management of Horses with Displacement of the Distal Phalanx

Andrew H. Parks

Introduction

In the acute and early chronic stages of laminitis, the mainstays of treatment are typically medical therapy and supportive measures to the hoof to prevent/limit displacement of the distal phalanx (DP). As the disease progresses, hoof care becomes more important, and this will form the main substance of this chapter. Hoof care only works when the initial lamellar insult is not so overwhelming that it is still possible to stabilize the DP within the hoof capsule. If the disease is so severe that hoof care cannot stabilize the DP, the only way forward is to reduce the weight on the foot, either by slinging the horse or by placing some apparatus on the limb (e.g., cast ± transmedullary pins) such that the force in the more proximal bones of the limb bypasses the foot. These latter practices are beyond the scope of this chapter.

The basic principles underlying hoof care of a laminitic horse are no different to the treatment of any other disease that requires hoof care. That is, it is first necessary to: (i) determine which tissues are injured/under excessive stress, (ii) to decide whether the affected tissue is stressed under tension or compression, and then (iii) to deduce what manipulation will reduce the excess stress in that tissue. Typically, this involves one of the four manipulations described below. It should be borne in mind that whenever one tissue is protected or unloaded, one or more others are going to be loaded more heavily unless the weight borne by the limb is reduced (which is rare). The evidence for which tissues are under excessive stress may be derived from examination of the hoof capsule, the way the animal moves, regional analgesia, radiographs, magnetic resonance imaging, or a combination of these techniques. Failure of a rational approach such as the one outlined above to result in a positive outcome may occur for at least one of two reasons. First, there are the unknowns, ranging from our general lack of understanding of normal function of the digital tissues to the veterinarian and/or farrier not realizing the nature/severity of the injury in a specific laminitis case. Second, even when rational principles are applied to hoof care, current knowledge regarding the impact of application of a principle is largely qualitative, because it is derived primarily by extrapolation from biomechanical studies on normal feet and from experience of their use on clinical cases, not from quantitative data (that could only be gleaned from basic research studying foot biomechanics in horses with laminitis). Therefore, even if the correct principle is applied, the procedure may fail by either not applying enough of it, or applying the principle in an excessive manner actually causing harm. For now, hoof care aspects of treating laminitis remain a balance of the underlying science and the art of application.

The Nature of Lamellar Injury and the Balance of Forces that Create Types of Displacement

In horses with laminitis, the initial injury is within the lamellae. The lamellae are normally under tension because they are responsible for suspending the DP [1]; when the stresses that they are subjected to exceed their capacity to withstand them (due to lamellar tissue dysregulation/injury), the DP moves within the hoof capsule. The lamellar stresses can exceed the tissue's load-bearing capacity for one of two reasons: (i) there is a dramatic increase in load; or (ii) the lamellae's tensile strength is reduced. The first possibility is not likely to commonly play an important role because the normal lamellae have vast reserve capacity; therefore, lamellar failure from dramatic increase in load would be a rare occurrence. The only possible cases resulting from this possibility would be the suspected cases of road founder/trauma-induced laminitis, where repetitive loads greater than normal magnitude, but less that that required to cause acute disruption, may cause damage to the lamellae. In the majority of instances, the second possibility is the biggest factor when laminitis follows an inflammatory, ischemic, or metabolic/endocrine process that results in the reduced tensile strength of the lamellae and potentially lamellar separation (partial or complete) with subsequent displacement of the DP. Why one pattern of digital displacement or another predominates is discussed in detail elsewhere in the book (see

Equine Laminitis, First Edition. Edited by James K. Belknap and Raymond Geor.

Chapters 5 and 20), but there are a few definitive statements that can be made about it. Of most importance in relation to the management of displacement is: (i) the anatomical attachment of the DP and ungula (collateral) cartilage to the hoof capsule, (ii) the dynamic nature of the forces imposed on the lamellae, and (iii) the distribution of lamellar injury. All three are important in reducing pain and further injury with therapeutic farriery. In horses with rotation, the displacement is occurring due to an imbalance in the flexor and extensor moments (see Fig. 41.1) acting on the DP about the distal interphalangeal joint; it would logically follow that the injury to the dorsal lamellar tissues is greater than elsewhere around the circumference of the foot. In symmetrical distal displacement, the alignment of the phalangeal axis in the sagittal plane is maintained. For this to occur, the nature of the injury must be such that the flexor and extensor moments must remain equal (see Fig. 41.1) when the displacement occurs (see Fig. 20.1c); symmetry of the medial and lateral aspects of the DP in the dorsal plane is maintained (see Fig. 20.1d). Asymmetrical distal displacement (commonly termed medial or lateral distal displacement (see Fig. 20.1e and f) occurs when the force sustained by the lamellae, the extent of lamellar injury, or both, are sufficiently greater on one side (medial or lateral) of the foot than the other that displacement only occurs on one side of the foot and not the other. Even though the distal interphalangeal joint is not typically thought of as rotating in the dorsal plane, there is normally significant movement in the dorsal plane, which is termed *collateromotion*. Therefore, in asymmetrical distal displacement, when lamellar injury is greater on one side than the other, the DP is not as well supported and so will move slightly to one side in relation to the middle phalanx; this causes one side of the joint to be compressed and the other side (the side with lamellar failure) will open. Why does all this matter? Given an understanding of how the forces within the digit change during the course of the disease provides a first line rationale for treatment.

Goals of Treatment

The goals of treating a horse with displacement of the DP are to stabilize the DP, to control pain, and to encourage the foot to return to the most normal shape possible. Stability of the DP is impossible to measure, but it is generally assumed that the more unstable the DP is, the more likely the degree of displacement is changing/prone to change. Whereas serial radiographic imaging is commonly used every few days to assess changes in digital displacement in horses with laminitis, the comfort of the horse is also often used as an indicator of lamellar stability in horses with acute laminitis. The more uncomfortable the horse is, the more likely the degree of displacement is changing. However, the use of pain to assess lamellar instability must be used with caution in the chronic case of laminitis, because secondary complications such as sole bruising (due to a chronically displaced DP applying pressure to a thin sole) and digital sepsis (which may lead to increased pain regardless of the degree of lamellar instability or ongoing digital displacement). Therefore, in the absence of painful complications such as bruising or infection, the degree of stability is inferred from the level of comfort of the horse and the lack of progression of displacement on radiographic imaging. The occasional horse will demonstrate progressive displacement, either with rotation or distal displacement, in which the severity of displacement is not reflected in the level of pain (the present authors have observed this phenomenon in the very slow, insidious displacement of endocrinopathic laminitis, but also post sepsis and post corticosteroid administration). The reason behind this phenomenon is not understood. Aside from

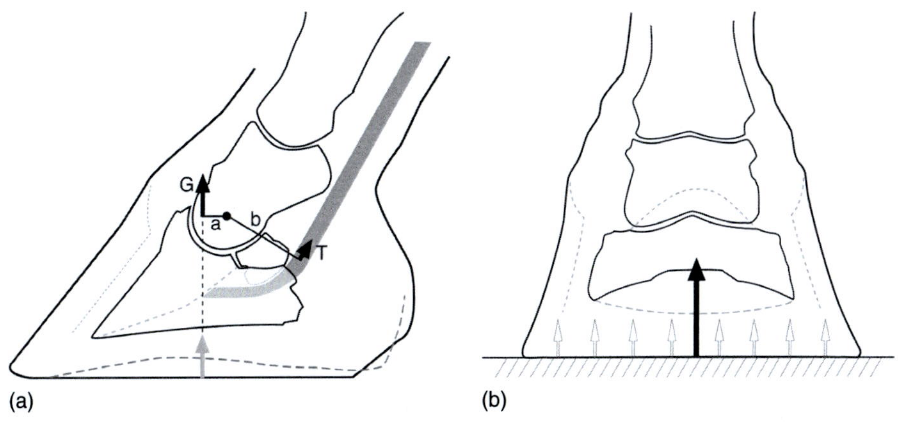

Figure 41.1 In the normal foot at rest the extensor moment and the flexor moment must be equal. The same is true if a horse is undergoing symmetrical distal displacement; that is, the alignment of the phalanges stays the same as the lamellae are disrupted. The extensor moment is the product of the ground reaction force (G) and the length of the Extensor Moment Arm (a). The ground reaction force is the force exerted by the ground on the foot (equal and opposite to the weight borne by the limb) and is a vector (panel (a) gray arrow; panel (b) black arrow) that represents the sum of all the forces across the ground surface of the foot (panel (b) open arrows). As a vector it has both magnitude, represented by arrow length, and direction, and it acts through the center of pressure (COP, located at point of arrows in a and b). The flexor moment is the product of the force in the tendon (T) and the length of the flexor moment arm (b). Illustration courtesy of Andrew Parks, University of Georgia, Athens, GA, USA.

the latter circumstance, the very act of increasing the stability of the DP should increase comfort. Additionally, it is important to avoid pressure on areas that are sensitive to hoof testers/digital compression (typically the dorsal sole in horses with dorsal rotation and the medial/lateral sole in horses with asymmetric distal displacement). Getting the foot back as close as possible to the normal shape varies with the type of displacement that has occurred.

Treatment and the Healing Process

Anyone who has examined horses with chronic rotation of the DP recognizes the secondary changes that occur with laminitis, including concavity of the dorsal hoof wall, the disparity in growth between the heels and toe, the flattened sole, and the very wide white line. Should it be possible to examine the inside of the foot, the following may be seen:

- Reorientation of the coronary papillae such that they are no longer parallel to the dorsal hoof wall, but rather projecting much more dorsally.
- The development of a large lamellar wedge.
- Distortion of the solear dermis around the dorsal solear margin of the distal phalanx.
- Changes in the dorsal and solear surfaces of the DP (see Fig. 27.5, which shows many of these changes radiographically) [2].

At the initial onset of laminitis, none of these points is present. During the course of the disease and its treatment, some horses' feet return to a relatively normal shape whereas others develop all of these secondary changes. Whilst it is unknown what determines which way a horse will respond, it seems reasonable to assume that the more rapidly the distracting forces are minimized by treatment, the less likely the secondary changes are to occur. When secondary changes do occur, the lamellae are less able to suspend the DP because of reduced functional surface area of interdigitating dermal and epidermal lamellae. Additionally, because it is thought that those forces are associated with weight-bearing (which are distributed across the sole and are transferred to the DP via the sole–wall junction; Chapter 5), damage and loss of function of the white line may further impede weight-bearing by the lamellae and increase compression of the subsolear dermis between the DP and the sole.

Only So Many Biomechanical Objectives

The present author encourages the reader to review the biomechanics of weight-bearing discussed in Chapter 5. The specific aspects of foot function that are important with regard to hoof care of the horse with laminitis are: (i) the distribution of force across the ground surface of the foot; (ii) the location of the center of pressure; (iii) the moments about the distal interphalangeal joint (creating torque); and (iv) the acceleration/deceleration of the digit associated with landing and breakover (at the walk in most horses with laminitis). As such, these are the principal variables that can be altered to change foot function/improve stability of the DP within the hoof capsule. However, while they will be considered individually, these different aspects of foot function are interrelated, so an action taken to change one is likely to affect another.

Distribution of Force Across the Ground Surface of the Foot

The distribution of force across the ground surface of the foot is determined by what parts of the ground surface of the foot are in contact with the ground (see Fig. 41.2), which itself is related to the nature of the ground surface, and the relative contribution to weight-bearing by the different parts of the foot that are in contact with the ground. The less the overall area of contact, the greater the pressure will be on those areas of the ground surface of the foot that do touch the ground. Recruiting a greater surface area of the ground surface of the foot is commonly achieved by the application of a material (e.g., silicone putty; other materials are discussed below and in Chapter 39) to the solear surface, with the express aim of loading the sole, frog, and bars (see Figs. 39.2 & 39.3) to reduce the stresses on the hoof wall and therefore the lamellae. Why it appears to work clinically in some horses and not in others is undetermined. However, part of the explanation may relate to the difference in the function of the sole of a healthy horse versus the function of the sole of a horse with laminitis. More specifically, it is hypothesized that a normal sole

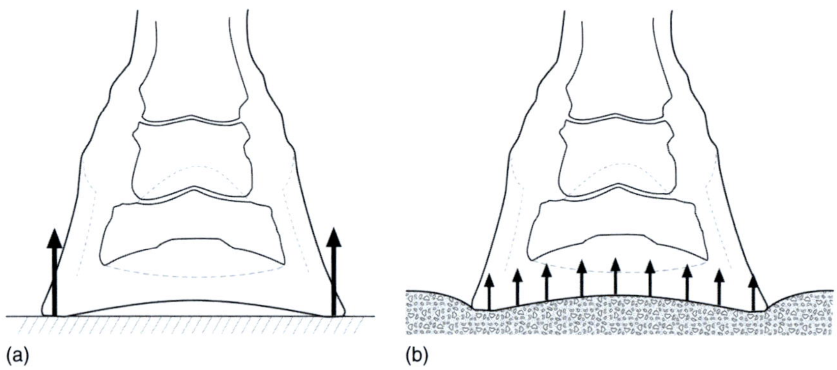

Figure 41.2 The distribution of force across the ground surface of the foot is determined by what parts of the foot are in contact with the ground. (a) If the foot is standing on a flat hard surface, the force from the ground opposing weight is distributed around the periphery of the foot (± the frog). (b) If the foot is standing on a readily deformable surface such as sand, the force from the ground opposing weight is broadly distributed across the ground surface of the foot. How these forces are summed in the ground reaction force vector is shown in Figure 41.1. Illustration courtesy of Andrew Parks, University of Georgia, Athens, GA, USA.

redistributes the forces of weight-bearing to the wall and thence to the lamellae, as discussed in Chapter 5 [3]. If this is the case, then should either the structure of the sole or the relationship between the wall and sole – that is, the white line – be changed, failure to transmit the forces on the sole (associated with weight-bearing) to the wall would make the sole more likely to compress the underlying soft tissues (i.e., solear dermis) against the solear surface of the DP. This would certainly explain why some laminitic horses can tolerate pressure over the entire ground surface of the foot while others cannot tolerate solear pressure (most commonly on the dorsal sole).

Locating the Center of Pressure

The center of pressure (COP) is the point about which the forces acting on the ground surface of the foot are evenly distributed (Fig. 41.1). Clearly, the COP and distribution of force across the ground surface of the foot are interrelated. If the area of contact of force is increased symmetrically, the COP may remain the same, but, if the area of contact of force is altered asymmetrically, this is likely to change the location of the COP. Changing the COP can move weight-bearing from its normal location towards the front or the back of the foot, or towards one side and away from the other, and can thereby be used to reduce the stresses on one part of the foot (at the expense of another).

Moments about the Distal Interphalangeal Joint

The moments about the distal interphalangeal joint of greatest interest in the digit are extensor and flexor moments (see Fig. 41.1a; see Chapter 5 for a full description). Of greatest interest in horses with laminitis is the development of an imbalance between these two moments, such that the flexor moment exceeds the extensor moment, possibly resulting in rotational displacement of the DP. These two moments may be altered for the horse standing at rest by changing the degree of flexion/extension of the distal interphalangeal joint (i.e., with a heel wedge). For horses with laminitis, this is most commonly done by increasing the degree of flexion of the distal interphalangeal joint. Inducing flexion of the distal interphalangeal joint shortens the deep digital flexor tendon, which reduces the tension in it. Reduced tension in the deep digital flexor tendon results in a decreased flexor moment. As the foot is stable on the ground, the corresponding extensor moment (needed to oppose the flexor moment) is also decreased. Assuming the weight on the limb hasn't changed, this means that the extensor moment *arm* (i.e., the distance from the center of pressure to the center of rotation of the distal interphalangeal joint) is decreased (Fig. 41.3). The moments about the distal interphalangeal joint during breakover are altered by changing the horizontal distance from the center of rotation of the distal interphalangeal joint to the most dorsal point of the foot in contact with the ground (e.g., by rolling the toe; Fig. 41.4a and b). Shortening this distance decreases the force needed to elevate the heels off the ground (i.e., the tension of the deep digital flexor tendon), thereby theoretically decreasing the stresses in the dorsal wall and lamellae. Furthermore, this benefit is enhanced by decreasing the radius of curvature of the ground surface from the point of breakover to the dorsal tip of the shoe/foot (for any given point of breakover). The reason is that the length of the extensor lever arm changes throughout the process of breakover (Fig. 41.4c and d). That is, immediately after the heel lifts off the ground, there is a new point of contact on the ground dorsally as the foot pivots about the toe and the new length of the lever arm is related to the curvature of the breakover surface. To get the maximal benefit of moving breakover in a palmar direction, the radius of curvature of the rounded toe should be such that the distance from the center of rotation to the point of breakover remains consistent or shortens throughout breakover (Fig. 41.4e and f).

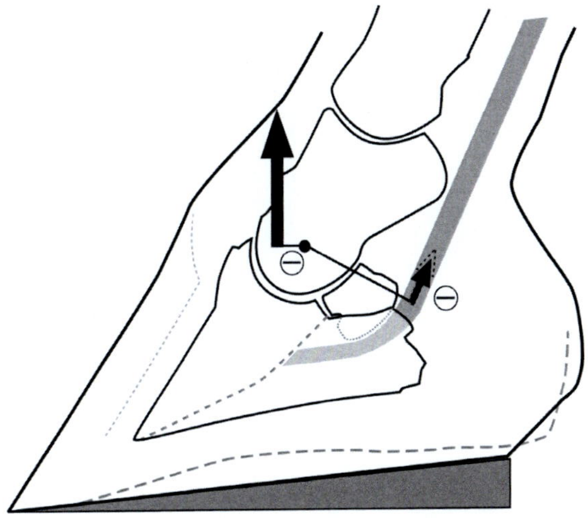

Figure 41.3 Elevating the heels causes the foot to rotate about the distal interphalangeal joint – that is, it partially flexes. In doing so, it moves the center of pressure closer to the center of rotation of the joint, which shortens the extensor moment arm. Because the flexor moment arm changes little (if any), this decreases the tension in the deep digital tendon required to oppose the ground reaction force. Illustration courtesy of Andrew Parks, University of Georgia, Athens, GA, USA.

Acceleration/Deceleration of the Digits

The rate at which the foot decelerates as it makes contact with the ground determines the peak force that is applied to the foot (i.e., the faster the foot slows down, the greater the force and vice versa). Modification of the rate of deceleration is best achieved by placing deformable material on the bottom of the foot that compresses during loading. This approach is not used very much once the foot is stable, but the use of the wooden shoe with a deformable ethyl vinyl acetate (EVA) base (as described below) is a good 'in-between' measure.

Many Ways to Accomplish Biomechanical Objectives

Having said that there are only so many ways to change foot function, there are innumerable ways to accomplish these changes. The area over which the ground reaction force is

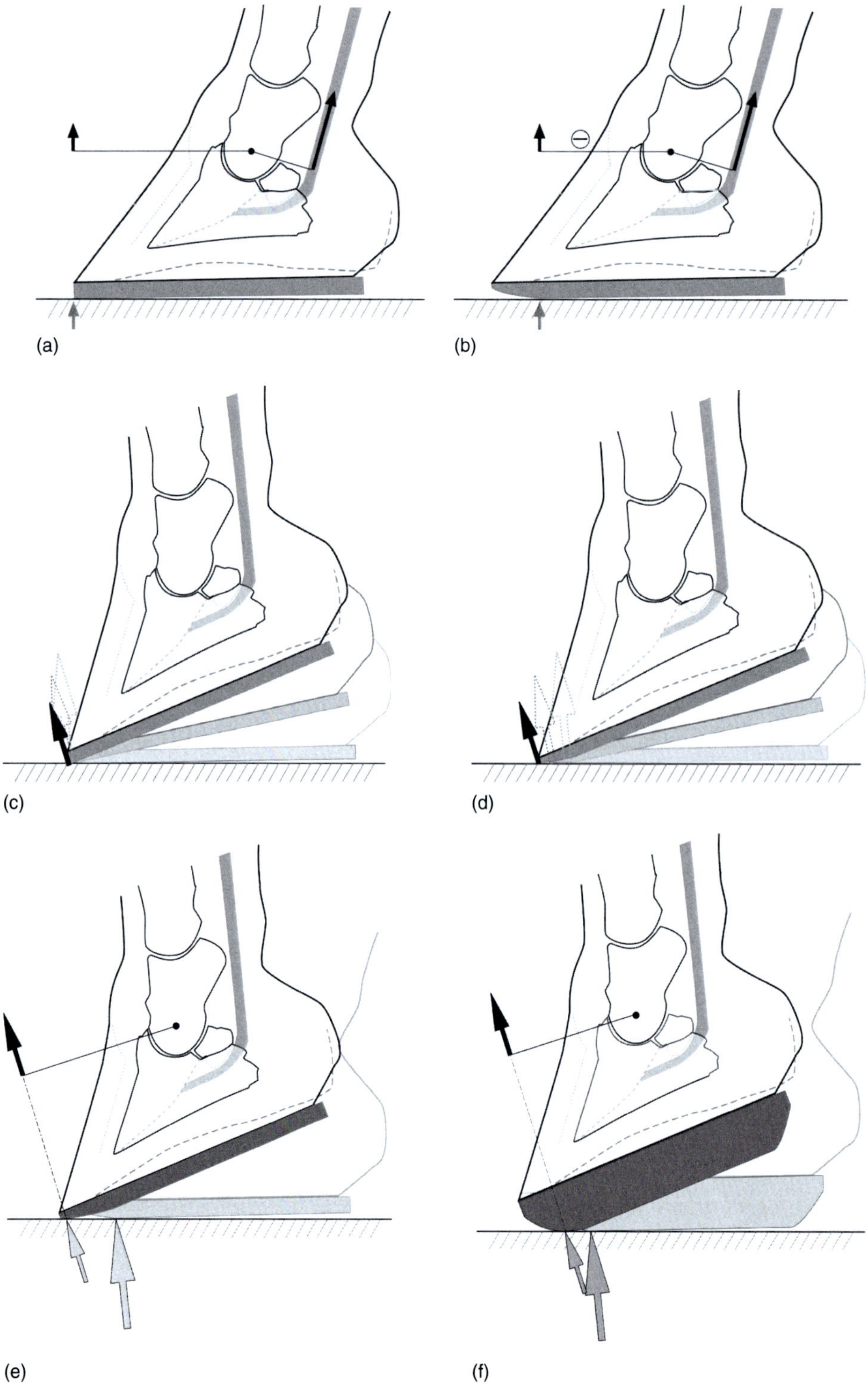

Figure 41.4 During breakover, the toe pivots about the toe. (a) At the moment of breakover the center of pressure moves to the most dorsal point of contact between the shoe and the ground; this is frequently referred to as the point of breakover. In a horse with a square shoe, this is at the dorsal most point of the toe. (b) By rolling the toe, the point of breakover is located in a more palmar position that it is with a standard flat shoe. This decreases the length of the extensor moment arm at the point of breakover, which means that breakover can occur slightly sooner. (c) As breakover progresses and the heels lift further off the ground, the foot continues to rotate. With a flat square shoe, the point of breakover does not change. (d) In a horse with a rolled toe, the point of contact changes, so that unrolling of the toe occurs in a smoother fashion. The forces associated with unrolling of the toe are further affected by the thickness of the shoe and radius of curvature of the rolled toe of the shoe. (e, f) Two shoes with the same point of breakover (large arrows), but with different radii of curvature of the toe. The thicker shoe means that there is greater flexibility in determining the radius of curvature at the toe; note how much shorter the extensor moment arm is in (f) than in (e) as breakover progresses. Of course, the thicker shoe would also make it possible to move the point of breakover even further in a palmar direction. Illustration courtesy of Andrew Parks, University of Georgia, Athens, GA, USA.

distributed is frequently increased to spread the load more widely over the ground surface of the foot, in order to decrease the load on the most severely affected positions of the foot. This can be done by either altering the nature of the substrate on which the horse is standing, or by applying a material to the bottom of the horse's foot. Common changes in the ground substrate include moving a horse from a relatively firm stall floor to a surface of sand, peat, or shavings. These conform to varying degrees to the ground surface of the foot, thereby increasing the area of contact. Sand appears to be significantly more effective than shavings in producing a greater degree of comfort, but it has its drawbacks and does not necessarily translate into survival.

Changing the Distribution of Pressure

Aside from changing the nature of the ground, several different materials have been used in alone or conjunction with shoes to spread the load over the ground surface of the foot, including Styrofoam, silicone putty (impression material), polyurethane, plaster of Paris, and even methyl methacrylate (Technovit[1]). These materials are of varying hardnesses, and have been used to distribute force across all of the ground surface or, more selectively, to load one area and relieve another area from load bearing. Many of these appear to help some horses, to hurt some, and make no difference to others. Until more is known about the role of the sole in weight-bearing, it would be wise to avoid the use of the more rigid/hard compounds such as the harder-setting polyurethanes and methyl methacrylate, and, even with the softer substances, the horse should be monitored carefully. Asymmetrical application of these products to the ground surface of the foot will also change the COP.

Changing the COP

The COP is manipulated to redistribute the overall distribution of stresses on the ground surface of the foot, and, by extension, to redistribute the stresses away from the lamellae. That is, moving the COP to one side of the foot increases the weight-bearing by that side of the foot and reduces weight-bearing by the opposite side. There are several ways to change the COP. The application of a wedge to the medial or lateral aspect of the foot (i.e., raising one side of the foot) causes the COP to be moved towards that side. The effect of elevating one side of the foot is too difficult to adjust, but a similar and more subtle/gentler effect can be obtained by extending the shoe in a lateral or medial direction, which will also change the COP towards the extended side (Fig. 41.5). The application of a wedge to raise the heel does not appear to change the COP in relation to the ground surface of the foot [4], but it does decrease the horizontal distance between the COP and center of rotation of the distal interphalangeal joint. Although a finite element analysis study suggests that wedging the heels increases the energy stored in the dorsal lamellae [5], this is in contrast to the present author's clinical observations

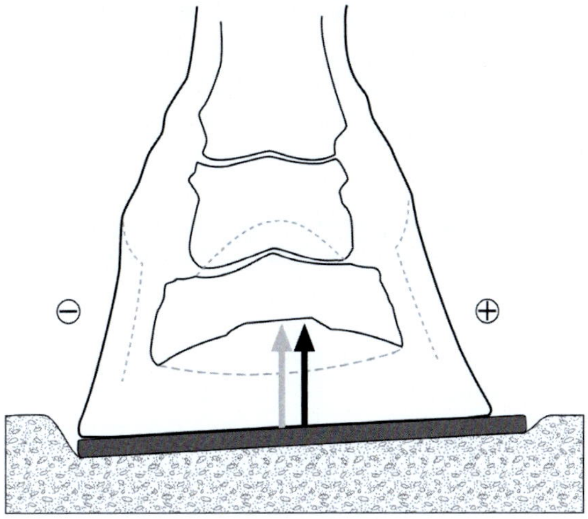

Figure 41.5 The center of pressure can potentially be moved by several therapeutic maneuvers. This schematic depicts the use of an extension on one side of the foot, which acts as a lever when a horse is standing on a deformable surface. The action of the lever is to cause the side with the extension to descend less into the substrate and move the center of pressure to the ipsilateral side. This increases the compression in the wall and the tension in the lamellae of the ipsilateral side while having the opposite effect on the contralateral side. Illustration courtesy of Andrew Parks, University of Georgia, Athens, GA, USA.

which indicate that raising the heels can be a benefit to many horses. Wedging is likely to have an effect regardless of the nature of the ground surface. There are several ways to elevate the heels, including placing a wedge between the shoe and the hoof, incorporating the wedge into the branches of the shoe (graduated branches), or placing rails on the ground surface of the shoe. Elevating the heels with wedge pads is usually done with a full pad that will also distribute some pressure across the entire ground surface of the foot. If shoes that incorporate a wedge through graduated branches or rails to elevate the heels are used without incorporating material (e.g., silicone putty) to distribute force to the frog bars, and sole, two deleterious events will occur: (i) the heels of the shoe may dig deeper into the ground substrate negating the effect of a heel wedge, and (ii) the unsupported solear surface (including the frog) between the bars of the shoe can move/"sink" distally between the branches of the shoe. For these reasons, such shoes are normally used in conjunction with synthetic polymers described above – typically silicone putty or less commonly polyurethane (e.g., pour-in pad) – to fill in any spaces between the solear surface of the foot and the ground surface of the shoe (see Chapter 39). There is also a commercial system of pads that can be used in conjunction with rail shoes,[2] which could just as easily be used with shoes that incorporate graduated branches.

Other methods of moving the COP include using an extension (that is, extending part of the shoe beyond the normal shoe perimeter in the horizontal plane), varying the width of the web

[1] Jorgensen Labs, Loveland, CO. USA.

[2] Equine Digit Support System, Inc., Penrose, CO, USA.

for different parts of the shoe, adding a bar at the heels (straight-bar, heart-bar, egg-bar)/using an open-toed shoe, and partially filling any space between the branches of the shoe with a synthetic polymer (e.g., filling the palmar half of the space between the branches of the shoe increases ground contact palmar to the COP). On a hard, flat surface, all of these latter techniques potentially have no effect on the COP; however, if the horse is standing on a surface that deforms, those parts of the shoe/ground surface of the foot with greatest contact area/furthest from the center of the foot will not sink as far into the substrate, thus acting functionally as a wedge. As noted above, in addition to changing the COP, any modification of the ground surface of the foot that involves a wedge – albeit physical or functional – also changes the moments about the distal interphalangeal joint.

Changing the Moments about the Distal Interphalangeal Joint

Elevating the heels decreases the flexor moment when the foot is bearing weight, as discussed previously. Changing breakover is usually accomplished by rounding or rockering the toe of the shoe (Fig. 41.4), but how effective this is depends on how far the point of breakover is moved in a palmar direction, and how that dorsal point of contact changes as the foot unrolls (the process by which the point of contact of a rolled toe changes between the time the heel lifts off and the toe leaves the ground). There is no well-defined 'best position' for the point of breakover, but it is frequently recommended to put the breakover 0–1 cm dorsal to the dorsal margin of the DP (see below; Radiographic Control of Shoe Placement). The full rocker shoe's ground surface forms a continuous curve such that the point of breakover is immediately dorsal to whatever point on the shoe the horse is resting on; the net result of this is that the point of breakover is functionally further palmar than flat shoes in which the toe has been rounded or rockered. The wooden shoe (see Fig. 41.4f) fits somewhere between a flat steel shoe with a rounded toe and the full rocker shoe, primarily due to the fact that the breakover can be brought further palmar than with a flat steel shoe due to the greater thickness of the wooden shoe.

With regard to unrolling (the pivoting about the most dorsal point (s) of ground contact of the foot during breakover as the heels lift off the ground) for any given initial point of breakover, the thicker the shoe the less the extensor moment arm is likely to change after initial heel lift off. For example, a steel shoe that is 9 mm thick and has a rounded toe is going to have a significantly greater radius of curvature than a wooden shoe that is 30 mm thick with the point of breakover in a comparable location with regards to the center of rotation of the distal interphalangeal joint. This means that the extensor moment arm for the thicker shoe will be shorter (resulting in less stress on the dorsal lamellae) for any comparable degree of heel elevation once the heels have begun to lift off of the ground.

Damping Forces Associated with Impact

Damping the forces associated with impact is readily apparent in horses with acute disease that are placed on compressible/deformable foam (most commonly closed-cell foam) pads; the pads usually result in an immediate improvement in comfort that is visible as the horse moves. Almost all shoes are made of metal, and regardless of whether this is steel or aluminum, they do not yield very much. It is difficult to achieve the same damping of impact with a regular shoe; rim pads may provide some damping, but it is likely minimal in comparison to foam materials. Some plastic shoes are available in a variety of configurations, including normal shape, straight-bar, heart-bar, and open-toed heart-bar. How much the shoe is able to enhance the damping of impact forces is to some extent inversely related to the hardness of the plastic; very hard plastics do not provide very much advantage over metal. In other respects, plastic shoes may be modified in a similar manner to steel shoes, but many of them are designed to be attached to the foot without nails (see below). More recently, shoes made of wood (typically plywood) have become relatively commonplace for the treatment of laminitis. The property of the wood would likely provide a greater damping of impact than metal. One commercially available wooden shoe has a plywood form to which is attached a base made from EVA,[3] a material that is slightly stiffer than most closed-cell foams and appears to offer comparable damping to foam or other materials commonly applied to the ground surface of the foot. The main advantage of this shoe over the direct application of a compressive material to the sole is that, when correctly applied, it avoids sole pressure due to the flat surface of the plywood, while taking advantage of EVA's damping quality.

Methods of Shoe Attachment

Though shoes are routinely attached to the hoof with nails, there are occasions when this is either not possible or not desirable. The principal reasons for attaching a shoe to a foot other than with nails is either because nailing the shoe to the foot is too painful, or because there is insufficient wall into which to drive the nails. The most common alternative to nailing is using glue. Shoes can either be glued on directly, where the glue is placed directly between the shoe and the ground surface of the wall, or the shoe may have a cuff that can be glued to the outer surface of the wall. Direct gluing limits expansion of the foot [6], but a cuffed shoe that is glued only to the wall should in theory restrict movement of the hoof against the adjacent surface of the shoe less than would direct gluing, so that expansion of the foot is theoretically more normal. Although any glue on the wall tends to cause the underlying wall to deteriorate, many horses have been shod in this way for periods of months or years. Due to the possibility of wall deterioration, some clinicians prefer not to glue a shoe on if possible, or to glue the shoes on for the shortest amount of time needed.

Shoes may also be attached with screws, in which case the shoes are almost always made of wood (though metal shoes have been attached with screws). The main advantage of screws is that

[3] Equicast, Southern Pines, NC, USA.

their application is relatively atraumatic compared to nails, and they do not cause the wall to deteriorate compared to glue. When attaching a wooden shoe with screws, the screws are applied through the hoof into the wooden shoe in a proximal-to-distal direction (though many veterinarians/farriers first make glide holes for the screws in a distal-to-proximal direction from the ground surface of the foot to ensure that the holes are in the keratinized horn of the hoof wall).

Lastly, shoes may be attached to the foot with casting material, typically after the shoe has been lightly stabilized in position with screws or tape to stop it shifting as the tape is applied. The casting tape is usually applied around the circumference of the ground surface of the hoof wall such that it covers 2–3 cm of the hoof wall and 2–3 cm of the immediately adjacent sole. At the heels, the casting tape may pass below the heel bulbs or over the top of them. The former is usually done when the tape is used as an adjunct to another form of attachment (e.g., one to two screws per side), and above the heel bulbs when it is the only form of attachment. In the latter instance, the heel bulbs must be protected from developing pressure sores by placing a strip of casting felt over them. Casting tape applied directly to the wall will also cause the quality of the hoof wall horn to deteriorate if it is kept in place for an extended period of time. However, this rarely becomes a problem during the two- to three-month period that is commonly needed for the application of shoes, especially those made from wood.

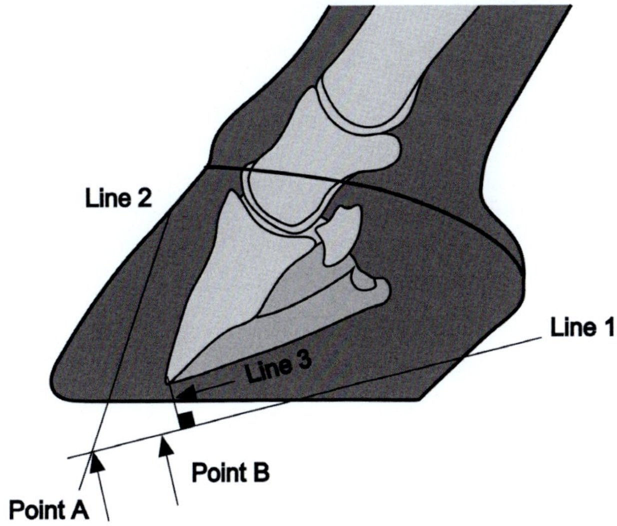

Figure 41.6 Schematic depicting guidelines for trimming a foot with dorsal rotation in preparation for shoeing. The object is to realign the ground surface of the foot with the solear margin of the distal phalanx and appropriately position the shoe in the sagittal plane. First, a line is drawn almost parallel to and 15 mm distal to the solear margin of the distal phalanx (Line 1). A second line is drawn parallel to and approximately 15–18 mm dorsal to the dorsal parietal surface of the distal phalanx. The point of intersection of these two lines (Point A) is the dorsal-most point a shoe should be placed (though it may be positioned in a more palmar position than this). Lastly, a line is drawn perpendicular to Line 1 from the dorsal margin of the distal phalanx to Line 1. This is used a as a guide to position breakover (Point B), typically 5–10 mm dorsal to the intersection of these two lines. Illustration courtesy of Andrew Parks, University of Georgia, Athens, GA, USA.

Radiographic Control of Shoe Placement

Radiography is the only way to definitively determine the position of the shoe in relation to the position of the DP. With practice using radiography, it should in time become possible to place shoes increasingly accurately without radiographic guidance, though this approach is not advised unless the owner cannot afford the cost. Shoe placement itself is subject to some degree of variability depending on clinician/farrier preference, but the following represents reasonable guidelines as a starting place. This description is directed primarily at horses that have dorsal rotation, but the positioning of a shoe (if needed) can be extrapolated for horses with distal displacement. As shown in Figure 41.6, it is first important to determine a plane for trimming the foot to return the solear margin of the DP to a near-normal angle to the ground while maintaining maximal sole depth. Therefore, a line is drawn approximately 15 mm distal and parallel to the solear margin of the DP for the plane of the trim (which may form two planes to the ground surface; see below). A second line is drawn parallel to and 15–18 mm dorsal to the dorsal surface of the DP (see Fig. 41.6). Where these two lines intersect is, in theory, the most dorsal position of the toe of the shoe, though it may well be somewhat palmar to this. Lastly, a line perpendicular to the first line is drawn from the dorsal solear margin of the DP distally to intersect with the first line. This point is used to position the point of breakover which typically is positioned 5–10 mm dorsal to this intersection, though others have positioned it in a more palmar location. Placing a shoe with two nails and then taking a radiograph, followed by repositioning as needed, offers the best approach to optimal shoe positioning.

Treatment Decisions

The most important determinant as to how a horse with displacement of the DP is to be treated is the type of displacement that has occurred, and the three main types will be discussed separately. However, within each pattern of displacement there is great variation that relates to the initial degree of injury to the lamellae duration of the disease, the severity of lameness, and secondary changes that have occurred in both the hoof capsule and the underlying soft tissues and bone. As it is clearly not possible to discuss every scenario, some extrapolation from the following descriptions is inevitably necessary. Additionally, it is common for horses that have displaced very recently to be managed in a similar manner to those that have not displaced. That is, medical management does not change just because a horse has begun to rotate, and the supportive foot care that is usually initiated is continued for a variable time until the foot is perceived as beginning to stabilize before more involved therapeutic shoeing is performed. The medical management and supportive care of these early cases of disease is discussed in Chapters 30–37.

Dorsal Rotation

The biomechanical event underlying the development of rotation of the DP is an imbalance between the extensor and flexor moments about the distal interphalangeal joints. This occurs because the level and distribution of injury to the lamellae has occurred in a manner that causes the flexor moment applied to the DP about the distal interphalangeal joint to exceed the extensor moment applied to the DP. Consequently, rotation of the DP about the distal interphalangeal joint ensues (see Fig. 20.1a). Macroscopically, in horses with dorsal rotation, the greatest injury occurs within the dorsal lamellae. In suspending the DP within the hoof capsule the lamellae are under tension. Any action that increases tension in the compromised lamellae in an unstable foot will tend to exacerbate the injury (i.e., anything that increases the load on the dorsal wall and anything that increases the flexor moment, and vice versa). To address this therapeutically, the flexor moment and the load on the dorsal wall should be minimized.

The objectives of trimming the foot of a horse with rotation of the DP is to realign the solear margin of the DP so that it assumes a normal angle with the ground, typically 3–6°, while preserving the full depth of the sole. The trimming technique is well described in Chapter 38. It is important to preserve as much sole as possible (at least up to a normal thickness) because reducing the thickness likely changes sole function and decreases the capacity of the sole to distribute weight to the wall and thence lamellae, and also increases the likelihood of compression of the soft tissues underlying the sole.

The flexor moment in a horse standing at rest can only be reduced by physically or functionally elevating the heels. The ways to elevate the heels have been described above. It appears counterintuitive to shorten the heels with the trim, only to then elevate them later with a corrective shoe. The rationale for doing so is, however, straightforward; shortening the heels moves the reflection of the wall at the heels in a palmar direction in relation to the center of rotation. Therefore, the application of a wedge after trimming the heels can restore the previous angle of the solear margin with the added benefit of more ground surface palmar to the center of rotation to bear weight. In another simplistic view, trimming the heels restores the normal (close to parallel) relationship of the solear margin of the DP to the sole which, once the heels have been extended/elevated with a wedge to decrease the tension in the deep digital flexor tendon (and hence decrease the flexor moment), decreases the deleterious pressure on the dorsal sole present with DP rotation. There are several measures on clinical examination by which the degree of heel elevation (if any) can be selected (these are discussed in detail in Chapter 38). In the case in which a deep digital flexor tenotomy has also been performed, radiographic assessment of subluxation of the coffin joint – and amelioration of the subluxation with a specific degree of heel wedge – is used to determine the degree of heel elevation needed.

In conjunction with shoeing ± elevating the heels, the ground surface of the foot is frequently packed to fill the space between the branches of the shoe, either completely or selectively with a silastic putty or polyurethane ('pour-in') material to not only provide sole support (possibly decreasing the chance of an unsupported sole 'sinking' between the bars of the shoe in the unstable foot) but also to change force distribution. Completely filling the space between the branches of the shoe distributes force over the entire ground surface of the foot; the larger ground surface area created by filling in the space between the bars of the shoe (vs. only having the bar of the shoes contacting the ground surface) also prevents the shoes from sinking into a soft substrate. However, many horses will not tolerate the additional pressure on the dorsal aspect of the sole, and so frequently only the palmar half of the space between the branches is filled (this may also increase the movement of the COP in a palmar direction, which is a further benefit if heel elevation is desired).

The flexor moment at breakover is reduced by moving the point of breakover in a palmar direction (see Fig. 41.4), and the thicker the shoe the greater the effect (as described above). This causes breakover to occur slightly earlier and lowers the moment arm length at breakover [7]. The latter would be expected to decrease the stresses in the dorsal hoof wall, and therefore presumably the stresses in the dorsal lamellae. In the present author's opinion, an additional advantage of this is that it also enhances sole growth, a phenomenon seen regularly following the application of either full rocker or wooden shoes. The mechanism for the enhanced sole growth is unknown, but it seems likely that the way these shoes roll at breakover decreases the pressure on the dermis of the dorsal sole because reduced pressure on any part of the hoof appears to enhance its growth.

Types of Shoe

In practice, many different shoe types [8] have been used to accomplish these goals, including egg-bar, heart-bar [9], rail shoes (the Equine Digital Support System[4]/4 Point Rail Shoe[5]) [10], full rocker shoes, glue-on cuffs with customizable plates and wedges (Sound Horse Series III[6]), and wooden shoes [11].

Metal Shoes

Flat metal shoes of any configuration may be modified to: (i) incorporate a shortened lever arm at breakover by beveling the toe (subject to limitations of the radius of curvature of the toe of the shoe because of the limited thickness of the metal); (ii) alter the distribution of pressure across any part of the sole by using one of the synthetic polymers between the branches of the shoe; and (iii) provide heel elevation by placing a wedge pad between the shoe and the foot. However, only a modest amount of mediolateral breakover can be incorporated into the shoe.

[4] Equine Digit Support System, Inc., Penrose, CO, USA.
[5] Nanric, Inc., Lawrenceburg, KY, USA.
[6] Sound Horse Technologies, Inc., Unionville, PA, USA.

The Equine Digital Support System (EDSS) and 4 Point Rail Shoe (4PRS)

The Equine Digital Support System (EDSS) and 4 Point Rail Shoe (4PRS) are commercial systems that are currently available and have the breakover built in at the time of manufacture. They both use rails to elevate the heels. Rails are made from narrow wedges of metal or plastic (with the tallest end at the heel of the shoe) that are attached to the inside of the branch of the shoe. As such, they provide heel elevation and a better mediolateral breakover than is feasible with a flat steel shoe. The EDSS is supplied with a series of wedges of different height that are attached to the shoe after it is nailed on. This permits the clinician to adjust the degree of heel elevation based on how the animal moves, both in terms of how it lands and how comfortable it is. The rails of the 4PRS are forged into the shoe and are of a height considered beneficial to the majority of horses by the manufacturer. The rails will sink into a soft substrate and/or the frog will displace distally relative to the heels unless pressure (e.g., via application of putty or a pad) is applied across the palmar structures between the ground surface of the shoe; the EDSS comes supplied with a system of pads to fulfill this function, but silicone putties are probably used more commonly with both systems.

Wooden Shoes

The wooden shoe is a remarkably simple device to build and apply, and seemingly has the biomechanical benefits of most of the other systems combined. It can essentially be built to incorporate whatever biomechanical concepts are desirable. Typically, it is constructed from two pieces of plywood so that it is between 25 and 35 mm thick, depending on the size of the horse, and the toe is beveled 30° and 40° to bring the breakover approximately under the dorsal aspect of the coronet; the sides and back of the shoe are beveled to 45° to provide breakover in other directions. A marked advantage of the wooden shoe is that, because of its thickness, the same angle of beveling which would result in a minor improvement in breakover in a thinner metal shoe will result in a much more marked change in breakover in the wooden shoe. Silicone putty may be placed between the solear surface and the shoe, typically just on the palmar ground surface, to increase weight-bearing by the palmar structures of the foot. Although this method was common during the early use of wooden shoes, many clinicians do not currently use putty with the wooden shoe due to concerns that this may cause undue pressure on the subsolear dermis which has commonly already been compromised by the distally displacing phalanx. The wooden shoe is usually attached with screws; pilot holes may be drilled from the ground surface entering the white line and exiting the outer hoof wall approximately 15 mm proximal to the ground surface. Depending on the number of screws used, it may need reinforcing with a rim cast; the cast encompasses the distal 20–25 mm of the wall and 20 mm of the shoe, and does not cover the heel bulbs. The foot surface of the shoe may be recessed (e.g., using a Dremel tool) to prevent the sole impinging on the wood in horses with solear prolapse, to decrease the pain secondary to sole pressure, particularly if the horse is found to be painful on digital pressure or hoof testers. There may be advantages of the wooden shoe associated with the properties of the wood itself.

Neither rail nor wooden shoes should be seen as a permanent solution, but rather as a means to stabilize the foot before transitioning to a more traditional shoe or to a barefoot state. Therefore, when transitioning back to normal hoof care in a more severely affected horse that initially required: (i) heel elevation, (ii) application of material (e.g., silicone putty) to the ground surface of the foot, and (iii) markedly enhanced breakover, the heel elevation should likely be reduced first (as soon as it is comfortable for the horse to do so), with subsequent removal of the material used to distribute forces across the ground surface of the foot. It is probably advantageous to maintain the horse with an enhanced breakover for a more extended period of time. As mentioned previously, because the variability of presentation is so great, the needs of each horse are somewhat different and should be tailored accordingly. However, the return to as near-normal as possible should be a similar process, but with the two procedures just starting at different points.

Distal Displacement (Symmetrical)

The biomechanical events that underlie symmetrical distal displacement of the DP occur in a manner such that the extensor and flexor moments about the distal interphalangeal joint are both reduced. This allows the balance between them to be maintained, allowing a symmetrical downwards movement of the DP that may occur due to the distribution of damage to the lamellae and or the recruitment of other structures to contribute to these moments. Therefore, there is no discernible benefit in moving the COP in the hope of removing the stresses of the most damaged lamellae and transferring them to other areas, because doing is unlikely to have a protective effect given that the lamellae around the full circumference of the foot are damaged (unless the distal displacement is later accompanied by dorsal rotation). Consequently, there are there are only three main alternative options: (i) to spread the load over a greater area; (ii) to decrease the shock of impact; and (iii) to improve the ease of breakover. Of these three options, the only one that is effective in a stationary horse is to attempt to redistribute the load – that is, to spread the load over more of (if not the entire) the ground surface of the foot, and this is given the previous caveats regarding weight-bearing by the sole. The results of these techniques are highly variable. Some horses with distal displacement are actually more comfortable with a regular shoe on applied because the shoe limits the contact of the sole with the ground (and therefore decreases any pain that would result by applying solear pressure). However, in doing so, the DP may push the sole further and further distally between the branches of the shoe, thus turning a temporary transient increase in comfort into a disastrous overall result. Providing a greater ease of breakover – much as in horses with rotation – will reduce stresses within the dorsal capsule and lamellae. For this reason, wooden shoes are commonly used for horses with distal displacement; however, if the DP continues to displace and cause the sole to contact the wood, the horse is likely to become more painful. Although dremelling out the wood that would contact painful areas of the sole (e.g., the dorsal sole) is commonly performed prior to appication of wooden shoes, the DP may sink into this dremmeled out region resulting in the animal exhibiting more pain when the displaced sole contacts the wooden surface of this dremelled out area.

In addition to these measures, phalangeal casts have also reportedly met with a measure of success (see Chapter 42) [12]. Phalangeal casts can be applied in a manner that distributes load across the bottom of the foot and enhances breakover in any direction. Additionally, it is postulated that the rigidity of the casts limits movement of the hoof capsule, which limits the length to which the lamellae are stretched to make the animal more comfortable.

Asymmetrical Displacement

Asymmetrical (also termed unilateral) distal displacement may occur as a single entity, but it is frequently accompanied by some degree of rotation. On other occasions, it is more a situation of distal displacement on both sides of the foot, except that displacement is more severe on one side. Therefore, whatever measures are most likely to be successful for rotation or symmetrical distal displacement should be incorporated. To address the asymmetrical distal displacement, it is both rational - and seemingly effective in some horses - to move the COP away from the affected/most severely affected side (most commonly the medial side). Although this can be accomplished several by using a wedge to elevate the least/unaffected side, this is difficult to adjust and potentially deleterious. Instead, it is more common to either set the shoe wide or to use a shoe with a wider web on the unaffected/less affected side; this will decrease the pressure on the most severely affected side (and increase it on the less affected side; Fig. 41.5). Typically, an extension of 4–6 mm on the unaffected side seems satisfactory, but results may vary depending on the severity of the injury and the substrate on which the horse is standing.

Conclusions

There seems to be little doubt that over the past twenty-five years, significant gains have been made in treating displacement of the DP. These improvements have come with a myriad of innovative products and techniques, and there is significant anecdotal testimony to their successes, but no controlled studies comparing different techniques. The lack of controlled studies is not surprising given the lack of uniformity of presentation of horses with laminitis, and the difficulty of persuading clinicians to use techniques with which they are less comfortable. It is almost certain that there will always be horses with disease of sufficient severity that no treatment is likely to be successful. Furthermore, there are still very significant gaps in the present understanding of the way in which the foot functions, particularly with respect to the role of the sole in weight-bearing and how the associated forces are transmitted from the ground to the DP. Further improvements will be achieved with greater understanding of foot function, a greater understanding of how the disease process affects the biomechanical properties of the tissues within the foot, and a more biomechanically oriented mindset of clinicians.

References

1. Pollitt, C.C. and Collins, S.N. (2016) The suspensory apparatus of the distal phalanx in normal horses. *Equine Vet. J.*, **48** (4), 496–501.
2. Collins, S.N., van Eps, A.W., Pollitt, C.C., *et al.* (2010) The lamellar wedge. *Vet. Clin. North Am. Equine Pract.*, **26**, 179–195. Available at: http://linkinghub.elsevier.com/retrieve/pii/S0749073910000052.
3. Thomason, J. (0000) Biomechanics of the Equine Foot, in *Equine Podiatry. The hoof as a smart structure: Is it smarter than us?* (eds A. Floyd and R. Mansmann), Elsevier Health Sciences, Philadelphia, PA, pp. 46–56.
4. Rogers, C.W. and Back, W. (2003) Wedge and eggbar shoes change the pressure distribution under the hoof of the forelimb in the square standing horse. *J. Equine Vet. Sci.*, **23**, 306–309.
5. Ramsey, G.D., Hunter, P.J., and Nash, M.P. (2011) The effect of hoof angle variations on dorsal lamellar load in the equine hoof. *Equine Vet. J.*, **43**, 536–542.
6. Yoshihara, E., Takahashi, T., Otsuka, N., *et al.* (2010) Heel movement in horses: comparison between glued and nailed horse shoes at different speeds. *Equine Vet. J.*, **42**, 431–435.
7. van Heel, M.C.V., van Weeren, P.R., and Back, W. (2006) Shoeing sound warmblood horses with a rolled toe optimises hoof-unrollment and lowers peak loading during breakover. *Equine Vet. J.*, **38**, 258–262.
8. Morrison, S. (2004) Foot management. *Clin. Tech. Equine Pract.*, **3**, 71–82.
9. Eustace, R.A. and Caldwell, M.N. (1989) The construction of the heart bar shoe and the technique of dorsal wall resection. *Equine Vet. J.*, **21**, 367–369.
10. Redden, R.F. (1997) Shoeing the laminitic horse. *Proc. Am. Assoc. Equine Pract.*, **43**, 356–359.
11. Steward, M.L. (2010) The use of the wooden shoe (Steward clog) in treating laminitis. *Vet. Clin. North Am. Equine Pract.*, **26**, 207–214.
12. Bras, R.J. (2011) How to use foot casts to manage horses with laminitis and distal displacement secondary to systemic disease. *Am. Assoc. Equine Pract.*, **57**, 415–423.

PART 7

Treatment of the Laminitis Case

Equine Laminitis, First Edition. Edited by James K. Belknap and Raymond Geor.

CHAPTER 42

The Use of Casts in Equine Laminitis

James K. Belknap and Raul J. Bras

Introduction

Reports of the use of cast material for laminitis cases includes both its use only around the hoof capsule itself, and its use in the more traditional coaptation form as either a foot cast (incorporating the pastern region) or half-limb cast. The different cast techniques have been used to treat different stages of laminitis (ranging from acute to chronic cases), and to treat complications such as solear prolapse.

With regards to techniques which incorporate only the hoof capsule itself, the two primary techniques that have been described include one using plaster cast material [1] and the other a combination of fiberglass cast material and impression material on the sole [2]. Whereas the plaster hoof cast was used primarily for acute laminitis cases [1], the fiberglass cast/impression material combination was used more for the chronic case with poor hoof wall integrity and sole bruising [2]. In both descriptions, the caudal aspect of the solear surface is incorporated into the weight-bearing surface using a roll of the plaster in the plaster cast and impression material in the fiberglass cast [1, 2]. In both techniques, it is stated that the palmar angle (e.g., the degree of heel wedging) can be adjusted with the techniques. Additionally, the author of the synthetic cast technique describes the ability of the circumferential cast material to decrease the normal expansion of the hoof wall that occurs with weight-bearing, possibly limiting further damage to the compromised lamellae (the same is likely true when cast material is used to apply a wooden shoe) [2]. Whereas the technique with plaster is described as more of a temporary technique to be used for the first one to three weeks in the acute phase of laminitis [1], the combination of synthetic cast material and impression material can reportedly be left on the foot for one to two months [2].

Few reports exist concerning the use of more traditional casts for external coaptation in the treatment of laminitis; in this chapter, attention will be focused on two types of casts used by the present authors in laminitis cases, namely a half-limb open-sole cast and a specially designed foot cast. The impetus for the use of casts in both techniques was somewhat similar, attempting to neutralize in part the distracting forces on the lamellae caused by: (i) decreasing the downward force of the weight of the horse on the distal phalanx (DP); (ii) decreasing the independent movement of the hoof capsule and bony column; and (iii) stabilizing the hoof capsule (decreasing the normal expansion and contraction that occurs with weight-bearing, as described for the hoof casts above). In addition to addressing these concerns, the cast must also deal with the usual concerns addressed by corrective shoeing in laminitis, including: (i) recruiting the palmar/plantar aspect of the sole and frog to help support the weight of the horse (taking some stress off of the hoof wall/lamellae); and (ii) decreasing the moments around the distal interphalangeal joint to further decrease distractive forces on the dorsal lamellae (see Chapter 5).

Foot Cast

One of the present authors (R.J.B.) has used a modified foot cast to primarily treat acute sepsis-related laminitis (SRL) cases with evidence of distal displacement of the DP (both cases of symmetrical and asymmetrical distal displacement) [3]. As applied (application described below), the foot casts address many of the principles discussed above for shoeing, including decreasing lamellar stress by: (i) incorporation of the sole and frog as weight-bearing entitities while providing cushioning to the solear surface; and (ii) decreasing the moment arms around the distal interphalangeal joint by easing breakover in all directions by beveling the solear surface of the cast. Additionally, the foot cast is likely to decrease lamellar stress and injury by properties not provided by corrective shoeing, including: (i) decreasing independent movement of the bony column and hoof capsule; (ii) decreasing expansion of the hoof capsule with weight-bearing; and (iii) providing some protection from the weight of the horse. One advantage of the foot cast (compared to the half-limb cast) is that it can be applied to two or all four feet, without severe consequences (cast sores, etc.). This is critical in animals with distal displacement of the DP in SRL as all four feet are commonly involved.

Equine Laminitis, First Edition. Edited by James K. Belknap and Raymond Geor.

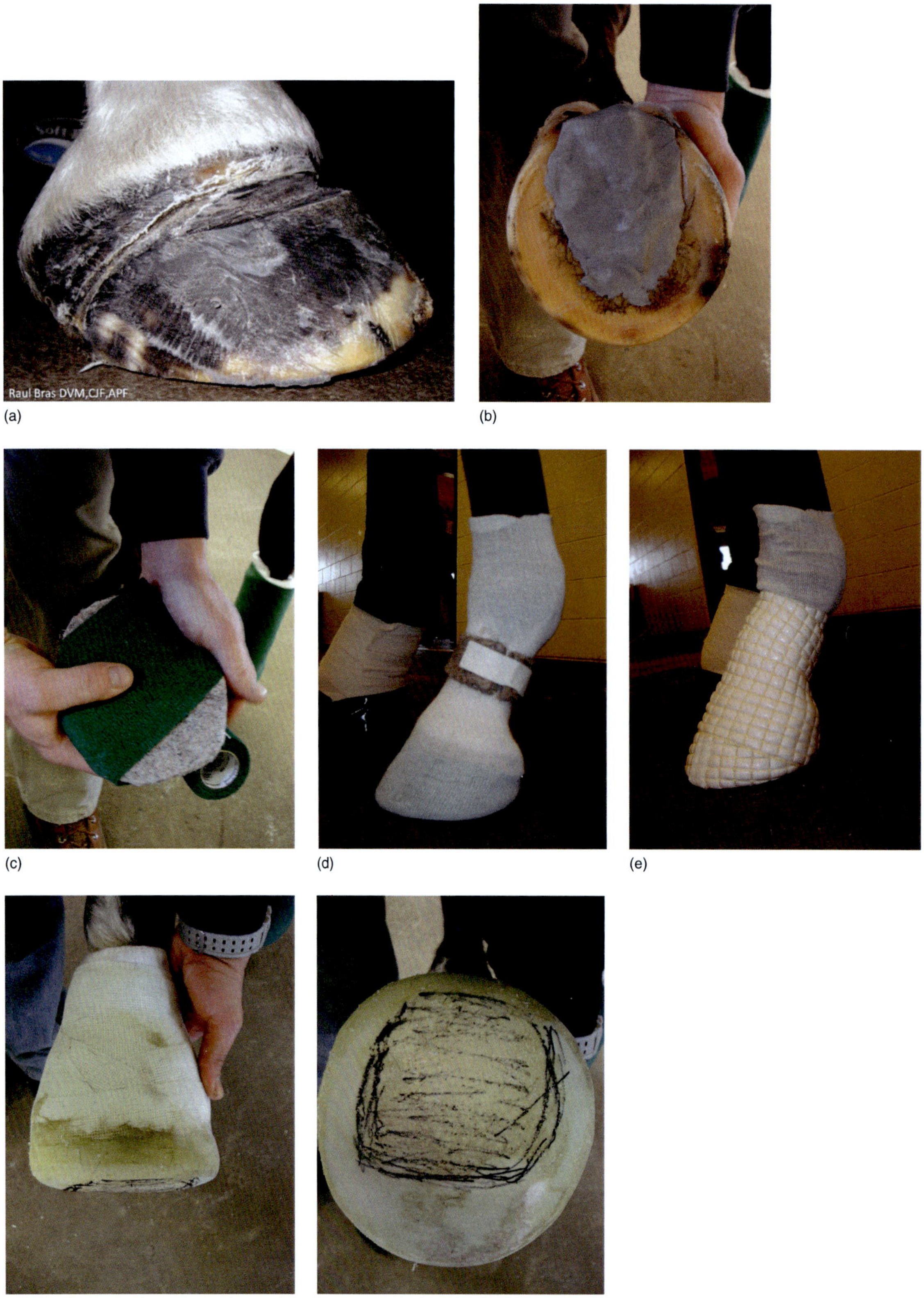

(a) (b) (c) (d) (e) (f) (g)

Figure 42.1 Modified foot cast. After grooving the proximal hoof wall and beveling the distal hoof wall (a), impression material (two parts putty) is placed on the caudal solear surface (b). A layer of felt is then applied to the solear surface (c), followed by stockinette and cast felt applied to the foot and distal limb (d). Cast padding is then applied to the distal limb (e), followed by the application of cast material (f) and methyl methacrylate acrylic (g), molded into a dome-like shape.

Prior to cast application, subcoronary band grooving is performed by the present author (R.J.B.), as is beveling of the entire distal border of the hoof wall (Fig. 42.1a). For application of the cast:

1 Impression material is placed in/over the sulci, frog, and adjacent sole to recruit the caudal surface for weight-bearing (Fig. 42.1b).
2 Felt (0.5-inch; 12 mm) is applied to the sole surface to allow some cushioning of the sole (Fig. 42.1c).
3 Stockinette and cast padding are applied as normally performed for a foot cast (Fig. 42.1d), followed by the application of cast padding around the entire distal limb (Fig. 42.1e).
4 Fiberglass cast material (ca. three rolls) is applied as normally performed for a foot cast (Fig. 42.1f), and the cast is placed on a flat surface with the animal weight-bearing to allow the cast to cure in the correct conformation for the limb. Methyl methacrylate (ca. 5 oz; 150 g) is applied to the solear surface to make a dome-like contour (beveled on all sides) (Fig. 42.1g).

In a study of 43 horses (most of which were suffering from SRL) with asymmetrical or symmetrical distal displacement in which the foot casts were applied (26 forelimbs only, 17 all four feet), the overall survival rate was 47% [3]. In addition to the distal displacement already present at the time of foot cast

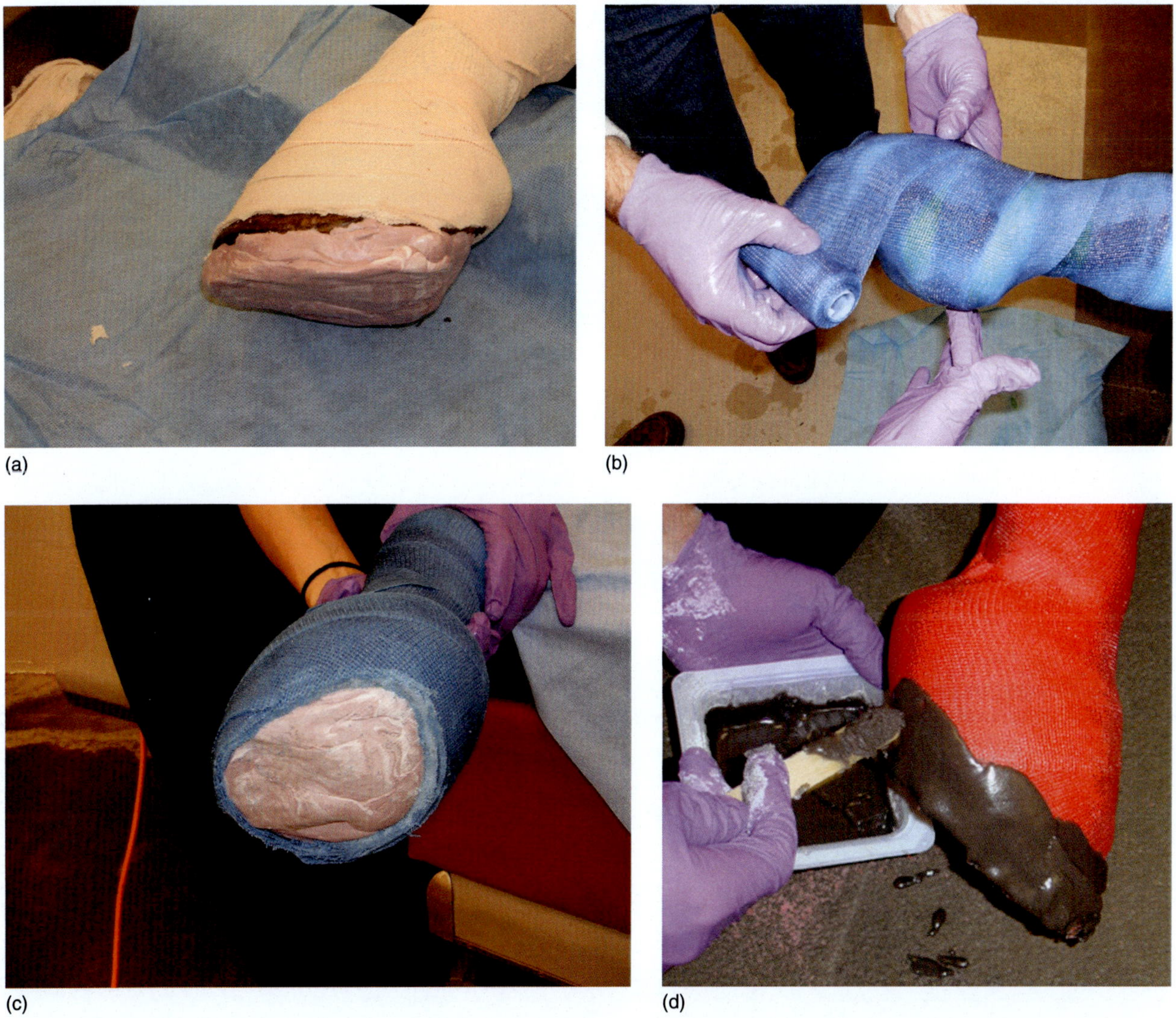

Figure 42.2 Open-sole cast. Stockinette is applied from the foot to the distal carpus; after application of cast felt at the proximal metacarpus, the stockinette is cut from the sole and adhered to the hoof wall with adhesive tape (a). Approximately 2.5–4 cm of impression/cushion support material is applied to the entire solear surface (a), followed by the application of a half-limb fiberglass cast (b). The bottom of the cast is removed with a cast saw to make a rim of cast material even with (or slightly proximal to) the ground surface of the impression material (c). Acrylic is applied to the distal 5–6 cm of the cast material to strengthen the rim (d), and impression material is removed from areas needing ongoing therapy or to protect from solear pressure (e). The cast commonly allows the full use of a limb (f) that is too painful to place weight on without the cast.

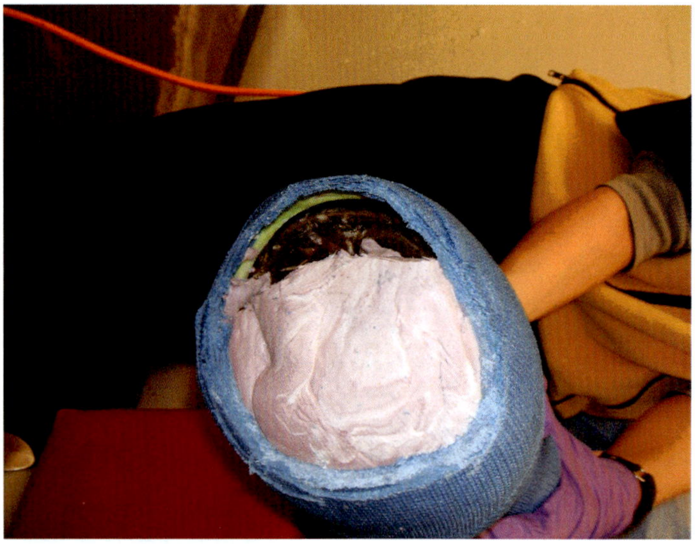
(e)

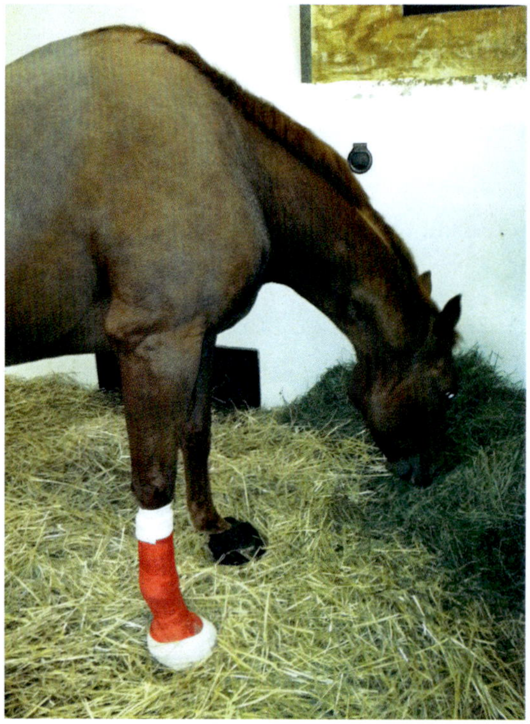
(f)

Figure 42.2 (*Continued*)

application, approximately half of the animals ($n = 23$) developed marked capsular rotation while either in the cast or after cast removal, and 13 of these horses were treated with deep digital flexor tenotomy after the casts were removed.

Open-sole Cast

The open-sole cast is a half-limb cast which provides support for the distal limb while allowing ongoing treatment of the solear surface. Although the open-sole cast has been used bilaterally in laminitis cases, it has primarily been used by the present author (J.K.B.) in chronic laminitis cases in which the animal has become severely lame in one forelimb due to complications that included subsolear sepsis and solear prolapse/perforation [4]. The urgency in this scenario is that the excess weight being borne by the opposite foot (which also is usually affected by chronic laminitis) is likely to re-exacerbate lamellar injury/instability in that foot. The main goal of the cast in these cases is to increase comfort/weight-bearing on the severely lame limb while still allowing access to the sole to treat the complication (e.g., lavaging an abscess [see Fig. 45.2 in Chapter 45]). In order to provide solear support, impression material is used in those areas of the sole not affected by the complication (i.e., the palmar half to two-thirds of the foot in animals with solear prolapse at the dorsal aspect of the sole). The technique has been modified since that previously described [4], primarily to address some problems with cast wall failure when using that technique. The technique is currently used as follows:

1. A stockinette is applied to the limb as normal for a half-limb cast, with cast felt applied tightly to the proximal metacarpus, as performed routinely for half-limb casts. The stockinette is removed from the solear surface of the foot, and elastic adhesive bandage material is applied to adhere the stockinette to the hoof (Fig. 42.2a). Cast padding can be applied to the coronary band and/or fetlock region.
2. Impression material (two parts acrylic putty) is applied to the entire solear surface of the foot to make a pad approximately 1–1.5 inches (2.5–3.8 cm) thick, ensuring that the pad is slightly wider than the solear hoof wall around the circumference of the digit (to reduce the purchase of the cast material on the distal hoof wall in an attempt to transfer more stress away from the hoof wall and lamellae; Fig. 42.2a). The impression material/pad will be cut out later from the areas of the sole in which the clinician either does not want solear pressure, wants access to the sole, or, commonly, both. Once hardened, the pad is taped to the hoof wall with two to three wraps of elastic adhesive bandage (this also creates some distance between the hoof wall and cast material in an attempt to transfer more stress away from the hoof wall and onto to the 'rim' of the cast material).
3. Fiberglass cast tape (4- to 5-inch rolls) is applied to the limb as normally performed for a half-limb cast, except that the

clinician needs to ensure that at least four to five layers of cast material cover the distal hoof wall and the solear impression material (Fig. 42.2b; this will be the wall of the cast that takes a great deal of the stress once the cast material covering the solear surface is removed).

4 When hardened, the ground surface of the cast material is removed with a cast saw to the level of the impression material pad, creating a 'rim' around the digit that extends 2–3 cm distal to the solear surface of the foot (and is even with ground surface of the impression material; Fig. 42.2c). Commercial acrylic resin (e.g., methyl methacrylate) is then applied to the 'rim' from the middle of the hoof wall to the ground surface of the cast (Fig. 42.2d) to provide ample strength to the rim of cast material so that it will not collapse.

5 The impression material is cut out from the areas in which the clinician does not want pressure (i.e., the dorsal aspect of the sole; Fig. 42.2e), but is left in as large an area as possible to support the digit.

The use of these casts can have dramatic immediate effects; the patient in Figure 42.2e was non-weight-bearing in the casted limb prior to cast application due to an acute perforation of the sole by the DP. In other horses, the response may be slower, depending on the severity of the laminitis or complication (e.g., sepsis). However, owners need to be warned that some horses do not tolerate the casts well, with a small number appearing to become more painful in the casts. Cast sores appear to occur more frequently with this type of cast than traditional half-limb casts, most likely due to more movement of the limb caused by the resilient putty on the ground surface instead of firm cast material. Although these sores are usually minor, the owner should be informed of this possibility. An increase in the severity of cast sores has been noted when casts are applied bilaterally, except when used in small horses [4]. To avoid cast sores, the present author (J.K.B.) has, in smaller horses, used the same type of open-sole cast with a half-limb bandage underneath the cast material from the coronary band proximally. Although this does appear to limit the incidence of cast sores, it does not seem to provide the same amount of relief to the digit as a regular open-sole cast.

Half-limb transfixation pin casts have been infrequently used to treat severe cases of laminitis; the more invasive nature of the technique and the complications (e.g., pin loosening prior to the healing of the foot and catastrophic fracture of a third metacarpus/metatarsus through the pin holes) are likely the reasons that this technique is not more commonly employed in laminitis cases [2].

References

1. Castelijns, H.H. (2008) How to apply a (plaster) cast in cases of acute laminitis. *Proc. Am. Assoc. Equine Pract.*, **54**, 225–227.
2. Hunt, R.J. and Werner, H.W. (2008) Equine laminitis: practical clinical considerations. *Proc. Am. Assoc. Equine Pract.*, **54**, 347–353.
3. Bras, R.J. (2011) How to use foot casts to manage horses with laminitis and distal phalanx displacement secondary to systemic disease. *Proc. Am. Assoc. Equine Pract.*, **57**, 415–423.
4. Belknap, J.K. and Gomez, J. (2008) How to use an open-sole cast in cases of laminitis. *Proc. Am. Assoc. Equine Pract.*, **54**, 219–224.

CHAPTER 43

Deep Digital Flexor Tenotomy

R. Wayne Waguespack, Jr

Introduction

Laminitis is a common and often debilitating cause of lameness in the horse, characterized by compromise to the lamellar tissue that acts as a suspensory apparatus between the distal phalanx (DP) and hoof capsule [1]. The objectives of treatment are to alleviate pain, to establish a more normal relationship between the DP and the hoof capsule, and to prevent further alterations in the orientation of the DP within the hoof capsule (e.g., rotation or distal displacement). Treatment options include the use of pharmaceutical agents, cryotherapy, corrective hoof trimming and shoeing, and tenotomy of the deep digital flexor tendon (DDFT) [2–6]. Despite the variety of available therapies, the treatment of refractory acute and chronic laminitis can be challenging.

The purpose of the DDFT tenotomy procedure as a surgical treatment for laminitis is to reduce the forces responsible for distopalmar (or distoplantar) rotation of the dorsodistal aspect of the DP and to attenuate the pain associated with lamellar separation. The proximopalmar traction of the DDFT on the DP exerts shearing forces on the dorsal lamellae that form the attachment between the DP and the hoof capsule. These forces, combined with the weight of the horse (and possibly the solear conformation acting as a fulcrum), are responsible for the separation of the digital lamellae and subsequent distraction of the DP from the hoof capsule in a laminitic foot [2,7,8]. By transecting the DDFT, the pull of the tendon – and therefore the forces that favor separation of the lamellae – are reduced. In addition, there is a reduction in pressure of the DP on the sole corium[2]. The final benefit, and the primary reason the procedure is performed, is the ability to aggressively perform corrective trimming (e.g., 'derotation') in the case of rotational displacement of the DP.

No clear guidelines dictate when and if this surgery should be performed. Although DDFT tenotomies were commonly performed in acute cases of laminitis during the 1980s, reports of poor results with the surgery have resulted in DDFT tenotomy being reserved as somewhat of a 'last-ditch' therapy for horses with severe refractory acute laminitis which are not responding to medical therapy and/or corrective farriery in the chronic case of laminitis. The surgery is currently most commonly being performed in chronic laminitis cases in which some lamellar stability has been re-established, but therapeutic farriery has not been successful in treating rotational displacement (usually phalangeal rotation) of the DP. Radiographs provide vital information for making the decision for performing the surgery. One report recommends a DDF tenotomy if a horse is presented with less than 10 mm of sole depth at the apex of the third phalanx and/or has greater than 15° of palmar angle to help restore realignment and perfusion of the digit [9]. Some clinicians use digital venograms to assist in their decision on whether or not to perform DDFT tenotomy. Venograms of the digit are performed by some clinicians to help determine the degree of vascular compromise, more specifically the submural lamellar circulation, coronary perfusion, and solear circulation [10] (as described in detail in Chapter 27). In the present author's opinion, if a veterinarian is questioning whether or not a DDF tenotomy would benefit a case based on survey radiographs, a venogram may be helpful in the decision-making by providing information regarding perfusion deficiencies not identifiable by other means.

Once the decision is made, a DDFT tenotomy may be performed either at the level of the mid-metacarpus or the proximal interphalangeal (PIP) joint [2, 3]. In the original description of the DDFT tenotomy, a 3-cm vertical incision is made on the palmar aspect of the flexor tendon sheath at the level of the PIP joint [2]. The surgery is performed with the horse under general anesthesia and with the limb surgically prepared and draped to maintain a sterile environment [2]. Subsequently, a DDFT tenotomy procedure was developed in which the surgery is performed at the level of the mid-metacarpus with the horse standing [3]. Due to the ease of performing the procedure at the mid-metacarpus, the potential increase in complications (i.e., increased instability/subluxation of the distal interphalangeal [DIP] joint) when the procedure is performed more distally at the level of the PIP joint, and the lack of need for general anesthesia, the mid-metacarpal tenotomy has been widely adopted as the best technique for performing tenotomies for the first time in the laminitic horse. However, the option of performing the tenotomy at the level of the PIP joint becomes an important option if DDFT tenotomy needs to be repeated with the

Equine Laminitis, First Edition. Edited by James K. Belknap and Raymond Geor.

recurrence of clinical signs following a tenotomy performed at mid-metacarpus. Although some clinicians will perform a second tenotomy in the mid-metacarpal region slightly distal to the original surgery, repeating the mid-metacarpal DDF tenotomy can be difficult due to significant scarring that occurs in response to the initial procedure. The presence of this scar tissue may make it difficult to identify the landmarks used to identify the DDFT, thereby resulting in inadvertent damage to surrounding soft tissue structures [3]. In addition, a greater separation between the tendon ends can be achieved after tenotomy at the level of the PIP joint because of the lack of attachments within the flexor tendon sheath, while separation after mid-metacarpal tenotomy is limited by peritendinous attachments to subcutaneous tissue [8]. Consequently, there are circumstances in which it is advantageous to perform the DDFT tenotomy at the level of the PIP joint if it needs to be repeated. Because many refractory laminitis cases are managed on the farm or already have been discharged from the veterinary hospital when a second tenotomy is required, the ability to perform a standing DDF tenotomy at the level of the PIP joint is beneficial in some cases. With this in mind, a standing mid-pastern DDF tenotomy has been described [11] in which the surgery allows a second transection of the DDFT in a location with normal anatomical landmarks, eliminates the need for general anesthesia, reduces the cost of the procedure, and bypasses the potential stress associated with transporting the horse to a veterinary hospital.

Mid-Metacarpal DDF Tenotomy

DDF tenotomy at the level of the mid-metacarpal region was originally described by Hunt *et al.* [3]. All procedures are performed standing with the horse sedated (i.e., using xylazine or detomidine, or one of these combined with butorphanol). The surgical site is locally anesthetized with a high palmar nerve block, commonly combined with the infiltration of mepivacaine HCl immediately proximal to the surgical site in somewhat of a ring block fashion to ensure total anesthesia of the cutaneous innervation. After routine clipping and aseptic preparation around the entire limb from distal carpus to the level of the fetlock, a vertical skin incision is made between the superficial digital flexor and DDF tendon in the middle one-third of the metacarpal region to allow transection immediately distal to the insertion of the check ligament on the lateral aspect of the limb. The paratenon is opened bluntly with a pair of mosquito hemostatic forceps. This opening is extended with sharp dissection using Metzenbaum scissors to end with a 2- to 3-cm incision in the paratenon. Two "tunnels" are created: one tunnel between DDFT and the superficial digital flexor tendon (SDFT), and the second tunnel between the DDFT (palmarly/plantarly) and neurovascular bundles/suspensory ligament (dorsally), mainly to separate the neurovascular bundles from the DDFT. Once the DDFT is isolated, either a guarded, single-edge, straight (or curved) tendon bistoury can be introduced, or two sterile broad-blade butter knives with curved tips, are inserted into the tunnels [3, 12]. Transection of the DDFT immediately distal to the inferior check ligament will allow the procedure to be repeated in a slightly more distal location (proximal to the tendon sheath palmar to the fetlock) if excessive scar tissue does not limit access to the DDFT.

If the veterinarian is utilizing a tendon bistoury, it is introduced between the SDFT and the DDFT. The bistoury is then rotated 90° so its cutting edge encounters the palmar aspect of the DDFT (Fig. 43.1). The tendon is transected by applying dorsal pressure and using a fine sawing motion. Prior to insertion of the bistoury knife, some surgeons insert a hemostat immediately dorsal to the DDFT, palpating to ensure that both neurovascular bundles are dorsal to the hemostat to protect these structures from inadvertent transection during the tenotomy. After transection, the tendon ends immediately retract approximately 2 cm. The paratenon is closed routinely using a simple continuous appositional suture pattern, while the skin is closed with a simple interrupted or horizontal mattress pattern (some clinicians only perform a skin closure).

If the curved butter knife technique is selected, the paired sterile broad-blade butter knives, with their tips curved, are inserted into the tunnels created between the DDFT and SDFT and the DDFT and neurovascular bundle/suspensory ligament. The handles are then separated from each other to form a 'V' shape. With the curved tips pointing toward each other, the butter knife tips isolate the DDFT, a #10 scalpel blade is inserted between the knives perpendicular to the DDFT and the tendon is transected [12] (Fig. 43.2). Prior to transection of the tendon, light overlapping of the curved portion of each knife deep to the DDFT protects the soft tissues and, with moderate tension, can bring the DDFT to the level of the incision. This can make transecting the tendon straight forward while minimizing any potential for iatrogenic trauma to surrounding soft tissues. The paratenon and skin are closed as previously described for the tendon bistoury technique.

Mid-Pastern DDFT Tenotomy

A DDFT tenotomy at the level of the PIP joint can be performed either under general anesthesia or, as recently described, with the horse standing [2, 11]. For the original description by Allen *et al.*, the horse is placed in lateral recumbency under general anesthesia. A 3-cm incision is made in the skin on the midline of the palmar aspect of the pastern, beginning 1 cm proximal to the heel bulbs and extending proximally (Fig. 43.3a). Dissection is continued through the subcutaneous tissue to expose the digital flexor tendon sheath, which is then incised along the same plane as the skin incision to expose the DDFT (Fig. 43.3b). Curved forceps are placed under the tendon to protect the surrounding soft tissue structures (Fig. 43.3c). Once the DDFT is isolated, it is usually transected with a scalpel. The surgical site is closed in three layers: the tendon sheath, subcutaneous tissue, and skin.

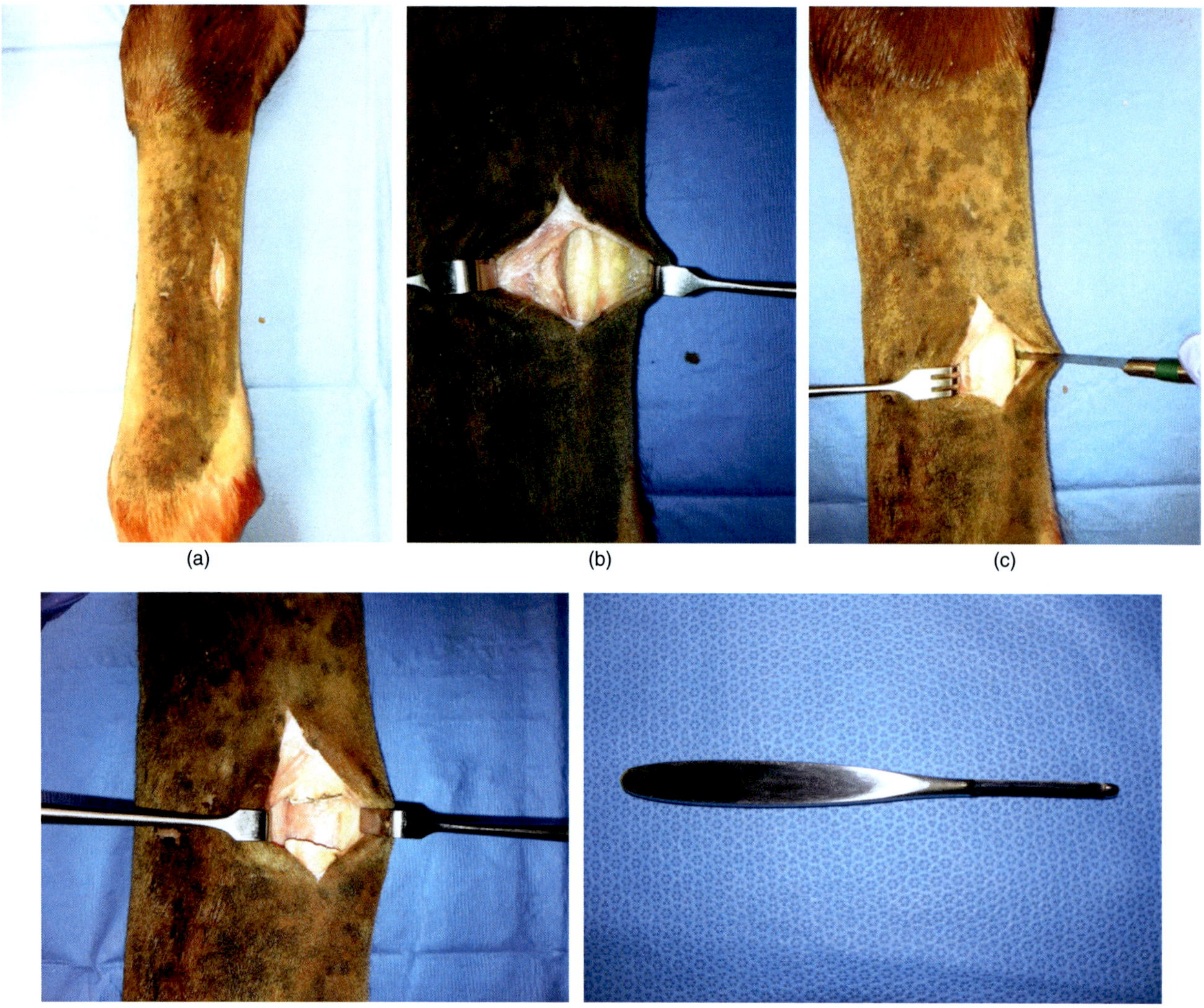

(a) (b) (c) (d) (e)

Figure 43.1 A mid-metacarpal deep digital flexor tendon (DDFT) tenotomy. (a) The mid-metacarpal incision to expose the paratenon. (b) Dissection planes isolating the DDF tendon. (c) The tendon bistoury is introduced between the superficial digital flexor tendon (SDFT) and DDF tendon. (d) A 2-cm release of the DDFT after successful transection. (e) An example of the tendon bistoury used to perform the DDF tenotomy.

The tendon sheath, as well as the subcutaneous tissue, is closed with a simple continuous appositional suture pattern, while the skin is closed in an interrupted appositional suture pattern.

For the standing procedure, the horse is sedated with detomidine HCl (0.02 mg kg^{-1}, intravenous), and an abaxial sesamoid nerve block is performed by injecting 3 ml of mepivacaine HCl over each palmar digital nerve. The skin is clipped circumferentially from just proximal to the abaxial sesamoid bones to the coronary band, and aseptically prepared. The limb is held in flexion by an assistant or the veterinarian performing the procedure; the nonholding hand is kept sterile to perform the procedure (Fig. 43.4).

The distal limb is flexed, and the DDFT is palpated within the flexor tendon sheath immediately proximal to the collateral cartilage. A 1-cm incision is made between the lateral branch of the SDFT and the DDFT on the palmar aspect of the limb, just proximal to the collateral cartilage (Fig. 43.5). Using a Kelly hemostatic forceps, blunt dissection is then used to enter the flexor tendon sheath. With the distal limb flexed, a straight bistoury knife is introduced into the flexor tendon sheath. Then, following placement of the bistoury knife with the side of the knife lying flat between the dorsal surface of the DDFT and the interior aspect of the flexor tendon sheath, the end of the knife is palpated through the skin to ascertain its correct position deep to the DDFT. The cutting edge of the bistoury knife is then rotated 90° to face palmarly to engage the dorsal aspect of the DDFT (Fig. 43.6). The distal limb is then extended and the DDFT transected, with transection of the tendon being confirmed by digital palpation. The skin incision is closed using a simple interrupted appositional suture pattern. The skin closure can be performed either with the limb being held by an assistant, or with the horse standing.

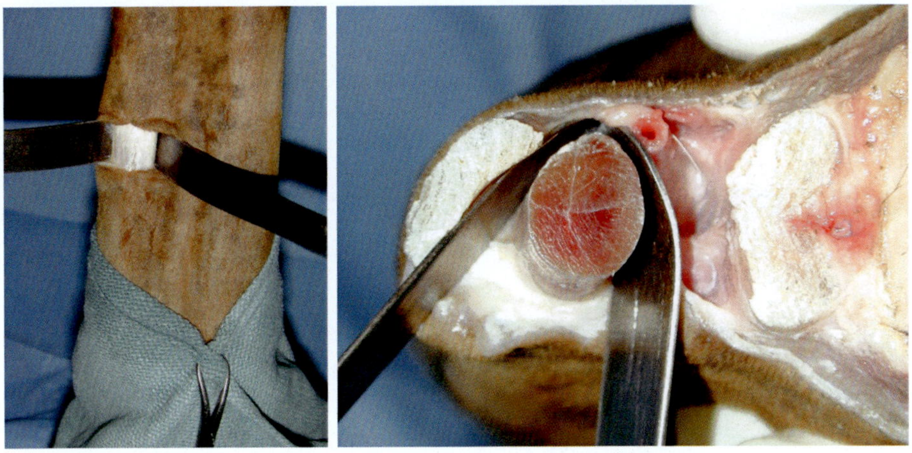

(a) (b)

Figure 43.2 (a) The curved butter knife technique and use of the paired butter knives to isolate the DDF tendon. (b) A cross-sectional image of how, prior to transection of the tendon, light overlapping of the curved portion of each knife deep to the DDF tendon protects the soft tissues. Illustrations courtesy of Daniel Burba.

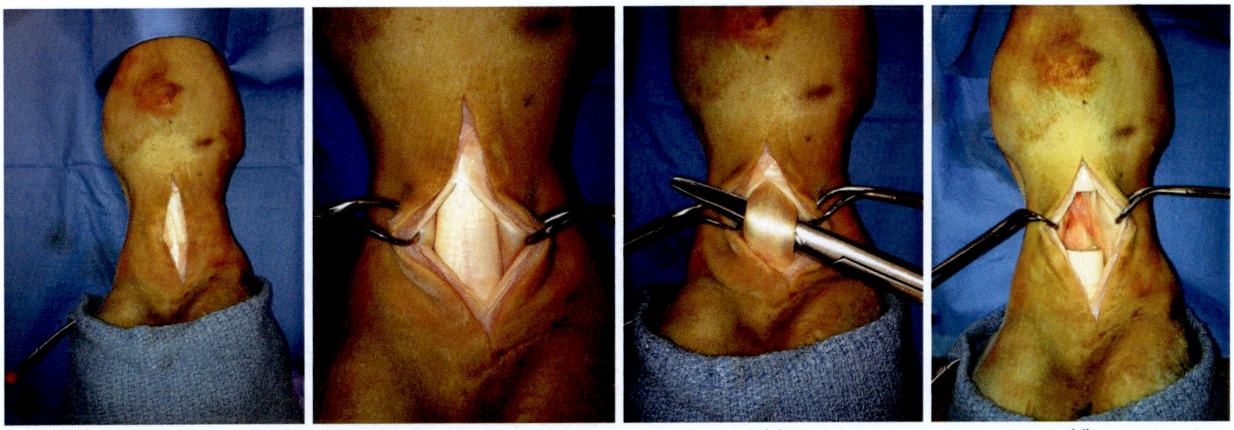

(a) (b) (c) (d)

Figure 43.3 (a) The 3-cm incision which is made for the mid-pastern approach to the DDF tendon on the palmar aspect of the pastern, beginning 1 cm proximal to the collateral cartilage and extending proximally. (b) The sheath is incised along the same plane as the skin incision to expose the DDFT. (c) An example of how a curved instrument is placed under the tendon to protect the surrounding soft tissue structures during sharp transection. (d) The 6–10 cm of release that can be achieved when the DDF tendon is transected at level of the pastern.

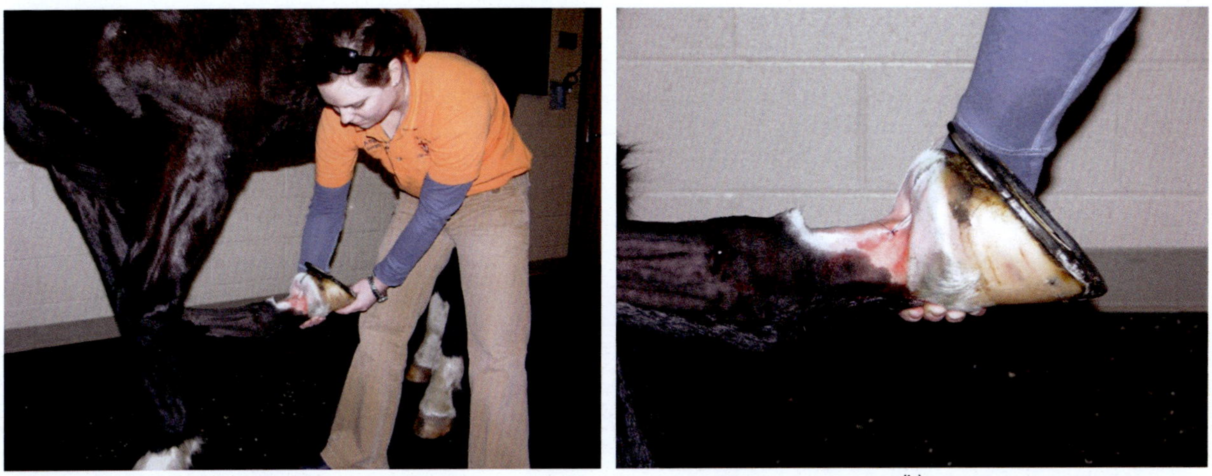

(a) (b)

Figure 43.4 (a) An assistant holding the limb in flexion during surgery. (b) The modified DDF tenotomy can be performed with either an assistant or the individual performing the procedure holding the limb during surgery.

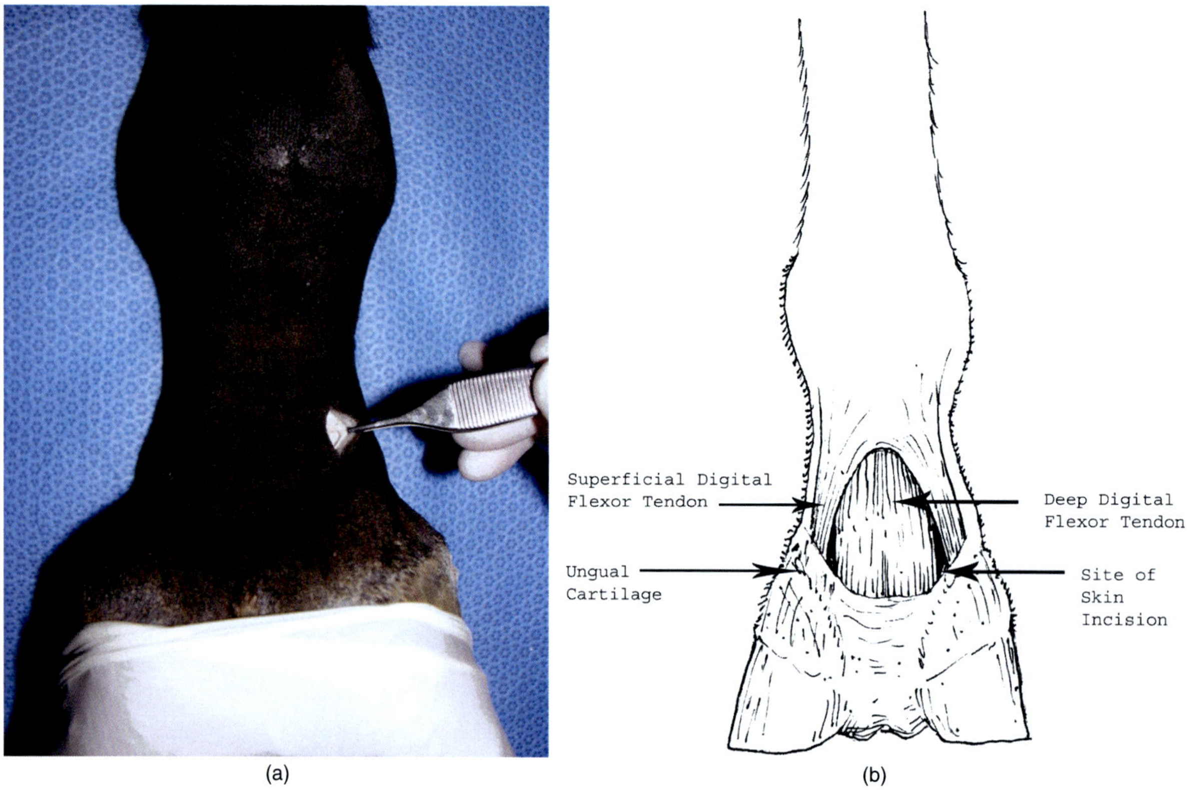

Figure 43.5 (a) The 1-cm incision that is made between the lateral branch of the superficial digital flexor tendon and the DDF tendon on the palmar aspect of the limb, just proximal to the collateral cartilage. (b) Sketch of the palmar surface of the digit, showing the anatomical landmarks for the modified standing DDF tenotomy procedure.

Postoperative Care

After DDF tenotomy, the limbs should be bandaged with a cotton support wrap to support the soft tissue structures of the distal limb and minimize swelling for a minimum of 8–12 weeks, with the horse confined to a stall for that entire period of time. This length of stall rest and support bandage is critical to decrease the degree of scarring when the procedure is performed at mid-metacarpus. As the majority of horses requiring this procedure are already confined to a stall or similar area due to the stage and severity of the disease that they are experiencing at the time, this is usually not a stressful situation for the owner or the animal. One author recommends that horses undergoing DDFT tenotomy should not have significant turnout for a minimum of six months [13].

Two significant concerns may be associated with the DDFT tenotomy techniques. The first of these is the fact that horses undergoing a DDF tenotomy can develop subluxation of the DIP joint (Fig. 43.7). Distal interphalangeal joint subluxation can be a critical issue to address during the first year after surgery, as it can result in significant lameness in the short term and degenerative joint disease of the DIP joint in the long term. Although one early study reported that spontaneous resolution of the DIP subluxation may occur six to eight weeks after DDFT tenotomy [2], most clinicians currently address DIP subluxation more aggressively, especially when the tenotomy is performed at the level of the mid-pastern as DIP subluxation is more exacerbated with this approach. Part of the reason for the greater impact on subluxation may be that an intact DDFT at the level of the distal limb provides stability to the caudal aspect of the DIP joint. The previously reported increased degree of tension release after the mid-pastern procedure compared with the mid-metacarpal technique is likely to play a major role in the increased subluxation (the mid-pastern technique reportedly provides 6–10 cm of release, while the mid-cannon procedure releases the tendon approximately 2 cm) [8]. In one of the present author's studies it was shown ultrasonographically that a mean separation of tendon ends of 10.7 ± 1.74 cm occurs after the modified standing mid-pastern DDF tenotomy [11]. Thus, transection of the DDFT at the mid-pastern level is usually considered by most surgeons to cause more instability than transection at the mid-metacarpus. It is recommended in some reports to apply an extended heel shoe before or after the procedure [11,14]. However, the addition of heel wedges is commonly sufficient by increasing the caudal support of the DIP joint and returning the middle and distal phalanges into alignment [8]. Although it has recently been stated that a 3° wedge is appropriate for most animals after DDF tenotomy, the present author

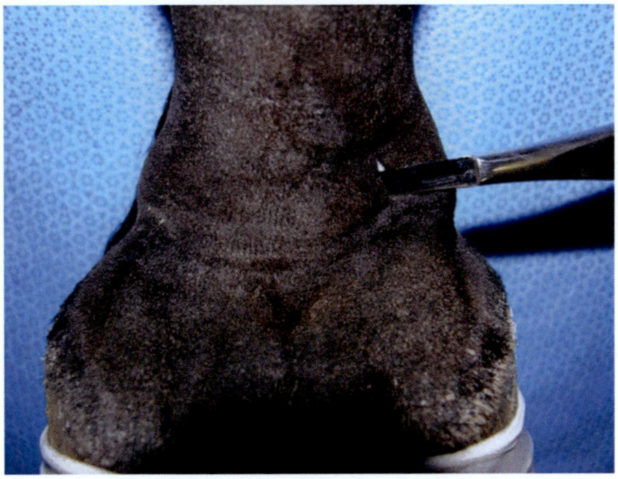

(a)

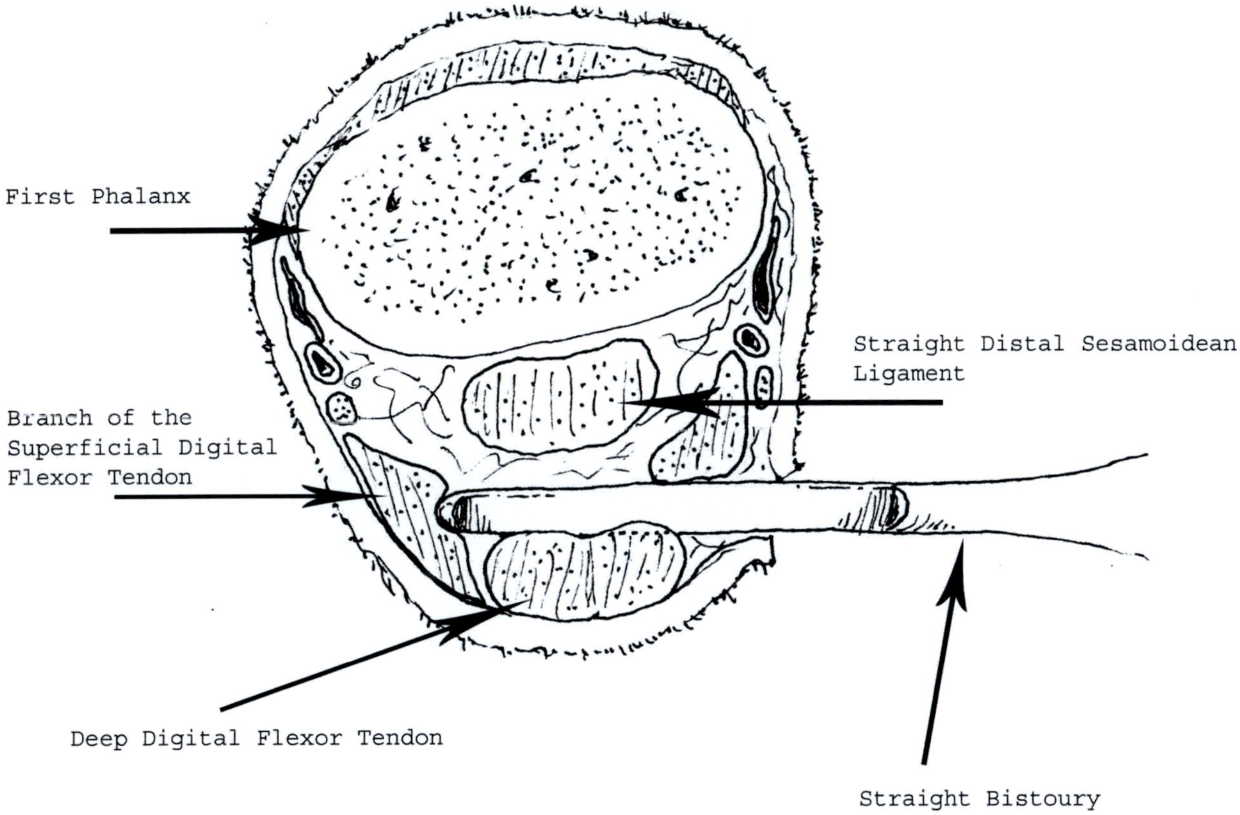

(b)

Figure 43.6 (a) Placement of the bistoury with the side of the knife lying flat between the DDF tendon and the interior aspect of the flexor tendon sheath. The end of the knife is palpated through the skin to ascertain its correct position deep to the DDF tendon. (b) Sketch of the cutting edge of the bistoury knife as it is turned in an outward direction to engage the DDF tendon.

finds that the degree of wedging needed is different for different animals. For that reason, it is probably best to shoe the animal immediately subsequent to the surgery, and to use concurrent radiographic assessment to determine the appropriate degree of elevation for each individual animal. Although it may seem counterintuitive to wedge the heel to counteract subluxation after lowering the heel by trimming, the relationship between the DP and the solear surface is changed by the combination of therapeutic trimming and DDF tenotomy. Finally, subluxation does not always occur when the surgery is performed on animals with chronic rotation of the DP. The aim should be to provide only the amount of wedging needed to limit subluxation,

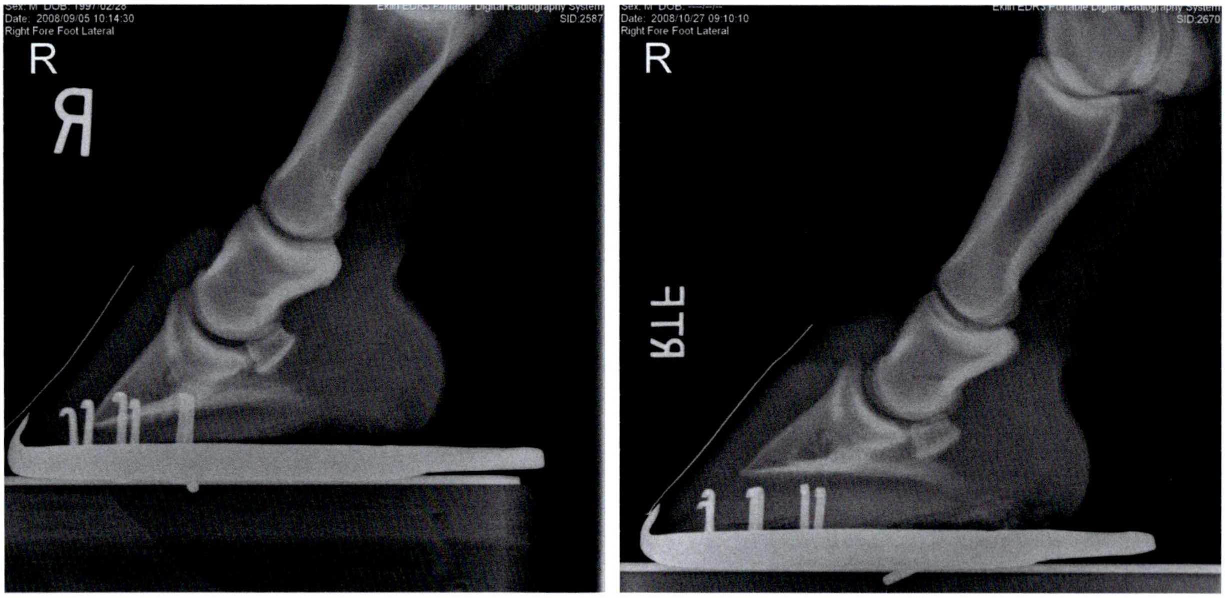

(a) (b)

Figure 43.7 Lateromedial radiographs demonstrating subluxation of the distal interphalangeal joint following DDF tenotomy. (a) The horse's boney column alignment prior to surgery. (b) Radiograph taken after the tenotomy in the same horse, showing evidence of palmar displacement of the distal aspect of middle phalanx, a negative palmar angle of the distal phalanx, and widening of the dorsal aspect of the distal interphalangeal joint space. These are all findings indicative of subluxation of the distal interphalangeal joint.

while allowing maximal separation of the tendon ends before firm adhesions form to the surrounding structures. Regardless of the type of shoeing used after the DDF tenotomy, it is essential that the DP be 'derotated' aggressively by removing as much heel as needed to obtain a normal palmar angle for the DP and return the relationship between the DP and the sole to a more normal orientation. In some animals, derotation cannot be accomplished by only trimming of the heel due to the severity of the rotational displacement. In these cases, the veterinarian and farrier need to decide whether it may be appropriate to apply a reverse wedge to obtain the normal angle; this cannot usually be done in the animal with substantial subluxation postoperatively, as the reverse wedge will usually worsen the subluxation. The other choice is to perform the first reshoeing earlier than normal (approximately three to four weeks) to allow more heel to be removed prior to the establishment of strong adhesions between the severed ends of DDF tendon and surrounding structures. The veterinarian and farrier should re-examine and reshoe the horse at approximately four- to six-week intervals. Corrective shoeing will need to be performed for approximately one year, with radiographic assessments at least every two to three shoeing cycles to address the degree of DIP joint subluxation and the orientation of the DP in relation to the hoof capsule. Realignment of the DP while addressing subluxation after a tenotomy is the most important aspect of this whole clinical process.

The second concern is associated with tenotomy at the level of the mid-pastern. With this procedure, the synovial sheath is entered at the time of surgery. Contamination of the surgical site could lead to sepsis of the flexor tendon sheath. With the traditional open approach described by Allen *et al.*, the limb is aseptically prepared and draped prior to surgery to minimize the potential for contamination. The minimally invasive nature of the modified standing technique may reduce the chance of contamination at the surgical site, as no horses developed infection of the tendon sheath or incision in the study by Waguespack *et al.* [11]

Lastly, one less significant concern is severance of the neurovascular bundle [3]. This usually only affects one side, so the overall innervation and vascular supply to the foot is not compromised. Simple ligation of the severed vasculature is acceptable, as ample circulation to the entire foot can be supplied by one digital artery. A neuroma could potentially develop at the transected end of the palmar nerve, but, to the present author's knowledge, this has not been reported.

Prognosis

The DDF tenotomy is a salvage procedure, although some horses may become sound for athletic activity. The intended goal should be limited to an improvement in comfort level and pasture soundness. In cases of severe chronic laminitis, coffin joint and surrounding soft tissue contracture may be to such a degree that the limb position may not improve significantly after the tenotomy and thus lead to a more guarded prognosis for the horse. Other causes of chronic pain may result from overloading the SDFT (usually in the first few months before healing of the severed DDFT has occurred), osteoarthritis of the DIP joint, or chronic infection of the digit [5, 9, 13, 14].

In the initial description by Allen *et al.*, 11 out of 13 horses improved significantly after mid-pastern DDF tenotomy, with five out of the 11 returning to some limited form of athletic activity [2]. These horses were chronic cases of laminitis, as compared with those described by Hunt *et al.*, where the mid-metacarpal tenotomy was reported in acute refractory laminitic cases and the prognosis was more guarded. In the latter study, five out of 20 horses were alive, with four remaining lame with chronic laminitis and one sound in the pasture [3]. The authors of this report hypothesized that the more guarded prognosis found in their study could be due to the severity of laminitis in the horses included. These horses had undergone a DDF tenotomy because they were refractory to all other forms of therapy at that time. In addition, distal displacement of the DP was detected in 11 of 20 horses, and was one of the most common reasons for euthanasia in the study [3]. In another study conducted by Eastman *et al.*, it was reported that 27 of 35 horses were alive at six or more months, and 19 of 32 survived for more than two years after undergoing a DDF tenotomy for the treatment of laminitis [5]. Of the horses surviving more than two years, the mean survival time was 4.5 years. The horses in this study were estimated to be in Obel grade 3(21/35) or Obel grade 4 (14/35) that were lame at the time of surgery, and the population consisted mainly of horses with chronic laminitis or acute exacerbations of chronic laminitis. Despite having chronic laminitis, none of the horses in that study had evidence of symmetrical (or assymetrical) distal displacement of the third phalanx, which might explain the difference in prognosis reported in this study compared to that by Hunt *et al.* [3, 5]. In a final report by Morrison, 124 horses out of 245 that underwent a DDF tenotomy and corrective shoeing survived for a minimum of one year after surgery, maintained a good body condition, and were no more than an Obel grade 2 lame [14]. Of the laminitic horses in this study with severe bone disease (i.e., significant demineralization characterized as a loss of density approaching the terminal arch of the third phalanx, as seen on the lateromedial radiograph), only 21 of 48 horses were successfully treated with a DDF tenotomy and digit realignment. The author hypothesized that the compromised third phalanx [14], due to either inflammation or infection, was a chronic source of pain leading to the horse's inability to mechanically load the limb normally [14]. This could result in the DDF tendon healing in a contracted position and with excessive scar tissue. The study's author believed that returning the horse to full weight-bearing after the tenotomy was important to the animal's overall outcome. Importantly, only 17 of the 95 horses with evidence of distal displacement who underwent a DDF tenotomy were treated successfully in this same study [14]. Thus, in two separate studies, the DDF tenotomy did not have a significant impact on the management of horses with distal displacement of the third phalanx [3, 14].

Refractory or chronic laminitis cases may require repeated DDFT tenotomy procedures with recurrence of clinical signs. The mid-metacarpal technique is most commonly utilized, but the mid-pastern approach is a viable alternative when multiple procedures have been performed in this region, or if significant fibrosis makes this approach difficult. The prognosis of horses with laminitis that undergo a DDFT tenotomy is not specifically related to the amount of release between the tendon ends or how the surgical site heals, but the impact of the surgery on the overall lamellar support of the DP, and the ability to maintain the DP in a 'derotated' position to allow the growth of a healthy sole and therefore avoid further bouts of bruising and subsolear sepsis. Due to the many complications that can occur in the laminitic foot, the veterinarian needs to be careful not to be overly optimistic when discussing this option with the horse's owners, and to describe it as an option which is likely to increase the comfort of the animal for a variable amount of time, but rarely allows animal to return to a previous level of athletics.

References

1. Furst, E.F. and Lischer, C.J. (2012) Foot, in *Equine Surgery*, 4th edition (eds J.A. Auer and J.A. Stick), Elsevier Saunders, St Louis, MO, pp. 1264–1299.
2. Allen, D., Jr, White, N.A., Foerner, J.F., *et al.* (1986) Surgical management of chronic laminitis in horses: 13 cases (1983–1985). *J. Am. Vet. Med. Assoc.*, **189**, 1604–1606.
3. Hunt, R.J., Allen, D., Baxter, G.M., Jackman, B.R., and Parks, A.H. (1991) Mid-metacarpal deep digital flexor tenotomy in the management of refractory laminitis in horses. *Vet. Surg.*, **20**, 15–20.
4. Pollitt, C.C. (2011) Medical therapy of laminitis, in *Diagnosis and Management of Lameness in the Horse*, 2nd edition (eds S.J. Dyson and M.W. Ross), Saunders, St Louis, pp. 372–374.
5. Eastman, T.G., Honnas, C.M., Hague, B.A., Moyer, W., and von der Rosen, H.D. (1999) Deep digital flexor tenotomy as a treatment for chronic laminitis in horses: 35 cases (1988–1997). *J. Am. Vet. Med. Assoc.*, **214**, 517–519.
6. Nickles, F.A. (2011) Hoof care of a laminitic horse, in *Diagnosis and Management of Lameness in the Horse*, 2nd edition (eds S.J. Dyson and M.W. Ross), Saunders, St Louis, pp. 379–382.
7. Coffman, J.R., Johnson, J.H., Finocchio, E.J., and Guffy, M.M. (1970) Biomechanics of pedal rotation in equine laminitis. *J. Am. Vet. Med. Assoc.*, **156**, 219–221.
8. Hunt, R.J. (2011) Deep digital flexor tenotomy for managing laminitis, in *Diagnosis and Management of Lameness in the Horse*, 2nd edition (eds S.J. Dyson and M.W. Ross), Saunders, St Louis, pp. 382–384.
9. Floyd, A.E. (2007) An approach to the treatment of the laminitic horse, in *Equine Podiatry* (eds A.E. Floyd and R.A. Mansmann), Saunders, St Louis, pp. 347–358.
10. Rucker, A. (2007) The digital venogram, in: *Equine Podiatry* (eds A.E. Floyd and R.A. Mansmann), Saunders, St Louis, pp. 328–346.
11. Waguespack, R.W. and Caldwell, F. (2009) How to perform a modified standing deep digital flexor tenotomy at the level of the

proximal interphalangeal joint. Proceedings American Association of Equine Practice, Las Vegas, NV, pp. 230–237.
12. Burba, D.J., Hubert, J.D. and Beadle, R. (2006) How to perform a mid-metacarpal deep digital flexor tenotomy on a standing horse. Proceedings American Association of Equine Practice, San Antonio, TX, pp. 547–550.
13. Kramer, J. (2006) Deep digital flexor tenotomy, in *Manual of Equine Field Surgery* (eds D.A. Wilson, J. Kramer, G.M. Constantinescu, and K.R. Branson), Saunders, St Louis, pp. 98–102.
14. Morrison, S. (2011) Long-term prognosis using deep digital flexor tenotomy and realignment shoeing for treatment of chronic laminitis. *J. Equine Vet. Sci.*, **31**, 89–96.

CHAPTER 44

Dorsal Hoof Wall Techniques

Amy Rucker

Historical

During the mid 1980s, shoeing in conjunction with a dorsal hoof wall resection was briefly in vogue as a treatment for acute and chronic laminitis [1–6]. In the majority of reports, a shoe incorporating frog support was applied to the foot prior to the wall resection. Shoes used in conjunction with dorsal hoof wall resections included a reverse shoe with a pad and silicone [1], a heart-bar shoe [2,4,5], a hospital plate shoe with positive frog pressure and clips that screwed into the medial and lateral walls to help prevent collapse [3], and pads with packing that were bandaged (not nailed) to the feet when used in acute cases [2,3]. The treatment concept involved the thinking that positive frog pressure would 'push' the distal phalanx (DP) dorsally. In theory, dorsal wall resection reduced resistance to the upward movement of the DP, removed the lamellar wedge, relieved compression of the coronary dermis, allowed drainage of fluid from beneath the wall or sole, and exposed diseased or necrotic lamellae allowing access for treatment [1–6]. Investigators varied in their methods of trimming the heel prior to shoeing (parallel to frog [1], no lowering of heel [2], and trimming to solid heel [4]). All were emphatic that no pressure be placed on the sole-only on the frog [1–6]. The proximal extent of the resection varied between clinicians. 'Unattached' dorsal epidermal horn was removed from the toe proximally to: (i) a solid attachment between the dermis and epidermis was perceived [4]; (ii) the proximal aspect of the radiographically apparent seroma beneath the wall was reached [3]; (iii) immediately below the coronary band [1]; or (iv) the proximal aspect of the coronary band (the dorsal wall or entire wall was removed, including the coronary band) [2]. Alternatively, if a depression was palpable behind the coronary band, the resection extended proximally until the wall was thinned over the coronary groove [4]. Aftercare involved local tissue therapies, bandaging, and occasionally casts, debridement of exuberant granulation tissue, and continued therapeutic shoeing [1–6].

Although initial reports indicated positive results, the dorsal wall resection quickly lost favor even among its initial proponents [6, 7]. Reportedly, the technique was associated with a painful recovery that included a further collapse of the hoof secondary to a loss of stability of the medial and lateral walls when the dorsal arch of the hoof capsule was removed. The initial reports on this topic included differences in technique between groups, as well as differences in case presentations and complications (cases ranged from distal displacement with septic osteitis to lamellar abnormalities secondary to endocrinopathic laminitis [8]). Subsequent reports touting the technique were published [8, 9], but success secondary to dorsal wall resection is now regarded overwhelmingly as poor [6,7,10–12].

During the 1990s, hoof wall grooving became a popular therapy that is still employed today. The groove was purported to achieve the following results: fluid drainage, relief of local dermal compression; and stimulation of hoof growth [11–13]. A 2 cm-wide full epidermal thickness groove was created parallel to the coronary band, 15 mm distal to the coronet, and extending from the medial to the lateral quarter [11–14]. Initially, the groove technique was used in chronic laminitis cases in an effort to improve the heel:toe growth ratio [13, 14]. Grooving is now more commonly used in an area of slow wall growth [15, 16]. The groove is commonly performed prior to lamellar failure in an effort to promote growth and prevent lamellar separation and coronary band shear lesions [15, 16]. In an area of constricted growth rings, 2 cm distal to the hair line, a 0.6 cm (1/4 inch)-diameter Dremel burr or the edge of a rasp is used to thin the wall until tiny areas of hemorrhage are evident [15,16]. In the present author's experience, if the groove is performed in the foot with lamellar instability, the walls collapse vertically, compressing the dermis beneath the groove, which is counterproductive. Thus, the technique is primarily for the chronic case after the lamellae have stabilized, but with abnormal hoof growth.

A more conservative type of hoof wall resection, most commonly involving resection of only the proximal portion of the hoof wall, was developed as a treatment technique for the prolapsed coronary band during the 1990s [17]. In this case, an area of the wall may be resected when displacement of the DP compresses the coronary dermis, when irregular/uneven growth of the hoof capsule compresses the sublamellar dermis, and/or secondary to inflammation associated with pedal osteitis. Therefore, a conservative/limited hoof wall resection may be employed to treat complications of laminitis.

Equine Laminitis, First Edition. Edited by James K. Belknap and Raymond Geor.

Growth of the Foot

Each coronary dermal papilla is 4–6 mm in length, and contains an artery, a vein, and their anastomosis [18, 19]. Epidermal basal cells cover the surface of the coronary groove and line the holes. The basal cells of the coronary epidermis undergo mitosis to produce keratinocytes, which keratinize and become the intertubular horn of the stratum medium. The basal cells lining the holes in the coronary band produce keratinocytes that are organized into tubules within the hoof wall. The tubules are oriented vertically while the intercellular matrix (the keratinized tissue making up the remainder of the hoof wall) is formed at right-angles and is the primary source of the mechanical strength of the hoof wall [18, 19]. The tubules are fused to the matrix, and the tubule density is highest in the external portion of the stratum medium. This design is thought to reduce energy at hoof landing and to dissipate the forces to prevent damage to the DP. The wall is thus able to withstand the forces of load bearing without breaking down and cracking [18, 19].

The epidermal cell proliferative index is highest in the coronet (12%) and proximal lamellae (7%), and almost nonexistent in the majority of the lamellae (0.11%), which have few mitotic figures [19–21]. The most distal lamellae, white line, and dorsal sole also have a high proliferative index. The investigators of these studies concluded that normal lamellae are nonproliferative, their primary function being to suspend the DP within the hoof capsule through the lamellar basal cell layer's attachment to the sublamellar dermal tissue (via the basement membrane) [20]. The lamellar tissue appears to have the potential to re-establish itself when injured. When the external hoof wall was pulled away ('stripped') from the underlying tissue in one investigation, epidermal lamellar tips, most of the epidermal lamellar basement membrane and some lamellar basal cells remained with the dermis [21]. Three days after removal of the wall, the investigators reported that the basement membrane was intact, with epidermal cells proliferating to create new epidermal lamellae. By day five, yellow epidermis covered the area. Eventually the epidermis thickened, hardened, and was replaced by new wall growing distally from the coronary band [21].

Mild laminitic insults, such as pasture-induced laminitis associated with insulin resistance, may result in lamellar attenuation and elongation [19, 22]. If more extensive pathology occurs to the lamellae and the basement membrane, it is hypothesized that the lamellar separation removes contact inhibition of the normally quiescent epidermal cells distal to the coronary band, resulting in the basal keratinocytes undergoing mitosis with subsequent increased lamellar epidermal cell numbers and horn (commonly aberrant horn) production [19, 23, 24]. Progressive degenerative and regenerative changes, complicated by hyperproliferative aberrant hoof horn production, results in the formation of a lamellar wedge (Fig. 44.1) [25–27]. Basal keratinocytes from secondary epidermal lamellae invaginate into the apical region of the primary dermal lamellae, forming a series of 'cap horn' papillae which produce metaplastic tubules and intertubular arcades [27]. The size, appearance, histopathology, and stability of the lamellar wedge depends on the severity (and recurrences) of the laminitic insult and the success of treatment [25, 27]. Structural failure of the lamellae may result in reorientation of the coronary and terminal dermal papillae (inset, Fig. 44.1), altering the direction of horn production which may contribute to further dermal and bone pathology [27].

In the present author's opinion, if the horse experiences repeated small bouts of endocrinopathic laminitis, the lamellar wedge has an insidious onset which may not be recognized by the owner for several years. Minor changes may include a gradual widening of the white line at the toe, widening of the growth rings at the heels, and flattening of the solear arch. The present author believes that eventually, when the lamellae are unable to maintain a strong attachment between the DP and the wall, the horse becomes significantly lame. Lateromedial radiographs reveal a moderate widening of the dorsal wall but often minimal remodeling of the DP. The management of endocrine disease and therapeutic shoeing often returns the horse to soundness, but the lamellar wedge commonly remains. In these cases, the wedge, although abnormal, is thought to be critical to stabilization and most do not attempt to alter it.

If a laminitic horse has a more singular laminitic insult (sepsis-related or supporting limb laminitis origins), the lamellar wedge may still form. However, if shoeing (with or without a deep digital flexor tenotomy) is successful in relieving the distractive forces, and the dermis is able to recover, the new wall growth at the coronet may be parallel to the parietal face of the DP. In these cases, the present author allows the wedge to grow down the foot, believing that the wedge and dorsal arch of the wall stabilize the capsule. As the capsule grows out, the wedge is trimmed away at the ground surface. When the most proximal aspect of the lamellar wedge reaches the distal margin of the DP, a rasp is used to dress the remaining dorsal toe until it is parallel to the proximal wall (and face of the DP). While the lamellar wedge is growing out, the toe can be rockered (beveling of the dorsal ground surface to unweight the toe and bring the breakover caudally) or a shoe can be used with no contact at the toe to keep the dorsal toe from being a weight-bearing structure.

Chronic Laminitis

Wall resection is indicated when lamellar instability results in dermal compression that cannot be alleviated by shoeing, or shoeing in conjunction with deep digital flexor tenotomy. In the present author's opinion, resection may be necessary in both acute and chronic cases. The area that requires resection may be delineated by voids of contrast on the venogram, a lack of wall growth in a focal area that results in distortion of the hoof capsule, or by the visualization of coronary band prolapse over the proximal hoof wall [28–38].

When imagining a foot, it is not only the symmetry in the hoof capsule that is visualized but also the internal load to

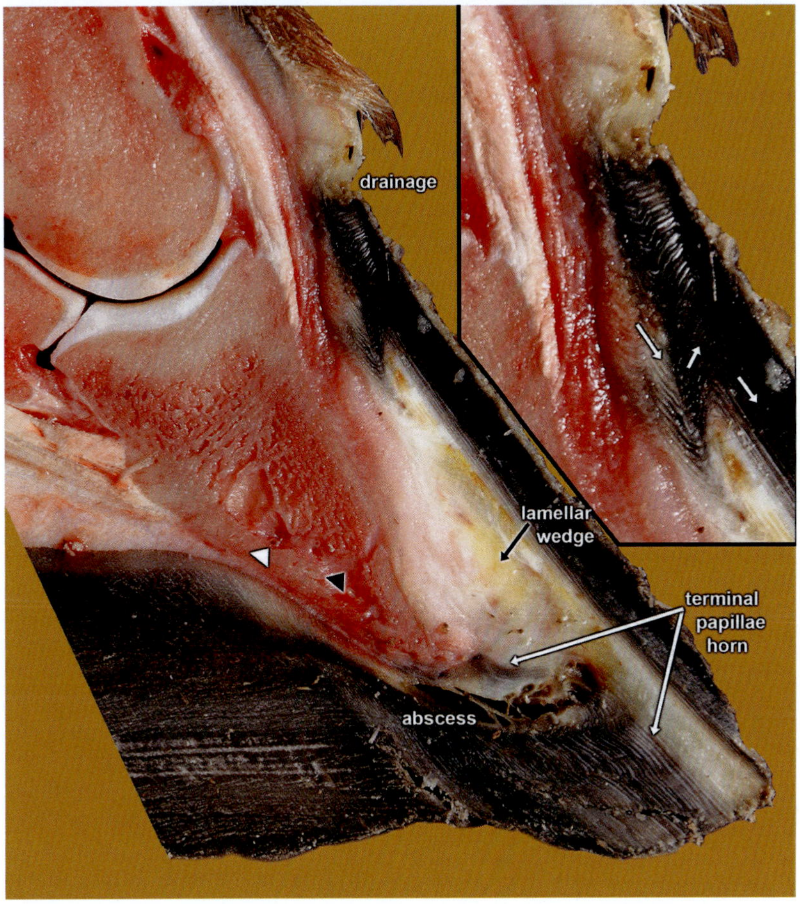

Figure 44.1 Lamellar wedge in an American Saddlebred euthanized after two bouts of laminitis over an 11-week period. The growth pattern of both coronary (inset, white arrows) and terminal papillae are altered as descent of the third phalanx distorts tubular horn production. The lamellar wedge contains both dysplastic horn tissue as well as transudate/exudate associated with the foot abscess. Bone modeling with enlargement of the terminal arch (white arrowhead) and vascular channels (black arrowhead) are apparent within the distal phalanx. At euthanasia, a subsolear foot abscess pocket had established drainage at the coronet.

the tissues of the foot within the hoof capsule. Limb conformation (e.g., angular and rotational deformities) influences the actual loading of the bones, dermis, and epidermis of the distal limb. Most horses' conformation contributes to a greater loading of the medial foot, complicating the laminitis-induced changes within the hoof. Lamellar attenuation and loss of stability of the dermal–epidermal attachment on the medial side (as occurs in asymmetrical distal displacement of the DP) may result in compression of the dermis. Medial wall and sole growth may slow, creating growth rings that are wider laterally (see Fig. 26.1 in Chapter 26). The hoof capsule grows asymmetrically and appears to twist (the sagittal plane of the dorsal toe appears to turn medially). Both, irregular hoof growth and the loss of medial lamellar attachment allow the DP to displace distally on the medial aspect of the foot within the hoof capsule. The resulting asymmetrical distal displacement of the DP (i.e., 'medial sinker') is most commonly diagnosed on a dorsopalmar radiograph (see Fig. 27.8 in Chapter 27). Eventually, loading forces and vascular compromise result in the bony remodeling of the DP (commonly termed osteitis; most commonly resorption, but increased bony production on the solear margin [commonly termed 'lipping'] is also possible). The present author uses venograms to confirm dermal compression, and comparisons are made between weight-bearing and non-weight-bearing dorsopalmar views (see Chapter 28). If contrast returns to an area in the non-weight-bearing image, then strategic shoeing may reduce the internal forces and wall resection is avoided. However, the venogram should be repeated within one to three weeks to confirm the resolution of dermal compression. Wall resection is indicated if compression is not resolved, or if compression is apparent on both weight-bearing and non-weight-bearing views. The wall may be removed at that time instead of waiting for a coronary band prolapse to occur as the dermis may become devitalized.

The combination of dermal compression and pathology to the DP may result in inflammation and occasionally fluid accumulation that is not apparent on radiographs (the radiolucency associated with lamellar and dermal injury most likely develops over time as the area filled initially with fluid dries resulting in a radiolucent 'gas density') [27]. The capsule limits dermal expansion, and the foot becomes very painful. If a drainage tract is not established distally at the white line, fluid may travel proximally to the coronary band, separating the coronary papillae and dermis from the hoof capsule. With mild injury/inflammation, the coronary band separation may be small and resolve with treatment (e.g., twice-daily application of AnimaLintex poultice[1] to

[1] Animalintex Poultice; 3M Animal Care Products, St Paul, MN, USA.

the coronary band). If the inflammation is not resolved within two to three days, in the present author's opinion, wall resection should be considered.

In more severe cases, the coronary band swells and prolapses over the proximal edge of the hoof capsule (Fig. 44.2). The sharp rim of the wall cuts into the coronary dermis, further contributing to the inflammation and potentially damaging the progenitor cells at the coronary band which are vital for future hoof wall growth. Inflammation and edema of the lamellar and coronary dermis beneath the rigid wall further compromises the circulation, creating somewhat of a 'vicious cycle.' In the present author's opinion, a conservative hoof wall resection is critical and timing is critical (Fig. 44.2c). Without prompt treatment, irreversible damage occurs to the growth centers of the coronary band. Furthermore, prolonged compression of the lamellar and coronary dermis may lead to cumulative damage of the tissue, preventing future recovery and epidermal attachment (Fig. 44.3).

In addition to addressing asymmetric (most commonly medial) displacement, other types of displacement resulting in coronary prolapse at the dorsal wall may occur and require the wall resection to extend distal to the extensor process. The prolapse may extend abaxially between the medial and lateral toe pillars. Only the proximal third to half of the wall is resected, allowing a horn bridge at the distal toe to stabilize the medial and lateral portions of the hoof wall. The present author commonly performs proximal dorsal wall resections with concurrent shoeing and deep digital flexor tenotomy (see Chapter 43 for a discussion of tenotomies).

Procedure

The extent of the hoof wall resection may be determined by visualization of the boundaries of a coronary prolapse, or an area of dermal compression on a venogram (Fig. 44.4). The palmar digital nerves (and dorsal branches) are anesthetized at approximately the level of the metacarpophalangeal joint (i.e., abaxial sesamoid nerve block). Usually, a resection does not require a tourniquet because the compressed dermis does not immediately hemorrhage when the wall is removed.

A sharpie marker is used to mark the area of resection, beginning at the coronary band, extending distally then transversely for the appropriate distances, and finally returning to the coronary band. The length of resection includes approximately 2 cm on either side (in a dorsopalmar direction) of the prolapse/separation/'wall pinch.' The resection is in the shape of a concave curve based proximally (curving distally, Fig. 44.5a) with no sharp angles. If a venogram was performed, the resection would extend distally to an area that contains contrast (i.e., is not compressed). When resecting the medial or lateral wall, there may be a need to extend the resection as far as the wall–sole junction (the distal margin of the DP). In the present author's opinion, it is important to carry the resection at least half-way down the wall to remove compression beyond the inflamed tissue. Most people err in being too conservative, only removing a small section of the proximal wall. If too little wall is removed, the dermis commonly swells over the proximal edge of the remaining wall within 24 h and the resection must then be extended.

Half-round nippers, a Dremel, or a die grinder can be used to make the approach through the wall. Care is taken not to excessively heat the dermis by friction if a grinder is used. The epidermis appears pigmented (stratum medium), then white (stratum internum), and finally yellow (stratum lamellatum) (Fig. 44.5a). Because the lamellae have usually separated from the dermis, a small space is commonly entered immediately underlying yellow epidermis. Extreme caution is used through the final layer of epidermis in an effort to avoid cutting or damaging the dermis. A hoof knife or surgical blade can be used to remove any sharp margin from the border of the remaining wall.

The area to be resected is grasped by the half-rounds and slowly peeled away from the dermis (Fig. 44.5b). A surgical blade is used to carefully excise any remaining epidermal attachment, with care being taken not to cut the dermis which, if bumped or cut, commonly begins to hemorrhage. The tissue may be edematous, but should hemorrhage when 'pumped' by gentle digital pressure. If the tissue is purple or necrotic, the prognosis is decreased (Fig. 44.3). It must also be considered that, if the lamellae are necrotic, the DP may not be viable. Any palpable bony spicules should be removed. Any DP that is left exposed must be vascular and healthy if it is to develop a strong lamellar attachment to the wall. If septic, dead bone is visible, it must be removed with a curette. However, the curetting bone of bone must be avoided unless it appears dead (yellowish/gray and waxy), and the curettage limited to the dead bone. Finally, curetting must not be extended into the terminal arch of the palmar digital vessels.

After the resection, the present author applies thick wool felt or cast-felt (at least 2 cm thick, soaked in 0.1% povidone iodine solution in saline) as a pressure bandage to the dermal bed. The felt mirrors the resection border and extends proximal to the coronary band. The felt is trimmed to mimic the proximal aspect of the remaining wall, and should protrude outwards beyond the hoof capsule so that bandaging will apply pressure to the dermis; multiple layers of felt may be necessary to achieve this.

To bandage the area, cover the dermal bed with the soaked felt, carefully applying it in a proximal-to-distal direction to point all coronary papillae distally, parallel to the face of the DP. Firmly tape the betadine/saline-soaked felt in place with 2-inch (5-cm) tape.[2] The tape must catch under the heel so that the bandage does not displace proximally. Pressure on the tissue bed is critical to prevent it from swelling outward. Apply a padded bandage over the foot to keep the area clean and protect it from

[2] Elastikon; Johnson & Johnson, Skillman, New Jersey, USA.

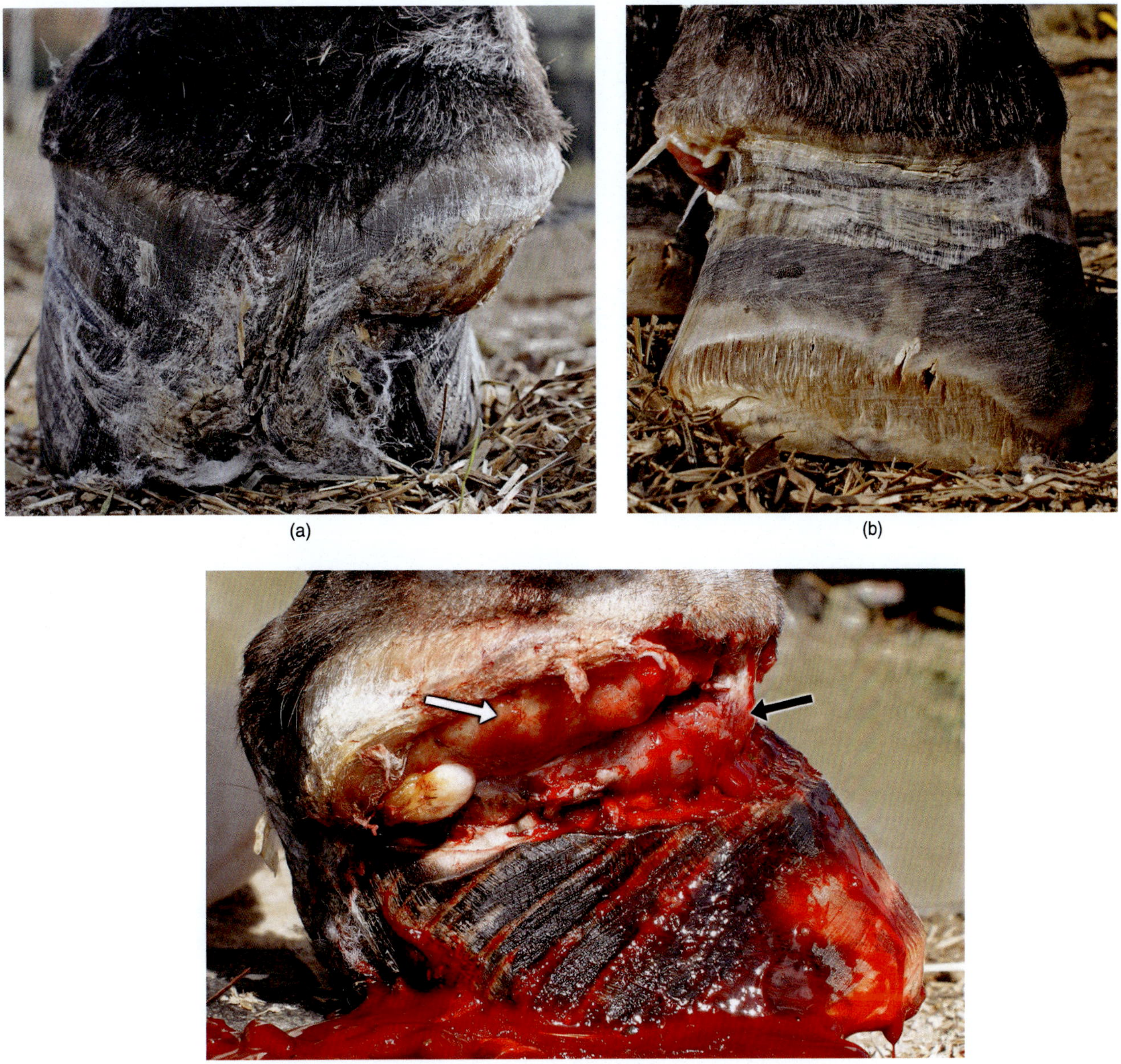
(a) (b) (c)

Figure 44.2 Chronic prolapse of coronary band. In both the palmodorsal (a) and dorsopalmar (b) views of the foot, the coronary band prolapses over the proximal edge of the hoof capsule. (c) Resection of the proximal wall reveals viable but edematous proximal lamellae (black arrow). Granulation tissue is present in the coronary dermis (white arrow), indicating chronicity of the prolapse and compromise of the tubular growth centers.

injury. The bandage should be changed daily and, if stuck to the tissue, loosened by irrigating with saline or additional dilute povidone iodine solution. Alternative therapies such as topically applied amniotic membrane [28] or products such as platelet-rich plasma may be used [33].

Within the first week, small islands of epithelialization are evident (Fig. 44.6), appearing as waxy yellow tissue on the granulation tissue covering the dermis. Epithelialization does not start at the coronary band and progress distally, but rather begins randomly across the tissue bed. During the second week, epithelialization continues to spread across the tissue bed and cornification begins. The entire bed should cornify within two weeks, including the distal margin at the junction of the old hoof wall. Once the bed has completely cornified, continue wrapping with dilute povidone iodine-soaked felt to protect the area as it thickens. By the fourth week, organized tubular horn is commonly visible growing at the coronary band. The entire wall should grow out in eight months (Fig. 44.6d and e). Ideally, the wall will be allowed to 'regrow' a second time before the horse is returned to work.

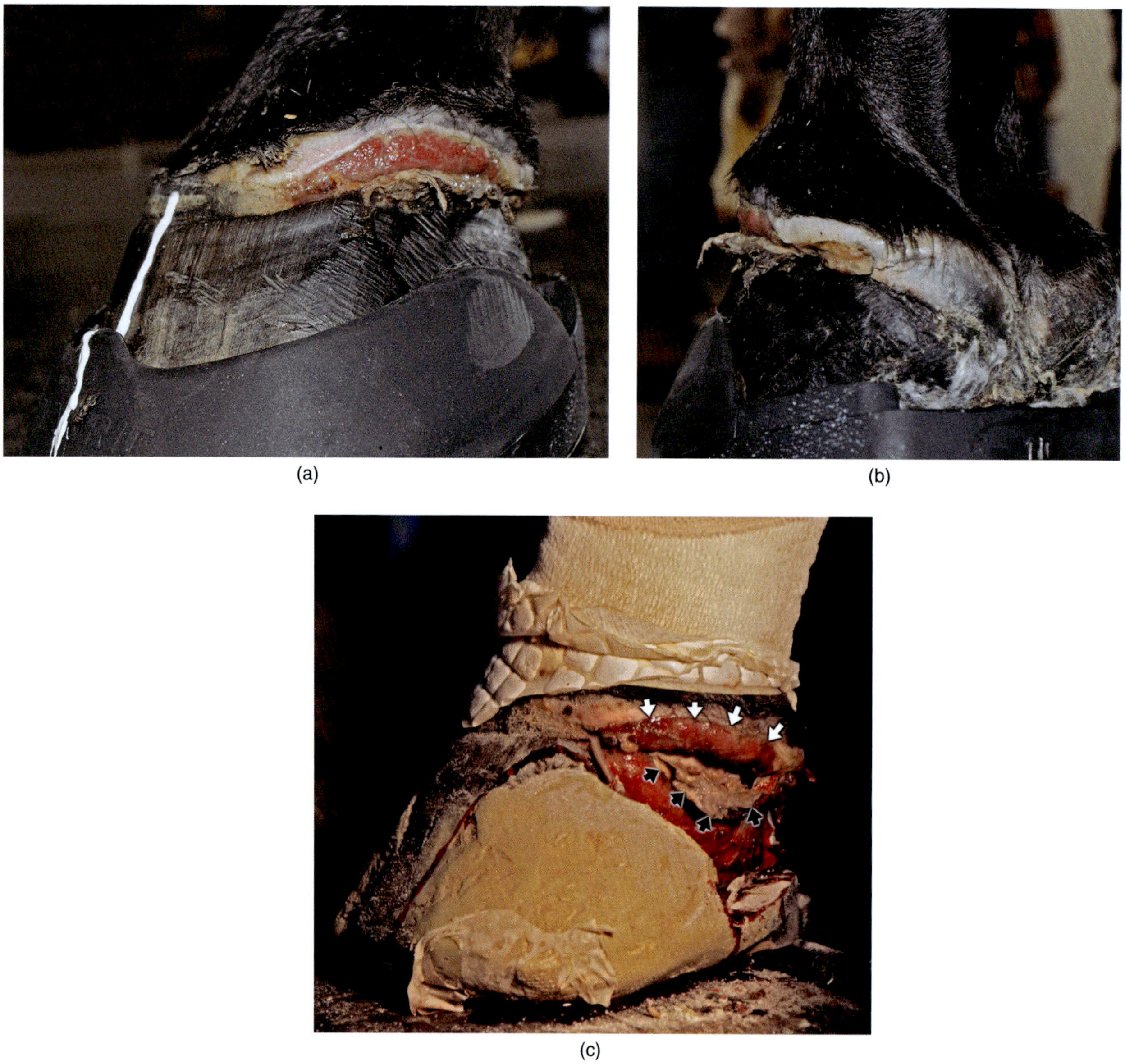

Figure 44.3 Laminitis of several weeks' duration with coronary prolapse treated by bandaging and systemic antibiotics. The horse presented with a coronary prolapse extending from the dorsomedial toe pillar (a) to the heel (b). When the proximal wall was removed, a sheet of gray tissue was visible (black arrows, panel c). That tissue originated at the coronary dermis, and included the papillae (white arrows, panel c). This indicates a poor prognosis for the return of strong tubular horn within a stable wall. (Prior to the wall resection, a rail shoe attached (glue[3] on dorsomedial wall), a deep digital flexor tenotomy performed, and the limb was bandaged in preparation for casting.)

If a large area of wall is resected, casting the limb may be utilized in an effort to stabilize tissue and support the weight of the horse (see Fig. 44.3). Casting the limb distal to the carpus/tarsus while leaving the shoe exposed to the ground surface seems to stabilize torque motion as the horse moves, improving the animal's comfort level. Butterfly catheters may be placed through the cast so that medication (betadine/saline solution) can be added to the felt over the lamellar bed. Alternatively, a treatment window may be cut into the cast. If the bone and dermis are viable, the dermis will epithelialize and cornify beneath the cast.

If the lamellar detachment is so extensive that the entire wall is involved (as can occur with distal displacement of the DP), an aggressive salvage option includes: (i) shoeing in conjunction with a deep digital flexor tenotomy; (ii) the use of transfixation pins placed in the metacarpus/metatarsus; and (iii) removal of the wall from the coronary band distal to the sole interface, leaving only the heels, distal wall, and sole [29, 30, 33, 37]. The

[3]Equilox; Equilox International, 110 NE 2nd Street, Pine Island, MN, USA.

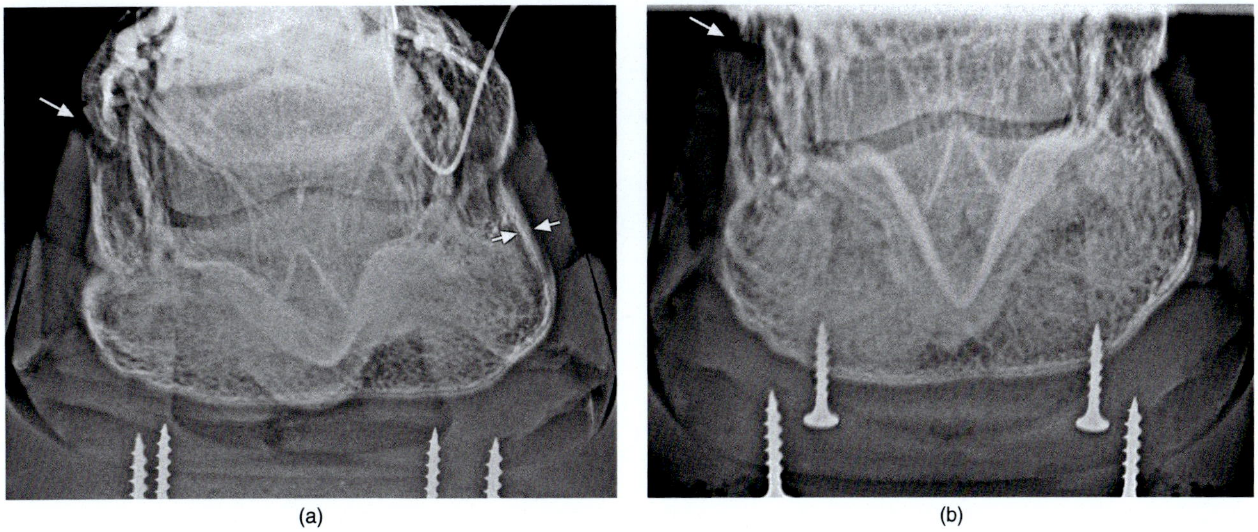

Figure 44.4 Venogram images of the foot in Figure 44.5. On the dorsopalmar weight-bearing (a) and non-weight-bearing view (b), widening of the lateral sublamellar vascular bed indicates instability of the lamellar tissue (arrowheads.) The medial dermis is compressed at the coronary band and proximal lamellae as evidenced as a void of contrast (arrow.) The distal medial sublamellar vascular bed and the circumflex and solear vessels are filled with contrast. In this case, the dermal compression is in the proximal third of the wall; hence, in the present author's opinion the resection should only be extended distally half-way down the wall.

limb is then placed in a cast for one to three months to allow the wall a chance to regrow with some attachment to the DP while in a partially suspended state. Considerations include the early identification of acute displacement with treatment within hours to days (not weeks) of onset. These cases are closely monitored with physical assessments, radiographs, and venograms, and may necessitate euthanasia if progress is not being made. As with any severe case of laminitis, a blunt discussion with the clients regarding humane issues should include the expected severity of pain suffered by the patient during the treatment process, the duration of protracted treatment (one year), the extensive nursing required during the prolonged recovery, the large financial expenditure, and the expected outcome.

If the extent of the lamellar attachment between the wall and the DP is difficult to ascertain, the present author commonly performs a venogram. A rule of thumb is that, at six months, "…the foot you have is the foot you are going to live with." In the present author's opinion, the lamellar attachment/wall quality will rarely improve after that time. Assessing the strength of the attachment will help the veterinarian and farrier guide the owner in long-term shoeing and turn-out recommendations (Fig. 44.7).

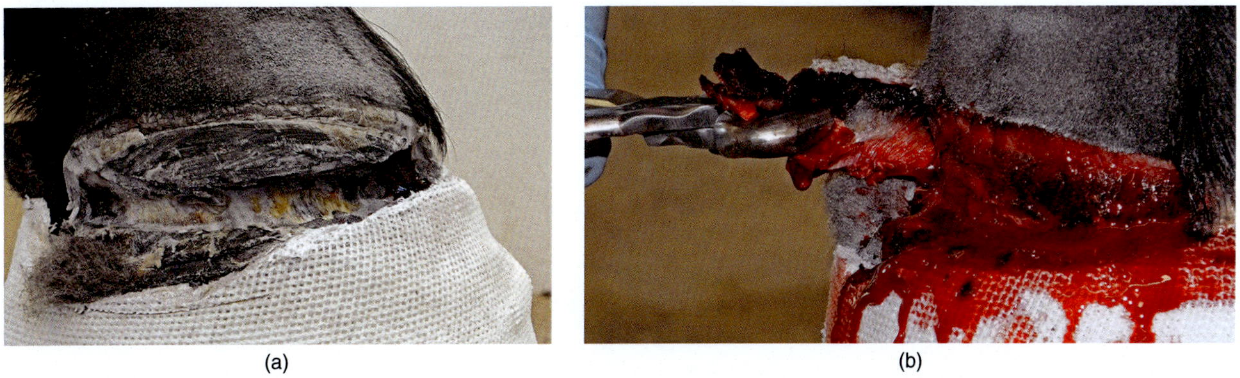

Figure 44.5 Wall resection. (a) A Dremel and small half-round nippers were used to remove the stratum externum and medium in a curved line that extends dorsal, palmar and distal to the area of wall constriction. (b) After completing the surgical approach, the dorsal edge of the wall to be resected is grasped with half-round nippers and then slowly and gently peeled away from the coronary dermis, allowing any dermal papillae and coronary germinal epithelium present underneath the periople to remain attached. The vascularity of the coronary and lamellar dermis with minimal edema indicates a good prognosis for recovery.

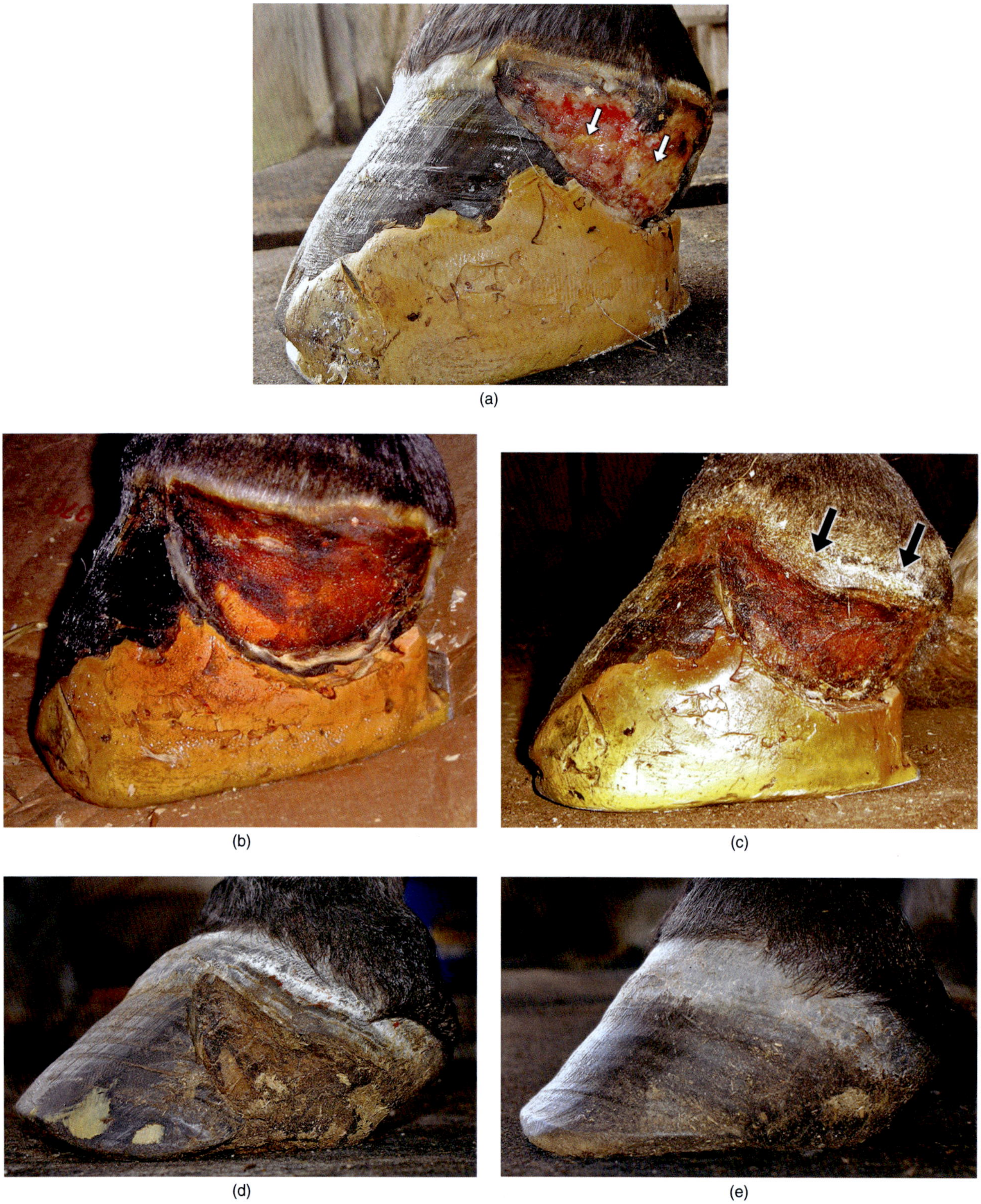

Figure 44.6 Wall resection one month post shoeing and deep digital flexor tenotomy. Note the islands of yellow epithelialization visible one week after wall resection (panel a, white arrows). At two weeks, cornification was complete (panel b). At three weeks new growth was evident at the coronet (panel c, black arrows) and the cornification had thickened. At three-and-a-half months, multiple new growth rings, evidence of proper hoof wall growth are evident proximal to the resection (panel d). Finally, at 11 months after wall resection the medial hoof was strong and functional (panel e), and the wall was symmetrical when viewed from the front. (The horse was sound for light riding.)

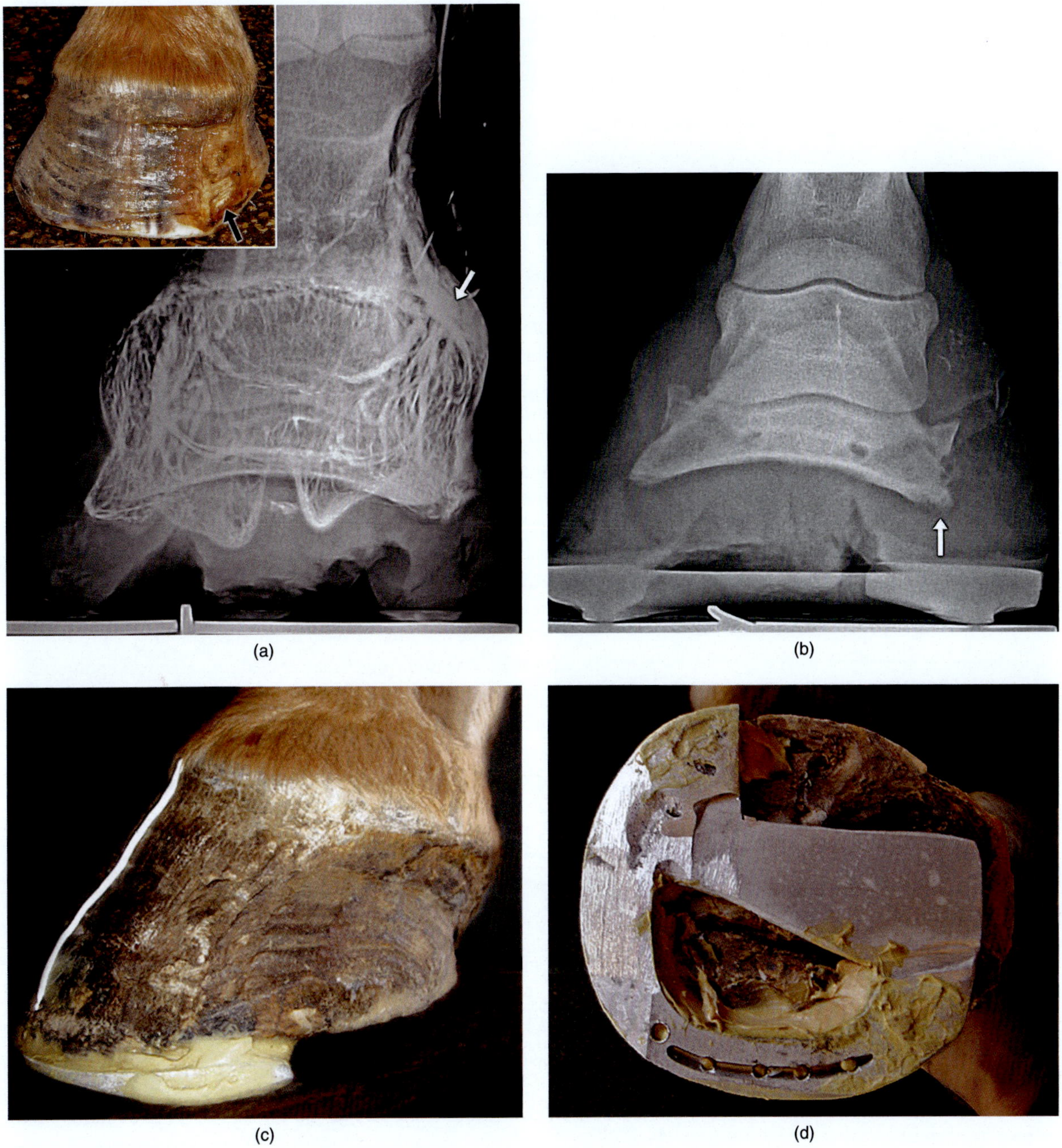

Figure 44.7 Note the poor-quality hoof wall (did not appear to have tubular horn within the medial wall) at 10 months (a, upper left insert) and at 15 months (c) following hoof wall resection. The dorsopalmar venogram confirmed that although the lateral coronary band, lamellar and circumflex vessels were organized, the medial sublamellar vascular bed remained widened (a). Contrast was reduced distal to the remodeled medial wing of the distal phalanx, and the lamellar–circumflex junction was distorted. The medial palmar digital vein had been catheterized, and a large venous structure was filled with contrast at the proximal aspect of the coronary band (arrow, panel a). Remodeling of the distal aspect of the medial wing of the distal phalanx (arrow) is apparent on a dorspalmar radiograph (b). Note the example of a Z bar shoe (c and d) to 'float' the affected hoof wall.

Incorrect Use of Wall Resection

Wall resection removes vascular and dermal compression, and is a complementary procedure when treating laminitis. Resection is not successful if underlying forces are not addressed via shoeing (± casting) with or without a deep digital flexor tenotomy.

Unsuccessful Outcome

If damage to the dermis and bone is so extensive that it is devitalized, complete epithelialization and cornification will not occur. When an area of the wall is resected, it should epithelialize and cornify within two weeks. However, if the distal border does not cornify then consideration should be given to extending the resection distally to the level of the sole. When the wall is removed, the quality of the dermis is explored, assessing the health of the DP. Alternatively, if the majority of the bed has epithelialized and started to cornify, a venogram can be performed. (Note that contrast will run out of any uncornified tissue, so a contrast volume deficit may create artifacts on the venogram.)

If the tissue bed does not heal and cornify, and if recurrent granulation tissue is a problem, it is possible that the DP may no longer be viable, necessitating euthanasia.

Partially Successful Outcome

If the coronary dermis and germinal epithelium are damaged, then resection may only be partially successful due to a loss of integrity or strength of the new wall growth. In this case it is probable that the wall lacks a strong lamellar attachment to the bone, and often the DP has also sustained some damage (Fig. 44.7). Some walls regrow, but visually appear to lack tubular horn (Fig. 44.7a). The farrier may find that the wall is 'soft' and easy to nail through, but difficult to clinch without tearing down the side of the wall (thereby commonly necessitating glue for the attachment of shoes). These horses may be sound at a walk and maintained without phenylbutazone, but are delicate to manage.

The unattached or soft wall can only sustain minimal weight-bearing. As the weather cycles, the horse with sole mass may be barefoot during wet seasons but shod to protect the foot during dry seasons. Some farriers will use a Z-Bar type of shoe to allow the compromised wall to 'float' and not bear the full weight (Fig. 44.7c and d). If ample unaffected hoof wall is present, others prefer to use a more traditional type shoe (e.g., a frog/heart/egg-bar or a shoe that utilizes sole packing material) and float the affected wall. These horses must be maintained in a small turnout with good footing (the size of the turnout depends on the strength of the wall and lamellar attachment, and the behavior of the horse). If a horse over-exercises, such as getting out and galloping, it may break down what little attachment was present (Fig. 44.7c and d). The wall can collapse and/or a submural seroma develop, resulting in lameness. With shoeing and local therapy (such as applying a poultice to the coronary band), the attachment may heal to some extent but never return to normal.

When a foot appears to have a compromised dermis at the time of a wall resection, the owners should be warned of this possible complication (see Figs 44.2 and 44.3). If cornification of the resection does not occur in a two-week time frame and new horn growth does not appear distal to the coronary band in the first month, the condition of the wall should again be discussed with the owners, who must be mentally, physically, and financially prepared to care for a horse that requires special shoeing and limited exercise for the rest of the animal's life. In the present author's experience, at the time of the initial laminitis crisis, most owners "...just want to save the horse." However, after a few years of care, they really want the horse to be 'normal' and return to 'normal' care, shoeing, and even riding.

Conclusions

Wall resection can be used to treat a complication of laminitis, and should not be considered a primary treatment for the disease. The procedure does not resolve forces on the dermis of the sole or the DP. Furthermore, once the exposed lamellae cornify, the original forces resume. Wall resections are not necessary for mild cases of laminitis. If a wall resection is performed, the clinician should also evaluate the effectiveness of her/his primary treatment. In the present author's opinion, indications to consider performing a wall resection include alterations on the venogram with or without uneven growth (which can cause a pinching or distortion of the hoof wall). If the coronary band swells and drains, treatment with a topical poultice[4] can be carried out for a few days while the need for a resection is evaluated. If the coronary band prolapses over the hoof wall, a resection should be considered/performed immediately.

The wall resection is only intended to remove compression from an area of dermis. If successful, the area will epithelialize and then cornify, with new growth becoming apparent at the coronary band four weeks after surgery. Once the wall grows out completely, there may be no evidence that a resection was performed. If the coronary dermis is damaged, the resection will only be partially successful. Without normal tubular horn, the wall is weak and usually lacks a strong lamellar attachment to the bone.

Complications include a lack of prompt epithelialization and cornification of the tissue bed. If the distal aspect of the resection remains moist, does not epithelialize, and the lamellae protrude over the edge of the distal wall, then the resection must be extended further distal (possibly to the sole–wall junction). If the bone remains viable, with epithelialization occurring over the dermal tissue covering the bone, the prognosis for survival is improved. If the bone and overlying tissue remain unhealthy with a failure to epithelialize, the prognosis is guarded to grave. Progress venograms can help to guide any treatment, but the veterinarian cannot perform regional limb perfusion or venograms until the tissue has cornified (in this case, fluid will run out of the dermis).

Acknowledgments

This chapter is a collaboration of investigations with Dr Justin Berger, Dr Mark Cassells, Chris Clark, Jeff Davis, Randy Holthusen, Dr Ric Redden, Dr Roger Shaw, and Howard Wilson.

[4] Animalintex Poultice; 3M Animal Care Products, St Paul, MN, USA.

References

1. White, N.A. and Baggett, N. (1983) A method of corrective shoeing for laminitis in horses. *Vet. Med. Small Anim. Clin.*, **78** (5), 775–778.
2. Chapman, B. and Platt, G. (1984) Laminitis in the horse. *Proc. Am. Assoc. Equine Pract.*, **30**, 99–109.
3. Redden, R.F. (1986) Hoof wall resection as a treatment in laminitis. *Proc. Am. Assoc. Equine Pract.*, **32**, 647–656.
4. Eustace, R.A. and Caldwell, M.N. (1989) The construction of the heart bar shoe and the technique of dorsal wall resection. *Equine Vet. J.*, **21** (5), 367–369.
5. Eustace, R.A. and Caldwell, M.N. (1989) Treatment of solar prolapse using the heart bar shoe and dorsal hoof wall resection technique. *Equine Vet. J.*, **21** (5), 370–372.
6. Moyer, W. and Redden, R.F. (1989) Chronic and severe laminitis: a critique of therapy with heart bar shoes and hoof wall resection. *Equine Vet. J.*, **21** (5), 317–318.
7. Redden, R.F. (1988) Complicated laminitis. *Proc. Am. Assoc. Equine Pract.*, **34**, 311–319.
8. Peremans, K., Verschooten, F., *et al.* (1991) Laminitis in the pony: conservative treatment vs. dorsal hoof wall resection. *Equine Vet. J.*, **23** (4), 243–246.
9. Wilford, S., Fowke, G.S., McKane, S., *et al.* (2011) Post-foaling laminitis: a case report. *Companion Animal*, **16**, 4–9.
10. Parks, A.H., Balch, O.K., and Collier, M.A. (1999) Treatment of acute laminitis: supportive therapy. *Vet. Clin. North Am.*, **15** (2), 363–374.
11. Curtis, S., Ferguson, D.W., Luikart, R., *et al.* (1999) Trimming and shoeing the chronically affected horse. *Vet. Clin. North Am.*, **15** (2), 463–480.
12. Parks, A.H. and O'Grady, S.E. (2003) Chronic laminitis: current treatment strategies. *Vet. Clin. North Am.*, **19** (2), 412–413.
13. Ritmeester, A.M. and Ferguson, D.W. (1996) Coronary grooving promotes dorsal hoof wall growth in horses with chronic laminitis. *Proc. Am. Assoc. Equine Pract.*, **42**, 212–213.
14. Ritmeester, A.M., Blevins, W.E., Ferguson, D.W., *et al.* (1998) Digital perfusion, evaluated scintigraphically, and hoof wall growth in horses with chronic laminitis treated with egg bar-heart bar shoeing and coronary grooving. *Equine Vet. J.*, **30** (26), 111–118.
15. Morrison, S. (2010) Chronic laminitis: foot management. *Vet. Clin. Equine*, **26**, 425–446.
16. Morrison, S. (2004) Foot management. *Clin. Tech. Equine Pract.*, **3** (1), 71–82.
17. Redden, R.F. (1998) Understanding laminitis, in *The Blood-Horse*. Lexington, Kentucky, p. 67.
18. Pollitt, C.C. (2004) Anatomy and physiology of the inner hoof wall. *Clin. Tech. Equine Pract.*, **3**, 3–21.
19. Pollitt, C.C. (2010) The anatomy and physiology of the suspensory apparatus of the distal phalanx. *Vet. Clin. North Am.*, **26** (1), 29–49.
20. Daradka, M. and Pollitt, C.C. (2004) Epidermal cell proliferation in the equine hoof wall. *Equine Vet. J.*, **36** (3), 236–241.
21. Pollitt, C.C. and Daradka, M. (2004) Hoof wall wound repair. *Equine Vet. J.*, **36** (3), 210–215.
22. De Laat, M., McGowan, C.M., Sillence, M.N., *et al.* (2010) Equine laminitis: induced by 48 h hyperinsulinemia in Standardbred horses. *Equine Vet. J.*, **42** (2), 129–135.
23. Pollitt, C.C. and Visser, M.B. (2010) Carbohydrate alimentary overload laminitis. *Vet. Clin. North Am.*, **26** (1), 65–78.
24. Budras, K.-D., Hullinger, R.L., and Sack, W.O. (1989) Light and electron microscopy of keratinization in the laminar epidermis of the equine hoof with reference to laminitis. *Am. J. Vet. Res.*, **50**, 1150.
25. Hood, D.M. (1999) The mechanisms and consequences of structural failure of the foot. *Vet. Clin. North Am.*, **15**, 437.
26. Kuwano, A., Katayama, Y., Kasashima, Y., *et al.* (2002) A gross and histopathological study of an ectopic white line development in equine laminitis. *J. Vet. Med. Sci.*, **64**, 893.
27. Collins, S.N., van Eps, A.W., Pollitt, C.C., *et al.* (2010) The lamellar wedge. *Vet. Clin. North Am.*, **26** (1), 179–195.
28. Long, C.G. and Schultz, L.A. (2006) How to use hoof-wall resection and amniotic membrane as a treatment for coronary-band prolapse. *Proc. Am. Assoc. Equine Pract.*, **52**, 501–504.
29. Floyd, A.E. (2007) An approach to the treatment of the laminitic horse, in *Equine Podiatry* (eds A.E. Floyd and R.A. Mansmann), Saunders, St Louis, Missouri, pp. 347–358.
30. Rucker, A. (2007) The digital venogram, in *Equine Podiatry* (eds A.E. Floyd and R.A. Mansmann), Saunders, St Louis, Missouri, pp. 339–345.
31. Morrison, S. (2008) Rehabilitating the laminitic foot. Proceedings of the North American Veterinary Conference - Large Animals, pp. 186–189.
32. Eustace, R.A. and Emery, S.L. (2009) Partial coronary epidermectomy (coronary peel), dorsodistal wall fenestration and deep digital flexor tenotomy to treat severe acute founder in a Connemara pony. *Equine Vet. Educ.*, **21** (2), 91–99.
33. Redden, R.F. (2004) How lacerum has improved the progress of high scale foot damage. Proceedings of the Annual Bluegrass Laminitis Symposium, 15–17 January, Lexington, Kentucky, vol. 17, pp. 37–40.
34. Redden, R.F. (2003) How to treat high scale laminitis with wall ablation and transcortical cast. Proceedings of the Annual Bluegrass Laminitis Symposium, 16–18 January, Lexington, Kentucky, vol. 16, pp. 65–68.
35. Orsini, J.A. (2010) Clinical updates in laminitis. *J. Equine Vet. Sci.*, **30** (9), 455–459.
36. Rucker, A. (2010) Clinical applications of digital venography. *J. Equine Vet. Sci.*, **30** (9), 491–503.
37. Rucker, A. (2010) Chronic laminitis: strategic hoof wall resection. *Vet. Clin. North Am.*, **26** (1), 197–205.
38. Eustace, R. and Emery, S.L. (2008) Partial separation of the hoof at the coronary band following acute founder – a review of twenty three cases. Proceedings of the International Laminitis Symposium, 11–13 November, Berlin, Germany, pp. 233–238.

CHAPTER 45

Complications of Laminitis

Robert J. Hunt and James K. Belknap

Introduction

Although laminitis itself is not a life-threatening disease, complications of the disease often result in the humane destruction of the animal. A horse should not be allowed to suffer and linger with no hope of a comfortable existence; conversely, it is unacceptable to wrongfully terminate a patient with a rectifiable or transient complication. Once laminitis has affected a patient to the point in which there is morphologic derangement of the internal structures of the hoof, there is lifetime potential for a myriad of complications to ensue. These complications may be a direct result of pathologic changes within the hoof capsule, or they may be indirect and occur from therapeutic intervention gone awry or other body system involvement. It is critical for the clinician to adopt a global or 'whole-horse' approach when confronted with a patient with laminitis in order to recognize complications early, to prevent complications in high-risk individuals, and to implement treatment changes at the appropriate time. The attending veterinarian should have enough knowledge of the stages of the disease to understand the abnormalities which occur within the laminitis complex. It is important to have realistic expectations of the clinical progress and to recognize complications or deterioration of the patient. In this chapter, attention will be focused on expected and predictable complications directly associated with changes that occur within the hoof, as well as those affecting other body systems and those which occur as a result of treatment.

Many of the events or changes within the digit during the onset of laminitis have been described and are continually being further defined at the molecular level. In-depth discussions of these events are available elsewhere in this book (see Chapters 6–19); however, primary common denominators of these events are loss of structural integrity of the lamellar epithelium and its adherence to the underlying basement membrane and lamellar dermis (see Chapters 15 and 19). The result is lamellar disruption allowing mechanical overload of the diseased as well as the normal lamellae and solear tissue. This has the potential to create a vicious cycle in that continual overload of the remaining lamellae perpetuates further damage and more disruption. The major biomechanical forces on the digit opposing the lamellar attachment of the distal phalanx (DP) to the hoof wall include the vertical load through the bony column and the pull of the deep digital flexor tendon (DDFT) (see Chapter 5) [1–3]. The magnitude and severity of the damage occurring as a result of the primary insult in conjunction with these forces is the major determinant of the prognosis and the potential ensuing complications.

Although the lamellae within the entire hoof capsule are susceptible to laminitis, the majority of the morphologic lamellar changes recognized clinically occur in the dorsal two-thirds of the hoof. Therefore, complications involving the foot after laminitis tend to involve this region of the foot. The normal foot is strongest in its natural state, and any disruption of the normal architecture of the foot associated with laminitis has the potential to permanently weaken the hoof, thereby making it more vulnerable to further damage to the wall and internal structures of the foot.

Events Leading to Complications

During the early stages of laminitis, the primary events are intracapsular and, whether of metabolic, toxic, vascular or mechanical origin, or medication-induced, the end result is varying degrees of disruption of lamellar function with an ensuing loss of suspension of the DP within the hoof capsule [4]. Subcapsular abnormalities associated with the onset and early stages of laminitis include hemorrhage and seroma formation beneath the wall as well as the sole, most likely resulting from rupturing of the sublamellar vasculature secondary to lamellar shearing and separation and possibly increased permeability of the vasculature. The DP becomes unstable with a loss of structural integrity of the lamellar bond, and displacement may occur. Displacement of the DP results in ischemia of the solear tissue due to compression and ischemia of the epidermal lamellae due to both injury to the dermal vasculature and physical separation of the epidermal lamellae from the vasculature in the dermis with displacement of the DP. Recognizable signs of digital pathology during this acute phase of the disease includes thickening or edema of the coronary band, followed by flattening and

Equine Laminitis, First Edition. Edited by James K. Belknap and Raymond Geor.

depression creating a ridge along the proximal hoof wall [4, 5]. This ridge differs depending on the type of bony displacement. Rotational displacement exhibits a ridge in the central dorsal one-third of the coronary band, whereas symmetrical distal displacement displays a complete circumferential ridge of the coronary band. Horses that undergo asymmetric distal displacement of the DP, or medial collapse, display a prominent ridge along the medial coronary band.

Other signs of early contour changes include a loss of the degree of concavity of the sole, progressing to a convex or prolapsed sole; these solear contour changes compound solear deterioration due not only to the increased pressure on the dermal side of the sole from the displaced digit but also result in an increased contact of the sole with the ground surface, which causes the already compromised solear tissue to become 'pinched' between the ground surface and displaced DP. This can result in solear perforation when the sole deteriorates to the point that it cannot withstand the downward pressure of the dorsodistal aspect of the phalanx. In cases where actual prolapse of the DP through the sole does not occur, seromas commonly form between the dorsodistal aspect of the DP and the solear epidermis from the injury to the solear dermis. Subsolear abscess formation can also frequently occur with solear compromise, due most likely to a loss of integrity of the sole allowing bacteria to traverse the normally protective solear epithelium and enter the solear dermis. Total digital collapse and sloughing of the hoof capsule occurs in extreme situations; this is most common in supporting limb laminitis and severe cases of sepsis-related laminitis (SRL). Interestingly, it can also occur in young septic animals (e.g., yearlings) which, although they do not have as high an incidence of laminitis as larger, mature animals, can undergo severe digital changes [6] including, in one of the present author's (J.K.B.) experience, exungulation when they do exhibit signs of laminitis.

Distortional disorders of the capsule which occur in chronic laminitis may be appreciated as changes in the external hoof wall; however, internal structures including the lamellar architecture, vasculature, and bone are also affected. A compromise of the germinal epithelium, combined with mechanical overload, may result in reorientation of the coronary papillae which further results in new lamellar growth perpendicular to the existing wall [1]. In cross-section, this appears as a proximal to distal sigmoid configuration at the coronary band. This directional change in horn production, along with lamellar damage, results in misoriented and dysfunctional growth culminating in a scarred, thickened horn material referred to as a lamellar wedge (see Fig. 44.1 in Chapter 44) [1]. Preservation of the orientation of the germinal layer and vasculature through the heel region in comparison to the region of collapse and impeded growth of the dorsal wall are well recognized clinically as a relative increased rate of growth in the heels compared to the toe.

Progressive developmental changes of the lamellae and hoof wall associated with lamellar dysplasia result in the development of an abnormal, thickened white line with poor structural

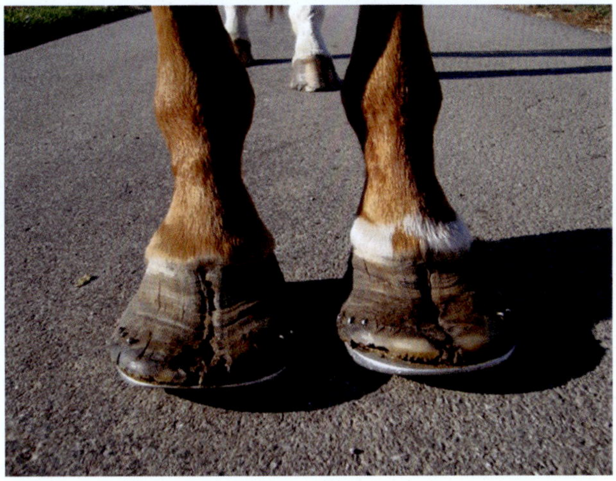

Figure 45.1 Cloven hooves are clearly visible in this chronic laminitis patient.

integrity on the solear surface and a dished shape of the dorsal hoof wall. This structure is biomechanically inferior and subject to further injury and degradation of the wall and sole. An abnormal, thickened white line commonly has poor structural integrity, allowing the entrance of bacteria through clefts in the ground surface and resulting in sepsis which can travel up the wall (i.e., 'seedy toe'), or possibly result in subsolear abscessation. The abnormally shaped and biomechanically inferior dorsal hoof wall can lead to a dorsal wall vertical fissure being formed, creating a cloven hoof (Fig. 45.1). In all cases of chronic laminitis with loss of lamellar integrity, ensuing pathology of the DP from inflammation, altered vasculature, and abnormal mechanical forces resulting from a combination of lack of support from damaged lamellae and increased concussion on the dorsodistal aspect of the DP from distal displacement commonly results in an aseptic pedal osteitis (discussed below). Ongoing insult to the distal phalanx can result in severe erosive changes, sepsis, multiple types of pathologic fracture, and osteoarthritis of the distal interphalangeal joint [1, 4, 5]. The time frame for the development of these changes varies on an individual basis, but is determined by the amount of initial structural damage, ongoing insults to the foot, the number of load cycles on an unstable foot, and hoof care. It is important to understand that, with appropriate management, horses can survive for years with severe changes within the foot.

Direct Complications of Laminitis

Pain

A common clinical sign of laminitis is *pain*, which may also be considered a complication of the disease and is present for a reason. This is a very important point to bear in mind, as pain has a protective function in the event of structural compromise of the digit. The clinician should be aware of the source of pain and the stability of the distal phalanx within the hoof capsule when medicating the patient in order not to propagate further mechanical failure. Different types of pain (see Chapter 33) manifest from a number of sources depending on the stage and severity of laminitis and accompanying problems [4, 5, 7]. An integral part of the management of a laminitic patient is the ability to localize and understand the source of pain and, commonly, its fluctuating nature. The source of pain varies with the stage of disease, and is likely multifactorial. The pathophysiology of pain in the initial stages is poorly understood in the acute patient and may be mild; it is likely associated with ischemia, intracapsular edema, and lamellar shearing forces (and tearing) associated with varying degrees of detachment. Pathologic events during this period include loss of structural integrity of both the lamellar epithelium and the underlying basement membrane and dermal matrix, commonly leading to mechanical failure. With increasing degrees of insult and lamellar instability, the severity of pain appears to increase. It is believed that there is a correlation between the outcome of the patient, the amount of lamellar disruption, and the severity of pain. There is often a reduction in the intensity of pain after several days of an acute onset which may be associated with tissue compromise or cell death. This is often mistaken as an improvement in the patient, which is then allowed more exercise with disastrous results.

Pain may also arise from secondary mechanical failure resulting in displacement of the DP [8]. This displacement creates pain by increasing pressure on the solear tissues from the DP within the hoof capsule. Rotational displacement may result in excessive pressure on the solear components dorsal to the apex of the frog. Resulting complications include hemorrhage, sole bruising, subsolear seroma formation, subsolear abscessation, solear prolapse, and possibly perforation of the sole by the DP. It is important to realize that, in the long-term chronic case in which there is lamellar stability but rotational displacement of the DP, the pain is more likely to be due primarily to solear pain, with minimal involvement of the lamellae.

Chronic recurring pain may arise from local inflammatory processes, which are integrally associated with chronic instability relating to the compromised lamellar interface. This predisposes the tissues to chronic bruising, degradation of soft tissue and bone, and eventual infection of these structures.

Subsolear Seroma/Abscess

Events which are often misconstrued as recurrent bouts of laminitis are commonly recurrent episodes of subsolear and lamellar bruising, abscessation or septic pedal osteitis. Intracapsular sepsis should be considered in any chronic laminitic patient which presents with an acute increase in severity of lameness in a single limb. On physical examination, these patients are commonly acutely painful to solear pressure, most commonly when applied in the toe region. In horses which display a convex bulge in the solear surface cranial to the apex of the frog, digital pressure alone may induce a pain response. Radiographs may be helpful in detecting a seroma or abscess if a gas density or other pathologic changes are present.

It is sometimes difficult to differentiate between subsolear seroma and subsolear abscessation. Although it is less than ideal to open and possibly contaminate a seroma, the possibility of the fluid being a subsolear abscess commonly dictates that the fluid pocket and sole be evaluated. In order to avoid inadvertent exposure or injury to the DP, a conservative approach of paring out the affected part of the sole should be taken. A lateral radiograph prior to exploration of the sole may aid as a guide to determine the thickness of solear tissue and its relationship to the DP. With appropriate treatment after entering a seroma or abscess, resolution is generally rapid. Most podiatrists would agree that the degree of exposure of the subsolear tissue should be minimized; a large granulating wound in the sole is extremely painful, and healing is often slow. Excessive exposure of solear tissue may be avoided by making a small 2–4 mm entry through the sole into the suspected pocket on either the dorsal, lateral, or medial aspect of the suspected abscess/seroma, assessing any fluid which drains from the sole, and using a narrow malleable probe to assess the dimensions of the undermined tissue (commonly after performing a short-acting nerve block with lidocaine). At that point in time, one or two other small 2–4 mm entries can be made at the far side of the undermined cavity to allow to and fro lavage (another option one of the present authors [R.H.] uses is to insert a 16–18-gauge needle into the suspect area; if purulent material is obtained, a larger opening may be established). A short 14-gauge intravenous catheter, teat cannula, or large needle (14- or 16-gauage with the end blunted) is then introduced into one of the entries, and the pocket is lavaged under pressure with saturated Epsom salts using a 60-ml syringe and a short intravenous extension set attached to the catheter, cannula, or needle (Fig. 45.2). The area is lavaged daily or every two days until all drainage subsides; daily lavage usually results in the seroma or abscess drying up within three to seven days. Lavage is required for varying lengths of time depending on an individual basis.

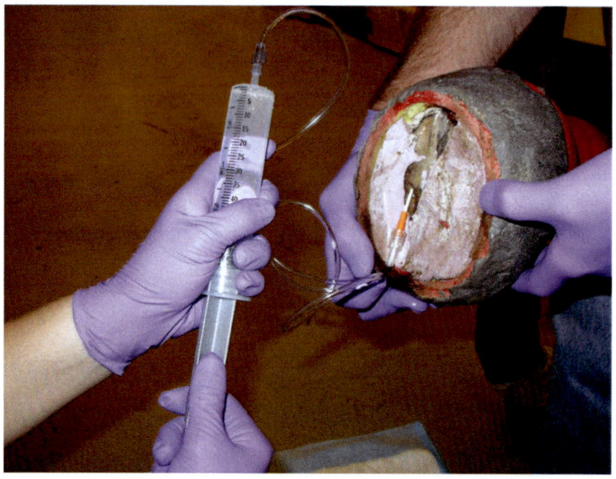

Figure 45.2 Flushing of a large under-run abscess with Epsom salts through small holes in which a shortened 14-gauge catheter is inserted. The foot was placed in an open-sole cast, as described in Chapter 42.

If an abscess is at least partially located near the hoof wall (and there is no disruption of the sole), it may be possible to enter the abscess and lavage it through the hoof wall, leaving the sole intact. In the rare case of subsolear/intracapsular sepsis that is unresponsive to Epsom salt lavage (commonly due to a large amount of tissue involvement), medical-grade maggots can be an effective option for the debridement of dead tissue [9].

Pedal Osteitis

Pedal osteitis (Fig. 45.3) is usually a radiographic diagnosis in which bony changes ranging from a mild, diffuse to focal, more extensive loss of bone at the solear margin of the DP indicates a nonseptic or septic pedal osteitis, respectively. Pedal osteitis is extremely common in the chronic laminitis case with displacement of the DP, with the latter exhibiting extensive bony changes indicative of pedal osteitis due to chronic inflammation and bruising of the dorsodistal tip of the DP (Fig. 45.3a). Thus, it is difficult at times to determine whether or not the bony changes are indicative of a nonseptic or septic pedal osteitis, especially due to the fact that subsolear abscesses in chronic laminitis cases usually originate immediately distal to the dorsal solear margin of the DP. However, in the majority of cases with subsolear sepsis in which a diffuse pedal osteitis is present radiographically (nonseptic pedal osteitis is shown in Fig. 45.3a), the bone is not septic and should not be curetted. A distinct lucent focus is most commonly present on a solear margin view if sepsis is present (arrowheads, Fig. 45.3b and c) [10]; sequestrae may also be present in some cases (Fig. 45.3c, black arrow).

The treatment of nonseptic pedal osteitis primarily consists of improving the physical displacement of the DP predisposing the horse to bruising, primarily by attempting to make the ground surface of the sole more parallel to the palmar surface of the DP by trimming the caudal foot (generally from the apex of the frog, caudally; see Chapter 38). If a large amount of heel is removed, the farrier may need to elevate the heels when shoeing, which will still allow a better (more parallel) relationship of the DP to the sole but decrease the tension on the DDFT (described in detail in Chapter 41). The only other option to neutralize the tension of the DDFT when 'derotating' the DP is to perform a deep digital flexor tenotomy at the same time that corrective trimming and shoeing are taking place (see Chapter 43). Other shoeing techniques used to protect the sole for pedal osteitis include the use of wide-webbed shoes, and either full pads or rim pads to increase the distance between the ground and sole. The only concern with these techniques in the chronic laminitis patient is that solear support may need to be applied in the caudal two-thirds of the foot if active laminitis/lamellar instability is present at the time of treatment.

Septic pedal osteitis is a surgical condition in which the affected parent bone needs to be debrided, and any sequestra removed. In most horses, this can be performed standing with sedation and an abaxial nerve block, while maintaining the opposite foot in some type of support shoe (e.g., a SoftRide boot) to minimize trauma to that digit during the surgery. In a horse still suffering pain and/or lamellar instability in the opposite limb due to laminitis, it may be indicated to perform the surgery under general anesthesia. A tourniquet may be placed either mid-cannon or at the level of the fetlock joint affected limb; it is usually more effective in the recumbent horse. Septic pedal osteitis can occur with or without a draining tract in the sole. If a tract is present, it is best to insert a malleable probe into the deepest extent of the tract and to obtain a radiograph (solear margin view) to determine if the focus of septic bone can be effectively reached from the draining tract (Fig. 45.4a). If so, the affected region of the DP can be debrided (normally using a curette) through the tract. Although the curette will have to be placed through a contaminated tract to reach the DP, this is usually an impractical concern as the DP is likely already to be contaminated with or infected by the same organisms present in the tract. Perioperative antibiotics are usually administered; these can be administered systemically, via regional limb perfusion, or both. The clinician should still aseptically prepare the sole and debride and lavage the tract prior to the curettage. It is important to thoroughly curette the entire area of affected bone. The clinician

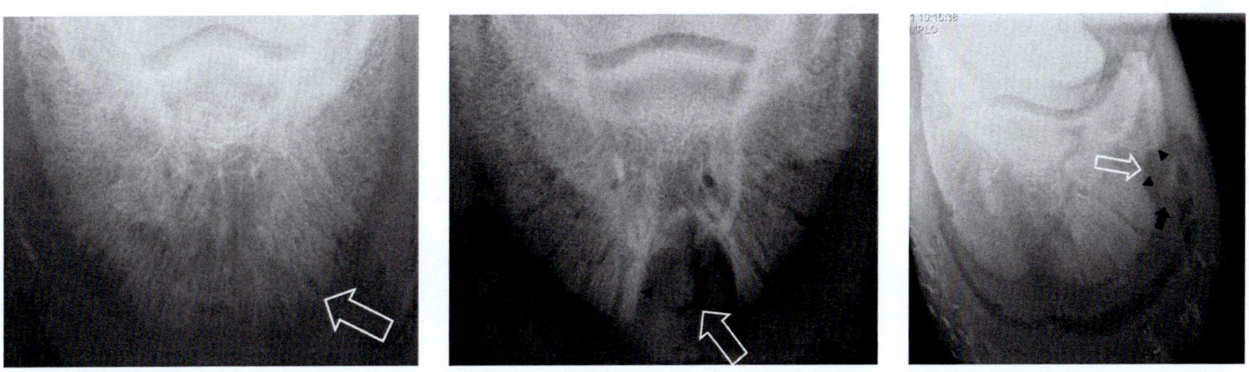

(a) (b) (c)

Figure 45.3 Radiographic evidence of pedal oseitis. (a) Note the 'moth-eaten' appearance of the solear margin (arrow, and inset at higher contrast) due to bone resorption from chronic bruising and inflammation. (b,c) Examples of septic pedal osteitis at (b) toe (open arrow, arrowheads indicating margins of sepsis), and (c) quarter (open arrow, arrowheads indicate margins, small closed black arrow indicates sequestrum).

will be able to ascertain when adequate curettage has occurred (only healthy bone is left) by the feel of the bone while curetting; a postoperative radiograph is indicated to ensure that all sequestrate and other bone fragments are removed. The owner needs to be warned that healing can be a slow process, taking several months [10]. If the sole is intact, the focus of septic osteitis can be approached through the hoof wall (Fig. 45.4b and c). In this case, a radiodense marker (the short screw in Fig. 45.4b) is placed at the anticipated site of entry in the hoof wall, and a radiograph is taken with the affected surface of the foot placed immediately adjacent to the radiographic screen to minimize magnification and distortion (Fig. 45.4b). A small hole is placed through the hoof wall (a Dremel bit or large drill bit works well) based on the radiographic findings, and the affected bone curetted and lavaged (Fig. 45.4c). The hoof defect is packed with a gauze soaked in mild antiseptic, and kept in place with adherent tape placed around the hoof wall. The gauze and bandage should be changed every two to four days, and the surgical site assessed for any evidence of ongoing sepsis. It may be necessary to lavage, or at least gently debride, the area with a sterile gauze sponge (or possibly again with a curette) if there is excessive exudate or any signs of ongoing sepsis (i.e., foul odor or purulence). The hoof wall normally heals by granulation followed by keratinization in a short period of time (two to four weeks).

Solear Perforation

One of the most difficult complications to assess and rectify is intracapsular instability of the DP. Presentation of changes at the coronet during the early stages of laminitis are indicative of intracapsular movement of the DP. The amount of instability is directly related to the number of compromised lamellae and applied load. In general, the greater the instability, the greater the pain in the acute phase. There are limited practical means of accurately determining the degree of instability of the bone to wall unit in a live animal. Plain and contrast radiographs taken of the digit under no load can be compared to one taken under full load in order to provide a means by which to assess movement of the bony column (see Chapter 28).

Excessive motion between the hoof capsule and bony column may be attenuated by applying the basic principles of podiatry providing uniform sole support, establishing appropriate angulation, and easing breakover of the foot. A variety of shoes and hoof appliances are available to facilitate the application of these principles. It is important to bear in mind the limitations of working through the distal surface of the hoof capsule to counteract the tremendous vertical force (from the horse's body weight) applied through compromised tissue. With extreme separation of lamellar tissue it is virtually impossible to prevent the distal movement of the DP with any hoof device. Other factors which must be considered as importantly as podiatry when addressing the unstable laminitic include the type of footing and bedding, activity restriction, the individual's body weight and condition, and the amount of time spent in recumbency.

Perforation of the sole by the DP most commonly occurs early in the disease process during the time of digital instability, but may occur later in the disease if the sole is compromised from chronic displacement of the DP. Solear perforation is a severe (but treatable) complication which needs to be addressed aggressively, especially in the early cases with ongoing instability. The physical dynamics that lead to perforation need to be addressed using an array of options including 'derotation' of the foot (trimming the heel in attempt to approximate a more normal relationship between the DP and sole; see Chapter 38), deep digital flexor tenotomy (see Chapter 43), and possibly the application of a cast to support the limb while neutralizing the forces leading to perforation. An open-sole cast can be applied to allow further treatment of the solear surface of the foot while applying support to the limb (see Chapter 42).

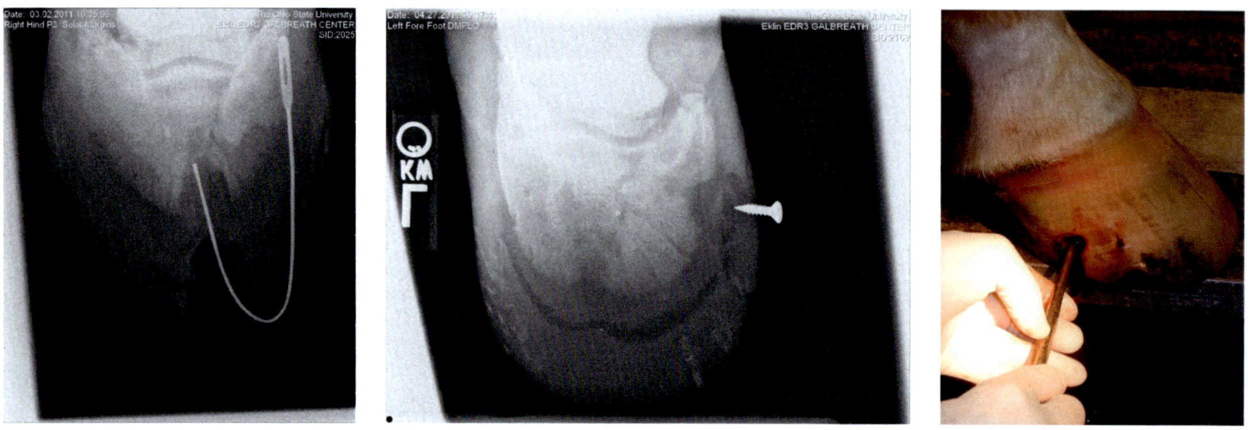

(a) (b) (c)

Figure 45.4 Surgical approach to pedal osteitis. (a) Note the use of a malleable probe to confirm that the draining tract in the sole leads to the septic focus. (b) Placement of a small screw in the hoof wall to determine access through the wall to a focus of septic osteitis with an intact sole. (c) Once the site was entered, a curette is used to debride the affected bone.

Complications of Other Body Systems and Treatment

Complications involving other body systems not directly related to the foot may result from the precipitating disease process, or from the long-term therapies employed to manage the patient. These complications may affect the integumentary, respiratory, reproductive, and gastrointestinal systems.

Prolonged recumbency frequently results in integumentary disruption. Decubital ulcers are most commonly seen and can be associated with cachectic body condition; this results in poor soft tissue coverage over bony prominences which combine to lead to pressure necrosis. The management of these ulcers can be challenging (see Chapter 30), and nonhealing wounds can lead to osteomyelitis and/or sepsis.

Respiratory system complications may also occur in recumbent animals, where oxygenation is decreased. In combination with depressed immunity and poor mucociliary clearance, pneumonia may develop. The same phenomenon may occur in patients undergoing prolonged suspension in a sling. Early recognition and treatment, as well as changes in management must be employed to reverse the lung pathology before end-stage pneumonia occurs.

Reproductive system complications can be varied, and may have the most significant impact on patients salvaged exclusively for breeding purposes. These occur in both sexes, although more are recognized in mares than in stallions. The catabolic state commonly present in severely affected laminitis patients is associated with a poor reproductive efficiency, including infertility in both mares and stallions. Within the equine breeding industry, this can have significant economic repercussions. Other common occurrences in the laminitic mare include stillbirth, abortion, and fetal dysmaturity; reduction in expected fetal body weight may also occur from poor *in-utero* nutrition and/or placentitis. In one of the presents authors' (R.H.) experience, once this occurs, a mare is unlikely to carry normal-weight foals to term in the future. The exception would be in cases of treatable bacterial placentitis, where intensive therapy may result in a favorable outcome.

Gastrointestinal system complications can range from mucosal ulceration to ileus or colic. Therapy with nonsteroidal anti-inflammatory drugs (NSAIDs) – particularly phenylbutazone – may contribute to gastric or large intestinal ulceration, although chronic pain may also create these conditions. The adverse effects on gastrointestinal motility in compromised patients (and also commonly from the prolonged use of opioids for analgesia) may result in many types of colic from a number of sources.

Complications of Diagnostic Procedures

The inability to correctly interpret diagnostic information in lameness examinations may contribute to an exacerbation of laminitis by creating a delay in the correct management of the disease. Local anesthesia may create complications; for example, failure of pain relief after local anesthesia may occur in the laminitis patient. Although the mechanism of failure is poorly understood, it is possibly associated with the intense level of inflammation in the tissue (see Chapter 33). Conversely, an increase in activity level when anesthesia occurs may also be detrimental. Other examples include a lack of response to hoof tester evaluation and the misinterpretation of digital pulse quality. Radiographic misinterpretation of both false-positive and false-negative "laminitics" may occur (see Chapter 27). Because of the dynamic and progressive nature of the disease, it is imperative to have serial radiographic and clinical evaluations in order to correctly interpret the pathologic processes.

Digital venography is a useful and commonly employed procedure in the diagnosis and management of laminitis (described in detail in Chapter 28) [23–26]. The most frequently observed technical complication is the perivascular administration of contrast media, which results in local pooling of contrast media at the injection site (Fig. 45.5a). Digital venography may also result in local tissue injury, inflammation and necrosis, and venous thrombosis. There are also variations created by techniques utilized in performing digital venography. Because there is a lack of standardization of technique regarding the amount of pressure used to insufflate the vasculature, variations in the

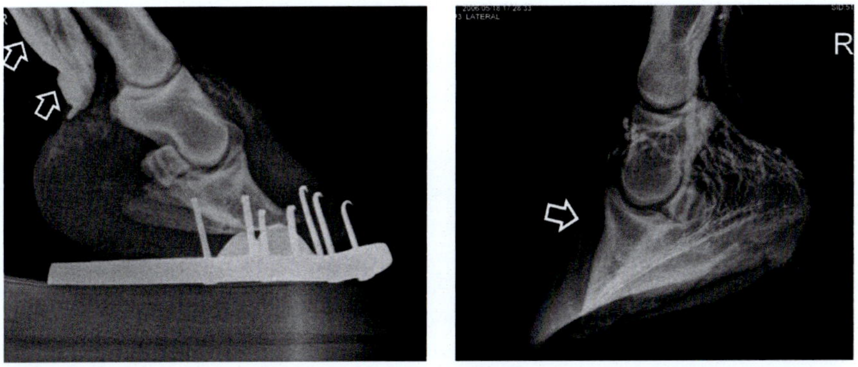

(a) (b)

Figure 45.5 (a) Perivenular pooling of contrast (arrow) with an inadvertent perivascular administration of contrast media. (b) Inadequate venular filling of the dorsal lamellae (arrow) due to poor injection technique, leading to the false interpretation of inadequate dorsal lamellar perfusion.

amount of contrast present may exist and may be interpreted as changes when none is present. Placement of the leg in a non-weight-bearing position while injecting the contrast media provides a lower resistance in the vascular space, allowing a more complete filling of the vasculature than when the limb is loaded, although operator preference may determine the technique used. Insufficient or asymmetrical filling of the vascular space may lead to an incorrect interpretation of the pathologic changes present (see Chapter 28). Inadequate filling of the dorsal lamellar space will occur with inadequate volume or pressure during injection, which may lead to the erroneous interpretation of the pathology (Fig. 45.5b). Likewise, a laterally injected foot with inadequate media filling may incorrectly be diagnosed as a 'medial sinker' (asymmetric distal displacement).

Complications of Hoof Care

Laminitis is not an exclusive trimming and shoeing problem, but rather a whole-horse management dilemma in which shoeing should be considered an adjunctive therapy. Essentially all of the physical therapies performed for the treatment of laminitis have the potential for complications. Commonly encountered problems are those associated with trimming, the application of shoes, or aggressively altering the mechanics of the foot.

Trimming complications generally arise from excessive changes in the angle (e.g., the solear margin/palmar angle), length, or balance of the foot, or from inadvertent perforation of the keratinized sole. It is critical to carefully evaluate the whole horse and to consider foot morphology and mechanics with regards to the stage of laminitis, the degree and reason for lameness, and to consider environmental and client factors when lining out a foot management program.

There should be a definitive indication for the application of shoes to a patient afflicted with acute laminitis, as the complications may be considerable. One of the most common problems with shoe application includes elevating the wall of the hoof without providing adequate solear support, thus propagating instability and DP displacement. Therefore, in the patient with early-stage laminitis in which digital instability is possible, a shoe may be of little benefit if there is a good-quality hoof capsule. As discussed earlier, the caregiver needs to bear in mind that there is not a type of shoe that can counteract severe intracapsular instability with excessive lamellar damage compounded by a vertical load of the weight of the horse. If an external device is required, the principles of uniform support should be adhered to, and may be accomplished with a variety of products that provide digital support and cushioning (see Chapters 39 and 40). If a shoe is applied, it must likewise adhere to these principles of uniform support, and not propagate instability nor apply too much solear pressure. If the patient is in a tenuous state in which instability is a concern, it should not be allowed access to excessive activity.

In chronic laminitis cases where intracapsular instability is not imminent, mechanical considerations such as breakover and the utilization of stable and more normal regions of the foot such as the heels and quarters are employed (see Chapters 38 and 41). These principles are more easily accomplished with the application of a therapeutic shoe, although it is imperative not to overload the heels and quarters or other normal regions of the foot, propagating further lamellar breakdown. For the long-term health of the foot, maintaining a bare foot state is ideal if the hoof is of adequate structural integrity.

Another complication of treatment can be excessive sole pressure resulting in solear bruising and pain. This may occur due to the direct application of a shoe over sensitive tissue, or it may arise from an excess amount of material used as sole support. This may also occur with intracapsular instability which allows displacement of the DP into the material, creating a relative increase in sole pressure. It best to err on the side of applying too-little material than an excessive amount and to remove material if there is a decline in the patient's condition after application.

Other complications are propagated from the use of hyperthermic composite/acrylic materials utilized in shoe application or hoof repair. Applying these materials over potentially contaminated horn without adequate drainage may result in abscess formation. Additionally, the chronic use of commonly used composite materials for shoe application or hoof reconstruction tends to trap moisture and contribute to degradation of the hoof wall over time. When utilizing these materials, it is vital to assess the condition of the underlying horn prior to the reapplication of any composite material. It may be necessary to allow the foot to undergo a drying period of several days or longer prior to reapplication in order to prevent deterioration of the horn.

Complications of Cryotherapy

Cryotherapy/digital hypothermia has been well documented as an effective preventive therapy for experimentally induced laminitis and in clinic patients in the developmental phase of sepsis-related laminitis, and even when the therapy is not initiated until the onset of clinical signs of laminitis (see Chapter 34) [27–32]. The distal extremity of the horse tolerates extreme cold for prolonged periods with few adverse effects, and therefore complications are not commonly reported in the literature. Anecdotal reports of adverse effects of locally applied ice therapy include blistering/maceration of the skin and coronary band, nerve damage, frostbite, and local immune-compromise associated with hypothermia. One possible cause of complications is when placing ice directly against the leg (i.e., without adequate water interface), due to the fact that ice from the freezer is at −20 °C to −30 °C (which may cause true frostbite) in comparison to exceeding 0 °C when it is mixed with water (A. van Eps, personal communication). Although normally used only for a few days in most cases, due in part to anecdotal reports of increased complications with prolonged use, one of the present authors (R.H.) has utilized the modality continuously after the onset of clinical signs for more than four weeks with favorable clinical results while arresting the progression of acute displacement.

Complications of Surgery

The most common surgical procedures performed in the patient with laminitis include curettage and debridement of the DP and deep digital flexor tenotomy [13–15, 33]. Deep digital flexor tenotomy complications include surgical errors of vascular transection, inadvertent transection of other tendons, sepsis at the surgery site, creation of instability in the palmar region of the foot, and distal interphalangeal joint subluxation (see Chapter 43). This procedure therefore may be contraindicated in patients that exhibit a negative palmar angle of the DP, underslung heels, or have palmar instability and lamellar overload. These conditions are indicative of compromised lamellar attachment through the palmar region of the foot, and deep digital flexor tenotomy may exacerbate the instability, resulting in further detachment of the hoof. Ideal surgical candidates are those which suffer from chronic stable laminitis with phalangeal rotation (rotation of the dorsal aspect of the DP away from the hoof wall with concurrent flexion of the distal interphalangeal joint) with recurrent lameness issues due to the pressure of the dorsodistal aspect of the DP on the solear surface (e.g., solear bruising, abscessation).

Inadequate foot management following tenotomy can result in either sub-luxation of the distal interphalangeal joint or contraction of the metacarpophalangeal joint. A greater release of tension of the DDFT – and greater palmar instability to the distal interphalangeal joint – may be achieved with the palmar pastern tenotomy; therefore, it is imperative to apply an elevated (and possibly extended) heel shoe or hoof device in order to prevent subluxation of the distal interphalangeal joint. The elevation is generally between 2° and 5°, but this varies based on the angle of the foot. A similar shoe should be applied prior to mid-metacarpal tenotomy, although the same degree of luxation is generally not experienced.

Conscientious aftercare and follow-up are required to prevent or recognize metacarpophalangeal contraction at its earliest occurrence. Contraction of the metacarpophalangeal joint occurs more commonly following the mid-metacarpal tenotomy. This contracture usually occurs secondary to recrudescence of pain and relative shortening of the DDFT following healing and scarring. The prolonged use of pressure wraps over the surgical area and extended stall rest (up to three months postoperatively) decreases the degree of scarring/excessive DDFT thickening, and may therefore decrease the incidence of contraction of the metacarpophalangeal joint. Treatment for postoperative metacarpophalangeal contraction generally involves transection of the DDFT at the mid-pastern level, along with the application of an appropriate shoe.

Complications encountered with curettage of the DP include no improvement or worsening of lameness due to inadequate removal of septic material, or removal of excess healthy bone/tissue (with possible entry into the distal interphalangeal joint).

Summary

The multitude of complications affecting horses suffering from laminitis commonly dictate the final outcome of the patient. Having an understanding of the mechanisms of these complications is paramount for enacting preventive strategies to obtain a successful outcome. Early recognition and intervention is critical to prevent progression of the complications, which can occur at all stages of the disease process. Unfortunately, many cases are beyond the current ability to successfully treat, and it is important that this is recognized and accurately conveyed to the client to prevent the inhumane suffering of the patient.

References

1. Pollitt, CC. (2010) The anatomy and physiology of the suspensory apparatus of the distal phalanx. *Vet. Clin. North Am. Equine Pract.*, **26**, 29–49.
2. Kyaw-Tanner, M.T., Wattle, O., Van Eps, A.W., *et al.* (2008) Equine laminitis: membrane type matrix metalloproteinase-1 (MMP-14) is involved in acute phase onset. *Equine Vet. J.*, **40**, 482–487.
3. Pollitt, C.C. (1994) The basement membrane at the equine hoof dermal epidermal junction. *Equine Vet. J.*, **26**, 399–407.
4. Van Eps, A.W. and Pollitt, C.C. (2009) Equine laminitis model: lamellar histopathology seven days after induction with oligofructose. *Equine Vet. J.*, **41**, 735–740.
5. Molyneux, G.S., Haller, C.J., Mogg, K.C., *et al.* (1994) The structure, innervation and location of arteriovenous anastomoses in the equine foot. *Equine Vet. J.*, **26**, 305–312.
6. Pollitt, C.C. (1996) Basement membrane pathology: a feature of acute equine laminitis. *Equine Vet. J.*, **28**, 38–46.
7. Johnson, P.J. (2002) The equine metabolic syndrome: peripheral Cushing's syndrome. *Vet. Clin. North Am. Equine Pract.*, **18**, 271–293.
8. Belknap, J.K. and Moore, J.N. (eds) (2009) Special issue: inflammatory aspects of equine laminitis. *Vet. Immunol. Immunopathol.*, **T3-4**, 149–262.
9. Pollitt, C.C. and Daradka, M. (1998) Equine laminitis basement membrane pathology: loss of type IV collagen, type VII collagen and laminin immunostaining. *Equine Vet. J. Suppl.*, **26**, 139–144.
10. French, K.R. and Pollitt, C.C. (2004) Equine laminitis: cleavage of key hemidesmosome proteins associated with basement membrane dysadhesion. *Equine Vet. J.*, **36**, 242–247.
11. Pollitt, C.C., Pass, M.A., and Pollitt, S. (1998) Batimastat (BB-94) inhibits matrix metalloproteinases of equine laminitis. *Equine Vet. J. Suppl.*, **26**, 119–124.

12. Collins, S.N., Van Eps, A.W., and Pollitt, C.C. (2010) The lamellar wedge. *Vet. Clin. North Am. Equine Pract.*, **26**, 179–196.
13. Hunt, R.J., Allen, D., Baxter, G.M., *et al.* (1991) Mid-metacarpal deep digital flexor tenotomy in the management of refractory laminitis in horses. *Vet. Surg.*, **20**, 15–20.
14. Morrison, S. (2011) Long-term prognosis using deep digital flexor tenotomy and realignment shoeing for treatment of chronic laminitis. *J. Equine Vet. Sci.*, **31**, 89–96.
15. Allen, D, Jr, White, N.A., II, Foerner, J.F., and Gordon, B.J. (1986) Surgical management of chronic laminitis in horses: 13 cases (1983–1985). *J. Am. Vet. Med. Assoc.*, **189**, 1604–1606.
16. Grosenbaugh, D.A., Morgan, S.J., and Hood, D.M. (1999) The digital pathologies of chronic laminitis. *Vet. Clin. North Am. Equine Pract.*, **15**, 419–436.
17. Hunt, R.J. and Wharton, R.E. (2010) Clinical presentation, diagnosis, and prognosis of chronic laminitis in North America. *Vet. Clin. North Am. Equine Pract.*, **26**, 141–154.
18. Collins, S.N., Pollitt, C.C., Wylie, C.E., and Matiasek, K. (2010) Laminitic pain: parallels with pain states in humans and other species. *Vet. Clin. North Am. Equine Pract.*, **26**, 643–72.
19. Hood, D.M. (1999) The mechanisms and consequences of structural failure of the foot. *Vet. Clin. North Am. Equine Pract.*, **15**, 437–462.
20. Morrison, S. (2010) Maggot debridement therapy for laminitis. *Vet. Clin. North Am. Equine Pract.*, **26**, 447–450.
21. Cauvin, E.R. and Munroe, G.A. (1998) Septic osteitis of the distal phalanx: findings and surgical treatment in 18 cases. *Equine Vet. J.*, **30**, 512–519.
22. Burnt, N.W., Baker, S.J., Wagner, I.P., *et al.* (1997) Digital instability as a potential prognostic indicator in horses with chronic laminitis, in *Proceedings of the Hoof Project* (eds D.M. Hood, I.P. Wagner, and A.C. Jacobson), Private Publishers, College Station, Texas, p. 105.
23. Redden, R.R. (2001) A technique for performing digital venography in the standing horse. *Equine Vet. J.*, **13**, 128–134.
24. Rucker, A. (2006) How to perform a digital venogram. *Proc. Am. Assoc. Equine Pract.*, **52**, 526–530.
25. Baldwin, G.I. and Pollitt, C.C. (2010) Progression of venographic changes after experimentally induced laminitis. *Vet. Clin. North Am. Equine Pract.*, **26**, 135–140.
26. Rucker, A. (2010) Equine venography and its clinical application in North America. *Vet. Clin. North Am. Equine Pract.*, **26**, 167–178.
27. Van Eps, A.W. and Pollitt, C.C. (2004) Equine laminitis: cryotherapy reduces the severity of the acute lesion. *Equine Vet. J.*, **36**, 255–260.
28. Van Eps, A.W. and Pollitt, C.C. (2009) Equine laminitis model: cryotherapy reduces the severity of lesions evaluated seven days after induction with oligofructose. *Equine Vet. J.*, **41**, 741–746.
29. Van Eps, A.W. (2010) Therapeutic hypothermia (cryotherapy) to prevent and treat acute laminitis. *Vet. Clin. North Am. Equine Pract.*, **26**, 125–133.
30. Van Eps, A.W. and Orsini, J.A. (2016) A comparison of seven methods for continuous therapeutic cooling of the equine digit. *Equine Vet. J.*, **48** (1), 120–124.
31. Burke, M., Tomlinson, J., Dallap-Schaer, B., *et al.* (2015) Measurement of digital lamellar and skin temperature during cryotherapy with a sleeve style ice boot in healthy horses. *Proc. Vet. Surg. Am. Coll. Vet. Surg.*, **44**, E47.
32. Pollitt, C.C. and Van Eps, A.W. (2004) Prolonged, continuous distal limb cryotherapy in the horse. *Equine Vet. J.*, **36**, 216–220.
33. Waguespack, R.W. and Caldwell, F. (2009) How to perform a modified standing deep digital flexor tenotomy at the level of the proximal interphalangeal joint. *Proc. Am. Assoc. Equine Pract.*, **55**, 230–237.

PART 8

Management of Chronic Laminitis

Equine Laminitis, First Edition. Edited by James K. Belknap and Raymond Geor.

CHAPTER 46
Management Changes in the Laminitis Case

Andrew Van Eps, Robert J. Hunt, James K. Belknap and Jeff Ridley

Introduction

This chapter is a compilation of the views of the authors (ranging from equine veterinary internists and surgeons to a certified journeyman farrier) regarding the judgment of changes in management, including medical therapies, approaches to foot care, the decision for euthanasia of the laminitis case and, importantly, the communication of these changes in management with the owner.

Client Communications in Treatment Decisions

Client communication is one of the most important but least discussed aspects of case management of laminitis; this is particularly important in laminitis due to the multiple changes in treatment commonly necessary to treat one animal, the likelihood of failures of some treatments, the multiple complications that can occur, and the degree of suffering that animals afflicted with the disease commonly endure. Client expectations at the onset of the disease process are often unrealistic, and the importance of explaining the possible outcomes cannot be overstated. Often, client expectations are based on a previous experience with laminitis, and it is important to understand that this can cause confusion. For example, if a client has previously owned a pony with mild chronic laminitis that was successfully managed over several years, they may have difficulty understanding that an acute severe sepsis-related laminitis (SRL) or supporting limb laminitis (SLL) case is quite different and carries a poorer prognosis. On the contrary, it is essential for the veterinarian and farrier to convey a good prognosis in some situations (e.g., the case of endocrinopathic laminitis likely to respond well to therapeutic and management changes), as some owners believe all types of laminitis carry a dismal prognosis. The accurate conveyance of information on a regular basis is critical not only for the animal's benefit, but also to avoid client dissatisfaction, unpaid debt, and possible litigation. A policy of open, honest communication must be observed, and it is also important to temper false expectations. Given the seriousness of a case of severe laminitis, clients will most likely inquire with other sources regarding management of their horse. It is imperative that the treating veterinarian and farrier are well versed in the common inquiries and that these are addressed prospectively.

A critical factor at the initiation of management of any laminitis case is open communication between the veterinarian and farrier, resulting in the presentation of a unified approach to case management. A vital component to the combined approach of farrier and veterinarian which should be discussed early in the course of treatment in the severe case is the guarded prognosis for the case; this needs to be clearly and plainly communicated, and includes: (i) the likelihood of failure to successfully treat the disease even with state of the art care; and (ii) what parameters will be assessed to determine when the humane concerns outweigh other concerns and will dictate the euthanasia of the animal. It is often necessary to reiterate with the client possible outcomes as the disease process continues. If these parameters are established early during the course of treatment, owners are usually much more amenable to making difficult decisions when the horse exhibits these parameters than when the owner feels that they have been 'blindsided' with a negative appraisal by the professional examining the patient at a later point in the treatment.

It is important to ensure that clients thoroughly understand several main points when managing a horse with laminitis. The first point to make is that, once afflicted with morphological changes within the foot, the horse is at risk for complications for the remainder of its life. The client also needs to understand that, even without serious complications, long-term management of these patients is a necessity and may encompass one year or even the remainder of the life of the horse. In severely affected patients, it is common for the final outcome to be a persistently unsound horse in which the only humane choice may eventually be euthanasia. Finally, the owner needs to understand that every patient is different, and that there is commonly a degree of trial and error involved to establish the best combination of therapies for their horse.

Accurately predicting the outcome of horses with laminitis is controversial and challenging. This is understandable given the number of variables associated with management of the clinical patient including not only the feet but also the rest of the

Equine Laminitis, First Edition. Edited by James K. Belknap and Raymond Geor.

patient, in addition to client variables. In the remainder of this chapter the authors will discuss their general views on the adjustment of medical and shoeing management through the course of therapy, and finally highlight the circumstance when humane euthanasia is the appropriate decision to make for a particular case.

Judging the Need for Adjustments of Medical Therapy

The two primary types of therapy that the clinician must continuously assess when treating the different types of laminitis case are those dealing with analgesia from digital pain, and therapies for the underlying disease process which led to laminitis. Although the most common form of analgesia used in practice is nonsteroidal anti-inflammatory drugs (NSAIDs), intramuscular opioids and constant rate infusions (CRIs) of different classes of drugs may also be used (primarily in the hospital setting). Medications for the predisposing disease processes are primarily a concern for SRL and endocrinopathic laminitis, although they play an important role in SLL if due to a septic condition in the originally affected limb.

Sepsis-Related Laminitis (SRL)

The use of NSAIDs in SRL is commonly to serve two purposes: (i) to provide analgesia; and (ii) to address systemic and local lamellar inflammation associated with endotoxemia/sepsis. As flunixin meglumine is regarded as the most effective NSAID for counteracting the systemic inflammation of sepsis (see Chapter 35), most clinicians continue the use of flunixin while the animals are exhibiting clinical signs of sepsis in either the septic horse at risk of laminitis or the horse exhibiting initial signs of laminitis. As signs of sepsis diminish, the clinician treating a septic horse at risk of laminitis will likely taper off the flunixin to lower doses and then discontinue NSAID therapy over the next few days. In the horse exhibiting clinical signs of lameness due to laminitis (which commonly begins as signs of sepsis subside in acute causes of sepsis such as grain overload or acute metritis), a change from flunixin to phenylbutazone is frequently performed due to anecdotal reports of superior musculoskeletal analgesia associated with phenylbutazone. The cases which are somewhat less straightforward are those that continue to exhibit signs of sepsis while exhibiting moderate to severe digital pain from laminitis (common in disease states such as enterocolitis). Some clinicians may combine the two NSAIDs in an attempt to achieve the 'anti-endotoxin effect' of flunixin and the 'musculoskeletal effect' of phenylbutazone. Although there is experimental evidence of increased musculoskeletal analgesia with a combination of these NSAIDs [1], using lower doses of both drugs is indicated if they are combined due to the likelihood of increased side effects [1]. There is probably no need to do this, as flunixin has been shown also to effectively decrease musculoskeletal pain [2, 3], just as phenylbutazone has been shown to mitigate the effects of endotoxin [4]. It is probably best to continue flunixin in the animal exhibiting moderate signs of both sepsis and digital pain, not only due to its increased efficacy in treating systemic inflammation but also due to its decreased incidence of renal side effects compared to phenylbutazone as, similar to kidneys being a target organ of human sepsis, equids with ongoing sepsis (commonly enterocolitis cases) are also at risk of renal injury. If flunixin therapy is not adequately addressing digital pain in these animals, it may be indicated to add intramuscular opioid therapy or a CRI of an opioid (see Chapter 33) or a mixture of analgesics (e.g., lidocaine, ketamine, and an opioid). The two primary reasons for adjusting NSAID dosages and intramuscular or CRI analgesia are the onset of complications associated with these drugs (e.g., large intestinal impaction due to decreased gastrointestinal motility with opioids) or inadequate control of digital pain. A large concern with the use of NSAIDs in the septic horse is renal or gastrointestinal (stomach or large intestine) injury, which may necessitate either the cessation of NSAIDS or a change to an NSAID with less detrimental effects on the kidney such as ketoprofen [5, 6] or the more cyclooxygenase-2 (COX-2)-selective NSAIDs (firocoxib or meloxicam). The primary complication with the use of opioids (especially in a CRI) is large intestinal impaction, which will require cessation of opioids until the impaction resolves.

Other medications used for the treatment of sepsis in SRL include intravenous fluid support, polymixin B, and antibiotics (see Chapter 35). All of these therapies are usually halted as soon as the animals are not exhibiting clinical signs of sepsis; polymixin B therapy should be halted earlier if indications of renal damage are present. Due to the robust clinical and experimental data supporting its efficacy, the use of digital hypothermia (cryotherapy) in septic animals has become a mainstay of treatment, both as a prophylactic treatment to avoid laminitis in equine cases of sepsis and in the treatment of laminitis in the animal exhibiting clinical signs of sepsis (see Chapter 34). Although most clinicians and researchers agree that cryotherapy should be applied constantly whilst the primary septic disease process runs its course, no data exists regarding when to stop the therapy; this results in variation between clinicians regarding the duration of the cryotherapy. When used as a prophylactic therapy in the septic horse, many clinicians halt cryotherapy soon after the animal is not demonstrating clinical signs of sepsis, whereas others continue cryotherapy for one to several days after recovery from sepsis. Most clinicians are likely to extend cryotherapy in those animals exhibiting clinical signs of laminitis past the point of resolution of systemic sepsis, as the therapy has been demonstrated to be effective in limiting lamellar injury in experimentally induced acute SRL cases, even when not initiated until after the development of lameness.

Endocrinopathic Laminitis

Horses with endocrinopathic laminitis commonly have more lamellar stability (than SRL or SLL cases) due in part to the insidious nature of this type of laminitis, and therefore are frequently not as painful (see Chapter 22) as the other two types of laminitis. Although there may be acute lamellar pain particularly in pasture-associated cases, due to an insidious, chronic displacement of the distal phalanx (DP) common to endocrine-related causes of laminitis, the pain commonly emanates from sole bruising more so than lamellar pain. Therefore, NSAID therapy is commonly the only analgesia needed for endocrinopathic laminitis, and can commonly be used at lower doses than with other types of laminitis. Even in endocrine-related cases of active lamellar pain, the pain frequently decreases more rapidly due to a greater degree of lamellar stability than that commonly present in SRL or SLL. Thus, it is not uncommon to be able to rapidly decrease the dose of NSAIDs once the animal's diet has been managed and shoeing performed to address solear bruising/injury as well as lamellar concerns. In horses with metabolic syndrome being treated with thyroxine, this treatment can commonly be stopped in approximately three to four months if dietary changes (and possibly mild exercise) are resulting in weight loss and increased insulin sensitivity (see Chapter 36). Although recent studies have indicated that pituitary pars intermedia dysfunction (PPID) may only exacerbate equine metabolic syndrome-associated laminitis and not be a cause of laminitis itself [7], treatment of the endocrinopathic laminitis case suffering from PPID with pergolide to ameliorate the effects of the benign functional pituitary tumor is usually long term (for the life of the horse), as the tumor will be active for the rest of the animal's life (see Chapter 37). In one of the present authors' (A.V.E.) experience, metformin administration to reduce the insulin response to ingested carbohydrates can make a dramatic difference in the management of endocrinopathic laminitis, even when foot pathology is advanced. Adjustments in the dosage and timing of metformin (i.e., targeted administration prior to feed or turnout) are commonly necessary in management of chronic endocrinopathic cases (see Chapter 36).

Supporting Limb Laminitis (SLL)

Due to the rapid catastrophic lamellar failure that commonly occurs with SLL once signs of laminitis are present (see Chapter 25), aggressive changes in management may be indicated in an attempt to halt a rapid progression to irreversible lamellar failure. If the horse's temperament will allow it, placement of the animal in a sling may be indicated if it does not respond to more conservative therapy. Increased doses of NSAIDs or additional analgesia may be indicated in the animal that is not responding, hopefully to allow some weight-bearing on the initially injured limb. Finally, although not experimentally assessed in SLL, cryotherapy is commonly started immediately to treat the limb affected with SLL.

Judging the Timing and Need for a Change in Foot Care

Foot care in the laminitis case requires a great deal of teamwork between the veterinarian and farrier, with constant communication with the owner and/or trainer. The two primary needs for a change in foot care/shoeing management are: (i) the case which is not responding well to the current shoeing; and (ii) the case which has responded well to therapy, where the veterinarian and farrier need to consider when to change the shoeing to a sustainable shoeing management which can be used for the long term. The veterinarian and farrier must work together from the onset. It is essential that there is an effort for either the farrier or veterinarian examining a laminitis case to immediately involve the other – both on the initial workup of the case and continuously as the case progresses. In a recent survey of over 500 farriers in the US and UK, one of the primary frustrations of farriers in farrier/veterinarian communication was a failure of veterinarians to immediately contact the farrier when the veterinarian is the first professional (versus the farrier) to be called to examine/treat a laminitis case (most farriers wanted to be called immediately regardless of whether it was during night/emergency hours). An accurate diagnosis of a specific cause for the onset of laminitis will contribute to the expectations of success or failure of the effort. Farriery becomes irrelevant in a laminitic case when an animal does not respond to the medical (or possibly surgical) treatment of the condition that brought upon the laminitis. It is also essential that the veterinarian and farrier respect each other's experience in designing a plan for the horse. Although both need to be open-minded regarding each other's views on each case, it is usually best to incorporate methods of foot care with which the farrier has extensive experience (i.e., not to have the veterinarian dictate a type of foot care with which the farrier has no experience and is uncomfortable using). It is also important to realize that there are multiple options that can be considered viable for the same case; one of the present authors (R.H.) commonly maintains his laminitis cases (even moderate to severe cases) barefoot for the entire treatment period, whereas the others are more likely to address the feet with different types of apparatuses (discussed below).

The frequency with which radiographs are used to guide the trim, as well as the choice of an appropriate selection of appliance for the feet, may depend not only on the cause of the onset of laminitis but also on the type of treatment prescribed. The environment in which the horse lives also becomes a major factor, along with the ability of the owner to provide daily follow-up treatment.

The first time that a change in foot care may be necessary is within the first few days of the onset of laminitis. At this point in time, the foot management will most likely consist of the initial removal of standard shoes and the application of some type of padding or temporary shoe (e.g., the Redden Ultimate or clog; see Chapter 40). If the animal worsens with the initial apparatus placed on the feet, the veterinarian/farrier team needs to contemplate whether a different type of apparatus should be applied. It is imperative for the veterinarian and farrier to both assess the horse upon changing management of the feet together without anesthetics (local or general), as the horse will often show an immediate indication whether or not the chosen apparatus offers relief or increases pain. For example, some horses may respond negatively to an increase in tension on the deep flexor apparatus when dressing heels to increase the ground surface of the foot. Additionally, repeat radiographs are commonly taken to assess whether the type or severity of DP displacement has changed over that period of time. If a flat pad is initially applied to the foot with minimal response over 24–48 h, the team may want to contemplate changing to a type of apparatus/shoe that does more than provide cushioning and support. A plastic shoe to change foot dynamics such (e.g., the Redden Ultimate with a 20° heel wedge) can be temporarily applied with tape for 12–24 h (to assess the response to the shoeing change) if the team feel that it is indicated. Another option is either a wooden or ethyl vinyl acetate (EVA) clog either early in the management or if the animal has not responded to the discussed options. In the latter case, the clogs can be taped on for a few minutes for an initial assessment, but need to be applied at least with a cast material if they are going to be used overnight. The team needs to bear in mind that any deterioration may be solely due to extensive lamellar injury resulting in severe lamellar instability for which no shoe is likely to be effective; this scenario is usually accompanied by severe pain and rapid changes on serial radiographs. At this point in time, the only options may be to decrease the downward forces on the DP by the application of a cast (see Chapter 42) or possibly to place the horse in a sling. As these animals are usually in extreme pain and the prognosis deteriorates immensely with rapid displacement of the DP, the contemplation of euthanasia should be part of the conversation at that point in time (this is discussed in detail later in the chapter).

In the equine patient that the team is successfully maintaining in relative comfort, and is halting the progression of displacement of the DP over the first three to four weeks, the veterinarian/farrier team needs to assess whether the lamellae have stabilized to the point that the application of a longer-term shoe is now possible.

After three to four weeks of management with the above type of treatments, the horse should be assessed for the possibility of therapeutic shoeing by placing either a metal shoe or wooden shoe at that point in time. A thorough examination of the foot, in addition to a radiographic assessment, should be performed to determine if the foot has stabilized adequately for shoe application. The degree of digital pain will hopefully have decreased from that observed during the first one to two weeks. On radiographic assessment, measurements taken from lateral and dorsopalmar radiographs should indicate a stabilization of the displacement when compared to earlier radiographs (i.e., no further displacement). Obtaining an adequate degree of stability over three to six weeks is going to be more likely in the animal without a severe loss of lamellar stability (and therefore not a severe degree of displacement of the DP); this is commonly the case in many equine metabolic syndrome cases and also in horses in which the systemic insult causing the lamellar injury was quickly resolved (e.g., pasture-associated laminitis, consumption of black walnut shavings). With severe displacement or longer-term systemic insult (e.g., enterocolitis cases or possibly severe endocrinopathic cases which require several months of therapy to control systemic derangements), the time point at which a shoe can be applied may be extended by several weeks. Many of the shoe types applied at the three- to six-week time point may also be considered temporary for only three to six months, at which time – if the horse continues to improve – the foot management may be changed more towards the type of foot care that the animal will employ long term for its expected use. Shoeing at this point in time is likely to incorporate the principles described in Chapter 38, decreasing stress on the affected hoof wall by beveling the toe or different aspects of the shoe under the affected wall (or by beveling all parts of the shoe, as seen in the wooden shoe and recently in more metal shoes). If the animal has been maintained in some type of flat pad (e.g., either a commercial system such as the SoftRide or a basic pad made from closed-cell foam), the first type of shoe may be either a flat shoe or clog, possibly combined with the application of putty to the foot to provide some digital support. If the animal has been comfortable for several weeks in a system such as the Redden Ultimate, in which a marked heel elevation has been used, then a shoe still incorporating a heel wedge such as a rail shoe or an adjustable system such as the EDSS natural balance shoe (Equine Digital Support System, Inc.) may be applied in which an adjustable wedge and silastic putty can be used (this is a good option for a farrier not well versed in therapeutic farriery).

After several months in therapeutic shoeing in which the horse has continued to improve, the team needs to reassess and attempt to make a transition back to a type of foot management consistent with the expected function of the horse in the future. In some horses (especially the broodmare or retired athlete) the team may contemplate managing the horse barefoot at this time, depending on the environment in which the horse lives and the reasonable expectation of soundness. A thorough examination by the veterinarian and farrier, including radiographic assessment, is critical at this time to aid in the decision, and to guide the farrier's trimming and possible shoe application. In the case of the horse which the owner would like to transition to barefoot, it is critical to obtain radiographs to assess the orientation of the DP to the sole, sole depth, and general health of the hoof capsule. With prior displacement and a thin sole, the animal will be prone to bruising and secondary seroma/abscess formation; these animals will likely require further therapeutic shoeing to protect the sole (primarily the toe) until a more normal relationship of the DP to the sole and greater sole depth are accomplished. In the case in which palmar rotation of the DP is resulting in recurring sole injury, a gradual derotation will be necessary before the animal will be able to be managed without shoes. In some horses (especially geriatric animals) the owner may request to maintain the animals in a pad in the long term (e.g., SoftRide) versus keeping the animal in shoes. This approach works well in many animals with minimal expectations regarding ambulation, but the animals often appear not to improve their sole thickness with this type of management.

Management of Chronic Laminitis: Determining when Further Treatment is No Longer Humane

Laminitis is commonly a debilitating disease that can cause crippling, persistent lameness. Since laminitis cannot be effectively cured, but will not lead directly to the death of the horse, euthanasia becomes an important consideration for horses that have progressive or persistent lameness or dysfunction, and when suffering due to pain is perceived as being too great. Laminitis, along with other causes of lameness such as arthritis, is a leading reason for euthanasia in geriatric horses [8]. Currently, the ability to effectively treat chronic laminitis is very limited, and the provision of adequate analgesia in severe or longstanding cases is very challenging. However, many horses with laminitis can recover and regain an excellent quality of life, and many return to athletic function despite an initial period of moderate to severe lameness. Thus, in coming to a recommendation for euthanasia, it is very important to consider the balance between prognosis and welfare/quality of life in the short and long term for the horse, as well as the expectations, resources, and goals (for the horse) of the owner. Horses cannot represent their own interests, and therefore the responsibility rests with the owner and the veterinarian/farrier team to decide what course of action is in the best interest of the horse. Owners are generally more familiar with the animal's history and normal behavioral traits, and are therefore commonly better equipped to assess changes in these factors when trying to ultimately estimate the horse's quality of life. Although the final decision generally rests with the owner, the veterinarian/farrier team is still best equipped to make informed judgments about the balance between prognosis and welfare in most cases; the veterinarian is most commonly expected to work with and guide the owner as to whether euthanasia is indicated.

Considering the Prognosis

Very little information is freely available on the prognosis for laminitis cases, and there is great variability in the findings and opinions related to such prognoses which may be due to multiple variables, including differences in the primary underlying causes of laminitis in different populations. When considering the prognosis, the veterinarian should take into account: (i) the underlying cause of laminitis; (ii) the severity, chronicity, and rate of progression of lameness and foot pathology; and (iii) other concurrent health concerns (e.g., ongoing sepsis, decubital sores, etc.). The owner's expectations in terms of the outcome and the current/intended usage of the horse may also be important factors in some cases. In more severe cases where there is likely to be a protracted convalescence, the availability of resources (funds, facilities and human resources) required to care for the horse must also be considered.

Horses that develop SLL have a poor prognosis due to the fact that this form of laminitis is often rapidly progressive and results in a widespread simultaneous failure of lamellar attachment [9]. Additionally, the primary problem in the opposite limb in SLL cases is also often not resolved (e.g., a fracture repair) at the time of development, and this factor alone can diminish the prognosis to an extent where euthanasia is often indicated. The pain of SLL development is often so intense that the horse preferentially shifts weight back onto the limb with the primary problem which can be detrimental to healing (possibly leading to failure of internal fixation) in many orthopedic cases.

Laminitis secondary to sepsis/systemic inflammatory conditions tends to also be rapidly progressive and can be severe enough to cause widespread lamellar failure. Similar to treating the originally injured limb in SLL, successful control of the primary disease causing systemic inflammation/sepsis may be an issue both for controlling laminitis progression and also in terms of overall prognosis. In a retrospective study of SRL, primarily of gastrointestinal origin, survival was approximately 50%, and only 25% of animals returned to an athletic career [10]. The importance of laminitis development to the overall prognosis in horses with sepsis was highlighted in a more recent study of clinical colitis cases, where survival for horses that developed laminitis was only 48% compared to 98% for those horses that did not develop laminitis [11].

In contrast, laminitis associated with endocrine dysfunction – either PPID or equine metabolic syndrome (EMS) – tends to be more slowly progressive, and although these horses may have periods of severe lameness (often associated with access to carbohydrate-rich feed or pasture) they can often recover remarkably well. Of 107 horses and ponies affected by pasture-induced laminitis in one study, survival was 95% at eight weeks after the onset of lameness, and approximately 60% of horses returned to riding usage [12]. Smaller-breed horses and ponies appeared to have a better prognosis for clinical outcome in that study [12]. The ability to control insulin resistance and insulin responses to dietary carbohydrates through nutritional management and/or pharmacological intervention in these cases is important for an ongoing good prognosis.

Although the severity of radiographic displacement of the DP relative to the hoof capsule may help to predict which horses might return to athletic function, the severity of lameness appears to be the most reliable prognostic indicator for survival [10, 13, 14]. The speed of progression of radiographic change may be more important to prognosis than the absolute severity of displacement [14], and the serial monitoring of clinical and radiographic parameters is therefore vital when attempting to prognosticate. It is well accepted that radiographic evidence of progressive distal displacement of the DP within the hoof capsule is associated with a poorer prognosis for survival (although there are still clinical exceptions to this rule) [10, 13–17].

The inability to control pain is the most important factor contributing to treatment failure and euthanasia in horses suffering from laminitis. However, laminitis is a somewhat unique situation in that pain itself plays an important role in promoting self-preservation, particularly in the acute and early chronic phases of the disease; without pain, weight-bearing and ambulation are not restricted and the consequence of this is an increase in the mechanical distractive forces acting on the lamellar tissue and progression of the lesion itself. When considering prognosis for severely affected horses, it is one of the present authors' (A.V.E.) experience that many cases may take at least seven days to show clinical improvement after the onset of lameness; however, horses experiencing clinical signs for more than two weeks without noticeable improvement have a greatly reduced probability of a favorable outcome [18].

Important Welfare Considerations Including Quality of Life

The treatment of horses with chronic laminitis always involves periods where the horse must endure not only varying degrees of pain but also stress associated with procedures and unnatural environments (e.g., confinement). When considering treatment options (including euthanasia) for laminitis cases, the prognosis should be balanced against welfare considerations, most importantly the current and likely future quality of life for the horse. Quality of life is determined not only by an assessment of the severity of pain but also by the presence of a range of other negative experiences related to disease pathology and husbandry (e.g., distress, frustration, anxiety, boredom), and also the presence of positive experiences (e.g., amusement, curiosity, social interaction) for the animal [19]. The expectation regarding longevity is also an important factor, particularly in older horses where, for example, a prolonged convalescent period characterized by constant lameness or prolonged confinement might dominate the remainder of the horse's life and there may be little likelihood of positive experiences in the future. According to the survey results of one study, a poor quality of life (as assessed by the owner) and not veterinary advice regarding prognosis contributed most to the owner's decision to euthanize in 34% of geriatric horses with chronic diseases (including laminitis) [8].

Quality of life assessment techniques have been developed for other companion animal species [20, 21], but very little published information is available for horses. Parker and Yeates [19] have suggested methods for quality of life assessment in horses, and they include a supplementary case example of quality of life assessment specifically in a chronic laminitis case. A description of the steps involved in decision making suggested by Parker and Yeates [19], adapted specifically to be relevant to the chronic laminitis case, is included in Table 46.1.

Table 46.1 Suggested steps in decision making when considering treatment options versus euthanasia in horses with chronic laminitis. Adapted from Ref. [19]; © Wiley.

Decision step and factors	Considerations
1. Decide which aspects affect the horse's quality of life.	• Chronic pain, ongoing confinement and the stress of procedures or treatments will negatively affect quality of life • Exercise, freedom and company of other horses will positively affect quality of life • What is the horse's age – how long is the horse expected to live for?
2. Identify useful information to assess these aspects.	• Owner assessment – the owner may be best able to evaluate changes in behavior that reflect deteriorating quality of life. • An assessment of the clinical condition of the horse, the quality of its environment, the level of care it receives. • Clinical measures including radiographic measurements, clinical pathology or other testing. • Veterinary assessment of behaviors (e.g., prolonged recumbency, standing at the back of the stall) may be useful indicators of pain in particular.
3. Develop appropriate assessment methods for the individual case.	• Clinical evaluation and diagnostic tests can be used to assess the current status and prognosis. • History provided by the owner may help to gauge progression. • If ongoing treatment, assessment methods must evaluate the response to treatment and detect any deterioration.
4. Infer the patient's expected quality of life.	• Using a combination of assessment methods and a combination of opinions (owner, carer, veterinarian, farrier), the expected quality of life may be predicted for the individual case under different circumstances or with different treatment options.
5. Make a decision about actions or recommendations.	• Compare the expected quality of life for each treatment option (including euthanasia and no treatment) and decide which is in the best interest of the horse.
6. Achieve that decision.	• Clear and tactful communication is necessary if euthanasia is the recommendation. • If further treatment is elected, then specific observations for monitoring deterioration and thresholds for euthanasia should be designated.

The careful monitoring of pain is an important aspect of quality of life assessment, and should be as objective as possible. Lameness evaluation is the primary means of evaluating laminitis pain, along with regular assessments of vital parameters such as heart rate. In a recent study, certain behaviors (including increased forelimb lifting and an increased proportion of time spent at the back of the stable) were consistently and significantly associated with laminitis-related pain [22]. A pain assessment scoring sheet that incorporates behavioral parameters as well as serial measurement of objective clinical parameters (e.g., heart rate, respiratory rate, blood pressure) can be very useful in a hospital environment, and also can be adapted for use by owners caring for horses at home [18]. Such a serial record can help to objectively demonstrate a trend of worsening pain (or a failure to improve) that may assist with decision making.

When faced with a chronic laminitis case that is likely to require ongoing care, it is also important to consider whether there is sufficient owner commitment present, as well as whether appropriate resources will be available for the animal, including nursing care, facilities/housing, finances, and the availability of a skilled farrier. In the present authors' experience, the combination of a committed owner, farrier, and veterinarian is vital to the care of chronic laminitis cases.

Guiding Owners Towards a Decision when Euthanasia is Indicated on Humane Grounds

Fortunately, in the majority of laminitis cases, the veterinarian, farrier, and owner will agree on an appropriate course of action, whether that be euthanasia or ongoing treatment. In some cases the owner may not realise or acknowledge the deterioration in their horse's quality of life (and/or they may refuse to accept a poor prognosis for improvement). In these cases, it is most often highly bonded owners who fail to first consider the animal's welfare interests when making decisions regarding ongoing treatment; these cases can be particularly challenging for the veterinarian [23]. The steps described in Table 46.1 can be used in difficult cases to help come to a resolution. In addition to these options, inviting a colleague to provide a second opinion may also help an owner to reach an appropriate decision. In any circumstance, ongoing treatment should always be compared with euthanasia as continued life is only beneficial if the resultant life is worth living [24].

In circumstances where the owner refuses to give permission for euthanasia, even when it is considered strongly indicated, the veterinarian should elect to either refer the matter to relevant authorities (depending on the jurisdiction) or provide palliative therapy with regular assessment and vigorous follow-up. However, it should be recognized that it may be difficult to strike a balance between palliating suffering and not perpetuating a poor quality of life for the horse [24].

References

1. Keegan, K.G., Messer, N.T., Reed, S.K., Wilson, D.A., and Kramer, J. (2008) Effectiveness of administration of phenylbutazone alone or concurrent administration of phenylbutazone and flunixin meglumine to alleviate lameness in horses. *Am. J. Vet. Res.*, **69**, 167–173.
2. Toutain, P.L., Autefage, A., Legrand, C., and Alvinerie, M. (1994) Plasma concentrations and therapeutic efficacy of phenylbutazone and flunixin meglumine in the horse: pharmacokinetic/pharmacodynamic modelling. *J. Vet. Pharmacol. Ther.*, **17**, 459–469.
3. Erkert, R.S., MacAllister, C.G., Payton, M.E., and Clarke, C.R. (2005) Use of force plate analysis to compare the analgesic effects of intravenous administration of phenylbutazone and flunixin meglumine in horses with navicular syndrome. *Am. J. Vet. Res.*, **66**, 284–288.
4. King, J.N. and Gerring, E.L. (1989) Antagonism of endotoxin-induced disruption of equine bowel motility by flunixin and phenylbutazone. *Equine Vet. J. Suppl.*, **7**, 38–42.
5. Owens, J.G., Kamerling, S.G., Stanton, S.R., and Keowen, M.L. (1995) Effects of ketoprofen and phenylbutazone on chronic hoof pain and lameness in the horse. *Equine Vet. J.*, **27**, 296–300.
6. MacAllister, C.G., Morgan, S.J., Borne, A.T., and Pollet, R.A. (1993) Comparison of adverse effects of phenylbutazone, flunixin meglumine, and ketoprofen in horses. *J. Am. Vet. Med. Assoc.*, **202**, 71–77.
7. Karikoski, N.P., Patterson-Kane, J.C., Singer, E.R., McFarlane, D., and McGowan, C.M. (2016) Lamellar pathology in horses with pituitary pars intermedia dysfunction. *Equine Vet. J.*, **48**, (4), 472–478.
8. Ireland, J.L., Clegg, P.D., McGowan, C.M., Platt, L., and Pinchbeck, G.L. (2011) Factors associated with mortality of geriatric horses in the United Kingdom. *Prev. Vet. Med.*, **101**, 204–218.
9. Van Eps, A., Collins, S.N., and Pollitt, C.C. (2010) Supporting limb laminitis. *Vet. Clin. North Am. Equine Pract.*, **26**, 287–302.
10. Hunt, R.J. (1993) A retrospective evaluation of laminitis in horses. *Equine Vet. J.*, **25**, 61–64.
11. Kullmann, A., Holcombe, S.J., Hurcombe, S.D., Roessner, H.A., Hauptman, J.G., Geor, R.J., and Belknap, J. (2014) Prophylactic digital cryotherapy is associated with decreased incidence of laminitis in horses diagnosed with colitis. *Equine Vet. J.*, **46**, 554–559.
12. Menzies-Gow, N.J., Stevens, K., Barr, A., Camm, I., Pfeiffer, D., and Marr, C.M. (2010) Severity and outcome of equine pasture-associated laminitis managed in first opinion practice in the UK. *Vet. Rec.*, **167**, 364–369.
13. Orsini, J.A., Parsons, C.S., Capewell, L., and Smith, G. (2010) Prognostic indicators of poor outcome in horses with laminitis at a tertiary care hospital. *Can. Vet. J.*, **51**, 623–628.
14. Hunt, R.J. and Wharton, R.E. (2010) Clinical presentation, diagnosis, and prognosis of chronic laminitis in North America. *Vet. Clin. North Am. Equine Pract.*, **26**, 141–153.
15. Eustace, R.A. (2010) Clinical presentation, diagnosis, and prognosis of chronic laminitis in Europe. *Vet. Clin. North Am. Equine Pract.*, **26**, 391–405.
16. Cripps, P.J. and Eustace, R.A. (1999) Factors involved in the prognosis of equine laminitis in the UK. *Equine Vet. J.*, **31**, 433–442.
17. Baxter, G.M. (1986) Equine laminitis caused by distal displacement of the distal phalanx: 12 cases (1976–1985). *J. Am. Vet. Med. Assoc.*, **189**, 326–329.
18. Van Eps, A.W. (2010) Acute laminitis: medical and supportive therapy. *Vet. Clin. North Am. Equine Pract.*, **26**, 103–114.
19. Parker, R.A. and Yeates, J.W. (2012) Assessment of quality of life in equine patients. *Equine Vet. J.*, **44**, 244–249.
20. Yeates, J. and Main, D. (2009) Assessment of companion animal quality of life in veterinary practice and research. *J. Small Animal Pract.*, **50**, 274–281.
21. Green, T.C. and Mellor, D.J. (2011) Extending ideas about animal welfare assessment to include 'quality of life' and related concepts. *N. Z. Vet. J.*, **59**, 263–271.
22. Jones, E., Vinuela-Fernandez, I., Eager, R.A., Delaney, A., Anderson, H., Patel, A., Robertson, D.C., Allchorne, A., Sirinathsinghji, E.C., Milne, E.M., MacIntyre, N., Shaw, D.J., Waran, N.K., Mayhew, J., and Fleetwood-Walker, S.M. (2007) Neuropathic changes in equine laminitis pain. *Pain*, **132**, 321–331.
23. Wensley, S.P. (2008) Animal welfare and the human-animal bond: considerations for veterinary faculty, students, and practitioners. *J. Vet. Med. Educ.*, **35**, 532–539.
24. Yeates, J.W. (2010) When to euthanase. *Vet. Rec.*, **166**, 370–371.

PART 9

Prevention of Laminitis

Equine Laminitis, First Edition. Edited by James K. Belknap and Raymond Geor.

CHAPTER 47

Overview of Laminitis Prevention

James K. Belknap and Andy E. Durham

Due to irreversible changes to the equine digit which commonly occur in laminitis (especially with displacement of the distal phalanx [DP]), there is a great deal of interest in both identification of the equid at risk of laminitis, and the establishment of preventive measures to avoid the onset of the disease. With knowledge gained from the extensive research performed during the past two to three decades, it has been possible not only to establish three primary types of laminitis – endocrinopathic, sepsis-related laminitis (SRL), and supporting limb laminitis (SLL) – but also to greatly expand the understanding of events leading to lamellar dysregulation/injury in these different types of laminitis. As the risk factors are vastly different for the different types of laminitis, they must be discussed separately. As preventive techniques for the individual components of endocrinopathic laminitis have been described in depth in Chapters 36, 37, and 50, only a brief general discussion will be provided in this overview.

Endocrinopathic Laminitis

Endocrinopathic laminitis primarily comprises equine metabolic syndrome (EMS, including pasture-associated laminitis) and pituitary pars intermedia dysfunction (PPID), although laminitis following exogenous glucocorticoid administration can also be included in this category. It should also be remembered that, when investigating endocrinopathic diseases, they are not mutually exclusive conditions and may serve as additive cofactors in increasing laminitis risk in the same individual. In marked distinction to SRL and SLL, animals with endocrinopathic laminitis commonly develop laminitis unexpectedly without apparently being noted to be at risk of the disease until there are already clinical signs of foot pain. There are several reasons for missing earlier signs indicative of laminitis risk prior to the onset of lamellar pathology, not the least of which is that the onset of both PPID and EMS is commonly much more subtle and gradual than the onset of sepsis or severe injury to one limb as seen with SRL or SLL. Indeed, although owners might be expected to readily appreciate externally detectable signs such as excessive adiposity, several studies have indicated a poor recognition of this state in horses by their caregivers [1, 2]. This is compounded by the unpredictable relationship between visible or palpable adiposity and insulin dysregulation [3, 4], with the consequence that other animals at the same facility may carry a similar amount of body fat as a herd mate diagnosed with EMS yet never exhibit any indication of insulin dysregulation or its clinical consequence of laminitis. This variability between animals may have acquired elements related to individual management, but is also influenced by: (i) the genetic makeup of that animal, or (ii) the genetic makeup of specific breeds which appear to put all members of the breed at particular risk of EMS (as discussed in Chapters 18 and 23). Similarly for PPID, clinical laminitis may arise prior to clinical suspicion of endocrinopathic disease. The classically described clinical signs of PPID (hypertrichosis, regional adiposity, muscle wasting, etc.; see Chapter 24) may not be apparent until later years. Although undoubtedly an age-related problem, PPID is well recognized in younger horses, with several well-described cases in animals as young as seven or eight years [5–7]. As a progressive disease, it is reasonable to assume that PPID is likely to have been present for quite some time prior to the development of classical clinical signs. Therefore, again, the first clinical signs noted may be those associated with the hoof wall (e.g., divergent growth lines, dishing of the dorsal aspect of the hoof) or lameness associated with laminitis in a not particularly elderly individual in the absence of further signs such as hypertrichosis. A unique aspect of lamellar pathology in laminitis cases associated with both EMS and PPID, and which further muddies the clinical picture, is that, in contrast to the acute nature of the pain associated with the onset of the disease in most cases of SRL and SLL (discussed below), endocrinopathic laminitis involves more commonly a slow, insidious process in which clinical signs of the disease process are not detected until after extensive displacement of the DP may have taken place [8]. Commonly, the digital pain appears more associated with subsolear bruising secondary to the displaced phalanx pressing on the dorsal aspect of a thinned sole than from lamellar pain.

Thus, prevention in the context of endocrinopathic laminitis entails maintaining targeted vigilance and surveillance with

Equine Laminitis, First Edition. Edited by James K. Belknap and Raymond Geor.

close assessment of any equid on an annual (or semi-annual) basis in regards to body condition score, soundness, hoof appearance, endocrine testing, and, optimally, radiographic imaging. Client education and support is crucial in facilitating access to susceptible individuals prior to their presentation as clinical laminitis cases. Due to the insidious nature of displacement of the DP, annual radiographs (with measurements performed; see Chapter 27) represent a valuable tool to detect minor changes in the relationship of the DP to the hoof before extensive displacement occurs. Liberal dietary provision and inadequate exercise which promote the development of EMS, may begin quite early in life (e.g., age 3–4 years), and the monitoring of susceptible breeds with body condition scoring and tests for insulin dysregulation should begin as early as possible. Finally, starting perhaps as early as 10 years of age (possibly earlier in breeds at risk of EMS or individuals exhibiting the EMS phenotype), adrenocorticotrophic hormone (ACTH) concentrations and tests for insulin dysregulation should be performed annually. In the animal found to be at risk of EMS due to changes in adiposity or endocrine testing, preventive measures such as increased exercise, dietary management, and possible pharmaceutical management should be instituted (see Chapters 36 and 50 for thorough discussions). For the animal with a high suspicion of PPID due to clinical signs and results of ACTH and insulin testing, the institution of pergolide treatment should be strongly considered (see Chapter 37). Strict dietary management and 'preventive' foot care should also be used, especially in those animals with radiographic and clinical hoof-related signs of lamellar dysregulation/injury (see later discussion of SRL and SLL).

Sepsis-Related Laminitis (SRL)

Due to the commonly rapid, catastrophic nature of lamellar failure in sepsis-related laminitis (SRL), and the availability of an effective prophylactic therapy for SRL (digital hypothermia; see Chapters 34, 35, and 49), it is vitally important to identify and treat the animal at risk of SRL. In SRL, the animals at risk of the disease are usually readily identifiable, allowing therapeutic intervention prior to clinical or radiographic signs of lamellar injury if the animal is examined early in the disease process. Unlike endocrinopathic laminitis, where the farrier or astute owner may be the first to note the clinical signs of the animal at risk of the disease, the veterinarian is more likely to identify the animal at risk for SRL due to being called to examine the horse for the original sepsis-related disease. Similar to organ injury (e.g., kidney, liver, or lung injury/failure) in human sepsis [9, 10], infections in multiple distant organs or tissues ranging from acute metritis, pleuropneumonia and, most commonly, gastrointestinal diseases (e.g., enterocolitis) can lead to lamellar injury in the horse (see Chapters 22 and 35 for further discussions). However, unlike humans, viral infections and Gram-positive bacterial infections rarely lead to laminitis in horses. Nonetheless, the high incidence of SRL in enterocolitis cases caused by rickettsial agents (e.g., Potomac Horse Fever) and nonseptic diseases such as myopathies indicate that other causes of systemic inflammation in addition to Gram-negative bacterial sepsis can induce SRL. In addition to the identification of the septic tissue or organ, risk factors for SRL include the following clinical signs (primarily those associated with systemic inflammatory response syndrome [SIRS] in sepsis): hyperthermia or hypothermia, elevated heart rate and mucous membrane changes (hyperemia or cyanosis); along with laboratory findings such as leucopenia and hyperlactemia (see Chapters 22 and 35 for further discussions). Preventive strategies (as discussed in Chapters 35 and 49) consist primarily of aggressively treating the source of sepsis (e.g., uterine or lung infection), treating the systemic inflammation, and local therapy targeted to the digit. Treatment of the source of the infection will most commonly include systemic (and possibly local) antibiotics (see Chapter 35 for an in-depth discussion), and physical removal of the organisms (e.g., uterine lavage in acute metritis) when possible. Medical therapy for systemic inflammation most commonly consists of nonsteroidal anti-inflammatory drugs (NSAIDS) such as meloxicam or flunixin meglumine. Polymixin B may be added if there is a high suspicion of endotoxemia (see Chapter 35 for discussion of its use and limitations). Finally, in the light of using evidence-based medicine, one therapy which is demonstrated consistently to be effective as both a prophylactic and therapeutic treatment in SRL is digital hypothermia (see Chapters 34 and 35) [11–13]. It is important to address the biomechanical concerns of the digit even with the use of cryotherapy; this can be accomplished by the attachment (usually with tape or fiberglass casting material) of some type of padding or cushion support to the bottom of the foot (e.g., an ethyl vinyl acetate [EVA] clog), or using the commercial ice boot (Soft-Ride Co.) which incorporates a support pad in the base of the boot. A more thorough discussion of padding/solear support is presented in Chapters 39 and 40.

Supporting Limb Laminitis (SLL)

Even more so than SRL, supporting limb laminitis (SLL; as described in detail in Chapters 25 and 48) is most commonly characterized by a rapid onset of catastrophic lamellar failure once signs of laminitis are present, with little opportunity for intervention during the clinical phase. Hence, there is a great deal of interest in establishing preventive therapies/management for the animal at risk of SLL. In SLL, identification of the animal at risk is overall fairly straightforward, being the animal with severe lameness on one limb, thereby putting the contralateral (supporting) limb at risk for lamellar failure. The only caveat to this group of animals is that the disease periodically occurs in an animal with what appears to be only a mild to moderate degree of lameness on one limb. The additional challenge is the range of time between the onset of lameness in the opposite limb and the onset of laminitis in the supporting limb (from two days to over two months; see Chapter 25 for more in-depth discussion); this not only requires constant vigilance by caregivers but also the use of treatments/management techniques which can be performed over an extended period of time. Although the 'at-risk' group is commonly associated with postoperative orthopedic patients, the animal with severe lameness from soft tissue sepsis (primarily sepsis in a joint or tendon sheath) is also at great risk. In a recent survey of equine surgeons in the US and Canada, the most commonly encountered case of SLL was that in an animal being treated for joint/tendon sheath sepsis. Recent research on SLL (some of it not yet published) suggests that the lamellar injury in this type of laminitis is due primarily to a decreased blood flow, most likely due to a combination of: (i) a lack of movement of the supporting limb (likely needed for distal limb blood flow); and (ii) a constant, excessive lamellar load in the supporting limb (X. Schneider, A. van Eps A, and J. Belknap, unpublished data). Thus, the primary goal of SLL preventive techniques should likely focus on techniques to increase digital blood flow. Due to disappointing data over the years regarding the lack of efficacy of vasoactive drugs in improving lamellar blood flow (see Chapter 32), it is likely that there is a need to concentrate on therapeutic techniques which encourage movement and periodic unweighting of the digit in the supporting limb in animals at risk of the disease. Interestingly, if a horse is made to stand on one limb for a few minutes, there appears to be a stimulus to move/lift that supporting limb which is sensed by the animal (similar to a human being forced to stand on one limb). Thus, it is likely that: (i) pain in the opposite limb; (ii) a total inability to use that limb (as in a radial nerve paralysis patient); and (iii) exhaustion of the animal (or a combination of these) overrides this stimulus and results in the animal standing on the supporting limb with minimal movement. In a recent study with microdialysis catheters [14, 15] placed in the lamellar tissue in Standardbred horses placing excessive weight on one limb (with minimal cycling due to constant local anesthesia of the limb), lamellar ischemia occurred between 48 and 72 h in the majority of horses (X. Schneider, A. van Eps, and J. Belknap, unpublished data). An interesting aspect of these results was that, with likely even less movement of the supporting limb in this model than occurs in the clinical case at risk of SLL, there was still a delay prior to the onset of lamellar ischemia; this fits well with the long period of time which can occur between the onset of severe lameness in the opposite limb and the onset of SLL in the supporting limb. One therapeutic option to encourage periodic movement of the supporting limb is an appropriate use of analgesics, which will encourage the animal to undertake limited ambulation while not overly stressing the other limb if there is internal fixation for a fracture. The most practical option is the use of NSAIDs, though opioids can also be used (see Chapters 31 and 33 for a discussion of these drugs). There are obvious concerns regarding adverse effects with both classes of drugs over long-term usage. Addressing the foot is also important both in regards to addressing biomechanical stress on the lamellae and possibly encouraging ambulation (as discussed in Chapter 48). Finally, a pneumatic device attached to the foot to constantly provide movement of the distal supporting limb is currently being tested (J. Belknap and A. van Eps, unpublished data). Although there are anecdotal reports regarding the efficacy of digital hypothermia/cryotherapy as a prophylactic therapy for SLL, no studies have yet been performed to substantiate the anecdotal information. A challenge to this type of work-intensive therapy is the reality that these therapies may be needed for multiple weeks if the animal remains lame on the opposite limb for that period of time. In addition to these therapeutic options, environmental management (bedding, etc.; see Chapter 30) to encourage the animal to lay down is also an important aspect of managing the clinical case at risk of SLL. Although placing a horse in a sling can also allow the animal to unweight the support limb, and may be a viable option in some hospitals, slings are not well tolerated by many horses [16]. Moreover, most current systems for slinging horses do not work well for the extensive period of time commonly necessary for management of the clinical case at risk of SLL.

References

1. Wyse, C.A., McNie, K.A, Tannahill, V.J., Murray, J.K., and Love, S. (2008) Prevalence of obesity in riding horses in Scotland. *Vet. Rec.*, **162** (18), 590–591.
2. Stephenson, H.M., Green, M.J., and Freeman, S.L. (2011) Prevalence of obesity in a population of horses in the UK. *Vet. Rec.*, **168** (5), 131.
3. Bamford, N.J., Potter, S.J., Harris, P.A., and Bailey, S.R. (2015) Effect of increased adiposity on insulin sensitivity and adipokine concentrations in horses and ponies fed a high fat diet, with or without a once daily high glycaemic meal. *Equine Vet. J.*, **48** (3), 368–373.
4. Durham, A.E. (2016) Insulin dysregulation and obesity: You are what you eat. *Vet. J.*, **213**, 90.
5. Heinrichs, M., Baumgartner, W., and Capen, C.C. (1990) Immunocytochemical demonstration of proopiomelanocortin-derived peptides in pituitary adenomas of the pars intermedia in horses. *Vet. Pathol.*, **27** (6), 419–425.
6. Beech, J., McFarlane, D., Lindborg, S., Sojka, J.E., and Boston, R.C. (2011) alpha-Melanocyte–stimulating hormone and adrenocorticotropin concentrations in response to thyrotropin-releasing hormone and comparison with adrenocorticotropin concentration after domperidone administration in healthy horses and horses with pituitary pars intermedia dysfunction. *J. Am. Vet. Med. Assoc.*, **238** (10), 1305–1315.
7. Couetil, L.L. (1996) New developments in equine Cushing's disease. *Equine Pract.*, **18** (9), 28–32.
8. Karikoski, N.P., McGowan, C.M., Singer, E.R., Asplin, K.E., Tulamo, R.M., and Patterson-Kane, J.C. (2015) Pathology of natural cases of equine endocrinopathic laminitis associated with hyperinsulinemia. *Vet. Pathol.*, **52** (5), 945–956.
9. Belknap, J.K. and Black, S.J. (2012) Sepsis-related laminitis. *Equine Vet. J.*, **44** (6), 738–40.
10. Belknap, J.K., Moore, J.N., and Crouser, E.C. (2009) Sepsis – From human organ failure to laminar failure. *Vet. Immunol. Immunopathol.*, **129** (3-4), 155–157.
11. Kullmann, A., Holcombe, S.J., Hurcombe, S.D., Roessner, H.A., Hauptman, J.G., Geor, R.J., *et al.* (2014) Prophylactic digital

cryotherapy is associated with decreased incidence of laminitis in horses diagnosed with colitis. *Equine Vet. J.*, **46** (5), 554–559.
12. Pollitt, C.C. and Van Eps, A.W. (2004) Prolonged, continuous distal limb cryotherapy in the horse. *Equine Vet. J.*, **36** (3), 216–220.
13. Van Eps, A.W., Pollitt, C.C., Underwood, C., Medina-Torres, C.E., Goodwin, W.A., and Belknap, J.K. (2014) Continuous digital hypothermia initiated after the onset of lameness prevents lamellar failure in the oligofructose laminitis model. *Equine Vet. J.*, **46** (5), 625–630.
14. Medina-Torres, C.E., Underwood, C., Pollitt, C.C., Castro-Olivera, E.M., Hodson, M.P., Richardson, D.W., *et al.* (2016) Microdialysis measurements of lamellar perfusion and energy metabolism during the development of laminitis in the oligofructose model. *Equine Vet. J.*, **48** (2), 246–252.
15. Medina-Torres, C.E., Underwood, C., Pollitt, C.C., Castro-Olivera, E.M., Hodson, M.P., Richardson, D.W., *et al.* (2016) The effect of weightbearing and limb load cycling on equine lamellar perfusion and energy metabolism measured using tissue microdialysis. *Equine Vet. J.*, **48** (1), 114–119.
16. Winfield, L.S., Kass, P.H., Magdesian, K.G., Madigan, J.E., Aleman, M., and Pusterla, N. (2014) Factors associated with survival in 148 recumbent horses. *Equine Vet. J.*, **46** (5), 575–578.

CHAPTER 48

Prevention of Supporting Limb Laminitis

Harry J. Markwell and Gary M. Baxter

Introduction

Supporting limb laminitis (SLL) has been reported as sequelae to any orthopedic, synovial, soft tissue or neurological condition in one limb that contributes to a period of excessive unilateral weight-bearing, in the opposite limb regardless of its duration. The prevalence or incidence of this complication is variable depending on the circumstances, but a recent study reported that up to 12% of horses treated with casts for a variety of conditions developed SLL. In that study, horses with fractures were at no greater risk than other causes such as synovial sepsis [1]. The most significant factors that are thought to contribute to SLL are the bodyweight of the horse, the duration and severity of the primary lameness, and the duration of casting/lameness during treatment [1, 2]. A direct mechanical overload of the contralateral limb, or a primary hypoperfusion of the lamellae from a lack of movement in the supporting foot, are proposed etiologies for this condition [1, 3, 4], with recent literature reporting that limb movement improves lamellar perfusion [5,6]. Data from a recent experimental study provide strong evidence of lamellar ischemia and lamellar energy failure in the supporting limb within 48–72 h of the onset of excessive weight-bearing on one forelimb, most likely due to a combination of a lack of movement of the limb and a constant, increased mechanical load upon the lamellar/sublamellar tissue (X. Schneider, A. van Eps, and J. Belknap, unpublished data). Preventive measures are usually directed toward these two events. Although a multitude of approaches exists to prevent SLL in horses, most should be based on the following five objectives:

1. Provide musculoskeletal and neuropathic analgesia.
2. Maintain adequate vascular perfusion of the at-risk digit.
3. Provide axial and external support to the at-risk digit.
4. Minimize the moment arm around the distal interphalangeal (DIP) joint.
5. Reduce effective bodyweight.

Musculoskeletal and Neuropathic Analgesia

The management of orthopedic and neuropathic pain of the primary (i.e., non-weight-bearing) limb should be the major objective in any horse with unilateral weight-bearing or during any period of severe lameness. A multimodel approach to analgesia is usually preferred, and it should be part of any postoperative orthopedic surgical plan. The goal is to prevent a variety of behavioral, neurophysiological, endocrine, metabolic, and cellular responses that will initiate, maintain, and amplify pain and associated inflammatory mediators [7] (see Chapter 33). Perioperative, intraoperative, and postoperative pain should be addressed aggressively to prevent the upregulation of nociceptor pathways and excessive nerve 'wind-up' (see Chapter 33). Most multimodal pain management strategies incorporate a nonsteroidal anti-inflammatory drug (NSAID), an opioid, an alpha-2 agonist, and some type of local therapy (epidural, or possibly perineural or local nerve blocks, or topical anti-inflammatories). Epidural analgesia can be particularly useful for hind limb SLL concerns; local anesthesia needs to be carefully contemplated to ensure, if used, that the animal does not place excessive weight on the affected limb (i.e., endangering internal fixation, etc.). Additional medications that may be used to provide analgesia include parenteral constant rate infusions and adjunctive therapies such as oral gabapentin or tramadol [4, 7, 8]. A variety of applicable medications for providing multimodal analgesia is listed in Tables 48.1 and 48.2.

Maintain Vascular Perfusion

The maintenance of adequate perfusion of the at-risk digit to minimize ischemic damage to the digit remains one of the hallmarks in managing an acute laminitic episode. Lamellar cells have been shown to possess a great need for glucose, likely

Equine Laminitis, First Edition. Edited by James K. Belknap and Raymond Geor.

Table 48.1 Common NSAIDs used to manage orthopedic pain in horses.

Drug	Route	Recommended dose	Comments
Phenylbutazone	PO or IV	2.2–4.4 mg/kg^{-1} SID–BID	Most common NSAID used for musculoskeletal pain. Increased dose above 4.4 mg/kg^{-1} has no increased analgesic effects.
Flunixin meglumine	PO or IV	1.1 mg/kg^{-1} SID–BID	Similar analgesic effects as phenylbutazone. No evidence of increased analgesia when used in combination with phenylbutazone.
Firocoxib	Oral	0.1 mg/kg^{-1} SID–BID	Similar analgesic effects as phenylbutazone.
Ketoprofen	IV	2.2 mg/kg^{-1} SID	Least commonly used NSAID.

IV, intravenous; PO, per os (oral); BID, twice daily; SID, once daily.

making them very susceptible to small reductions in vascular supply to the digit [9]. In horses with SLL, a lack of lamellar blood flow due to decreased digital movement is thought to occur during extended periods of weight-bearing (prolonged dorsiflexion of the fetlock). The reduced frequency of cyclic loading and forward ambulation has recently been reported to contribute to lamellar hypoperfusion and to be a major risk factor in the development of SLL [5]. In addition, prolonged tension on the deep digital flexor tendon (DDFT) has been proposed to contribute to both reduced lamellar perfusion and increases in the shear forces over the dorsal lamellae. In one study which used digital venograms to assess lamellar perfusion in normal horses, unloading the DDFT by buckling the carpus dorsally was reportedly necessary to achieve adequate perfusion of the dorsal lamellae [10]. The DDFT can be effectively unloaded by elevating the heel, and heel elevation of 5–10° to relax the DDFT has been purported to improve lamellar perfusion and is recommended by many clinicians to prevent laminitis in at-risk horses with unilateral lameness. However, a recent *in-vitro* study [11] using a computer model showed that heel elevation from 0 to 15° might actually increase the shearing forces on the dorsal lamella.

Other methods to promote more equal weight-bearing – and therefore improve digital perfusion – include small periods of hand walking, intermittent periods of slinging, and addressing the solear surfaces to ensure that the limbs are of similar length [3, 12, 13]. An elevated wooden block, shoe (e.g., clog), or padding material can be placed on the contralateral limb to counteract differences in limb length in horses with casts on their primary (lame) limb [12]. This promotes even weight-bearing between the limbs, thus minimizing the preferential weight-bearing on the shorter, non-casted limb. Small periods of hand walking may not be possible in some cases, but can effectively give the supporting limb 'a break' in horses with severe lameness. The results of recent studies also suggest that limb movement may be helpful to maintain perfusion of the lamellae. Intermittent periods of slinging may accomplish the same objective, which is to promote more cyclic loading and unloading of the digit.

Table 48.2 Recommended doses of opioid analgesics in horses.

Drug	Analgesia dose and route
Morphine	0.1–0.3 mg/kg^{-1} IV or IM
Meperidine	0.3–0.6 mg/kg^{-1} IV 1–2 mg/kg^{-1} IV/IM
Methadone	0.05–0.1 mg/kg^{-1} IV 0.1–0.2 mg/kg^{-1} IV or IM
Butorphanol	0.01–0.02 mg/kg^{-1} IV 0.02–0.1 mg/kg^{-1} IM
Buprenorphine	10–20 $\mu g\ kg^{-1}$ IV 60 $\mu g\ kg^{-1}$ IV or IM

IM, intramuscular; IV, intravenous.

Other systemic therapies that may be used to potentially improve lamellar perfusion in horses with laminitis include acepromazine, heparin, isoxsuprine, pentoxifylline, and aspirin [3, 14,15]. The efficacy of these systemic drugs to improve perfusion in horses with SLL is highly debatable and most likely not effective. Recent investigations have indicated that acepromazine, a sedative commonly used by clinicians in an attempt to increase lamellar blood flow, actually decreases blood flow by reducing limb movement in the sedated animal (A. van Eps, unpublished data). In addition, local cryotherapy, the only therapy proven effective for prophylaxis or treatment of sepsis-related laminitis (SRL) [16, 17] which likely does not work through enhanced blood flow, has been anecdotally found to be more effective than any systemic medication in the treatment of SLL.

Axial and External Foot Support

Axial forces on the digit are considered to be the weight-bearing forces that propagate distally through the boney column of the limb. Providing axial or internal support is an attempt to counteract these downward forces on the at-risk digit, and usually entails one or more of the following: (i) recruiting the sole, bars, and frog in weight-bearing; (ii) unloading the lamellar interface of the entire perimeter of the hoof wall; and (iii) reducing strain over the dorsal hoof wall [3, 18]. These are often achieved through a combination of hoof management, direct sole support, corrective shoeing, external coaptation with support shoes or casts, or changes in the stall surface to recruit a larger weight-bearing surface. Each of these approaches will be discussed below.

Targeted Trimming

Pre-emptive hoof management is thought to be fundamental in the prevention of SLL, and may also serve to limit displacement of the distal phalanx (DP), control pain, and optimize new hoof wall growth [19]. Removing the shoe (if present), performing a light balanced trim, and removing the loose sole and long toe (if present) should be the mainstays to redistribute weight from the most stressed wall to the least stressed wall [3, 19]. This also helps to decrease the moment arm around the DIP joint and redistributes stress from the dorsal digital lamellae to the weight-bearing surfaces of the ground surface of the foot (discussed in Chapters 5, 6, and 38) [3, 19]. Heel elevation may reduce tension on the DDFT and can be accomplished with either shoes or possibly sole/frog support. However, heel elevation (either through shoeing or trimming) for an extended period of time may also be undesirable, leading to bruising of the digital cushion and crushing of the bars and heels, which results in pain over the caudal foot and a reluctance to bear weight over this surface.

Direct Sole Support

Direct sole support can be achieved by a number of products on the market such as silicone, polyurethane, and elastomers (see Chapter 39). Many of these products are malleable and create an impression of the sole and frog whilst providing a cushion that matches the consistency of the frog. When placing malleable sole/frog support, the material should be applied from the cranial tip of the frog caudally over the sole, bars and frog; and may be shaped so that the ground surface is slightly convex, reducing load over the hoof wall [3,4]. Although most clinicians apply a variable degree of heel elevation with malleable sole/frog support, heel elevation is not mandatory and it has been reported that a reduction in breakover alone may cause a similar reduction in tension of the DDFT [10]. Other materials such as foam and rubber pads can also be utilized, and have been found to increase the total contact surface area and move the center of pressure (COP; the center of the ground reaction force acting on the foot) in a palmar/plantar direction [20] (see Chapter 5). These products are generally effective if they are approximately 2.5–3 cm thick, do not compress to more than 50% during weight-bearing, and allow ease of breakover to the foot [3].

Conventional Shoeing Modifications

Standard metal or aluminum shoes concentrate weight-bearing over the periphery of the foot and limit the breakover (both increasing stress on the lamellae), and generally should be removed from the at-risk foot in horses with severe unilateral lameness. Most interventions that involve shoeing increase the shock waves of impact as the animal ambulates, and the natural damping mechanisms within the digit almost always function better in a healthy horse if it is barefoot [18]. However, if shoeing is required for the particular patient for a known pre-existing condition, it should follow the general principles of improving axial support and relieving tension on the DDFT. If metal shoes are required, ideally a commercial wide-webbed aluminum shoe or a customized wide-webbed steel shoe with or without bars should be used [3, 21]. Hanson *et al.* [22] reported that a steel bar shoe combined with a malleable direct sole support product was able to reduce dorsal hoof wall strain by up to 23%. Once axial support is provided, the use of an adjustable wedge slipper-type shoe, wooden shoe, or interchangeable support boots can be incorporated if deemed appropriate.

Commercial Support Shoes and External Coaptation

An adjustable wedge slipper-type shoe (e.g., Ultimate/Redden Ultimate) may help to reduce tension on the DDFT of the at-risk foot, and is used by many clinicians as a preventative measure for SLL. The shoe elevates the heels, reduces breakover and, when combined with a malleable impression material, facilitates significant arch support [10]. The device can be secured to the hoof wall using an adhesive bonding material or an adhesive bandage.

The wooden shoe/clog (Steward clog) has the ability to provide a solid base with the cushioning ability of wood protecting the lamella from shearing forces, while also providing a height adjustment for horses with a disparity in limb length commonly due to casting [23]. Shoe modifications are easy to achieve using regular farrier tools to improve breakover, reduce the lever arm (moment) around the DIP joint, and unload pressure from the DP. Wooden shoes (Fig. 48.1) can be placed with or without digital sole/frog support, with many clinicians choosing to use minimal amounts of impression material to minimize excessive solear pressure on the foot [3, 23].

Commercially available reuseable products (e.g., SoftRide™ Equine Comfort Boot) have gained increasing popularity in recent years for the prevention of SLL. Current products combine a rubber sole with interchangeable frog supports, and can be secured to the foot with Velcro attachments. Axial support

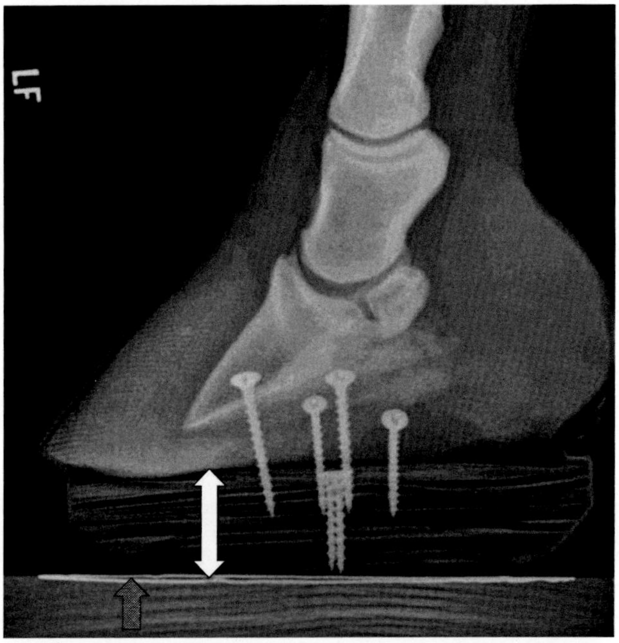

Figure 48.1 Lateral radiogram of a foot with a modified wooden clog for the prevention of supporting limb laminitis. Note the reduced breakover (shaded arrow) and slight heel elevation provided by the shoe in addition to substantially increasing the working length of the leg (open arrow).

of the sole can be provided by interchangeable rubber cushions with variable wedge angles and firmness of support available, depending on the requirement of the case or clinician preference. The use of an interchangeable support boot with a patient-specific customized insert made from malleable silicone/polyurethane/elastomers may be useful in providing flexible approaches for axial support in at-risk horses.

Hoof casts with a heel wedge have been reported *in vitro* to cause a reduction in compression of the dorsal hoof wall by up to 60% [22]. This is thought to be achieved through a combination of vertical load reduction to the palmar/plantar structures and a reduction of the tension on the DDFT. By unloading the tension over the dorsal hoof walls, casting may also reduce the occurrence of crushed heels that is experienced with prolonged use of wedges [10]. The clinical effectiveness of hoof casts has yet to be determined.

Changes in Footing/Stall Surface

It is generally accepted that horses at risk of developing SLL should not be housed in stalls with hard surfaces (i.e., concrete). This is related to weight-bearing and the COP of the digit, which determines the relative load-bearing of the different parts of the foot. Hooves on hard surfaces are thought to bear weight primarily through the hoof wall, with little weight-bearing forces transferred to the sole or frog regions of the foot [18]. In contrast, hooves on sand, soft dirt, peat moss, shavings or tan bark/mulch are thought to 'sink in' to the soft surface, therefore recruiting the sole and frog regions of the foot to help support the weight of the horse. The main rationale for distributing part of the load of weight-bearing over more of the sole and frog is to reduce load-bearing by the lamellae and wall. Acceptable stall flooring includes sand or soft dirt, deep shavings, tan bark/mulch or straw, concrete covered with rubber matting (some type of deformable bedding usually used over matting), or any combination of these. Although the importance of the flooring material may be questioned since the same type of resilient/cushioning sole support has already been applied to the foot, it is critical to providing a comfortable surface to encourage the animal to lay down as much as possible while minimizing the chance of decubital sores.

Reduce the Distal Interphalangeal (DIP) Joint Extensor Moment Arm

It is important to address the foot to decrease the forces that may cause more physical stress to the injured lamellae and therefore exacerbate lamellar failure and displacement of the DP. The center of the DIP joint can be used to approximate forces acting on the foot. For example, a long toe moves the COP dorsally (forwards), and therefore increases the extensor moment arm of the DIP joint; this increases the torque/stress (and thus the damaging forces) on the dorsal lamellae of the foot during breakover [18] (see Chapter 5). Increasing the height of the heel or shortening the length of the toe will move the COP towards the center of rotation of the DIP joint, respectively, and, in doing so can shorten the extensor moment arm around the joint and therefore the torque/stress on the dorsal lamellae. This is important in horses at risk for SLL, because any method that moves the COP towards the heels can help reduce tensile stress on the DDFT and dorsal lamellae, and potentially prevent destructive displacement of the DP in laminitis. This is especially true in horses with a combination of long toes and low heels, which may be at the greatest risk to develop SLL. Minimizing toe length and providing adequate heel height are the fundamentals in laminitis prevention. These dynamic changes to the foot are most commonly accomplished with the use of shoes which can both be beveled (to decrease the functional length of the toes and therefore breakover) and can apply heel elevation if necessary.

Reduction of Effective Body Weight

It has been shown recently in a retrospective study of horses with unilateral limb casting that body weight was a significant risk factor for SLL [1]. There are several methods that can be used to reduce the effective body weight in horses, and therefore the load on the at-risk foot. These include placing the horse in soft bedding or sand, external support of the foot with a cast or shoe, encouraging the horse to lie down if appropriate, and slinging [22,24]. The most effective method to limit limb loading is slinging, because it can completely unweight the at-risk digit as well as the contralateral primary diseased limb. However, slinging is labor-intensive and requires appropriate equipment, expertise, and monitoring. Patient tolerance of the sling can also be problematic, although many horses will tolerate intermittent slinging quite well. Slinging is probably used too late in the disease process in many at-risk horses; it is usually less effective as a treatment for SLL than as a preventive measure.

Conclusions

The prevention of SLL primarily revolves around two principles: (i) decreasing the forces sustained by the digital lamellae on the supporting limb; and (ii) maintaining adequate digital/lamellar perfusion to the overburdened digit when the animal is standing. Techniques used to decrease the forces on the digital lamellae include analgesia, therapeutic shoeing and trimming, management of the environment (e.g., bedding material for foot support and to encourage recumbency), and intermittent slinging to assist the animal to unload the supporting limb. Because many of the animals at risk for SLL spend extended periods of time standing, recent evidence indicating the need for limb motion to maintain adequate lamellar perfusion, combined with the limited efficacy of currently availiable vasodilator drugs, suggests that methods should be investigated to promote more physical movement of the supporting digit and limb. Unfortunately, this may be difficult in horses that are severely lame.

References

1. Virgin, J.E., Goodrich, L.R., Baxter, G.M., and Rao, S. (2011) Incidence of support limb laminitis in horses treated with a half limb, full limb, or transfixation pin casts: a retrospective study of 113 horses (2000–2009). *Equine Vet. J. Suppl.*, **40**, 7–11.
2. Peloso, J.G., Cohen, N.D., Walker, M.A., Watkins, J.P., Gayle, J.M., and Moyer, W. (1996) Case-control study of risk factors for the development of laminitis in the contralateral limb in Equidae with unilateral lameness. *J. Am. Vet. Med. Assoc.*, **209** (10), 1746–1749.
3. Baxter, G.M. and Morrison, S. (2008) Complications of unilateral weight bearing. *Vet. Clin. North Am. Equine Pract.*, **24** (3), 621–642.
4. Van Eps, A.W. (2010) Acute laminitis: medical and supportive therapy. *Vet. Clin. North Am. Equine Pract.*, **26** (1), 103–114.
5. Medina-Torres, C.E., Underwood, C., Pollitt, C.C., Castro-Olivera, E.M., Hodson, M.P., Richardson, D.W., *et al.* (2016) The effect of weight bearing and limb load cycling on equine lamellar perfusion and energy metabolism measured using tissue microdialysis. *Equine Vet. J.*, **48** (1), 114–119.
6. Medina-Torres, C.E., Pollitt, C.C., Underwood, C., Castro-Olivera, E.M., Collins, S.N., Allavena, R.E., *et al.* (2014) Equine lamellar energy metabolism studied using tissue microdialysis. *Vet. J.*, **201** (3), 275–282.
7. Goodrich, L.R. (2008) Strategies for reducing the complication of orthopedic pain perioperatively. *Vet. Clin. North Am. Equine Pract.*, **24** (3), 611–620.
8. Clutton, R.E. (2010) Opioid analgesia in horses. *Vet. Clin. North Am. Equine Pract.*, **26** (3), 493–514.
9. Van Eps, A.W., Leise, B.S., Watts, M., Pollitt, C.C., and Belknap, J.K. (2012) Digital hypothermia inhibits early lamellar inflammatory signaling in the oligofructose laminitis model. *Equine Vet. J.*, **44** (2), 230–237.
10. Redden, R.F. (2004) Preventing laminitis in the contralateral limb of horses with nonweight-bearing lameness. *Clin. Tech. Equine Pract.*, **3**, 57–63.
11. Ramsey, G.D., Hunter, P.J., and Nash, M.P. (2011) The effect of hoof angle variations on dorsal lamellar load in the equine hoof. *Equine Vet. J.*, **43** (5), 536–542.
12. Carpenter, R.S., Wallis, T.W., Baxter, G.M., Zubrod, C.J., and Hague, B.A. (2007) How to apply a half limb cast and elevated support limb shoe in the standing patient. *Proc. Am. Assoc. Equine Pract.*, **53**, 403–408.
13. Morrison, S. (2004) Foot management. *Clin. Tech. Equine Pract.*, **3**, 71–82.
14. Belknap, J.K. (2010) The pharmacological basis for the treatment of developmental and acute laminitis. *Vet. Clin. North Am. Equine Pract.*, **26** (1), 115–124
15. Ingle-Fehr, J.E. and Baxter, G.M. (1999) The effect of oral isoxsuprine and pentoxifylline on digital laminar blood flow in healthy horses. *Vet. Surg.*, **28** (3), 154–160.
16. Van Eps, A.W. and Pollitt, C.C. (2004) Equine laminitis: cryotherapy reduces the severity of the acute lesion. *Equine Vet. J.*, **36** (3), 255–260.
17. Van Eps, A.W., Pollitt, C.C., Underwood, C., Medina-Torres, C.E., Goodwin, W.A., and Belknap, J.K. (2014) Continuous digital hypothermia initiated after the onset of lameness prevents lamellar failure in the oligofructose laminitis model. *Equine Vet. J.*, **46** (5), 625–630.
18. Parks, A.H. (2011) Therapeutic Trimming and Shoeing, in *Adams and Stashak's Lameness in Horses*, 6th edition (ed. G.M. Baxter), Wiley-Blackwell Publishing, Ames, IA, pp. 980–989.
19. Parks, A.H. and O'Grady, S.E. (2003) Chronic laminitis: current treatment strategies. *Vet. Clin. North Am. Equine Pract.*, **19** (2), 393–416.
20. Schleining, J.A., McClure, S.R., Derrick, T.R., and Wang, C. (2011) Effects of industrial polystyrene foam insulation pads on the center of pressure and load distribution in the forefeet of clinically normal horses. *Am. J. Vet. Res.*, **72** (5), 628–633.
21. O'Grady, S.E. (2010) Farriery for chronic laminitis. *Vet. Clin. North Am. Equine Pract.*, **26** (2), 407–423.
22. Hanson, N., Buchner, H.H., Haller, J., and Windischbauer, G. (2005) Evaluation using wall strain gauges of a therapeutic shoe and hoof cast with a heel wedge as potential supportive therapy for horses with laminitis. *Vet. Surg.*, **34** (6), 630–636.
23. Steward, M.L. (2010) The use of the wooden shoe (Steward clog) in treating laminitis. *Vet. Clin. North Am. Equine Pract.*, **26** (1), 207–214.
24. Parks, A.H. (2007) How to: prevent and/or manage distal phalanx displacement in the acute stages of laminitis. *Proc. Br. Equine Vet. Assoc.*, **46**, 206–207.

CHAPTER 49

Prevention of Sepsis-Related Laminitis

Samuel D. Hurcombe and Susan J. Holcombe

Introduction

Horses with sepsis (including endotoxemia) are at risk for acute laminitis, and proactive measures aimed at attenuating the inflammatory events within the lamellae are believed to help reduce this risk of clinical lamellar failure. Laminitis can have catastrophic consequences, ranging from acute lamellar inflammation and pain without lamellar failure to complete mechanical lamellar failure often necessitating humane euthanasia of the animal. The onset of laminitis in some disease processes causing systemic sepsis can be sudden with a rapid onset of clinical signs of foot pain. For example, the present authors have observed some horses with typhlocolitis caused by *Neorickettsia risticii* (Potomac Horse Fever) to develop laminitis at a spectacularly rapid rate (Fig. 49.1).

Few therapies, shoeing recommendations and other preventive measures have been suspected or proven to prevent laminitis in these 'at-risk' patients; however, treatments aimed at: (i) ameliorating the primary disease process; (ii) reducing inflammation and systemic inflammatory response syndrome (SIRS) in the horse; and (iii) providing basic foot support make logical sense.

Medical management of the equine patient with sepsis/endotoxemia was addressed specifically in Chapter 36, where important aspects of treating the primary disease process as well as specific anti-endotoxemia therapies were discussed. The focus of the present chapter is to review important concepts aimed at preventing the development of lamellar inflammation in horses with clinical evidence of endotoxemia.

Reducing Inflammation

Digital Hypothermia/Cryotherapy

Methods aimed at reducing the local temperature of the foot have been evaluated as potential therapies and preventive measures to reduce laminitis development and the severity of the acute lesion. Distal limb hypothermia/cryotherapy has been proposed to be a therapeutic tool in cases of inflammation-induced laminitis, as is associated with endotoxemia.

Acute laminitis is characterized by lamellar injury, including destruction of the lamellar basement membrane [1]; this has been theorized to occur through the enhanced delivery of 'laminitis trigger factors' (LTFs), resulting in increases in the levels of matrix metalloproteinases (MMPs) in the lamellar tissue [2]. Endotoxemia and the resultant upregulation of proinflammatory mediators is characterized by an early hyperdynamic phase in which the cardiac output increases, causing hyperperfusion of tissue capillary beds. This stage may be recognized in the endotoxemic patient by tachycardia, brisk capillary refill time, injected and bright red mucous membranes (see Fig. 22.1), and warm extremities. Digital pulses in the feet may be 'bounding' or, at the very least, more prominent and palpable. It is theorized that such patients may actually have increased blood flow to the foot, as has been shown in an alimentary carbohydrate overload (CHO) model of laminitis [3–5] and therefore may result in an enhanced delivery of LTFs.

By cooling the digit, a decrease in lamellar tissue metabolic rate occurs which is believed to ameliorate protease destruction of the tissue. In addition to possibly reducing the delivery of LTFs to the foot, cryotherapy has been shown to reduce MMP (specifically MMP-2) mRNA expression and markedly reduce expression of multiple types of inflammatory mediators in cryotherapy-treated feet in CHO models of acute laminitis [6,7].

Several studies have shown that, by surrounding the feet in ice and/or ice with water, digital temperatures are significantly decreased to a mean hoof temperature of 11.9 °C by 2 h after initiating cryotherapy [8,9]. More recently, three constructs for delivering cryotherapy to the digit were evaluated, and showed that ice bags made from used 5-liter fluid bags filled with ice and water and a wader-style boot [Jack's Whirlpool boot; Jack's Manufacturing, Inc., Washington, Ohio, USA] filled with ice and water were each superior in reducing lamellar and digital venous temperatures compared to a frozen gel-filled boot [Grand Circuit Gel Products LLC, Louisville, KY, USA] (Mean

Equine Laminitis, First Edition. Edited by James K. Belknap and Raymond Geor.

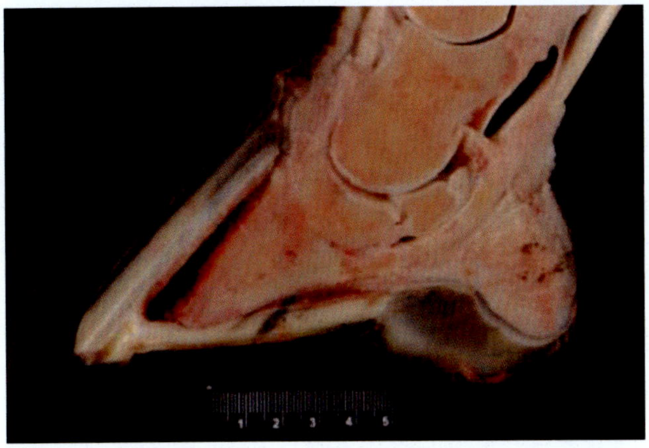

Figure 49.1 Post-mortem specimen of the digit cut in the sagittal plane from a horse with severe acute laminitis secondary to *Neorickettsia risticii* infection. This horse developed quadripedal severe laminitis and lamellar failure that resulted in separation from the hoof wall and sinking 24 h after hospital admission.

digital lamellar temperatures: 11.14 °C (wader boot), 11.41 °C (ice bag), 33.4 °C (gel boot)). The magnitude of cooling did not differ between the ice bags and wader boot, however, making the use of ice bags an inexpensive and effective method for cooling the digit (Fig. 49.2) [10].

Experimentally, cryotherapy has been evaluated over a longer duration following the induction of laminitis with oligofructose. In one study it was shown that, in horses which had received continuous cryotherapy for 72 h, clinical lameness and laminitis histopathology scores were significantly decreased compared to control horses who did not receive distal limb cryotherapy [8]. Cryotherapy also appears to be safe, well-tolerated, cheap, and practicably feasible.

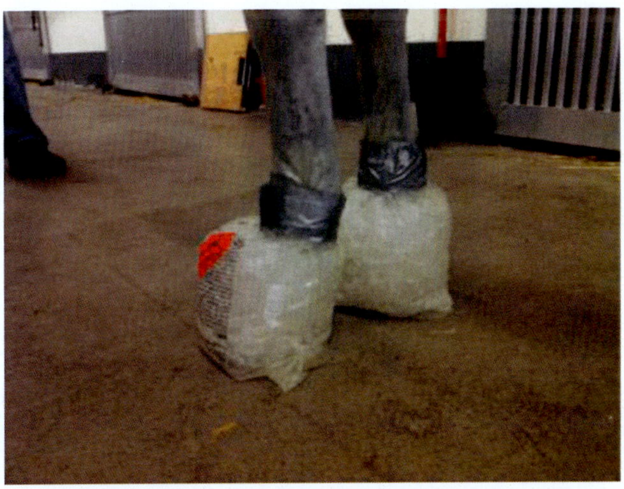

Figure 49.2 Pony gelding wearing ice boots on all four feet (front feet shown) made from 5-liter intravenous fluid therapy bags filled with ice and secured to the limbs using duct tape. This horse wore ice boots continuously for 72 h following exploratory celiotomy and correction of a strangulating lipoma and small bowel resection.

Clinical Use of Digital Cryotherapy

The present authors routinely apply ice boots to critically ill horses at risk of developing laminitis. These patients typically include (but are not limited to) horses with typhlocolitis, colitis, enteritis, postoperative surgical colic, fever of unknown origin, and endometritis/retained placenta. Essentially, used 5-liter fluid bags are applied to the feet ± frog support, and pour in ice (it is best always to have water present with ice to avoid injury to the skin). The bags are secured to the distal limb using duct tape, and are changed every 1–4 h, depending on the rate at which the ice melts but ensuring that ice is continually present. The 5-liter fluid bags are ideal because they are readily available, will fit over most horse's feet (draft horses excluded; feed sacks have been used for draft horses), and are durable when the horse ambulates around its stall. Typical ice boots used by the present authors are shown in Figure 49.2. Recently, ice boots with digital cushions have become commercially available (SoftRide Inc.).

The time to institute and apply cryotherapy is considered to be whenever the clinician identifies a horse at risk of laminitis, rather than waiting until the onset of clinical signs of laminitis. The aim is to prevent the onset of clinical lameness by attenuating the inflammatory events that are ongoing during the developmental stages of laminitis.

If a horse shows signs of SIRS, has a clinical disease that is known to cause laminitis, or is a critically ill breed of horse at risk of other forms of laminitis (i.e., a horse of an at-risk breed for endocrinopathic laminitis – for example, a Morgan horse with equine metabolic syndrome that presents with inflammatory gastrointestinal disease such as enteritis), cryotherapy is recommended sooner rather than later.

The duration of cryotherapy is debatable. Cryotherapy should be continued until the risk of laminitis development is low – that is, when the primary disease process has been treated, the horse is stable, and the clinical signs of SIRS are no longer evident. However, if cryotherapy is used, it should be applied constantly and not intermittently (i.e., every 2–4 h). Recently, the present authors evaluated digital cryotherapy in a population of 115 horses with SIRS due to enterocolitis. Continuous digital cryotherapy was significantly associated with a decreased prevalence of laminitis (7%) compared to horses that did not have ice applied to their feet (12%). The use of intermittent digital cryotherapy (ice on/ice off every 2–4 h) was associated with the highest prevalence of laminitis ($n = 5/9$; 55%) [11].

Other Therapies

Treatments for endotoxemia and sepsis have been outlined in Chapter 36, and are important to consider when the goal is to prevent laminitis development. Some specific therapies and their effectiveness on lamellar inflammation have been evaluated, at least experimentally.

Lidocaine, a local anesthetic agent, has been reported to have attenuating effects on systemic inflammation, including the inhibition of neutrophil phagocytic activity and free radical production [12, 13]. The main uses of lidocaine in clinical equine practice include management of pain, postoperative ileus, cardiac dysrrhythmia, and laminitis prevention. Lidocaine did not, however, reduce proinflammatory cytokine mRNA expression in the lamellae of horses given black walnut extract (BWE) compared to control horses [14], bringing into question its utility in ameliorating or preventing lamellar inflammatory events in endotoxemic horses. Moreover, when horses were given BWE, Loftus *et al.* showed that lamellar neutrophils were activated as determined by cluster differentiation (CD) surface markers and lidocaine did not attenuate this activation [15].

The use of low-molecular-weight heparin to specifically prevent the onset of laminitis has also been advocated in horses following colic surgery [16] by inhibiting the development of microthrombi in the digit, as has been documented in horses with laminitis previously [17, 18].

In a similar vein, rheologic agents aimed at improving erythrocyte deformability and movement through the digital lamellae vasculature have been advocated for maintaining lamellae vitality by enhancing nutrient delivery to the tissues and effectively removing metabolic waste products. BAY TG 1000, a dihydropyridine with these qualities, was reportedly effective at decreasing the severity of laminitis and improved clinical recovery in horses with experimentally induced laminitis [19]. Drugs with a similar mechanism of action (e.g. pentoxifylline [typically administered at 8.8 mg kg^{-1}, oral, q. 12 h]) have been used in endotoxemic horses.

Footing and Bedding for the At-Risk Patient

Limited data exist informing the clinician as to the best footing for horses with laminitis. Most practitioners would agree that no bedding is probably not ideal in terms of support of the frog or weight-bearing hoof wall. Concrete flooring or hard stone is unlikely to provide much support for the foot and is likely deleterious. Deep sand bedding, soft composite synthetic material, tan bark material, peat moss or deep straw might offer some support to the foot. Rubber mats that are easy to clean and offer some 'spring' or 'give' might be an attractive option for hospitals. Currently, no data are available for horses as to the 'ideal' surface for those animals with laminitis or at risk of laminitis; however, there is some evidence in dairy cows that deep sand bedding offers improved comfort to cattle with lameness, as well as having low bacterial counts compared to other surfaces [20]. This might hold true for horses in which lying down is often encouraged, particularly if already clinically affected with laminitis. As some horses appear to resist lying down on sand, it can be covered with other types of bedding to encourage the animals to lay down. For horses at risk of sepsis-related laminitis (SRL), the provision of bedding offering support makes intuitive sense. Bedding should be kept clean and dry, and urine/fecal material should be removed often to minimize the risk of thrush and abscess development.

Conclusions

In the prevention of SRL, many therapies have been tried clinically but their success is unproven. To date, there has been no 'silver bullet' in preventing laminitis in endotoxemic/septic patients. Therapies aimed at treating the primary disease process, including antimicrobials (if indicated), 'anti-endotoxin' therapies (e.g., polymixin B), anti-inflammatories, and antithrombotic medications should each be considered when the clinician is faced with the septic patient. Cryotherapy should be instituted in at-risk patients as it is the only proven therapy that specifically decreases inflammatory mediator expression and may prevent the onset of clinical laminitis in horses.

References

1. Pollitt, C.C. (1996) Basement membrane pathology: a feature of acute equine laminitis. *Equine Vet. J.*, **28** (1), 38–46.
2. Johnson, P.J., Tyagi, S.C., Katwa, L.C., Ganjam, V.K., Moore, L.A., Kreeger, J.M., *et al.* (1998) Activation of extracellular matrix metalloproteases in equine laminitis. *Vet. Rec.*, **142**, 392–396.
3. Robinson, N.E., Scott, J.B., Dabney, J.M., and Jones, G.A. (1976) Digital vascular responses and permeability in equine alimentary laminitis. *Equine Vet. J.*, **37**, 1171–1176.
4. Pollitt, C.C. and Davies, C.T. (1998) Equine laminitis: its development coincides with increased sublamellar blood flow. *Equine Vet. J. Suppl.*, **26**, 125–132.
5. Trout, D.R., Hornof, W.J., Linford, R.L., and O'Brien, T.R. (1990) Scintigraphic evaluation of digital circulation during the developmental and acute phases of equine laminitis. *Equine Vet. J.*, **22** (6), 416–421.
6. Van Eps, A.W. and Pollitt, C.C. (2004) Equine laminitis: cryotherapy reduces the severity of the acute lesion. *Equine Vet. J.*, **36** (3), 255–260.
7. Van Eps, A.W., Leise, B.S., Watts, M., Pollitt, C.C., and Belknap, J.K. (2012) Digital hypothermia inhibits early lamellar inflammatory signalling in the oligofructose laminitis model. *Equine Vet. J.*, **44** (2), 230–237.
8. Van Eps, A.W. and Pollitt, C.C. (2009) Equine laminitis model: cryotherapy reduces the severity of lesions evaluated seven days after induction with oligofructose. *Equine Vet. J.*, **41** (8), 741–746.
9. Pollitt, C.C. and Daradka, M. (0000) Prolonged, continuous distal limb cryotherapy in the horse. *JOURNAL*, **00**, 00–00.
10. Reesink, H.L., Divers, T.J., Bookbinder, L.C., Van Eps, A.W., Soderholm, L.V., Mohammed, H.O., *et al.* (2012) Measurement of digital laminar and venous temperatures as a means of comparing three methods of topically applied cold treatment for digits of horses. *Am. J. Vet. Res.*, **73** (6), 860–866.
11. Kullman, A., Holcombe, S.J., Hurcombe, S.D., Roessner, H.A., Hauptman, J.G., Geor, R.J., *et al.* (2014) Prophylactic digital cryotherapy was associated with decreased incidence of laminitis in horses diagnosed with colitis. *Equine Vet. J.*, **46** (5), 554–559.

12. Hollmann, M.W. and Durieux, M.E. (2000) Local anesthetics and the inflammatory response: a new therapeutic indication? *Anesthesiology*, **93** (3), 858–875.
13. Hyvonen, P.M. and Kowolik, M.J. (1998) Dose-dependent suppression of the neutrophil respiratory burst by lidocaine. *Acta Anaesthesiol. Scand.*, **42** (5), 565–569.
14. Williams, J.M., Lin, Y.J., Loftus, J.P., Faleiros, R.R., Peroni, J.F., Hubbell, J.A., *et al.* (2010) Effect of intravenous lidocaine administration on laminar inflammation in the black walnut extract model of laminitis. *Equine Vet. J.*, **42** (3), 261–269.
15. Loftus, J.P., Williams, J.M., Belknap, J.K., and Black, S.J. (2010) In vivo priming and ex vivo activation of equine neutrophils in black walnut extract-induced equine laminitis is not attenuated by systemic lidocaine administration. *Vet. Immunol. Immunopathol.*, **138** (1-2), 60–69.
16. de la Rebiere de Pouyade, G., Grulke, S., Detilleux, J., Salciccia, A., Verwilghen, D.R., Caudron, I., *et al.* (2009) Evaluation of low-molecular-weight heparin for the prevention of equine laminitis after colic surgery. *J. Vet. Emerg. Crit. Care (San Antonio)*, **19** (1), 113–119.
17. Weiss, D.J., Geor, R.J., Johnston, G., and Trent, A.M. (1994) Microvascular thrombosis associated with onset of acute laminitis in ponies. *Am. J. Vet. Res.*, **55** (5), 606–612.
18. Weiss, D.J., Trent, A.M., and Johnston, G. (1995) Prothrombotic events in the prodromal stages of acute laminitis in horses. *Am. J. Vet. Res.*, **56** (8), 986–991.
19. Hood, D.M., Brumbaugh, G.W., and Wagner, I.P. (2002) Effectiveness of a unique dihydropyridine (BAYTG 1000) for prevention of laminitis in horses. *Am. J. Vet. Res.*, **63** (3), 443–447.
20. Van Gastelen, S., Westerlan, B., Houwers, D.J., and Eerdenburg, F.J. (2011) A study on cow comfort and risk for lameness and mastitis in relation to different types of bedding materials. *J. Dairy Sci.*, **94** (10), 4878–4888.

CHAPTER 50

Nutritional Management for Avoidance of Pasture-Associated Laminitis

Pat Harris

Introduction

As farms have diversified and ponies/horses are kept more often on 'improved' pastures established for dairy or beef production, there appears to have been an increased recognition of the importance of pasture-associated laminitis (PAL). Turning certain ponies or horses out onto 'lush' (i.e., green, actively photosynthetic) or 'stressed' (i.e., where environmental conditions are suboptimal for growth) pastures is a common predisposing and/or triggering factor for laminitis. Currently, it is thought that high levels of water-soluble carbohydrates (WSC) and/or starch are involved in the development of laminitis in horses at pasture (see Chapters 18 and 23). Although research has shown that a bolus of inulin-type fructan (oligofructose; after a short adaptation phase) at between 5 g and 12.5 $g\,kg^{-1}$ bodyweight can induce laminitis [1, 2], this protocol may not be a good model for PAL because:

- The clinical signs of gastrointestinal disease observed after bolus administration of oligofructose are much more severe than those typically seen in cases of PAL (or are not observed in PAL cases).
- Temperate-grass fructans are complex in nature and very different from the type of fructans that have been used in the experimental studies.
- Grazing animals cannot achieve an equivalent intake of fructan from pasture within such a short period of time.

Even though this model is unlikely to mimic PAL, recent studies have shown that ponies can ingest substantially more dry matter (DM) per day (up to ~5% of body weight) than previously suggested, both when fed *ad libitum* short-chopped fiber feeds [3] or when out at grass [4]. In one study, ponies were observed to ingest more than 30% and up to 41% of their daily DM intake within a 3-h turnout period [5], while investigations evaluating the effect of grazing muzzles showed that ponies can ingest up to 1% of body weight as DM within a 3-h period [6]. With the knowledge that the fructan and WSC contents of some grasses can be very high at certain times of the year (e.g., the *average* fructan content of ryegrass can be as high as 27–28% DM basis when harvested in May; A. Longland personal communication), a 250-kg pony turned out to pasture forage with a 27.5% fructan content would only need to ingest 4.5 kg DM grass (~1.8% body weight as DM) in order to achieve a fructan intake equivalent to that used by Kalck and coworkers [2] to induce laminitis in healthy horses. A pony could potentially ingest this amount over a 6-h period, and certainly over the course of a day, even when lower pasture forage WSC is present. A key question, therefore, is whether pasture intake is just the final trigger for laminitis in an animal that is predisposed to developing the condition, or whether exposure to pasture *per se* predisposes an individual to laminitis. Grazing pasture with high nonstructural carbohydrate (NSC; comprising simple sugars, fructans and starch) content could, for example, promote the development of insulin resistance and/or persistent hyperinsulinemia. Grazing high-NSC pastures may result in peaks of insulin similar to those following a high-starch diet [7]; this in turn may lower the threshold for laminitis to be triggered.

A number of risk factors have been identified that are believed to increase the risk of PAL, including obesity (or recent gain in body weight) and insulin resistance/dysregulation (see Chapter 23 and Fig. 50.1). It is possible that the various predisposing events and/or threshold lowering factors may be additive in nature (see Fig. 50.2). However, it should also be recognized that pasture turnout can be a trigger factor for laminitis in lean, nonobese animals that do not have elevated basal plasma insulin concentrations. Therefore, regardless of the specific pathophysiology, PAL by definition occurs in association with being out on pasture, and, consequently, the most obvious way to prevent episodes is to prevent access to pasture. There are, however, a number of issues with this recommendation:

- Pasture-based systems arguably are the most welfare friendly management system for horses, as they allow animals (especially when kept in herds) to express 'natural' behaviors and feeding patterns.
- Pasture often is the most economical management system.

Equine Laminitis, First Edition. Edited by James K. Belknap and Raymond Geor.

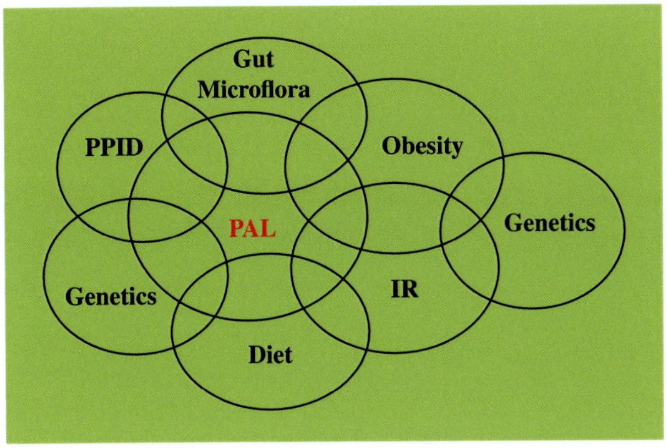

Figure 50.1 Inter-relationship between various factors that impact risk for pasture-associated laminitis (PAL). Diet and genetics may influence the risk of several other factors. PPID, pituitary pars intermedia dysfunction; IR, insulin resistance/insulin dysregulation.

- The majority of animals out on pasture do not develop laminitis – and even those that are prone to laminitis can often be kept at pasture for a substantial part of the day/year.
- Animals not out at pasture but fed purely/predominantly on preserved pasture forages can suffer from laminitis (although this circumstance could be taken to reflect PAL).

A more pragmatic approach is to decide whether an individual animal is at low, moderate, or high risk of having an episode of PAL. For example:

  - *Low-risk* animals (e.g., non-obese, Thoroughbred type horses in full work) can be allowed unrestricted access to appropriate grazing as required for their management.
  - *Moderate-risk* animals (e.g., an obese or insulin-resistant pony) may require restricted access to pasture, especially at certain times of the year. In addition, the implementation of countermeasure strategies that target laminitis risk factors (e.g., insulin resistance, obesity) may be indicated.
  - *High-risk* animals (recent episode of PAL or animals that have suffered recurrent episodes of PAL) may require limited or no access to pasture.

This approach has its own limitations. For example how would an obese, insulin-resistant Thoroughbred or a moderately conditioned pony of unknown laminitis history be classified? Until more information is available on the pathophysiology of PAL, and the means are provided to identify accurately animals at low, moderate and high risk, it is only possible to 'best guess' into which risk category an individual animal may fall.

Nutritional Management After an Episode of PAL

Affected animals must be removed from pasture, housed either in a dry lot (mild signs of laminitis) or a box stall with deep bedding (more severe signs of laminitis indicative of possible lamellar instability), and introduced to a low-NSC, preserved forage-based ration with an appropriate forage balancer [8]. The duration of confinement and restricted diet, as well as decisions regarding a return to pasture grazing, will depend on the severity and time course of the laminitis and the presence of underlying endocrine and metabolic problems. The following are suggestions for management depending on the clinical state of the equid:

- The horse or pony should be held off pasture until there has been complete resolution of the acute laminitis episode and, where indicated, diagnostic testing for equine metabolic syndrome (EMS) and pituitary pars intermedia dysfunction (PPID). If there is no evidence of EMS or PPID, a gradual reintroduction to pasture may be considered. Start with 1–2 h of grazing, once or twice per day, or turn out for longer periods if the horse is fitted with a grazing muzzle (fitted appropriately and which allows limited grazing but access to water; see Table 50.1). More caution may be required under a number of circumstances – that is, when the pasture is green and growing rapidly (e.g., in spring) or is 'stressed' (through drought/inappropriate management, etc.) or where clover has become dominant.
- Obese, insulin-resistant animals should be held off pasture for a longer period (e.g., two to three months), allowing time for the implementation of management changes (i.e., dietary

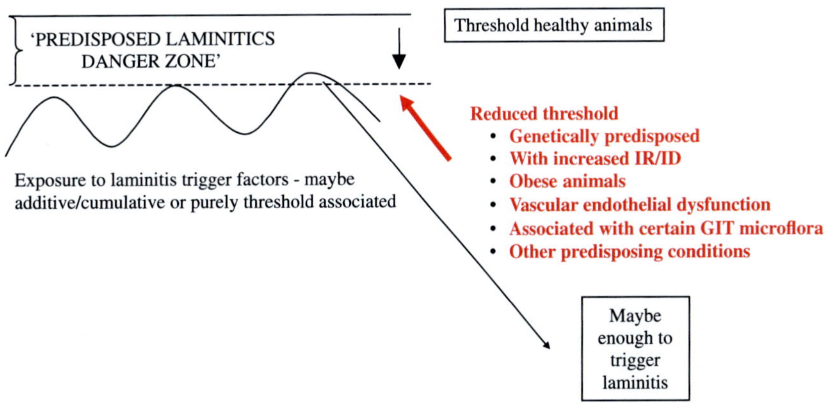

Figure 50.2 Illustration of how a theoretical threshold for laminitis induction can be lowered under certain situations. Adapted from Harris & Geor 2007 by kind permission of WALTHAM Centre for Pet Nutrition). IR, insulin resistance; ID, insulin dysregulation; GIT, gastrointestinal tract.

Table 50.1 Practical tips on using grazing muzzles see 6 and 9.

Tip no.	Procedure(s)
1	Muzzles need to be fitted carefully and checked regularly to ensure they are not causing chaffing injury to the muzzle area. Muzzles should not be tight-fitting and should be designed so that they will break away if the horse gets into difficulties.
2	The horse should have constant access to water; therefore total restriction muzzles (that prevent access to water) should not be used.
3	It is important to ensure that grass can be accessed through the base of the muzzle. If the grass is too short or too long, then it may be impossible or extremely difficult for the horse or pony to access the grass, and this may result in abnormal/'stressed' behavior.
4	For muzzles with a central access hole, the muzzle should be positioned such that there is at rest a ca. 1-inch (25-mm) gap between the base of the muzzle and the horse's nose (this enables the muzzle hole to be positioned below the incisors). There needs also to be a gap (ca. 0.5 in; 12 mm) around the edge of the muzzle to allow movement of the jaw. The fitting will need to be amended depending on the individual. Watch the horse grazing with the muzzle and adjust as required.
5	An adaptation period will usually be required – do not leave horses/ponies for long periods of time when first fitted with a muzzle. Some horses even need to be positively encouraged to use the hole/slats to graze; try introducing cut blades of grass through the hole or providing a treat (mint/carrot) in a similar way. Horses/ponies should not be left unsupervised while wearing muzzles until they have been observed to graze and drink.
6	All feed and water vessels that may be used by horses wearing muzzles need to be smooth to minimize the risk of the muzzle getting snagged.
7	The use of grazing muzzles can disturb herd social dynamics, sometimes necessitating the separation of horses in the group.
8	All animals should have regular periods of time without a muzzle to enable them to groom themselves, and so on.
9	Muzzles should not be used when there is no or very limited grass available. These muzzles are designed to restrict grass intake – not to totally inhibit grazing. When minimal or no grass is present, muzzles should be removed and controlled amounts of an alternative suitable forage should be provided.
10	Ensure that the animal's teeth are checked regularly, typically every six months.
11	The author's current recommendation is that grazing muzzles should only be used as an adjunctive method for restricting grass intake, for example to further restrict grass intake during short periods of turnout – with the at-risk animal being fed a controlled amount of an alternative suitable forage for the majority of the day.

restriction, increased physical activity) that result in weight loss and improved insulin sensitivity. Similarly, horses with PPID should be held off pasture pending improvement in clinical signs, for example, treatment with pergolide.

- Some EMS- and PPID-affected animals with a history of repeated episodes of laminitis require permanent housing in a dry lot because they appear to be susceptible to further episodes of laminitis in the face of even small variations in pasture availability and nutrient content.
- Whilst there are no specific data to support the increased provision of certain vitamins and trace elements, it may be helpful to provide additional biotin (with total biotin intake of 3–5 mg per 100 kg body weight) in a ration providing sufficient amino acids, zinc, and calcium and so forth, in order to help support optimal hoof growth and quality.
- The use of bran mashes is likely to be contraindicated (particularly when fed just with forage), especially in animals unaccustomed to bran within their diet. Apart from being potentially an irritant to the gastrointestinal tract, bran has an unbalanced Ca:P ratio and is deficient in many key nutrients such as lysine.
- Although the relevance of oxidative stress in the pathophysiology of laminitis is unclear, the author currently recommends that laminitic animals are provided with higher than maintenance intake of vitamin E (e.g., a minimum of 200 IU kg^{-1} diet DM or 3 IU kg^{-1} bodyweight if the horse is on a restricted diet).

Nutritional Recommendations to Reduce the Risk of PAL

In the future, genetic as well as blood and/or microbiome screening tests may enable the identification of certain animals within the high-risk category, so that more targeted preventive strategies can be implemented. Current recommendations for avoidance of PAL focus on the management of grass intake, the NSC content of the grass being ingested, and animal-related risk factors such as obesity and insulin resistance.

Managing Grass Intake

As discussed above, the rate and/or magnitude of grass intake are potentially central to the pathophysiology of PAL. Methods of reducing grass intake include:

- *Restricting time out at pasture*: in this circumstance, grass intake will depend on herbage yield, time out at pasture, and the individual animal's rate of intake. Ponies may adapt to a restricted time regimen so that they maximize the amount of grass ingested within a given turnout period [5]. There is evidence that ponies can ingest approximately 1% of their body weight as DM during a 3-h turnout period [6].
- *Strip grazing*: allowing a laminitis-prone animal to graze a small strip of land (typically delineated by means of electric fencing), commonly after another animal has removed most of the grass, can reduce intake. Overgrazed grass can,

however, have a high fructan content when compared to unstressed grass.

- *Use of dirt paddocks or dry lots*: this approach allows interaction with other equids, as well as opportunity for voluntary exercise. Weed control and the potential for the development of conditions such as 'mud fever' need to be considered.
- *Use of 'pasture-free' alternative turn out areas*: these may include sand arenas and woodchip-covered areas. As with dirt/dry lots, this approach is highly effective for the restriction of grass intake. The use of sand lots will increase the risk of sand colic, especially if forage intake is restricted.
- *Use of grazing muzzles*: the application of grazing muzzles can reduce grass DM intake by approximately 80% in ponies provided 3 h of pasture turnout, regardless of season [6]. Further research is needed, including an evaluation of the effects of grazing muzzles over longer periods of time, to provide more detailed information on the utility of grazing muzzles in different management systems [9]. In the meantime, some practical tips on the use of grazing muzzles are provided in Table 50.1.

Managing Pasture Forage

It is currently thought that the incidence of PAL can be reduced if at-risk animals only have access to pasture when the levels of forage starch, sugar, and fructans are low. Unfortunately, it is very difficult to predict pasture forage NSC content, which varies markedly from season to season, location to location, and even within a location during a particular day, depending on plant species, environmental conditions, field topography, and the grazing patterns of individual animals among other factors. The availability of methods that quickly identify 'high-risk pastures,' or the presence of factors that can result in a high-NSC pasture, might enable an owner to determine when is the best time to restrict access to pasture for avoidance of PAL [8]. As this methodology is currently not available, only very general advice can be given. It is also worth noting that it is currently not known whether the ingestion of large amounts of grass containing moderate amounts of NSC is more or less risky than ingesting small amounts of grass with a high NSC content.

The following recommendations can be made for at-risk equids based on current knowledge:

- Consider a total restriction on grazing (whilst providing the horse with suitable diet [e.g., low-NSC forage with a forage balancer]) if it is essential that the horse ingests minimal levels of sugar, starch, and fructans, or a strict weight-management program is required. Voluntary exercise and socializing aspects need to be considered, such as periods of turnout with companions in dry lots.
- Turn horses out to pasture when fructan/WSC levels are likely to be at the lowest. For temperate grasses in the Northern hemisphere, this tends to be from very late at night to early morning, removing the horse/pony from the pasture by mid-morning.
- More mature, stemmy grasses may contain more fructan (as it is stored in the stem) than younger growing grasses (that are using the sugars for growth). In general, therefore, at-risk animals should be grazed on actively growing pastures with a predominance of young, leafy grass. However, even if the WSC content per blade of grass is low, the amount that may be ingested per day could still be an issue if there is a moderate to large quantity of grass available. Pending further research on whether total daily intake versus the WSC/NSC concentration of forage is most important in regards to laminitis risk, the author currently suggests that restriction of grass intake is often indicated when the pasture is actively growing.
- Do not allow horses to graze on pastures that have not been properly managed by regular grazing or cutting.
- Pastures should receive an appropriate amount and type of fertilizer to support growth. In general, fructan levels are lower in growing grass (sward). As mentioned above, however, herbage yield of the pasture (which will affect grass intake) may be as or more important than the NSC or WSC content per blade of grass. Some restriction to grazing (e.g., time or use of a grazing muzzle) may therefore be required for moderate- to high-yielding pastures. Alternatively, the pasture should be cut ('topped') and allowed to rest for a few days before the at-risk horse or pony is allowed to graze.
- Avoid grazing pastures when the grass is changing from a vegetative (i.e., leaf growth and expansion) to reproductive (ear emergence) state because WSC/fructan levels are likely to be high. In general, avoid/restrict turnout in spring (before flower development) and also in autumn (during flowering and early seed development).
- Cold temperatures and drought will reduce grass growth, resulting in the accumulation of fructan. Do not allow horses to graze on pastures that have been exposed to low temperatures (e.g., frosts overnight) followed by warm, bright sunny weather, or to graze pastures that have been 'stressed' through drought.
- Rotate the use of paddocks regularly; consider grazing by other species such as sheep or cattle, to keep the grass/sward at an appropriate height and also to avoid the pastures from becoming 'stressed' through either under- or over-grazing.
- Actively manage the composition of pastures. For example, clover (high in starch) tends to become more predominant in overgrazed pastures. Weeds/other non-grass species can be high in fructans and are commonly found in some pastures (e.g., dandelions).
- Consider grazing animals on specific pastures that contain grass species which tend to produce lower levels of WSCs and also fructans with a higher molecular weight than ryegrass (e.g., timothy and cocksfoot/orchard grass) that may be fermented less rapidly [10–12]. This advice, however, will need to be adjusted based on the grass species that grow in the local environment [11, 12].

Providing Alternative Forage Sources

For those animals which require restricted access to pasture, preserved forage (e.g., hay) or forage replacers (e.g., pelleted/cubed/chopped hay, complete fiber-based diets; see below) are required to ensure that they receive [13] at least 1.5 kg per 100 kg body weight per day of forage on a DM basis (and ≥1 kg per 100 kg body weight even when feeding obese animals on an energy restricted diet). However, preserved forage with a high NSC content may also result in laminitis which, although not directly linked to time out on pasture, can be considered to be a variant of PAL. Accordingly it is recommended to:

- Analyze any forage fed to animals at risk of laminitis and only provide forage with <12% NSC and preferably <10% NSC (i.e., starch, sugar, and fructan) content on a DM basis. Many hays will have NSC content >10–12% DM. Soaking hay in clean water (>8 °C and perhaps more ideally at approximately 16 °C [i.e., U.K. summer tap water]) for approximately 3 h may help to reduce the WSC content [14]. However, as the results from soaking are [15, 16] variable (between and even within forage species) [15], it is advisable to ensure that the original forage has a low NSC content (or feed an appropriate forage replacer). Soaking also potentially reduces the hygienic quality of the hay [15,16], and, therefore, current advice is that hay should not be soaked for >3 h in hot weather. Ideally, the NSC and DM content (especially when energy-restricted rations are being fed) should be assessed after soaking to determine whether or not the target NSC and DM intake will be achieved [14, 16, 17].
- Feed a broad-spectrum vitamin and mineral supplement (i.e., an appropriate forage balancer) when forage is the only or primary component of the diet. Ensure an adequate intake of magnesium. There is no current evidence, however, to suggest that magnesium intake above recommended levels will reduce the risk of laminitis.
- Choose low-NSC feedstuffs when the horse or pony requires additional calories; options include:
  - The use of more digestible forage (i.e., less mature grass hay) provided that the WSC/NSC content is <10–12% DM. The author currently does not recommend feeding alfalfa or haylage to animals that are prone to laminitis.
  - Highly digestible fiber sources such as sugar beet pulp (*without* added molasses) or soya hulls. These feeds provide a means to increase energy intake without increasing starch or sugar intake. To minimize the provision of WSC (including fructose) when feeding sugar beet pulp, the author currently recommends that the ration is soaked (according to manufacturer's guidelines) with removal of the water before feeding.
  - The use of vegetable oil as an energy source rather than cereal starch – especially for those animals not being exercised (the level of oil feeding should be increased gradually and it is advisable to add vitamin E at 100–150 IU per 100 ml oil). Do not add more than 1 ml oil per kg body weight without obtaining advice from a qualified nutritionist or veterinarian.
  - The use of smaller, more frequent meals per day (rather than one or two feedings) in order to minimize the insulin response to feeding.
  - The use of a low-starch and low-sugar, high-fiber and high-oil commercial feed which ideally has been shown to elicit a low to low–moderate insulin response.

Managing Animal Risk Factors

The management of animal-related risk factors for laminitis, including obesity and insulin resistance ('insulin dysregulation'), is also important in the overall approach to the avoidance of PAL. A detailed discussion of this topic is provided in Chapter 36.

Conclusions

Pasture turnout can be a cause of laminitis even in the lean, non-obese animal that does not have evidence of insulin dysregulation (e.g., increased basal plasma insulin concentrations). However, obesity and insulin resistance/hyperinsulinemia, as well as turning animals out to pasture with a high NSC content (or feeding preserved forage with high NSC), appears to increase the risk of PAL. Management changes that reduce the intake of high-NSC forage and other feedstuffs can help to reduce the risk of laminitis, especially when combined with strategies to reduce the impact of other risk factors such as obesity.

References

1. Van Eps, A.W. and Pollitt, C.C. (2006) Equine laminitis induced with oligofructose. *Equine Vet. J.*, **38**, 203–208.
2. Kalck, K.A., Frank, N., Elliott, S.B., and Boston, R.C. (2009) Effects of a low-dose oligofructose treatment administered via nasogastric intubation on induction of laminitis and associated alterations in glucose and insulin dynamics in horses. *Am. J. Vet. Res.*, **70**, 624–632.
3. Dugdale, A., Curtis, G.C., Cripps, P., Harris, P., and Argo, C.McG. (2011) Effects of season and body condition on appetite, body mass and body composition in ad libitum fed pony mares. *Vet. J.*, **190**, 329–337.
4. Longland, A.C., Ince, J., and Harris, P. (2011) Estimation of pasture intake by ponies from liveweight change during six weeks at pasture. *J. Equine Vet. Sci.*, **31**, 275–276.
5. Ince, J., Longland, A.C., Newbold, J.C., and Harris, P. (2011) Changes in proportions of dry matter intakes by ponies with access to pasture and haylage for 3 and 20 hours per day respectively for six weeks. *J. Equine Vet. Sci.*, **31**, 283.
6. Longland, A., Barfoot, C., Harris, P. (2016) Effects of grazing muzzles on intakes of dry matter and water-soluble carbohydrates by ponies grazing spring, summer and autumn swards, as well as autumn swards of different heights. *J. Equine Vet. Sci.*, **40**, 26–33.
7. Byrd, B.M., Treiber, K.H., Staniar, W.B., Kronfeld, D.S., and Geor, R.J. (2006) Circadian and seasonal variation on pasture NSC and circulating insulin concentrations in grazing horses. *J. Animal Sci.*, **84** (Suppl.1), 330–331 (abstract).
8. Geor, R.J. and Harris, P. (2013) Laminitis, in *Equine Clinical and Applied Nutrition* (eds R.J. Geor, P. Harris, and M. Coenen), Elsevier, pp. 469–486.

9. Longland, A., Barfoot, C., Harris, P. (2016) Efficacy of wearing grazing muzzles for 10 hours per day on controlling bodyweight in pastured ponies. *J. Equine Vet. Sci.*, **45**, 22–27.
10. Longland, A.C. and Byrd, B.M. (2006) Pasture nonstructural carbohydrates and equine laminitis. *J. Nutr.*, **136**, 2099S–2102S.
11. Chatterton, N., Harrison, P., Bennett, J., and Assay, K. (1989) Carbohydrate partitioning from 185 accessions of gramineae growth under warm and cool conditions. *J. Plant Physiol.*, **134**, 169–179.
12. Ince, J., Longland, A., Moore-Colyer, M., and Harris, P. (2005) In vitro fermentation of three species of fresh grass differing in water soluble carbohydrate content with an equine faecal inoculum. Proceedings of the Equine Nutrition Conference, Hanover, Germany, Pferdeheilkunde, vol. 21, pp. 66–67.
13. Harris, P.A., Coenen, M., and Geor, R.J. (2013) Controversial areas in equine nutrition and feeding management: the editors' views, in *Equine Clinical and Applied Nutrition* (eds R.J. Geor, P. Harris, and M. Coenen), Elsevier, pp. 455–468.
14. Longland, A., Barfoot, C., and Harris, P.A. (2014) Effect of water temperature and agitation on loss of water-soluble carbohydrates and protein from grass hay: implications for equine feeding management. *Vet. Rec.*, **174**, 68.
15. Longland, A.C., Barfoot, C., and Harris, P.A. (2011) Effects of soaking on the water-soluble carbohydrate and crude protein content of hay. *Vet. Rec.*, **168**, 618.
16. Moore-Colyer, M.J.S., Lumbis, K., Longland, A., and Harris, P. (2014) The effect of five different wetting treatments on the nutrient content and microbial concentration in hay for horses. *PLoS ONE*, **9** (11), e114079.
17. Argo, C.M., Dugdale, A.H.A., and McGowan, C.M. (2015) Considerations for the use of restricted, soaked grass hay diets to promote weight loss in the management of equine metabolic syndrome and obesity. *Vet. J.*, **206.2**, 170–177.
18. Harris, P.A. and Geor, R. (2007) The latest findings in laminitis research The 1st WALTHAM-Royal Veterinary college Laminitis Conference, in *Nutritional Countermeasures to laminitis* (eds P.A. Harris, S.J. Hill, J. Elliott, and S.R. Bailey), WALTHAM, published by Equine Veterinary Journal, pp. 29–38.

Glossary

ADAMTS: A disintegrin and metalloproteinase with thrombospondin motifs – a family of protease enzymes primarily known for their function in processing/cleaving matrix proteoglycans (e.g., aggrecan, versican).

Apoptosis ('programmed cell death'): A type of cell death occurring both in health and disease in which a 'programmed' sequence of events occurs (e.g., fragmentation of nuclear DNA) which leads to the elimination of cells without the release of cellular proteins which can cause an inflammatory response (in distinction to necrosis).

Asymmetrical distal displacement: Displacement on the distal phalanx which can occur in horses with laminitis (and white line disease) in which there is distal displacement of either the lateral or medial aspect of the distal phalanx (most commonly the medial aspect).

Basement membrane: A thin connective tissue layer made up primarily of laminin, collagen IV, nidogen and perlecan which, in the parietal (lamellar) integument, is situated between the basal epithelial cell layer and the lamellar dermis. It provides a critical structural interface due to its relationship with both epithelial cells (via integrins) and extracellular matrix components of the dermis.

Breakover point: The most dorsal part of the ground surface, either the hoof capsule in the unshod horse or the shoe in the shod horse that is in contact with the ground at the moment the heels begin to rise off the ground.

Capsular rotation: Divergence of the dorsal parietal surface of the distal phalanx from the dorsal hoof wall.

Center of Pressure: The point of action of the Ground Reaction Force. At rest it is close to the center of the ground surface of the foot, but changes during the course of the stride. Also called the Point of Zero Moment and the Point of Force.

Chemokine: A class of cytokines that control cell functions including directed chemotaxis (migration of cells towards a substance) of different cell types (esp. leukocytes).

Chronic laminitis: The phase of laminitis that follows the acute phase. It is associated with displacement of the distal phalanx relative to the hoof capsule and the ensuing changes in shape of the hoof capsule. Its onset has been said to coincide with the displacement of the distal phalanx; however, from a temporal perspective, this is commonly not useful because displacement can occur at markedly different times after the development of acute disease (or even without evidence of acute disease).

Coronary band: A circumferential band of integument at the proximal aspect of the hoof from which the hoof wall grows distally.

Coronary band-extensor process distance (C–E distance; syn. founder distance): The vertical distance between the dorsoproximal border of the coronary band and the proximal extent of the extensor process of the distal phalanx (measured on a lateral radiograph of the digit; it is used to assess displacement of the distal phalanx).

Coronet: The junction of the pastern and the foot.

Cuneate: Pertaining to the frog.

Cryotherapy: See Digital hypothermia.

Cushion support material: See Impression material.

Cyclo-oxygenase (COX): The enzyme, predominantly present as two forms, COX-1 (the 'constitutive form' normally present) and COX-2 (the 'inducible form'), which are the therapeutic target of non-steroidal anti-inflammatory drugs (NSAIDs). Both COX-1 and COX-2 use arachidonic acid as a substrate to produce a central prostanoid, PGH2, which is then used as a substrate by different prostaglandin and thromoboxane synthases to make specific prostanoids (e.g., thromboxane, prostacyclin, prostaglandin PGE2 [PGE2]).

Cytokine: A broad group of small signaling proteins produced by multiple cell types which can have a wide range of effects on other cells, a large number of which are related to inflammation/immunoregulation.

Damage-associated molecular pattern (DAMP): Endogenous products from host cells which are either passively released though non-physiologic cell death (primarily nuclear and mitochondrial proteins and nucleotides) or actively released from live cells (alarmins) and activate an innate immune response, primarily through the activation of pattern recognition receptors. Examples of DAMPs include nuclear histones, host RNA and DNA (mitochondrial and nuclear), calprotectin, and formyl peptides.

Dermis: A layer of tissue deep to the epidermis, which is continuous with the basement membrane superficially made up primarily of matrix proteins (e.g., collagens and proteoglycans) to provide mechanical support. The dermis also contains vasculature, lymphatics, and nerves to sustain the epidermis.

Desmosome: Multiprotein complexes in epithelial and muscle cells responsible both for intercellular adhesion and for tethering the intermediate cytoskeleton to the cell membrane.

Digital hypothermia: The therapeutic technique of maintaining the distal limbs of equids in an ice slurry to provide protection of the digital lamellae against further injury and failure in animals at risk of or suffering from clinical laminitis. Primarily used in sepsis-related laminitis.

Distal: Situated farthest from the point of attachment or origin of a limb (away from the trunk and towards the ground surface in the standing horse).

Dorsal: Pertains to the cranial (anterior) surface of anatomic structures distal to the carpus and tarsocrural joint in the forelimbs and hindlimbs.

Equine Laminitis, First Edition. Edited by James K. Belknap and Raymond Geor.

Endocrinopathy: A disease associated with dysfunction of one or more members of the endocrine system (e.g., thyroid gland, pituitary gland, beta-cells of the pancreas, hypothalamus, adrenal gland). The diseases are commonly associated with abnormal concentrations of circulating hormones (e.g., hyperinsulinemia).

Endotoxemia: The presence of endotoxin in the bloodstream; the term is commonly used interchangeably with sepsis in the literature.

Endotoxin (lipopolysaccharide): A PAMP present in the outer membrane of Gram-negative bacteria.

Epidermis: The outer layer of the skin/integument/hoof containing all epithelial cells from the inner basal layer to the outermost dead cornified/keratinized layer. This layer not only provides protection from the environment, but also, in the hoof, plays a vital structural role in the suspension of the distal phalanx, both through the attachment of the LBECs to the basement membrane and through the normal 'stiffness' of the lamellar epithelial cells (most likely due to cytoskeletal integrity) resisting deformation from the tension and shear forces placed on the lamellar epidermis. The epidermis has no blood vessels, lymphatics, or nerves; its cellular components in the epidermal lamellae rely on the dermal vasculature for oxygenation and nutrient supply.

Equine metabolic syndrome (EMS): A cluster of risk factors in horses linked to increased risk of endocrinopathic laminitis. These include obesity, regional adiposity, thriftiness and insulin dysregulation (commonly hyperinsulinemia or excessive insulin response to a carbohydrate diet).

Extensor moment: The product of the ground reaction force (and possibly the pull of the digital extensor tendon) and the length of the extensor moment arm; results in a tendency to raise the toe (dorsiflex the distal interphalangeal joint) if greater than the flexor moment.

Extracellular matrix: A collection of extracellular molecules (e.g., structural proteins [collagens], glycoproteins [laminins], proteoglycans [perlecan, decorin]) secreted by neighboring cells that provides mechanical and biochemical support to the surrounding cells.

Flexor moment: Product of the force in the deep digital flexor tendon and the length of the flexor moment arm.

Founder distance: See Coronary band–extensor process (C–E) distance.

Ground reaction force: The force exerted on a body by the ground, equal to the weight of the object on the surface of the Earth. With regards to the horse's foot, it is the sum of all the forces exerted by the ground on the entire surface on that hoof as the horse stands or moves.

Hemidesmosome: A multiprotein complex responsible for the adherence of epithelial cells to the underlying basement membrane. The complexes are attached to the intermediate filament cytoskeleton (e.g., keratin) on the cytoplasmic side, and primarily adhere to the laminin component of the basement membrane via integrins on the extracellular side.

Hoof: All integumentary tissues (including the epidermal, dermal, and subcutaneous [commonly termed deep dermis or sublamellar dermis] tissues) distal to the coronet.

Hoof capsule: Keratinized epidermis (also termed 'horn') providing the protective hard exterior of the coronary band, hoof wall, sole, frog and heel bulbs.

Hoof wall: Keratinized epidermis/'horn' consisting of the stratum externum, stratum medium, and the stratum internum.

Hypoxia: Deprivation of an adequate oxygen supply to a tissue.

Impression material: A two-part silicone putty which is mixed together and applied to the solear surface of the foot (most commonly used with therapeutic shoeing), usually to incorporate the sole as a weight-bearing surface in attempt to provide support to the distal phalanx in cases of laminitis.

Innate immune system: The cells and proteins which provide an immediate defense to infection, the components of which include the epidermis, leukocytes (primarily neutrophils, eosinophils, basophils, and monocytes/macrophanges), pattern recognition receptors, and pro-inflammatory cytokines and chemokines.

Integument: The outer protective layer of a tissue; it includes the epidermis and dermis when used to describe anatomic features of the equine foot.

Ischemia: Insufficient supply of blood to a tissue or organ, usually resulting in the disruption of cellular metabolism (i.e., due to inadequate oxygen and nutrient delivery and decreased waste removal) and possible cell death.

Keratinocyte: Epithelial cells making up the predominant cell type of the epidermis in the skin and hoof.

Lamella/lamellae (syn. lamina/laminae): Interdigitating folds of epidermal tissue (epidermal lamellae) and dermal tissue (dermal lamellae) critical to the suspension of the distal phalanx by the hoof wall.

Lamellar basal epithelial cell layer: The innermost layer of epidermal cells responsible for attachment of the epidermal lamellae to the underlying basement membrane and dermis of the dermal lamella.

Lamellar junction: The interface of the epidermal lamellae and the dermal lamellae which is the point of lamellar separation (between the LBECs and the basement membrane attached to the lamellar dermis) in lamellar failure.

Limbic integument: That layer of the integument that forms the junction between the skin of the pastern and the foot. It forms the stratum externum of the hoof wall.

Matrix metalloproteinase/metalloprotease: A zinc-containing enzyme (of the endopeptidase family) which hydrolyzes (breaks down) matrix proteins (e.g., collagens).

Moment (moment of force): The tendency of a force to rotate an object (distal phalanx in this text) around an axis/reference point (center of rotation of the distal interphalangeal joint in this text). The moment is a product of both the force and the distance from the axis (similar to torque).

Moment arm: The shortest distance between an axis/reference point (center of rotation of the distal interphalangeal joint in this text) and the line of action of the force causing the body to rotate.

Necrosis: Cell death due to cell injury from external factors (e.g., infection, ischemia, trauma), which results in an uncontrolled release of cellular products which can induce inflammation (i.e., DAMPs) into the extracellular environment (in distinction to apoptosis).

Non-steroidal anti-inflammatory drug (NSAID): A drug which inhibits cyclo-oxygenase enzymes (primarily COX-1 and COX-2). NSAIDs which primarily inhibit COX-2 are termed COX-2-selective NSAIDs (e.g., firocoxib), whereas NSAIDs which inhibit COX-1 and COX-2 to similar degrees are termed non-selective NSAIDs (e.g., flunixin meglumine, phenylbutazone).

Non-structural carbohydrate (NSC): A carbohydrate that occurs either as simple sugars in the horse's feed or that can be broken down by enzymes produced by the horse (include glucose, fructose, sucrose and starch). These are the target nutrients that most diets limit for the management of metabolic syndrome.

Palmar: Pertains to the caudal (posterior) surface of anatomic structures distal to the carpus in the forelimbs.

Palmar angle: See Solear margin angle.

Parietal: Pertaining to the wall of a cavity or hollow structure. Refers to the wall of the hoof (e.g., parietal dermis) or to the anatomic relationship of a structure to the hoof (e.g., parietal surface of the distal phalanx) in equine podiatry.

Pathogen-associated molecular pattern (PAMP): A molecular motif associated with pathogens (e.g., bacteria), which is recognized by and can activate cells of the innate immune system. Examples include endotoxins, lipoproteins, flagellin, peptidoglycans, bacterial/viral DNA.

Pattern recognition receptor (PRR): Receptors (e.g., Toll-like receptors, C-type lectin receptors, intracytoplasmic NOD-like receptors) on immune cells and other cell types of the host which bind PAMPs and DAMPs, resulting in the activation of downstream signaling pathways associated with the innate immune response.

Pituitary pars intermedia dysfunction (PPID): A slowly progressive disorder primarily in aging equids in which a functional adenoma (or adenomatous hyperplasia) of the pars intermedia develops as a result of loss of inhibitory factor, dopamine, due to the neurodegeneration of dopaminergic hypothalamic neurons. This results in an excessive secretion of proopiomelanocortin-derived hormones from the endocrine cells of the pars intermedia (melanotropes).

Plantar: Pertains to the caudal (posterior) surface of anatomic structures distal to the tarsocrural joint in the hindlimbs (synonymous with palmar in forelimbs; opposite of dorsal).

Pour-in pad: A liquid material (usually a polyurethane) which is applied to the solear surface after the application of a shoe, usually to incorporate the sole as a weight-bearing surface in an attempt to provide support to the distal phalanx in cases of laminitis.

Proximal: Situated nearest the point of attachment or origin of a limb (towards the trunk).

Rotation of the Distal Phalanx: Displacement of the dorsodistal aspect of the distal phalanx in a palmarodistal direction resulting always in divergence of the dorsal aspect of the distal phalanx from the dorsal aspect of the hoof capsule (capsular rotation), and commonly divergence of the dorsal aspect of the distal phalanx from the normal axis of the phalanges (phalangeal rotation, indicated by 'flexion' of the distal interphalangeal joint).

Sepsis: A dysregulated host response (primarily of the immune system) culminating in organ or tissue dysfunction resulting from the presence of pathogenic organisms and/or their toxins (i.e., PAMPs) in the bloodstream.

Sepsis-related laminitis: Laminitis secondary to disease states in equids associated with sepsis (e.g., enterocolitis, pleuropneumonia, retained fetal membranes/septic metritis, grain overload).

Solear margin angle (syn. Palmar angle): The angle formed by the palmar surface of the distal phalanx and the ground surface (assessed on a lateromedial radiograph of the digit).

Solear prolapsed: A convexity of the sole that develops distal to the dorsal solear margin of the distal phalanx; it occurs most commonly dorsal to the apex of frog with rotation of the distal phalanx.

Solear perforation: Perforation of the full thickness of the sole that develops most commonly with either rotation or asymmetrical distal displacement of the distal phalanx.

Stratum externum: The thin outer layer of the wall derived from the limbic (perioplic) integument.

Stratum internum: The thin layer of the wall derived from parietal (lamellar) integument that connects the stratum medium with the underlying dermal lamellae.

Stratum medium: The thick central layer of the hoof wall derived from the coronary integument that provides the rigidity of the wall responsible for most of the weight-bearing properties of the wall.

Supporting limb laminitis (syn. Support limb laminitis): Laminitis secondary to excessive weight-bearing on one limb due to decreased weight-bearing on the contralateral limb due to either pain (i.e., from sepsis of a synovial cavity or a fracture) or injury to the innervation of the limb (i.e., from a brachial plexus avulsion).

Suspensory apparatus of the distal phalanx (SADP): The combination of cellular components of the epidermal lamellae and matrix components of the basement membrane, dermal lamellae, and sublamellar dermis/corium that functions to suspend the distal phalanx within the hoof wall.

Symmetrical distal displacement: Distal displacement of the distal phalanx in which the entire palmar surface of the distal phalanx (dorsal, medial and lateral aspects) displace distally to the same degree in relation to the hoof capsule; that is, the flexor and extensor moments are in equilibrium while the displacement occurs.

Systemic inflammatory response syndrome (SIRS): A systemic inflammatory response to infection or trauma involving activation of the horse's innate immune system. The inflammatory response is primarily due to the activation of pattern recognition receptors (PRRs) on cellular components of the immune system (e.g., leukocytes) to PAMPs and DAMPs, resulting in activation on inflammatory pathways and release of inflammatory mediators (e.g., cytokines and chemokines) into the systemic circulation.

Tissue inhibitors of metalloproteinases (TIMPs): A family of four proteins (TIMP1–4) which, overall, inhibit the active forms of different metalloproteinases and ADAMTSs. TIMPS have also been found to have other roles independent of metalloproteinases.

Index

Equine Laminitis, First Edition. Edited by James K. Belknap and Raymond Geor.